Perioperative Medicine

SECOND EDITION

Perioperative Medicine

The Medical Care of the Surgical Patient

Editors:

David R. Goldmann, M.D.
Associate Professor of Medicine
University of Pennsylvania School of Medicine
Philadelphia, Pennsylvania

Frank H. Brown, M.D.
Associate Professor of Medicine
University of Pittsburgh School of Medicine
Pittsburgh, Pennsylvania

David M. Guarnieri, M.D.
Instructor in Anesthesiology
Jefferson Medical College
Thomas Jefferson University
Philadelphia, Pennsylvania

McGraw-Hill, Inc.
Health Professions Division
New York St. Louis San Francisco Auckland Bogotá Caracas
Lisbon London Madrid Mexico City Milan Montreal New Delhi
Paris San Juan Singapore Sydney Tokyo Toronto

PERIOPERATIVE MEDICINE, Second Edition

1234567890   MALMAL   9876543

ISBN 0-07-023702-6

This book was set in Times Roman by R/TSI, Inc., which also performed the project supervision.
The editors were J. Dereck Jeffers, Mariapaz Ramos Englis;
the production supervisor was Clare Stanley;
the cover designer was N.S.G. Design;
the indexer was Alexandra Nickerson.
Malloy Lithographic was printer and binder.
This book was printed on acid-free paper.

Library of Congress Cataloging-in-Publication Data

Perioperative medicine : the medical care of the surgical patient :
  [edited by] David R. Goldmann, Frank H. Brown, David M.
  Guarnieri. — 2nd ed.
      p.   cm.
    Rev. ed. of: Medical care of the surgical patient. Philadelphia :
  Lippincott, c1982.
    Includes bibliographical references and index.
    ISBN 0-07-023702-6
    1. Therapeutics, Surgical.   2. Surgery—Complications.
  I. Goldmann, David R.   II. Brown, Frank H.
  III. Guarnieri, David M.   IV. Medical care of the surgical
  patient.   V.   Title: Medical care of the surgical patient.
    [DNLM: 1. Intraoperative Care.   2. Postoperative Care.
  3. Preoperative Care.   WO 178 P4452 1994]
  RD49.M4   1994
  617—dc20
  DNLM/DLC   93-20975
  for Library of Congress   CIP

To our wives
Bonnie, Maura, and Kathy

CONTENTS

Part III
PREOPERATIVE
ASSESSMENT AND
MANAGEMENT OF
THE SURGICAL
PATIENT WITH
COEXISTING DISEASE

Part IV
PROPHYLACTIC THERAPY AND THE PREVENTION OF POSTOPERATIVE PROBLEMS

Part V
POSTOPERATIVE COMPLICATIONS: A PROBLEM-ORIENTED APPROACH

CONTRIBUTORS

ELIAS ABRUTYN, M.D. [44]

Professor and Associate Chairman of Medicine
Medical College of Pennsylvania
Associate Chief, Medical Service
Chief, Infectious Diseases
Veterans Affairs Medical Center
Philadelphia, Pennsylvania

RICHARD A. BANKOWITZ, M.D. [4]

Adjunct Assistant Professor of Medicine
University of Pittsburgh School of Medicine
Pittsburgh, Pennsylvania
Director, Clinical Evaluative Sciences Program
University Hospital Consortium
Oak Brook, Illinois

WILLIAM M. BATTLE, M.D. [7]

Clinical Assistant Professor of Medicine
University of Pennsylvania School of Medicine
Director of Gastrointestinal Endoscopy
Jeanes and Nazareth Hospitals
Philadelphia, Pennsylvania

LAURENCE H. BECK, M.D. [63]

Professor of Medicine
Jefferson Medical College
Thomas Jefferson University
Philadelphia, Pennsylvania
Executive Vice President
Geisinger Clinic
Danville, Pennsylvania

GENE B. BISHOP, M.D. [38]

Clinical Assistant Professor of Medicine
University of Pennsylvania
Director, Medical Clinics
Presbyterian Medical Center
Philadelphia, Pennsylvania

CLIFFORD A. BRASS, M.D., Ph.D. [69]

Assistant Professor of Medicine, Biochemistry and Biophysics
University of Pennsylvania School of Medicine
Medical Director, Liver Transplantation Program
Hospital of the University of Pennsylvania
Philadelphia, Pennsylvania

SETH BRAUNSTEIN, M.D., Ph.D. [24]

Associate Professor of Medicine
University of Pennsylvania School of Medicine
Philadelphia, Pennsylvania

JAMES R. BRORSON, M.D. [35]

Assistant Professor of Neurology
University of Chicago
Chicago, Illinois

FRANK H. BROWN, M.D. [10, 13, 14, 34, 43, 48]

Associate Professor of Medicine
University of Pittsburgh School of Medicine
Pittsburgh, Pennsylvania

LOUIS L. BRUNETTI, M.D., J.D. [4]

Assistant Professor of Medicine
University of North Carolina
Carolinas Medical Center
Charlotte, North Carolina

DONALD L. BUDENZ, M.D. [10]

Assistant Professor of Ophthalmology
University of Pennsylvania School of Medicine
Philadelphia, Pennsylvania

CONNIE CAMPBELL [9]

Temple University School of Medicine
Philadelphia, Pennsylvania

JAIME CARRIZOSA, M.D. [44]

Chairman, Department of Medicine
Florida Hospital
Orlando, Florida

JEFFREY L. CARSON, M.D. [3]

Associate Professor of Medicine
Chief, Division of General Internal Medicine
Robert Wood Johnson Medical School
University of Medicine and Dentistry of New Jersey
New Brunswick, New Jersey

ARNOLD W. COHEN, M.D. [40]

Professor of Obstetrics and Gynecology
University of Pennsylvania School of Medicine
Director, Obstetrics and Maternal-Fetal Medicine
Hospital of the University of Pennsylvania
Philadelphia, Pennsylvania

ALICIA M. CONILL, M.D. [24]

Assistant Professor of Medicine
University of Pennsylvania School of Medicine
Philadelphia, Pennsylvania

MALCOLM COX, M.D. [60]

Professor of Medicine
University of Pennsylvania School of Medicine
Vice-Chairman, Department of Medicine
Chief, Medical Service
Veterans Affairs Medical Center
Philadelphia, Pennsylvania

GARY W. CROOKS, M.D. [67]

Assistant Professor of Medicine
University of Pennsylvania School of Medicine
Philadelphia, Pennsylvania

PAUL G. CURCILLO II, M.D. [16]

Instructor in Surgery
Jefferson Medical College
Thomas Jefferson University
Philadelphia, Pennsylvania

JOHN M. DALY, M.D. [42]

Jonathan E. Rhoads Professor of Surgery
University of Pennsylvania School of Medicine
Philadelphia, Pennsylvania

HORACE M. DeLISSER, M.D. [22]

Assistant Professor of Medicine
University of Pennsylvania School of Medicine
Philadelphia, Pennsylvania

DANIEL DEMPSEY, M.D. [7]

Associate Professor of Surgery
Temple University School of Medicine
Philadelphia, Pennsylvania

TUSAR K. DESAI, M.D. [61]

Attending Physician
North Oakland Medical Center
Pontiac, Michigan

FRANCIS J. DuFRAYNE, M.D. [67]

Clinical Associate in Medicine
University of Pennsylvania School of Medicine
Philadelphia, Pennsylvania

HOWARD J. EISEN, M.D. [19]

Assistant Professor of Medicine
University of Pennsylvania School of Medicine
Medical Co-Director, Cardiac Transplantation Program
Director, Nuclear Cardiology
Hospital of the University of Pennsylvania
Philadelphia, Pennsylvania

JOHN M. EISENBERG, M.D. [3]

Professor and Chairman of Medicine
Georgetown University School of Medicine
Washington, DC

JEFFREY FINKELSTEIN, M.D., D.M.D. [11]

Assistant Professor of Otorhinolaryngology and
*   Bronchoesophagology*
Temple University School of Medicine
Philadelphia, Pennsylvania

STEVEN J. FISHMAN, M.D. [41]

Fellow in Pediatric Surgery
Children's Hospital
Boston, Massachusetts

KEVIN R. FOX, M.D. [29]

Assistant Professor of Medicine
University of Pennsylvania School of Medicine
Director, Hematology-Oncology Inpatient Unit
Philadelphia, Pennsylvania

JOSEPH FRANCIS, JR., M.D., M.P.H. [39]

Assistant Professor of Medicine and Preventive Medicine
University of Tennessee
Memphis, Tennessee

LOREN M. FREIMUTH, M.D. [70]

Director, Child Psychiatry Unit
Eastern State School and Hospital
Trevose, Pennsylvania

DAVID F. FRIEDMAN, M.D. [51]

Assistant Professor of Pediatrics and Pathology
University of Pennsylvania School of Medicine
Associate Director, Blood Bank
Children's Hospital of Philadelphia
Philadelphia, Pennsylvania

GREGG J. FROMELL, M.D. [23]

Associate Director, Clinical Research
Rhone-Poulenc Rohrer
Collegeville, Pennsylvania

STEPHEN L. GALETTA, M.D. [36]

Assistant Professor of Neurology
University of Pennsylvania School of Medicine
Philadelphia, Pennsylvania

MICHAEL A. GEHEB, M.D. [61]

Professor of Medicine and Associate Dean for Clinical Affairs
State University of New York at Stony Brook
Stony Brook, New York

CHRISTOPHER C. GETCH [13]

Instructor in Neurosurgery
Temple University School of Medicine
Philadelphia, Pennsylvania

STEPHEN J. GLUCKMAN, M.D. [52]

Professor of Clinical Medicine
Robert Wood Johnson Medical School at Camden
University of Medicine and Dentistry of New Jersey
Camden, New Jersey

BONNIE J. GOLDMANN, M.D. [28]

Senior Director, Regulatory Liaison Domestic
Merck Research Laboratories
West Point, Pennsylvania

DAVID R. GOLDMANN, M.D. [1, 16, 26, 67]

Associate Professor of Medicine
University of Pennsylvania School of Medicine
Director, General Internal Medicine Consultation Service
Hospital of the University of Pennsylvania
Philadelphia, Pennsylvania

FRANCISCO A. GONZALEZ-SCARANO, M.D. [35]

Associate Professor of Neurology
University of Pennsylvania School of Medicine
Philadelphia, Pennsylvania

GARY L. GOTTLIEB, M.D., M.B.A. [37]

Associate Professor and Executive Vice-Chairman of
*   Psychiatry*
University of Pennsylvania School of Medicine
Philadelphia, Pennsylvania

ERNEST M. GRAHAM, M.D. [40]

Fellow in Maternal-Fetal Medicine
Department of Obstetrics and Gynecology
Hospital of the University of Pennsylvania
Philadelphia, Pennsylvania

ROSANNE GRANIERI, M.D. [9, 17]

Assistant Professor of Medicine
University of Pittsburgh School of Medicine
Pittsburgh, Pennsylvania

ARTHUR GREENBERG, M.D. [62]

Associate Professor of Medicine
University of Pittsburgh School of Medicine
Pittsburgh, Pennsylvania

MICHAEL A. GRIPPI, M.D. [22]

Associate Professor and Vice-Chairman of Medicine
University of Pennsylvania School of Medicine
Philadelphia, Pennsylvania

DAVID M. GUARNIERI, M.D. [6, 8]

Instructor in Anesthesiology
Jefferson Medical College
Thomas Jefferson University
Philadelphia, Pennsylvania

KATHLEEN M. GUARNIERI, M.D. [49]

Instructor in Anesthesiology
Jefferson Medical College
Thomas Jefferson University
Philadelphia, Pennsylvania

DAVID H. HENRY, M.D. [30, 65]

Clinical Associate Professor of Medicine
University of Pennsylvania School of Medicine
Philadelphia, Pennsylvania

MARGARET TREXLER HESSEN, M.D. [44]

Clinical Assistant Professor of Medicine
Medical College of Pennsylvania
Philadelphia, Pennsylvania

ROBERT A. HIRSH, M.D. [2]

Chief, Department of Anesthesiology
Memorial Hospital of Burlington County
Mount Holly, New Jersey

JOHN W. HIRSHFELD, JR., M.D. [20]

Professor of Medicine
University of Pennsylvania School of Medicine
Director, Cardiac Catheterization Laboratory
Hospital of the University of Pennsylvania
Philadelphia, Pennsylvania

KURT P. HOFMANN, M.D. [42]

Staff Surgeon
Pocono Medical Center
East Stroudsburg, Pennsylvania

DAVID A. HOROWITZ, M.D. [24]

Instructor of Medicine
University of Pennsylvania School of Medicine
Philadelphia, Pennsylvania

SUSAN C. HUNT, M.D. [31]

Associate Professor of Medicine
University of Pittsburgh School of Medicine
Medical Director, Pittsburgh AIDS Center for Treatment
Pittsburgh, Pennsylvania

HOWARD I. HURTIG, M.D. [35]

Professor of Neurology
University of Pennsylvania School of Medicine
Chief, Department of Neurology
Graduate Hospital
Philadelphia, Pennsylvania

JOSEPH IANNOTTI, M.D. [14]

Assistant Professor of Orthopedics
University of Pennsylvania School of Medicine
Philadelphia, Pennsylvania

VALLUVAN JEEVANANDAM, M.D. [8]

Associate Professor of Surgery
Temple University School of Medicine
Surgical Director, Heart Failure and Transplant Program
Temple University Hospital
Philadelphia, Pennsylvania

LEIGH C. JEFFERIES, M.D. [66]

Assistant Professor of Pathology and Laboratory Medicine
University of Pennsylvania School of Medicine
Philadelphia, Pennsylvania

DAVID F. JIMENEZ, M.D. [13]

Assistant Professor of Neurosurgery
University of Missouri Hospital and Clinic
Columbia, Missouri

MARC J. KAHN, M.D. [28]

Fellow in Hematology-Oncology
Hospital of the University of Pennsylvania
Philadelphia, Pennsylvania

KEITH T. KANEL, M.D. [11, 64]

Assistant Professor of Medicine
University of Pittsburgh School of Medicine
Pittsburgh, Pennsylvania

JOHN KELLY, M.D. [14]

Assistant Professor of Orthopedics
Temple University School of Medicine
Philadelphia, Pennsylvania

KAREN G. KELLY, M.D. [18]

Clinical Assistant Professor of Medicine
Jefferson Medical College
Thomas Jefferson University
Philadelphia, Pennsylvania

MARK A. KELLY, M.D. [59]

Professor of Medicine
University of Pennsylvania School of Medicine
Vice Dean, Clinical Affairs
University of Pennsylvania Medical Center
Philadelphia, Pennsylvania

A. RICHARD KENDALL, M.D. [12]

Professor of Urology
Temple University School of Medicine
Philadelphia, Pennsylvania

MATTHEW N. KLAIN, M.D. [31]
Clinical Assistant Professor of Medicine
University of Pittsburgh School of Medicine
Staff Physician, Pittsburgh AIDS Center for Treatment
Pittsburgh, Pennsylvania

WILHELMINA C. KOREVAAR, M.D. [72]
Director, Pain Relief and Relief and Rehabilitation
Bala Cynwyd, Pennsylvania

FRANK KROBOTH, M.D. [50]
Professor of Medicine
University of Pittsburgh School of Medicine
Pittsburgh, Pennsylvania

JAMES A. KRUSE, M.D. [61]
Associate Professor of Medicine
Wayne State University School of Medicine
Director, Medical Intensive Care Unit
Detroit Receiving Hospital
Detroit, Michigan

MARGARET L. LANCEFIELD, M.D., Ph.D. [25]
Assistant Professor of Clinical Medicine
Robert Wood Johnson School of Medicine
University of Medicine and Dentistry of New Jersey
Medical Director, Outpatient Clinics
Princeton, New Jersey

PAUL N. LANKEN, M.D. [58]
Associate Professor of Medicine
University of Pennsylvania School of Medicine
Medical Director, Medical Intensive Care Units
Hospital of the University of Pennsylvania
Philadelphia, Pennsylvania

GARY L. LEVINE, M.D. [68]
Professor of Medicine
Temple University School of Medicine
Chief, Division of Gastroenterology and Nutrition
Albert Einstein Medical Center
Philadelphia, Pennsylvania

WILLIAM K. LEVY, M.D. [18]
Staff Cardiologist
Abington Memorial Hospital
Abington, Pennsylvania

JAMES D. LUKETICH, M.D. [41]
Fellow in Cardiothoracic Surgery
New York Hospital–Cornell Medical Center
New York, New York

DAVID S. MACPHERSON, M.D. [12]
Assistant Professor of Medicine
University of Pittsburgh School of Medicine
Pittsburgh, Pennsylvania

BRIAN F. MANDELL, M.D., Ph.D. [27]
Clinical Assistant Professor of Medicine
University of Pennsylvania School of Medicine
Philadelphia, Pennsylvania

FRANCIS E. MARCHLINSKI, M.D. [21]
Co-Director, Philadelphia Heart Institute
Presbyterian Medical Center
Philadelphia, Pennsylvania

WILLIAM H. MATTHAI, JR., M.D. [45]
Assistant Professor of Medicine
Robert Wood Johnson School of Medicine at Camden
University of Medicine and Dentistry of New Jersey
Camden, New Jersey

BERNADETTE PASTEWSKI McKEON, Pharm.D. [49]
Adjunct Assistant Professor of Pharmacy
Philadelphia College of Pharmacy and Science
Philadelphia, Pennsylvania

THOMAS A. MICKLER, M.D. [5]
Assistant Professor of Anesthesia
University of Pennsylvania School of Medicine
Philadelphia, Pennsylvania

JOHN MIKUTA, M.D. [15]
Professor of Obstetrics and Gynecology
University of Pennsylvania School of Medicine
Philadelphia, Pennsylvania

MARK MORGAN, M.D. [15]
Assistant Professor of Obstetrics and Gynecology
University of Pennsylvania School of Medicine
Philadelphia, Pennsylvania

WADIA R. MULLA, M.D. [40]
Fellow in Maternal-Fetal Medicine
Department of Obstetrics and Gynecology
Hospital of the University of Pennsylvania
Philadelphia, Pennsylvania

JAMES L. MULLEN, M.D. [41]
Associate Professor of Surgery
Director, Nutrition Support Service
Hospital of the University of Pennsylvania
Philadelphia, Pennsylvania

MICHAEL J. NEARY, M.D. [53]
Co-Director, Surgical Intensive Care Unit
Department of Anesthesiology
Deborah Heart and Lung Center
Browns Mills, New Jersey

CONSTANCE F. NEELY, M.D. [54]
Assistant Professor of Anesthesia
University of Pennsylvania School of Medicine
Philadelphia, Pennsylvania

CHARLES W. NICHOLS, M.D. [10]
Professor of Ophthalmology
University of Pennsylvania School of Medicine
Philadelphia, Pennsylvania

GREGORY R. OWENS, M.D. [57]
Associate Professor of Medicine and Anesthesiology
University of Pittsburgh School of Medicine
Pittsburgh, Pennsylvania

THOMAS D. PAINTER, M.D. [48]
Professor of Medicine
University of Pittsburgh School of Medicine
Pittsburgh, Pennsylvania

PAUL M. PALEVSKY, M.D. [60]
Assistant Professor of Medicine
University of Pittsburgh School of Medicine
Chief, Hemodialysis Unit
Veterans Affairs Medical Center
Pittsburgh, Pennsylvania

REYNOLD A. PANETTIERI, JR., M.D. [47]
Assistant Professor of Medicine
University of Pennsylvania School of Medicine
Director, Pulmonary Diagnostic Services
Hospital of the University of Pennsylvania
Philadelphia, Pennsylvania

RONNIE C. PARKER, M.D. [34]
Assistant Professor of Medicine
University of Pittsburgh School of Medicine
Pittsburgh, Pennsylvania

ERIC C. RAPS, M.D. [36, 71]
Assistant Professor of Neurology
University of Pennsylvania School of Medicine
Philadelphia, Pennsylvania

JAMES C. REYNOLDS, M.D. [46]
Associate Professor of Medicine
University of Pittsburgh School of Medicine
Pittsburgh, Pennsylvania

MAX RONIS [11]
Professor and Chairman of Otorhinolaryngology and
*   Bronchoesophagology*
Temple University School of Medicine
Philadelphia, Pennsylvania

ERNEST F. ROSATO, M.D. [16]
Professor of Surgery
University of Pennsylvania School of Medicine
Philadelphia, Pennsylvania

MARK E. ROSENTHAL, M.D. [56]
Clinical Assistant Professor of Medicine
University of Pennsylvania School of Medicine
Philadelphia, Pennsylvania
Director, Cardiac Electrophysiology and Cardiac Pacing
Abington Memorial Hospital
Abington, Pennsylvania

ROBERT H. ROSENWASSER, M.D. [13]
Associate Professor of Neurosurgery
Temple University School of Medicine
Philadelphia, Pennsylvania

RAYMOND A. RUBIN, M.D. [69]
Clinical Instructor of Medicine
University of Pennsylvania School of Medicine
Philadelphia, Pennsylvania

JOSEPH S. SAVINO, M.D. [55]
Assistant Professor of Anesthesia
University of Pennsylvania School of Medicine
Philadelphia, Pennsylvania

E. JAMES SEIDMON, M.D. [12]
Associate Professor of Urology
Temple University School of Medicine
Philadelphia, Pennsylvania

MICHAEL E. SELZER, M.D., Ph.D. [36, 71]
Professor of Neurology
University of Pennsylvania School of Medicine
Philadelphia, Pennsylvania

TIMOTHY SHAPIRO, M.D. [20]
Fellow in Cardiology
Hospital of the University of Pennsylvania
Philadelphia, Pennsylvania

NEIL SHUSTERMAN, M.D. [32]
Adjunct Assistant Professor of Medicine
University of Pennsylvania School of Medicine
Philadelphia, Pennsylvania

STEVEN A. SILBER, M.D. [70]
Clinical Assistant Professor of Medicine
University of Pennsylvania School of Medicine
Director, Internal Residency Training Program
Presbyterian Medical Center
Philadelphia, Pennsylvania

LESLIE E. SILBERSTEIN, M.D. [51, 66]
Associate Professor of Pathology and Laboratory Medicine
University of Pennsylvania School of Medicine
Director, Blood Bank
Hospital of the University of Pennsylvania School of Medicine
Philadelphia, Pennsylvania

PETER J. SNYDER, M.D. [16]
Professor of Medicine
University of Pennsylvania School of Medicine
Philadelphia, Pennsylvania

KURT P. SPINDLER, M.D. [14]
Assistant Professor of Orthopedics
Vanderbilt University School of Medicine
Nashville, Tennessee

JAMES L. STINNETT, M.D. [70]
Professor of Psychiatry
University of Pennsylvania School of Medicine
Philadelphia, Pennsylvania

JOEL E. STREIM, M.D. [37]
Assistant Professor of Psychiatry
University of Pennsylvania School of Medicine
Philadelphia, Pennsylvania

HAROLD M. SZERLIP, M.D. [60]
Associate Professor and Associate Chairman of Medicine
Tulane University School of Medicine
Chief, Tulane Medical Service
Medical Center of Louisiana
New Orleans, Louisiana

GEORGE H. TALBOT, M.D. [52]

Associate Director, Clinical Research
Rhone-Poulenc-Rorer
Collegeville, Pennsylvania

GREGORY TINO, M.D. [47]

Assistant Professor of Medicine
University of Pennsylvania
Assistant Director, Pulmonary Diagnostic Services
Hospital of the University of Pennsylvania
Philadelphia, Pennsylvania

BARBARA TODD, CRNP [8]

Department of Surgery
Temple University Hospital
Philadelphia, Pennsylvania

STUART J. WEISS, M.D., Ph.D. [55]

Assistant Professor of Anesthesia
University of Pennsylvania School of Medicine
Philadelphia, Pennsylvania

JOHN WHITE, M.D. [9]

Associate Professor of Surgery
Temple University School of Medicine
Philadelphia, Pennsylvania

SANKEY V. WILLIAMS, M.D. [33]

Sol Katz Professor of General Internal Medicine
University of Pennsylvania School of Medicine
Chief, Division of General Internal Medicine
Hospital of the University of Pennsylvania
Philadelphia, Pennsylvania

FOREWORD

Perioperative Medicine, edited by Goldmann, Brown, and Guarnieri, represents in several ways a maturation of its predecessor, *The Medical Care of the Surgical Patient*, published in 1982. Whereas the earlier book was written chiefly by junior faculty at the University of Pennsylvania, this new volume is the work of many of the original contributors who have advanced substantially in their careers and new contributors from several other academic institutions. In addition, the system-oriented structure of the older book has been expanded and reorganized into five sections covering an overall introduction to surgery and anesthesia, issues arising from specific procedures, details of medical disease, preventive strategies, and common complications. The organization of the new book should therefore make it much easier to use.

In *Surgery, Principles and Practice*, published in 1957, Carl Moyer wrote:

Ideally, the assessment of operative risk should be approached as a statistical problem and the risk expressed as the probability of dying during an operation and convalescence. However, the statistical approach demands accurate data pertaining to the effects of many factors such as age, starvation, heart disease, etc., upon the operative risk. These data are practically nonexistent. . . . Obviously, because of these factors, the accurate assessment of the operative risk for an individual case is impossible today. All we can do is guess.

Much has been observed and recorded since Moyer wrote this statement. In discussing all aspects of medical care of the surgical patient, *Perioperative Medicine* brings our current knowledge up to date and makes us realize that perioperative care is much less of a guessing game than it was a quarter of a century ago.

It is always an honor to be asked to contribute a Foreword to an important book, and I believe that this volume, written as it is by men and women who are active participants in perioperative care, is the most comprehensive and authoritative book that I know of in this field.

Jonathan E. Rhoads, MD
Professor of Surgery
University of Pennsylvania School of Medicine

PREFACE

Perioperative Medicine is a comprehensive textbook designed to help physicians and other health care providers care for patients undergoing surgery. Like its predecessor, *Medical Care of the Surgical Patient*, which appeared in 1982, it seeks to provide medical professionals with the body of knowledge necessary to manage underlying medical illness during the perioperative period, assess operative risk, and deal with complications. Its recommendations remain grounded in critical review of as much quantitative data as are available in the medical literature. We have again attempted to avoid reiteration of basic material found in standard textbooks of medicine, surgery, and anesthesia and to produce instead a comprehensive but well-focused and easily accessible guide for the clinician, textbook for the trainee, and database for the investigator.

Perioperative Medicine is, however, not just a second edition of an earlier book. It has grown from 38 to 72 chapters and represents the work of 117 contributors from across the country. New topics include the medical-legal implications of consultation, a primer of anesthesiology for the internist, surgery in patients with cancer, surgery in patients with HIV and other communicable diseases, surgery in the pregnant patient, alternatives to homologous transfusion, and management of postoperative pain. Many of the former chapters dealing with specific organ systems have been subdivided and expanded for clarity. An entirely new section of ten chapters (Part II) is devoted to important issues specific to different types of surgery and covers over 70 individual surgical procedures.

The organization of the book is designed to facilitate its use as an accessible reference and a well-focused teaching tool. It is divided into five parts covering (1) the art and science of consultation and an overview of the effects of surgery and anesthesia on human physiology and disease; (2) the essentials of the individual procedures and their impact on patients with and without underlying disease; (3) more detailed treatment of the broad range of medical illness, how it is affected by surgery and anesthesia, and how it contributes to surgical risk; (4) the issues of prevention important in minimizing risk; and (5) the common postoperative complications of surgery and anesthesia. Although the new organization requires that some issues be considered in more than one chapter, undue repetition has been minimized by extensive cross-referencing. It is hoped that this design will provide readers with a clear conceptual framework for mastering the substance of perioperative medicine and enable them to find answers to specific questions rapidly.

In designing this book, we have drawn upon contributors from the fields of internal medicine and its subspecialties, surgery, anesthesia, nursing, and law. In so doing, we have increasingly realized that optimal perioperative care depends on input from a variety of health care providers with their own individual expertise. However, effective patient care requires cooperation among caregivers not only in effectively communicating with one another but also in acquiring a common vocabulary and mastering the body of knowledge of perioperative medicine. We sincerely hope that *Perioperative Medicine* will provide the impetus to achieve these goals and, in so doing, to forge an important new discipline.

Special thanks go to Daniel Dempsey, MD, for coordinating the new section on specific surgical procedures. In addition, we thank C. Donald Weinberg, Suzanne Maiorano, Sue Galvin, and Alice Kuller for their editorial assistance and Ellen Klein for her tireless work over many months in tending to the multitude of details required in transforming a manuscript into a finished book.

David R. Goldmann
Frank H. Brown
David M. Guarnieri

PREFACE TO THE FIRST EDITION

Patients undergoing surgery frequently have medical problems that influence their course in the perioperative period. The interactions of medical and surgical illnesses are complex and may complicate management. Many questions, even those that arise most commonly, remain unanswered. What are the risks of surgery and general anesthesia in patients with a given set of medical illnesses? What are the predictors of those risks? Can they be reduced by preoperative measures? How should medical problems be managed before and after surgery? What complications might be expected? How should problems common to the perioperative period be approached diagnostically and therapeutically?

The information necessary to answer these questions is scattered throughout the literature and is never systematically addressed during medical school or house-staff training. *Medical Care of the Surgical Patient: A Problem-Oriented Approach to Management* began with a critical review of this literature to help senior residents at the Hospital of the University of Pennsylvania who serve as consultants to surgical services. Although the book was originally conceived to meet the needs of the training program, its potential usefulness to all those caring for surgical patients became apparent. It is not a textbook of medicine dealing with diagnosis and treatment of medical illnesses or a textbook of surgery discussing indications for surgery or techniques and complications. Rather, it is our intention to assemble existing data from diverse sources in readily accessible form, to review critically what is known, to indicate deficiencies in current knowledge, and to identify areas for future research. Internists, surgeons, anesthesiologists, family practitioners, and trainees can use this book to formulate a comprehensive approach to perioperative patients.

Medical Care of the Surgical Patient: A Problem-Oriented Approach to Management stands as the concerted effort of many physicians and pharmacologists, nearly all of whom are or were affiliated with the Department of Medicine at the University of Pennsylvania School of Medicine. We gratefully acknowledge the contributions of our medical and surgical colleagues. We acknowledge the generous support of the Robert Wood Johnson Foundation. We thank Barbara Mihatov and Pamela Wagner for their technical assistance and our publishers for their invaluable advice. Finally, we thank Dr. Lawrence Earley and Dr. Arnold S. Relman, present and past Chairman of the Department of Medicine, respectively, for their inspiration.

David R. Goldmann, M.D.
Frank H. Brown, M.D.
William K. Levy, M.D.
Gail B. Siap, M.D.
Elliot J. Sussman, M.D.

Perioperative Medicine

INTRODUCTION TO PERIOPERATIVE MEDICINE

I

1 WHAT IS PERIOPERATIVE MEDICINE?

David R. Goldmann

The term *perioperative*, literally meaning "around the operation," is used loosely in the literature to refer to the period just before, during, and after a surgical procedure. Kroenke defines perioperative medicine in a similarly time-centered way to refer to management of the patient during surgery and in the forty-eight hours thereafter.[1] More often than not, this term is equated with consultation by internists or other nonsurgical physicians in the surgical setting. Consulting internists evaluate health status before surgery, define medical issues, and attempt to anticipate the effects of anesthesia and surgery. Sometimes they are called in after the procedure to help in the management of an unexpected complication. In their role of consultant, they sometimes uncover undiagnosed medical problems, often provide continuity of care, and frequently use the opportunity to initiate preventive screening measures. Up to 60 percent of surgical patients have symptoms or signs of concurrent systemic disease with an even higher prevalence in the elderly. Most are due to cardiovascular disease followed by respiratory and metabolic conditions.[2] Perioperative medical care is also provided by surgeons, anesthesiologists, and other health care providers, who bring their own expertise and the perspectives of their disciplines to the management of patients undergoing surgery. Thus, perioperative medicine can be considered more broadly as embracing intersecting subsets of several different fields directed toward the common goals of managing the patient at a particular point in his medical history and defining a common body of knowledge.

Defining perioperative medicine in this way blurs the lines of jurisdiction among caregivers and threatens traditional roles. Surgeons, internists, and anesthesiologists are frequently limited by their disciplines and interact in well-established patterns. Internists perform preoperative evaluations to assess the short-term effects of surgery and anesthesia and offer management advice. They are most often asked to "clear patients for surgery," an impossible task which assumes that they can predict and avoid all possible risks. In addition to their role in the operating room, anesthesiologists also do preoperative evaluation in an effort to tailor the anesthetic technique to the patient's health status and medication history and to provide appropriate respiratory and hemodynamic management in the recovery room. Surgeons generally focus on the major problem requiring surgery and traditionally assume man-

agement of postoperative matters like wound care, drain management, and parenteral nutrition.

Lee et al.[3] describe this "interesting tension" among caregivers and their resistance to change. In their study, consultations which were most valued (as defined by compliance rates in following consultants' recommendations) were those requesting performance of a special procedure. The limited focus of such consultations thus predicts the greatest compliance. Attending physicians tend to reject recommendations that go beyond a specific request, introduce new issues, or impact on other disciplines. Moreover, consultants run the risk of alienating others if they step beyond the bounds of their expected role. When Choi[4] admonishes "the prudent medical consultant is wise enough to choose the anesthesiologist rather than the agent of choice of anesthesia," he is describing the division of labor among differentially informed specialists and missing the importance of creating consensus among commonly informed care providers. Fragmentation of concerns and definitions of "turf" make the development and acceptance of a common body of knowledge in perioperative medicine difficult to achieve. However, common knowledge should provide the background and vocabulary to create the teamwork necessary for more effective communication and better and more cost-effective patient care. As stated in the preface, the purpose of this book is to define that common body of knowledge to increase collaboration among all those providing perioperative care.

Medical consultation for surgical patients, what might be considered the forerunner of perioperative medicine, developed as a new area of interest within the field of general internal medicine in the early 1980s. Early work was largely descriptive, dealing with developing general internal medicine consultation services in teaching hospitals and concentrating on what internists should do as consultants.[5-9] A number of articles extend these descriptions to psychiatric, geriatric, cardiac, and pulmonary consultation services. In this regard, Lee Goldman's often-quoted "Ten Commandments for Effective Consultation"[9] enunciate rules of etiquette for the consultant and have come to define a standard of practice from a medical-legal point of view (see Chap. 4). He advised consultants to (1) clarify the question; (2) determine the urgency of the consultation; (3) gather data independently without relying only on that previously obtained; (4) be brief and avoid recapitulation; (5)

state the differential diagnosis concisely and be specific in all recommendations; (6) anticipate potential problems and provide therapeutic options; (7) honor the roles of other caregivers; (8) teach with tact; (9) maintain direct personal contact with the consulting physician; and (10) follow up with periodic notes and recommendations.

In the mid-1980s, the emphasis in the literature turned to the effectiveness of consultation.[10–21] However, in these studies, effectiveness was equated with compliance with recommendations rather than patient outcome. Consultations were judged effective if the recommendations contained in them were followed by the requesting physician. These studies examined factors which affected compliance and suggested that consultants could be more effective if they were more cognizant of them. In general, these studies indicated that compliance was better when recommendations (1) numbered five or fewer, (2) were restricted to the question asked of the consultant, (3) were offered after rather than before surgery, (4) concerned medication rather than diagnostic tests, (5) did not require appreciable extra work, (6) were communicated in person, (7) were made within twenty-four hours, (8) were specific, and (9) involved consultant follow-up. The factors involve focus, clarity, and communication and largely correspond to the issues raised in Goldman's ten commandments. None of these studies considered quality of overall care or quantitative outcome measures.

Several studies considered compliance in relation to the expectations of the physician requesting the consultation. Ballard et al. evaluated compliance with recommendations based on the surgeon's view of them as either essential or nonessential. In their discussion, "essential" was defined as "germane to current management issues" and "nonessential" as included "for the sake of completeness." Approximately 75 percent of these essential recommendations were followed as opposed to 44 percent of those considered nonessential. They concluded that "recommendations peripheral to current patient care issues are unlikely to be implemented by our surgical colleagues."[11]

Klein et al. also found that "centrality" was a significant factor in determining compliance.[12] However, they noted that emphasis on centrality can sometimes lead to a negative outcome. As part of the consultation process, internists often identify previously unrecognized medical issues and make relevant recommendations. The authors found this to be particularly true when general internists rather than subspecialists were asked to do preoperative consultations. Unfortunately, the advantage was frequently negated by the low compliance of surgeons in following their recommendations. Mackenzie et al. similarly documented low compliance with recommendations in cardiology consultation but examined the variables from a different perspective.[13] They found that concordance with consultants' drug recommendations was 82 percent but only 64 percent when recommendations involved diagnostic studies. Among general surgeons, the compliance rate for diagnostic recommendations was even lower at 50 percent. The authors attributed low rates of compliance with diagnostic recommendations not to judgments regarding the risk, expense, or inconvenience of following the recommendations but to the "more general phenomenon . . . that consultations were requested principally for assistance in management rather than diagnosis."

Robie's study points out the potential significance of diagnostic recommendations in perioperative medical consultations and their importance in delivering better care.[14] He reviewed the cases of 162 patients seen by a general medicine consultation service in a university teaching hospital and found that consultants made 361 new diagnoses. As a result, twenty-six patients required transfer to another service. Although the impact of establishing diagnoses on overall care and referring physician satisfaction were not studied, Robie suggested that limiting consultants only to questions raised by the surgical service can lead to "missed diagnoses and to a potentially lower quality of patient care." In so doing, Robie shifts the emphasis for consultants from following procedural norms to assure greater compliance to offering recommendations that embrace the quality of the entire range of patient care in the perioperative period.

Compliance with consultants' recommendations may be higher outside the university hospital setting but with significant trade-offs. Clearly compliance alone does not assure quality consultative care. In their study of consultation in a community hospital setting, Ferguson and Rubinstein found the compliance rate to be 95 percent.[23] They found that 46 percent of consulting internists and 64 percent of the surgeons emphasized continuity of prior care as a major factor in justifying perioperative medical care and follow-up. In 86 percent of the cases, consultants had previously cared for the patients. Moreover, they judged the need for preoperative consultation to be appropriate in 92 percent of the cases and for postoperative follow-up to be indicated in 94 percent. However, despite the appropriateness of the consultation and the high rate of compliance with recommendations, these consultations were often anything but effective. The researchers found "shortcomings in the depth and thoroughness of the written documentation, . . . deficiencies related to poor evaluation, . . . lack of attention to abnormal laboratory and ECG findings, and lack of attention to therapeutic issues." The consultants had ignored one of the keys to good consultation by not looking for themselves and had missed important issues. Although patients in community hospitals may not have as many complex problems as those in tertiary care facilities, only 8 percent of the consults in this study resulted in new diagnoses, and in only 7 percent of the cases did the consultant have significant impact on the decisions.

Rates of compliance with consultants' recommendations may not only serve as poor indicators of effectiveness and quality of care but may also increase already-existing rifts between different disciplines and even interfere with patient care. Although they do not specifically deal with surgical patients, the studies of Popkin et al. in psychiatric consultation serve as a case in point.[15] These investigators accept compliance as a measure of effectiveness, find it to be low, and ascribe it to bias against psychiatry in general. In one study, recommendations for diagnostic action were followed in only 59 percent of the cases. In a second study, they even found compliance rates with medication recommendations to be in the 60 percent range.[16] Only those suggesting continuation of a medication or adjustment of dose commanded rates of over 80 percent. Popkin et al. believe that "psychiatric consultation in the general hospital is predominantly viewed by consultees as nonmedical intervention" and state that "once the functional category has been invoked to account for psychiatric features, consultees appear to consider medical aspects and approaches concluded." Moreover, in further attempts to explain low compliance, the authors ascribe an inappropriate attitude toward the use of psychotropic medication and even speculate on issues of turf and character, stating that differences in compliance levels may indicate that "consultees perceive recommendations to start or discontinue as a criticism of or an insult to their clinical judgment. These recommendations may more readily evoke issues of control and narcissistic injury in consultees."

The language in this last statement clearly indicates the absence of a true team approach by the community of health care providers to serve the best interests of the patient. When fostered by poor communication and lack of a shared body of knowledge, such sometimes adversarial relationships deprive the patient of treatment and leave the principal caregivers without a solution to the problem. In a letter to the editor accompanying the study of Popkin et al., Kramer et al. postulate that noncompliance may not be due solely to the nature of consultants' recommendations on their own grounds.[17] They assert that psychiatric consultation may be requested for unspoken reasons. "If the primary physician is angry with the patient, wishes to 'dump' him on the psychiatric ward or is looking for a magical solution to a difficult problem, it is unlikely that . . . recommendations will make much of an impact." Other investigators in psychiatric consultation have taken a more positive approach in an effort to meet the needs of physicians requesting consultation. One group has developed a psychiatric consultation checklist to be used in place of the standard consultation request form.[22] Such instruments may allow a better mutual understanding of patient stressors and behavior and go a long way toward improving communication and providing the patient with focused comprehensive care.

Only recently has perioperative consultation been seriously confronted by the exigencies of cost-containment strategies posed by third-party payors such as limitations on the number of consultations or the possibility of physician diagnostic related group (DRG) reimbursement.[24] Gluck et al. approached the issue of cost-effectiveness in medical consultation in perioperative patients by studying the impact of consultation on patients with varying disease severity.[25] They concurred with the role of the consulting internist in using preoperative medical evaluation to prevent or manage potential problems that may contribute to surgical morbidity and mortality but stress his importance in "managing certain medical diseases . . . [and] interpreting the more complex medical problems." Therefore, patients in the American Society of Anesthesiologists (ASA) Class I and II may gain little to justify the cost of medical consultation while those in Class III benefit most in terms of cost-effective outcome. Similarly, Levinson has shown that, although internists uncover previously undiagnosed disease, most of the benefit of their efforts is realized in patients over 50.[26] The process of consultation itself may have varying effects on cost. One study of consultation on a surgical service has shown that delay in requesting and performing a consultation and implementing its recommendations extends hospital length of stay.[27] Another has documented a significant increase in the number of additional studies resulting from the input of consultants on a medical service.[28] On the other hand, services providing mandatory guideline–based consultation for clinicians instituting anticoagulant therapy or platelet transfusions have been shown to reduce the incidence of drug-induced bleeding in the former case and use of precious resources in the latter.[29,30] Investigators are thus beginning to discard compliance as a measure of effectiveness and recognize outcome as a more defendable basis for consultation if for no other reason than cost.

Further studies of the effect of medical consultation on quantifiable measures of outcome and efforts to make the consultation process more efficient are clearly needed to improve quality and justify expense. Many uncertainties remain regarding the efficacy

and validity of what physicians do in the perioperative setting, and many traditional practices demand rigorous scientific scrutiny.[31] Otherwise, therapeutic decisions may continue to rely on the consultant's "power of personal rather than statistical persuasion."[32] Research beyond descriptive articles and compliance studies requires agreement among all those involved in perioperative care on a common purpose for their efforts. At present, many surgeons still see consultation solely as the process by which patients are cleared for surgery. Internists most often view themselves as patient advocates providing definition and management of underlying medical problems in the perioperative period and continuity of care thereafter. Anesthesiologists use preoperative evaluation largely for their own purposes to choose the safest and most effective anesthetic technique and to anticipate possible complications during and just after the procedure. Would not research be facilitated and overall care improved if caregivers shared a common purpose and knew enough about each other's perspective to further that purpose together? In truth, it is this collaboration and shared knowledge that best defines the term perioperative medicine.

True collaboration among caregivers has further implications. Given current pressure to reduce cost and increase the efficiency of medical care, cooperation and the use of a common knowledge base may allow physicians to develop more specific criteria for consultation. The preliminary work of Gluck described above indicates that patients in ASA Classes I and II probably may not require the input of medical consultants. In less complex cases, familiarity with an expanded well-defined knowledge base may allow surgeons to understand disease-related risk better, assume elements of perioperative care formerly requested of consulting internists, and obviate the need for the input of multiple subspecialists. Similarly, appreciation of this knowledge base may help internists to open the "black box" of the operating room and understand procedure-related risk more fully in preparing patients for surgery, managing them postoperatively, and arranging long-term follow-up for them. If prospective payment systems more tightly limit the number of consultants for a given case, internists may be required to subsume the role of some subspecialists. In one study, 60 consecutive consultations to the cardiology service from noncardiac surgery services were reviewed in order to focus curriculum planning for generalists training in perioperative consultation.[33]

Cost constraints and pressure to reduce hospital length of stay have shifted a significant portion of preoperative consultation and surgery to the outpatient setting. Studies show that many patients, including the elderly and those with stable medical problems, can successfully undergo ambulatory surgery after appropriate preparation.[34,35] The likelihood of unanticipated admission to the hospital after ambulatory surgery appears to be related more to the type of anesthesia and procedure rather than to patients' clinical characteristics.[36] Outpatient consultation theoretically allows more time for careful evaluation and effective communication with the referring physician. In many cases, it obviates unnecessary hospitalization for those admitted for surgery who are subsequently found to be unsuitable to undergo the procedure. However, outpatient preoperative evaluation may require even greater efforts at collaboration and cooperation to avoid fragmentation of care especially when it is performed by those who may have no continuing relationship with the patient and are unaware of previous care rendered by other physicians.[26] Clearly a common body of knowledge in perioperative medicine would facilitate such efforts.

In recent years, both patient needs and economic forces have led to significant changes in the organization and delivery of medical care. One such change has been the development of fields of expertise that cross the boundaries of traditional disciplines. Interdisciplinary specialities like critical care and geriatrics are examples of organized collaboration among caregivers who bring different perspectives to solving problems peculiar to subsets of patients in specific settings. As broadly defined, perioperative medicine may be similarly conceived as an important interdisciplinary area. Over the years, a number of textbooks including this one have laid out the boundaries of the area and filled in parts of it. It only lacks additional research and the commitment of those who participate in it to give perioperative medicine the recognition it deserves.

SUMMARY

1. Up to 60 percent of surgical patients have symptoms or signs of concurrent systemic disease with an even higher prevalence in the elderly. Most are due to cardiovascular disease followed by respiratory and metabolic problems.

2. Consulting internists traditionally assume the task of identifying and treating underlying disease to minimize surgical risk, participate in management of complications, and assure continuity of care after surgery. Perioperative medicine also encompasses the activities of surgeons, anesthesiologists, and other health care providers.

3. The effect of these contributions on patient care in the perioperative setting has not been rigorously studied. Effectiveness of consultation has largely been measured by determining compliance with consultants' recommendations rather than patient outcome.

4. Limited data suggest that the contribution of medical consultation to overall care in the surgical setting is most likely to be significant for older patients with more serious underlying disease.

5. Effective consultation requires active collaboration and cooperation among members of different disciplines fostered by agreement on a common purpose and familiarity with a common body of knowledge.

6. Rigorous investigation involving the role of medical consultation on patient outcome is essential to improve patient care and determine cost-effectiveness.

REFERENCES

1. Kroenke K: Preoperative evaluation: The assessment and management of surgical risk. *J Gen Intern Med* 2:257, 1987.
2. Wijesurendra RJ, Norihan AA, Millar RA: Incidence of concurrent systemic disease in the surgical population of a tertiary care hospital. *Canad Anaesth Soc J* 28(1):67, 1981.
3. Lee T, Pappius EM, Goldman L: Impact of inter-physician communication on the effectiveness of medical consultations. *Am J Med* 74:106, 1983.
4. Choi JJ: An anesthesiologist's philosophy on 'medical clearance' for surgical patients. *Arch Intern Med* 147:2090, 1987.
5. Charlson ME, Cohen RP, Sears CL: General medicine consultation. Lessons from a clinical service. *Amer J Med* 75:121, 1983.
6. Deyo RA: The internist as consultant. *Arch Intern Med* 140:137, 1980.
7. Bomalaski JS, Martin GJ, Webster JR Jr: General internal medicine consultation. The last bridge. *Arch Intern Med* 143:875, 1983.
8. Anonymous: Contrasts in Academic Consultation (Editorial Note). *Ann Intern Med* 94(4):537, 1981.
9. Goldman L, Lee T, Rudd P: Ten commandments for effective consultation. *Arch Intern Med* 153:1753, 1983.
10. Sears CL, Charlson ME: The effectiveness of a consultation. *Am J Med* 74:870, 1983.
11. Ballard WP, Gold JP, Charlson ME: Compliance with the recommendations of medical consultants. *J Gen Intern Med* 1:221, 1986.
12. Klein LE, Moore RD, Levine DM et al: Effectiveness of medical consultation. *J Med Ed* 58:149, 1983.
13. Mackenzie TB, Popkin MK, Callies AL et al: The effectiveness of cardiology consultation. *Chest* 79:16, 1981.
14. Robie PW: The service and educational contributions of a general medicine consultation service. *J Gen Intern Med* 1:227, 1986.
15. Popkin MK, Mackenzie TB, Callies AL: Consultees' concordance with consultants' recommendations for diagnostic action. *J Nerv Mental Dis* 168:9, 1980.
16. Popkin MK, Mackenzie TB, Hall RCW et al: Consultees' concordance with consultants' psychotropic drug recommendations. *Arch Gen Psychiatry* 37:1017, 1980.
17. Kramer BA, Spikes J, Strain JJ: Compliance with psychiatric consultant's recommendations. *Arch Gen Psychiatry* 37:1082, 1980.
18. Klein LE, Levine DM, Moore RD et al: The preoperative consultation. Response to internists' recommendations. *Arch Intern Med* 143:743, 1983.
19. Pupa LE Jr, Coventry JA, Hanley JF et al: Factors affecting compliance for general medicine consultations to non-internists. *Amer J Med* 81:508, 1986.
20. Horwitz RI, Henes CG, Horwitz SM: Developing strategies for improving the diagnostic and management efficacy of medical consultations. *J Chron Dis* 36(2):213, 1983.
21. Popkin MK, Mackenzie TB, Hall RCW et al: Physicians' concordance with consultants' recommendations for psychotropic medication. *Arch Gen Psychiatry* 36:386, 1979.
22. Zigun, JR: The psychiatric consultation checklist: A structured form to improve the clarity of psychiatric consultation requests. *Gen Hosp Psych* 12(1):36–44, 1990.
23. Ferguson RP, Rubinstein E: Preoperative medical consultations in a medical hospital. *J Gen Intern Med* 2:89, 1987.
24. Lowenstein SR, Iezzoni LI, Moskowitz MA: Prospective payment for physician services. Impact on medical consultation practices. *JAMA* 54(18):2632, 1985.
25. Gluck R, Munoz E, Wise L: Preoperative and postoperative medical evaluation of surgical patients. *Am J Surg* 155:730, 1988.
26. Levinson W: Preoperative evaluations by an internist—are they worthwhile? *West J Med* 141:395, 1984.
27. Kelley DC, Weng J-S, Watson A: The effect of consultation on hospital length of stay. *Inquiry* 16:158, 1979.
28. Braham RL, Ron A, Ruchlin HS et al: Diagnostic test restraint and the specialty consultation. *J Gen Med* 5(2):95–103, 1990.
29. Landfeld CS, Anderson PA: Guideline-based consultation to prevent anticoagulant-related bleeding. A randomized, controlled trial in a teaching hospital. *Ann Intern Med* 116:829–837, 1992.
30. Simpson MB: Prospective-concurrent audits and medical consultation for platelet transfusions. *Transfusion* 27:192–195, 1987.
31. Goldman L: The art and science of perioperative consultation: Where we are and where we should be going. *J Gen Intern Med* 2:284, 1987.
32. Burack RC: Beta error and the consultant. *Ann Intern Med* 98(6):1031, 1983.
33. Golden WE, Lavender RC: Preoperative consultations in a teaching hospital. *South Med J* 82:292–295, 1989.

34. Lieber CP, Seinige UL, Sataloff DM: Choosing the site of surgery. An overview of ambulatory surgery in geriatric patients. *Clin Geriatr Med* 6:493–497, 1990.

35. Davis JE, Sugioka K: Selecting the patient for major ambulatory surgery. Surgical and anesthesiology evaluations. *Surg Clin N Am* 67:721–732, 1987.

36. Gold BS, Kitz DS, Lecky JH et al: Unanticipated admission to the hospital following ambulatory surgery. *JAMA* 262:3008–3010, 1989.

2 AN APPROACH TO ASSESSING PERIOPERATIVE RISK

Robert A. Hirsh

Operative risk is the probability of adverse outcome and death associated with surgery and anesthesia. Implicit in the decision to accept risk is the possibility of benefit from a therapeutic intervention resulting in amelioration or cure of disease, restoration of function, or relief of pain. Decisions to proceed are based on conceptualized risk-benefit ratios. The possibility of gain or benefit, whether in an elective or urgent situation, is central to whether or not a given risk is acceptable. Estimates of risk are accurate only when they are applied to groups of comparable patients undergoing similar procedures. Estimates of risk for individuals within a group are not reliable.[1]

Death, a well-defined clinical outcome, has frequently been used in studies of anesthesia risk. In 1954, Beecher and Todd ascribed 78 percent of postoperative deaths on surgical services in ten university hospitals to patients' underlying diseases, 18 percent to surgery, and 3 percent to anesthesia. The overall death rate related to anesthesia was 3.7 in 10,000.[2] In the 1970s and 1980s, the contribution of anesthesia to perioperative death decreased markedly. The death rate from anesthesia in healthy patients with American Society of Anesthesiologists (ASA) physical status ratings of I and II may be as low as 1 in 200,000 (see Table 2–1).[3,4] The rate of permanent major sequelae is 1 in 90,000.[3]

Medical consultation is often requested to assess patients, prepare them for surgery, and assist in their postoperative management. The objective is to reduce risk and increase the probability of a good outcome. The anesthesiologist and surgeon look to the medical consultant to answer the following questions: (1) Does the patient have significant underlying systemic disease? (2) If so, has he had maximum benefit from medical therapy? (3) If further improvement is possible, what additional therapy is indicated? These questions should be explicitly asked by the consulting physician and specifically addressed by the consultant. Written statements by the medical consultant providing vague estimates of risk or medical clearance for surgery serve no useful purpose. Recommendations regarding the type of anesthesia or details of surgery

TABLE 2–1. The American Society of Anesthesiologists' Physical Status Classification

Class I. No organic, physiologic, biochemical, or psychiatric disturbance. The pathologic process for which operation is to be performed is localized and does not entail a systemic disturbance. Examples: inguinal hernia in a fit patient; fibroid uterus in an otherwise healthy woman.

Class II. Mild to moderate systemic disturbance caused either by the condition to be treated surgically or by other pathophysiologic processes. Examples: non- or only slight limiting organic heart disease; mild diabetes; essential hypertension; anemia. Some might choose to list the extremes of age here, the neonate and the octogenarian, even though no discernible systemic disease is present. Extreme obesity and chronic bronchitis may be included in this category.

Class III. Severe systemic disturbance or disease from whatever cause, even though it may not be possible to define the degree of disability with finality. Examples: severely limiting organic heart disease; severe diabetes with vascular complications; moderate to severe degrees of pulmonary insufficiency; angina pectoris; healed myocardial infarction.

Class IV. Severe systemic disorders that are already life-threatening and not always correctable by operation. Examples: organic heart disease with marked signs of cardiac insufficiency, persistent anginal syndrome, or active myocarditis; advanced degrees of pulmonary, hepatic, renal, or endocrine insufficiency.

Class V. Moribundity with little chance of survival. Examples: burst abdominal aneurysm with profound shock; major cerebral trauma with rapidly increasing intracranial pressure; massive pulmonary embolus. Most patients of this class require operation as a resuscitative measure with little if any anesthesia.

Emergency Operation (E). Any patient in one of the classes listed above who is operated upon as an emergency is considered to be in poorer physical condition than normal. The letter E is placed beside the numeric classification. Thus, the patient with a hitherto uncomplicated hernia now incarcerated and associated with nausea and vomiting is classified as IE.

Source: After Hallen B: *Acta Anesthesiol Scand* [Suppl] 52:5, 1973. © 1973 Munksesard International Publishers Ltd., Cophenhagen, Denmark.

are similarly inappropriate. However, plans for surgery and anesthesia are certainly legitimate topics for discussion among internist, anesthesiologist, and surgeon. They can often reach consensus regarding timing of surgery, relative merits of different anesthetic and surgical techniques, and anticipated perioperative complications and management.

DETERMINANTS OF PERIOPERATIVE RISK

The risks associated with anesthesia and surgery can be classified as *patient-related*, *procedure-related*, *provider-related*, and *anesthetic agent–related*.

Patient-Related Risks

Age, gender, race, socioeconomic status, surgical disease, concurrent medical disease(s), medication history, and nutritional state are significant factors in estimating risk. Many of these variables are interdependent, such as age and prevalence of cardiovascular disease requiring specific drug therapy. Some, such as socioeconomic status, may determine the characteristics of the institution and its physicians from whom the patient obtains medical care.[5] Ewy et al. devised a logistic function to estimate operation-specific mortality on the basis of such patient-control variables.[6] More recently, Cohen et al. found that perioperative mortality could be predicted by factors of advanced age, male gender, ASA physical status, and the need for major or emergency surgery. Factors not predictive of mortality were duration of anesthesia, experience of the anesthesiologist, and use of an inhalational anesthetic agent.[7]

Most investigators have found that age-related perioperative mortality is a U-shaped function with a nadir in death rate in the 15- to 25-year old age group.[8-11] Dripps and Deming made a similar observation regarding the association between age and the incidence of postoperative atelectasis and pneumonia after upper abdominal surgery.[12] In three major studies of anesthesia-related deaths, women had lower death rates than men.[2,7,11] Beecher and Todd found no relation between perioperative death rate and race.[2]

The patient's overall physical status can be described by the American Society of Anesthesiologists (ASA) Physical Status Scale (PSS) seen in Table 2–1. Although this classification was not originally designed as a predictor of risk, it does correlate with surgical outcome. Both anesthesia-related mortality (Table 2–2) and postoperative mortality (Table 2–3) rise from PSS classification I to V.[7,9,11,13-15] Anesthetic and surgical mortality double in the case of emergency surgery for patients in PSS categories I, II, and III. Emergency surgery does not add to the risk of death for patients in physical status groups IV and V.[16,17]

Drug therapy may also be associated with specific perioperative risks. Diuretic drugs may produce hypokalemia. This can potentiate the effects of nondepolarizing neuromuscular blocking agents and sometimes result in prolonged postoperative muscle weakness. Hypokalemia has been thought to increase the risk of intraoperative cardiac arrhythmias. However, this long-held belief has been challenged in both healthy patients and those with significant heart disease undergoing major surgery.[18,19] Aminoglycoside antibiotics, particularly neomycin, may also potentiate the effect of nondepolarizing neuromuscular blocking agents. Ecothiophate eye

TABLE 2–2. Anesthetic Death Rate by Physical Status

Physical Status	Death Rate [Number of Deaths/ 10,000 Operations (%)]*	
	Dripps et al[13]	Marx et al[10]
I	0/16,192 (0)	2/18,320 (0.01)
II	12/12,154 (0.1)	1/10,609 (0.01)
III	27/4070 (0.66)	11/3820 (0.29)
IV	33/720 (4.58)	9/1073 (0.84)
V	8/87 (9.20)	5/323 (1.55)
Total	80/33,224 (0.24)	27/34,145 (0.08)

*Includes "definite" and "possible" anesthetic deaths. There were 0, 7, 11, 17, and 4 "definite" anesthesia deaths among class I, II, III, IV, and V patients, respectively.

drops impair plasma pseudocholinesterase activity and prolong the neuromuscular blockade of succinylcholine, a commonly used short-acting depolarizing muscle relaxant. Chronic steroid therapy may compromise the patient's ability to respond to the stress of surgery and anesthesia.

Most drug therapies pose no significant risks in anesthetic management beyond those determined by the disease for which they are prescribed. However, the two exceptions to this generalization are insulin and monoamine oxidase inhibitors. Potentially fatal hypoglycemia may go unnoticed in anesthetized diabetic patients, and strategies to avoid it are discussed in Chap. 24. Monoamine oxidase inhibitors may have unpredictable cardiovascular effects when given in conjunction with meperidine or vasopressors and are discussed in Chap. 37.

Procedure-Related Risks

The nature of the operative procedure itself is an important determinant of perioperative mortality.[7] In the National Halothane Study, mortality level was determined for various procedures in patient groups standardized for age, gender, and physical status (Table 2–4).[20] Procedures associated with a high death rate included craniotomy, cardiac procedures, exploratory laparotomy, and large bowel surgery. Those with a low death rate were cystoscopy, dilatation and curettage, hysterectomy, herniorrhaphy, procedures involving the eye or mouth, and plastic surgery in general. There was, however, significant variation in mortality rate within each category. It should also be noted that this study included patients receiving general anesthesia only. Other investigators have found higher death rates associated with intraabdominal, intrathoracic, and cardiac procedures and those involving the head and neck.[10,11,13] Crude operation-specific death rates based on over 4 million hospital discharges in the United States in 1969 have been published for the 50 most common operations.[21]

Provider-Related Risks

Institutional differences in perioperative death rate have been documented for both university medical centers and comparable nonuniversity medical centers.[2,20] Moses and Mosteller found a 3- to 24-fold difference in postoperative death rate among 34 participat-

TABLE 2–3. Postoperative Death Rate per 10,000 Operations by ASA Physical Status (Total Number of Operations Shown in Parentheses)

ASA Physical Status	Author/Years Studied					
	Vacanti[15]		Marx et al/[10]		Cohen et al/[7]	
	48-hour mortality		1965–1969 7-day mortality		1975–1984 7-day mortality	
I	8.5	(50,703)	6	(18,320)	7.2	(38,980)
II	27	(12,601)	47	(10,609)	19.7	(38,506)
III	182	(3,616)	440	(3,820)	115	(18,073)
IV	780	(1,850)	2345	(1,073)	766	(3,276)
V	940	(608)	5080	(323)	3358	(405)
Total Cases		(68,378)		(34,145)		(99,240)

TABLE 2–4. Death Rate by the Mortality Level of Operation Standardized for Physical Status, Age, and Gender*

Mortality Level of Operation	Death Rate
Low	0.27%
Middle	1.76%
High	9.48%
All operations	1.91%

*These data from the National Halothene Study include patients who had general anesthesia only.
Source: After Moses LE, Mosteller F.[22]

ing institutions in the National Halothane Study. They concluded that such differences could not be attributed entirely to patient characteristics, procedural factors, or sampling error and implied that differences in quality of medical care may be one explanation. Other noted factors included differing nutritional levels in the population, willingness of surgeons to operate on poor-risk patients, and the percentage of referred cases.[22]

Beecher and Todd noted a threefold difference in surgical death rates among ten university medical centers which could not be accounted for by case mix.[2] Ament et al. found that mortality for cholecystectomy was higher than expected in small hospitals with fewer than 5000 annual discharges and lower than expected in large hospitals with more than 15,000 annual discharges with an overall difference between the two groups of 40 percent (Table 2–5).[23] They do not discuss the underlying reasons for these observed differences and do not comment on the patterns of operative mortality with respect to etiology.

Ewy reported a fourfold difference in standardized mortality rate among 1213 hospitals but found no relationship between hospital size and postoperative death rate.[24] He reported a clearcut correlation between good surgical outcome and the amount of money expended per patient-day within each size class, and this association was stronger for smaller than for larger hospitals. Similarly, hospitals with greater emphasis on nursing care had lower mortality rates.

Experience of hospitals and providers with particular surgical procedures also correlates with outcome. Mortality for coronary artery bypass surgery decreases as institutional experience increases. Hotchkiss found that teaching hospitals have lower mortality rates in procedures for patent ductus arteriosus (PDA) than nonteaching hospitals (Table 2–6)[25] Four times as many PDA ligations and 11 times as many PDA divisions were performed in teaching hospitals. Luft et al. found that mortality rates for openheart, major vascular, and transurethral surgery were 25 to 41 percent lower in institutions performing 200 or more of these operations annually than in hospitals with lower volumes.[26] Hannan et al. found significantly lower mortality rates in New York state hospitals for physicians who performed higher numbers of coronary artery bypass procedures, resections of abdominal aortic aneurysms, partial gastrectomies, and colectomies.[27] Hospital volume itself had less effect on mortality but was associated with significantly lower mortality following cholecystectomy.

TABLE 2–5. Cholecystectomy Mortality

Hospital Size Group	Number of Hospitals	Number of Patients	Actual Mortality Rate*	Expected Mortality Rate*	Difference
Small	353	10,672	21.3	16.5	+4.8
Medium-Small	278	23,673	17.4	16.5	+0.9
Medium-Large	201	27,653	14.7	15.7	−1.0
Large	144	29,972	14.1	15.7	−1.6
All Hospitals	976	91,970	16.0	16.0	0.0

*Per 1000 patients.
Source: After Kinkaid WH: *PAS Reporter* 9 (12):1, 1971.

TABLE 2–6. Mortality from Ligation and Division of Patient Ductus Arteriosus in Teaching and Non-Teaching Hospitals

	Ligation No. of deaths/ No. of patients (%)		Division No. of deaths/ No. of patients (%)	
Teaching Hospitals	38/1476	(2.6)	63/2212	(2.75)
Non-Teaching Hospitals	12/320	(3.75)	18/188	(9.55)

Source: After Ament RP, Gustafson PG, Holtz CL: *PAS Reporter* 8:1, 1970.

Anesthetic Agent–Related Risks

Until recently, no study of perioperative death had established that any one of the major modes of anesthesia—regional (spinal, epidural, and nerve block) or general—is safer than any other. Indeed, Dornette reported anesthetic deaths associated with overdoses of local anesthesia,[28] and the Baltimore Anesthesia Study Committee ascribed two deaths to anesthetic management when no anesthetic agent was used.[8] In the latter cases, the committee felt that "more adequate preparation and the contribution of an anesthetic might have enhanced the patient's chances of surviving the operative intervention."

Similar conclusions have been drawn for postoperative pulmonary morbidity. Greene concluded that the incidence of postoperative pulmonary complications is higher following general anesthesia than following spinal anesthesia if prophylactic measures are not taken or if anesthesia is administered by lesser-trained personnel. However, if the quality of medical care is high, there is no difference that can be ascribed to the type of anesthesia.[29]

A number of studies support the belief that spinal and epidural anesthesia are associated with better surgical outcome. The incidences of thromboembolism and overall mortality are lower with these techniques compared with general anesthesia in hip surgery.[30,31] Other investigators, however, find that, while mortality within two weeks of surgery is less in those patients receiving spinal anesthesia, there is no difference after one to two months.[32,33]

Yeager et al. found mortality, morbidity, and costs to be lower in a group of high-risk surgical patients receiving epidural anesthesia and postoperative epidural local anesthesia and/or narcotic analgesia compared with a control group receiving general anesthesia and conventional postoperative parenteral narcotic analgesia.[34] This study was a randomized prospective controlled clinical trial but involved a relatively small number of patients in each group. However, the overall complication rate was so much higher in patients receiving general anesthesia (19/25) when compared with those receiving epidural anesthesia (9/28) that the authors felt it necessary to terminate the study.[35] These results have not been confirmed by other investigators.

The experience of anesthesiologists with new drugs has also been shown to affect mortality. Dripps and his associates showed that deaths associated with the use of muscle relaxants were often related to physician error.[13] This finding and three decades of subsequent experience refute the hypothesis of Beecher and Todd that such deaths are due to the inherent toxicity of the drugs themselves. This controversy demonstrates that it is sometimes difficult to determine the cause of adverse outcomes and that associations do not necessarily imply causation.

Most anesthetic deaths are due to failure to ventilate, unsuspected hypoxemia, or overdose of anesthetic.[36-38] Deaths attributable to anesthesia management have decreased markedly in recent years. The reasons for these improvements are many and include improved understanding of the pharmacology of anesthetic agents, better drugs, more qualified practitioners, safer anesthesia equipment, and intraoperative monitoring of oxygen saturation and expired carbon dioxide levels.[39,40]

Emergency Surgery

Patients undergoing emergency surgery have a higher risk of death than those undergoing elective surgery.[13,15] Intravascular hypovolemia potentiates the renal, cardiac, and cerebral hypoperfusion resulting from the myocardial depressant and vasodilatory effects of anesthetic agents. Emergency patients are more likely to vomit or regurgitate gastric contents and aspirate. These patients often have acid-base, extracellular fluid volume, and electrolyte abnormalities for any number of reasons.

It is important that these abnormalities be corrected and that appropriate monitoring of central blood volume and left ventricular function as well as timely pertinent blood studies be carried out. Ideally, a full stomach should be decompressed before surgery. However, if there is uncontrolled blood loss, as from a ruptured aorta or ectopic pregnancy, delaying surgery is unjustified since control of the bleeding vessel is the definitive resuscitative measure.

In addition, high-risk patients are more sensitive to the effects of hypotension, cardiac depression, and acid-base derangements. It may be advisable to transfer high-risk patients to tertiary care centers before surgery when the need for specialized measures like prolonged respiratory or hemodynamic support, hemodialysis, or specific care of spinal cord injury or head trauma is anticipated.

Sound patient care necessitates not only satisfactory physiologic evaluation and monitoring but also provision for communication among physicians rendering concurrent care. Treatment strategies should be established before surgery and before the development of the crises that frequently beset high-risk surgical patients.

SUMMARY

1. Most operative illness and death result from the patient's concurrent underlying physiologic dysfunction.

2. Anesthetic deaths are most often due to human error. However, anesthetic deaths account for only one to four percent of the total perioperative mortality rate.

3. The goal of preoperative preparation is to achieve the optimal level of function for a particular patient. Disease states and medications which may cause problems should be identified so that complications can be anticipated and treated in a timely fashion in both elective and emergency surgery.

REFERENCES

1. Goldstein A, Keats AS: The risk of anesthesia. *Anesthesiology* 33:130, 1970.
2. Beecher HK, Todd DP: A study of the deaths associated with anesthesia and surgery. *Ann Surg* 140:2, 1954.
3. Eichhorn JH: Prevention of intraoperative anesthesia accidents and related severe injury through safety monitoring. *Anesthesiology* 70:572, 1989.
4. Lunn JN, Devlin HB: Lessons from the confidential inquiry into perioperative deaths in three NHS regions. *Lancet* 2:1384, 1987.
5. Egbert LD, Rothman IL: Relation between the race and economic status of patients and who performs their surgery. *N Engl J Med* 279:90, 1977.
6. Ewy W: Important patient control variables in outcomes of surgery and anesthesia, in Hirsh RA, Forrest WH, Orkin FK et al (eds): *Health Care Delivery in Anesthesia*. Philadelphia, George F. Stickley, 1980, p 85.
7. Cohen MM, Duncan PG, Tate RB: Does anesthesia contribute to operative mortality? *JAMA* 260:2859–2863, 1988.
8. Graff TD, Phillips OC, Benson DW et al: Baltimore Anesthesia Study Committee: Factors in pediatric mortality. *Anesth Analg* 43:407, 1964.
9. Hallen B: Computerized anesthesia record-keeping. *Acta Anaesthesiol Scand* [Suppl] 52:5, 1973.
10. Marx GF, Mateo CV, Orkin LR: Computer analysis of postanesthesia deaths. *Anesthesiology* 39:54, 1973.
11. Phillips OC, Frazier TM, Graff TD et al: The Baltimore Anesthesia Study Committee: Review of 1024 postoperative deaths. *JAMA* 174:2015, 1960.
12. Dripps RD, Deming MV: Postoperative atelectasis and pneumonia. *Ann Surg* 124:94, 1946.
13. Dripps RD, Lamont A, Eckenhoff JE: The role of anesthesia in surgical mortality. *JAMA* 778:261, 1961.
14. Lewin I, Lerner AG, Green SH et al: Physical class and physiologic status in the prediction of operative mortality in the aged sick. *Ann Surg* 174:2, 1971.
15. Vacanti CJ, Van Houten RJ, Hill RC: A statistical analysis of the relationship of physical status to postoperative mortality in 68,388 cases. *Anesth Analg* 49:564, 1970.
16. Dripps RD, Eckenhoff JE, Vandam LD: *Introduction to Anesthesia*, 5th ed. Philadephia, Saunders, 1977.
17. Gibert JP: Outcome—experience and training of the anesthetist, in Hirsh RA, Forrest WH, Orkin FK et al (eds): *Health Care Delivery in Anesthesia*. Philadephia, George F. Stickley, 1980, p 143.
18. Vitez TS, Soper LE, Wong KC et al: Chronic hypokalemia and intraoperative dysrhythmias. *Anesthesiology* 63:130–133, 1988.
19. Hirsch IA, Tomlinson DL, Slogoff S et al: The overstated risk of preoperative hypokalemia. *Anesth Analg* 67:131–136, 1988.
20. Bunker JP, Forrest WH, Mosteller F et al: *The National Halothane Study*. NIH, NIGMS, Bethesda, U.S. Government Printing Office, 1969.
21. Kinkaid WH (ed): Hospital deaths following surgery. *PAS Reporter* 9(12):1, 1971.
22. Moses LE, Mosteller F: Institutional differences in postoperative death rates. *JAMA* 203:492, 1968.
23. Ament RP, Gustafson PG, Holtz CL et al: Cholecystectomy mortality. *PAS Reporter* 8:1, 1970.
24. Ewy W: Hospital death and morbidity studies, in Hirsh RA, Forrest WH, Orkin FK, et al (eds): *Health Care Delivery in Anesthesia*. Philadelphia, George F. Stickley, 1980, p 49.
25. Hotchkiss WS: Patent ductus arteriosus and the occasional cardiac surgeon. *JAMA* 173:244, 1960.
26. Luft HS, Bunker JP, Enthoven AC: Should operations be regionalized? The empirical relation between surgical volume and mortality. *N Engl J Med* 301:1364, 1979.
27. Hannan EL, O'Donnell JF, Kilburn H et al: Investigation of the relationship between volume and mortality for surgical procedures performed in New York State hospitals. *JAMA* 262:503–510, 1989.
28. Dornette WHL, Ortho OS: Death in the operating room. *Anesth Analg* 35:545, 1956.
29. Greene N: *Physiology of Spinal Anesthesia*, 2d ed. Baltimore, Williams & Wilkins, 1969, p 130.
30. Modig J, Borg T, Karstrom G, et al: Thromboembolism after total hip replacement: Role of epidural and general anesthesia. *Anesth Analg* 62:174, 1983.
31. McKenzie PJ, Wishart HY, Smith G: Long-term outcome after repair of fractured neck of femur. *Br J Anaesth* 56:581, 1984.
32. McLaren AD, Stockwell MC, Reid VT: Anesthetic techniques for surgical correction of fractured neck of femur. *Anaesthesia* 33:10–14, 1978.
33. Davis FM, Woolner DF, Frampton C et al: Prospective multicentre trial of mortality following general or spinal anesthesia for hip fracture surgery in the elderly. *Br J. Anaesth* 59:1080–1088, 1987.
34. Yeager MP, Glass DD, Neff RK et al: Epidural anesthesia and analgesia in high-risk surgical patients. *Anesthesiology* 66:729–736, 1987.
35. McPeek B: Inference, generalizability, and a major change in anesthetic practice. *Anesthesiology* 66:723–724, 1987.
36. Keenan RL, Boyan CP: Cardiac arrest due to anesthesia. *JAMA* 253:2373, 1985.
37. Caplan RA, Ward RJ, Posner K et al: Respiratory mishaps: Principal areas of risk and implications for anesthetic care (abstract). *Anesthesiology* 67:A469, 1987.
38. Caplan RA, Wark RJ, Posner K et al: Unexpected cardiac arrest during spinal anesthesia: a closed claims analysis of predisposing factors. *Anesthesiology* 68:5–11, 1988.
39. Pierce EC: The development of anesthesia guidelines and standards. *Q Rev Bull* 16:61, 1990.
40. Orkin FK: Practice standards: the Midas touch or the emperor's new clothes? *Anesthesiology* 70:567–571, 1989.

3 THE PREOPERATIVE SCREENING EXAMINATION

Jeffrey L. Carson

John M. Eisenberg

Although it is generally agreed that a medical history and physical examination should be obtained before surgery, there is controversy about the additional benefit of preoperative screening tests. This chapter assesses the utility of such tests in the asymptomatic patient. Concepts of sensitivity, specificity, and predictive value as they apply to screening tests are reviewed, and recommendations are offered as to which tests are indicated in the preoperative evaluation.

In this context, the term *screening* refers to the search for unsuspected disease in preoperative patients who, aside from their surgical problems, are otherwise clinically well. A more appropriate term might be *case finding,* implying a search for disease in an individual already under the care of a physician or surgeon. In contrast, the traditional definition of screening refers to search for disease in large unselected general populations of asymptomatic people. Obtaining a chemistry profile in a patient undergoing an appendectomy is an example of case finding, while performing such a profile for every person in a community constitutes screening. However, this chapter conforms to the common use of the term screening to describe multiphasic testing in the hospitalized patient. It should be noted that this chapter does not address the evaluation of patients who have specific symptoms or who require emergency surgery.

PRINCIPLES OF SCREENING

The characteristics of an ideal screening test should include the following:

1. The patient must offer no evidence on history or physical examination of the condition for which he is being screened.
2. The condition can potentially alter the outcome of surgery.
3. Preoperative diagnosis will affect perioperative management.
4. The prevalence and severity of the condition are great enough to warrant the expense of screening.
5. The test is sufficiently sensitive to allow detection and specific enough to avoid over-diagnosis.[1-3]

The term *sensitivity* is defined as that percentage of patients with a disease who have an abnormal test. *Specificity* is that percentage of healthy patients who have a normal test. Hence, an ideal test will give positive results in all diseased subjects (100 percent sensitivity) and negative results in all healthy subjects (100 percent specificity).[4] *Prevalence* is that percentage of patients with the disease at the time of the study, whereas *incidence* is the number of new cases over a given period of time.

The *predictive value* of a positive test is the percentage of positive results obtained that are true positives, i.e., that are obtained from patients who have the disease in question. Positive results may also be seen in some patients who do not have the disease, and such results are called false positives. In contrast, the predictive value of a negative or normal test is defined as the percentage of negative results that are true negatives, i.e., that are obtained from patients who are free of the disease in question. False negative results may also be obtained from some patients who have the disease in question.

The predictive value of a test varies directly with the prevalence of the disease in the population studied. Table 3–1 shows that, if the sensitivity and specificity of a test are both 95 percent, the predictive value of the test varies considerably with different levels of prevalence. When the test is applied to a population with a prevalence of disease of 50 percent, the predictive value is 95 percent. However, if the prevalence is one percent, the positive predictive value is only 16 percent, implying that 84 percent of all positive test results will be false-positive ones.

The routine partial thromboplastin time (PTT) determination serves to illustrate the clinical relevance of predictive value. Because surgery may be postponed in patients with abnormal results, the proportion of true positives and false positives is important. The prevalence of hemostatic disease is low in asymptomatic patients. Therefore, although some people may actually have hemostatic abnormalities, most are normal, and the number of

TABLE 3–1. Predictive Value and Prevalence for a Test with 95% Sensitivity and Specificity

Prevalence of Disease (%)	Predictive Value of a Positive Test (%)
0.1	1.9
1	16.1
2	27.9
5	50.0
50	95.0

false-positive tests is relatively high. This means that the positive predictive value of the test is low, and surgery may be postponed or cancelled unnecessarily. Thus, an abnormal test inconveniences both patient and surgeon and leads to additional expense by necessitating further evaluation.

In an asymptomatic healthy population, the prevalence of disease is low, and most tests will be of little value. However, the prevalence of some diseases increases with age, making the test increasingly more valuable in older populations. Hence, the value of a test is directly proportional to the likelihood of finding disease.

Because the normal limits of a test are often defined as those values two standard deviations above and below the mean in a population of healthy people, a small proportion of normal individuals (about 4.5 percent) will have an abnormal result. Some false-positive results are therefore inevitable. The greater the number of tests carried out in a healthy individual, the greater the likelihood that a false-positive result will be found (Table 3–2).

Do screening tests provide information that would not have been obtained from the history and physical examination? Do they uncover new problems necessitating a change in patient managements? One study assessed the diagnostic yield of the medical history alone in 200 preoperative patients.[5] Answers to a set of simple questions predicted fitness for operation in 96 percent of the cases. A more extensive history, physical examination, and laboratory investigation provided little additional useful information. This said, the remainder of this chapter addresses the utility of several common preoperative screening tests in elective surgical patients.

TABLE 3–2. Probability of Obtaining an Abnormal Result in a Screening Battery

Number of Independent Tests	Abnormal Results Found (%)
1	5
2	10
4	19
6	26
10	40
20	64
50	92
90	99

Source: Galen RS, Gambino SR: *Beyond Normality: The Predictive Value and Efficiency of Medical Diagnosis.* New York, John Wiley & Sons, 1975.

PREOPERATIVE CARDIAC EXAMINATION AND THE ELECTROCARDIOGRAM

Cardiac disease is the most common cause of postoperative morbidity and mortality.[6] A preoperative electrocardiogram (ECG) may be used to assess the risk of cardiac complications, to guide management in order to reduce the risk of such complications, and to provide a baseline for comparison if problems arise after surgery.[6]

Assessing Risk

Goldman's prospective study of cardiac risk factors and complications in 1001 consecutive patients undergoing noncardiac surgery includes data on the utility of the electrocardiogram.[7] All patients age 40 or older admitted for elective procedures had a history and physical examination, an electrocardiogram, and a chest x-ray. All had routine postoperative electrocardiograms five days after surgery and were evaluated postoperatively if cardiac symptoms developed.

Five factors were associated with a significantly higher risk of developing a postoperative myocardial infarction: (1) age greater than 70; (2) history of dyspnea, orthopnea or edema; (3) murmur of mitral regurgitation of grade 2/6 or louder; (4) more than five premature ventricular contractions per minute; and (5) tortuous or calcified aorta on chest radiograph. Postoperative heart failure was associated with a variety of murmurs but not with findings dependent on the preoperative ECG. Factors correlated with postoperative death included age greater than 70, history of myocardial infarction within the six months before surgery, jugular venous distention, an S_3 gallop, cardiac rhythm other than sinus, more than five premature ventricular contractions per minute, the need for emergency surgery, and intraoperative hypotension.

By weighting each of these factors, Goldman developed an index to predict cardiac risk. This index, however, succeeded in identifying only about 40 percent of patients who developed postoperative cardiovascular events. Moreover, nearly all of its significant component factors could be identified by a thorough history and physical examination. Although confirmation of premature ventricular contractions or a rhythm other than sinus may require electrocardiographic confirmation, a regular rhythm on cardiac auscultation should be adequate screening for nearly all arrhythmias. Three additional studies have largely confirmed most of Goldman's findings.[8,9,10]

Other studies investigating the value of the preoperative ECG are flawed in design. In 1958, Wang and Howland studied 482 patients who had preoperative ECG's and found "little definitive" correlation between preoperative electrocardiographic abnormalities and postoperative complications.[11] Twenty years later, Cooperman et al. retrospectively analyzed cardiovascular risk factors in 566 patients undergoing certain major vascular procedures and identified five risk factors correlated with postoperative complications:[12] (1) a prior myocardial infarction; (2) congestive heart failure; (3) arrhythmia; (4) an abnormal electrocardiogram (including bundle-branch block); and (5) a previous cerebrovascular accident. Most of these risk factors could have been detected by careful history and physical examination. Although an abnormal electrocardiogram was considered a risk factor in the study, the criteria for abnormality were not defined. In contrast, two other studies have found that, in patients with right bundle-branch block and left axis deviation, the risk of developing complete heart block after surgery is nearly zero.[13,14] McCleane and McCoy evaluated the proportion of abnormal ECGs in 877 patients admitted to the hospital for elective surgery. More abnormalities were noted in older patients and in those with ASA classifications of II or higher. However, the clinical significance of these abnormalities was not considered.[15]

Knowledge of past myocardial infarction may be important in guiding management in the perioperative period. The utility of an ECG in detecting myocardial infarction has been assessed in the Framingham and other studies.[16-18] In the former, the ECG served as the only means of detecting a past myocardial infarction in 28 percent of patients, but its success in doing so was limited and mostly confined to elderly patients. However, the yield is age-dependent and very low. Since evidence of myocardial infarction occurring within the six months preceding surgery affects decision making, a former comparison tracing is most often needed in an attempt to time the event.

Three recent studies confirm that most important abnormalities occur in patients over age 50. Jakobsson found abnormal ECGs in 247 of 731 patients, but only 8 percent were unexpectedly so.[19] All patients with evidence of unsuspected past myocardial infarction on ECG were age 50 or older. Elston and Taylor found abnormal ECG's almost exclusively confined to patients over age 60.[20] In 1068 surgical patients, Ferrer found most abnormalities in those age 71 to 85.[21] Most were T-wave changes which did not correlate with clinical outcome.

Establishing the Baseline

Another reason to perform a preoperative ECG is to provide a baseline comparison should problems develop postoperatively. Approximately 67 percent of patients with proven acute myocardial infarction develop characteristic electrocardiographic changes while 10 percent of such patients have normal ECGs. In the remaining 23 percent, ECG findings are nonspecific, and a comparison tracing may be useful.[22]

There are no studies assessing the utility of a baseline ECG in the setting of postoperative myocardial infarction. However, two studies have examined this issue in the emergency room setting. Rubenstein and Greenfield evaluated 236 patients and found that a baseline tracing would have been useful in five percent of patients in deciding whether to admit a patient to the hospital.[23] In a second study, Hoffman and Igarashi asked house officers if a baseline ECG would influence their decision about admission to the hospital.[24] The decision process was influenced in 25 percent of the patients but did not ultimately change disposition of the patient. These two studies do not support the value of a baseline ECG in an emergency room, but it is not clear if these data are transferable to the perioperative setting.

Guiding Management

The preoperative ECG is useful in guiding management if it shows evidence of ischemic heart disease or ventricular arrhythmias. If the preoperative ECG demonstrates a pattern consistent with an old myocardial infarction, the time of the infarction in relation to the proposed surgery should be determined. If it occurred within six months, elective surgery should be postponed until six months have passed. When surgery cannot be delayed, intensive medical therapy and monitoring should be instituted. When the time of the

infarction cannot be determined, postponement of surgery for six months should be considered when possible. Stress testing is probably indicated in all patients to assess cardiac function.

If new ventricular ectopy is noted on the ECG, further evaluation to identify the cause of the rhythm disturbance is indicated. Electrolyte abnormalities, hypoxia, and drug-induced disease should be excluded. Coronary artery disease and ventricular dysfunction should be excluded with a stress test and echocardiogram. Specific therapy should be directed at the underlying cause of the arrhythmia. (See Chap. 21.)

In summary, current evidence suggests that an ECG is not routinely indicated before noncardiac surgery. The data support the thoughtful recommendations of Goldberger and O'Konski suggesting that an ECG be performed in

Patients with history and physical examination suggestive of cardiovascular disease,

Patients with systemic disease or other conditions that may be associated with unrecognized heart disease such as hypertension or diabetes,

Patients taking medications which might have cardiac toxicity,

Patients at risk for electrolyte disturbances, and

Patients undergoing major surgical procedures.[25]

They also suggest that routine ECGs be performed in men 40 to 45 years of age or older and in women 55 or older. They concede that the choice of these specific ages is necessarily arbitrary. One could reasonably argue that, in patients having no cardiovascular risk factors and a normal history and physical examination, the yield is too low to warrant the expense at any age.

CHEST RADIOGRAPH

The chest radiograph is the most frequently performed x-ray in the Untied States[26] and is often included in the preoperative evaluation. In patients undergoing cardiopulmonary surgery for known disease in the thorax, the chest radiograph confirms the diagnosis, aids in assessing operative risk, and provides a baseline for postoperative comparison. It does not serve as a screening test in these patients.

The value of the screening preoperative chest radiograph in other surgical settings has been questioned by many investigators. In a large study from the Royal College of Radiologists, 10,619 patients undergoing elective surgery other than cardiopulmonary procedures were studied.[27] Radiographs were ordered in 29.7 percent of these patients for no apparent clinical reason. The films did not alter the choice of anesthesia or the decision to operate and were of little value as a baseline study against which to judge subsequent radiographs. In a study of 607 patients undergoing elective surgery, Rees et al. reported 126 significant abnormalities.[28] However, they found that the history and physical examination were more sensitive than chest x-rays in detecting disease other than tuberculosis. Finally, Petterson and Janover found that the routine chest film led to postponement of surgery in only two of 1393 preoperative patients.[29]

Rucker et al. studied the utility of preoperative screening chest radiographs in patients with and without risk factors detected by history and physical examination.[30] Risk factors included findings consistent with cardiac or pulmonary disease and age over 60 years. Of 905 preoperative patients, 368 had no risk factors. Only one patient had a serious abnormality on chest x-ray which did not affect perioperative management. None of these patients had postoperative cardiac or pulmonary complications. Of 504 with risk factors, 114 had serious chest x-ray abnormalities, but outcomes in these patients were not assessed. The authors concluded that the chest radiograph should be used only as an adjunct to a careful history and physical examination.

The frequency of chest x-ray abnormalities is related to age. In 1000 preoperative radiographs, Loder found abnormalities in only five under the age of 30.[31] Rees et al. found normal chest radiographs in all patients under 20 years of age and nothing on chest x-rays in patients under 30 which altered the clinical diagnosis.[28] Similarly, Sagel et al. discovered no new abnormalities on chest x-rays in 521 patients under 20 and only nine abnormalities in 894 patients under 30.[32] In patients age 65 and older undergoing non-cardiopulmonary surgery, Seymour et al. noted that 40.3 percent of 233 patients had a clinically significant abnormality on chest x-ray.[33] Patients with a cardiac abnormality on chest x-ray were twice as likely to have a perioperative myocardial infarction or heart failure. However, there was no correlation between preoperative pulmonary abnormalities on chest radiograph and postoperative pulmonary complications.

Only one study addressed the value of the preoperative chest x-ray as a baseline for comparison in those developing postoperative pulmonary problems. In Seymour's study of patients over age 65, 32.2 percent of patients required a postoperative radiograph, and in all of these cases the preoperative study was considered invaluable.[33] However, the study did not examine independent readings with and without comparison to the preoperative radiograph to assess accurately the contribution of the preoperative study.

It is therefore recommended that the chest radiograph be abandoned as a routine preoperative test. However, a preoperative chest x-ray should be obtained in patients with suspected cardiac or pulmonary disease and in those 60 years of age or older. Moreover, while the value of a baseline preoperative chest radiograph is uncertain, it seems reasonable to recommend one for patients with an increased risk of postoperative pulmonary complications. Such patients include cigarette smokers, obese patients, and those undergoing cardiothoracic or upper abdominal surgery. A single view is

sufficient and the lateral view may be eliminated. Further discussion of the preoperative evaluation of patients with pulmonary disease is found in Chap. 22.

CHEMICAL AND HEMATOLOGIC PROFILES

Although multiphasic blood profiles are convenient for the physician and less expensive for the patient, their value depends upon their ability to detect disease in the asymptomatic patient and thereby influence perioperative care. The true cost of such profiles often includes that of follow-up testing to explain abnormal screening tests.

Three studies examine the usefulness of screening laboratory tests in preoperative surgical patients. Kaplan et al. reviewed the impact of a complete blood count, a chemistry panel (SMA-6), a prothrombin time (PT), a partial thromboplastin time (PTT), a platelet count, and a serum glucose determination on the management of 2000 patients undergoing elective surgery.[34] A mere 0.22 percent of the results might have influenced the management of the patient but were not acted upon and did not affect outcome (Table 3–3).

Turnbull and Buck examined the value of preoperative screening tests in 1010 patients undergoing cholecystectomy with an otherwise normal history and physical examination.[35] Of 5003 tests performed, 225 were abnormal, but only 104 were of potential importance. Preoperative action was taken in the case of only 17 abnormalities, and only four patients may have actually benefited from having been tested. The authors concluded that the laboratory tests provided little additional help beyond the history and physical examination. This study did not examine outpatient tests or consider how abnormalties might have affected perioperative monitoring.

Blery et al. prospectively tested a preconceived protocol for selective preoperative testing in 3866 consecutive surgical patients.[36] Only 0.2 to 0.4 percent of unincluded but otherwise routine presurgical tests would have been potentially useful. The authors concluded that a protocol limiting preoperative testing has little adverse effect on patient care but should be modified by clinical judgment.

The specific utility of inpatient screening clinical chemistry profiles has been extensively studied. Daughaday et al. found at least one abnormal test in 60 percent of all hospitalized patients studied.[37] Abnormalities were found in 14 percent of patients un-

TABLE 3–3. Summary of Preoperative Test Study

Test	No. of Tests	No. (%) of Abnormal Results in Sample	No. (%) of Unindicated Abnormal Results	No. (%) of Unindicated SSA* Results	95% Confidence Interval**
Prothrombin time	650	2 (1.0)	0 (0)	0 (0)	0–1.8
Partial thromboplastin time	650	1 (0.5)	0 (0)	0 (0)	0–1.8
Plalelet count	1320	3 (0.7)	2 (0.5)	1 (0.2)	0–1.4
Complete blood cell count	4660	22 (3.6)	2 (0.3)	0 (0)	0–0.6
Differential cell count	1480	2 (0.5)	1 (0.3)	0 (0)	0–0.9
Six-factor automated multiple analysis	3200	41 (8.0)	1 (0.2)	0 (0)	0–1.1
Glucose level	3100	25 (5.4)	4 (0.9)	2 (0.4)	0–1.6

*Unindicated SSA results indicates unindicated (potentially) surgically significant abnormal results.
**Confidence limits: 95% upper and lower confidence for the true fraction of unindicated surgically significant abnormal results.
Source: Modified from Kaplan et al. *JAMA*, 1985

der 40 and in 43 percent of patients over 70. Newman uncovered new disease on the basis of screening serum calcium levels in 0.4 percent of patients, cholesterol in 0.5 percent, glucose in 5.5 percent, alkaline phosphatase in 1.9 percent, uric acid in 1.8 percent, and serum glutamic oxaloacetic transaminase (SGOT) in 3.9 percent.[38] In 31,439 tests done in 2071 patients, Whitehead and Wootton found only 0.7 percent to be unexpectedly abnormal and to provide new diagnostic information.[39]

Finding an abnormal test result or making a new diagnosis may not necessarily be beneficial to the patient. Korvin et al. evaluated 1000 patients undergoing 20 chemical and hematologic tests.[40] Of the 2223 abnormal results obtained, 675 were predictable on clinical grounds, 1325 yielded no new information, and the remaining 223 led to 83 new diagnoses. In the authors' opinion, recognition of only one of these diagnoses proved beneficial to the patient. Durbridge et al. compared a group of 500 patients undergoing admission testing with two control groups for which admission multiphasic testing was not available.[41] They found no significant difference in the quality of care provided these patients. The use of routine admission testing did not shorten the length of hospital stay but did increase the total cost of hospitalization by five percent, probably because of a greater number of follow-up tests and consultations.

Glucose

Levels of serum glucose outside the reference range are the most frequently detected abnormalities on biochemical profiles. Of 57 new diagnoses made in Korvin's series, 17 were diabetes mellitus.[40] In a series reported by Galloway and Shuman, the initial diagnosis of diabetes mellitus was made on the basis of a preoperative glucose test in 100 of 467 patients, and 40 of the 100 had serum glucose levels greater than 200 mg/dl.[42] However, the diagnosis of diabetes mellitus might have been suspected in 70 of the 100 patients from careful review of the history and physical examination. Most other studies document a two to five percent prevalence of abnormal glucose levels, but few abnormalities were deemed clinically significant enough to pursue.[36] None of these studies considered how knowledge of an abnormal preoperative glucose level may have affected postoperative monitoring.

Serum glucose levels may rise postoperatively as a result of the stress of anesthesia and surgery and from the administration of intravenous fluids.[43,44] Significant postoperative hyperglycemia may cause osmotic diuresis and dehydration or impair white-cell function. Although the preoperative serum glucose level is of undecided value, it may influence postoperative patient monitoring and obviate such problems.

Creatinine

The ability of the kidney to metabolize and excrete drugs and anesthetic agents is important in the clinical course of the surgical patient. Although the serum creatinine level generally does not rise until renal function has been compromised by more than 50 percent,[45] this test is less expensive and more easily obtained than a 24-hour creatinine clearance. However, the prevalence of renal insufficiency among asymptomatic patients with no history of renal disease is only 0.2 percent.[34,35] A creatinine or serum blood urea nitrogen level should be considered before surgery in patients undergoing operations associated with acute renal failure, e.g., ab-

dominal aortic aneurysm repair. In all other patients, a test for renal function is not indicated.

Urinalysis

Richter et al. found that preoperative evaluation of the urine was useful in 150 patients undergoing prostatectomy. Wound infections were more common in patients with infected urine than in those with sterile urine. Organisms obtained from infected wounds were identical to those isolated from the urine in 84 percent of the patients. The investigators concluded that urinalysis should be performed before prostatectomy and the procedure postponed until the urine is sterile. However, in this case preoperative urinalysis should not be considered a screening test because it is performed in patients with a known abnormality of the urinary tract.[46]

In contrast, preoperative screening urinalysis has not been demonstrated to be valuable in other studies. Gold and Wofersberger found that about one percent of 3375 patients undergoing ambulatory oral and maxillofacial surgery had proteinuria and that one patient had hematuria.[47] Glynn and Sheehan analyzed the significance of asymptomatic bacteriuria in patients undergoing hip and knee arthroplasty.[48] Of 299 patients, a significant number had urine cultures growing > 100,000 colonies of bacteria. These abnormalities did not correlate with postoperative infection, although all of the patients were treated after cultures results were known. In a study of all hospital admissions, Heimann et al. examined the records of 400 patients and found that 116 patients or 29 percent had abnormalities on routine urinalysis.[49] Physicians recognized these abnormalities in only 51 percent of the cases, and it is not clear whether care was influenced by the findings. In the asymptomatic patient, the value of a routine preoperative urinalysis must be questioned.[50]

Liver Enzyme Tests

Liver enzyme determinations may be important in detecting underlying hepatic disease which may influence the metabolism of drugs or anesthetic agents, increase their toxicity, or affect coagulation. Two studies have examined the value of preoperative liver enzyme tests. Schemel examined the yield in 7620 elective surgical patients.[51] The incidence of elevated liver enzymes was 1 in 700 and that of jaundice was 1 in 2540. Similar results were found in a study by Wataneeyawech and Kelley.[52] Both studies concluded that screening liver enzymes should be performed in all preoperative patients, but it is unclear whether any of these patients would have been adversely affected by their liver disease.

In Korvin's study, 22 of 1000 patients had unsuspected elevated serum bilirubin levels, and 19 had elevated liver enzyme levels leading to information possibly important to their care.[40] Similarly, Daughaday et al. suspected liver enzyme abnormalities and subsequently confirmed liver function impairment in 5 of 1869 patients.[37] Although Belliveau et al. did not assess ultimate changes in outcome, they found abnormalities in serum alkaline phosphatase in 4.8 percent of patients, SGOT in 13.5 percent, lactic dehydrogenase in 12.3 percent, and total bilirubin in 5.8 percent.[53] On the basis of these abnormal results, six new cases of cirrhosis were discovered among 1046 patients admitted to a community hospital.

These data suggest that liver enzyme determinations are not indicated in most patients since the prevalence of liver disease is low. However, in patients undergoing procedures likely to compromise hepatic function, it is reasonable to obtain a serum glutamic oxaloacetic transaminase (SGOT) or serum glutamic pyruvate transaminase (SGPT) level before surgery.

Complete Blood Count

A complete blood count is traditionally performed before surgery. Low white blood cell counts are found in only 0.02 percent of preoperative patients.[34,35] The prevalence of thrombocytopenia in asymptomatic patients is similarly only 0.04 percent.[35] Although thrombocytopenia is potentially important, the history and physical examination are usually sufficient to predict risk of perioperative bleeding.

A hematocrit of at least 30 percent or a hemoglobin level of 10 g/dl or greater has been a traditional prerequisite for elective surgery. A survey of 1249 American hospitals suggested that nine g/dl is the minimum acceptable hemoglobin level in preoperative patients.[54] This criterion is based on the fact that patients with chronic anemia normally increase cardiac output when the hemoglobin level falls below eight g/dl. Transient hypoxia in the perioperative period is common, and the induction of anesthesia may cause a 20 to 30 percent reduction in cardiac output. These factors decrease the delivery of oxygen to peripheral tissues and further increase cardiac workload.

Despite these theoretical considerations, a recent National Institutes of Health consensus conference has challenged the common clinical practice of transfusing all patients to a hemoglobin level of 10 g/dl.[55] It remains unknown below what level of hemoglobin surgical morbidity and mortality rise. Studies in man are either seriously flawed[56,57] or too small[58] to answer this question. Rawstron retrospectively analyzed 145 surgical patients with hemoglobin levels below 10 g/dl and compared them to a control group of 412 with normal levels.[56] He concluded that there was no difference in perioperative complications in the two groups. However, others believe that these data suggest that the frequency of major complications is 15 percent in the anemic patients and only 6 percent in the control group.[59] Lunn and Elwood examined the relationship between the preoperative hemoglobin level and the risk of death in 1584 patients.[57] They noted an increased risk of death in patients with hemoglobin levels less than 10 g/dl. Neither of these two studies controlled for co-morbid conditions which might have resulted in death. Finally, Carson et al., in a small study of 125 surgical patients refusing blood transfusion, found that death rates did not correlate with preoperative hemoglobin levels below 10 g/dl but did demonstrate an association between death and operative blood loss.[58] No data document that giving blood to anemic patients will eliminate or lower the risk associated with surgery.

The value of obtaining a preoperative hemoglobin level has been assessed in several studies. Kaplan et al. believe that a hemoglobin level is indicated if a blood type and antibody screen are ordered.[34] Turnbull and Buck found that a low hemoglobin level was the most common laboratory abnormality, but the lowest hemoglobin found was 9.9 g/dl.[35] Of the seven patients with a low hemoglobin level, 29 percent developed "relevant" complications such as postoperative hypotension compared to 1.4 percent of patients with a normal hemoglobin. Blery found that it would have been desirable to obtain preoperative hemoglobin levels in 1.6 percent of those in whom they had not been ordered.[36] In contrast,

Gold and Wofersberger found hemoglobin levels less than 10 g/dl in only 0.33 percent.[47]

It is difficult to make the diagnosis of anemia clinically until the hemoglobin level drops below seven g/dl. In addition, the prevalence of anemia in an asymptomatic population is approximately one percent. A hemoglobin determination is clearly indicated in patients undergoing a surgical procedure associated with significant blood loss. The relatively high prevalence of anemia and the limited sensitivity of the physical examination speak in favor of routinely ordering a preoperative hemoglobin level in all patients.

Prothrombin Time, Partial Thromboplastin Time, and Bleeding Time

The value of the prothrombin time (PT) and partial thromboplastin time (PTT) to detect coagulation disorders has been evaluated in several recent studies. Clark and Eisenberg studied the prevalence of prolonged PT and PTT in surgical patients without evidence of a bleeding disorder on history or physical examination and assessed the consequences of abnormalities not being detected.[60] They defined patients with an increased risk of bleeding as those with: (1) a history of anticoagulant use; (2) a history or physical examination suggestive of liver disease; (3) active bleeding; or (4) a history or physical examination indicative of a bleeding disorder. In 467 patients with no risk of bleeding, they found 13 (2.8%) abnormal coagulation tests in contrast to 25 (18%) of 139 with defined risk. Of the 13 patients with abnormal results but no risk, five had repeat tests that were normal, and eight underwent surgery without further investigation and experienced no bleeding complications. The investigators concluded that preoperative testing is necessary only in those patients previously identified with an increased risk of bleeding.

Eika et al. studied 101 patients undergoing elective surgery in whom a platelet count, bleeding time, and a variety of other coagulation tests (including PT and PTT) were obtained.[61] Two hematologists subsequently assigned each patient to one of three groups according to bleeding risk. Despite small numbers, stratification by coagulation tests did not correlate with bleeding.

Robbins and Rose studied 1025 patients in whom PTT testing was done and found 143 or 14 percent with abnormal values.[62] On chart review it was found that each of these patients had an underlying process that could explain the abnormality. The authors concluded that abnormal results occur in patients who have a clinically predictable bleeding risk.

Suchman and Mushlin extended these observations by evaluating the PTT in predicting hemorrhage in hospitalized patients undergoing invasive diagnostic or therapeutic procedures.[63] High-risk groups were defined for patients with known coagulopathy, trauma, active hemorrhage, or potential factor deficiency (as in liver disease, malabsorption, and malnutrition), while others were considered low risk. The PTT poorly predicted bleeding in low-risk groups but did somewhat better in high-risk groups. Several other studies have examined the PT and PTT. None of Kaplan's 154 subjects without indications for these tests bled.[34] Turnbull and Buck found only one elevated PT or PTT in 213 patients.[35] Blery found that only 0.1 percent of omitted tests may have been useful.[36]

The bleeding time has been examined as a screening test in two studies. Harris and Nilsson suggested performing the bleeding time in patients undergoing microsurgery.[64] In 300 undergoing microsurgery of the ear, bleeding times were prolonged in 25 or 8.3 percent, although in 17 patients there were easily identifiable reasons. The authors provided no evidence that abnormal test results were related to postoperative bleeding.

Barber et al. studied the value of the bleeding time in approximately 1800 preoperative patients.[65] Of 110 or 6 percent abnormal tests, 75 could have been suspected from a history of drug use, abnormal platelet count, or renal dysfunction. In 25 percent of the patients, no etiology was identified to explain the abnormality. The test was repeated for 17 patients and was normal in 12. Of the 58 patients with abnormal bleeding times undergoing surgery, bleeding complications occurred in 10. Only 2 of 27 in whom abnormalities might not have been suspected had bleeding times greater than 20 minutes. The authors concluded that this small number does not justify routine bleeding time determinations in all preoperative patients.

In a more recent study, Bolger et al. found that, among 31 patients undergoing tonsillectomy, the PT and PTT were prolonged in 5.8 percent and 11.5 percent, respectively, and the bleeding time was prolonged in 9.6 percent.[66] After evaluation, 11.5 percent were felt to have important hemostatic abnormalities despite a negative personal and family history of bleeding. However, it is unclear how many of these patients would have had increased bleeding.

The clinical utility and cost-effectiveness of the PT and PTT has been evaluated by Bushnick et al.[67] Of more than 600 patients undergoing elective orthopedic procedures, nine percent had an abnormal PT and 5.8 percent had an abnormal PTT. However, fewer than one percent of these were considered significant enough to require additional action. The authors concluded that these tests had little influence on clinical care but more significant impact on its cost.

Overall consideration of these data suggests that the PT, PTT, and bleeding time are not valuable in predicting bleeding in asymptomatic patients undergoing surgery if they do not have a prior personal or family history of bleeding.

HIV Testing

Since the acquired immune deficiency syndrome (AIDS) can be transmitted by blood, screening surgical patients for antibodies to the human immunodeficiency virus (HIV) has been suggested as a way to protect surgical personnel from acquiring the infection. Recently, Hagen et al. attempted to address this issue by considering the risk of infection after skin puncture, the frequency of suffering a skin puncture at surgery, the sensitivity and specificity of the HIV test, and the prevalence of infection in the population tested.[68] Based upon these variables, they calculated that HIV testing will falsely label 130,000 patients in preventing transmission of one infection to a surgeon. They concluded that testing is not indicated in patients with no known risk factors.

Others argue that knowledge of HIV status would result in extra care to prevent puncture wounds and that seropositive patients may be more prone to postoperative infections and require more careful monitoring.[69] It may not be possible to identify high-risk behavior by history alone in 33 to 50 percent individuals with HIV infection. Despite these arguments, current data support screening only patients with known risk factors for HIV infection.

Other Miscellaneous Tests and Repeat Testing

The RPR and other serologic tests for syphilis have no relevance in perioperative management, and preoperative screening is not indicated.[70] Blood alcohol level and drug screening may be appropriate for trauma patients, but this issue has not been examined. Pregnancy testing has been suggested in women of child-bearing age[71] since unknown pregnancy does occur in ill patients.[72] Although pregnancy is not a contraindication to surgery, it is important for both mother and fetus that the surgeon and anesthesiologist be aware of this condition.

Many hospitals require that preoperative testing be performed within several weeks of surgery. However, Macpherson et al. demonstrated that patients with normal tests within four months of the procedure do not require repeat studies.[73] Of 3096 duplicated tests performed within one year of surgery in 1109 patients undergoing elective procedures, only 0.4 percent were significantly abnormal. All of the abnormalities could be explained by the patients' histories. However, of 461 previously abnormal tests, only 17 percent were abnormal when repeated. Over 70 percent of the tests examined were performed within four months of surgery, and retesting was thus considered unnecessary.

COST AND MEDICAL–LEGAL IMPLICATIONS

It is clear that if all of the recommendations in this chapter are followed, there will be a rare adverse outcome which might have been prevented by performing a preoperative test. Furthermore, it is likely that some of these cases may result in malpractice litigation. For these reasons, surgeons sometimes prefer to perform all of these diagnostic tests in all of their preoperative patients even if the clinical situation does not justify them.

The cost of medical care is no longer an issue which the medical profession can ignore. Pressure from patients, employers, and government is mounting to reduce cost.[74] Despite the fact that most of these tests are relatively inexpensive, performing them in millions of patients undergoing surgery will result in a large national expenditure. Based upon the yield in their study, Kaplan et al. estimate that it will cost approximately $4.2 million to save one life.[34]

The medical-legal issues also need to be addressed. The definition of malpractice includes deviation from the standard of care.[75,76] This standard can be established at a hospital by agreement among surgeons, anesthesiologists and internists that blanket routine preoperative testing is not required in surgical patients. Instead, thoughtful guidelines based upon the data in the medical literature can be established.

SUMMARY

1. A detailed medical history and physical examination are the most important factors in the evaluation of the surgical patient. They constitute the best possible screening process and provide nearly all the clinical data necessary for detection of diseases that may affect surgical outcome. Additional preoperative testing should be obtained based upon these clinical data, the nature of the surgical procedure, and known information in the medical literature.

2. *Electrocardiogram.* Available data fail to demonstrate that an electrocardiogram is more effective in predicting cardiovascular morbidity or mortality than a history and physical examination. The electrocardiogram is a poor predictor of ischemic heart disease and is therefore not routinely recommended in most patients. However, it may be useful for patients over the age of 50 or in those undergoing cardiovascular procedures.

3. *Chest radiograph.* A chest radiograph should be performed in patients age 60 or older, in patients undergoing cardiopulmonary or upper abdominal surgery, and in those with cardiopulmonary risk factors. There is little evidence to support the usefulness of preoperative chest radiographs in other patients.

4. *Hemoglobin or hematocrit.* This simple inexpensive test should be carried out for all patients undergoing surgery. The one percent prevalence of anemia in asymptomatic patients is relatively high, and the physical examination is limited in its sensitivity in detecting anemia.

5. *Creatinine or blood urea nitrogen.* One of these tests should be considered in patients receiving drugs excreted by the kidneys or in those undergoing surgery associated with possible postoperative renal failure. However, the very low prevalence of renal insufficiency and the subsequent high cost of detecting a significant abnormality argue against performing this test routinely.

6. *Serum glucose.* It is uncertain how management or surgical outcome is affected by knowledge that the serum glucose level is elevated preoperatively. However, because the prevalence of diabetes mellitus is relatively high and the test is inexpensive, serum glucose determination is recommended.

7. *Platelet count.* A platelet count is not recommended for preoperative screening because of the very low prevalence of unsuspected thrombocytopenia in the asymptomatic population.

8. *Prothrombin time, partial thromboplastin time, and bleeding time.* PT, PTT, and bleeding time determinations are of no demonstrated value in the preoperative patient. A careful history and physical examination can identify nearly all patients with an increased risk of bleeding.

9. *Urinalysis.* The available data suggest that, despite the high prevalence of abnormalities, a urinalysis is unlikely to contribute significantly to the care of the patient.

10. *Liver enzyme tests.* Hepatic dysfunction has significant implications for perioperative care, but the prevalence of liver enzyme abnormalities is low. Tests of hepatocellular function, such as SGOT or SGPT levels, are reasonable but of uncertain value in the patient undergoing surgery where liver function may be compromised postoperatively.

11. *HIV testing.* The very low prevalence of disease in patients without risk factors for HIV infection and the significant false labeling of many normal patients suggest that routine testing for HIV is not indicated.

REFERENCES

1. World Health Organization: Mass health examinations. *Public Health Pap* 45:50, 1971.
2. Robbins JA, Mushlin AI: Preoperative evaluation of the healthy patient. *Med Clin North Am* 63:1145, 1979.
3. Frame PS, Carlson SJ: A critical review of periodical health screening using specific screening criteria. *J Fam Prac* 2:29, 1975.
4. Galen RS, Gambino SR: *Beyond Normality: The Predictive Value and Efficiency of Medical Diagnosis.* New York, John Wiley & Sons, 1975, pp 10–11.
5. Wilson ME, Williams NB, Baskett PJF et al: Assessment of fitness for surgical procedures and the variability of anesthetists' judgments. *Br Med J* 1:509, 1980.
6. American College of Surgeons: *Surgery in the U.S.* Chicago, 1976, p 2132.
7. Goldman L, Caldera DL, Southwick FS et al: Cardiac risk factors and complications in non-cardiac surgery. *Medicine.* 57:375, 1978.
8. Detsky AS, Abrams HB, McLaughlin JR et al: Predicting cardiac complications in patients undergoing non-cardiac surgery. *J Gen Intern Med* 1:211–219, 1986.
9. Zeldin RA, Math B: Assessing cardiac risk in patients who undergo noncardiac surgical procedures. *Can J Surg* 27:402–40, 1984.
10. Jeffrey CC, Kunsman J, Cullen DJ, Brewster DC: A prospective evaluation of cardiac risk index. *Anesthesiology* 58:462–464, 1983.
11. Wang KC, Howland WS: Cardiac and pulmonary evaluation in elderly patients before elective surgical operations. *JAMA* 166:993, 1958.
12. Cooperman M, Pflug B, Martin EW et al: Cardiovascular risk factors in patients with peripheral vascular disease. *Surgery* 85:505–509, 1978.
13. Rooney SM, Godinger PL, Muss E: Relationship of right bundle branch block and marked left axis deviation to complete heart block during general anesthesia. *Anesthesiology* 44:64, 1976.
14. Pastore JO, Yurchak PM, Janis KM et al: The risk of advanced heart block in surgical patients with right bundle branch block and left axis deviation. *Circulation* 57:677, 1977.
15. McCleane GJ, McCoy E: Routine preoperative electrocardiography. *BJCP* 44:92, 1990.
16. Kannel WB, Abbott RD: Incidence and prognosis of unrecognized myocardial infarction: An update on the Framingham study. *N Engl J Med* 311:1144–1147, 1984.
17. Rosenman RG, Friedman M, Jenkins CD et al: Clinically unrecognized myocardial infarction in the western collaborative group study. *Am J Cardiol* 19:776–782, 1967.
18. Medasle JH, Goldbourt U: Unrecognized myocardial infarction: Five year incidence, mortality, and the risk factors. *Ann Intern Med* 84:526–531, 1976.
19. Jakobsson A, White T: Routine preoperative electrocardiograms. *Lancet* 1:972, 1984.
20. Elston RA, Taylor DJE: The preoperative electrocardiogram. *Lancet* 1:349, 1984.
21. Ferrer MI: The value of obligatory preoperative electrocardiograms. *J Am Med Wom Assoc* 33:459, 1978.
22. Sox HC, Garber AM, Littenberg B: The resting electrocardiogram as a screening test. A clinical analysis. *Ann Intern Med* 111:489–502, 1989.
23. Rubenstein LZ, Greenfield S: The baseline ECG in evaluation of acute cardiac complaints. *JAMA* 244:2536, 1980.
24. Hoffman JR, Igarashi E: Influence of electrocardiographic findings on admission decisions in patient with acute chest pain. *Am J Med* 79:699–707, 1985.
25. Goldberger AL, O'Konski J: Utility of the routine electrocardiogram before surgery and on general hospital admission. *Ann Int Med* 105:552–557, 1986.
26. Bureau of Radiological Health: *Chest x-ray screening practices: An annotated bibliography.* Washington DC, HEW Publication (FDA) 78–8067, 1978.
27. Royal College of Radiologists: Preoperative chest radiology. *Lancet* 2:83, 1979.

28. Rees NM, Roberts CJ, Bligh AS et al: Routine preoperative chest radiography in noncardiopulmonary surgery. *Br Med J* 1:1333, 1976.

29. Petterson SR, Janover ML: Is the routine preoperative chest film of value? *Appl Radiol* 6:70, 1977.

30. Rucker L, Frye EB, Staten MA: Usefulness of screening chest roentgenograms in preoperative patients. *JAMA* 250:3209–3211, 1983.

31. Loder RE: Routine preoperative chest radiography. *Anaesthesia* 33:972, 1978.

32. Sagel SS, Evans RG, Forrest JV et al: Efficacy of routine screening and lateral chest radiographs in a hospital-based population. *N Engl J Med* 291:1001, 1974.

33. Seymour DG, Pringle R, Shaw JW: The role of the routine preoperative chest x-ray in the elderly general surgical patient. *Postgrad Med J* 58:741–745, 1982.

34. Kaplan ED, Sheiner LB, Boeckmann AJ et al: The usefulness of preoperative laboratory screening *JAMA* 253:3576–3581, 1985.

35. Turnbull JM, Buck C: The value of preoperative screening investigations of otherwise healthy individuals. *JAMA* 147:1101–1105, 1987.

36. Blery C, Charpak Y, Szatan M et al: Evaluation of a protocol for selective ordering of preoperative tests. *Lancet* 1:139–141, 1986.

37. Daughaday WH, Erickson MM, White W et al: Evaluation of routine 12-channel chemical profiles on patients admitted to a university general hospital. In Benson ES, Standjord PE (eds): *Multiple Laboratory Screening*. New York, Academic Press, 1969, p 18.

38. Newman HF: Chemical screening. *NY State J Med* 78:2172, 1978.

39. Whitehead TP, Wootton IDP: Biochemical profiles for hospital patients. *Lancet* 2:1439, 1974.

40. Korvin CC, Pearce RH, Stanley J: Admissions screening: Clinical benefits. *Ann Intern Med* 83:197, 1975.

41. Durbridge TC, Edwards F, Edwards RG et al: An evaluation of multiphasic screening on admission to hospital. *Med J Aust* 1:703, 1976.

42. Galloway JA, Shuman CR: Diabetes and surgery. *Am J Med* 34:177, 1963.

43. Clark RSJ: Anesthesia and carbohydratic metabolism. *Br J Anaesth* 45:237, 1973.

44. Fletcher J, Langman MJS, Kellock TD: Effect of surgery on blood sugar levels in diabetes mellitus. *Lancet* 1:52, 1965.

45. Brenner BM, Hostetter TH: Disturbances of renal function, in Wilson JD, (ed): *Harrison's Principles of Internal Medicine*. New York, McGraw-Hill, 1991, p 1134.

46. Richter S, Lang R, Zur F, et al: Infected urine as a risk factor for postprostatectomy wound infection. *Infect Control Hosp Epidemiol* 12:147–149, 1991.

47. Gold BD, Wofersberger WH: Findings from routine urinalysis and hematocrit on ambulatory oral and maxillofacial surgery patients. *J Oral Surg* 38:677–678, 1980.

48. Glynn MK, Sheehan JM: The significance of asymptomatic bacteriuria in patients undergoing hip/knee arthroplasty. *Clin Ortho and Related Research* 185:151–154, 1984.

49. Heimann GA, Frohlich J, Bernstein M: Physicians' response to abnormal results of routine urinalysis. *Can Med Assoc J* 115:1094, 1974.

50. Lawrence VA, Gafni A, Gross M: The unproven utility of the preoperative urinalysis: economic evaluation. *J. Clin Epidemiol* 42:1185–1192, 1989.

51. Schemel WH: Unexpected hepatic dysfunction found by multiple laboratory screening. *Anesth Analg* 55:810–812, 1976.

52. Wataneeyawech M, Kelley KA: Hepatic diseases unsuspected before surgery. *NY State J Med* 75:1278–1281, 1975.

53. Belliveau RE, Fitzgerald JE, Nikerson DA: Evaluation of routine profile chemistry screening of all patients admitted to a community hospital. *Am J Clin Pathol* 53:447, 1970.

54. Kowalyshyn TJ, Prager D, Young J: A review of the present status of preoperative hemoglobin requirements. *Anesth Analg* 51:75, 1972.

55. NIH Consensus Conference: Perioperative red blood cell transfusion. *JAMA* 260:2700–2703, 1988.

56. Rawstron ER: Anemia and surgery. A retrospective clinical study. *Aust NZ J Surg* 39:425–432, 1970.

57. Lunn JN, Elwood PC: Anaemia and surgery. *Br Med J* 3:71–73, 1970.

58. Carson JL, Poses RM, Spence RK, et al: Anemia and surgery: the relationship between the severity of anemia and surgical mortality and morbidity. *Lancet* 1:727–729, 1988.

59. Gillies IDS: Anemia and anesthesia. *Br J Anaesth* 46:589, 1974.

60. Clark JR, Eisenberg JM: Screening for coagulation disorders in surgical patients. *Clin Res* (in press).

61. Eika C, Havig D, Godal HC: The value of preoperative hemostatic screening. *Scand J Haematol* 21:349, 1978.

62. Robbins JA, Rose SD: Partial thromboplastin time as a screening test. *Ann Intern Med.* 90:796, 1979.

63. Suchman AL, Mushlin AI: How well does the activated partial thromboplastin time predict postoperative hemorrhage? *JAMA* 256:750–753, 1986.

64. Harris S, Nilsson IM: Preoperative test of bleeding time in ear surgery. *Acta Otolaryngol* 89:474–478, 1980.

65. Barber A, Green D, Galluzzo T, et al: The bleeding time as a preoperative screening test. *Am J Med* 78:761–764, 1985.

66. Bolger WE, Parsons DS, Potempa L: Preoperative hemostatic assessment of the adenotonsillectomy patient. *Otolaryngol Head Neck Surg* 103:396–405, 1990.

67. Bushnick JB, Eisenberg JM, Kinman , et al: Pursuit of abnormal coagulation screening tests generates modest hidden preoperative costs. *J Gen Intern Med* 4:493–497, 1989.

68. Hagen MD, Meyer KB, Pauker SG: Routine preoperative screening for HIV. Does the risk to the surgeon outweigh the risk to the patient? *JAMA* 259:1357–1359, 1988.

69. Routine preoperative screening for HIV [letter]. *JAMA* 260:179–181, 1988.

70. Boren SD: The usefulness of the RPR. *JAMA* 254:3421, 1985.

71. Robbins JA: Preoperative evaluation of the healthy patient, in Bolt RJ (ed): *Medical Evaluation of the Surgical Patient*. Mount Kisco, Futura, 1987, pp 55–65.

72. Laubach GE, Wilchins SA: Ill patient with unknown or hidden pregnancy. *Postgrad Med J* 58:115–118, 1975.

73. Macpherson DS, Snow R, Lofgren RP: Preoperative screening: Value of previous tests. *Ann Intern Med* 113:969–973, 1990.

74. Lundberg GD: Is there a need for routine preoperative laboratory tests? *JAMA* 253:3589, 1985.

75. Gebhard PG, Feingold SG: Legal aspects of mammography screening. *Cancer* 60:1692–1693, 1987.

76. Black HC: *Black's Law Dictionary*, rev. 4th ed. St. Paul, West, 1968, p 1111.

4 LEGAL IMPLICATIONS OF MEDICAL CONSULTATION

Louis L. Brunetti

Richard A. Bankowitz

Medical consultation constitutes 15 to 50 percent of an internist's total practice and provides referring physicians with focused assessment of patients' medical problems and strategies for perioperative management.[1,2,3] Guidelines for effective consultation have been developed over the years by Goldman[4,5,6] and others[7,8,9] and have helped to define standards for care in this important area of medicine.

Significant changes have taken place in the practice of hospital-based medicine with the advent of diagnostic related groups (DRGs), peer review, and quality assessment programs. In an effort to lower health care costs and improve the overall quality of medical care, these developments have created an environment of intense cost control and risk awareness.[10-14] These innovations may eventually affect standards of care and physician liability. It is therefore increasingly important that consultants understand the general principles of medical-legal responsibility to their patients.

The legal and ethical duties of the consultant to the patient are similar to those of the primary physician. However, the patient management roles of these two physicians are often different and therefore give rise to somewhat different questions of liability. Consulting physicians generally do not have complete authority in making management decisions. Although there are instances in which the referring physician may need to delegate some measure of autonomy to the consultant—as in requesting that he perform a certain procedure—the role of the consultant remains primarily advisory. This relationship requires clear and timely communication between the referring and the consulting physicians in coordinating patient care.

The consultant's responsibilities are, however, influenced by legal obligations, ethical duties, and practical business considerations. Therefore, there can be no single "best" strategy for practicing consultative medicine. Good consultative strategy is often a function of perspective. From the point of view of a defense attorney or risk manager, this may mean providing only patient evaluation, diagnosis, and recommendations for treatment or further study. In this context, this does not include writing orders or active patient management. From the practitioner's perspective,

however, this role may be impractical and unrealistic because it fails to take into account the expectations of many referring physicians who may want medical consultants to both diagnose and manage problems.

In view of the inherent differences in the perceived role of the consultant, this chapter attempts to furnish the practitioner with a review of legal principles of professional responsibility, to emphasize those aspects of consultative medicine that may pose difficulties for the practitioner, and to provide guidelines for minimizing risk of liability.

PRINCIPLES OF LIABILITY

There are several different theories of liability upon which a cause of action for alleged physician error may be initiated. Much of the law pertaining to medical malpractice falls within the category of negligence. *Negligence* refers to conduct not intended to bring harm to others but which exposes others to an unreasonable risk of injury.[15] Simply stated, negligence is careless conduct.[16] Other less common but equally important bases for physician liability include *vicarious liability*, *breach of contract*, and *abandonment*. Breaches in the doctrine of informed consent fall into the general category of negligence. However, it is useful to consider this form of action separately from other more common negligence actions involving questions of inadequate treatment or failure to make a timely diagnosis.

Negligence

According to the law of negligence, we all have a duty to refrain from careless conduct in all of our daily activities. We owe a duty to anyone we can reasonably foresee might be injured by our conduct if we do not exercise reasonable care and prudence.[17,18] In order for a plaintiff to prove negligence, four criteria must be met:

1. *Duty*. It must be shown that the defendant owed a duty of care to the plaintiff, requiring the defendant to conform to a

25

certain standard of conduct. Existence of a duty is established by showing that the physician agreed to accept the patient for treatment. The medical consultant owes the same duty of care to the patient as does the primary physician and must act in a non-negligent manner in accordance with the accepted standard of medical care. However, the consultant's precise role may not be clear, and it is important that he ascertain his role in the case and determine the expectations of the primary physician at the outset.

One important exception to this general rule is embodied in "good samaritan" statutes that apply in certain specific circumstances. In most states, a physician who in good faith renders first aid or emergency treatment to a person who is unconscious, ill, or injured and who receives no compensation for his services will not be held to the same standard of duty.[19] In this situation, a different patient-physician relationship is established which limits the liability of the physician.[20] Grossly negligent acts or omissions or those intentionally designed to harm are not included within the scope of immunity.[21] Because of the variability in good samaritan laws from state to state, the physician should review the law in his own state to determine the extent of immunity provided for emergency treatment.

2. *Breach of Duty.* It must be demonstrated that the defendant breached his duty of care by failing to exercise reasonable care and prudence. Breach of duty is shown by proof that the physician failed to conform to a recognized standard of care during the course of treatment. This standard is not a static predetermined concept. Instead it must be established in each case by the jury after evaluating competing evidence introduced by expert testimony for the plaintiff and defendant. The starting point in determining the physician's standard of care is the reasonable person standard. This rule asks the jury to compare the conduct of the defendant physician with that of similarly trained members of the profession in good standing. If the defendant represents himself as having greater skill, as is the case with a specialist, the standard is modified accordingly.[22,23]

The standard of care must be determined in all malpractice cases except in circumstances in which negligence may be inferred from circumstantial evidence. These latter cases fall under the doctrine of *res ipsa loquitur*, or the thing speaks for itself. Typical cases in which this doctrine applies involve circumstances in which foreign objects, such as sponges or surgical instruments, have been left inside the patient's body after surgery.[24,25]

The standard of care can be determined in any one of three ways: (1) that standard prevalent in the community in which the physician practices (sometimes referred to as the strict locality rule); (2) that standard prevalent in a community similar to the one in which the physician practices (sometimes referred to as the general locality rule); or (3) by reference to a national standard. The precise rule to be applied is governed by the jurisdiction in which the physician practices and by other factors such as the expertise of the defendant, representations made by him to the patient, and his prior training and board certification, if any.[26,27]

In establishing the standard of care, it is not unusual for several "schools of thought" to exist regarding the management of a specific medical problem. If multiple opinions exist, the physician is free to choose from among the acceptable modes of practice. However, despite the fact that the standard of care is based upon the level of care of similarly trained physicians, the practice of substandard care in a given community does not lower the stand-

ard to which a practitioner will be held. For example, if a physician fails to prescribe appropriate prophylactic antibiotic therapy to a patient with mitral valvular disease, the fact that other physicians in a particular hospital do not follow the appropriate guidelines for endocarditis prophylaxis cannot be used as an argument that the practitioner had followed the standard of care in that community.

3. *Proximate Cause.* It also must be shown that the breach of duty was the proximate cause of the plaintiff's injury. In other words, there is a reasonably close causal connection between the physician's conduct and the resulting injury such that the harm would have been avoided if the physician had conformed to the standard of care. Depending upon the jurisdiction, one of two types of causal tests may be applied. The first is a "but for" argument, i.e., "but for" the breach in care by the physician, the plaintiff's injuries would not have occurred. Some courts instead use the substantial factor test. This requires that the patient prove that the negligence of the physician was a material element and substantial factor in causing the injury.

4. *Damages.* Finally, it must be established that the injury resulted in actual loss or damage to the plaintiff.[28,29] Malpractice actions, as civil actions, seek to recover monetary damages from those who have negligently caused the plaintiff's injury. Secondary motivations include use of a lawsuit as a general deterrent against negligent conduct by the medical profession, redress by the patient as compensation for a sense of wrongdoing or injustice suffered at the hands of the physician, or sometimes in response to poor communication between the physician and the patient and family.

Monetary damages are awarded as compensation to the plaintiff for losses incurred as a result of the physician's negligence. These damages vary among jurisdictions but generally fall into two broad categories: *compensatory damages* and *exemplary or punitive damages*. Compensatory damages are intended to compensate the plaintiff for pecuniary losses suffered as a result of the injury. These damages often include past and future medical expenses, loss of wages and earning capacity, pain and suffering, embarrassment and humiliation, disfigurement, loss of enjoyment of life, and loss of consortium to the plaintiff's spouse.[30] Exemplary or punitive damages are intended to penalize the wrongdoer. These damages are awarded only in cases involving intentional or particularly outrageous conduct, and mere negligence does not justify punitive damages.[31,32]

Damages resulting from the alleged negligence of the physician are not usually difficult to establish. Damages must, however, be real, and negligent care alone is not sufficient for recovery. Indeed, it is not enough to show that the physician's negligence subjected the patient to the potential of harm; proof of actual harm is required to sustain an award for damages.

Informed Consent

According to the doctrine of informed consent, a physician may be held liable for damages from treatment complications independent of the adequacy of treatment. The principle for this is grounded in the patient's right to refuse medical treatment or his right of self-determination.[33] The physician is obliged to inform the patient of the nature of the treatment, its known risks and expected benefits, and details of alternatives to the proposed therapy.[34] In the event of complications, liability is based upon the adequacy of disclosure by the physician.

Difficulties arise in trying to determine what risks must be disclosed for the patient to make an informed decision. Two standards of disclosure are currently used, the *professional standard* and the *material risk standard*. Under the professional standard, the disclosure is assessed in relation to the customary information other reasonable physicians would provide in the same or similar circumstances.[35] Increased recognition of patient autonomy led to the adoption of the material risk standard in 1972.[36] Courts have reasoned that continued use of a professional standard left the right of choice for the content of the disclosure to the medical community, often in derogation of the patient's right of self-determination. Extent of disclosure is therefore defined in terms of what a reasonable person in the patient's position would want to know before deciding whether to accept the planned therapy.

Vicarious Liability

Vicarious liability is the extension of liability from a negligent first party to a seemingly uninvolved second party. The second party is not involved in the negligent act but is nevertheless responsible for the actions of the first party and must therefore assume legal responsibility for the consequences.[37] This form of liability is expressed within the law of agency under the doctrine of *respondeat superior*, which holds that a principal (e.g., employer or master) is responsible for the wrongful acts (torts) of his agent (e.g., employee or servant) which occur within the scope of the agency.[38,39]

In the context of medical consultation, this form of liability is most often seen when the consultant relies on evaluations by others in arriving at a diagnosis or recommendations for treatment, or when other health care professionals provide care under his direction.[40,41] This commonly occurs in teaching hospitals where the consultant supervises resident physicians on a consult service, thereby rendering them agents acting on his behalf.

Breach of Contract

A patient may rarely bring a claim against a physician solely under the theory of contract law. In such claims, compensation is more limited than that available under negligence theory. In a breach of contract action, the plaintiff must show that a contract to deliver specific care existed and that the promise to deliver such care was not kept.[42,43] Compensation is limited to damages that flow from the breach[44] and may consist of the cost of obtaining medical care elsewhere or for out-of-pocket expenses incurred by the patient because of the "loss of the bargain." If a physician "guarantees" a particular result from a given procedure and fails to achieve the result, a court could find that a contract for a specific outcome existed and was breached, providing sufficient grounds for compensation.

Abandonment

Abandonment is a tort unique to the health care professional and is always a source of potential liability for the consultant. Because of the nature of the physician's duty to the patient and because of the dependence of the patient on the physician for continued care, a physician may not unilaterally terminate this relationship except under certain limited circumstances. The physician can be held liable for actively withdrawing from a case or for leaving the

patient when his services are required.[45,46] As a consultant, the physician would not be liable for abandoning the patient after a procedure or medical intervention if he or she were only consulted to perform a specific service which was completed in the expected manner. If, however, the referring physician expected and so indicated that the consultant would deliver continued follow-up or treatment, then failure to do so could represent abandonment.

The consultant can also be held liable for abandonment at a time when medical circumstances require further monitoring. If the consultant orders a particular laboratory test and does not return to check the results or decide on further action, he may be liable to suit for abandonment. The law does not specify a particular time period during which a consultant is required to follow a patient. A reasonable approach would be to follow the patient until he is stable and has no unresolved problems and if necessary until discharge from the hospital.[47] At that time, the consultant should clearly sign off the case by communicating with the referring physician and confirming it in writing in the patient's chart.

Other Areas of Potential Liability for the Consultant

Because of his special role as advisor, the consultant may face issues which would not ordinarily arise if he were the patient's primary caregiver. One such problem is disagreement on management of the patient and authority over issues of patient care. The referring physician, as "captain of the ship," must assume ultimate responsibility for diagnostic and treatment decisions. Referring and consulting physicians may disagree about optimal management strategies, but such disagreements are usually minor and are easily resolved.

If the consulting physician strongly objects to the current management, he has several ethical, if not legal, obligations. First, he should avoid an open argument with the referring physician and should not criticize him to the patient or family. Second, the consultant should not engage in a "chart war." The medical record is a legal document, and argumentative entries will only serve to undermine the credibility of both physicians in a legal action. Third, if the consultant believes that the primary physician's management is harmful, he should withdraw from the case and suggest that he seek another opinion.[48]

If he chooses to withdraw, the consultant must avoid allegations of abandonment by not doing so at a time when his care is critically needed. In addition, it is wise to provide a mechanism or recommendations for a competent replacement consultant. Furthermore, if the consultant believes that the primary physician is acting unprofessionally or unethically, he should seek the advice of the risk management department or the chief of the medical staff at the hospital.

Another important issue is that of authority to obtain consultations. Unless there is an emergency requiring prompt action to protect the well-being of a patient, all consults should be initiated by the attending physician. Other health professionals should communicate new data, findings, or recommendations for additional medical evaluation to the attending physician and refrain from taking it upon themselves to request a consultation. A medical consultant should not see the patient unless specifically requested to do so by the patient's primary attending physician.

DUTIES OF THE CONSULTANT: RECOMMENDATIONS

Referring physicians have a duty to seek consultation whenever they are confronted with medical problems beyond their expertise, when they believe that it would be helpful in the care of the patient, or if requested by the patient or his representative.[49-51] As discussed above, consulting physicians have specific duties as well. By incorporating the following rules[52] into daily practice, the consultant can adequately fulfill these duties and reduce the risk of legal liability.

1. *Delineate the responsibilities of the consulting and referring physicians.* The consultant should have a clear understanding of which aspects of the case he will manage. It is best to define the scope of his consultation in the medical record in order to reflect his understanding of his responsibilities accurately.

2. *Determine the urgency of the request and respond in a timely manner.* The consultant should assess the patient as quickly as possible, particularly when successful outcome depends upon prompt treatment.

3. *Become familiar with the patient's medical history and current symptoms* through a careful review of the patient's chart or other pertinent records. Indicate what information was available from these records and perform a directed history and physical examination of the patient.

4. *Maintain clear and direct communication.* Do not communicate solely through the progress notes in the medical record. Keep the referring physician informed about the patient's care and document this in writing. The written consultative report should include a brief outline of the findings, probable or differential diagnosis, suggested further studies, recommended treatment or referral, and prognosis. It is advisable to keep a copy of your consultation report in your records.

5. *Clearly sign off the case when you are certain that your services are no longer needed.* Make it clear that you will not return to see the patient but will remain available if further consultation is needed. If follow-up is needed after the initial consultation, provide it in a consistent manner. Avoid random or haphazard return visits to the patient and adequately document follow-up visits.

6. *Do not make guarantees or imply them* with phrases such as "the patient is cleared for surgery." It is more appropriate to make an assessment of risks and to suggest measures to reduce the risks as much as feasible before surgery.

7. *If there are management disagreements, do not argue with the referring physician in the presence of the patient or his family.* Do not criticize the referring physician's care to the patient.

8. In cases of possible medical negligence or when thorny medical-legal issues arise, *seek the advice of the hospital risk management department.*

REFERENCES

1. Ferguson RP, Rubinstien E: Preoperative medical consultations in a community hospital. *J Gen Intern Med* 2:89–92, 1987.
2. Mendenhall RC, Tarlov AR, Girard RA et al: A national study of internal medicine and its subspecialties: II. Primary care in internal medicine. *Ann Intern Med* 91:275–287, 1979.
3. Robie PW: The service and educational contributions of a general medicine consultation service. *J Gen Intern Med* 1:225–227, 1986.
4. Goldman L, Caldera DK, Nussbaum SR et al: Multifactorial index of cardiac risk in non-cardiac surgical procedures. *N Engl J Med* 297:845–850,1977.
5. Goldman L, Caldera DK, Southwick FS et al: Cardiac risk factors and complications in non-cardiac surgery. *Medicine* 57:357–370, 1978.
6. Goldman L, Lee T, Rudd P: Ten commandments for effective consultations. *Arch Intern Med* 143:1753–1755, 1983.
7. Ballard WP, Gold JP, Charlson ME: Compliance with the recommendations of medical consultants. *J Gen Intern Med* 1:220–224, 1986.
8. Detsky AS, Abrams HB, McLaughlin JR et al: Predicting cardiac complications in patients undergoing non-cardiac surgery. *J Gen Intern Med* 1:211–219, 1986.
9. Goldberger AL, O'Konski M: Utility of the routine electrocardiogram before surgery and on general hospital admission: Critical reviews and new guidelines. *Ann Intern Med* 105:552–557, 1986.
10. Relman AS: Changing the malpractice liability system. *N Engl J Med* 322:626–627, 1990.
11. Manuel BM: Professional liability: A no-fault solution. *N Engl J Med* 322:627–630, 1990.
12. Brook RH: Practice guidelines and practicing medicine: are they compatible? *JAMA* 262:3027–3030, 1989.
13. Eddy DM: Practice policies—what are they? *JAMA* 263:877–880, 1990.
14. Lomas J, Anderson GM, Domnick-Pierre K et al: Do practice guidelines guide practice? The effect of a consensus statement on the practice of physicians. *N Engl J Med* 321:1306–1311, 1989.
15. Hirshfeld EB: Practice parameters and the malpractice liability of physicians. *JAMA* 263:1556–1562, 1990.
16. 57A Am Jur 2p, *Negligence*, sec 6 at 67.
17. *A.E. Investment Corporation v. Link Builders, Inc.*, 62 Wis. 2d 479, 483, 214 N.W. 2d 764, 766 (1974).
18. Hirshfield, op. cit., p 1556.
19. Cf. N.C. Gen. Stat., sec 90-21.14. First aid or emergency treatment; liability limitation.
20. *Kearns v. Rader*, 252 Cal. Rptr. 4, 204 Ca. 3d 1325 (1988).
21. 42. Pa. Cons. Stat., sec 8331.
22. Keeton W, Dobbs D, Keeton R et al: *Prosser & Keeton on the Law of Torts*, 5th ed. St. Paul, West, 1984, pp 186–187.
23. *McPherson v. Ellis*, 305 N.C. 266, 287 S.E. 2d 892 (1982).
24. Louisell DW, Williams H: *Medical Malpractice*. New York, Matthew Bender, 1960, vol 1, ch 14, sec 14.02.
25. 57B Am Jur 2d, *Negligence*, sec 1819 et seq.
26. *Kubrick v. United States*, 435 F. Supp. 166 (E.D. Pa. 1977).
27. Post BL, Peters BM, Stahl SP et al: *The Law of Medical Practice in Pennsylvania and New Jersey*. Rochester, The Lawyers Co-Operative, 1984, p 345.
28. Prosser & Keeton, op. cit., pp 164–165.
29. Hirshfeld, op. cit., p 1556.
30. Pa. Standard Jury Instruction (Civil), sec 6.01 A & B (1981).
31. *Medvecz v. Choi*, 569 F. 2d 1221 (CA3 Pa. 1977).
32. *Restatement of Torts*, St. Paul, MN, American Law Institute, 1979, sec 908.
33. *Schloendorff v. Society of New York Hospital*, 211 N.Y. 125, 105 N.E. 92 (1914).
34. *Canterbury v. Spence*, 464 F. 2d 772 (D.C. Cir. 1972), *cert. denied*, 409 U.S. 1064.
35. *Natanson v. Kline*, 350 P. 2d 1093 (Kan. 1960).
36. *Canterbury v. Spence, supra.*
37. 57B Am Jur 2d, *Negligence*, sec 1759 at 451, et seq.
38. 57B Am Jur 2d, *Negligence*, sec 1752 at 446, et seq.
39. *Restatement of Agency 2d*, St. Paul MN, American Law Institute, 1950, sec 140, p 359.
40. Cf. *Connell v. Hayden*, 443 N.Y.S. 2d 383 (App. Div. 1981).

41. Cf. *Young v. Carpenter*, 694 P. 2d 861 (Colo. App. 1984).
42. Prosser & Keeton, op. cit., pp 186–187.
43. Cf. *Scarzella v. Saxon*, 436 A. 2d 358 (D.C. App. 1981).
44. *Noel v. Proud*, 367 P. 2d 61 (Kan. 1962).
45. *Capps v. Valk*, 189 Kan. 287, 369 P. 2d 238 (1962).
46. *Johnson v. Vaughn*, 370 S.W. 2d 591 (Ky. Ct. App. 1963).
47. Wolinsky H: Preoperative evaluation: The next malpractice battleground. *ACP Observer* 7:11:1,14–16, 1987.

48. Diosegy AJ: *Body medical, body legal: a look at health care in North Carolina*. Raleigh, NC, Fasion & Brown and the North Carolina Medical Society, 1989, vol III, p 18.
49. Council on Ethical and Judicial Affairs of the American Medical Assocation, *Current Opinions*, sec. 8.04 (1986).
50. Prosser & Keeton, op. cit., p 29 (pocket part).
51. *Philips v. United States*, 566 F. Supp. 1, 14 (D.S.C. 1981).
51. Risk Management Review, *Minn Med* 71:638–639, 1988.

5 THE PHYSIOLOGIC RESPONSE TO SURGERY AND ANESTHESIA

Thomas A. Mickler

The physiologic response to surgery is identical to the "stress response" of the human body to emotional or environmental change. This response is largely mediated by the neuroendocrine system and is produced by the outpouring of a wide array of hormonal substances which significantly alter metabolism, hemodynamics, and fluid balance. The metabolic changes are those of a general hypermetabolic state in which there is increased glucose production (gluconeogenesis) with hyperglycemia, lipolysis, and protein breakdown. The hyperdynamic state is characterized by increased cardiac output and redistribution of blood flow to vital organs.

Anesthetic agents have three effects on the stress response. First, they attenuate the nociceptive signals which cause the central nervous system to respond to stress. Second, they exert a direct effect on the secretion of certain hormones. Finally, they affect organs like the heart and lungs directly. During surgery, it is difficult to determine which aspects of the overall physiologic picture are due to the endogenous stress response and which are due to the direct effects of the anesthetic agents. In general, the direct effects of the anesthesia are minimal compared with those of surgery itself. In fact, the overall purpose of anesthesia might be defined as an attempt to reduce the response of the body to that stress.

The nidus of the stress response is hormonal secretion. This chapter describes the salient hormones in the context of their effects on organ system function and outlines the effects of anesthetic agents on the secretion of these hormones during surgery. The direct effects of these agents on the cardiovascular and pulmonary systems are discussed separately. It is important to realize that the effects of anesthesia and surgery are intimately intertwined and often difficult to separate completely.

DIRECT EFFECTS OF ANESTHETIC AGENTS ON HORMONAL SECRETIONS

ACTH and Cortisol

The hypothalamic-pituitary-adrenal axis is the major regulator of the stress response. Nociceptive signals are transmitted to the ventral posterior nucleus of the thalamus by way of afferent fibers in the substantia gelatinosa of the dorsal horn of the spinal cord. These signals cause the hypothalamus to secrete corticotropin releasing factor (CRF) which in turn stimulates the anterior pituitary to produce adrenocorticotropin hormone (ACTH). ACTH stimulates the adrenal cortex to produce glucocorticoids, primarily cortisol, and to a lesser extent the mineralocorticoid aldosterone. In addition to the stress-induced stimulation, ACTH secretion is regulated by two other mechanisms: circadian rhythm mediated by CRF secretion and a negative feedback mechanism mediated by plasma cortisol levels.

Cortisol is the most important glucocorticoid produced by the adrenal cortex. Normally, ACTH secretion peaks shortly after awakening and subsequently declines through the day. Since cortisol secretion is controlled by ACTH, it too peaks in the morning. This rhythm is dependent on a normal sleep cycle, and abnormal sleep will alter the time of peak secretion.

Cortisol has many physiologic effects, including the regulation of protein, carbohydrate, and lipid metabolism. Increased cortisol levels result in decreased utilization of glucose by skeletal muscle and adipose tissue, increased triglyceride catabolism to free fatty acids, and increased protein breakdown to amino acids. Cortisol also has anti-inflammatory effects and causes suppression of cellular immunity.

Hemodynamic status is critically dependent on adequate circulating cortisol levels, and hemodynamic collapse is a recognized phenomena in patients who have an inadequate cortisol response to stress. Approximately 20 to 30 mg of cortisol are produced by the adrenal cortex each day. During stress, cortisol secretion can reach 100 mg per day.[1] Although the goal of anesthesia is to blunt the endocrine effects of surgical stimuli, total absence of cortisol response can lead to a hypotensive crisis. Therefore, patients who have been on chronic steroid therapy or those with known adrenal insufficiency must have exogenous perioperative steroid coverage.[2]

The timing and magnitude of the increase in ACTH and cortisol levels caused by surgery are related to the intensity of the surgical stimulus.[3] Major abdominal procedures cause a rapid increase in these levels beginning with the skin incision and persisting throughout the procedure.[4,5] More minor procedures may cause no increase in levels until the end of the procedure at which time they rise dramatically.[6,7] Administration of volatile anesthetics without surgical stimulation has no effect on ACTH and cortisol secretion.[8] Neurolept anesthesia with droperidol, narcotic, oxygen, and nitrous oxide also has no significant effect on cortisol levels. Ketamine is unique among the intravenous agents because it significantly stimulates adrenocortical activity.[9]

The ACTH response to stress can be temporarily blunted with opioids. Premedication with morphine combined with diazepam and scopolamine decreases the ACTH response to operation in children.[10] High-dose fentanyl in doses of 50 to 200 µg/kg, often used in cardiac surgery, can transiently inhibit ACTH and cortisol production. Once cardiopulmonary bypass begins, these inhibitory effects disappear.[11,12] However, if cortisol has already been stimulated, fentanyl in doses of 50 µg/kg does not reverse it.[13]

Etomidate, a sedative-hypnotic agent, deserves special note. It selectively inhibits the adrenocortical response to surgery in a dose-dependent fashion and acts by inhibiting both 17-alpha and 11-beta hydroxylase activity, resulting in an overall decrease in cortisol synthesis. ACTH levels are elevated whereas plasma cortisol levels are depressed, implying a generalized lack of cortisol production in response to ACTH.[14,15] Etomidate, even in a single dose, may therefore be contraindicated in patients with adrenocortical hypofunction.[16] Clinical doses of propofol, midazolam, and thiopental do not suppress the adrenocortical response to the stress of surgery.[17,18]

The effects of neural blockade in epidural and intrathecal anesthesia on the adrenocortical response prior to the start of surgery are minimal. Several studies show that neural blockade does inhibit the usual rise in ACTH and cortisol during lower extremity and lower abdominal procedures.[19-21] However, a very high neural block is required to abolish the rise in cortisol level completely.[22] This inhibitory effect is less marked during thoracic and upper abdominal procedures[23] and is probably related to a lesser degree of afferent blockade.[24] As the level of blockade decreases, both ACTH and cortisol levels rise markedly and approach values similar to those seen in patients who receive general anesthesia. Intrathecal narcotics have also been shown to attenuate the increase in cortisol levels induced by surgery.[25]

Catecholamines

Catecholamines exert cardiovascular, pulmonary, and metabolic effects by way of alpha and beta receptors in the tissues. The two most important catecholamines are epinephrine and norepinephrine, and their effects are somewhat different. The cardiovascular effects of epinephrine include increased myocardial contractility and increased heart rate which lead to increased cardiac output. Blood flow to the skin, mucosa, and kidney are reduced while flow to skeletal muscle is increased. Epinephrine is a potent bronchodilator and increases respiratory rate and tidal volume. The metabolic effects of epinephrine lead to an elevated blood glucose level from decreased uptake of glucose by the tissues, increased glycogenolysis, and inhibition of insulin secretion. The effects of norepinephrine are less diverse. Its major action is to cause peripheral vasoconstriction in most vascular beds.

The adrenal medulla produces epinephrine and can produce norepinephrine, but the majority of norepinephrine is synthesized in peripheral autonomic nerve terminals. Epinephrine is synthesized only in the adrenal medulla, the site of an enzyme necessary for the methylation of norepinephrine to epinephrine. The control of catecholamine secretion resides in the hypothalamus. However, serum cortisol can affect the production of epinephrine because it regulates the enzyme which facilitates the conversion of norepinephrine to epinephrine. Thus, plasma levels of catecholamines do not always increase in parallel. The half-lives of catecholamines are less than one minute, and they are quickly broken down on a single pass through the liver or kidney.

There is a marked surge of catecholamine release in response to surgical stimulation which generally parallels the increases in ACTH and cortisol levels. However, epinephrine and norepinephrine increases follow different patterns depending on the anesthetic agents. Epinephrine levels remain stable or actually decrease after induction of general anesthesia with volatile agents and rise only at the end of the procedure.[5,6,26] When neurolept anesthesia is used, epinephrine levels vary throughout the procedure depending on the intensity of the surgical stimulus.[25] Changes in levels of norepinephrine also vary according to the surgical stimulus. Halothane causes no change in norepinephrine levels before the beginning of surgery or only a transient increase that returns to baseline after an hour.[27,28] The overall effect of halothane is to inhibit or attenuate the sympathetic nervous system response to surgery and blunt the release of catecholamines once surgery has begun. Increasing the concentration of halothane does not diminish these changes in catecholamine levels.[29] The effects of enflurane on catecholamine release in response to surgical stimulation are similar to those of halothane, but no evidence suggests that enflurane alone alters baseline catecholamine levels prior to surgery. Isoflurane has been less well studied, but its effect on catecholamine release at the beginning of surgery is similar to that of other volatile agents.[30]

High-dose opiates are effective in attenuating the release of catecholamines in response to surgery. However, this effect does not persist long into the postoperative period. For example, when fentanyl in a dose of 25 µg/kg is used in cardiac procedures, plasma levels of epinephrine and norepinephrine do not change in response to endotracheal intubation. When a dose of 75 µg/kg is used, catecholamine levels decrease during the period before bypass but rise significantly 15 minutes after bypass begins.[10,11] Even when 100 µg/kg is given, the decrease in plasma catecholamine levels persists for only 60 minutes after surgical incision.[31] In comparing halothane to halothane with fentanyl, the combination of halothane with fentanyl is more effective in preventing the release of norepinephrine than halothane alone.

Regional anesthesia can decrease the stress-induced release of catecholamines for longer periods of time. Effects are greater with spinal anesthesia to higher dermatomal levels. Neural blockade can completely abolish the epinephrine response to lower abdominal surgery, but its effect on changes in plasma norepinephrine levels is controversial.[5,32] Neural blockade is more effective in blocking catecholamine release in lower abdominal than in upper abdominal procedures.

Renin-Angiotensin-Aldosterone System

Aldosterone is the principal mineralocorticoid secreted by the adrenal gland. It acts on the kidney to maintain fluid and electrolyte homeostasis. Although ACTH may cause a moderate increase in the secretion of aldosterone, its regulation is not dependent on the pituitary gland or secretion of ACTH. Aldosterone secretion can be stimulated by a decrease in serum sodium concentration, a fall in the serum sodium-to-potassium ratio, and a decrease in blood volume. Juxtaglomerular cells in the kidney are sensitive to decreases in arteriolar volume and pressure and respond by releasing renin, a proteolytic enzyme which cleaves angiotensinogen to produce angiotensin I. Converting enzymes present in the vascular endothelium rapidly convert angiotensin I to the active entity angiotensin II. Angiotensin II causes arteriolar vasoconstriction and stimulation of the adrenal cortex to produce aldosterone. Aldosterone causes the renal tubules to reabsorb sodium while promoting excretion of potassium, leading to an increase in intravascular volume. Increased pressure is sensed by the juxtaglomerular cells which decrease renin secretion, completing the feedback loop.

With halothane and enflurane anesthesia, aldosterone levels rise at the beginning of surgery, increase even further once surgery has begun, and remain elevates in the postoperative period.[4,33] No general anesthetic agents are known to inhibit increases in renin and aldosterone, but neural blockade may attenuate or abolish the increases. Limited data suggest that plasma aldosterone and renin levels are decreased both intraoperatively and postoperatively during hysterectomy and pelvic surgery performed under regional anesthesia.[33] The actual effect on water and electrolyte balance remains unclear since neural blockade can directly influence glomerular filtration rate, block sympathetic innervation to the kidneys, and indirectly influence hormones that regulate salt and water balance.

Antidiuretic Hormone

Arginine vasopressin or antidiuretic hormone (ADH) is synthesized in the hypothalamus and transported to the posterior pituitary gland where it is stored for later release. ADH release is regulated by serum osmolality and circulating blood volume, and a fall in blood volume or a rise in osmolality stimulates its release. ADH causes a decrease in free water clearance in the kidney. It also has vasopressor and clotting effects. Vasopressor activity is greatest in the splanchnic, coronary, and renal vascular beds. Its effect on clotting has been inferred from the finding that an ADH analog, ddAVP, increases the level of factor VIII and von Willebrand's factor in hemophiliac patients.[34,35] Moreover, ddAVP has been used to reduce bleeding in patients undergoing open heart surgery with cardiopulmonary bypass[36] but its benefit has been questioned.[37]

The decrease in urine output seen during abdominal procedures may be caused by indirect effects of volatile agents on the kidney and increased circulating levels of ADH induced by the stimulation of surgery. Halothane, enflurane, and isoflurane cause dose-dependent decreases in renal blood flow in the absence of hypotension even when corrected for cardiac output.[38] Anesthetics alone do not alter plasma levels of ADH, but surgical stimulation causes marked increases. Patients who receive relatively light anesthesia during surgery can have very large increases in plasma ADH concentration[39], and greater depth of anesthesia appears to reduce these increases. This is supported by a study of patients receiving halothane, morphine at a dose of 1 mg/kg, or morphine at a dose of 2 mg/kg.[40] There was no increase in plasma ADH in any group until surgery began. With the beginning of surgery ADH levels increased most in the halothane group and least in those receiving higher dose morphine. Similarly, no increases in ADH level occur with enflurane or fentanyl anesthesia until an incision is made.[4,41] Blocking afferent neural stimuli with high epidural blockade does not inhibit the increases in serum ADH levels induced by cholecystectomy.[42] However, others have found that neural blockade reduces the increases expected with surgical stimulation.[43,44] After surgery, elevated plasma ADH levels persist for up to four days, but the elevation can be attenuated with epidural narcotics used for pain control.[45]

Insulin and Glucose Metabolism

Insulin is a polypeptide anabolic hormone secreted by the beta cells of the pancreas. Its physiologic and metabolic effects include glucose transfer across cell membranes into cells, increased glycogen formation, inhibition of lipolysis and glycolysis, transport of glucose into fat tissue for conversion and storage as fatty acids, and facilitation of potassium influx into cells with glucose. Growth hormone, glucagon, cortisol, and catecholamines all have anti-insulin effects, and during stress all of these hormones play a part in determining the metabolic state. However, it is the glucagon-to-insulin ratio which is the major determinant of gluconeogenesis activity.

Insulin secretion is increased by the stress of surgery, but the countervailing effects of cortisol, glucagon, and catecholamines lead to hyperglycemia during surgery. In the past, hyperglycemia was most marked with ether anesthesia. Commonly used general anesthetic agents like halothane and enflurane also result in elevated plasma glucose levels, but the effects of these agents are less marked.

High-dose fentanyl anesthesia at a dose of 75 µg/kg prevents the hyperglycemia response associated with cardiac surgery but only in the period before bypass.[11] Neural blockade attenuates the hyperglycemia that would otherwise occur with volatile agents. When continuous spinal or epidural anesthesia is combined with general anesthesia under enflurane, the response is significantly attenuated but not abolished.[46] The attenuating effect is less with epidural than with spinal anesthesia but is more marked if the epidural is placed in the thoracic spine.[47,48] The attenuation of the hyperglycemic response by epidural anesthesia is probably due to inhibition of catecholamine and cortisol responses rather than to a direct effect on insulin release.[49]

Thyroid Hormones

The two major physiologically active thyroid hormones are tetraiodothyronine (thyroxine or T_4) and the more potent deiodinated hormone triiodothyronine (T_3). Circulating T_3 and T_4 are more than 99 percent bound to serum proteins, mostly to thryroxine-binding globulin (TBG) and thyroxine-binding prealbumin, but the metabolic effects of these hormones are determined by the amount of free hormone available. The effects of thyroid hormones are complex and the significance of changes in thyroid hormone levels in the face of acute stress is unclear. In adults, circulating thyroid hormone regulates the basal rate of metabolism, oxygen consumption, and heat production, but the exact mechanisms by which they act remain unknown.

T_3 and T_4 are both produced in the thyroid gland, but 80 percent of T_3 is produced in peripheral tissues, especially in the kidneys and liver, by monodeiodination of T_4. Production and release of T_3 and T_4 from the thyroid are regulated by thyroid stimulating hormone (TSH) produced by the anterior pituitary. Circulating levels of thyroid hormones alter the secretion of TSH by way of a negative feedback mechanism in which high levels of thyroid hormone reduce the secretion of TSH. In addition, thyrotropin releasing hormone (TRH) produced by the hypothalamus stimulates the pituitiary to increase TSH secretion. Somatostatin is also produced by the hypothalamus and exerts a negative effect on pituitary production of TSH.

Until recently, it was thought that plasma levels of TSH remain unchanged with surgical stress, general anesthesia, or regional blockade. However, sensitive radioimmunoassay techniques reveal that TSH levels do rise abruptly at the time of skin incision. This increase can be attenuated by epidural blockade.[50] The stress of surgery usually produces a "euthyroid sick syndrome" in which TSH and T_4 levels are normal, T_3 levels are reduced, and reverse T_3 levels are elevated. The combination of nitrous oxide and narcotics or enflurane anesthesia has no effect on serum T_4 levels.[4,51] Serum T_4 levels, however, increase significantly with the use of halothane. It has been proposed that halothane anesthesia in combination with surgery may cause a shift of T_4 from the liver into the circulation.[52,53] Isoflurane, spinal, and epidural anesthesia have no effect on plasma T_4 levels.[54] Plasma T_3 levels are decreased by surgery, inhalational anesthetics, and most intravenous agents. Neural blockade is not thought to influence this decrease in T_3.

DIRECT EFFECTS OF ANESTHETIC AGENTS ON THE PULMONARY AND CARDIOVASCULAR SYSTEMS

Pulmonary

Anesthesia may contribute to preoperative, intraoperative, and postoperative pulmonary dysfunction by significantly impairing the mechanisms of gas exchange and the control of ventilation. Moreover, surgery itself may impair the mechanical function of the bellows mechanism of the lungs. Postoperative pain can lead to atelectasis by causing patients to take only shallow tidal volumes and limiting effective cough.

Even before the induction of anesthesia, the respiratory system can be adversely affected by premedications. In one study, patients scheduled for cardiac surgery given morphine, lorazepam, and droperidol suffered persistent arterial oxygen desaturation greater than that induced by sleep.[55] One-third of them developed new electrocardiographic changes with desaturation. Supplemental oxygen may circumvent this problem, but the benefits of heavy preopera-

tive sedation must be balanced against the risks. Even commonly used agents like diazepam can blunt the ventilatory response to carbon dioxide.[56]

Induction of general anesthesia causes changes in ventilatory patterns that can result in hypoxemia and hypercarbia. A 15 to 20 percent reduction in the functional residual capacity (FRC) can occur, and this effect continues into the postoperative period.[57] Reduction in FRC is caused by cephalad movement of the diaphragm induced by loss of inspiratory tone and an increase in end-expiratory tone. The position of the patient also affects pulmonary mechanics, and a change from the upright to the supine position decreases the FRC by 0.5 to 1.0 liters.[58,59] The effects of Trendelenburg and lateral decubitus positions are even more marked. The ultimate effects of a reduction in FRC are atelectasis and hypoxemia.

Volatile agents and narcotics depress the sensitivity of the respiratory control center to hypercarbia and hypoxia.[60-62] This effect is dose-dependent and can lead to a rising PCO_2. If a patient is allowed to breathe spontaneously while under a volatile general anesthetic, a mild respiratory acidosis may occur, depending upon the depth of anesthesia. These effects may be mitigated by surgery itself, which causes an increase in minute ventilation. However, intubation and mechanical ventilation allows complete control over ventilation, making reduced sensitivity to carbon dioxide only a factor after extubation.

Inhalation anesthetics, even at subtherapeutic concentrations, markedly blunt the normal ventilatory response to hypoxia. This is usually of little importance in the operating room when ventilation is controlled and high inspired concentrations of oxygen are used. However, this effect combined with reduced sensitivity to carbon dioxide can be deleterious in the immediate postoperative period and makes supplemental oxygen necessary.[63] Despite oxygen, many patients still experience hypoxemia. Continuous pulse oximetry is useful in alerting caregivers to this situation.[64] After thoracotomy, postoperative hypoxemia can persist up to four days after the procedure.[65]

Dry anesthetic gases can depress mucociliary function.[66] This effect, when combined with endotracheal intubation, positive pressure ventilation, and the use of high inspired oxygen concentrations, may contribute to postoperative pulmonary atelectasis and infection. All volatile agents, in blunting pulmonary vasoconstriction in response to hypoxia, can exacerbate ventilation-perfusion abnormalities. This can be especially problematic during one-lung ventilation in thoracic procedures.[67]

Respiratory function is usually not impaired with low-level spinal and epidural anesthesia. With spinal anesthesia, tidal volume, respiratory rate, minute ventilation, and mean inspiratory flow rate do not change, but there can be decreases in end-tidal carbon dioxide concentrations and increased breath-to-breath variability.[68] Ventilatory responsiveness to carbon dioxide may actually increase.[69,70] With ascending levels of spinal or epidual anesthesia, intercostal muscle paralysis occurs. However, even total intercostal muscle paralysis has little effect on resting ventilatory mechanics as long as the phrenic drive to the diaphragm is preserved.[71,72] On the other hand, intercostal muscle paralysis does interfere with the ability to cough and clear secretions and can continue to do so in the postoperative period.

Pre-existing respiratory dysfunction, surgical positioning, massive blood loss, and surgical retraction on the lung will also have significant effects on intraoperative and postoperative pulmonary dynamics. Obese, bronchitic, or emphysematous patients may already have a decreased FRC-to-closing capacity ratio. If anesthesia causes a further decrease in FRC, serious ventilation-perfusion (V/Q) mismatching and/or atelectasis may occur. Patients with chronic bronchitis and copious airway secretions may suffer even more from an anesthetic-induced decrease in mucociliary clearance. Acute pulmonary infections, chest trauma, chest wall deformities, and age also alter pulmonary dynamics during anesthesia and surgery.

Cardiovascular

Commonly used intravenous induction agents like sodium thiopental and propofol decrease myocardial contractility. After a bolus dose, these effects are transient and generally do not cause concern in healthy individuals. However, precipitous hypotension may occur in patients who are hypovolemic at the time of induction or who already have poor left ventricular function. The synthetic narcotics fentanyl and sufentanil have very little effect on myocardial contractility when used alone in high doses and are commonly used in cardiac surgery. However, at high doses, their long duration of action precludes their use for relatively short procedures since central nervous system and respiratory depression persist.

Two major effects on the cardiovascular system common to all the volatile agents are decreased myocardial contractility and dilatation of the arterial and venous vasculature. The circulatory effects of enflurane, halothane, and isoflurane have been studied in healthy volunteers. Isoflurane and halothane both reduce stroke volume by 20 percent. Isoflurane increases heart rate to maintain cardiac output, but halothane does not. Enflurane increases heart rate but decreases stroke volume by nearly 40 percent and results in a decrease in cardiac output similar to that seen with halothane. Along with reduced cardiac output is a 10 to 15 percent reduction in myocardial oxygen consumption.[73] Halothane, enflurane, and isoflurane relax smooth muscles in vascular beds and cause a reduction in systemic vascular resistance. Halothane causes the least decrease in systemic vascular resistance, and isoflurane causes the most.

Volatile anesthetics can significantly alter regional blood flow. They increase flow to the brain, muscle, and skin and decrease flow to the liver, kidneys, and gut. Halothane is reported to result in a greater depression of hepatic blood flow than isoflurane. Even though volatile agents decrease blood pressure, autoregulatory mechanisms in the kidney usually serve to keep renal blood flow constant. With increasing duration of anesthesia, there is gradual recovery from the circulatory depressant effects of halothane, to a lessor degree with enflurane, and much less so with isoflurane. This recovery may involve beta-adrenergic stimulation leading to increases in cardiac output and stroke volume and decreases in systemic vascular resistance.[74,75]

Nitrous oxide is commonly used as an adjunct to general anesthesia because it produces minimal myocardial depression. Animal data have recently raised the question of a detrimental effect in the presence of coronary artery disease,[76,77] but clinical data in humans do not support this conclusion even in patients with poor left ventricular function.[78,79]

The effects of the volatile agents on coronary circulation have been studied in animals, and the results have been extrapolated to humans.[80] Most agents are thought to cause coronary artery dilatation but decrease coronary artery blood flow regulation, possibly resulting in a coronary "steal" phenomenon. Halothane has the least effect on coronary vascular tone and autoregulation. Enflurane causes coronary vasodilatation in dogs but has not been shown to cause coronary steal in humans. Isoflurane has been shown to cause "steal" phenomena in some animal studies but not in others.[81] These studies call into question its use in patients with known or suspected coronary artery disease. However, clinical studies fail to show that isoflurane increases the risk of ischemia in patients.[82]

Spinal and epidural anesthesia cause hypotension as a direct result of preganglionic sympathetic blockade. This venodilatation causes decreased cardiac output and stroke volume. It may be accompanied by tachycardia if compensatory reflexes are intact or by a bradycardia if the blockade extends high enough to block the cardio-accelerator fibers at the T_1–T_4 level.[83] Hypotension can theoretically compromise coronary perfusion but, because of decreased afterload, oxygen requirements of the myocardium are reduced, and coronary perfusion is usually adequate.[84]

SUMMARY

1. The physiologic response to the stress of surgery and anesthesia is predominantly mediated by the neuroendocrine system. Surgery affects the secretion of a variety of hormones while anesthesia modulates both their secretion and actions.

2. Hormones induced by the stress of surgery exert important effects on metabolism, hemodynamics, and fluid balance. The changes mimic those typically seen in the human "fight or flight" response. Anesthesia generally blunts this stress response of the body.

3. Anesthetics also have direct effects on end organs and particularly affect cardiac and pulmonary function.

4. A knowledge of the physiologic effects of surgery and anesthesia enables the clinician to monitor patients with underlying disease more effectively.

REFERENCES

1. Kehlet H, Binder C: Alterations in distribution volume and biological half-life of cortisol during major surgery. *J Clin Endocrinol Metab* 36:330–333, 1973.
2. Napolitano LM, Chernow B: Guidelines for corticosteroid use in anesthetic and surgical stress. *Int Anesth Clinics* 26:226–232, 1988.
3. Chernow B, Alexander RH, Smallridge RC et al: Hormonal responses to graded surgical stress. *Arch Intern Med* 147:1273–1278, 1987.
4. Naito Y, Tami S, Shingu K et al: Response of plasma adrenocorticotropic hormone, cortisol and cytokines during and after upper abdominal surgery. *Anesthesiology* 77:426–431, 1992.
5. Omayama T, Taniguchi K, Ishihara H et al: Effects of enflurane anesthesia and surgery on endocrine function in man. *Br J Anaesth* 51:141–148, 1979.
6. Engquest A, Fog-Moller F, Christiannsen C et al: Influence of epidural analgesia on the catecholamine and cyclic AMP response to surgery. *Acta Anaesth Scand* 24:17–21, 1980.
7. Udelsman R, Norton JA, Jelenich SE et al: Response of the hypothalamic-pituitary-adrenal and renin-angiotensin axes and the sympathetic system during controlled surgical and anesthetic stress. *J Clin Endocrinol Metab* 64:986–994, 1987.

8. Frieling B, Brandt L: The influence of inhalation anesthetics on human plasma cortisol without superimposed stress (Abstract). *Anesthesiology* 63:A288, 1985.

9. Oyama T: Influence of anaesthesia on the endocrine system, in Stoeckel H, Oyama T (eds): *Endocrinology in Anaesthesia and Surgery.* Berlin, Springer-Verlag, 1980, pp. 39–51.

10. Sigurdsson G, Lindahl S, Norden N: Influence of premedication on plasma ACTH and cortisol concentrations in children during adenoidectomy. *Br J Anaesth* 54:1075–1080, 1982.

11. Stanley TH, Berman L, Green O et al: Plasma catecholamine and cortisol response to fentanyl-oxygen anesthesia for coronary artery operations. *Anesthesiology* 55:250–253, 1980.

12. Walsh ES, Paterson JL, O'Rioradan JBA et al: Effect of high-dose fentanyl anaesthesia on the metabolic and endocrine response to cardiac surgery. *Br J Anaesth* 53:1155–1165, 1981.

13. Bent JM, Paterson JL, Mashiter K et al: Effects of high-dose fentanyl anaesthesia on the established metabolic and endocrine response to surgery. *Anaesthesia* 39:19, 1984.

14. Fragen RJ, Shanks CA, Molteni A et al: Effects of etomidate on hormonal responses to surgical stress. *Anesthesiology* 61:652–656, 1984.

15. Oyama T, Wakayama S: The endocrine responses to general anesthesia. *Intern Anesth Clin* 26:176–181, 1988.

16. Wagner RL, White PF: Etomidate inhibits adrenocortical function in surgical patients. *Anesthesiology* 61:647–651, 1984.

17. Crozier TA, Beck D, Schlaeger M et al: Endocrinological changes following etomidate, midazolam, or methohexital for minor surgery. *Anesthesiology* 66:628–635, 1987.

18. Fragan RJ, Weiss HW, Moleteni A: The effect of propofol on adrenocortical steroidogenesis: A comparative study with etomidate and thiopental. *Anesthesiology* 66:839–842, 1987.

19. Brandt MR, Kehlet H, Binder C et al: Effect of epidural analgesia on the glucoregulatory endocrine response to surgery. *Clin Endocrinol* 5:107, 1976.

20. Cosgrove DO, Jenkins JS: The effect of epidural anaesthesia on the pituitary-adrenal response to surgery. *Clin Sci Mol Med* 46:403, 1974.

21. Davis FM, Laurenson VG, Lewis J et al: Metabolic response to total hip arthroplasty under hypobaric subarachnoid or general anesthesia. *Br J Anaesth* 59:725–729, 1987.

22. Engquist A, Brandt MR, Fernandes A et al: The blocking effect of epidural analgesia on the adrenocortical and hyperglycemia responses to surgery. *Acta Anaesth Scand* 21:330–335, 1977.

23. Tsuji H, Shirasaka C, Asoh T et al: Effects of epidural administration of local anaesthetics or morphine on postoperative nitrogen loss and catabolic hormones. *Br J Surg* 74:421–425, 1987.

24. Kehlet H: Epidural analgesia and the endocrine-metabolic response to surgery. Update and perspectives. *Acta Anaesth Scand* 28:125–127, 1984.

25. Downing R, Davis I, Black J et al: Effect of intrathecal morphine on the adrenocortical and hyperglycemic responses to upper abdominal surgery. *Br J Anaesth.* 58:858–861, 1986.

26. Hamberger B, Jarnberg PO: Plasma catecholamines during surgical stress; differences between neurolept and enflurane anaesthesia. *Acta Anaesth Scand* 27:307–310, 1983.

27. Joyce JT, Roizen MF, Gerson JI et al: Induction of anesthesia with halothane increases plasma norepinephrine concentrations. *Anesthesiology* 56:286, 1982.

28. Price HL, Linde HW, Jones RE et al: Sympatho-adrenal responses to general anesthesia in man and their relation to hemodynamics. *Anesthesiology* 20:563–574, 1959.

29. Lacoumenta S, Paterson JL, Burrin J et al: Effects of two differing halothane concentrations on the metabolic and endocrine responses to surgery. *Br J Anaesth* 58:844, 1986.

30. Gelmann S, Rivas JE, Erdemir H et al: Hormonal and haemodynamic responses to upper abdominal surgery during isoflurane and balanced anaesthesia. *Can Anaesth Soc J* 31:509, 1984.

31. Kono K, Philbin DM, Coggins CH et al: Renal function and stress response during halothane and fentanyl anesthesia. *Anesth Analg* 60:552–556, 1981.

32. Pflug AE, Halter JB: Effect of spinal anesthesia on adrenergic tone and the neuroendocrine response to surgical stress in humans. *Anesthesiology* 55:120, 1981.

33. Brandt MR, Olgaard K, Kehlet H: Epidural analgesia inhibits the renin and aldosterone response to surgery. *Acta Anaesthesiol Scand* 23:267, 1979.

34. Richardson DW, Robinson AG: Desmopressin. *Ann Int Med* 103:228–239, 1985.

35. Holmberg L, Nilsson IM, Borge L et al: Platelet aggregation induced by 1-deamino-8-D-arginine vasopressin (DDAVP) in type IIB von Willebrand's disease. *N Eng J Med.* 309:816–821, 1983.

36. Salzman EW, Weinstein MJ, Weintraub RM et al: Treatment with desmopressin acetate to reduce blood loss after cardiac surgery: A double blind randomized trial. *N Eng J Med* 314:1402–1406, 1986.

37. Hackman T, Gascoyne RD, Naiman SC et al: A trial of desmopressin (1-desamino-8-*d*-arginine vasopressin) to reduce blood loss in uncomplicated cardiac surgery. *N Eng J Med* 321:1437–1443, 1989.

38. Groves ND, Leach KG, Rosen M: Effects of halothane, enflurane and isoflurane anaesthesia on renal plasma flow. *Br J Anaesth* 65:796–800, 1990.

39. Oyama MD, Wakayama S: The endocrine responses to general anesthesia. *Int Anesth Clinics* 26:176–181, 1988.

40. Philbin DM, Coggins CH: Plasma antidiuretic hormone levels in cardiac surgical patients during morphine or halothane anesthesia. *Anesthesiology* 49:95–98, 1978.

41. Stanley TH, Philbin DM, Coggins CH: Fentanyl oxygen anesthesia for coronary artery surgery. *Can Anaesth Soc J* 26:168–172, 1979.

42. Cochrane JPS, Forsling ML, Gow NM et al: Arginine vasopressin release following surgical operations. *Br J Surg* 68:209–213, 1981.

43. Bonnet F, Harari A, Thibonnier M et al: Suppression of antidiuretic hormone hypersecretion during surgery by extradural anesthesia. *Br J Anaesth* 54:29, 1982.

44. Punnonen R, Viinamaki O: Vasopressin release following operation upon the vagina performed under general anesthesia or epidural analgesics. *Surg Gynecol Obstet* 156:781, 1983.

45. VonBroman B, Weidler B, Dennhardt R et al: Influence of epidural fentanyl on stress-induced elevation of plasma vasopressin (ADH) after surgery. *Anesth Analg* 62:727–732, 1983.

46. Webster J, Barnard M, Carli F: Metabolic response to colonic surgery: Extradural versus continuous spinal. *Br J Anaesth* 67:467–469, 1991.

47. Lund J, Stjernstrom H, Jorfelt L et al: Effect of extradural analgesia on glucose metabolism and gluconeogenesis. *Br J Anaesth* 58:851–857, 1986.

48. Asoh A, Tsuji H, Shirasaka C et al: Effect of epidural analgesia on metabolic response to major upper abdominal surgery. *Acta Anaesth Scand* 27:233–237, 1983.

49. Uchida I, Asoh T, Shirasak C et al: Effect of epidural analgesia on postoperative insulin resistance as evaluated by insulin clamp technique. *Br J Surg* 75:557–562, 1988.

50. Noreng MF, Jensen P, Tjellden NJ: Pre- and postoperative changes in the concentration of serum thyrotropin under general anaesthesia, compared to general anaesthesia with epidural analgesia. *Acta Anaesth Scand* 31:292–294, 1987.

51. Chan V, Wang C, Yeung RTT: Pituitary-thyroid responses to surgical stress. *Acta Endocrinologica* 88:490–498, 1978.

52. Oyama T: Thyroid, in Oyama T (ed): *Anaesthetic Management of Endocrine Disease.* Berlin, Springer-Verlag, 1973, pp 92–97.

53. Harland WA, Horton PW, Strang R et al: Release of thyroxine from the liver during anaesthesia and surgery. *Br J Anaesth* 46:818–820, 1974.

54. Matsuki A, Oyama T: The thyroid and anesthesia, in Oyama T (ed): *Endocrinology and the Anaesthetist.* Amsterdam, Elsevier, 1983, pp 65–79.

55. Marjot R, Valentine SJ: Arterial oxygen saturation following premedication for cardiac surgery. *Br J Anaesth* 64:737–740, 1990.

56. Bailey PL, Andriano KP, Goldman M et al: Variability of the respiratory response to diazepam. *Anesthesiology* 64:460–465, 1986.

57. Don H: The mechanical properties of the respiratory system during anesthesia, in Kafter ER (ed): *International Anesthesiology Clinics*, vol 15: *Anesthesia and Respiratory Function*. Boston, Little Brown, 1977, pp 113–136.

58. Craig DB, Whaba WM, Don HF et al: Closing volume and its relationship to gas exchange in seated and supine positions. *J Appl Physiology* 31:717, 1971.

59. Lumb AB, Nunn JF: Respiratory function and ribcage contribution to ventilation in body positions commonly used in anesthesia. *Anesth Analg* 73:422–466, 1991.

60. Bellville JW, Seed JC: The effect of drugs on the respiratory response to carbon dioxide. *Anesthesiology* 21:727–741, 1960.

61. Weil JV, McCullough RE, Kline JS et al: Diminished ventilatory response to hypoxia and hypercarbia after morphine in normal man. *N Eng J Med* 292:1103–1106, 1975.

62. Keats AS: The effects of drugs on respiration in man. *Ann Rev Pharmacol Toxicol* 25:41–65, 1985.

63. Hempenstall PD, DePlater RMH: Oxygen saturation during general anesthesia and recovery for outpatient oral surgical procedures. *Anaesth Intens Care* 18:517–521, 1990.

64. Brown LT, Purcell GH, Traugott FM: Hypoxemia during postoperative recovery using continuous pulse oximetry. *Anaesth Intens Care* 18:509–516, 1990.

65. Entwistle MD, Roe PG, Sapsford DJ et al: Patterns of oxygenation after thoracotomy. *Br J Anaesth* 67:704–711, 1991.

66. Chalon J, Patel C, Ali M et al: Humidity and the anesthetised patient. *Anesthesiology* 50:195–198, 1979.

67. Benumof JL: One-lung ventilation and hypoxic pulmonary vasconstriction: Implications for anesthetic management. *Anesth Analg* 64:821–833, 1985.

68. Steinbrook RA, Concepcion M: Respiratory effects of spinal anesthesia: Resting ventilation and single-breath CO_2 response. *Anesth Analg* 72:182–186, 1991.

69. Steinbrook RA, Concepcion M, Topulos GP: Ventilatory responses to hypercapnia during bupivicaine spinal anesthesia. *Anesth Analg* 67:247–252, 1988.

70. Steinbrook RA, Topulos GP, Concepcion M: Ventilatory responses to hypercapnia during tetracaine spinal anesthesia. *J Clin Anesth* 1:75–80, 1988.

71. Askrog VF, Smith TC, Eckenhoff JE: Changes in pulmonary ventilation during spinal anesthesia. *Surg Gynecol Obstet* 119:563, 1964.

72. Pikanen MT: Body mass and spread of spinal anesthesia with bupivacaine. *Anesth Analg* 66:127–131, 1987.

73. Theye RA, Michenfelder JD: Whole body and organ $\dot{V}O_2$ changes with enflurane, isoflurane and halothane. *Br J Anaesth* 47:813, 1975.

74. Eger EI, Smith NT, Stoelting RT: Cardiovascular effects of halothane in man. *Anesthesiology* 32:396, 1970.

75. Ritter JW, Shigezawa GY, Roe SD et al: Increasing myocardial oxygen demand during prolonged halothane anesthesia in dogs. *Anesth Analg* 62:788, 1983.

76. Philbin DM, Foex P, Drummond G et al: Postsystolic shortening of canine left ventricle supplied by stenotic coronary artery when nitrous oxide is added in the presence of narcotics. *Anesthesiology* 62:166–174, 1983.

78. Nathan HJ: Nitrous oxide worsens myocardial ischemia in isoflurane-anesthetized dogs. *Anesthesiology* 68:407–415, 1988.

78. Cahalan MK, Prakash O, Rulf ENR et al: Addition of nitrous oxide to fentanyl anesthesia does not induce myocardial ischemia in patients with ischemic heart disease. *Anesthesiology* 67:925–929, 1987.

79. Mitchell MM, Prakash O, Rulf ENR et al: Nitrous oxide does not induce myocardial ischemia in patients with ischemic heart disease and poor ventricular function. *Anesthesiology* 72:526–534, 1989.

80. Hickey RF, Sybert PE, Verrier ED et al: Effects of halothane, enflurane, and isoflurane on coronary blood flow autoregulation and coronary vascular reserve in the canine heart. *Anesthesiology* 68:21–30, 1988.

81. Buffington CW, Romson JL, Levine A et al: Isoflurane induces coronary steal in a canine model of chronic coronary occlusion. *Anesthesiology* 66:280–292, 1987.

82. O'Young J, Mastrocostopoulos G, Hilgenberg A et al: Myocardial circulatory and metabolic effects of isoflurane and sufentanil during coronary artery surgery. *Anesthesiology* 66:653–658, 1987.

83. Caplan RA, Ward RJ, Posner K et al: Unexpected cardiac arrest during spinal anesthesia: A closed claims analysis of predisposing factors. *Anesthesiology* 68:5–11, 1988.

84. Hackel DB, Sancetta SM, Kleineman J: Effect of hypotension during spinal anesthesia on coronary blood flows and myocardial metabolism in man. *Circulation* 13:92, 1956.

6 A PRIMER IN ANESTHESIOLOGY FOR THE INTERNIST

David M. Guarnieri

The primary function of the anesthesiologist in the operating room is to provide relief from pain for patients undergoing surgery. To do this safely and effectively, the anesthesiologist must consider a number of factors in order to make an appropriate choice of anesthetic agent and technique. These factors include knowledge of the patient's current disease status; review of past medical, surgical, medication, and allergy history; results of the physical examination and laboratory tests; understanding of the surgical procedure and the patient's preferences; and consideration of requirements for postoperative pain relief. A well-planned and well-executed anesthetic involves balancing the perioperative concerns of the patient, surgeon, anesthesiologist, and often a consulting internist. The anesthetic scenario may be one of many, and the various anesthetic techniques are detailed in Table 6–1. This chapter outlines the process by which an anesthesiologist plans a safe and effective anesthetic for the individual patient.

TABLE 6–1. Anesthetic Techniques

Local Anesthesia
  Administered by the surgeon without IV sedation
  May or may not involve a premedication

Monitored Anesthesia Care
  Combination of local anesthesia and IV sedation with appropriate monitoring
  May or may not involve a premedication

Regional Anesthesia
  Major conduction block such as spinal or epidural
  Peripheral nerve block
  May or may not involve premedication or IV sedation

General Anesthesia
  May be administered via mask or endotracheal tube
  May be based primarily on inhalational or intravenous agents
  May require skeletal muscle relaxation
  May be combined with a local or regional anesthetic for intraoperative and postoperative analgesia
  May or may not involve a premedication

All Forms
  Choice of premedication, local anesthetics, regional anesthetics, IV sedatives, and general agents should reflect operative and postoperative concerns

PREMEDICATION

Preparation for anesthesia and surgery includes both psychological and pharmacologic components. In the initial visit with the patient, the anesthesiologist should discuss anesthetic options and risks in a manner that allays apprehension. The value of a comforting, informative preoperative visit cannot be overestimated as a means of relieving anxiety and potentially reducing drug requirements (see Table 6–2). However, relief of pain, amnesia, and decreased anxiety cannot be consistently guaranteed by a preoperative visit alone, and pharmacologic agents are commonly given as premedication. An appropriate premedication will provide relief of anxiety, sedation, analgesia, and amnesia. In addition, an appropriately chosen agent can reduce anesthetic requirements, prevent sympathetic reflex responses, increase the pH and reduce the volume of gastric fluid, and provide prophylaxis against allergic reactions. Other considerations in choosing premedication include prevention of postoperative nausea and vomiting, facilitating induction of anesthesia, and reducing cardiac vagal tone.

There are several classes of drugs available to accomplish these goals (see Table 6–3). Variables such as age, weight, physical status, tolerance to depressant drugs, and previous experience of the patient should be considered in choosing an appropriate premedication. Sometimes patients at the extremes of age suffering from severe cardiac, pulmonary, or neurologic disease are better served if no depressant premedication is given. The nature of the

TABLE 6–2. Comparison of Preoperative Visit and Pentobarbital (2 mg/kg IM) (% of Patients)

	Felt Drowsy	Felt Nervous	Adequate Preparation
Control Group	18	58	35
Pentobarbital Only	30	61	48
Preoperative Visit	26	40	65
Pentobarbital and Preoperative Visit	38	38	71

Source: Data from Egbert LD et al: The value of the preoperative visit by the anesthetist. *JAMA* 185:553, 1963.

TABLE 6–3. Drugs and Doses Used for Pharmacologic Premedication Before Induction of Anesthesia

Classification	Drug	Typical Adult Dose (mg)*	Route of Administration
Barbiturates	Secobarbital	50–150	Orally, IM
	Pentobarbital	50–150	Orally, IM
Opioids	Morphine	5–15	IM
	Meperidine	50–100	IM
Benzodiazepines	Diazepam	5–10	Orally, IM
	Lorazepam	2–4	Orally, IM
	Midazolam	2.5–5	IM
	Flurazepam	15–30	Orally
	Temazepam	15–30	Orally
	Triazolam	0.125–0.25	Orally
Antihistamines	Diphenhydramine	25–75	Orally, IM
	Promethazine	25–50	IM
	Hydroxyzine	30–100	IM
Anticholinergics	Atropine	0.3–0.6	IM
	Scopolamine	0.3–0.6	IM
	Glycopyrrolate	0.2–0.3	IM
H$_2$ antagonists	Cimetidine	300	Orally, IM, IV
	Rantitidine	150	Orally, IM
Antacids	Particulate	15–30 ml	Orally
	Nonparticulate	10–20 ml	Orally
Stimulants of gastric motility	Metoclopramide	10–20	Orally, IM, IV

*Except for antacids.
IM, intramuscularly; IV, intravenously.
Source: Stoelting RK, Miller RD: *Basics of Anesthesia*, 2d ed. New York, Churchill Livingstone, 1989, p 124.

surgical procedure and its duration are also important factors. It may be unwise to premedicate a patient before a brief outpatient procedure if it will delay recovery from anesthesia or discharge from the hospital. The peak effect of the medication should coincide with the patient's arrival in the operating room. All drugs, doses, routes of administration, and effects of premedications should be noted in the anesthesia record.

LOCAL ANESTHESIA AND MONITORED ANESTHESIA CARE

Local anesthetics are used as the primary form of analgesia if the patient can comfortably tolerate the procedure when only the area of surgical interest is anesthetized. This method is simple, appropriate for brief and superficial procedures, free of the side effects of general anesthesia, and requires only minimal postoperative care. A common misconception concerning the use of local anesthetics is that this technique is appropriate for patients who have recently eaten and are at risk for aspiration of gastric contents. If the local anesthetic does not provide sufficient relief of pain, general anesthesia may need to be administered midway through a partially successful local block. At this point the risk to the patient is increased due to the emergent nature of the induction.

Local anesthetics may seem better for patients who are too critically ill for general anesthesia, but overall risk may not be reduced. In a study of over 34,000 patients, mortality was highest in those given local anesthesia.[1] This was most likely due to a greater percentage of poor-risk patients in the group receiving local anesthesia. This underscores the common misbelief that the less complicated anesthetic techniques are safer for sicker patients.

Guidelines for the use of local anesthetics with or without sedation include:

1. Some parts of the body are inaccessible or impractical for local anesthetics. When the number of injections and the dose of anesthetic required near toxicity, reactions including drowsiness, convulsions, and cardiovascular collapse are possible (see Table 6–4). Preventing complications requires using minimal effective drug concentrations in the smallest volume and avoiding vascular injection sites. Addition of epinephrine will help slow the rate of systemic absorption but carries its own hazards. Tremor, sweating, tachycardia and palpitations occur frequently and should be avoided in patients with hypertension, coronary artery disease, malignant arrhythmias, and hyperthyroidism.

2. Many local anesthetics are available and differ greatly in their onset and duration of action (see Table 6–4). Lidocaine is widely used because of its rapid onset of action and would be adequate for intraoperative repair of an inguinal hernia. However, bupivicaine would be better for infiltrating the wound prior to closure to provide postoperative pain relief.

3. The common adjunctive practice of giving intraoperative intravenous sedation is not without risk. When it produces apparent sleep, unappreciated hypoxia and hypercarbia may develop and precipitate cardiac arrest if the patient is not closely monitored.

TABLE 6–4. Comparative Pharmacology of Local Anesthetics

Classification	Potency	Onset	Duration After Infiltration (Minutes)	Maximum Single Dose for Infiltration (Adult, mg*)	Toxic Plasma Concentration ($\mu g \cdot ml^{-1}$)
Esters					
Procaine	1**	Slow	45–60	500	—
Chloroprocaine	4	Rapid	30–45	600	—
Tetracaine	16	Slow	60–180	100	—
Amides					
Lidocaine	1***	Rapid	60–120	300	5
Mepivacaine	1	Slow	90–180	300	5
Bupivacaine	4	Slow	240–480	175	About 1.5
Etidocaine	4	Slow	240–480	300	About 2
Prilocaine	1	Slow	60–120	400	5

*Increased if solution contains epinephrine.
**Standard of comparison for esters.
***Standard of comparison for amides.
Source: Stoelting RK, Miller RD: *Basics of Anesthesia,* 2d ed, New York, Churchill Livingstone, 1989, p 85.

REGIONAL ANESTHESIA

Regional anesthesia includes spinal, epidural, and peripheral nerve blocks. Spinal anesthesia is accomplished by injecting local anesthetic into the subarachnoid space to temporarily interrupt nerve transmission to the spinal cord and higher centers. Epidural block is achieved by injecting local anesthetic into the epidural space from which it diffuses into the nerve roots, subarachnoid space, and outer layers of the spinal cord. Peripheral nerve blocks require deposition of anesthetic near bundles of nerve fibers elsewhere in the body. Regional anesthesia can be selective for the surgical site, allows for catheter placement to facilitate continuation of analgesia, provides skeletal muscle relaxation, and permits patients to remain awake.

Regional anesthesia may have other advantages. One is to favorably modify the endocrine stress response to surgery and anesthesia (see Chap. 5). In addition, rates of intraoperative blood loss, thromboembolic complications, cardiopulmonary complications, and postoperative recovery are better when regional anesthesia is compared to general.[2] Finally, the ability to inject opioids into the epidural and subarachnoid spaces has continuously expanded available options for postoperative analgesia and chronic pain therapy as well (see Chap. 72).

Both spinal and epidural blocks interrupt sensory, motor, and sympathetic nervous system innervation. Spinal anesthesia requires a smaller amount of local anesthetic solution than epidural blockade given the lesser need for diffusion. A total dose of 75 to 100 mg of lidocaine will generally produce a T_4 sensory level if given intrathecally, but 300 to 400 mg may be needed to achieve this same level of block if injected into the epidural space. The onset of action of spinal anesthesia is two to three times faster than that of epidural. Rapid production of sympathetic block causes decreased venous return and bradycardia and therefore a spinal anesthetic can cause more abrupt hypotension.

The dermatomal sensory level achieved in either case depends upon the distribution of the local anesthetic in the cerebrospinal fluid and at the spinal nerve roots. When local anesthetics are placed directly into the cerebrospinal fluid, the baricity of the solution and position of the patient in the first few minutes after injection are key determinants. When the epidural space is injected, diffusion becomes more important, and dose (mg/dermatomal segment), volume, and concentration of the anesthetic become critical. In both cases, the duration of action is affected most by the choice of agent. Addition of epinephrine will prolong the duration of the block. Placement of a soft plastic catheter allows for intermittent bolus dosing with either block or continuous infusion in epidural blocks. Incremental dosing facilitates gradual production of sensory and sympathetic block and titration to a specific level of anesthesia. The catheter can be left in place to administer opioids for postoperative pain relief, making for a highly adaptable technique.

Guidelines for the use of spinal or epidural anesthesia include:

1. The nature of the surgical procedure may dictate whether or not a spinal or epidural anesthesic may be used (see Table 6–5).

2. The patient must be receptive to the idea of spinal or epidural anesthesia. Concerns about being awake in the operating room and fears of needle sticks must be addressed preoperatively. Sedation may be helpful but must not interfere with the patient cooperation needed for placement of the block or result in respiratory compromise.

3. There are some contraindications to spinal and epidural anesthesia. Absolute contraindications are localized infection at the puncture site, severe uncorrected hypovolemia, and untreated coagulation defects. Relative contraindications are anatomic abnormalities of the spine, some neurologic disorders, and generalized infection (e.g., bacteremia). In the case of relative contraindications, risk must be weighed against benefit in each individual patient.

4. There are many potential complications of spinal and epidural anesthesia, and some can be serious. These include total spinal blockade, postdural puncture headache, major neurologic injury, local anesthetic toxicity, catheter-related prob-

TABLE 6–5. Surgical Procedures Often Performed Under Spinal or Epidural Anesthesia

1. Any intraabdominal procedure
2. Gynecological procedures
   a. Hysterectomy
   b. Cone biopsy
   c. D & C
   d. Ovarian cystectomy
3. Obstetrical procedures
   a. Cesarean section
   b. Circlage
   c. Vaginal delivery
4. Herniorraphies
5. Lower limb procedures
   a. Orthopedic
   b. Vascular
   c. Amputations
6. Urological procedures
   a. Transurethral resections
   b. Cystoscopy
   c. Open prostatectomies
   d. Penile implant
   e. Orchiectomy
7. Perineal and rectal surgery
   a. Bartholin cyst
   b. Rectal fissures
   c. Hemorrhoids
8. Others

Source: Corrino BG, Lembert DH: Epidural and spinal anesthesia, in Barash PG, Cullen BF, Stoelting RK (eds): *Clinical Anesthesia*, 1st ed, Philadelphia, Lippincott, 1989, p 762.

lems, backache, and nausea. Generally, the potential drawbacks are predictable and acceptable, considering the merits of the technique.

5. Sometimes spinal and epidural blocks are unsuccessful from the outset or fail to provide continued adequate analgesia. In all cases, there must be plans formulated and provisions available for general anesthesia. Even if regional anesthesia is chosen to avoid a difficult airway situation, contingency plans for general anesthesia must be made in advance.

Peripheral nerve blocks of the trunk and extremities provide alternatives to or adjuncts to general anesthesia (see Table 6–6). Preoperative selection and preparation of patients for these blocks is similar to that discussed above. Each block has its own specific risks and complications dependent on its site and degree of invasiveness. Systemic toxicity from absorption of local anesthetic varies with the site of the block and the choice of agent.

GENERAL ANESTHESIA

The goal of general anesthesia is depression of consciousness sufficient to allow tolerance of painful stimuli. Classically, there are four components of general anesthesia: hypnosis, amnesia, analgesia, and autonomic stability. A fifth component, skeletal muscle relaxation, is a variable requirement. Anesthetic agents can be administered in inhalational or intravenous form, but commonly, both approaches are used in nearly every case. General anesthesia is achieved in two phases—induction and maintenance. During

TABLE 6–6. Peripheral Nerve Blocks

Cervical plexus
Brachial plexus

Interscalene
Supraclavicular
Axillary

Median nerve
Ulnar nerve
Radial nerve
Intercostal nerves
Sciatic nerve
Femoral nerve
Lateral femoral cutaneous nerve
Obturator nerve
Stellate ganglion
Celiac plexus
Lumbar sympathetic nerves
Intravenous regional block

Source: Stoelting RK, Miller RD: *Basics of Anesthesia*, 2d ed, New York, Churchill Livingstone, 1989, p 190.

induction, the awake patient achieves a plane of surgical anesthesia. This can be accomplished with inhalational drugs alone. However, this technique is usually reserved for patients with a compromised airway in whom spontaneous ventilation allows optimal gas-flow patterns to be maintained, for children whose lack of cooperation makes establishing intravenous access difficult, and for patients with endotracheal or tracheostomy tubes already in place. The intravenous route is quick and comfortable for most patients, and it presumes no airway management problems.

Induction may or may not involve intubation of the trachea. Only a face mask may be used if a relatively brief procedure with no ventilation problems is foreseen. There may be a need to protect the patient's lungs from aspiration of gastric contents. In this case a rapid-sequence induction is performed using quick-acting intravenous agents, posteriorly directed pressure on the cricoid cartilage, and tracheal intubation. It is not uncommon to secure the airway prior to induction. Under these circumstances, intubation is performed in the awake patient in whom all airway reflexes are intact. This is done when the patient has a high risk of aspiration and is expected to pose problems for intubation during a rapid-sequence induction, when the patient has a compromised airway and an inhalational approach is not appropriate, and when the patient is in acute respiratory failure and needs positive pressure ventilation.

In the maintenance phase of anesthesia, inhalational or intravenous agents are chosen based on their relative merits for the individual patient and surgical procedure. When the intravenous route is the primary mode, drugs may be given as a large bolus prior to surgical incision, in smaller intermittent boluses as needed, or by titrating a constant infusion to produce the desired effect. Blood levels and drug effect depend upon the process of elimination which may be redistribution within the body or by hepatic or renal metabolism and excretion. An inhalational drug is taken up and eliminated primarily through alveolar ventilation. Because of the large absorptive surface of the lung, blood concentrations and drug effect can be regulated on a moment to moment basis as the demands of the operation dictate. In a majority of cases, combinations of intravenous and inhalational drugs are used to reap the advantages and minimize the side effects of each.

Two trends are becoming more prevalent in current anesthesia practice. First, it is becoming increasingly common to use a regional technique for analgesia and a "light" general anesthetic for hypnosis and amnesia during the maintenance phase. This combination provides many of the benefits of both techniques in the operating room as well as into the recovery phase. Second, a large number of surgical procedures are now done in a "day surgery" setting in which the patient is never admitted to the hospital. This demands that patients be appropriately screened prior to their procedure, the procedure and the patient's disease allow for return home the same day, and the anesthetic and its effects be designed to produce an alert, comfortable and ambulatory patient.

Currently used inhaled anesthetics include the gas nitrous oxide and the volatile liquids—halothane, enflurane, isoflurane, desflurane, and sevoflurane. Examples of intravenous agents are barbiturates, benzodiazepines, opioids, and miscellaneous drugs such as ketamine, etomidate, and propofol. Planning safe anesthesia requires an understanding of these drugs when used in varying doses and combinations in patients who are premedicated, undergoing the stress of surgery, and perhaps suffering from a variety of disease states requiring multiple medications. A discussion of adverse drug reactions and interactions to the anesthetic agents may be found in Chap. 49.

Skeletal muscle relaxation is a variable requirement of general anesthesia. Relaxation or paralysis can be achieved with high doses of volatile anesthetics, regional anesthetics, or specific drugs which interrupt transmission at the neuromuscular junction. Muscle relaxants facilitate intubation of the trachea and provide optimal surgical exposure. Use of a relaxant in the anesthetic plan is based on several factors (see Table 6–7). Choice of a neuromuscular blocking agent is influenced by speed of onset, duration of action, route of elimination, and associated side effects. When rapid onset and brief duration of paralysis are needed as in the case of tracheal intubation, succinylcholine, a depolarizing neuromuscular blocker, is an excellent choice. When longer duration of action is necessary and an immediate onset is not imperative, any of the nondepolarizing muscle relaxants are acceptable (e.g., pancuronium or vecuronium). Intraoperative assessment of the degree of neuromuscular blockade is performed with the assistance of a peripheral nerve stimulator.

TABLE 6–7. Factors Involved in the Decision to Use a Muscle Relaxant as Part of the Anesthetic

I. Surgical procedure
  A. Anatomic location
  B. Intensity and duration
  C. Patient position
II. Anesthetic technique
  A. Primary agent (inhalational vs. N_2O and opioid)
  B. Airway management (mask vs. endotracheal)
  C. Ventilatory pattern (spontaneous/assisted vs. controlled)
III. Patient factors
  A. Body habitus (lean vs. obese)
  B. ASA status
    1. Respiratory
    2. Cardiovascular
    3. Neuromuscular
    4. Neurologic
  C. Age

Source: Lebowitz PW, Ramsey FM: Muscle relaxants, in Barash PG, Cullen BF, Stoelting RK (eds): *Clinical Anesthesia,* 1st ed, Philadelphia, Lippincott, 1989, p 340.

Guidelines for the use of neuromuscular blocking agents include:

1. The use of muscle relaxants allows lesser concentrations of potentially toxic anesthetic drugs to be used to keep patients immobile. Many patients will not tolerate deep levels of anesthesia for circulatory reasons.
2. Muscle relaxants are devoid of analgesic properties and should not be administered to inadequately anesthetized patients. Patient movement usually means that additional anesthetic agent is required.
3. Some procedures like intracranial operations require there to be no patient movement throughout the procedure, while others demand intense neuromuscular blockade only at certain points such as during a delicate vascular anastomosis. Relaxants do provide improved exposure but are usually not absolutely necessary for this reason alone.

The reversal of competitive neuromuscular blockade is complicated and requires administration of an anticholinesterase like edrophonium, neostigmine, or pyridostigmine. These inhibit acetylcholinesterase, resulting in accumulation of acetylcholine at the neuromuscular junction. Peripheral side effects of anticholinesterases can be minimized by simultaneous administration of an anticholinergic muscarinic blocker like atropine or glycopyrrolate. Wide swings in parasympathetic activity may occur, and proper choice of agent and dosage is imperative. Reversal of neuromuscular blockade assumes that removal of the endotracheal tube will be attempted. There are numerous ways to assess neuromuscular function before extubation, but none is perfect in helping to judge the patient's ability to sustain a patent airway.

The decision to use invasive monitoring, including Swan-Ganz and arterial catheters, and management of intraoperative fluids usually lie with the anesthesiologist. Invasive monitoring allows assessment of key physiologic parameters, determination of the effects of therapeutic interventions, and early recognition of adverse effects. There are definite risks during placement and maintenance of these catheters. Moreover, no controlled prospective study has documented that the use of pulmonary artery catheters improves outcome. Use of invasive monitoring should be decided on a case-by-case basis in which anesthesiologist, surgeon, and consulting internist all have appropriate input.

The management of intraoperative fluid therapy depends upon clinical judgment and knowledge of how to calculate requirements for maintenance fluids, deficit replacement, third spacing, and blood loss. One suggested regimen for determining hourly fluid therapy is presented in Table 6–8. The numbers in the table are only guidelines and may need to be adjusted depending upon the type of patient, the medical history, type of surgical procedure, and changes in blood pressure, urine output, and central venous or pulmonary artery wedge pressure measurements.

A consulting internist or surgeon may need to review the anesthesiologist's record to answer a specific question about intraoperative care. Though appearing unnecessarily complicated at first glance, a good anesthesia record provides important information about the patient's condition at any moment. The contents of any anesthesia record are detailed in Table 6–9. Data are recorded at frequent intervals and charted graphically. The record should allow determination of the anesthetic and adjuvant drugs given, the patient's response, and fluid status at any point in time. Space is

TABLE 6–8. Intraoperative Fluid Therapy

Maintenance Fluid
  4 cc/kg/hr for first 10 kg of body weight
  2 cc/kg/hr for second 10 kg of body weight
  1 cc/kg/hr for each additional kg of body weight
Maintenance fluids are to be administered each hour the patient is in the operating room.

Fluid Deficit
  Deficit = Maintenance Requirement × Number of Hours NPO
    (assuming no IV fluids prior to arrival in operating room)
  Deficit fluids are replaced ½ over the first hour and ¼ over each successive hour × 2

Third Space Losses
  2–10 cc/kg/hr (depending on the size and location of the incision)
Third space losses are replaced each hour the operation is in progress

Calculation of Allowable Blood Loss (ABL)
  Estimated Blood Volume = 60–70 cc/kg
  $ABL = EBV \times \dfrac{H(initial) - H(final)}{H(initial)}$
  H(initial) = Initial Hemoglobin
  H(final) = Final Hemoglobin

Suggested Approach to Intraoperative Fluid Therapy
  Replace maintenance fluids, deficit, and third space losses with crystalloid
  Replace first third of ABL with crystalloid 3 ml for each 1 ml of blood loss
  Replace second third of ABL with colloid 1 ml for each 1 ml of blood loss
  Replace final third of ABL with packed RBCs diluted to 500 ml with normal saline

Source: Suggested Approach from Dodge C, Glass DD: Crystalloid and colloid therapy. *Seminars in Anesthesia* 1(4):293–301, 1982.

TABLE 6–9. Contents of the Anesthesia Record

Biographical data (name, hospital number, age, height, weight)
Preoperative diagnosis
Name of surgical procedure
Physical status
Premedication (drug, dose, route, time) and effect
Current medications
Allergy history
Verification of operative permit
Documentation of NPO status
Nature and location of IV access and invasive monitors
Continuous monitoring of vital signs*
Anesthetic induction**
Details of airway management***
Mode of ventilation****
Concentration of supplemental oxygen
Anesthetic agents (dose, route, time of administration)
Fluids (IV, blood loss, blood products, urine output)
Position
Level of spinal or epidural block (if appropriate)
Anesthetic and operative start and termination times

  *May include heart rate, heart rhythm, blood pressure, oxygen saturation, end-tidal carbon dioxide, temperature, central venous pressure, pulmonary artery pressure, cardiac output, systemic vascular resistance, mixed venous oxygen saturation, arterial or venous laboratory values
  **Satisfactory or unsatisfactory (reasons for unsatisfactory such as vomiting, laryngospasm, or hypotension are cited)
  ***May include use of oropharyngeal or nasopharyngeal airway; route, method, and number of attempts at intubation; diameter, depth of insertion, and cuff inflation of endotracheal tube; confirmation of breath sounds; evidence of trauma; comments concerning technical ease and degree of visualization
  ****Spontaneous versus controlled (may include rate, tidal volume, peak airway pressures, minute ventilation)

usually reserved for specific notes concerning the course of the anesthesic, aspects of the patient's condition, treatments given during the procedure, and details of the surgical procedure. A complete and accurate anesthesia record is invaluable to all those involved in the patient's care.

DRUG-DISEASE INTERACTIONS

Malignant hyperthermia and pseudocholinesterase deficiency are two disease states which are generally considered to be specific to anesthesia-related drugs. This section discusses these entities and their implications for anesthesia and makes recommendations for perioperative drug management.

Malignant Hyperthermia

Malignant hyperthermia is a disease of skeletal muscle occurring in one in 50,000 anesthetic cases in adults and one in 15,000 cases in children.[3] Studies support an autosomal dominant inheritance pattern carried by a single gene with variable penetrance. All potent inhalational anesthetics, succinylcholine, and decamethonium can trigger malignant hyperthermia. The presumed mechanism of action involves prevention of calcium reuptake by the sarcoplasmic reticulum which results in generalized muscle contraction followed by a hypermetabolic state with increased oxygen consumption, increased carbon dioxide production, rapidly rising temperature, and respiratory and metabolic acidosis. Ventricular arrhythmias are common.[4] A history of hyperthermia, muscle rigidity during previous procedures, or a family history of malignant hyperthermia is useful in identifying susceptible patients, but a negative history does not exclude the possibility of it developing.

  The clinical manifestations are usually evident during anesthesia but may not appear until several hours after the procedure. Masseter muscle rigidity after administration of succinylcholine is a valuable early warning sign but is not always present.[5] Muscle biopsy testing with caffeine and halothane suggests that about 50 percent of patients with masseter muscle rigidity are susceptible to malignant hyperthermia.[3] Tachycardia and arrhythmias occur earlier, followed by tachypnea, respiratory and metabolic acidosis, hyperkalemia, and hyperglycemia. Hyperthermia, pulmonary edema, consumption coagulopathy, and acute renal failure from myoglobinuria follow.[5]

Management includes immediate cessation of anesthesia, vigorous hyperventilation with 100% oxygen, core and surface cooling, and correction of acidosis.[3,6,7] Dantrolene sodium is recommended in a dose of 2.5 mg/kg with repeated doses as needed up to a total of 10 mg/kg. Intravenous procainamide is useful in managing arrhythmias.[3]

Induction agents considered safe in patients susceptible to malignant hyperthermia include barbiturates, narcotics, benzodiazepines, and nitrous oxide. Other drugs like propofol, local anesthetics, vecuronium, atracurium, and antihistamines are also considered safe.[3] Oral dantrolene is not recommended to prevent malignant hyperthermia because of variability in blood levels and clinical reports of prophylaxis failures.[3,8]

Pseudocholinesterase Deficiency

Cholinesterases can be categorized as true cholinesterases present at nerve endings and in erythrocytes, and pseudocholinesterases found in the liver and serum. Succinylcholine is usually rapidly inactivated by serum pseudocholinesterase. However, in patients with pseudocholinesterase deficiency, ineffective inactivation results in prolonged postoperative apnea. This enzymatic defect is inherited as an autosomal recessive trait and is found in 1 in 3000 individuals in the homozygous state. Management of succinylcholine-induced apnea consists of mechanical ventilation until the respiratory depressant effects dissipate.

Serum cholinesterase activity can be measured in patients suspected of pseudocholinesterase deficiency. Plasma cholinesterase activity is inhibited in vitro by the local anesthetic dibucaine to a greater degree in normal individuals than in those lacking the enzyme. On the basis of this measurement, patients can be assigned a dibucaine number representing the percentage of enzyme inhibition by the local anesthetic. Normal individuals have numbers between 70 and 85, heterozygotes for atypical enzyme have numbers between 30 and 65, and homozygotes with only atypical enzyme have numbers between 16 and 25.[10–12] Homozygous patients experience significantly prolonged paralysis (three to four hours) after usual doses of succinylcholine, but heterozygotes experience only slight prolongation (20 minutes).[9,11]

SUMMARY

1. In order to deliver a safe anesthetic, the anesthesiologist must choose the proper technique and agents based on the patient's medical diseases and preferences, the surgical procedure, and expectations for postoperative function. More frequently, anesthesiologists are now performing their task in an outpatient setting or combining several anesthetic techniques for an individual procedure.

2. Local anesthesia is still a popular choice because of its simplicity. However, it may not always be the best choice for very ill patients or those who have recently eaten.

3. Regional anesthesia is appropriate for a large number of procedures. In experienced hands, the benefits outweigh the potential complications. The use of spinal, epidural, or peripheral nerve block is expanding due to favorable modification of the endocrine stress response and the use of opioids in the epidural or subarachnoid space.

4. General anesthesia can involve both inhalational and intravenous drugs. Ventilation may be delivered via face mask or endotracheal intubation. The specific agents chosen for induction and maintenance depend upon the patient's age, airway status, and coexisting diseases; the demands of the surgical procedure; and postoperative pain requirements.

5. Provisions for general anesthesia should always be available in the event of a failed local or regional technique.

6. Fluid management and decisions regarding intraoperative monitoring usually lie with the anesthesiologist. Since no precise guidelines exist for either, clinical judgment is needed in conjunction with generally accepted guidelines or approaches.

7. Malignant hyperthermia and pseudocholinesterase deficiency are genetically transmitted disease states which generally become manifest upon exposure to specific anesthesia-related drugs. Prompt recognition and treatment are essential to providing a good outcome.

REFERENCES

1. Marx GF, Mateo CV, Orkin LR: Computer analysis of postanesthetic deaths. *Anesthesiology* 39:54–58, 1973.
2. Covino BG, Lambert DH: Epidural and spinal anesthesia, in Barash PG, Cullen BF, Stoelting RK (eds): *Clinical Anesthesia*, 1st ed. Philadelphia, Lippincott, 1989, pp 755–757.
3. Rosenberg H, Seitman D: Pharmacogenetics, in Barash PG, Cullen BF, Stoelting RK (eds): *Clinical Anesthesia*, 1st ed. Philadelphia, Lippincott, 1989, pp 459–472.
4. Morley J: Muscular connective tissue diseases and malignant hyperthermia, in *Manual of Anesthesia and the Medically Compromised Patient*. Philadelphia, Lippincott, 1990, pp 576–580.
5. Britt. BA: Etiology and pathophysiology of malignant hyperthermia. *Fed Proc* 38:44, 1979.
6. Ryan JF: Treatment of acute hyperthermia crisis. *Int Anesth Clin* 17:153, 1979.
7. Gronert GA, Thompson RL, Onofrio BM: Human malignant hyperthermia: Awake episodes and correction by dantrolene. *Anesth Analg* 59:377, 1980.
8. Rosenberg H, Seitman D: Pharmacogenetics, in Barash PG, Cullen BF, Stoelting RK (eds): *Clinical Anesthesia*, 1st ed. Philadelphia, Lippincott, 1989, p 469.
9. Whittaker M: Plasma cholinesterase variants and the anesthetist. *Anaesthesia* 35:174, 1980.
10. Lebowitz PW, Ramsey FM: Muscle relaxants, in Barash PG, Cullen BF, Stoelting RK (eds): *Clinical Anesthesia*, 1st ed. Philadelphia, Lippincott, 1989, p 344.
11. Whitby LG: Biochemical screening tests for the anesthetist. *Br J Anaesth* 46:564, 1974.

EVALUATION OF THE PATIENT UNDERGOING SURGERY: A PROCEDURE-ORIENTED APPROACH

II

INTRODUCTION TO THE SURGICAL SECTION

This section is divided into ten chapters largely on the basis of surgical specialty. Each chapter contains an initial section discussing common comorbid conditions usually seen in patients undergoing the included surgical procedures, appropriate diagnostic and therapeutic measures to decrease surgical risk, and complications specific to the particular set of procedures. The most common procedures or families of procedures within that specialty are then presented in uniform outlines designed to provide an overview of the operation(s) followed by indications, details of the surgery itself, expected hospital course, complications, and follow-up. The initial discussions are designed to orient the reader within the surgical specialty, and the uniform outline format is designed to provide easy reference for practical details about individual procedures. Our goal is to help the reader assess procedure-related risk.

The initial discussions are extensively cross-referenced to specific chapters in the book for additional information. References have been kept to a minimum in this section of the book since cross-referenced chapters already contain extensive bibliographies. We believe that we have covered the majority of surgical procedures commonly performed in the United States today. In some cases, particular procedures could not be easily classified. For example, breast surgery is covered in Chap. 7 on abdominal surgery because most breast operations are performed by general surgeons. Similarly, although many endocrine procedures are performed by different surgical specialists, we have grouped them together in Chap. 16 in order to present important perioperative principles that pertain to most endocrine surgery.

For each procedure, we have included a qualitative measure of "surgical stress" designed to give the reader a general measure of the degree of alteration in hemodynamic, metabolic, and fluid balance that a particular operation causes in patients independent of their underlying medical condition. Because overall surgical stress is impossible to quantitate, these measures are simply designated minimal, low, moderate, or severe. These terms allow the reader to group operations into broad categories according to the overall demands they impose. Although we have attempted to avoid abbreviations in the procedure outlines, some were necessary to conserve space. Among those most often used are EBL for estimated blood loss and POD for postoperative day.

The editors gratefully acknowledge the efforts of Daniel Dempsey, MD, section coordinator.

7 EVALUATION OF THE PATIENT UNDERGOING ABDOMINAL SURGERY

Daniel Dempsey

William Battle

Abdominal surgical procedures vary greatly in duration, scope, and complexity. Nonetheless, in order to facilitate appropriate preoperative evaluation and preparation of the patient, it is important for the clinician to have an understanding of common comorbid illnesses and medical conditions known to be risk factors in abdominal surgery. Moreover, a brief review of anesthetic options, surgical techniques, and the pathophysiology of conditions requiring abdominal surgery is essential in understanding potential complications and avoiding them. Breast surgery is included in this chapter since it is most often performed by general surgeons.

COMMON COMORBID CONDITIONS

Abdominal operations, both elective and emergent, are often performed for neoplastic, infectious, inflammatory, or traumatic conditions which exert significant impact on the overall health of the patient. Infection often accompanies conditions requiring abdominal surgery and may lead to bacteremia, critical organ dysfunction, and wound infection or abscess. Malignancy, a common indication for abdominal surgery, is frequently complicated by anemia, malnutrition, increased risk of thromboembolic disease, and compromise of organ function by metastatic disease (see Chap. 29). Anemia is commonly caused by gastrointestinal cancers or nonmalignant inflammatory conditions such as gastroduodenal ulcer or inflammatory bowel disease and may be due to blood loss, nutritional deficiency, or chronic disease. Many patients suffer from intravascular volume depletion due to poor oral intake, fluid loss after bowel preparation, or third-space losses, all of which can lead to hemoconcentration. Thus, anemic patients may experience a further fall in the hematocrit level with rehydration. The significance of preoperative anemia and indications for preoperative transfusion are discussed in Chaps. 28 and 51. Diseases requiring abdominal surgery are commonly associated with malnutrition, a well-recognized risk factor in postoperative complications which may not always be clinically obvious. Significant malnutrition should be suspected in patients with unintentional weight loss of 10 pounds or 10 percent of body weight, a serum albumin level under 3.5g/dl when well-hydrated, or anergy to common antigen skin tests. Although preoperative enteral or parenteral alimentation may decrease the risk of surgery in severely malnourished patients, it may actually increase risk in those with mild to moderate malnutrition and should therefore only be initiated when indicated.[1] Most experts feel that three to five days of full preoperative support is adequate to produce anabolism in severely malnourished patients and reduce the incidence of preoperative complications (see Chap. 41).

RISK FACTORS IN ABDOMINAL SURGERY

Emergency surgery carries a higher risk of postoperative mortality and morbidity than elective procedures. This may be due in part to the nature and severity of the surgical problem, a higher risk of aspiration, and inadequate time to assess and prepare patients with acute or chronic medical conditions. Although most acute or chronic medical conditions may increase the risk of abdominal surgery, cardiac, pulmonary, and hepatic disease as well as underlying coagulopathies are of special concern.

A number of studies have shown that various forms of heart disease substantially increase the risk for noncardiac surgery.[2] A recent myocardial infarction, evidence of congestive heart failure, and hemodynamically significant aortic stenosis pose the greatest risks (see Chaps. 18–20).

Patients with significant obstructive or restrictive pulmonary disease may tolerate poorly the increased respiratory demands of abdominal surgery.[3] Splinting and atelectasis induced by incisional pain may cause decompensation in tenuous patients. Inadequate clearance of increased secretions may predispose patients to pneumonia. Those with pulmonary hypertension due to primary lung disease or cardiac disease have an especially high mortality rate. (see Chap. 22).

Cirrhosis is probably the single most overlooked risk factor in abdominal surgery, especially when accompanied by portal hypertension and compromise of hepatic synthetic function.[4,5] Significant blood loss and postoperative intraabdominal infections are common and poorly tolerated in patients with cirrhosis. Even an otherwise well-tolerated small anastomotic leak may lead to overwhelming sepsis, hepatic failure, and death. Surgery in the patient with acute viral or alcoholic hepatitis may result in fulminant hepatic failure (see Chap. 34). Patients with coagulopathy have increased operative risk for several reasons. First, significant intraoperative blood loss may cause hemodynamic embarrassment. Second, surgically unrelated bleeding may supervene postoperatively. Finally, intraabdominal hematomas can form after surgery and, if contaminated at the time of the procedure, can lead to abscess formation (See Chap. 30).

ANESTHETIC TECHNIQUE

Most abdominal operations are performed under general anesthesia for patient comfort and adequate muscle relaxation. Many procedures such as appendectomy, ventral hernia repair, and colon resection can be safely done with spinal or epidural anesthesia. However, upper abdominal surgery involving dissection near the diaphragm is poorly tolerated with these latter techniques. Local anesthesia and intravenous sedation can often be used for small abdominal procedures near the peritoneal surface. These include repair of inguinal and small ventral hernias, gastrostomy, cholecystostomy, and placement of peritoneovenous shunts. Although local or spinal anesthesia is frequently recommended for patients with severe pulmonary disease and other serious medical problems, there is little documentation that the type of anesthesia is a major determinant of operative risk in such patients.[6]

OPERATIVE APPROACH AND PATHOPHYSIOLOGY

Laparoscopic versus Open Procedures

An increasing number of abdominal procedures are being performed utilizing laparoscopic techniques. Avoiding a large incision results in a lower incidence of ileus, decreased need for analgesia, a quicker return to daily activities, and perhaps less stress on the cardiac and respiratory systems. However, in some cases, laparoscopic procedures take longer and usually require general anesthesia because of the discomfort caused by the pneumoperitoneum required for most operations. Laparoscopic surgery may not be as effective as open procedures in some circumstances. For example, in surgery for colon cancer, less mesentery may be resected by laparoscopic resection. Some complications like bile spillage associated with cholecystectomy are more common with laparoscopic surgery. Because laparoscopic techniques may be unsuccessful and require immediate subsequent open procedures, preoperative assessment and preparation should be no less diligent.

Incision and Wound Care[7]

Most open abdominal operations are done through a vertical or transverse incision. Upper abdominal incisions usually compromise respiratory function and cause more pain than lower abdominal incisions. Transverse incisions are thought to be stronger and less prone to dehiscence and herniation than midline vertical incisions. However, vertical midline incisions are preferred in trauma or when the diagnosis is uncertain because they can be extended to allow access to the entire peritoneal cavity. Occasionally, a thoracic incision must be performed with an abdominal incision for adequate exposure or emergency control of bleeding. When significant intraoperative contamination occurs, the skin and subcutaneous tissue of the abdominal wound are frequently not closed in an effort to avoid formation of wound abscesses. Such wounds may be allowed to granulate (secondary closure) or can be closed with suture under sterile conditions several days later if they appear healthy.

Gastrointestinal Function

Operations involving manipulation of intraperitoneal contents and/or the use of a general anesthetic are generally associated with ileus. The duration of ileus is proportional to the magnitude of the procedure. Paralysis of normal gastrointestinal function ranges from less than 24 hours after a laparoscopic cholecystectomy to five to seven days after a total pancreatectomy. Gastrointestinal function returns to normal sooner after laparoscopic procedures than after open procedures of the same type. Small bowel activity normalizes first, followed by that of the stomach and finally the colon. Return of normal bowel sounds accompanies the return of gastric function because air from the stomach is necessary for audible peristalsis in the small bowel. Passage of a significant bowel movement and/or flatus signals resumption of colonic function. Prolonged postoperative ileus may lead to delay in resuming feeding and complicate the administration of medications for coexisting medical conditions. Although the benefits of the practice have been questioned, nasogastric tubes are frequently left in place for gastric decompression after operations on the stomach and small intestine. Careful measurement and adequate replacement of fluid lost through nasogastric suction are necessary to prevent development of hypokalemic metabolic alkalosis.

Well-nourished patients rarely require more than 5% dextrose and electrolyte solutions after most uncomplicated abdominal procedures. Administering exogenous nutrients in large quantities to well-nourished perioperative patients may actually be harmful. Nasogastric feeding or oral feeding is usually started when bowel sounds are present and abdominal distention is absent. Although a progression of diet from clear liquids to full liquids and finally to a regular diet is often followed by rote, there are no clear data indicating that the practice is necessary or even beneficial.

If prolonged gastric decompression is necessary or the patient is unable to eat, a gastrostomy tube may be placed at the time of surgery. A feeding jejunostomy is frequently inserted during a complex procedure involving the proximal gastrointestinal tract because jejunostomy feedings can be started earlier than gastric feedings. Total nutritional support should be considered in moderately malnourished patients when a week or more of fasting is anticipated. If discontinuation of a medication in the perioperative period is deemed dangerous, an acceptable parenteral substitute can usually be found for one to five days until gut activity returns. If no acceptable substitute can be found, the necessary drug may be given orally with a sip of water or administered through a nasogastric tube. Most oral medications can be given through a jejunostomy 12 to 24 hours after surgery.

Pulmonary Function

Abdominal surgery and particularly upper abdominal procedures adversely affect pulmonary function. Incisional pain causes splinting, decreased lung volumes, and atelectasis. Inhibition of effective cough results in decreased clearance and pooling of secretions. These changes can cause ventilation-perfusion mismatching, hypoxia, and an increased risk of pneumonia. For these reasons, careful preoperative assessment of patients with existing lung disease and the use of prophylactic measures such as incentive spirometry and adequate analgesia are important.

PROPHYLAXIS

Antibiotics[8]

Prophylactic antibiotics are administered intravenously before induction of anesthesia and continued for no more than 24 hours after the procedures. They should be targeted against common pathogens encountered in infections which commonly complicate the specific procedure. Prophylactic antibiotics are given to all patients undergoing abdominal vascular surgery, colorectal operations, hernia repairs using prosthetic materials, and procedures to relieve small bowel or gastric outlet obstruction. They are also given routinely before surgery involving the common bile duct and in many other procedures determined by surgeons' preferences. When given for only a short time, complications are rare. However, allergic reactions, coagulation problems, renal insufficiency, and pseudomembranous colitis have been attributed to antibiotics used for surgical prophylaxis (see Chaps. 44, 63, 65, and 67).

Antibiotic prophylaxis against endocarditis is also warranted in susceptible patients undergoing most abdominal operations, including cholecystectomy and procedures involving intestinal incision or infected tissues. The AHA regimens, consisting of ampicillin and gentamicin or vancomycin and gentamicin, are formulated to provide protection against a broad range of pathogens including enterococcus species (see Chap. 43).

Thromboembolism[9]

The use of prophylactic measures to prevent postoperative thromboembolic disease should be considered in all patients over age 40 undergoing abdominal surgery. The incidence of deep venous thrombosis in this population is significant, and pulmonary embolism remains a major cause of postoperative death. The risk of thrombosis is related to patient age, type and duration of surgery, and the presence of one or more additional risk factors including obesity, malignancy, or prior history of venous thrombosis. Low dose heparin (LDH) and external pneumatic compression devices (EPC) have been shown to be safe and effective for most general surgery patients. For those with a particularly high risk, a number of empiric recommendations have been made including the concomitant use of LDH and EPC (see Chap. 48).

Pulmonary[10]

All patients undergoing abdominal surgery should be instructed in the use of incentive spirometry before the procedure. Elective abdominal operations should be postponed in patients with upper respiratory infections, especially if general anesthesia is planned. Smoking should be discontinued one to two months before elective surgery. In the postoperative period, pulmonary complications can be minimized with judicious use of narcotics, early ambulation, and frequent proper use of an incentive spirometer (see Chap. 47). Occasionally, instillation of a local anesthetic into the wound or a regional block will decrease splinting and aid respiratory effort.

Stress-Related Mucosal Disease[11]

All patients undergoing major or complex abdominal operations should be given adequate prophylaxis against stress gastritis. While antacids given in sufficient quantity to increase intragastric pH are effective, H_2 blockers and sucralfate are more convenient and equally effective if given properly. These agents may be discontinued when a regular diet is resumed (see Chap. 46).

POSTOPERATIVE COMPLICATIONS[12]

A wide array of complications can occur early in the postoperative period or as long-term sequelae of abdominal surgery. A brief review of some of the most common early postoperative problems follows.

Wound

Infection, dehiscence, and herniation are the most common wound complications following abdominal surgery. Postoperative wound infection may be superficial, as in the form of cellulitis or a subcutaneous abscess, or deep, as in fascitis or a subfascial abscess. Deep wound infections are sometimes the result of a significant intraabdominal complication such as an anastomotic leak. Both subcutaneous and deep wound infections predispose patients to the subsequent development of incisional herniation which usually becomes apparent within the first few months after surgery. Fascial dehiscence in the first week after the procedure is heralded by copious serous wound drainage and is best managed with reoperation.

Infection

Fever is common after abdominal surgery and may be the result of infection or noninfectious causes. Common infections involve the wound or operative bed, lungs, urinary tract, or intravenous catheter sites. Cholangitis may complicate biliary operations. Noninfectious causes include atelectasis, hematomas, drugs, and pulmonary embolism (see Chap. 52).

Cardiac

Supraventricular arrhythmias and unifocal premature ventricular contractions are frequently observed after abdominal surgery but rarely cause major morbidity (see Chap. 56). Congestive heart failure is also common and usually results from volume overload in patients with preexisting cardiac disease. Perioperative myocardial infarction and sustained ventricular arrhythmias are the most serious cardiac complications but are fortunately less common.

Pulmonary

Atelectasis is one of the most frequent complications of abdominal surgery, particularly after upper abdominal operations. When associated with tachypnea or hypoxia, therapeutic bronchoscopy may be indicated. Pneumonia can develop as a result of aspiration, retained secretions, or atelectasis and is especially common in the elderly and debilitated patients and in those with significant pulmonary disease (see Chap. 57). Pulmonary embolism should be considered in all postoperative patients with chest pain or unexplained tachycardia, tachypnea, hypoxia, or fever (see Chap. 59). Pneumothorax may become obvious only days after attempted central venous catheter placement.

Gastrointestinal

Most major abdominal procedures are associated with transient ileus. In some patients, it may be prolonged and may suggest postoperative mechanical bowel obstruction. Mechanical obstruction is sometimes due to anastomotic edema or a small leak. Reoperation should be avoided whenever possible in the otherwise stable patient. Anastomotic leak is a major complication of abdominal surgery. In patients recovering from biliary or pancreatic surgery, drains placed at the time of surgery may suffice for treatment. Computerized tomography-guided drainage is often necessary, and reoperation is rarely required. However, leaks from a gastrointestinal anastomosis may require surgical diversion, decompression, and repair. It is especially important to recognize this condition in patients who are deteriorating to avoid multisystem involvement. Postoperative gastrointestinal bleeding is increasingly rare now that adequate prophylaxis against stress gastritis is administered. Other causes of bleeding include an undiagnosed or inadequately treated gastroduodenal ulcer, anastomotic hemorrhage, intestinal ischemia, and anastomotic dehiscence with erosion of a major vessel. Some intermittent diarrhea is common when a regular diet is resumed after surgery. Persistent diarrhea should prompt an evaluation for antibiotic-associated enterocolitis (see Chap. 67).

Metabolic

Electrolyte disorders and acid/base imbalance often complicate major abdominal surgery. The most frequent are hyponatremia, hypokalemia, and metabolic alkalosis or acidosis (see Chaps. 60, 61, and 62). Hypomagnesemia is common in malnourished alcoholic patients.

Renal

Uncomplicated surgery should not cause deterioration of renal function. A postoperative diuresis normally occurs about the third day. Deterioration of renal function may be caused by renal hypoperfusion, sepsis, drugs, or operative injury (see Chap. 63).

Hepatic

Transient elevation of liver function tests is common after surgery in the region of the right upper quadrant. Progressive postoperative elevation suggests biliary obstruction, focal hepatic ischemia, or sepsis.

Neurologic

Postoperative delirium, manifested by obtundation, confusion and agitation, is most common in elderly patients with underlying cognitive dysfunction. Alterations in mental status may be caused by hypoxia, sepsis, dehydration, metabolic disturbances, drug and alcohol withdrawal, and medications like analgesics (see Chap. 70).

REFERENCES

1. The VA Total Parenteral Nutrition Cooperative Study Group: Preoperative total parenteral nutrition in surgical patients. *N Eng J Med* 325:525–532, 1991.
2. Goldman, L: Cardiac risks and complications of noncardiac surgery. *Ann Surg* 198:780–791, 1983.
3. Smith PK, Sabiston DC: Physiologic aspects of respiratory function and management of respiratory insufficiency in surgical patients, in Sabiston DC (ed): *Essentials of Surgery.* Philadelphia, Saunders, 1987, pp 969–980.
4. Aranha GV, Greenlee HB: Intra-abdominal surgery in patients with advanced cirrhosis. *Arch Surg* 121:275–277, 1986.
5. Garrison RN, Cryer HM, Howard DA et al: Clarification of risk factors for abdominal operations in patients with hepatic cirrhosis. *Ann Surg* 199:648–655, 1984.
6. Cohen MM, Duncan PG, Tate RB: Does anesthesia contribute to operative mortality? *JAMA* 260:2859–2863, 1988.
7. Rout WR: Abdominal incisions; drainage of abdominal wounds; complications of incision; closure of wound, in Zuidema GD (ed): *Shackelford's Surgery of the Alimentary Tract*, 3d ed. Philadelphia, Saunders, 1991, pp 284–34.
8. Antimicrobial prophylaxis in surgery. *Med Letter* 31(806):105–108.
9. Goldhaber SZ: Practical aspects of venous thromboembolism prevention—an overview, in Goldhaber SZ (ed): *Prevention of Venous Thromboembolism*. New York, Marcel Dekker, 1993, pp 129–144.
10. Hall JC, Tarala R, Harris J et al: Incentive spirometry versus routine chest physiotherapy for prevention of pulmonary complications after abdominal surgery. *Lancet* 337(8747):953–956, 1991.
11. Miller TA, Tornwall MS, Moody FG: Stress erosive gastritis. *Curr Prob Surg* XXVIII(7):459–509, 1991.
12. Hardy JD: *Complications in Surgery and their Management*, 4th ed. Philadelphia, Saunders, 1981.

PROCEDURE: APPENDECTOMY

Overview: Appendectomy is usually a small operation and is now frequently performed laparoscopically. Occasionally it becomes a larger more difficult operation if the surgeon suspects a carcinoma or if another serious disease such as a perforated duodenal ulcer or cholecystitis is masquerading as appendicitis.

1. *Operation*
    a. Indications:
        (1) Appendicitis (or suspected appendicitis) with and without abscess.
        (2) Tumor.
    b. Operative Steps: The blood supply is ligated. The base of the appendix is ligated. The appendix is removed.
    c. Incision: Right lower quadrant transverse or lower midline.
    d. Anesthesia: General or spinal.
    e. Intraoperative Monitoring: Routine.
    f. Operative Positioning: Supine.
    g. Duration: 30 to 60 minutes.
    h. EBL/Transfusions: Transfusion rarely required for routine cases.
    i. "Surgical Stress": Low to moderate.

2. *Expected Hospital Course/Treatment*
    a. Postoperative Monitoring
        (1) ICU Stay: Necessary only for those with general peritonitis, septic shock, recent myocardial infarction.
        (2) Invasive/Special Monitoring: Only for rare ICU cases.
        (3) Parameters To Be Monitored:
            i. Vital signs.
            ii. Urine output.
            iii. CBC.
            iv. GI function.
    b. Positioning/Activity: Out of bed on evening of surgery or POD 1.
    c. Alimentation: Liquids begun on POD 2. Regular diet begun on POD 3 or 4. Diet may be advanced sooner in laparoscopic cases.
    d. Would Care/Drains: Occasionally nasogastric tube necessary for complicated cases. Abdominal drain placed if appendiceal abscess found.
    e. Respiratory Care: Incentive spirometry encouraged.
    f. Analgesia/Postop Meds: Narcotics are generally necessary up to POD 5. Narcotics may not be required for laparoscopic cases.
    g. Length Of Hospital Stay: 2 to 4 days in uncomplicated cases and up to 10 days in those complicated by peritonitis, abscess, or fistula.

3. *Postoperative Complications*
    a. In Hospital
        (1) Morbidity:
            i. Wound infection.
            ii. Abscess.
            iii. Fistula.
            iv. Bowel injury.
            v. Injury to retroperitoneal structures (e.g., ureter, iliac vein) in complicated cases.
            vi. Bowel obstruction/ileus.
        (2) Mortality: 0.1% to 0.3% in uncomplicated cases with no perforation; 1% with perforation; 5% in complicated high-risk elderly patients.
    b. After Discharge:
        (1) Bowel obstruction.
        (2) Incisional hernia.

4. *Follow-up*
    a. Suggested Follow-up: Patients are seen at 3 weeks, 6 months, then as needed.

PROCEDURE: BILIARY SURGERY

Overview: Cholecystectomy, the most common biliary tract procedure (> 500,000/yr in the United States), is now performed laparoscopically in the majority of cases. There is a broad spectrum of biliary surgery from simple cholecystectomy or tube cholecystostomy to complex biliary tract resection or reconstruction.

1. *Operation*
   a. Indications:
      (1) Biliary colic.
      (2) Choledocholithiasis.
      (3) Cholecystitis.
      (4) Gallstone pancreatitis.
      (5) Stricture.
      (6) Tumor.
   b. Operative Steps: Cholecystectomy is performed by isolation of the cystic duct and artery along with dissection of the gallbladder from the liver bed. Common bile duct (CBD) exploration is indicated for evidence of common duct stones or obstruction and is usually performed by opening the CBD and removing the stones or biopsying the area of obstruction. Choledochoscopy is frequently performed, and the choledochotomy is closed around a t-tube. Resection of all or part of the extrahepatic biliary tree (including pancreaticoduodenectomy) may be indicated for malignant disease. Benign strictures are generally handled by segmental resection. Continuity is reestablished by biliary enteric anastomosis, usually Roux-en-Y choledochojejunostomy. Primary duct stones are another indication for the latter procedure or choledochoduodenostomy. Obstructive jaundice due to unresectable pancreatic carcinoma may be handled with cholecystojejunostomy or choledochojejunostomy.
   c. Incision: Transverse or vertical abdominal.
   d. Anesthesia: General or high spinal/epidural. Tube cholecystostomy may be performed under local anesthesia in the sedated patient.
   e. Intraoperative Monitoring: Routine unless high-risk patient or large operation (e.g., resection of a cholangiocarcinoma).
   f. Operative Positioning: Supine.
   g. Duration: 1 hour for routine cholecystectomy with cholangiogram to 6 hours for complicated biliary reconstruction.
   h. EBL/Transfusions: < 300 cc for elective cholecystectomy to 1000 cc for difficult cholecystectomy to 5000 cc for difficult resection of cholangiocarcinoma.
   i. "Surgical Stress": Low for elective uncomplicated laparascopic cholecystectomy to high for complex biliary procedures.

2. *Expected Hospital Course/Treatment*
   a. Postoperative Monitoring
      (1) ICU Stay: Usual for biliary reconstruction or resection.
      (2) Invasive/Special Monitoring: Arterial line, CVP, Foley catheter while in ICU.
      (3) Parameters To Be Monitored:
         i. Vital signs. ii. Urine output. iii. CBC, platelet count. iv. LFT's. v. Amylase. vi. Electrolytes. vii. PT, PTT
   b. Positioning/Activity: Out of bed same day or next morning at latest.
   c. Alimentation: Regular diet within 24 hours after routine cholecystectomy. In complex cases, liquids started on POD 3 and advanced to regular diet by POD 7.
   d. Wound Care/Drains: None for routine cholecystectomy. Abdominal drains and stents are common in complex or difficult cases.
   e. Respiratory Care: Incentive spirometry encouraged.
   f. Analgesia/Postop Meds: Narcotics required usually only for open cases.
   g. Length Of Hospital Stay: 1 day for routine laparoscopic cholecystectomy to 2 weeks for complex biliary reconstruction.

3. *Postoperative Complications*
   a. In Hospital
      (1) Morbidity:
         i. Duodenal, colonic, or major vascular injury. ii. Wound infection. iii. Biliary fistula. iv. Jaundice. v. Bleeding. vi. Ileus. vii. Pancreatitis. viii. Pulmonary embolus.
      (2) Mortality: 0.1% for elective cholecystectomy to > 5% for complex biliary procedure.
   b. After Discharge:
      (1) Post-cholecystectomy pain.
      (2) Retained stones.
      (3) Biliary stricture.
      (4) Incisional hernia.
      (5) Recurrent tumor.

4. *Follow-up*
   a. Suggested Follow-up:
      Routine: Patients are seen at 3 weeks, 6 months, then as needed.
      Complex: Patients are seen at 3 weeks, every 3 months for 4 visits, then every 4 to 6 months.

PROCEDURE: BREAST SURGERY

Overview: Operations on the female breast are among the most commonly performed general surgical procedures. Either a dominant mass or suspicious mammogram mandates an excisional biopsy. If the lesion is palpable, this is easily done under local anesthesia. If not, needle localization directs the surgeon to the suspicious site for excision. Specimen mammography is performed to assure adequate excision. Lumpectomy and axillary dissection is performed in patients with documented invasive breast cancer who have been deemed good candidates for local regional irradiation. Decisions regarding chemotherapy are made on the basis of nodal and menopausal status of the patient. Patients with large tumors and bulky axillary nodes are best treated by a modified radical mastectomy (MRM). One percent of breast cancers occur in males in whom the most common indication for breast surgery is gynecomastia.

1. *Operation*
   a. Indications:
      (1) Breast cancer.
      (2) Dominant mass.
      (3) Infection.
      (4) Gynecomastia.
   b. Operative Steps: Lumpectomy and axillary dissection involve local wide excision of the tumor, and through a separate incision, removal of some ipsilateral level 1 and 2 axillary nodes. Modified radical mastectomy involves incontinuity removal of the involved breast along with the level 1 and 2 nodes.
   c. Incision: For biopsy, small incision over lesion. Transverse axillary incision for axillary sampling. Elliptical incision to include nipple/areolar complex and previous biopsy site in modified radical mastectomy.
   d. Anesthesia: Breast biopsy: local. Lumpectomy and axillary dissection: general. MRM: general.
   e. Intraoperative Monitoring: Routine.
   f. Operative Positioning: Supine with arm extended.
   g. Duration: Biopsy: 20 to 30 min. Lumpectomy and axillary sampling: 60 to 90 min. MRM: 90 to 120 min.
   h. EBL/Transfusions: 300 to 700 ml for MRM.
   i. "Surgical Stress": Low to moderate.

2. *Expected Hospital Course/Treatment*
   a. Postoperative Monitoring
      (1) ICU Stay: Not necessary.
      (2) Invasive/Special Monitoring: None.
      (3) Parameters To Be Monitored:
         i. Drain output.
         ii. CBC.
         iii. Arm function.
   b. Positioning/Activity: Out of bed same day.
   c. Alimentation: Advance as tolerated.
   d. Wound Care/Drains: Suction catheters placed in all cases of axillary dissection and under skin flaps for MRM.
   e. Respiratory Care: Incentive spirometry encouraged.
   f. Analgesia/Postop Meds: Narcotics are needed for several days in axillary dissection and MRM patients.
   g. Length Of Hospital Stay: Biopsy: outpatient. Lumpectomy and axillary sampling: 2 days. MRM: 3 to 5 days.

3. *Postoperative Complications*
   a. In Hospital
      (1) Morbidity:
         i. Bleeding.
         ii. Seroma.
         iii. Winged scapula from long thoracic nerve damage.
         iv. Flap necrosis.
         v. Wound infection.
         vi. Axillary vein injury.
         vii. Injury to brachial plexus or thoracodorsal nerve.
      2. Mortality: 0.1% to 1%.
   b. After Discharge:
      (1) Shoulder dysfunction.
      (2) Lymphedema.
      (3) Recurrent cancer.

4. *Follow-up*
   a. Suggested Follow-up: Patients are seen every 6 to 12 months.

PROCEDURE: COLORECTAL RESECTION

Overview: Segmental colon resection is usually performed for tumor, diverticulitis, or trauma. Total colectomy or proctocolectomy are commonly performed for ulcerative colitis, ischemia, or lower GI bleeding. Often the patients have multiple medical problems which, when combined with the risk of infection from operating on a nonsterile viscus, make the morbidity appreciable. Laparoscopic technology is making inroads into this area as well.

1. *Operation*
   a. Indications:

   (1) Neoplasm.
   (2) Diverticulitis.
   (3) Inflammatory bowel disease.
   (4) Trauma.
   (5) Ischemia.
   (6) Lower GI bleeding.

   b. Operative Steps: The diseased segment is mobilized, devascularized, and transected proximally and distally. In emergency operations (e.g., diverticulitis with abscess, toxic megacolon, massive colonic bleeding), unstable patients (e.g., recent myocardial infarction or shock from GI bleeding), or for disease of the rectum (i.e., below the peritoneal reflection), anastomosis may not be attempted and an ostomy is performed. Complete removal of the rectum requires a combined abdominal/perineal approach.
   c. Incision: Vertical or transverse abdominal.
   d. Anesthesia: General or high spinal/epidural. Decompressing (blow hole) colostomy may on occasion be performed under local anesthesia in the sedated patient.
   e. Intraoperative Monitoring: Invasive hemodynamic monitoring is advisable in the unstable patient, the patient with cardiopulmonary disease, and for many total proctocolectomy or proctectomy patients.
   f. Operative Positioning: Supine. If the distal rectum is to be removed or anastomosed, a modified lithotomy position allows simultaneous operating on the abdomen and perineum.
   g. Duration: 1 hour for short segmental colectomy to 6 hours for total proctocolectomy with ileoanal anastomosis.
   h. EBL/Transfusions: For elective segmental colectomy, blood loss is usually below 1000 cc. However, bleeding may be precipitous and voluminous during any major colon resection. Blood loss is greater in total proctocolectomy, proctectomy, or in operations for large or recurrent tumors.
   i. "Surgical Stress": Moderate in uncomplicated segmental reaction to high in emergency or complicated cases.

2. *Expected Hospital Course/Treatment*
   a. Postoperative Monitoring

   (1) ICU Stay: Usually not needed for uncomplicated partial colon resection in healthy patients. Sick patients or those recovering from complicated operations generally require 1 to 3 days in the ICU.
   (2) Invasive/Special Monitoring: As needed while in ICU.
   (3) Parameters To Be Monitored:

   i. Vital signs. ii. Urine output. iii. CBC. iv. Electrolytes. v. Nasogastric/stoma output. vi. Bowel activity.

   b. Positioning/Activity: Out of bed and ambulate next day.
   c. Alimentation: Clear liquids can usually be started on POD 3 to 5, regular diet by POD 7.
   d. Wound Care/Drains: Subcutaneous tissue may be left open and packed in contaminated cases. Abdominal drains if placed are usually removed by POD 5 to 7. For cases with pelvic dissection (proctectomy), Foley catheter may be left in for several days.
   e. Respiratory Care: Incentive spirometry encouraged.
   f. Analgesia/Postop Meds: Parenteral narcotics required. Occasionally anti-emetics or H_2 blockers are needed.
   g. Length Of Hospital Stay: 5 days for uncomplicated right hemicolectomy to 14 days for complicated total colectomy or proctectomy.

3. *Postoperative Complications*
   a. In Hospital

   (1) Morbidity:
       i. Wound infection.
       ii. Abdominal abscess.
       iii. Anastomotic leak.
       vi. Fistula.
       v. Bleeding.
       vi. Atelectasis/pneumonia.
       vii. Urinary retention/infection.
       viii. Pulmonary embolus.
       ix. Injury to ureter, duodenum, spleen, major vessels, bladder, vagina.
   (2) Mortality: 2% for elective partial colectomy to 10% for complicated or emergent proctectomy or total colectomy.

   b. After Discharge:
       i. Incisional hernia.   ii. Anastomotic stricture.   iii. Recurrent cancer.

4. *Follow-up*
   a. Suggested Follow-up: Patients are seen every 6 to 12 months.

PROCEDURE: ESOPHAGOGASTRECTOMY

Overview: Total esophagectomy generally refers to complete removal of the esophagus from the neck to the gastroesophageal junction. If part of the stomach is resected with part of the esophagus, the procedure is termed a esophagogastrectomy. Both are large operations, frequently performed in older patients with significant medical problems.

1. *Operation*
   a. Indications:
      (1) Esophageal or proximal gastric malignancy.   (2) Complicated gastroesophageal reflux disease.
      (3) Failed antireflux operations.
   b. Operative Steps: For distal esophageal or proximal gastric disease, the entire operation may be done through a left thoracotomy. For mid or proximal esophageal disease, an abdominal and right thoracotomy approach is preferred. An alternative approach (which may be dangerous if the diseased segment is the midesophagus) is the transhiatal esophagectomy in which the thoracic esophagus is bluntly and often blindly dissected from its bed through an abdominal and cervical incision. Continuity may be reestablished by using the stomach or hemicolon as a conduit, both of which will easily reach the cervical esophagus. Shorter distal gaps may be bridged with a segment of jejunum.
   c. Incision: Left thoracotomy, left thoracoabdominal, or combined abdomen/right thoracotomy. Cervical incision may be added to latter and is always made for transhiatal resection.
   d. Anesthesia: General. Epidural anesthesia for postoperative pain control. Double lumen endotracheal tube is helpful if thoracotomy is planned.
   e. Intraoperative Monitoring: Arterial line and CVP or Swan-Ganz catheter are preferred, especially for transhiatal (blunt) esophagectomy.
   f. Operative Positioning: For left thoracotomy, full right lateral decubitus position. For combined abdomen/right thoracotomy, most surgeons do abdominal dissection first in the supine position, close the abdomen, then turn patient into full left lateral decubitus position. Others prefer a partial lateral decubitus position with the lower torso supine so both incisions can be open simultaneously. Transhiatal esophagectomy is done in the supine position.
   g. Duration: 4 to 8 hours.
   h. EBL/Transfusions: EBL usually ranges from 500 to 1500 ml, but occasionally massive bleeding may be encountered (> 5000ml). Transfusion is necessary in at least 50% of patients.
   i. "Surgical Stress": Severe. This is a very large operation with significant cardiopulmonary changes intraoperatively. The transhiatal esophagectomy causes hypotension during the mediastinal dissection, and although this approach obviates thoracotomy, it should probably be avoided in patients with tenuous cardiac status.

2. *Expected Hospital Course/Treatment*
   a. Postoperative Monitoring
      (1) ICU Stay: 1 to 3 days.
      (2) Invasive/Special Monitoring: Arterial line, CVP, and Swan-Ganz are usually left in for the duration of the ICU stay.
      (3) Parameters To Be Monitored:
         i. Vital signs. ii. Urine output. iii. Arterial blood gases. iv. CBC. v. Electrolytes. vi. ECG.
   b. Positioning/Activity: Out of bed to ambulate in room on POD 1 is ideal.
   c. Alimentation: Oral intake is usually not started until POD 5 to 10, depending upon the operation and clinical progress. Usually anastomotic integrity is checked radiologically first.
   d. Wound Care/Drains: If anastomosis is done in the neck, a Penrose drain is left in until oral intake is begun. If a thoracotomy is made, one or two thoracostomy catheters (chest tubes) are left in for 5 to 7 days.
   e. Respiratory Care: Extubation in operating room unless there is large blood loss or in complicated case. Incentive spirometry encouraged.
   f. Analgesia/Postop Meds: Parenteral narcotics or epidural analgesia required. H_2 blockers usually begun. Medications may be given through a nasogastric or jejunostomy tube.
   g. Length Of Hospital Stay: 2 to 3 weeks.

3. *Postoperative Complications*
   a. In Hospital
      (1) Morbidity:

i. Atelectasis/pneumonia.	v. Empyema.	ix. Injury to adjacent organs (i.e., spleen, liver, pancreas, lung, aorta).
ii. Wound infection.	vi. Vocal cord paralysis.	x. Cardiac arrhythmias.
iii. Anastomotic leak.	vii. Chylothorax or lymph fistula.	
iv. Hemorrhage.	viii. Tracheal and bronchial injury.	

2. Mortality: 3 to 5%.
   b. After Discharge:
      (1) Anastomotic stricture.   (3) Recurrent cancer.   (5) Malnutrition.
      (2) Incisional hernia.   (4) Gastrointestinal dysfunction.

4. *Follow-up*
   a. Suggested Follow-up: Patients with malignancy are seen every 3 months and monitored for recurrence with studies obtained on the basis of clinical course. Patients with benign disease are seen every 3 to 6 months.

PROCEDURE: HEPATIC RESECTION

Overview: Improvements in anesthesia and critical care along with surgical technique based on sound anatomic principles have decreased the morbidity and mortality of major hepatic resection. Adequate preoperative evaluation (often multidisciplinary) and planning is essential for safe and appropriate elective hepatic resection. An experienced team of surgeons, anesthesiologists, and internists is most helpful for optimal patient safety.

1. *Operation*
   a. Indications:
      (1) Tumor.
      (2) Trauma.
   b. Operative Steps: Ranges from small nonanatomic wedge resection of the liver to major hepatic lobectomy or trisegmentectomy. In the former, the liver is mobilized, the tumor cut out, and the bleeding controlled with pressure and then suture ligation. Formal hepatic resection involves complete mobilization of the lobe involved, isolation of the portal structures, and identification of the main hepatic vein draining the involved segment. Transection of the parenchyma is performed after ligation of the appropriate portal structures with suture control of bleeding vessels and bile ductules.
   c. Incision: Transverse or midline. Most liver surgery can be done adequately through the abdomen, but occasionally a right thoracoabdominal incision is necessary. The chest and sternum should always be prepped.
   d. Anesthesia: General. Epidural anesthesia for postoperative pain control is optional.
   e. Intraoperative Monitoring: Arterial line and CVP or Swan-Ganz catheter for major resections.
   f. Operative Positioning: Supine. Occasionally an oblique right side up may be requested if a right thoracoabdominal approach is planned.
   g. Duration: 1 to 8 hours, shorter for small accessible nonanatomic wedge resections, longer for major resection for large or multiple tumors.
   h. EBL/Transfusions: 1000 to 5000 cc for major hepatic resection. Transfusion very often necessary.
   i. "Surgical Stress": Moderate to severe.

2. *Expected Hospital Course/Treatment*
   a. Postoperative Monitoring
      (1) ICU Stay: 1 to 3 days for major resection.
      (2) Invasive/Special Monitoring: Invasive monitoring remains in place for duration of ICU stay.
      (3) Parameters To Be Monitored:
         i. Vital signs.
         ii. Urine output.
         iii. CBC, platelets.
         iv. Electrolytes.
         v. PT, PTT.
         vi. Liver function.
         vii. Serum glucose.
         viii. Arterial blood gasses.
   b. Positioning/Activity: Out of bed POD 1 or 2.
   c. Alimentation: Most patients can start clear liquids on POD 2 or 3.
   d. Wound Care/Drains: Abdominal drains are common. Biliary stents are placed for complex cases.
   e. Respiratory Care: Extubation in operating room unless large blood loss. Incentive spirometry encouraged.
   f. Analgesia/Postop Meds: Parenteral narcotics or epidural analgesia required. H_2 blockers usually begun.
   g. Length Of Hospital Stay: 1 to 2 weeks.

3. *Postoperative Complications*
   a. In Hospital
      (1) Morbidity:
         i. Bile leak.
         ii. Liver failure.
         iii. Hypoglycemia.
         iv. Massive bleeding.
         v. DIC.
         vi. Abscess.
         vii. Atelectasis/pneumonia.
         viii. Inadvertant injury or ligation of structures supplying or draining the remaining liver.
      (2) Mortality: 3 to 5% for major resection in experienced centers.
   b. After Discharge: 1. Incisional hernia. 2. Recurrent tumor.

4. *Follow-up*
   a. Suggested Follow-up: Patients are seen every 3 to 6 months.

PROCEDURE: HERNIA REPAIR

Overview: A hernia is a defect in the musculofascial (usually abdominal) wall. It may be congenital or acquired (e.g., after surgery). The peritoneal sac with its contents, often including viscera, protrudes through the defect. The purpose of the operation is reduction or removal of the sac and obliteration of the musculofascial defect, either with permanent sutures or permanent prosthetic material.

1. *Operation*
   a. Indications: Unless the patient is very high risk, the presence of a hernia in and of itself is adequate indication for repair. In the vast majority of cases, the risk of repair is lower than the potential for incarceration and strangulation.
   b. Operative Steps: For inguinal hernia repairs, the sac is excised and the floor of the inguinal canal is repaired with a variety of techniques. Prosthetic is commonly used in large hernias, recurrent hernias, or when inadequate autologous tissue is present for tension-free repair. In abdominal wall hernias (e.g., ventral, incisional, umbilical), the sac is excised, and the fascia is closed primarily or with the aid of prosthetic. Inguinal herniorrhaphy is now being performed laparoscopically.
   c. Incision: Inguinal: low transverse. Ventral: vertical or transverse.
   d. Anesthesia: Local with sedation, spinal, or general.
   e. Intraoperative Monitoring: Routine.
   f. Operative Positioning: Supine.
   g. Duration: 30 min to 2 hrs.
   h. EBL/Transfusions: Minimal for inguinal hernia repair. Usually < 500 ml for ventral hernia repair.
   i. "Surgical Stress": Low to moderate.

2. *Expected Hospital Course/Treatment*
   a. Postoperative Monitoring
      (1) ICU Stay: Only for very large ventral hernia in high-risk patients.
      (2) Invasive/Special Monitoring: While in ICU.
      (3) Parameters To Be Monitored:
         i. Vital signs.
         ii. Urine output.
   b. Positioning/Activity: Ambulate on day of operation. No heavy lifting or straining for 1 to 6 weeks, depending on size of hernia.
   c. Alimentation: Inguinal: Regular diet that day. Ventral: Advance as tolerated.
   d. Wound Care/Drains: Suction catheters often necessary to decompress large subcutaneous "dead space" following repair of large abdominal hernias. Sterile technique is imperative if mesh in place.
   e. Respiratory Care: Incentive spirometry encouraged for ventral hernia.
   f. Analgesia/Postop Meds: Oral narcotics as needed.
   g. Length Of Hospital Stay: Most inguinal repairs done as outpatient. Large ventral hernia repairs generally require 1 to 3 days of hospitalization.

3. *Postoperative Complications*
   a. In Hospital
      (1) Morbidity:
         i. Hematoma.
         ii. Swelling.
         iii. Nerve entrapment.
         iv. Ischemic orchitis.
         v. Wound infection (especially significant if mesh in place).
         vi. Bowel obstruction.
         vii. Inguinal: Injury to femoral vessels or visceral contents of hernia sac.
         viii. Ventral: Injury to bowel.
      (2) Mortality: < 0.1% uncomplicated inguinal. 2 to 3% large ventral hernia in elderly.
   b. After Discharge:
      (1) Recurrent hernia.
      (2) Infected prosthetic material.
      (3) Nerve entrapment.

4. *Follow-up*
   a. Suggested Follow-up: Patients are seen yearly or sooner if recurrence occurs.

PROCEDURE: PANCREATIC RESECTION

Overview: If the disease process is to the right of the neck of the pancreatic gland or involves the distal common bile duct (CBD) or periampullary duodenum (e.g., pancreatic cancer, duodenal carcinoma at the ampulla), a pancreaticoduodenectomy ("Whipple operation") is done. If the disease is to the left of the pancreatic neck (e.g., a cystadenoma of the tail or focal chronic pancreatitis of the tail), a distal pancreatectomy with or without splenectomy is done.

1. *Operation*
   a. Indications:
      (1) Neoplasm.
      (2) Chronic pancreatitis.
      (3) Trauma.
   b. Operative Steps: Pancreaticoduodenectomy involves several steps: mobilization of the duodenum and pancreatic head, determination of resectability, cholecystectomy and transection of the CBD, transection of the pancreatic neck, and ligation of the gastroduodenal artery. The specimen is then removed by ligating the multiple vessels supplying it. Three anastomoses are required to reestablish alimentary tract continuity: pancreaticojejunostomy, choledochojejunostomy, and gastrojejunostomy. Gastrostomy and/or jejunostomy may be added. Vagotomy is usually not done. Distal pancreatectomy involves mobilization of the gland, ligation of blood supply, and transection of the gland. Removal of the spleen with the specimen may simplify the procedure. If the pancreatic duct in the remaining gland is large, a pancreaticojejunostomy may be done in a Roux-en-Y fashion.
   c. Incision: Transverse or vertical.
   d. Anesthesia: General. Epidural anesthesia for postoperative pain control desirable for Whipple operation.
   e. Intraoperative Monitoring: Arterial line and CVP or Swan-Ganz catheter.
   f. Operative Positioning: Supine.
   g. Duration: 2 hours for a straightforward distal pancreatectomy to 8 hours for a difficult Whipple.
   h. EBL/Transfusions: Approximately 1000 ml for pancreaticoduodenal resection, but may be much more in difficult cases. Transfusion is necessary about 50% of the time for major pancreatic resection.
   i. "Surgical Stress": Severe.

2. *Expected Hospital Course/Treatment*
   a. Postoperative Monitoring
      (1) ICU Stay: 1 to 3 days for major pancreatic resection.
      (2) Invasive/Special Monitoring: Invasive monitors remain in place while in ICU.
      (3) Parameters To Be Monitored:
         i. Vital signs. ii. Urine output. iii. CBC, platelet count. iv. Arterial blood gasses. v. Electrolytes. vi. Liver function tests. vii. Amylase. viii. Drain and nasogastric tube output. ix. PT, PTT.
   b. Positioning/Activity: Out of bed on POD 1.
   c. Alimentation: TPN or jejunostomy feedings commonly needed in perioperative period. The alimentary tract is generally not used for 3 to 5 days after which time liquids may be started. Regular diet is begun by POD 7 to 10, sooner for distal pancreatectomy.
   d. Wound Care/Drains: Nasogastric and/or gastrostomy, jejunostomy, biliary stent, pancratic stent, abdominal drains are all common.
   e. Respiratory Care: Extubation in operating room unless large blood loss. Incentive spirometry encouraged.
   f. Analgesia/Postop Meds: Parenteral narcotics or epidural analgesia required. H_2 blockers usually begun.
   g. Length Of Hospital Stay: 2 to 3 weeks for Whipple operation, less for distal resection.

3. *Postoperative Complications*
   a. In Hospital
      (1) Morbidity:
         i. Bleeding. ii. Fistula (pancreatic, biliary, intestinal). iii. Abscess. iv. Pancreatitis. v. Liver dysfunction/jaundice. vi. Ileus/gastric stasis/bowel obstruction. vii. Inadvertant injury to hepatic or superior mesenteric artery compromising blood supply to liver or small bowel. viii. Atelectasis/pneumonia/adult respiratory distress syndrome. ix. Deep venous thrombosis/pulmonary embolism.
      (2) Mortality: 2 to 10% for Whipple operation, lower for distal resection.
   b. After Discharge:
      (1) Pancreatic insufficiency (exocrine or endocrine).
      (2) Recurrent tumor.
      (3) Incisional hernia.
      (4) Cholangitis.
      (5) Gastrointestinal dysfunction.
      (6) Peptic ulcer.

4. *Follow-up*
   a. Suggested Follow-up: Patients are seen every 3 to 6 months.

PROCEDURE: PORTO-SYSTEMIC SHUNT

Overview: The goal of porto-systemic shunting is to decrease the pressure in the portal venous system. This in turn decreases the likelihood of bleeding from varices which form wherever there are anastomoses between the portal circulation and systemic venous circulation, most commonly at the gastroesophageal junction. These operations are done less frequently because of better nonoperative techniques to manage bleeding varices, mainly pharmacotherapy and sclerotherapy.

1. *Operation*
   a. Indications:
      (1) Bleeding esophageal varices.
   b. Operative Steps: In central complete shunts, a large anastomosis is made between a proximal portal venous branch and the vena cava or its branches. Examples include a portocaval shunt, mesocaval shunt, and central splenorenal shunt. Selective shunt attempts to preserve nutrient portal blood flow while decompressing the varices around the gastroesophageal junction. Examples include the distal splenorenal shunt in which the splenic vein is transected and the distal end anastomosed to the left renal vein or the small caliber side-to-side portocaval shunt. The exposure of vessels shunted can be difficult and tedious.
   c. Incision: Vertical or transverse.
   d. Anesthesia: General.
   e. Intraoperative Monitoring: Arterial line and CVP or Swan-Ganz catheter.
   f. Operative Positioning: Supine or oblique.
   g. Duration: 3 to 8 hours.
   h. EBL/Transfusions: 1000 to 5000 ml. Transfusion is usually necessary.
   i. "Surgical Stress": Severe.

2. *Expected Hospital Course/Treatment*
   a. Postoperative Monitoring
      (1) ICU Stay: 2 to 5 days.
      (2) Invasive/Special Monitoring: Invasive monitors remain in place while in ICU.
      (3) Parameters To Be Monitored:
         i. Vital signs.
         ii. Urine output.
         iii. CBC, platelet count.
         iv. PT, PTT.
         v. Liver function tests.
         vi. Electrolytes, BUN, creatinine.
         vii. Ammonia.
         viii. Mental status.
   b. Positioning/Activity: Out of bed as soon as possible.
   c. Alimentation: TPN often necessary. Oral intake can be started on POD 3 in uncomplicated cases but is often inadequate.
   d. Wound Care/Drains: Care should be taken to avoid ascitic fluid leaks. Wounds with small ascitic leaks should be handled with sterile technique. Large ascitic leaks should be closed surgically. Drains are relatively contraindicated. Paracentesis or peritoneovenous shunt may be necessary for massive postoperative ascites.
   e. Respiratory Care: Extubation in operating room unless hemodynamically unstable or unresponsive. Incentive spirometry thereafter.
   f. Analgesia/Postop Meds: Narcotics should be used sparingly. H_2 blockers usually begun.
   g. Length Of Hospital Stay: 10 to 20 days.

3. *Postoperative Complications*
   a. In Hospital
      (1) Morbidity:
         i. Massive bleeding (i.e., intraabdominal; recurrent variceal bleeding suggests shunt thrombosis).
         ii. Infection.
         iii. Encephalopathy.
         iv. Intractable ascites.
         v. Ileus.
         vi. Liver failure.
         vii. Renal failure.
      (2) Mortality: 3 to 30%, depending on hepatic reserve.
   b. After Discharge:
      (1) Hepatic encephalopathy.
      (2) Spontaneous peritonitis.
      (3) Shunt occlusion.
      (4) Incisional hernia.

4. *Follow-up*
   a. Suggested Follow-up: Patients are seen every 3 months.

PROCEDURE: SMALL BOWEL RESECTION

Overview: Operations on the small bowel may be simple or very difficult, especially in cases of reoperation for Crohn's disease or in those involving previously irradiated tissue. Some cases are now done with laparoscopic techniques.

1. *Operation*
   a. Indications:
      (1) Tumor.
      (2) GI bleeding.
      (3) Obstruction with infarction or ischemia.
      (4) Crohn's disease.
      (5) Mesenteric ischemia.
   b. Operative Steps: Essential steps of the operation are to isolate the diseased segment, ligate the blood supply, divide the bowel and reanastomose.
   c. Incision: Vertical or transverse.
   d. Anesthesia: General is usually preferred, although spinal or epidural may be feasible.
   e. Intraoperative Monitoring: Usually routine measures are adequate. In high-risk patients or in patients in whom a difficult operation is anticipated, an arterial line and CVP may be indicated.
   f. Operative Positioning: Supine.
   g. Duration: 1 to 5 hours, depending on the indication and difficulty.
   h. EBL/Transfusions: In straightforward cases, EBL should be < 500 ml and transfusion unnecessary. Bleeding may be significantly greater (2000 to 3000 ml) in more difficult cases or in reoperations, and transfusion may be necessary.
   i. "Surgical Stress": Moderate.

2. *Expected Hospital Course/Treatment*
   a. Postoperative Monitoring
      (1) ICU Stay: For long and difficult operations, or in patient with significant cardiac or pulmonary disease.
      (2) Invasive/Special Monitoring: Invasive monitors remain in place while in ICU.
      (3) Parameters To Be Monitored:
         i. Vital signs.
         ii. Urine output.
         iii. CBC.
         iv. Electrolytes.
         v. Nasogastric tube output.
         vi. Bowel function.
   b. Positioning/Activity: Out of bed POD 1.
   c. Alimentation: Liquids usually begun on POD 4 to 6, regular diet by POD 7.
   d. Wound Care/Drains: Abdominal drains are usually not necessary. Gastrostomy and/or jejunostomy may be placed in selected cases. Nasogastric tube usually removed around POD 3 or after return of gastrointestinal function and clinical evidence of functional anastomotic patency.
   e. Respiratory Care: Incentive spirometry encouraged.
   f. Analgesia/Postop Meds: Parenteral narcotics required. H_2 blockers usually begun.
   g. Length Of Hospital Stay: 1 to 2 weeks.

3. *Postoperative Complications*
   a. In Hospital
      (1) Morbidity:
         i. Anastomotic leak (possibly leading to abscess and/or fistula).
         ii. Wound infection.
         iii. Hemorrhage.
         iv. In difficult reoperative cases, major vascular or ureteral injury.
         v. Bowel obstruction/ileus.
         vi. Atelectasis/pneumonia.
         vii. Pulmonary embolus.
      (2) Mortality: Depends on indications for operation and clinical risk factors. In healthy young patients undergoing first resection for Crohn's disease, mortality should be < 2%. In debilitated patients with massive infarction of bowel, mortality may approach 50%.
   b. After Discharge:
      (1) Malabsorption.
      (2) Recurrent disease.
      (3) Incisional hernia.

4. *Follow-up*
   a. Suggested Follow-up: Patient is seen every 6 months.

PROCEDURE: SPLENECTOMY

Overvew: The spleen is an important part of the immune system and should not be removed unless necessary. Prior to elective splenectomy, the patient should be given commercially available vaccines against pneumococcus and hemophilus species. The difficulty of this commonly performed procedure is related to the size of the spleen and the pathology. Laparoscopic splenectomy has been reported.

1. *Operation*
    a. Indications:
        (1) Trauma or rupture.
        (2) Hypersplenism.
        (3) Hemolytic anemia.
        (4) Idiopathic thrombocytopenic purpura (ITP).
        (5) Gastric varices ("left-sided portal hypertension" due to splenic vein thrombosis).
        (6) Malignancy.
        (7) Tumor (i.e., pseudocyst, lymphoma, large hemangioma).
        (8) Myelofibrosis.
    b. Operative Steps: The spleen is mobilized by cutting attachments to the diaphragm, colon, and kidney. The blood supply is divided in the hilum and gastrosplenic ligament containing the short gastric vessels. When the spleen is very large or in cases of splenic vein thrombosis or severe ITP, the splenic artery and short gastric vessels are often ligated prior to splenic mobilization.
    c. Incision: Vertical or transverse.
    d. Anesthesia: General.
    e. Intraoperative Monitoring: Routine unless patient is high risk patient or massive bleeding is anticipated.
    f. Operative Positioning: Supine.
    g. Duration: 1 to 3 hours. Routine splenectomy about 1 hour. Removal of large spleens with portal hypertension longer.
    h. EBL/Transfusions: In elective splenectomy for ITP, platelets are often given after the spleen is removed. In trauma or cases of severe splenomegaly or portal hypertension, transfusion of red blood cells is often necessary.
    i. "Surgical Stress": Moderate.

2. *Expected Hospital Course/Treatment*
    a. Postoperative Monitoring
        (1) ICU Stay: Not necessary in routine cases but may be necessary following cases involving large blood loss, in some cases of severe ITP, or in high-risk patients.
        (2) Invasive/Special Monitoring: Invasive monitors remain in place while in ICU.
        (3) Parameters To Be Monitored:
            i. Vital signs.
            ii. Urine output.
            iii. CBC, platelet count.
            iv. Amylase.
            v. Electrolytes.
    b. Positioning/Activity: Out of bed on POD 1.
    c. Alimentation: Clear liquids started on POD 2 to 3, advancing to regular diet by POD 5 for routine cases.
    d. Wound Care/Drains: Abdominal drainage indicated for complicated cases.
    e. Respiratory Care: Incentive spirometry encouraged.
    f. Analgesia/Postop Meds: Parenteral narcotics required. H_2 blockers usually begun.
    g. Length Of Hospital Stay: 5 to 10 days.

3. *Postoperative Complications*
    a. In Hospital
        (1) Morbidity:
            i. Bleeding.
            ii. Thrombocytosis.
            iii. Leukocytosis.
            iv. Injury to pancreas, stomach, or colon.
            v. Pancreatitis or pancreatic fistula.
            vi. Atelectasis/pneumonia.
        (2) Mortality: < 2%.
    b. After Discharge:
        (1) Recurrence of hematologic disorder or malignancy.
        (2) Incisional hernia.
        (3) Postsplenectomy sepsis (rare in adult).

4. *Follow-up*
    a. Suggested Follow-up: The patient is seen every 6 months. Aggressive antibiotic treatment of upper respiratory infections is warranted. A medical alert bracelet is recommended.

PROCEDURE: VAGOTOMY/GASTRECTOMY

Overview: Gastrectomy is now less common because of the impressive effectiveness of available ulcer medications. The trend in surgical therapy for duodenal ulcer is toward nonresective operations (e.g., parietal cell vagotomy or truncal vagotomy and drainage). Gastrectomy remains the mainstay of surgical therapy for gastric ulcer and gastric cancer.

1. *Operation*
   a. Indications:
      (1) Duodenal ulcer disease: highly selective vagotomy (HSV), vagotomy and drainage (i.e., pyloroplasty or gastrojejunostomy), or vagotomy and antrectomy.
      (2) Gastric ulcer: partial gastrectomy with or without vagotomy.
      (3) Gastric malignancy: subtotal or total gastrectomy.
   b. Operative Steps: HSV is performed by severing the branches from the anterior and posterior vagus which innervate the proximal two-thirds of the stomach while the branches to the antropyloric mechanism are left intact. Vagotomy and drainage is performed by cutting the main vagal trunks at the level of the gastroesophageal junction and facilitating gastric drainage by rendering the pylorus incompetent (pyloroplasty) or bypassing it (gastrojejunostomy). Optimal acid suppression may be attained by truncal vagotomy and antrectomy which involves a resection of the distal one-third of the stomach. GI continuity is reestablished by gastroduodenostomy (Billroth 1) or gastrojejunostomy (Billroth 2). For gastric ulcer, a hemigastrectomy to include the ulcer usually is sufficient, although some surgeons add vagotomy in patients with a high risk of recurrence, such as consumers of alcohol or nonsteroidal anti-inflammatory drugs. For cancer, an 80 to 100% gastrectomy is performed, sometimes with resection of adjacent involved organs (e.g., spleen or distal pancreas).
   c. Incision: Upper midline or transverse.
   d. Anesthesia: General.
   e. Intraoperative Monitoring: In patients with significant cardiac or pulmonary risk and in patients with large tumors, invasive hemodynamic monitoring should be considered.
   f. Operative Positioning: Supine.
   g. Duration: 1 to 6 hours, the lesser ulcer operations taking the shortest and the extensive cancer operations the longest.
   h. EBL/Transfusions: Transfusion rarely necessary for elective ulcer operations. EBL for gastrectomy for cancer is 300 to 2000 ml. Transfusion is necessary about 40% of the time.
   i. "Surgical Stress": Ranges from minimal for HSV and vagotomy and drainage to severe for radical total gastrectomy.

2. *Expected Hospital Course/Treatment*
   a. Postoperative Monitoring
      (1) ICU Stay: 1 to 2 days for radical subtotal or total gastrectomy.
      (2) Invasive/Special Monitoring: Invasive monitors remain in place while in ICU.
      (3) Parameters To Be Monitored:
         i. Vital signs. ii. Urine output. iii. CBC. iv. Electrolytes. v. Nasogastric tube output. vi. GI function.
   b. Positioning/Activity: Out of bed evening of surgery or next day.
   c. Alimentation: NPO for 3 to 5 days after ulcer surgery and 7 after total gastrectomy. In the latter group, TPN or jejunostomy tube feeding may be essential.
   d. Wound Care/Drains: Closed suction drainage for 3 to 7 days in uncomplicated cases. Drain not necessary for HSV or vagotomy and drainage.
   e. Respiratory Care: Incentive spirometry encouraged.
   f. Analgesia/Postop Meds: Parenteral narcotics required. H_2 blockers usually begun.
   g. Length Of Hospital Stay: 5 days for HSV to 14 days for total gastrectomy.

3. *Postoperative Complications*
   a. In Hospital
      (1) Morbidity:
         i. Delayed gastric emptying. ii. Anastomotic leak. iii. Fistula. iv. Hemorrhage. v. Wound infection.
         vi. Injury to surrounding viscera (spleen, pancreas, liver, esophagus). vii. Inadvertant ligation of the common bile duct, middle colic artery, or aberrant left hepatic artery. viii. Atelectasis/pneumonia.
      (2) Mortality: HSV 0%; vagotomy and drainage 1%; vagotomy and antrectomy 2%; subtotal gastrectomy for cancer 4 to 5%; total gastrectomy for cancer 8 to 10%. Mortality higher in patients requiring emergency surgery.
   b. After Discharge:
      (1) Recurrent ulcer.
      (2) Dumping/vagotomy-associated diarrhea.
      (3) Gastric stasis and weight loss.
      (4) Wound hernia.
      (5) Recurrent disease in cancer patients.

4. *Follow-up*
   a. Suggested Follow-up: If the indication for operation is benign ulcer, the patient is seen every 3 months for 2 visits, then every 6 months. If the operation is for cancer, the patient is seen every 3 months. Vitamin B_{12} is administered every 6 months for patients undergoing > 50% gastrectomy.

8 EVALUATION OF THE PATIENT UNDERGOING CARDIOTHORACIC SURGERY

David M. Guarnieri

Valluvan Jeevanandam

Barbara Todd

Successful management of the patient undergoing a cardiothoracic surgical procedure involves knowledge of the patient's functional cardiac status, evaluation and appropriate treatment of noncardiac diseases that may have significant impact on cardiac or pulmonary function, and an understanding of the special requirements of the proposed surgery. In most cases, the principles underlying the preoperative evaluation of patients with cardiac and pulmonary disease are the same for both cardiothoracic and noncardiothoracic surgery and are discussed elsewhere in this book. Additional management issues, pathophysiologic considerations, and risk-benefit analyses specific to cardiothoracic operations are discussed below.

CARDIAC STATUS

The major factor affecting patient outcome in cardiothoracic surgery is the functional status of the cardiovascular system.[1-5] Limited cardiac reserve, due to either congestive heart failure or recent myocardial infarction, is a significant predictor of cardiac morbidity for all types of surgery. Cardiothoracic operations place more excessive demands on cardiac function than most other surgical procedures. Those include cardiopulmonary bypass with extracorporeal circulation in open heart surgery and one-lung ventilation in thoracotomy. Outcome studies for coronary artery bypass graft (CABG) and valvular procedures uniformly rank patients with poor left ventricular function in a high-risk subgroup.[1-7] The New York Heart Association classification for heart failure, ejection fraction, measurement of left ventricular end-diastolic pressure, and wall motion abnormalities have all been used to predict outcome. However, assessment of ventricular function with contrast ventriculography remains the gold standard.[3,4] Decisions to proceed with surgery and those determining hemodynamic support and monitoring, anesthetic techniques, and intensive care unit stay are often based upon proper evaluation of cardiac reserve. When patients with severe left ventricular dysfunction (as evidenced by an ejection fraction below 20%) were studied before CABG,[4] none of the traditionally accepted risk factors discussed below predicted operative mortality. The only significant predictor of risk in this population was the urgency of surgery. Possible explanations for this finding include the presence of cardiogenic shock, ongoing ischemia, or lack of time for adequate preparation and comprehensive monitoring. In this specific population, the risks of operation may be modified by intensive medical therapy to permit some patients with unstable angina to undergo elective or semi-elective surgery or placement of an intraaortic balloon to stabilize hemodynamics. Thus, although operative risk for patients with severe ventricular dysfunction is high, strategies to improve outcome can be focused on aspects of their clinical situation amenable to intervention.

NONCARDIAC DISEASES

Comorbid conditions affecting cardiac function are listed in Table 8–1. In varying degrees they serve as risk factors in all procedures because they affect cardiac performance, oxygen supply and demand requirements, vascular perfusion, and circulatory blood volume. A recent attempt to stratify outcome according to preoperative risk factors in cardiac surgery concluded that emergency surgery, preoperative serum creatinine levels above 1.8 mg/dl, preoperative hematocrit levels below 34 percent, increasing age, chronic pulmonary disease, prior vascular surgery, reoperation, and mitral valve insufficiency were significant predictors of mortality.[5] To a lesser

TABLE 8–1. Noncardiac Diseases Affecting Cardiac Function

Hypertension

Vascular Disease
  Cerebral, aortic, peripheral

Pulmonary Disease
  Asthma, chronic bronchitis, emphysema, pneumonia, tuberculosis, alveolar diseases, pulmonary embolism, pulmonary hypertension

Hepatic Disease
  Cirrhosis, portal hypertension, ascites

Renal Disease
  Nephrotic syndrome, dialysis dependence

Endocrine Disease
  Diabetes mellitus, hypothyroidism and hyperthyroidism, pheochromocytoma, aldosteronism, adrenocortical insufficiency

Psychiatric Disease
  Drug dependence, alcoholism, tobacco smoking

Connective Tissue Diseases

Nutritional Deficiencies, Obesity

Infections and Fever

Source: Modified from Hug CC: Anesthesia for adult cardiac surgery, in Miller RD (ed): *Anesthesia,* 3d ed. New York, Churchill Livingstone, 1990, p 1608.

degree, diabetes mellitus, body weight of 65 kg or more, aortic stenosis, and cerebrovascular disease also predicted poor outcome. A history of smoking, high serum cholesterol and triglyceride levels, and hypertension failed to reach significance in this study. While controlled trials confirming that optimizing a patient's preoperative condition decreases morbidity in cardiothoracic surgery have not been performed for most of these diseases, it is generally assumed that this is the case.

Certain preoperative medical conditions present management dilemmas in cardiothoracic surgery. These include:

Coexistent carotid and coronary artery disease. Carotid artery disease is found in up to 38 percent of patients undergoing CABG.[8] The incidence of significant disease necessitating carotid endarterectomy (CEA) ranges from 1.3 to 6.0 percent.[9] Performing a CEA either as a staged or combined procedure with CABG has been extensively debated (see Chaps. 18 and 35).

Renal insufficiency and cardiac surgery. Patients with renal disease are known to have accelerated atherosclerosis and present a significant challenge when faced with the need for cardiac surgery. Hypertension, volume overload, anemia, platelet dysfunction, and electrolyte abnormalities require skillful management. Cardiopulmonary bypass itself may worsen renal function. Opinion is divided as to whether patients on dialysis are likely to suffer increased mortality during cardiac surgery (see Chap. 32).

Hypothyroidism and ischemic heart disease. Treatment of hypothyroid patients with symptomatic coronary artery disease poses a significant risk. Restoring the normal intravascular fluid volume, body temperature, respiratory function, and electrolyte balance of the euthyroid state may not be possible without exacerbation of anginal symptoms. Careful initiation of thyroid replacement therapy before or after coronary artery revascularization is a decision that must be individualized for each patient (see Chap. 25).

Chronic obstructive pulmonary disease (COPD) and intrathoracic surgery. Patients with COPD present conflicts in management in two ways. First, in those with severe disease, the question often arises whether or not compromised pulmonary function poses prohibitive risk for the proposed surgery. Second, when lung resection is deemed necessary, residual lung function may not be adequate. In such patients, lung function must be appropriately assessed and treated prior to making any judgments. The degree of impairment as well as the need and magnitude of the procedure are critical factors to be weighed (see Chap. 22).

OPERATIVE PATHOPHYSIOLOGY

Cardiac Surgery

CABG and valvular replacement procedures require the use of an extracorporeal circuit to bypass the heart and lungs. The goals of cardiopulmonary bypass (CPB) are to provide adequate ventilation and oxygenation, maintain circulation to the rest of the body while the heart is arrested, provide hypothermia to decrease body metabolism, and assure hypothermic myocardial preservation. The essential components of a CPB system are large catheters for venous drainage, an oxygenator/heat exchanger, a pump, and a cannula for arterial return. Additional elements such as separate circuits for cardioplegia administration or suction catheters, filters, alarms, blood gas monitors, and vaporizers for volatile anesthetics may be included in the system.

Most commonly, blood is drained into a reservoir from a cannula inserted into the right atrium. Additional blood is retrieved by suction of shed blood from the operative field and/or a "vent" cannula inserted into the heart to decompress the left ventricle. Oxygenated blood is returned to the patient through a cannula generally placed in the ascending aorta. The cannula can be placed in the femoral artery in emergency situations or "redo" operations. During the period of cardiac arrest, a clamp is placed across the ascending aorta to prevent retrograde flow into the heart and coronary circulation. Complications of establishing and maintaining CPB include aortic dissection, superior vena cava obstruction, air embolism, and mechanical equipment failure.

CPB circuits use either a bubble or membrane oxygenator to effect transfer of oxygen and carbon dioxide. A heat exchanger adjusts the temperature of the perfusate to provide moderate systemic hypothermia (28°C) during cardiac repair. Deliberate hypothermia reduces metabolic requirements and provides protection during periods of hypoperfusion and potential tissue ischemia. The CPB circuit is usually primed with an asanguineous crystalloid/colloid solution of 1500 to 2500 ml for adults. Acute normovolemic hemodilution to achieve hematocrit levels of 20 to 30 percent is customary. Systemic anticoagulation is initiated with heparin to prevent thrombus formation when blood is exposed to artificial surfaces. Reversal of anticoagulation with protamine is performed after the conclusion of CPB but before closure of the sternal incision. While the coronary circulation is interrupted, myocardial protection is accomplished with hypothermic (4°C) hyperkalemic cardioplegia injected either anterograde into the aortic root or retrograde through the coronary sinus to maintain a temperature of 10 to 15°C in the myocardium.

When the surgical repair is nearly complete, the patient is gradually rewarmed. Flow to the coronary circulation is reestablished by removing the aortic crossclamp. After defibrillation, the empty heart is allowed to beat. Discontinuation of CPB involves gradual decrease in bypass flow, restoration of cardiac function, and return of ventilation to the lungs. Inadequate cardiac performance may be due to ischemia, uncorrected structural defects, excess cardioplegia, arrhythmias, or preexisting ventricular dysfunction.[10] Pharmacologic support with inotropic or vasodilator drugs or mechanical support with an intraaortic balloon pump may be needed if cardiac output is inadequate. There are many algorithms for recognizing and treating low cardiac output syndrome after CPB.

Preservation of central nervous system function is a major concern when CPB is used. The occurrence of neurologic injury after CPB involves many factors, including age, preexisting cerebrovascular disease, history of diabetes mellitus, duration of CPB, hypoperfusion, postoperative arrhythmias, and the presence of mural thrombi.[11,12] The potential for emboli is increased when a cardiac chamber is opened, as in valve replacement or aneurysmectomy procedures. One study has shown that massive doses of thiopental (40 mg/kg) to suppress electroencephalographic activity completely have resulted in fewer neuropsychiatric complications.[13] However, high doses of barbiturates increased the need for inotropic support and prolonged the time to extubation in many cases.

Renal function may be compromised during CPB. Mechanisms include decreased tubular function due to hypothermia and CPB itself, decreased renal perfusion and loss of pulsatile flow, and hemoglobinuria from intravascular hemolysis.[14] Efforts to improve renal perfusion and urine output with low-dose dopamine infusion and osmotic or loop diuretics have not been consistently shown to decrease the incidence of postoperative renal dysfunction.

Postoperative considerations in patients undergoing cardiac surgery include bleeding, hypertension, prolonged intubation, weight gain, and arrhythmias.

Bleeding. Inadequate surgical hemostasis, incomplete heparin reversal, reduced platelet count or function, dilutional coagulopathy, and activation of the fibrinolytic system are the usual causes of bleeding after CPB. Reexploration necessitated by persistent blood loss or the likelihood of cardiac tamponade occurs in 4 to 10 percent of cases.[15]

Hypertension. Hypertension occurs in 30 to 80 percent of patients undergoing CABG and 8 to 37 percent of those undergoing valve replacement surgery (see Chap. 54). Prompt assessment and treatment of postoperative systolic hypertension are required to prevent increased myocardial work and strain on newly created anastomoses. Pain, hypoxia, hypoventilation, and excessive use of inotropic drugs are easily treatable causes.

Prolonged intubation. High-dose opioid anesthetic techniques to maintain hemodynamic stability require mechanical ventilation for 12 to 24 hours after surgery.

Weight gain. Patients routinely gain two to four kg because of accumulation of extravascular fluid primarily as a result of CPB-induced derangements in capillary permeability. Spontaneous diuresis occurs on the second or third postoperative day as normal homeostatic mechanisms bring body fluids into balance.

Rhythm disturbances. Atrial and ventricular dysrhythmias and intermittent or persistent conduction block are common. Cannulation of the heart, electrolyte abnormalities due to cardioplegia, acid-base changes, inotropic drugs, hypothermia, myocardial ischemia, and direct surgical trauma are likely causes. Epicardial pacemaker wires are routinely implanted as part of the procedure because of the frequency of early arrhythmias and conduction abnormalities. Cardiac rhythm monitoring is necessary for at least five days following surgery.

Thoracic Surgery

Patients undergoing thoracic surgery often have preexisting lung disease. Both intraoperative and postoperative events can cause additional impairment of lung function. For the majority of procedures, patients are positioned in the lateral decubitus position for a posterior lateral skin incision, usually in the fifth interspace. In order to gain access to all areas of the lung, the hilum, and most of the mediastinum, one-lung ventilation to the dependent lung is provided, and the nondependent lung undergoing surgery is collapsed. Significant respiratory changes are predictable both during and after surgery.

The indications for one-lung ventilation are listed in Table 8–2. A double-lumen endotracheal tube is used to separate lung function. Changes in ventilation and perfusion of the lungs are due to a variety of factors. Although blood flow is gravity dependent, any blood flow to the unventilated nondependent collapsed lung creates an obligatory right-to-left shunt. Dependent lung function is impaired because of reduced lung volume and functional residual capacity induced by general anesthesia, pressure of mediastinal and abdominal contents, formation of fluid transudate, accumulation of secretions, and suboptimal positioning on the operating

TABLE 8–2. Indications for One-Lung Ventilation

Absolute
1. Isolation of each lung to prevent contamination of a healthy lung
   a. Infection (abscess, infected cyst, etc.)
   b. Massive hemorrhage
2. Control of distribution of ventilation to only one lung
   a. Bronchopleural fistula
   b. Unilateral cyst or bullae
   c. Major bronchial disruption or trauma
3. Unilateral lung lavage

Relative
1. Surgical exposure—high priority
   a. Thoracic aortic aneurysm
   b. Pneumonectomy
   c. Upper lobectomy
2. Surgical exposure—low priority
   a. Esophageal surgery
   b. Middle and lower lobectomy
   c. Thoracoscopy under general anesthesia

Source: Modified from Benumof J: Physiology of the open chest and one-lung ventilation, in Kaplan JA (ed): *Thoracic Anesthesia,* 1st ed. New York, Churchill Livingstone, 1983, p 299.

table. Widening of the A-a gradient is therefore almost inevitable during one-lung ventilation. Standard procedures to increase oxygenation include use of a high inspired oxygen concentration (FiO_2 = 1.0); selective continuous positive airway pressure (CPAP) to the nondependent lung to decrease the shunt fraction; selective positive end-expiratory pressure (PEEP) to the dependent lung to improve ventilation-perfusion mismatching; intermittent reinflation of the nondependent lung; and, depending on the stage of the surgical procedure, temporary ligation of the pulmonary artery to the nondependent lung to eliminate any shunt.

Postoperative respiratory impairment is the result of resection of functional lung tissue and/or trauma to remaining parenchyma, atelectasis due to pain-induced inhibition of deep breathing and coughing, and increased secretions from airway manipulation. The decision whether to extubate the patient in the operating room or later in the intensive care unit depends on the nature of the underlying disease and the procedure. Continuing positive pressure ventilation in the postoperative period increases the likelihood of disrupting the bronchial stump when lung tissue has been resected. Methods to decrease postoperative pain and improve respiratory function include patient-controlled administration of intravenous narcotics, intercostal nerve blocks and epidural anesthesia. Routine use of epidural anesthesia has had a tremendous impact on decreasing postoperative pulmonary dysfunction and has added significantly to patient comfort.

Recently, thorascopic surgery has become an acceptable alternative to some open procedures. Thoracoscopy involves insertion of an endoscope into the thoracic cavity and pleural space. It is most commonly used for diagnosis of pleural and parenchymal disease when other diagnostic modalities like thoracentesis and closed-chest pleural or lung biopsy have failed; staging of neoplastic disease to determine resectability; and chemical pleurodesis. Thoracoscopy provides good visualization of the hemithorax, and fluid and biopsy specimens can be easily obtained with minimal trauma to the patient. Anesthesia can be provided with local agents, supplemented with intercostal nerve blocks two interspaces above and below the insertion site, or general anesthesia. Since positive pressure ventilation with general anesthesia interferes with visualization, one-lung ventilation is required.

PROPHYLACTIC ISSUES

Antibiotics

Although cardiac surgery is considered "clean," the devastating effects of infections like those of the mediastinum and prosthetic valves justify the use of prophylactic antibiotics. Generally, a first- or second-generation cephalosporin is administered before surgery and adequate tissue levels are maintained for 48 hours. Vancomycin is usually chosen for patients allergic to penicillin. Additional intraoperative dosing may be required for long procedures. Lifelong prophylaxis against endocarditis is necessary in all patients undergoing valve replacement, according to the recommendations of the American Heart Association (see Chap. 43). The use of prophylactic antibiotics before elective pulmonary resection is controversial (see Chap. 44). Most surgeons follow the guidelines outlined above for cardiac surgery.

Thromboembolism

The risk of thromboembolism in patients undergoing cardiac surgery is greatest for those who have had a prosthetic valve implanted. The risk is strongly correlated with the type of valve (mechanical or bioprosthetic), location (aortic, mitral, or combined), atrial fibrillation, proximity to surgery, and adequacy of anticoagulation.[16] General guidelines for anticoagulation after valve replacement include lifelong full anticoagulation for patients with mechanical valves and three months of anticoagulation for those with bioprosthetic valves. In the latter case, this may be optional for patients in sinus rhythm with bioprosthetic valves in the aortic position.

In thoracic surgery, the risk of postoperative thromboembolism correlates with prevention of deep venous thrombosis and pulmonary embolism. Guidelines for patients undergoing general surgical procedures apply here. Recommendations favor the use of prophylactic measures in all patients over age 40. Both low-dose heparin (LDH) and external pneumatic compression devices (EPC) are efficacious. Additional recommendations for high-risk patients are found in Chap. 48.

POSTOPERATIVE COMPLICATIONS

Cardiac Surgery

Complications of cardiac surgery may be general in nature or specific to a certain procedure. Problems related to procedures requiring CPB include mediastinal wound infection, post-CPB pulmonary dysfunction, postpericardiotomy syndrome, and heparin-induced thrombocytopenia.

Mediastinal wound infection. Infections of the sternal wound occur in 1 to 10 percent of patients undergoing sternotomy.[17,18] Factors associated with an increased incidence of infection are diabetes mellitus, prolonged CPB, combined CABG and valve replacement, excessive blood loss, reexploration for bleeding, prolonged low-output syndrome, and the need for prolonged ventilatory support.[17,18] Treatment usually includes intravenous antibiotics, wound irrigation, and serial debridement. Vascularized pedicle flaps of omentum or myocutaneous tissue have been used for reconstruction of deep sternal infections.

Post-CPB pulmonary dysfunction. Pulmonary dysfunction following CPB may range from mild decreases in PaO_2 to respiratory failure resembling that in adult respiratory distress syndrome. Although most patients exhibit some increase in the A-a gradient immediately after surgery, some may rarely develop full-blown respiratory failure. Events during CPB contributing to the development of pulmonary dysfunction include decreased pulmonary blood flow due to emboli or localized vasoconstriction, edema from complement activation and vasoactive compounds released from leukocytes, and edema from increased hydrostatic pressure due to inadequate left ventricular venting or increased bronchial blood flow.[19]

Postpericardiotomy syndrome. The incidence of postpericardiotomy syndrome is reported to be 0 to 28 percent.[20] Symptoms and signs vary and include low-grade fever with or without elevation in the white blood cell count, pericardial and pleural friction rubs, profound pain, lassitude, myalgias, and temperature as high as 104°F. The syndrome commonly develops two to three weeks after surgery and is treated with aspirin and steroids.

Heparin-induced thrombocytopenia.
Heparin-dependent antibodies to platelet membranes may develop in any patient receiving the drug and cause platelet activation and aggregation. Clinical manifestations range from asymptomatic thrombocytopenia to severe intravascular coagulation. Thrombotic complications include stroke, pulmonary embolus, limb loss, graft occlusion, and myocardial infarction. Management consists of early recognition of the syndrome, appropriate antibody studies, and cessation of all heparin-containing solutions.

CABG may be complicated by perioperative myocardial infarction and issues related to graft patency. The risk of developing a perioperative infarction is approximately 6 percent[21,22] and is related to the severity of underlying coronary artery disease and the duration of CPB. Other factors include the presence of left main coronary artery disease, depressed preoperative ejection fraction, and technical difficulties with anastomoses. Bypass graft occlusion may occur early within the first month or late after the first year. Technical factors related to the procedure exert their influence early and include inadequate graft size, mechanical occlusion due to kinking, thrombosis, and focal intimal hyperplasia. Late manifestations of occlusion are usually due to the development of atherosclerosis in the graft. Many surgeons currently use internal mammary arteries for bypass whenever possible because they remain patent longer than saphenous vein grafts.

Problems inherent in valve surgery are related to the length and severity of the preoperative condition, technical issues associated with open chamber procedures, and choice of prosthetic valve.[23] Decompensated cardiac function with pulmonary hypertension, atrial thrombus formation in patients with chronic atrial fibrillation, and severe calcification of the valve with the potential to shower emboli when removed adversely affect outcome. Factors to be considered in choosing a prosthesis are the thrombogenicity and durability of the valve; hemodynamic considerations including obstruction to flow and valve incompetence; hemolysis; the risk of endocarditis; and the suitability of anticoagulation for the individual patient.

Thoracic Surgery

Complications of thoracic surgery occurring in the immediate postoperative period require prompt diagnosis and treatment. The major entities include hemorrhage, bronchial disruption, and right heart failure.

Hemorrhage.
Bleeding of more than 200 cc/hr into chest tubes necessitates reexploration. Slippage of surgical ligatures on pulmonary vessels, diffuse hemorrhage from raw surfaces, or bleeding from bronchial or intercostal arteries may be found.

Bronchial disruption.
Communication between the tracheobronchial tree and the pleural cavity can result from dehiscence of the bronchial stump, rupture of an inflammatory lesion, erosion by neoplasm, or trauma. Signs and symptoms are variable and depend on the size of the communication and the presence or absence of chest tubes. Large leaks are signaled by bubbles of air in the chest tube drainage. Obstructed or absent chest tubes may result in tension pneumothorax.

Right heart failure.
Major pulmonary resection results in an increase in right ventricular afterload. Patients with preexisting pulmonary hypertension or a previous inferior-posterior myocardial infarction involving the right ventricle are more likely to develop right heart failure. Diagnosis is confirmed by pulmonary artery catheterization showing elevated right atrial pressure, decreased pulmonary artery wedge pressure, and reduced cardiac output. Treatment consists of optimizing preload, inotropy, and afterload, and initiating measures to reduce pulmonary artery vasoconstriction such as administering oxygen, normalizing acid-base balance, and treating bronchospasm and infection to reduce hypoxia.

Arrhythmias.
Supraventricular arrhythmias are common after major pulmonary resection. Contributing factors include age, underlying cardiac disease, surgical trauma, right atrial distention, poor gas exchange, and increased catecholamine secretion due to pain. Conventional treatment measures are appropriate after specific contributing factors have been addressed.

Neural injuries.
The phrenic, vagus, and recurrent laryngeal nerves may be injured during extensive dissection. The brachial plexus may be inappropriately stretched due to malpositioning of the patient on the operating table.

REFERENCES

1. Kuan P, Bernstein SB, Ellestad MH: Coronary artery bypass surgery morbidity. *J Am Coll Cardiol* 3:1391–1397, 1984.
2. Foster ED, Fisher LD, Kaiser GC et al: Comparison of operative mortality and morbidity for initial and repeat coronary artery bypass grafting: The Coronary Artery Surgery Study (CASS) registry experience. *Ann Thorac Surg* 38:563–570, 1984.
3. Royster RL, Butterworth JF, Prough DS et al: Preoperative and intraoperative predictors of inotropic support and long-term outcome in patients having coronary artery bypass grafting. *Anesth Analg* 72:729–736, 1991.
4. Christokis GT, Weisel RD, Fremes SE et al: Coronary artery bypass grafting in patients with poor ventricular function. *J Thorac Cardiovasc Surg* 103:1083–1091, 1992.
5. Higgins TL, Estafanous FG, Loop FD et al: Stratification of morbidity and mortality outcome by preoperative risk factors in coronary artery bypass patients. *JAMA* 267:2344–2348, 1991.
6. Davis EA, Gardner TJ, Gillivov M: Valvular disease in the elderly: Influence on surgical results. *Ann Thorac Surg* 55:333–338, 1993.
7. Craver JM, Goldstein J, Jones EC et al: Clinical, hemodynamic, and operative descriptors affecting outcome of aortic valve replacement in elderly versus young patients. *Ann Surg* 199:733–741, 1984.
8. Rosenthal D, Caudill DR, Lamis PA et al: Carotid and coronary arterial disease: A rational approach. *Ann Surg* 50:233–235, 1984.
9. Lezler DC: Uncommon diseases and cardiac anesthesia, in Kaplan JA (ed): *Cardiac Anesthesia*, 2d ed. Orlando, Grune & Stratton, 1987, p 812.
10. Andriakos PG, Hughes CW, Thomas SJ: Anesthesia for cardiac surgery, in Barash PG, Cullen BF, Stoelting RK (eds): *Clinical Anesthesia*, 1st ed. Philadelphia, Lippincott, 1989, p 1000.
11. Lynn GM, Stefanko K, Reed JF et al: Risk factors for stroke after coronary artery bypass. *J Thorac Cardiovasc Surg* 104:1518–1523, 1992.

12. Tuman KJ, McCarthy RJ, Najofi H et al: Differential effects of advanced age on neurologic and cardiac risk of coronary artery operations. *J Thorac Cardiovasc Surg* 104:1510–1517, 1992.

13. Nussmeier NA, Arlund C, Slogoff S: Neuropsychiatric complications after cardiopulmonary bypass: Cerebral protection by a barbiturate. *Anesthesiology* 64:165–170, 1986.

14. Hild PG: Pathophysiology of cardiopulmonary bypass, in Hensley FA, Martin DE (eds): *The Practice of Cardiac Anesthesia*, 1st ed. Boston, Little, Brown, 1990, p 617.

15. Andriakos PG, Hughes CW, Thomas SJ: Anesthesia for cardiac surgery, in Barash PG, Cullen BF, Stoelting RK (eds): *Clinical Anesthesia*, 1st ed. Philadelphia, Lippincott, 1989, p 1003.

16. Khan SS, Czer LS: Antithrombotic therapy after cardiac surgery, in Gray RJ, Matloff JM (eds): *Medical Management of the Cardiac Surgical Patient*, 1st ed. Baltimore, Williams & Wilkins, 1990, pp 226–227.

17. Grossi EA, Culliford AT, Kreiger KH et al: A survey of 77 major infectious complications of median sternotomy: A review of 7949 consecutive operative procedures. *Ann Thorac Surg* 40:214–223, 1985.

18. Miholic J, Hudec M, Domanig E et al: Risk factors for severe bacterial infections after valve replacement and aortocoronary bypass operations: Analysis of 246 cases by logistic regression. *Ann Thorac Surg* 40:224–228, 1985.

19. Hild PG: Pathophysiology of cardiopulmonary bypass, in Hensley FA, Martin DE (eds): *The Practice of Cardiac Anesthesia*, 1st ed. Boston, Little, Brown, 1990, p 619.

20. Engle MA, Gay WA, McCabe J et al: Postpericardiotomy syndrome in adults: Incidence, autoimmunity, and virology. *Circulation* 64:58–60, 1981.

21. Schaff HV, Gersh BJ, Fisher LD et al: Detrimental effect of perioperative myocardial infarction on late survival after coronary artery bypass. *J Thorac Cardiovasc Surg* 88:972–981, 1984.

22. Roberts AJ: Perioperative myocardial infarction and changes in left ventricular performance related to coronary artery bypass graft surgery. *Ann Thorac Surg* 35:208–225, 1985.

23. Conahan TJ: Complications of cardiac surgery, in Kaplan JA (ed): *Cardiac Anesthesia*, 2d ed. Orlando, Grune & Stratton, 1987, pp 1110–1111.

PROCEDURE: AORTIC VALVE REPLACEMENT

Overview: Valve replacement options include mechanical valve, porcine xenograft, or homograft (cadaver). Mechanical valves have the lowest incidence of failure but require permanent anticoagulation. Xenograft valves do not require anticoagulation but will deteriorate after 8 to 10 years. The homografts require no anticoagulation, are the valves that are least likely to become infected, and are useful for small aortic roots. Disadvantages of homografts are limited supply and inconclusive long-term results. In a novel operation, some surgeons have moved the autologous pulmonic valve to the aortic position, replacing the pulmonic valve with a prosthetic. Percutaneous balloon valvuloplasty has been performed in selected circumstances to avoid open-heart surgery, but the morbidity is high as is recurrence of disease. Aortic valve repair is usually not possible in the presence of significant calcific disease.

1. *Operation*
    a. Indications:
        (1) Aortic stenosis (i.e., valve area < 0.6 cm2) with angina, congestive heart failure, or syncope.
        (2) Aortic insufficiency with progressive cardiac enlargement, left ventricular hypertrophy, or dyspnea on exertion. It is especially important to operate on these patients before the development of irreversible myocardial dysfunction.
        (3) Emergency valve replacement for acute aortic dissection or bacterial endocarditis.
    b. Operative Steps: See text for details regarding cardiopulmonary bypass. After the aortic root is opened and explored, the valve is excised and the annulus decalcified. If the root is too small to accept a valve, it is enlarged by extending the aortotomy across the root of the mitral valve or across the right ventricular outflow tract. The new valve is sewn in place with figure-of-eight sutures or with pledgets, depending on the state of the root. The aortotomy is closed and the patient removed from cardiopulmonary bypass.
    c. Incision: Median sternotomy.
    d. Anesthesia: General.
    e. Intraoperative Monitoring: Arterial line; Swan-Ganz catheter; and temperature probes in the esophagus, bladder, or rectum. Transesophageal echocardiography is used as indicated.
    f. Operative Positioning: Supine.
    g. Duration: 4 to 6 hours.
    h. EBL/Transfusions: Same as coronary artery bypass grafting (CABG).
    i. "Surgical Stress": Severe.

2. *Expected Hospital Course/Treatment*
    a. Postoperative Monitoring
        (1) ICU Stay: 3 to 4 days.
        (2) Invasive/Special Monitoring: Same as CABG.
        (3) Parameters To Be Monitored: Same as CABG.
    b. Positioning/Activity: Same as CABG.
    c. Alimentation: Same as CABG.
    d. Wound Care/Drains: Same as CABG.
    e. Respiratory Care: Same as CABG.
    f. Analgesia/Postop Meds: Pain relief/sedation as in CABG. Anticoagulation with warfarin started on all patients POD 2 to achieve elevation in PT to 1.5 times normal. Mechanical valves require anticoagulation indefinitely, porcine valves for 3 to 6 months. Homograft valves do not require anticoagulation.
    g. Length Of Hospital Stay: 7 to 10 days.

3. *Postoperative Complications*
    a. In Hospital
        (1) Morbidity: Similar to CABG. A higher incidence of cerebrovascular events and heart block are seen in valve surgery. Bacterial prosthetic valve endocarditis and thromboembolism are additional risks.
        (2) Mortality: 3%, higher in patients requiring emergency surgery and reoperation.
    b. After Discharge
        (1) Endocarditis of the prosthetic valve.
        (2) Valve dysfunction due to mechanical failure or thrombosis.
        (3) Progressive left ventricular failure.

4. *Follow-up*
    a. Suggested Follow-up: The PT is monitored in patients who require anticoagulation (e.g., mechanical valve or atrial fibrillation). The patient is seen in the office at 6 weeks by the surgeon. Cardiac rehabilitation and periodic visits to the cardiologist are routine. Lifetime prophylaxis for endocarditis is needed.

PROCEDURE: ATRIAL SEPTAL DEFECT REPAIR

Overview: There are three types of atrial septal defects (ASD): (1) secundum—most common, middle of atrial septum, can be closed primarily or with pericardial or dacron patch; (2) primum—low septum involving AV valves, closed with patch along with frequent VSD; and (3) sinus venosus—high on septum at the superior vena cava junction, associated with anomalous drainage of pulmonary veins, repair may require baffle to left atrium. All repairs of ASDs require cardiopulmonary bypass. Inotropic agents are needed infrequently after bypass.

1. *Operation*
    a. Indications: ASD repair is indicated when calculated pulmonary blood flow is greater than 1.5 times systemic blood flow. Contraindication to repair is increased pulmonary vascular resistance (PVR) to > 50% of systemic values.
    b. Operative Steps: See description above. Exposure is through a right atriotomy. After repair is complete, careful deairing of left atrium and placement of temporary pacing wires are required.
    c. Incision: Median sternotomy. Submammary bilateral incisions for cosmetic purposes are possible but not optimal.
    d. Anesthesia: General.
    e. Intraoperative Monitoring: Arterial line; CVP with or without Swan-Ganz catheter depending on patient's age and condition of right heart; temperature probes in esophagus, bladder, or rectum. Transesophageal echocardiography helpful to check repair.
    f. Operative Positioning: Supine.
    g. Duration: 2 to 3 hours, depending on right heart function and pulmonary hypertension.
    h. EBL/Transfusions: Blood conservation with cell saver and reinfusion of shed mediastinal blood. Transfusion is usually unnecessary in straightforward cases.
    i. "Surgical Stress": Moderate to severe depending on pulmonary vascular resistance.

2. *Expected Hospital Course/Treatment*
    a. Postoperative Monitoring
        (1) ICU Stay: 1 to 2 days.
        (2) Invasive/Special Monitoring: Arterial line and CVP catheter for 1 to 2 days. Telemetry after discharge from ICU.
        (3) Parameters To Be Monitored: Same as CABG.
    b. Positioning/Activity: Same as CABG.
    c. Alimentation: Same as CABG.
    d. Wound Care/Drains: Same as CABG.
    e. Respiratory Care: Same as CABG.
    f. Analgesia/Postop Meds: Anticoagulation for atrial fibrillation and sometimes with use of dacron patch for 3 months.
    g. Length Of Hospital Stay: 7 days.

3. *Postoperative Complications*
    a. In Hospital
        (1) Morbidity:
            i. Low cardiac output from right heart failure and pulmonary hypertension.
            ii. Bradycardia or AV block.
            iii. Cerebrovascular accident from air embolus.
            iv. Others similar to CABG.
        (2) Mortality: < 1.0% with low PVR, 6 to 10% with elevated PVR.
    b. After Discharge: Thromboembolism with atrial fibrillation.

4. *Follow-up*
    a. Suggested Follow-up: The patient is seen by the surgeon at 4 weeks. Cardiac rehabilitation and periodic visits with the cardiologist are routine. Lifetime bacterial endocarditis prophylaxis.

PROCEDURE: CORONARY ARTERY BYPASS GRAFTING (CABG)

Overview: Ischemic cardiac disease is a major health problem in the United States, accounting for one-third of adult deaths. Blood supply to ischemic myocardium can be improved by bypassing the obstructing coronary lesions with an aortocoronary conduit, either internal mammary artery, or saphenous vein. From 1 to 5 bypasses are commonly done, depending on coronary anatomy and the distribution of atherosclerosis. The risks and benefits of medical management, percutaneous angioplasty, and CABG must be evaluated and individualized for each patient by a multidisciplinary team. Survival benefit for CABG has been demonstrated in patients with left main coronary artery obstruction or triple vessel disease and decreased ventricular function.

1. *Operation*
   a. Indications: Angina or anginal equivalents (e.g., pulmonary edema, mitral valve insufficiency due to ischemic papillary muscles, or arrhythmias) not responsive to maximal medical management in patients with occlusive coronary artery disease (CAD).
   b. Operative Steps: See text for details regarding cardiopulmonary bypass. Conduits used for CABG include left internal mammary artery (preferred), saphenous vein, right internal mammary artery, epigastric arteries, or gastroepiploic arteries. Distal anastomoses are performed end-to-side or side-to-side in sequential fashion. Proximal anastomoses are done to the ascending aorta after the crossclamp is released.
   c. Incision: Median sternotomy with elevation of the left or right side of the chest to dissect the internal mammary arteries.
   d. Anesthesia: General.
   e. Intraoperative Monitoring: Arterial line; Swan-Ganz catheter; temperature probes in esophagus, bladder, or rectum; transesophageal echocardiography if available.
   f. Operative Positioning: Supine with the arms at the side.
   g. Duration: 5 to 8 hours.
   h. EBL/Transfusions: Blood is salvaged intraoperatively through a cell-saver device. Shed mediastinal blood can be autotransfused. Depending on starting hematocrit, 30% of patients will need tranfusions. Platelets and fresh frozen plasma may be required if the patient develops a coagulopathy.
   i. "Surgical Stress": Severe.

2. *Expected Hospital Course/Treatment*
   a. Postoperative Monitoring
      (1) ICU Stay: 2 to 4 days.
      (2) Invasive/Special Monitoring: Arterial line and Swan-Ganz catheter remain in place for 2 to 3 days. Telemetry after discharge from ICU.
      (3) Parameters To Be Monitored:

i. Vital signs.	v. Electrolytes, BUN, creatinine.
ii. Urine output.	vi. PT, PTT.
iii. Arterial blood gases.	vii. ECG.
iv. CBC.	viii. Chest x-ray.

   b. Positioning/Activity: Patients may be out of bed with progressive ambulation after central monitoring lines and chest tubes are removed.
   c. Alimentation: Oral intake may begin one day after extubation and advanced as tolerated.
   d. Wound Care/Drains: Mediastinal and pleural chest tubes are continued until output is less than 100 cc in an 8-hour period. Epicardial pacing wires, if placed at surgery, are removed on POD 5 if arrhythmias are absent. Sternal incision site is undressed on POD 3. The patient is not allowed to shower until POD 7.
   e. Respiratory Care: Mechanical ventilation is required overnight. Extubation is performed on POD 1 in uncomplicated cases.
   f. Analgesia/Postop Meds: Parenteral narcotics and benzodiazepines are administered for pain relief and sedation while in the ICU. Some surgeons begin patients on enteric-coated aspirin and continue this medication indefinitely as tolerated.
   g. Length Of Hospital Stay: 7 to 10 days.

3. *Postoperative Complications*
   a. In Hospital
      (1) Morbidity:

i. Myocardial infarction.	vii. Phrenic nerve paresis.
ii. Low cardiac output syndrome.	viii. Brachial plexus injury due to positioning of retractor during internal mammary artery mobilization.
iii. Bleeding.	
iv. Graft thrombosis.	ix. Sternal wound infection.
v. Arrhythmias.	x. Postpericardiotomy syndrome.
vi. Cerebrovascular accident.	

      (2) Mortality: 2 to 3%, depending on left ventricular function.
   b. After Discharge
      (1) Vein graft occlusion.　(2) Progressive coronary artery disease.

4. *Follow-up*
   a. Suggested Follow-up: The patient is seen at 4 weeks by the surgeon. Cardiac rehabilitation and periodic visits to the cardiologist are routine. Activities that can stress the sternal closure (i.e., driving, swimming, lifting) are restricted for 6 weeks.

PROCEDURE: INTERNAL CARDIOVERTER DEFIBRILLATOR IMPLANTATION

Overview: Implantation of an internal cardioverter defibrillator (ICD) is a rapidly changing technique. Currently, rate-sensing leads are placed transvenously into the right ventricle through the left subclavian vein. Two conducting electrodes are required and are placed around the heart through a subxiphoid, thoracotomy, or median sternotomy incision. A transvenous electrode coil placed in the superior vena cava can be substituted for one of the patches. The ICD is placed in a subcutaneous pocket in the left upper quadrant of the abdomen. The system is tested by inducing ventricular fibrillation and checking for appropriate system firing. Total transvenous systems are currently being developed. Cardiopulmonary bypass is not needed for ICD implantation.

1. *Operation*
    a. Indications: Patients at high risk for sudden death from ventricular arrhythmias refractory to either pharmacological or electrophysiological interventions. Exclusion criteria include life expectancy less than 6 months, recent myocardial infarction, or drug toxicity.
    b. Operative Steps: See description above.
    c. Incision: Incisions are left deltopectoral groove, ICD pocket in abdomen, and thoracotomy if necessary.
    d. Anesthesia: General.
    e. Intraoperative Monitoring: Arterial line with or without access to the central venous circulation.
    f. Operative Positioning: Supine with chest elevated slightly.
    g. Duration: 3 to 4 hours.
    h. EBL/Transfusions: EBL < 500 ml. Transfusions are not required.
    i. "Surgical Stress": Mild to moderate depending on number of defibrillations required to check function.

2. *Expected Hospital Course/Treatment*
    a. Postoperative Monitoring
        (1) ICU Stay: 1 to 2 days.
        (2) Invasive/Special Monitoring: Telemetry after discharge from the ICU.
        (3) Parameters To Be Monitored:
            i. Vital signs.
            ii. ECG.
            iii. Chest x-ray to check lead placement and for hemo/pneumothorax.
            iv. CBC.
    b. Positioning/Activity: Full ambulation as tolerated.
    c. Alimentation: As tolerated.
    d. Wound Care/Drains: Chest tubes, if present, are removed on POD 2.
    e. Respiratory Care: Extubation in the operating room.
    f. Analgesia/Postop Meds: Parenteral narcotics initially. Oral narcotics afterward.
    g. Length Of Hospital Stay: 5 to 10 days.

3. *Postoperative Complications*
    a. In Hospital
        (1) Morbidity:
            i. Right ventricular perforation.
            ii. Hemo/pneumothorax.
            iii. Lead displacement.
            iv. Phrenic nerve injury.
            v. Air embolism.
        (2) Mortality: 4 to 6%, depending on preoperative ventricular function.
    b. After Discharge
        (1) ICD lead malfunction.
        (2) ICD life: 50 shocks or 18 months.
        (3) Infection.

4. *Follow-up*
    a. Suggested Follow-up: ICD check at regular intervals. Generator change every 18 to 24 months. The patient is unable to drive or swim after ICD implantation. The family should be instructed in CPR emergency procedures.

PROCEDURE: MITRAL VALVE REPLACEMENT

Overview: Patients with mitral regurgitation should undergo surgery prior to the development of irreversible ventricular dysfunction. Mitral commissurotomy can be performed in most patients with mitral stenosis, but this option may be limited by technical factors (e.g., extensive calcification) or associated disease (e.g., mitral regurgitation). Commissurotomy carries a 20% reoperation rate after 5 years. Mitral annuloplasty may be appropriate for some patients with mitral regurgitation if calcification is not present. For valve replacement, mechanical or porcine xenograft valves are used. Right ventricular function is critical in weaning patients from bypass, especially in patients with pulmonary hypertension. Inotropic agents and afterload reduction are often needed.

1. *Operation*
   a. Indications: Replacement is performed when commissurotomy or repair is not possible. Mitral stenosis is primarily rheumatic in origin. Mitral regurgitation is due to myxomatous degeneration, chordae or papillary muscle dysfunction from ischemic disease, or endocarditis unresponsive to medical management.
   b. Operative Steps: See text for details regarding cardiopulmonary bypass. Exposure of the mitral valve is accomplished through the left atrium or through the atrial septum from the right atrium. The valve is excised, and calcium debrided. The posterior leaflet is left in place to decrease the incidence of myocardial dysfunction. Careful placement of pledgeted sutures is needed to avoid the conduction system, circumflex artery, and atrioventricular groove.
   c. Incision: Median sternotomy.
   d. Anesthesia: General.
   e. Intraoperative Monitoring: Arterial line and Swan-Ganz catheter; temperature probes in the esophagus, bladder, or rectum. Transesophageal echocardiography is especially important in deciding if the attempted repair was successful.
   f. Operative Positioning: Supine. It is also possible to use right lateral decubitus position and left thoracotomy for reoperations or difficult exposure.
   g. Duration: 4 to 6 hours, depending on the difficulty of exposure and right heart function.
   h. EBL/Transfusions: Same as CABG.
   i. "Surgical Stress": Severe.

2. *Expected Hospital Course/Treatment*
   a. Postoperative Monitoring
      (1) ICU Stay: 3 to 4 days.
      (2) Invasive/Special Monitoring: Same as CABG.
      (3) Parameters To Be Monitored: Same as CABG.
   b. Positioning/Activity: Same as CABG.
   c. Alimentation: Same as CABG.
   d. Wound Care/Drains: Same as CABG.
   e. Respiratory Care: Same as CABG.
   f. Analgesia/Postop Meds: Anticoagulation with warfarin is started in all patients on POD 3 to achieve elevation of the PT to 1.5 times normal. Mechanical valves require anticoagulation indefinitely, porcine valves for 3 to 6 months, mitral valve repair with normal sinus rhythm for 3 months.
   g. Length Of Hospital Stay: 7 to 10 days.

3. *Postoperative Complications*
   a. In Hospital
      (1) Morbidity:
         i. Right heart failure.
         ii. Bradycardia or AV block.
         iii. Cerebrovascular accident.
         iv. Atrioventricular disassociation with fatal posterior rupture.
         v. Others similar to CABG.
      (2) Mortality: 4 to 6%, higher with reoperations and ischemic dysfunction.
   b. After Discharge: Same as aortic valve replacement.

4. *Follow-up*
   a. Suggested Follow-up: Same as aortic valve replacement.

PROCEDURE: PERICARDIECTOMY

Overview: Pericardiectomy for effusion can be performed through a left thoracotomy (open or videoscopic) with removal of as much pericardium as possible and drainage to the pleural space. It can also be done through a subxiphoid approach between the phrenic nerves. Constrictive pericarditis requires median sternotomy with standby cardiopulmonary bypass if perforation should occur. The pericardium is usually densely adherent and may require removal of the top layer of epicardium. The left side is done first and then the right to prevent pulmonary edema. Underlying cardiomyopathic processes may necessitate support with inotropes or mechanical assistance.

1. *Operation*
    a. Indications:
        (1) Significant effusion with tamponade due to trauma, infections, neoplasms, uremia, or idopathic.
        (2) Significant hemodynamic compromise from chronic constrictive pericarditis.
    b. Operative Steps: See description above.
    c. Incision: Left anterior thoracotomy, subxiphoid, or median sternotomy.
    d. Anesthesia: General.
    e. Intraoperative Monitoring: Arterial line, CVP with or without Swan-Ganz catheter.
    f. Operative Positioning: Supine. Patient discomfort due to dyspnea may require head elevation to 30 degrees.
    g. Duration: 1 hour for effusive pericarditis, 2 to 3 hours for constrictive pericarditis depending on degree of adherence of the pericardium to the heart.
    h. EBL/Transfusions: Blood conservation with cell saver and reinfusion of shed mediastinal blood are used. EBL should be < 500 ml. Constrictive pericarditis may require blood transfusion.
    i. "Surgical Stress": Moderate to severe depending on difficulty of case.

2. Expected Hospital Course/Treatment
    a. Postoperative Monitoring
        (1) ICU Stay: 1 to 2 days.
        (2) Invasive/Special Monitoring: Arterial line and CVP catheter for 1 to 2 days. Telemetry after discharge from ICU.
        (3) Parameters To Be Monitored:
            i. Vital signs.
            ii. Urine output.
            iii. Chest x-ray.
            iv. ECG.
            v. CBC.
            vi. Arterial blood gases.
    b. Positioning/Activity: Out of bed with progressive ambulation after invasive monitoring lines are removed.
    c. Alimentation: Oral intake is started one day after extubation and increased as tolerated.
    d. Wound Care/Drains: Chest tubes removed on POD 1 to 2 when drainage is decreased.
    e. Respiratory Care: Extubation in operating room, if possible.
    f. Analgesia/Postop Meds: Parenteral narcotics followed by oral agents as soon as possible.
    g. Length Of Hospital Stay: 7 to 10 days.

3. *Postoperative Complications*
    a. In Hospital
        (1) Morbidity:
            i. Congestive heart failure from inability of heart to handle increased blood return.
            ii. Bleeding.
            iii. Atrial arrhythmias.
            iv. Postpericardiotomy syndrome.
            v. Mediastinitis.
        (2) Mortality: 1 to 2%, higher with constrictive pericarditis.
    b. After Discharge:
        (1) Arrhythmias.
        (2) Persistent pericarditis.

4. *Follow-up*
    a. Suggested Follow-up: Echocardiogram as indicated to check for evidence of tamponade. Periodic visits with cardiologist.

PROCEDURE: PERMANENT PACEMAKER IMPLANTATION

Overview: Permanent pacemakers may be transvenous endocardial or epicardial systems. Simplistically, they consist of an afferent sensing lead and an efferent stimulating lead. These are very short in the epicardial variety and incorporated into a single long cable in the transvenous variety. The computer/battery pack senses the cardiac rate, firing at a nonexcitable time when the rate is too low and remaining in a sensing mode when the rate is above the set threshold. The output of the pacemaker is set at a level which ensures capture.

1. *Operation*
   a. Indications:
      (1) Symptomatic sick sinus syndrome.
      (2) Varying degrees of heart block.
      (3) Atrial fibrillation with slow ventricular response.
   b. Operative Steps: Endocardial access is gained to the right atrium and ventricle through the cephalic, subclavian, jugular, or femoral veins. Leads are placed in the appropriate chambers (i.e., ventricle, atrium, or both). Threshold and sensing data are obtained, and, when satisfactory, the leads are secured. The pacemaker is inserted into a subcutaneous pocket. Epicardial access is used when there are anomalous connections that prevent right atrium and ventricular access. Leads are screwed onto the heart, and are brought into a subcutaneous pocket and secured.
   c. Incision: Endocardial: right or left delto-pectoral groove. Epicardial: thoracotomy or subxiphoid approach.
   d. Anesthesia: Endocardial: local with IV sedation. Epicardial: general.
   e. Intraoperative Monitoring: Routine.
   f. Operative Positioning: Supine.
   g. Duration: 1 to 2 hours.
   h. EBL/Transfusions: EBL should be < 500 ml. Transfusion is not required.
   i. "Surgical Stress": Low.

2. *Expected Hospital Course/Treatment*
   a. Postoperative Monitoring
      (1) ICU Stay: 1 to 2 days for epicardial approach.
      (2) Invasive/Special Monitoring: Telemetry to monitor pacemaker function.
      (3) Parameters To Be Monitored:
         i. ECG.
         ii. Chest x-ray to check lead placement and for hemo/pneumothorax.
   b. Positioning/Activity: Full ambulation as tolerated.
   c. Alimentation: As tolerated.
   d. Wound Care/Drains: No drains are required.
   e. Respiratory Care: Routine.
   f. Analgesia/Postop Meds: Oral agents are satisfactory.
   g. Length Of Hospital Stay: 1 day.

3. *Postoperative Complications*
   a. In Hospital
      (1) Morbidity:
         i. Right ventricular perforation and/or tamponade.
         ii. Ventricular fibrillation.
         iii. Lead displacement.
         iv. Hemo/pneumothorax.
      (2) Mortality: < 0.5%.
   b. After Discharge
      (1) Exit block (increasing threshold as electrodes cause fibrosis).
      (2) Pacemaker syndrome.
      (3) Pacemaker dysfunction.
      (4) Infection of pacemaker leads.

4. *Follow-up*
   a. Suggested Follow-up: Pacemaker check at regular intervals. Lifetime bacterial endocarditis prophylaxis.

PROCEDURE: PNEUMONECTOMY

Overview: It is now recognized that many lung tumors previously treated with pneumonectomy are adequately treated with lobectomy or even nonanatomic wedge resection. Pneumonectomy is currently performed when an otherwise resectable primary tumor involves the hilar structures. In most cases, pneumonectomy is not indicated simply as a means of increasing the extent of nodal resection. Preoperative pulmonary function tests (PFT's) are essential prior to a planned pneumonectomy. Right pneumonectomy removes more functioning parenchyma than left pneumonectomy and carries a higher mortality rate. Patients with borderline PFT's or a history of pulmonary hypertension have an especially high risk.

1. *Operation*
   a. Indications:
      (1) Malignant neoplasms involving hilar structures making lobectomy not feasible.
      (2) Rarely for benign lesions such as tuberculosis, trauma, or persistent bronchopleural fistula after lobectomy.
   b. Operative Steps: The pleural space is entered either after resection of a rib or through an interspace. Control of the main pulmonary artery and venous branches is obtained. Intrapericardial dissection may be required. The mainstem bronchus is stapled and divided. Mediastinal lymph node dissection may be required for staging neoplasms. Chest tubes are usually not placed. Air is added to or removed from the hemithorax depending on the position of the mediastinum on chest x-ray. A chest tube may be placed with balanced drainage to allow escape or entry of air to keep the mediastinum midline.
   c. Incision: Posteriolateral or lateral thoracotomy.
   d. Anesthesia: General with double lumen endotracheal tube. Epidural anesthesia for postoperative pain control optional.
   e. Intraoperative Monitoring: Arterial line.
   f. Operative Positioning: Lateral decubitus with lesion side anterior.
   g. Duration: 2 to 3 hours.
   h. EBL/Transfusions: EBL should be < 500 ml. Transfusion is not required.
   i. "Surgical Stress": Moderate.

2. *Expected Hospital Course/Treatment*
   a. Postoperative Monitoring
      (1) ICU Stay: 1 to 2 days.
      (2) Invasive/Special Monitoring: Invasive monitors remain in place while in ICU.
      (3) Parameters To Be Monitored:
         i. Chest x-ray to follow mediastinal position and status of pneumonectomy space.
         ii. Arterial blood gases.
         iii. CBC.
         iv. ECG.
         v. Fluid balance (should be negative in the first 24 to 48 hours to avoid pulmonary edema).
   b. Positioning/Activity: Full ambulation as tolerated.
   c. Alimentation: As tolerated.
   d. Wound Care/Drains: Chest tubes not routinely placed after pneumonectomy. Based on postoperative chest x-ray and mediastinal shift, it may be necessary to inject or aspirate air into the operated chest.
   e. Respiratory Care: Extubation in operating room, if possible. Change to single-lumen endotracheal tube if mechanical ventilation needed. Chest physiotherapy encouraged.
   f. Analgesia/Postop Meds: Epidural analgesia or parenteral narcotics are required initially. Oral narcotics may be substituted in 2 to 3 days.
   g. Length Of Hospital Stay: 7 to 14 days.

3. *Postoperative Complications*
   a. In Hospital
      (1) Morbidity:
         i. Cardiac herniation through pericardial defect.
         ii. Atrial arrhythmias.
         iii. Phrenic/vagus nerve injury.
         iv. Thoracic duct injury.
         v. Empyema.
         vi. Bronchopleural fistula.
      (2) Mortality: 5 to 10%.
   b. After Discharge
      (1) Bronchopleural fistula.
      (2) Empyema.
      (3) Arrhythmias.

4. *Follow-up*
   a. Suggested Follow-up: 1 month with surgeon. Oncology follow-up if neoplasm is present.

PROCEDURE: PULMONARY LOBECTOMY

Overview: Pulmonary lobectomy is most commonly performed for nonsmall cell lung cancer. It is usually an adequate cancer operation and preserves significant pulmonary parenchyma. Stapling instruments have made the operation easier and safer. Preoperative pulmonary function tests are helpful because a pneumonectomy may be required for technical reasons. This operation has been done laparoscopically.

1. *Operation*
    a. Indications:
        (1) Benign and malignant neoplasms.
        (2) Refractory lung abscess.
        (3) Residual bronchiectasis.
        (4) Pulmonary sequestration.
        (5) Persistent pulmonary tuberculosis.
        (6) Hemoptysis of multiple etiologies.
    b. Operative Steps: The pleural space is entered either after resection of a rib or through an interspace. Control of the arterial and venous structures of the respective lobe is obtained, and the bronchus is stapled and divided. Mediastinal lymph node dissection may be required for staging neoplasms. Chest tubes are placed to evacuate air and blood and allow lung expansion.
    d. Anesthesia: General with double-lumen endotracheal tube. Epidural anesthesia for postoperative pain control optional.
    e. Intraoperative Monitoring: Arterial line.
    f. Operative Positioning: Lateral decubitus with lesion side anterior.
    g. Duration: 2 to 3 hours.
    h. EBL/Transfusions: EBL should be < 500 ml. Transfusion is not required.
    i. "Surgical Stress": Low to moderate depending on length of procedure and underlying illness.

2. *Expected Hospital Course/Treatment*
    a. Postoperative Monitoring
        (1) ICU Stay: 1 to 2 days.
        (2) Invasive/Special Monitoring: Telemetry after discharge from the ICU.
        (3) Parameters To Be Monitored:
            i. Chest x-ray to follow lung expansion, presence of infiltrates, or effusions.
            ii. Arterial blood gases.
            iii. ECG.
            iv. CBC.
    b. Positioning/Activity: Full ambulation as tolerated.
    c. Alimentation: As tolerated.
    d. Wound Care/Drains: Chest tubes removed after air leak stops and less than 100 ml drainage accumulates over 8 hours.
    e. Respiratory Care: Extubation in operating room, if possible. Change to single-lumen endotracheal tube if mechanical ventilation is needed. Chest physiotherapy encouraged.
    f. Analgesia/Postop Meds: Epidural analgesia or parenteral narcotics are required initially. Oral narcotics may be substituted in 2 to 3 days.
    g Length Of Hospital Stay: 7 to 10 days.

3. *Postoperative Complications*
    a. In Hospital
        (1) Morbidity: Same as pneumonectomy.
        (2) Mortality: 1 to 3%, higher if done as emergency for massive hemoptysis.
    b. After Discharge: Same as Pneumonectomy.

4. *Follow-up*
    a. Suggested Follow-up: 1 month with surgeon. Oncology follow-up if neoplasm is present.

9 EVALUATION OF THE PATIENT UNDERGOING VASCULAR SURGERY

Rosanne Granieri

John White

Connie Campbell

Atherosclerotic vascular disease of the lower extremity affects 10 to 15 percent of patients in the United States over age 50, although only approximately 3 percent are symptomatic. Approximately 2 percent of elderly persons have abdominal aortic aneurysms (AAA) with a prevalence rate of 350/100,000 in those over 60. The incidence of AAA in patients with lower extremity atherosclerotic vascular disease is five times higher than in the general population. Cerebrovascular disease is the third leading cause of death in the United States with an overall prevalence of 794/100,000.

Though the majority of patients with lower extremity atherosclerotic occlusive disease do not require reconstructive vascular surgery, the sheer magnitude of the problem and the inevitable presence of common comorbid medical conditions often require medical evaluation. Approximately 40,000 AAAs are resected annually. Carotid endarterectomy is gaining more support in the treatment of both symptomatic and asymptomatic cerebrovascular disease, based on recent data from ongoing clinical trials. Alternatively, percutaneous peripheral balloon angioplasty has become more popular in managing some patients with advanced peripheral vascular disease. In selected patients, it may be the procedure of choice and has proven relatively effective and safe.[1]

Patients undergoing vascular surgery usually fall into one of three categories. The first includes asymptomatic patients with incidentally discovered disease, e.g., asymptomatic AAA or carotid artery stenosis. The second category includes those with known peripheral vascular disease who remain symptomatic despite medical treatment or modification of risk factors, e.g., intermittent claudication or a nonhealing vascular ulcer. The third involves patients who present with threatened life or limb, e.g., ruptured aortic aneurysm, acute lower extremity arterial occlusion, or vascular trauma. Careful risk-benefit analysis more often enters into the preoperative evaluation of the first two groups and forms the bulk of the discussion in this chapter.

Preoperative evaluation and postoperative care of patients with vascular surgery must consider not only the specific medical problems of the individual patient but also the reason for the surgery, the details of the surgical procedure, and the complications associated with preoperative invasive testing. All of these issues must be weighed in choosing the optimal course, and patients should be actively involved in the decision process whenever possible. Data are available to guide some strategies, but individual variation frequently reflects the practice style and expertise of the internist, surgeon, and/or anesthesiologist as well as the available technology at a given institution.

COMORBID MEDICAL CONDITIONS

Cardiovascular Disease

Cardiovascular disease is the leading cause of postoperative and long-term mortality in patients requiring surgery for atherosclerotic peripheral vascular disease. In the largest series of patients undergoing routine preoperative coronary angiography before vascular surgery, only 8 percent of patients had normal coronary arteries.[2] The presence or absence of cardiac symptoms or ECG changes did not absolutely predict the presence or absence of significant coronary artery disease as revealed by catheterization. Thus, patients requiring peripheral vascular surgery constitute a selected population with a high risk of significant coronary artery disease.

Pulmonary Disease

About 80 percent of patients with peripheral vascular disease are past or current smokers.[3] Smoking is the strongest independent risk factor in the development of atherosclerotic peripheral vascular disease of the lower extremities. Smoking is also a well-recognized risk factor in the development of chronic obstructive pulmonary disease and postoperative pulmonary complications. Pulmonary risk is increased in patients who require an upper abdominal incision for certain aortic procedures. This clinical scenario may explain the high rate of major and minor postoperative pulmonary complications. In a recent study, 53 percent of 151 patients undergoing aortic, carotid, and lower extremity vascular procedures developed major and minor postoperative respiratory complications.[4]

Hypertension

Hypertension significantly increases the risk of developing peripheral vascular disease.[3] The risk of perioperative complications imposed by elevated blood pressure is discussed in Chap. 17.

Diabetes Mellitus

Approximately 20 percent of patients with peripheral vascular disease have previously diagnosed diabetes mellitus.[3] Though the contribution of diabetic control during the perioperative period to operative risk is controversial, diabetic-related end-organ dysfunction is important in perioperative management. For example, patients with diabetes and especially those with preexisting renal insufficiency have an increased risk of contrast media–induced nephropathy.[5] This becomes a major issue since the evaluation of peripheral arterial disease usually requires preoperative visualization with contrast media.

Cerebrovascular Disease

One study estimates that 10 percent of patients with lower extremity arterial disease have concurrent cerebrovascular disease,[3] but prevalence rates vary depending on the definition of disease. The approach to surgical patients with cerebrovascular disease is fully discussed in Chap. 35 and its relationship to peripheral vascular disease below.

Hyperlipidemia

Hyperlipidemia is present in about one-third of patients with peripheral vascular disease.[3] Though the importance of hyperlipidemia centers around its long-term role in the pathogenesis of atherosclerosis, identification is helpful to guide postsurgical risk modification with dietary and/or pharmacologic measures.

Age

The incidence of atherosclerotic peripheral vascular disease increases with advancing age. In some studies, age over 70 years is an independent risk factor for postoperative cardiac complications.[6] Age-associated changes in the cardiovascular system may be responsible for subclinical cardiac disease which is often unmasked by the stresses of surgery. Insufficient cardiovascular compensatory mechanisms in the elderly are well-described,[7] and these may make them more vulnerable to hemodynamic changes associated with vascular procedures like aortic crossclamping.

Surgical Procedures

Abdominal Aortic Crossclamping. In patients with impaired cardiac reserve, hemodynamic changes associated with abdominal aortic crossclamping may contribute to cardiac complications. Aortic crossclamping may cause increased systemic vascular resistance, decreased cardiac output, and decrease in stroke volume.[8,9] These changes may be exaggerated in patients with coronary artery disease[9] and tilt the balance unfavorably with respect to myocardial oxygen supply/demand, ultimately leading to myocardial ischemia. However, clamp time has not been identified as an independent predictor of postoperative renal failure.[10]

Mesenteric Traction. Decreases in systemic vascular resistance and mean arterial pressures have been documented with mesenteric traction.[11] These hemodynamic changes may lead to adverse cardiac outcomes.

Abdominal Incision. Vertical upper abdominal incisions necessary for aortic procedures increase the risk of postoperative pulmonary complications.

Location of Surgical Field. Abdominal aneurysms may involve the main or accessory renal arteries, and concomitant renal artery stenosis may exist in 5 percent of patients with AAA. In a recent review, 7 percent of patients undergoing extensive thoracoabdominal aneurysm resection and 17 percent of those with preexisting renal insufficiency developed acute renal failure requiring hemodialysis.[10] Since renal blood flow is pressure-dependent, preventive strategies center on volume expansion and optimization of perioperative hemodynamics. Renal hypothermia, mannitol, vasodilatory prostaglandins, angiotensin-converting enzyme inhibitors, and intraarterial verapamil have also been used. Invasive hemodynamic monitoring is justified in certain individuals, especially if preoperative renal insufficiency exists.

PREOPERATIVE EVALUATION OF PATIENTS UNDERGOING VASCULAR SURGERY

A good history and physical examination are essential in all patients being considered for peripheral vascular surgery with emphasis on elucidation of signs and symptoms of cardiopulmonary disease. Concerns specific to peripheral vascular surgery follow.

Cardiac Disease

Because of the high probability of underlying coronary artery disease and its impact on surgical morbidity and mortality, further cardiac evaluation beyond the history, physical examination, and resting electrocardiogram should always be considered. Clinical indices like those developed by Goldman and Detsky are less sensitive in predicting postoperative cardiac complications in patients with vascular disease.[6,12] These indices, derived and validated in patients with variable risk of coronary artery disease, underestimate cardiac complications in those undergoing vascular surgery. Detsky et al. attempted to compensate for this by factoring in the probability of postoperative complications based on the type of procedure.

Additional noninvasive cardiac testing successfully identifies patients with low cardiac risk. Those without clinical coronary artery disease or significant ventricular impairment on noninvasive testing experience relatively low surgical mortality. Identifying these patients is therefore helpful in assessing risk/benefit, counseling patients, and planning perioperative care. Noninvasive testing can identify patients with high risk who may benefit from preoperative cardiac catheterization and, if needed, coronary artery revascularization. Patients who survive coronary artery bypass grafting have a low mortality rate when undergoing subsequent peripheral vascular surgery, and some have a lower long-term mortality rate. Noninvasive testing may also identify patients with "prohibitive risk" and provide a rationale for more conservative management.

Though several diagnostic modalities are available, the most widely studied in patients undergoing vascular surgery is intravenous dipyridamole-thallium scintigraphy (DTS).[13–18] Adenosine performs as well as dipyridamole but is less well-studied. DTS does not require exercise and can therefore be useful in patients with claudication or prior lower extremity amputation. Reperfusion abnormalities on DTS imply ischemic myocardium ("myocardium at risk") and identify patients with a higher risk of postoperative cardiac events.

Pharmacologic stress testing with thallium has high negative predictive value. However, because its positive predictive value ranges only from 10 to 40 percent, a positive result is less useful. Quantification of reperfusion deficits may aid in enhancing positive predictive value.[15,16] Recently, Lette et al. developed a model designed to improve the accuracy of DTS in predicting postoperative events in patients undergoing vascular and nonvascular surgery.[17] A normal study conferred a 1.3 percent risk of cardiac events. Reversible defects in three segments, transient ventricular dilation, or more than one severe reversible defect were associated with a rate of 52 percent. Patients over 70 with two segments showing reperfusion abnormalities had a rate of 36 percent, and those under 70 with diabetes had a rate of 17 percent. Patients under 70 without diabetes had a lower rate of 8 percent.

Eagle et al. developed clinical criteria that identified a subgroup of patients in whom DTS was most useful, including patients with one or two of the following predictors: age over 70, diabetes mellitus, angina, ventricular ectopy requiring treatment, and Q-waves on the electrocardiogram.[18] Patients with only one or no criteria did well in surgery despite whatever was found on DTS, and those with three or more had a postsurgical cardiac event rate of 50 percent. Selective use of DTS has also been advocated by Madsen et al. who found DTS helpful in stratifying operative risk only in patients with clinical markers of ischemic heart disease.[19]

Contraindications to the use of dipyridamole or adenosine scintigraphy include unstable angina and severe bronchospastic lung disease. The elevated adenosine levels caused by either of these drugs can precipitate bronchospasm in predisposed individuals. Bronchospasm is promptly relieved by intravenous aminophylline. Aminophylline preparations should be discontinued 24 to 36 hours before the test, and caffeine should be omitted two to four hours beforehand.

In the 1990s, studies challenging the diagnostic accuracy of DTS in predicting postoperative cardiac complications in patients undergoing vascular surgery have appeared. Mangano et al. reported that seven of 13 postoperative cardiac events occurred in patients with a normal DTS.[20] Discrepancies among studies may be due to differences in study populations (referral bias), differences in the observer blinding, and small numbers of patients and adverse events.

Other modalities used to assess preoperative risk include radio-nuclide ventriculography;[21,22] ambulatory or perioperative electrocardiography;[23–26] thallium imaging after atrial pacing;[27] stress echocardiography with adenosine, dipyridamole, and dobutamine;[28] and perioperative transesophageal echocardiography.[29,30] Though all different, they share with DTS an impressive negative but weaker positive predictive value. Routine exercise testing obviously has a limited role in the preoperative evaluation of these patients because of the inability of most of them to perform adequately on the treadmill. Large-scale randomized controlled clinical trials comparing various testing modalities are lacking, and choice of initial study is influenced significantly by availability and expertise. However, the strongest data support the selected use of dipyridamole scintigraphy, using clinical criteria to select those patients most likely to benefit.

A negative test assures the physician of lower risk. Reperfusion abnormality on DTS, significant ischemic changes on ambulatory monitoring, or persistent wall motion abnormalities on stress echocardiography suggest a higher risk of postoperative cardiac complications. With this information the clinician can reassess the risks and benefits of surgery and consider continued conservative management; consider the feasibility of a less-extensive surgical procedure; proceed with cardiac catheterization to determine the extent of coronary artery disease and the need for coronary artery bypass grafting (CABG) or percutaneous transluminal coronary angioplasty (PTCA); or proceed with surgery with intense hemodynamic and electrocardiographic monitoring and intravenous anti-ischemic therapy.

The decision to proceed with cardiac catheterization and possible CABG or PTCA in the patients contemplating aortic or infraaortic peripheral vascular or carotid surgery must balance the benefits of further cardiac evaluation and treatment against the risk of delaying vascular surgery, the morbidity and mortality of the catheterization, and the morbidity and mortality of CABG or PTCA itself. In favor of further invasive evaluation is the fact that patients who survive CABG tolerate subsequent vascular surgery well, with mortality rates of 0 to 1 percent compared with 0 to 17 percent in those with coronary artery disease who do not undergo CABG.[31] Long-term survival may be improved in patients with vascular disease who undergo CABG.[32] Those with three-vessel or left main coronary artery disease and mild left ventricular impairment who undergo CABG have improved long-term survival.

Prophylactic PTCA of significant coronary artery lesions is an attractive option, but its role remains unclear in the preoperative management of patients with peripheral vascular disease. It often obviates major cardiac surgery and allows the nonvascular surgery to proceed more quickly. In a recent study, 50 patients with coronary artery disease underwent successful PTCA and then noncardiac surgery with a mortality rate of 1.9 percent. Perioperative myocardial infarctions occurred in 5.6 percent of the patients, but none occurred in patients who had undergone vascular surgery.[33] The long-term benefits of PTCA in these patients are still uncertain.

There are several disadvantages to performing an invasive cardiac evaluation in patients with peripheral vascular disease. First, delaying vascular surgery risks advancing symptomatic peripheral vascular disease including possible cerebrovascular accident and, in patients with abdominal aortic aneurysms, spontaneous rupture. In one series, 3 percent of patients had spontaneous rupture of an AAA while undergoing CABG.[2] Second, limited data support an increase in mortality after cardiac catheterization in patients with peripheral vascular disease.[34] Morbidity may also be increased and is most likely related to generalized atherosclerosis. For example, five of eight patients who developed cholesterol emboli syndrome after coronary artery angiography had known peripheral vascular disease.[35] Those who have diabetes have a higher risk of contrast media–induced renal failure.[5] Finally, larger studies show that mortality rates during CABG are higher in patients with peripheral vascular disease than those without. In a recent retrospective analysis of 5051 patients undergoing CABG, prior vascular surgery was one of nine independent risk factors for increased operative mortality.[36] Finally, the risks of PTCA in this population are those associated with any arterial catheterization and include cholesterol emboli, contrast media–induced renal failure, and occlusion of the angioplasty site sometimes requiring emergency CABG.

In summary, the data indicate that the mortality from prophylactic CABG offsets the improved survival expected from subsequent vascular surgery. However, if one survives the CABG, the prognosis of subsequent vascular surgery is better. It is therefore reasonable to consider CABG if the patient meets traditional criteria for improved long-term survival or if angina is refractory to medical therapy. PTCA holds promise in the preoperative management of selected patients, but further study is required.

Cerebrovascular Disease

Several studies document an increased risk of cerebrovascular accident (CVA) in patients undergoing major vascular and coronary artery bypass surgery independent of the presence or absence of carotid bruit. Most of these studies place the risk of CVA in these patients at about 15 percent.[37–39] A notable exception is the prospective study of Barnes in which 31 of 314 asymptomatic patients with a carotid stenosis of more than 50 percent detected by noninvasive means underwent coronary or peripheral arterial surgery without prophylactic endarterectomy.[40] None of those with significant disease had a postoperative stroke. However, total mortality was higher in the affected patients because of an increased incidence of myocardial infarction.

The etiology of many postoperative cerebrovascular accidents in these patients is thought to be embolic from polyvinyl tubing, silicone, air, or atheromas.[39] The role of carotid endarterectomy to decrease the risk of CVA is unclear in this population. Newer surgical techniques may decrease embolic phenomena and improve outcome. The decision to proceed with prophylactic staged carotid surgery before CABG or major vascular surgery should probably be based on evolving criteria for carotid endarterectomy discussed in Chap. 35.[40] Simultaneous carotid and coronary artery bypass surgery in one multicenter retrospective review was associated with a combined stroke-death rate of 13.3 percent and is now rarely performed.[41]

Pulmonary Disease

Patients with vascular disease have a high risk of underlying pulmonary disease and postoperative pulmonary complications. A recent study found that patients with vascular disease with $FEV_1 < 2.0$ liters or $FEV_1/FVC < 0.65$ had a higher risk of complications.[42] Prophylactic measures including smoking cessation and incentive spirometry before and after surgery are recommended as discussed in Chaps. 22 and 47.

Prophylactic Issues

Endocarditis Prophylaxis. The American Heart Association recommends antibiotic prophylaxis for patients who undergo placement of prosthetic intravascular materials.[43] A first-generation cephalosporin is usually recommended. In addition, certain cardiac conditions merit prophylaxis regardless of whether prosthetic material is inserted. These recommendations are discussed in Chap. 43.

Surgical Infection Prophylaxis. Postoperative infections are reduced in patients undergoing arterial reconstructive surgery of the abdominal aorta, lower extremity arterial reconstruction with a groin incision, lower extremity amputation due to arterial ischemia, and insertion of vascular prostheses by the prophylactic administration of a parenteral first-generation cephalosporin before surgery.[44]

Deep Venous Thrombosis (DVT) Prophylaxis. Most patients requiring peripheral vascular surgery have at least one risk factor for the development of postoperative thromboembolic disease. Vascular surgery itself has not been identified as a risk factor. If vascular hemostasis has been achieved, prophylaxis with subcutaneous heparin is reasonable. If hemostasis cannot be assured after placement of a prosthesis, low-dose heparin should be used with caution. The risk of infection may be increased in the presence of a hematoma. DVT prophylaxis is discussed in detail in Chap. 48.

Intraoperative Hemodynamic Monitoring and Vasodilator/Antianginal Therapy

Since myocardial ischemia increases the risk of postoperative cardiac events, several therapeutic regimens have been recommended to manage perioperative ischemia. Beta-blockers may reduce ischemic episodes in patients undergoing peripheral vascular and coronary artery bypass surgery, probably by preventing tachycardia-induced ischemia.[45,46] Whether this effect translates into reduced rates of cardiac death or postoperative myocardial infarction is unknown. Calcium channel blockers do not appear to reduce the incidence of ischemic episodes in these patients,[46,47] and the role of nitrates is unclear. Some data suggest that intraoperative invasive monitoring allowing minute-to-minute maintenance of hemodynamic stability may reduce mortality.

POSTOPERATIVE COMPLICATIONS

Cardiac Complications

The leading cause of death in patients undergoing peripheral vascular surgery is cardiac arrest, usually due to myocardial infarction. The most sensitive and specific strategy for diagnosing myocardial infarction in the postoperative period is to obtain electrocardiograms on the day of surgery, the first and second postoperative day, and when symptoms suggesting ischemia occur.[48] CPK isoenzyme levels should be checked when suspicious electrocardiographic changes are noted or episodes of chest pain occur.

Cholesterol Crystal Emboli

Cholesterol emboli syndrome can occur after any invasive procedure of the vascular tree. Cholesterol crystal emboli should be suspected in those undergoing vascular procedures who later develop acute renal failure and cutaneous lesions resembling livedo reticularis. Other visceral, gastrointestinal, and central nervous system manifestations may occur. Laboratory abnormalities are often nonspecific[35,49] and include an elevated sedimentation rate in many cases. Biopsy of an affected organ is usually diagnostic. Treatment with various modalities including stopping or starting heparin, steroids, or antiplatelet agents is usually unsatisfactory. Mortality is high and largely due to multiorgan failure. Supportive therapy may include dialysis.

Renal Failure

Postoperative renal failure in patients undergoing vascular surgery has multiple etiologies. Relevant considerations include intraoperative renal artery ligation, cholesterol emboli (as discussed above), and intravenous contrast media injury. The role of decreased renal artery perfusion pressure in patients undergoing thoracoabdominal aortic aneurysm surgery is discussed above.[10]

Contrast media–induced renal failure is particularly common in patients with diabetes mellitus and preexisting renal insufficiency. Compiled data reveal a risk of 3.6 percent in diabetics with serum creatinine level peaks within four days after the procedure and generally returns to normal within 10 days. Dialysis may be needed temporarily. Contrast procedures should be avoided whenever possible or spaced appropriately in high-risk patients. Assuring adequate hydration and discontinuing nonsteroidal anti-inflammatory agents are prudent adjunctive measures. The use of mannitol is controversial and not universally recommended. The risk of low-osmolality contrast media appears to be similar to that of high-osmolality agents except possibly in patients with preexisting renal insufficiency.[50] Although routine use of low-osmolality agents is not recommended because of its high cost, targeted use in high-risk patients should be considered.

Other

Other

Infection of artificial prostheses is a serious complication of vascular surgery usually caused by *S. aureus* and may require removal of the prosthetic material. Data on the effectiveness of prophylactic antibiotics is discussed above and in Chap. 44. Mesenteric ischemia and ischemic injury of the spinal cord are rare but potentially catastrophic complications of aneurysm repair. Impotence may occur in up to 15 percent of patients after repair of abdominal aortic aneurysms and is presumed due to dissection of the periaortic and peri-iliac sympathetic nerves.

REFERENCES

1. Belli AM, Cumberland DC, Know AM et al: The complication rate of percutaneous peripheral balloon angioplasty. *Clin Rad* 41:380–383, 1990.
2. Hertzer NR, Beven EG, Young JR et al: Coronary artery disease in peripheral vascular patients. *Ann Surg* 199:223–233, 1984.
3. Criqui MH, Browner D, Fronerk A et al: Peripheral arterial disease in large vessels is epidemiologically distinct from small vessel disease; an analysis of risk factors. *Am J Epidemiol* 129:1110–1119, 1989.
4. Vodinh J, Bonnet F, Rouboul C et al: Risk factors of postoperative pulmonary complications after vascular surgery. *Surgery* 105:360–365, 1989.
5. Berns AS: Nephrotoxicity of contrast media. *Kid Int* 36:730–740, 1989.
6. Goldman L, Caldera DL, Nussbaum SR et al: Multifactorial index of cardiac risk in noncardic surgical procedures. *N Engl J Med* 297:845–850, 1977.
7. Wiei JY: Age and the cardiovascular system. *N Engl J Med* 327:1735–1739, 1992.
8. Attia R, Murphy JD, Snider M et al: Myocardial ischemia due to infrarenal aortic crossclamping during aortic surgery in patients with severe coronary artery disease. *Circulation* 53:961–965, 1976.
9. Gooding JM, Archie JP, McDowell H: Hemodynamic response to infrarenal aortic crossclamping in patients with and without coronary artery disease. *Crit Care Med* 8:382–385, 1980.
10. Miller DC, Myers BD: Pathophysiology and prevention of acute renal failure associated with thoracoabdominal or abdominal aortic surgery. *J Vasc Surg* 5:518–523, 1987.
11. Seltzer JL, Ritter DE, Starsnic MA et al: The hemodynamic response to traction on the abdominal mesentery. *Anesthesiology* 63:96–99, 1985.
12. Detsky AL, Abrams HB, McLaughlin JR et al: Predicting cardiac complications in patients undergoing noncardiac surgery. *J Gen Intern Med* 1:211–219, 1986.
13. Boucher CA, Brewster DC, Darling RC et al: Determination of cardiac risk by dipyridamole-thallium imaging before peripheral vascular surgery. *N Engl J Med* 312:389–394, 1985.
14. Leppo J, Plaja J, Cirnet M et al: Noninvasive evaluation of cardiac risk before elective vascular surgery. *J Am Coll Cardiol* 9:269–276, 1987.
15. Lette J, Waters D, Lapointe J et al: Usefulness of the severity and extent of reversible perfusion defects during thallium-dipyridamole imaging for cardiac risk assessment before noncardiac surgery. *Am J Cardiol* 64:276–281, 1989.
16. Lane SE, Lewis SM, Pippin JJ et al: Predictive value of quantitative dipyridamole-thallium scintigraphy in assessing cardiovascular risk after vascular surgery in diabetes mellitus. *Am J Cardiol* 64:1275–1279, 1989.
17. Lette J, Waters D, Cerino M et al: Preoperative coronary artery disease risk stratification based upon dipyridamole imaging and a simple three-step, three-segment model for patients undergoing noncardiac vascular surgery or major general surgery. *Am J Cardiol* 69:1553–1558, 1992.
18. Eagle KA, Coley CM, Newell JB et al: Combining clinical and thallium data optimizes preoperative assessment of cardiac risk before major vascular surgery. *Ann Intern Med* 110:859–866, 1989.
19. Madsen PV, Vissing M, Munck O et al: A comparison of dipyridamole thallium-201 scintigraphy and clinical examination in the determination of cardiac risk before arterial reconstruction. *Angiology* 43:306–311, 1992.
20. Mangano DT, London MJ, Tubau JF et al: Dipyridamole thallium-201 scintigraphy as a preoperative screening test. A reexamination of its predictive potential. *Circulation* 84:493–502, 1991.
21. Kazmers A, Moneta GL, Cerqueira MD et al: The role of preoperative radionuclide ventriculography in defining outcome after revascularization of the lower extremity. *Surg Gynecol Obstet* 171:481–488, 1990.
22. Mosely JG, Clarke JMF, Ell PH et al: Assessment of myocardial function before aortic surgery by radionuclide angiocardiography. *Br J Surg* 72:886–887, 1985.

23. Raby KE, Goldman L, Creager MA et al: Correlation between preoperative ischemia and major cardiac events after peripheral vascular surgery. *N Engl J Med* 321:1296–1300, 1989.

24. Pasternack PR, Grossi EA, Baumann FG et al: The value of silent myocardial ischemia monitoring in the prediction of perioperative myocardial infarction in patients undergoing peripheral vascular surgery. *J Vasc Surg* 10:617–625, 1989.

25. Ouyang P, Gerstenblith G, Furman WR et al: Frequency and significance of early postoperative myocardial ischemia in patients having peripheral vascular surgery. *Am J Cardiol* 64:1113–1116, 1989.

26. Raby KE, Barry J, Creager MA et al: Detection and significance of intraoperative and postoperative myocardial ischemia in peripheral vascular surgery. *JAMA* 268:222–227, 1992.

27. Stratmann HG, Mark AL, Walter KE et al: Preoperative evaluation of cardiac risk by means of atrial pacing and thallium-201 scintigraphy. *J Vasc Surg* 10:385–391, 1989.

28. Martin TW, Seaworth JF, Johns JP et al: Comparison of adenosine, dipyridamole and dobutamine in stress echocardiography. *Ann Intern Med* 116:190–196, 1992.

29. Eisenberg MJ, London MJ, Leung JM et al: Monitoring for myocardial ischemia during noncardiac surgery. A technology assessment of transesophageal echocardiography and 12-lead electrocardiography. *JAMA* 268:210–216, 1992.

30. Gewertz BL, Kremser PC, Zarins CK et al: Transesophageal echocardiographic monitoring of myocardial ischemia during vascular surgery. *J Vasc Surg.* 5:607–613, 1987.

31. Granieri R, Macpherson DS: Perioperative care of the vascular surgery patient. *J Gen Intern Med* 7:102–113, 1992.

32. Hertzer N, Young JR, Beven EG et al: Late results of coronary bypass in patients with peripheral vascular disease. *Cleve Clin J Med* 53:133–143, 1986.

33. Huber KC, Evans MA, Bersnahan JF: Outcome of noncardiac operations in patients with severe coronary artery disease successfully treated preoperatively with coronary angioplasty. *Mayo Clin Proc* 67:15–21, 1992.

34. Kennedy JW: Registry Committee of the Society for Cardiac Angiography. Complications associated with cardiac catheterization and angiography. *Cathet Cardiovasc Diag* 8:5–11, 1982.

35. Colt HG, Begg RJ, Saportio J et al: Cholesterol emboli after cardiac catheterization. Eight cases and a review of the literature. *Medicine* 67:379–390, 1988.

36. Higgins TL, Estafanous FG, Loow FD et al: Stratification of morbidity and mortality outcome by preoperative risk factors in coronary artery bypass patients. *JAMA* 267:2344–2348, 1992.

37. Turnipseed WE, Berkoff HA, Belzer FO: Postoperative stroke in cardiac and peripheral vascular disease. *Ann Surg* 192:365–368, 1980.

38. Reed GL, Singer DE, Picard EG et al: Stroke following coronary artery bypass surgery. *N Engl J Med* 319:1246–1250, 1988.

39. Bojar RM, Najafi H, De Laria GA et al: Neurologic complications of coronary revascularization. *Ann Thorac Surg* 36:427–432, 1983.

40. Barnes RW, Marszalke PB: Asymptomatic carotid disease in the cardiovascular surgical patient: is prophylactic endarterectomy necessary? *Stroke* 12:497–500, 1982.

41. Fode NC, Sundt TM, Robertson JT et al: Multicenter retrospective review of results and complications of carotid endarterectomy in 1982. *Stroke* 17:370–376, 1986.

42. Kispert JF, Kasmers A, Roitman L: Preoperative spirometry predicts perioperative pulmonary complications after major vascular surgery. *The American Surgeon* 158:491–495, 1992.

43. Dajani AS, Bisno AL, Chung KJ et al: Prevention of bacterial endocarditis. Recommendations by the American Heart Association. *JAMA* 264:2919–2922, 1988.

44. Anonymous: Antimicrobial prophylaxis in surgery. *Med Lett* 31:105–108, 1989.

45. Pasternack PF, Grossi EA, Baumann FG et al: Beta blockade to decrease silent myocardiac ischemia during peripheral vascular surgery. *Am J Surg* 158:113–116, 1989.

46. Slogoff S, Keats AS: Does chronic treatment with calcium entry blocking drugs reduce perioperative myocardial ischemia? *Anesthesiology* 68:676–680, 1988.

47. Chung F, Houston PL, Cheng DCH et al: Calcium channel blockade does not offer adequate protection from perioperative myocardial ischemia. *Anesthesiology* 69:343–347, 1988.

48. Charlson ME, MacKenzie R, Ales K et al: The postoperative electrocardiogram and creatine kinase: Implications for diagnosis of myocardial infarction after noncardiac surgery. *J Clin Epidemiol* 42:25–34, 1989.

49. Fine MJ, Kapoor W, Falanga V: Cholesterol crystal embolization: A review of 221 cases in the English literature. *Angiology* 38:769–784, 1980.

50. Moore RD, Steinberg EP, Powe NR et al: Nephrotoxicity of high-osmolality versus low-osmolality contrast media: Randomized clinical trial. *Radiology* 182:649–655, 1992.

PROCEDURE: ABDOMINAL AORTIC ANEURYSM

Overview: Because aneurysmal disease of the infrarenal aorta is progressive and frequently fatal, all patients with aneurysms should be considered for surgical replacement. In the absence of symptoms, patients with aneurysms 4-cm or greater in diameter should be considered for elective surgical resection. The risk of rupture is directly proportional to diameter, with a five-year risk of rupture of a 4 cm aneurysm being approximately 4 to 5% per year, rising to a greater than 70% likelihood of rupture for aneurysm greater than 7 cm in diameter. Symptomatic aneurysms are an indication for urgent or emergent resection.

1. *Operation*
    a. Indications: See description above.
    b. Operative Steps: Resection of an infrarenal abdominal aortic aneurysm requires visualization of the aorta from the level of the renal arteries distally to the femoral arteries. Once the aneurysm is completely exposed, the type of resection is determined. A tube graft replacing the aorta from just below the renal arteries to just above the aortic bifurcation is most frequently used for aneurysm replacement. Alternatively, an aortobifemoral bypass graft can be used if the aneurysm extends beyond the bifurcation into the common iliac arteries. Once the proximal and distal extents of resection are isolated, the patient is given 5000 units of heparin intravenously. After an appropriate circulating time, the aneurysm is excluded from blood flow by placement of proximal and distal aortic crossclamps, and the aneurysm is opened throughout its length. The orifices of the lumbar arteries along the posterior wall of the aorta are sewn shut and the graft, generally Dacron or PTFE (polytetrafluoroethylene), is sewn end-to-end to the aorta just below the level of the renal arteries using a continuous suture. For the placement of a tube graft, the distal anastomosis is then created, and clamps are removed. If an aortobifemoral bypass graft is to be fashioned, the aorta just above the bifurcation is sewn shut with continuous suture, and the graft limbs are routed through retroperitoneal tunnels along the anatomic course of the iliac vessels. The graft limbs are then sewn in end-to-end fashion to the femoral arteries. Once the anastomoses are completed, flow to the legs is restored. The aneurysm wall is then wrapped around the graft in the area of the abdominal aorta to enclose it and prevent contact of the graft with bowel.
    c. Incision: The transabdominal approach is performed through a midline xiphoid-to-pubis incision. A retroperitoneal approach is accomplished through a curvilinear incision extending from the tip of the left eleventh rib laterally to a point midway between the umbilicus and pubis in the midline.
    d. Anesthesia: General. Epidural anesthesia as adjunct for postoperative pain control is desirable.
    e. Intraoperative Monitoring: Arterial line and CVP or Swan-Ganz catheter are required.
    f. Operative Positioning: Transabdominal: supine. Retroperitoneal: 30-degree right lateral decubitus position.
    g. Duration: 2 to 4 hours.
    h. EBL/Transfusions: EBL 200 to 800 ml. The vast majority of this shed blood can be recycled through a cell-saver device. Transfusion is generally limited to 1 to 2 units.
    i. "Surgical Stress": There is severe stress associated with aortic crossclamping and lower extremity ischemia.
2. *Expected Hospital Course/Treatment*
    a. Postoperative Monitoring
        (1) ICU Stay: 1 to 3 days.
        (2) Invasive/Special Monitoring: Invasive monitors remain in place while in ICU.
        (3) Parameters To Be Monitored:
            i. Vital signs. ii. Femoral and distal pulses. iii. Urine output. iv. CBC, platelet count.
            v. ECG. vi. Chest x-ray. vii. Arterial blood gases. viii. Electrolytes, BUN, creatinine.
            ix. PT, PTT.
    b. Positioning/Activity: Supine position in bed for 24 to 48 hours. After that time, the patient is generally permitted to get out of bed to a chair if comfortable. Ambulation can be undertaken by POD 3 to 5.
    c. Alimentation: Retroperitoneal approach: Patients can generally resume liquid intake by POD 1 and solids by POD 2 or 3. Transabdominal: Patients require nasogastric suctioning for 24 hours and can resume oral intake by POD 3 and solid foods by POD 5.
    d. Wound Care/Drains: Generally no drains are placed.
    e. Respiratory Care: Extubation may be attempted in the operating room for the more straightforward cases. Otherwise, overnight mechanical ventilation is needed. Incentive spirometry encouraged.
    f. Analgesia/Postop Meds: Parenteral narcotics or epidural analgesia are required. Oral narcotics may be begun when bowel function returns.
    g. Length Of Hospital Stay: 7 to 10 days.
3. *Postoperative Complications*
    a. In Hospital
        (1) Morbidity: i. Bleeding. ii. Graft thrombosis. iii. Myocardial ischemia/infarction. iv. Ischemia of the left colon. v. Renal dysfunction. vi. Infection. vii. Atelectasis/pneumonia.
        (2) Mortality: < 4% overall. Rates are slightly higher in patients over 80. Mortality is 40 to 60% for emergency resection for a leaking or ruptured aneurysm.
    b. After Discharge
        (1) Retrograde ejaculation in the male. (2) Aortoenteric fistula.
4. *Follow-up*
    a. Suggested Follow-up: The patient is seen at 2 and 4 weeks, at 3 and 6 months, then every 6 months thereafter.

PROCEDURE: AORTOBIFEMORAL BYPASS GRAFTING

Overview: The purpose of aortobifemoral bypass grafting is to provide a nonobstructed conduit for blood flow from the infrarenal aorta to the common femoral arteries. The operation is usually performed electively, although acute thrombosis may occur and produce significant lower extremity ischemia necessitating urgent intervention.

1. *Operation*
    a. Indications: Extensive occlusive disease of the infrarenal aorta and/or both iliac arterial systems associated with claudication and frequently impotence.
    b. Operative Steps: Once the aorta is isolated at the infrarenal level, dissection is carried distally to evaluate the inferior mesenteric artery. If this vessel is transmitting pulsatile flow from the aorta, it should be preserved and reimplanted into the graft. Significant dissection along the left common iliac artery should be avoided to reduce the likelihood of impotence postoperatively. At the level of the bifurcation of the aorta, a retroperitoneal tunnel is made along the course of the iliac vessels. The common femoral arteries are isolated bilaterally through 7 cm vertical incisions centered above them. If there is significant disease in the common femoral artery, the origin of the profunda femoris artery should be exposed for a distance of approximately 2 cm to enable the distal anastomoses to be created as profundaplasties. Once complete vascular isolation has been created, the patient is given 5000 units of heparin intravenously, and the graft is placed. The right graft limb is sewn first in end-to-side fashion to the recipient vessel. The aortic anastomosis is created next and sewn in end-to-end fashion. Once this anastomosis is completed and secured, the graft is flushed of all air and debris through the left graft limb. Flow is restored to the right leg. The left femoral or profunda anastomosis is completed in the same fashion as on the right.
    c. Incision: Transabdominal approach: midline xiphoid-to-pubis incision. Retroperitoneal approach: curvilinear incision extending from the tip of the left eleventh rib laterally to a point midway between the umbilicus and pubis in the midline.
    d. Anesthesia: General. Epidural anesthesia for postoperative pain control is desirable.
    e. Intraoperative Monitoring: Arterial line and CVP or Swan-Ganz catheter.
    f. Operative Positioning: Transabdominal: supine. Retroperitoneal: Partial right lateral decubitus position.
    g. Duration: 2.5 to 4 hours.
    h. EBL/Transfusions: EBL 400 to 600 ml. Transfusions can be avoided by the use of cell-salvage devices.
    i. "Surgical Stress": There is severe stress associated with aortic crossclamping and lower extremity ischemia.

2. *Expected Hospital Course/Treatment*
    a. Postoperative Monitoring
        (1) ICU Stay: 1 to 3 days.
        (2) Invasive/Special Monitoring: Invasive monitors remain in place while in ICU.
        (3) Parameters To Be Monitored: Same as abdominal aortic aneurysm (AAA) resection.
    b. Positioning/Activity: Same as AAA resection.
    c. Alimentation: Same as AAA resection.
    d. Wound Care/Drains: Generally no drains are placed.
    e. Respiratory Care: Extubation may be attempted in the operating room unless blood loss is large or cardiovascular status is unstable. Mechanical ventilation may be needed overnight. Incentive spirometry encouraged.
    f. Analgesia/Postop Meds: Parenteral narcotics or epidural analgesia required for several days.
    g. Length Of Hospital Stay: 7 to 10 days.

3. *Postoperative Complications*
    a. In Hospital
        (1) Morbidity:
            i. Graft-related problems including bleeding, thrombosis, or distal embolization.
            ii. Cardiac dysfunction manifested as myocardial ischemia or congestive heart failure.
            iii. Atelectasis/pneumonia.
        (2) Mortality: < 4%.
    b. After Discharge:
        (1) Graft infection.
        (2) Anastomotic dehiscence.

4. *Follow-up*
    a. Suggested Follow-up: The patient is seen at 2 and 4 weeks, 3 and 6 months, then every 6 months thereafter.

PROCEDURE: ARTERIOVENOUS FISTULA

Overview: The purpose of a surgically created arteriovenous fistula is to provide easy access to the arterial system for hemodialysis by arterializing the superficial veins of the forearm or by placing a piece of prosthetic graft as a bridge between the arterial and venous systems. This requires that the arterial inflow into the arm be sufficient to permit some diversion of blood flow and that the capacitance of the venous system of the extremity be adequate to accommodate the increase in venous outflow. If the superficial venous system of the forearm, including the cephalic vein, is patent, an autologous fistula may be created. The attachment of the cephalic vein to the radial artery at the level of the wrist is the most common type of AV fistula created for dialysis and is known as the Brescia-Cimino fistula. If the superficial veins are not in continuity or patent, as often occurs if the patient has been hospitalized for a prolonged period with indwelling venous catheters, a prosthetic bridge graft carrying flow from the radial artery to the basilic or deep venous system of the arm is preferred.

1. *Operation*
   a. Indications:
      (1) The anticipation or presence of complete renal failure.
      (2) Rarely fistulae are created for the chronic delivery of intravenous medications such as chemotherapy.
   b. Operative Steps: The radial artery just proximal to the wrist is surrounded with silastic vessel loops. The cephalic vein or a deep vein just distal to the antecubital fossa is isolated and connected to the artery in an end-to-side, side-to-side, or end-to-end fashion. A subcutaneous tunnel may need to be created to connect the arterial and venous incisions. A length of PTFE graft material, 6 mm in diameter, can then be placed into the tunnel and sewn in end-to-side fashion to the artery and vein. Upon release of the vascular clamps, there should be a slight thrill or pulse in the vein beyond the anastomosis.
   c. Incision: The artery and vein are isolated through small incisions made directly over them.
   d. Anesthesia: Local with IV sedation, axillary or interscalene block, or general.
   e. Intraoperative Monitoring: Patients may have multiple medical problems, but routine monitors are generally sufficient.
   f. Operative Positioning: Supine position with the appropriate arm extended outward onto a lateral arm support.
   g. Duration: 1 to 2 hours.
   h. EBL/Transfusions: EBL minimal. No transfusion therapy is necessary.
   i. "Surgical Stress": Low.

2. *Expected Hospital Course/Treatment*
   a. Postoperative Monitoring
      (1) ICU Stay: No ICU stay is routinely required.
      (2) Invasive/Special Monitoring: None.
      (3) Parameters To Be Monitored:
          i. The pulse or thrill in the venous outflow tract.
          ii. Evaluation of the hand for ischemia or swelling.
          iii. CBC.
          iv. Electrolytes.
   b. Positioning/Activity: As tolerated.
   c. Alimentation: As tolerated.
   d. Wound Care/Drains: None.
   e. Respiratory Care: Routine.
   f. Analgesia/Postop Meds: Acetaminophen with or without codeine or a nonsteroidal anti-inflammatory agent is generally adequate.
   g. Length Of Hospital Stay: 1 to 2 days.

3. *Postoperative Complications*
   a. In Hospital
      (1) Morbidity:
          i. Hyperdynamic congestive heart failure from excessive flow through the fistula.
          ii. Hand ischemia.
          iii. Arm edema due to venous overload.
      (2) Mortality: Mortality related directly to the procedure is minimal. However, some patients requiring creation of a fistula are critically ill and may succumb to other medical problems in the postoperative period.
   b. After Discharge
      (1) False aneurysm formation.
      (2) Graft infection.
      (3) Graft thrombosis.

4. *Follow-up*
   a. Suggested Follow-up: Patients are seen at 3- to 6-month intervals.

PROCEDURE: CAROTID ENDARTERECTOMY

Overview: The purpose of carotid endarterectomy is to reduce the likelihood of thromboembolic stroke by directly removing the intima and portions of the media containing atheromatous debris from the carotid artery. Controversy exists over which patients have the highest risk of cerebral infarction and should undergo this operation (see Chap. 35). Currently, most surgeons utilize continuous electroencephalographic (EEG) monitoring to detect hypoperfusion of the brain. Should slowing of the EEG occur at any time after placement of the carotid crossclamps, an intraluminal shunt is placed to direct blood around the endarterectomy site. Measurements of stump pressure in the distal common carotid artery or an awake patient have been used as alternatives to assess cerebral perfusion.

1. *Operation*
   a. Indications:
      (1) Asymptomatic carotid artery stenosis narrowing the origin of the internal carotid artery more than 80%.
      (2) Symptomatic carotid artery lesions narrowing the origin of the internal carotid more than 70%.
   b. Operative Steps: The carotid artery is isolated beyond the distal extent of the plaque. The patient is given 5000 units of heparin in an IV bolus, and the crossclamps are placed. The common carotid is opened at the proximal extent of the palpable plaque which is generally within 2 to 3 cm of the carotid bifurcation. An arteriotomy is made extending from this area of the common carotid artery up through the orifice of the internal carotid artery into the internal carotid artery distal to the palpable plaque. The intima containing the plaque is elevated from the media. This dissection plane is then followed distally to the origin of the external carotid artery. The endarterectomized surface of the carotid artery is carefully examined and cleared of any remaining debris. Closure is begun either directly in elderly males with large internal carotid arteries or with a patch in younger patients or women with smaller carotid arteries. When approximately 1 cm of arteriotomy remains to be closed, the shunt, if placed, is removed. The vessels are flushed of all air and debris, and the closure is completed. The clamps are removed first from the external and then from the common carotid artery so that any remaining intraluminal debris will be flushed through the external carotid system. After several seconds of flow through the external system, the internal carotid artery is opened. Once flow is restored, Doppler interrogation of the internal carotid artery should confirm diastolic flow.
   c. Incision: An oblique incision along the anterior border of the sternocleidomastoid muscle.
   d. Anesthesia: General or regional. Regional techniques assure an awake patient and allow for continuous mental status assessment during periods of crossclamping.
   e. Intraoperative Monitoring: Arterial line. Swan-Ganz catheter, if the patient has significant cardiovascular disease. Continuous EEG monitoring.
   f. Operative Positioning: Supine position with the neck hyperextended by a roll placed underneath the scapulae.
   g. Duration: 2 to 2.5 hours.
   h. EBL/Transfusions: EBL is minimal. No transfusions are generally required.
   i. "Surgical Stress": Moderate to severe because some patients may experience significantly compromised cerebral blood flow with carotid clamping.

2. *Expected Hospital Course/Treatment*
   a. Postoperative Monitoring
      (1) ICU Stay: 1 to 2 days.
      (2) Invasive/Special Monitoring: Invasive hemodynamic monitors remain in place while in ICU.
      (3) Parameters To Be Monitored:
         i. Neurologic status, including movement of the contralateral arm and leg, visual fields, and midline extension of the tongue.
         ii. Vital signs, especially blood pressure.
         iii. CBC.
         iv. ECG.
   b. Positioning/Activity: For the first 24 hours, activity is limited to bed or chair. Thereafter the patient can move about as tolerated.
   c. Alimentation: Regular diet is resumed on POD 1.
   d. Wound Care/Drains: A Jackson-Pratt drain may be placed in the wound. If so, it is removed on POD 1.
   e. Respiratory Care: Extubation in the operating room. Routine care afterward.
   f. Analgesia/Postop Meds: Analgesic requirements vary, but an oral analgesic is usually adequate.
   g. Length Of Hospital Stay: 3 to 4 days.

3. *Postoperative Complications*
   a. In Hospital
      (1) Morbidity: i. Intraoperative or postoperative cerebrovascular accident. ii. Bleeding and airway compromise. iii. Myocardial ischemia/infarction. iv. Lower cranial or peripheral nerve injury. v. Carotid sinus dysfunction.
      (2) Mortality: 1%.
   b. After Discharge: See suggested follow-up below.

4. *Follow-up*
   a. Suggested Follow-up: All patients are evaluated at 1 week, then at 1 and 6 months with duplex imaging. If the patient demonstrates myointimal hyperplasia at the endarterectomy site, they are followed every 2 to 6 months for assessment of the residual lumen. Follow-up should continue for 2 years at which time the hyperplastic response generally begins to recede.

PROCEDURE: FEMOROPOPLITEAL BYPASS GRAFTING

Overview: Femoropopliteal bypass grafting is performed to reduce the symptoms of calf claudication or distal ischemia due to superficial femoral artery occlusion. The exact operation depends on the results of preoperative angiography demonstrating the location and degree of the blockages as well as the arterial inflow and distal runoff of the vessels to be bypassed. The graft of choice for this bypass is the greater saphenous vein. If this vein is inadequate or absent, a prosthetic graft such as PTFE or umbilical vein can be used. The saphenous vein is prepared for *in situ* grafting by lysis of valves and ligation of all tributaries. For placement in an anatomic tunnel as a reverse saphenous vein, the appropriate length of saphenous vein is harvested, reversed, and placed into the anatomic tunnel following the course of the superficial femoral artery. If prosthetic material is used, it is simply placed into the anatomic tunnel running along the superficial femoral artery from groin to knee.

1. *Operation*
   a. Indications:
      (1) Severe disabling claudication.
      (2) Limb-threatening ischemia with rest pain, ulceration, or gangrene of the foot due to superficial femoral artery occlusion.
   b. Operative Steps: To create the bypass, the common femoral artery is isolated in the groin just proximal to its bifurcation into the superficial and deep femoral branches. The popliteal artery is isolated at the level of the knee. After intravenous heparinization with 5000 to 7000 units of heparin, the femoral artery is crossclamped proximally and distally. The saphenous vein or the prosthetic graft is sewn in an end-to-side fashion for both anastomoses. The distal anastomosis can then be evaluated intraluminally with angioscopy or angiography in the operating room. Angiography should demonstrate a technically precise result at the level of the distal anastomosis with good runoff to the foot.
   c. Incision:
      (1) A 7-cm vertical incision centered over the common femoral artery.
      (2) A medial incision placed just above or below the knee to isolate the popliteal artery.
      (3) The saphenous vein is isolated along its course with an incision placed along the medial aspect of the thigh.
   d. Anesthesia: General or epidural.
   e. Intraoperative Monitoring: Arterial line with or without CVP or Swan-Ganz catheter depending on cardiovascular status.
   f. Operative Positioning: Supine with external rotation of the leg to expose the medial aspect of the knee.
   g. Duration: With a prosthetic graft, 1.5 to 2 hours. With the greater saphenous vein, 3 to 4 hours.
   h. EBL/Transfusions: EBL is 100 to 200 ml. Transfusions are not usually required.
   i. "Surgical Stress": Moderate.

2. *Expected Hospital Course/Treatment*
   a. Postoperative Monitoring
      (1) ICU Stay: None in the absence of significant cardiac disease.
      (2) Invasive/Special Monitoring: While in ICU.
      (3) Parameters To Be Monitored:
         i. Pedal pulses and the appearance of the toes.
         ii. Vital signs.
         iii. Urine output.
         iv. CBC.
         v. ECG.
   b. Positioning/Activity: Once adequate analgesia has been established, progressive ambulation may begin as early as POD 1.
   c. Alimentation: Regular diet is resumed by POD 1.
   d. Wound Care/Drains: Usually none.
   e. Respiratory Care: Routine.
   f. Analgesia/Postop Meds: Parenteral then oral narcotics are required for 3 to 7 days.
   g. Length Of Hospital Stay: 7 to 9 days for uncomplicated cases.

3. *Postoperative Complications*
   a. In Hospital
      (1) Morbidity:
         i. Bleeding.
         ii. Graft thrombosis, infection, and distal embolization.
         iii. Lower extremity edema.
         iv. Myocardial ischemia/infarction.
      (2) Mortality: 2%.
   b. After Discharge
      (1) Graft infection.
      (2) Thrombosis.
      (3) Anastomotic dehiscence.

4. *Follow-up*
   a. Suggested Follow-up: The patient is seen at 2 weeks; 1, 3, and 6 months; and every 6 months thereafter.

PROCEDURE: LOWER EXTREMITY AMPUTATION

Overview: The purpose of lower extremity amputation is to remove ischemic, necrotic, or infected tissue. The level of amputation can be determined preoperatively by physical examination of the lower extremity, noting obvious changes in temperature, texture, and turgor of the skin in the region of demarcation; by transcutaneous oxygen tension measurements along the lower extremity; or by obtaining peak systolic pressures in the major arteries at the site of amputation. If absolute pressures exceed 10 mmHg, the likelihood of healing is greater than 80%.

1. *Operation*
   a. Indications:
      (1) Severe ischemia associated with rest pain, nonhealing ulcer, progressive infection, or ischemic gangrene.
      (2) Neoplasm.
      (3) Nonhealing bone fractures.
   b. Operative Steps: Once the appropriate level of amputation has been confirmed, all soft tissue should be divided with clean passes of the scalpel to avoid devitalizing tissue. The major neurovascular bundles in the area should be identified, ligated, and transected individually. The nerve should be transected at a level higher than the artery and vein and well beyond any area of weight bearing. A bone saw is then used to transect the bone, and the marrow space is made hemostatic with bone wax. The bone is shortened so that it is 1 to 2 cm shorter than the most proximal extent of the skin incision. In noninfected amputations, the muscles and subcutaneous tissues can be closed around the bone. In infected cases, the incision may be left open. If the use of a prosthesis is anticipated, a rigid dressing using cast material can be applied immediately upon conclusion of the operation.
   c. Incision: For below-knee amputation (BKA), the incision transects the upper third of the tibia with a posterior flap significantly longer so that it can be brought forward to meet with the anterior flap. For above-knee amputations (AKA), an elliptical fish mouth incision is chosen which will permit creation of a muscle and fat pad over the bone for protection of the bone stump during weight bearing.
   d. Anesthesia: General or regional.
   e. Intraoperative Monitoring: In critically ill patients, arterial line and/or Swan-Ganz catheter monitoring may be required.
   f. Operative Positioning: Supine.
   g. Duration: 30 to 60 minutes.
   h. EBL/Transfusions: EBL is 50 to 200 ml. Transfusions are usually not required.
   j. "Surgical Stress": Moderate.

2. *Expected Hospital Course/Treatment*
   a. Postoperative Monitoring
      (1) ICU Stay: May be required for critically ill patients.
      (2) Invasive/Special Monitoring: While in ICU.
      (3) Parameters To Be Monitored:
         i. Vital signs.   iii. CBC.
         ii. Urine output.   iv. ECG.
   b. Positioning/Activity: The patient refrains from weight bearing with the leg elevated while in bed or sitting in a chair for the first 7 days. At that time, the patient should begin physical therapy for upper-body strengthening and range-of-motion exercising of the lower extremity.
   c. Alimentation: Regular diet may be resumed on POD 1.
   d. Wound Care/Drains: The amputation site should be inspected daily. It should be dressed with sterile gauze and an Ace wrap compression dressing for 7 days. Drains are usually avoided in lower extremity amputations.
   e. Respiratory Care: Routine.
   f. Analgesia/Postop Meds: Patients who experience severe rest pain preoperatively generally have a reduction in analgesic requirements. However, an oral or parenteral narcotic may be required in the immediate postoperative period.
   g. Length Of Hospital Stay: 6 to 12 days at which time the patient should be discharged to a physical therapy unit.

3. *Postoperative Complications*
   a. In Hospital
      (1) Morbidity:
         i. Wound infection.
         ii. Deep-vein thrombosis.
         iii. Myocardial ischemia/infarction.
         iv. Cerebrovascular accident.
      (2) Mortality: BKA: 8 to 10%. AKA: 12 to 15%.
   b. After Discharge
      (1) Blunt trauma to the amputation site with subsequent wound dehiscence.

4. *Follow-up*
   a. Suggested Follow-up: Patients are seen at monthly intervals until gait training with a final prosthesis has been completed. Thereafter the patient is followed every 3 to 6 months with particular attention to preservation of the contralateral extremity.

10 EVALUATION OF THE PATIENT UNDERGOING OPHTHALMIC SURGERY

Donald L. Budenz

Charles W. Nichols

Frank H. Brown

Ophthalmic procedures vary from ten-minute corneal scrapings with topical anesthesia to six-hour vitrectomies with retinal membrane peeling under general anesthesia. However, ophthalmic procedures share many common features that differ markedly from other forms of surgery. These include anesthetic techniques, risk assessment, comorbid conditions and their implications, and the effects of topical and systemic medication used in the perioperative period.

ANESTHESIA AND OPHTHALMIC SURGERY

Most eye procedures are now performed in the ambulatory setting using local anesthesia and intravenous sedation. Inpatient hospitalization is usually only necessary for eye trauma surgery requiring intravenous antibiotics, some vitreoretinal operations, and orbital procedures requiring postoperative intravenous steroids. Patients requiring postoperative eye patching with contralateral blindness are also admitted to the hospital. Patients with confounding medical conditions requiring perioperative management and those who are unable to resume self-care promptly may also require inpatient management.

Anesthesia requirements differ for each type of ophthalmic procedure. If the procedure is relatively short, the patient calm and cooperative, and adequate anesthesia and akinesis of the eye and periocular tissues can be obtained, local anesthesia is preferred. With this technique, the facial nerve is blocked by injection of carbocaine or a similar local anesthetic to ensure akinesis of the orbicularis muscle. Anesthesia of the eye and periocular skin and akinesis of the extraocular muscles are achieved by retrobulbar injection of lidocaine, mepivacaine, or bupivacaine into the ex-traocular muscle cone or, more recently, into the anterior peribulbar tissue. Retrobulbar injection may uncommonly lead to central nervous system complications including seizures, central nervous system depression including coma, or respiratory depression if the anesthetic is inadvertently injected into the intravascular space. Additionally, hypotension, reduced myocardial contractility, or bradycardia may rarely occur. General anesthesia is preferred in children, patients who are too anxious to undergo surgery while awake, those who may not be able to lie still for an hour or longer, and those in whom mental status prohibits cooperation. Patients with chronic cough or a movement disorder also require general anesthesia to avoid jeopardizing the delicate maneuvering required in ophthalmic surgery. General anesthesia may also be required in patients with a bleeding diathesis, those with significant allergies to local anesthetics, and those in whom satisfactory local block cannot be obtained.

SPECIAL CONSIDERATIONS IN OPHTHALMIC SURGERY

Risk of Bleeding

Relatively small amounts of bleeding can affect outcome and jeopardize vision after ophthalmic surgery. Retrobulbar hemorrhage during administration of local anesthesia can result in proptosis; increased intraocular pressure; and extension of hemorrhage anteriorly to the subconjunctival and subcutaneous spaces, a complication that can potentially cause blindness. Likewise, a serious intraocular hemorrhage such as a suprachoroidal hemorrhage or hyphema may occur during surgery and threaten vision. Therefore, all patients undergoing ophthalmic surgery should be assessed for an increased risk of bleeding.

Risk of the Open Globe

Under local anesthesia, any intraoperative movement can cause hemorrhage and risk extruding intraocular contents. Patients with agitation, cough, orthopnea, or seizure disorders must be carefully assessed and treated before surgery to minimize this possibility, or general anesthesia may be required. Likewise, coughing, emesis, and the Valsalva maneuver can cause sudden congestion of the orbital veins and an acute rise in intraocular pressure. These situations must be avoided during the intraoperative and postoperative periods to prevent prolapse of intraocular tissue through a traumatic or surgical wound.

The Oculocardiac Reflex

The oculocardiac reflex is a vagal response induced by trigeminal stimulation occurring when tension is placed on the extraocular muscles. Bradycardia, hypotension, or other cardiac rhythm disturbances may occur. The reflex may be interrupted by decreasing tension on the extraocular muscles or administering a small dose of intravenous atropine or its equivalent. Similarly, acute increases in intraocular pressure, pressure on the globe, and retrobulbar injection can increase vagal tone and result in nausea, vomiting, bradycardia, and hypotension.[1]

Effects of Topical Drugs in Ophthalmic Surgery

Topical ophthalmic drops run through the lacrimal drainage system into the nasopharynx immediately after instillation and are rapidly absorbed into the bloodstream by the nasal mucosa. Several drugs used before and after eye surgery may have cardiovascular and other systemic side effects.

Phenylephrine, used preoperatively to produce pupillary dilation and vasoconstriction, may be associated with acute hypertension, tachycardia, palpitations, nervousness, and, occasionally, myocardial infarction and cerebrovascular accidents. These side effects are rare but occur more frequently when a 10% solution of phenylephrine is used.

Epinephrine, used topically in the management of glaucoma, intraocularly during cataract surgery, and subcutaneously as an adjunct to local anesthetic agents, may cause tachycardia, hypertension, palpitations, headache, and an increased frequency of ventricular premature beats. Its tendency to produce cardiac irritability is enhanced by halothane which increases myocardial sensitivity to catecholamines.[2] However, the intraocular concentration of epinephrine used in eye surgery is very low, and systemic complications are rare. Timolol, the beta-adrenergic blocking agent most widely used to lower intraocular pressure in patients with glaucoma, is sometimes used before and after surgery to prevent increases in intraocular pressure after cataract surgery. Timolol or other beta-blockers may cause bronchospasm in patients with asthma or chronic obstructive pulmonary disease. Additionally, bradycardia, palpitations, and decreased cardiac contractility may occur in patients with congestive heart failure.

The anticholinergic drug atropine is often used for dilation of the pupil and cycloplegia before and after surgery for retinal detachment and following glaucoma filtration procedures. Each drop of a 1% solution contains 0.5 mg of atropine. Systemic side effects include delirium in elderly patients, tachycardia, dry mouth, and flushing.

Parasympathomimetic agents like acetylcholine or corbamycholine are injected intraocularly during cataract surgery to produce rapid constriction of the pupil and have occasionally produced hypotension, bradycardia, and bronchospasm. Atropine sulfate may be given intramuscularly or intravenously to counteract these effects.

Echothiophate iodide is an irreversible cholinesterase inhibitor now rarely used to treat glaucoma, but commonly used in accommodative esotropia, a type of strabismus in children. Systemic absorption of the drug suppresses pseudocholinesterase and cholinesterase activity for prolonged periods. Since pseudocholinesterase is needed to hydrolyze the muscle relaxant succinylcholine, the use of these drugs together may result in prolonged muscle paralysis and respiratory failure.

Topical steroids used after surgery have no significant systemic side effects and have not been shown to suppress the hypothalamic-pituitary-adrenal axis.

Effects of Systemic Medications in Ophthalmic Surgery

Systemic medications used in patients undergoing ophthalmic surgery include intravenous mannitol, carbonic anhydrase inhibitors, and systemic steroids. The hyperosmotic agent mannitol is used to lower intraocular pressure before cataract surgery, corneal transplantation, glaucoma filtration surgery, and retinal detachment procedures. Mannitol is given over 30 to 40 minutes just before the operation. It causes an acute rise in intravascular volume and may precipitate congestive heart failure in patients with impaired cardiac or renal function. Angina may also occur, and blood pressure may rise in hypertensive patients. Since mannitol causes dehydration of the central nervous system, nausea, vomiting, and severe headache may develop. It produces a significant diuresis in all patients. Bladder distention requiring catheterization and occasionally urologic surgery may be necessary in those with bladder outlet obstruction.

Carbonic anhydrase inhibitors like acetazolamide are frequently used to reduce the transient rise in intraocular pressure that occurs after cataract surgery. Although usually necessary only for a short period, they may be required for extended therapy. Gastrointestinal disturbances, frequent urination, and paresthesias of the distal extremities are the most common side effects of acetazolamide. Potassium depletion, sometimes occurring during the first two weeks of therapy with acetazolamide, can be corrected if a normal diet is maintained.[3] Methazolamide causes less gastrointestinal upset and diuresis but more fatigue and drowsiness than acetazolamide.[3] Both may cause renal stones and a nonanion gap metabolic acidosis when used chronically.

Intravenous or oral steroids are occasionally used after orbital surgery to decrease orbital edema and after any ophthalmic surgery to reduce excessive postoperative inflammation. Usually only a short course of steroids is necessary, and systemic side effects are few and transient. However, some diabetic patients who receive even a brief course of steroids can experience loss of glycemic control and may require hospitalization.

MEDICAL RISKS OF OPHTHALMIC SURGERY

Ophthalmic surgery is remarkably safe with postoperative mortality rates between 0.06 and 0.18 percent.[4,5] A number of older studies have compared mortality rates with local and general anesthesia,[4,6-8] but they are difficult to interpret because most are retrospective and suffer from selection bias because more high-risk patients received local anesthesia. Newer data suggest that the risks of complications are approximately the same for both local and general anesthesia. One study has documented differences in mortality rates among specific types of ophthalmic procedures. The mortality rate for strabismus correction was 0.10 percent, for cataract surgery 0.19 percent, and for retinal detachment repair 0.24 percent.[6] The reason for these differences is not entirely clear. The frequency of general anesthesia was the same in all categories, but there were important differences in patient age and underlying medical condition. The presence of coexisting medical problems may therefore be the most important determinant of mortality following ophthalmic surgery. Another large study showed a clear correlation between perioperative death and ASA class.[7]

Because most ophthalmic surgery is elective, coexisting medical conditions should be fully assessed and treated before the procedure. However, in urgent and emergency situations such as cases of penetrating trauma and particularly those involving an intraocular foreign body, surgery should be performed as soon as the patient is medically stable. Processes which threaten the optic nerve such as orbital or optic nerve hemorrhage and retinal detachments posing an imminent threat to the macula should be handled emergently. Eyelid lacerations involving the marginal lid or the canaliculus should be repaired in the operating room within 24 hours. Certain glaucoma cases in which the intraocular pressure threatens ocular blood flow and cannot be reduced medically also require urgent surgery. In addition, vitrectomies are sometimes performed urgently when endophthalmitis is present. In these situations, emergency surgery may be sight-saving, particulary if useful vision in the other eye has been lost. Surgery should therefore not be unnecessarily delayed given the low overall risks associated with ophthalmic procedures. Medical input should be directed toward rapidly stabilizing the patient and assuring appropriate perioperative monitoring and treatment.

Coexisting Medical Problems and Ophthalmic Surgery

In a recent survey, patients undergoing ophthalmic surgery had a mean age of 64, and the majority had one or more chronic medical conditions.[9] As noted above, these conditions constitute the major risk factors for postoperative death and can contribute to postoperative morbidity and mortality. Thus, although ophthalmic surgery carries low risk, careful preoperative assessment and preparation of patients with underlying medical problems are important.

Hypertension is the most common chronic medical problem in eye patients, occurring in 52 percent in one series.[9] Preoperative blood pressure control is important because intraoperative complications like suprachoroidal hemorrhage are more common if the pressure is elevated. Except for diuretics, hypertensive patients should be given their antihypertensive medications with a sip of water on the morning of surgery. Topical nitroglycerine and sublingual nifedipine have both been used successfully to lower elevated blood pressure when surgery is urgent.

Diabetes mellitus is common among eye patients since it increases the risk of cataracts, glaucoma, and retinal disorders. Because most ophthalmic procedures are brief, cause little surgical stress, and allow rapid resumption of oral intake, severe derangements of glycemic control are uncommon unless high doses of systemic steroids are required. Diabetic patients on insulin or oral hypoglycemic agents should undergo surgery in the early morning to avoid hypoglycemia. If the procedure is short, the morning insulin or medication can be withheld until immediately thereafter. If insulin-dependent patients are scheduled later in the morning or afternoon, or if the anticipated procedure is long, one-third to one-half of the morning insulin dose can be given. In such cases, an intravenous glucose infusion is most frequently maintained, and blood sugars are monitored carefully throughout the perioperative period.

Coronary artery disease is found in approximately one-third of patients undergoing eye surgery,[9] but few data exist regarding the risk it poses. A single study of stable patients with prior myocardial infarction documented no cases of reinfarction after ophthalmic procedures.[10] Patients with coronary artery disease should be assessed in the usual way, and all antianginal medications except aspirin should be continued up to the time of surgery and resumed promptly thereafter. Phenylephrine, epinephrine, atropine, and mannitol can cause tachycardia or hypertension and can precipitate angina in patients with ischemic heart disease. Assessment of volume status is important in patients with congestive heart failure because orthopnea may cause movement during surgery. Transient volume expansion caused by mannitol or myocardial depression due to systemic absorption of timolol can precipitate overt failure in marginally compensated patients. Conversely, patients who are relatively volume-depleted due to excessive diuretic therapy may become hypotensive with an increase in vagal tone or the addition of osmotic diuretics or carbonic anhydrase inhibitors.

Acute or chronic pulmonary disease is an important consideration because of the risk of cough to an open eye. Elective surgery should be postponed to allow resolution of upper respiratory tract infection. Smoking cessation should be encouraged, and short courses of antibiotics may be beneficial in selected patients. Cough suppressants may provide alternatives to general anesthesia in these patients. Bronchospasm may be precipitated in patients with asthma or chronic obstructive lung disease by the systemic absorption of topical beta-blockers and parasympathomimetic agents. Patients with inherited or acquired bleeding diatheses require careful assessment and preoperative preparation as described in Chap. 30. Many patients take aspirin or other nonsteroidal anti-inflammatory agents, and some require long-term anticoagulation. Aspirin should be discontinued seven to 10 days before surgery. Although the correlation between the bleeding time and bleeding is not entirely reliable, it is often used as a guide in scheduling eye surgery for such patients. Nonsteroidal anti-inflammatory drugs are reversible inhibitors of platelet aggregation, and surgery may be performed after one dosing interval has passed.

Most patients on coumadin can discontinue it three days before surgery and resume it the day thereafter. This regimen has not been shown to increase the incidence of thrombotic complications even in patients with prosthetic heart valves.[11] Several studies have reported an increased risk of hemorrhagic complications when cataract surgery is performed without discontinuing coumadin, but the complications are relatively insignificant clinically.[12–14] Heparin should be discontinued six hours before surgery and restarted the next morning.

Elective surgery should be deferred in patients with thrombocytopenia to allow appropriate diagnosis and treatment. Urgent ophthalmic surgery can be safely performed if the platelet count is above 50,000/mm³.[15]

Prophylactic Issues

The eye is normally sterile, and most ophthalmic surgery poses no risk of bacteremia. Therefore, prophylaxis against endocarditis is not required even in high-risk patients. Bacteremia can theoretically occur during surgery involving infected ocular or orbital tissue but has not been demonstrated. Although some have recommended the standard AHA regimen for high-risk patients in this setting, it may not cover the bacterial flora involved. Moreover, many such patients are already receiving appropriate systemic antibiotics for their eye infection.

The risk of deep venous thrombosis following ophthalmic surgery is unclear. One study demonstrated that pulmonary embolism was the most common cause of death after ophthalmic surgery,[16] but it was done at a time when surgery was performed in the hospital and involved periods of bed rest. Most patients are now ambulatory within hours of surgery, and the risk of thrombosis may therefore be lower. However, in selected high-risk patients (such as those with a history of deep venous thrombosis) undergoing long procedures under general anesthesia, prophylactic measures should be considered. Although standard low-dose heparin has been recommended by some, there are no studies documenting its safety in this setting. External pneumatic compression devices pose no risk of bleeding and are probably a better alternative.

POSTOPERATIVE PROBLEMS

The differential diagnosis of common problems after ophthalmic surgery is somewhat different from that requiring consideration after other surgical procedures. Postoperative hypertension may be due to the systemic effects of topical sympathomimetic drugs or epinephrine used with local anesthetics. Acute urinary retention induced by anticholinergic drugs, analgesics, and diuretics can cause acute elevations in blood pressure, most often in men with prostatic hypertrophy. Catheterization is therapeutic.

Postoperative nausea and vomiting may result from vagal stimulation due to increased intraocular pressure or the effects of general anesthesia or other drugs such as carbonic anhydrase inhibitors. In ketosis-prone diabetics, nausea and vomiting may herald the onset of ketoacidosis. The cause should be identified rapidly and the symptoms treated to prevent rapid increases in intraocular pressure.

Bradycardia and hypotension may also result from increased vagal tone or systemic absorption of topical beta-blockers or parasympathomimetic agents. Hypotension can also be caused by intravascular volume depletion from diuretics.

Because many patients undergoing ophthalmic surgery are elderly, postoperative delirium is common. Many procedures require eye patching and frequent instillation of drops and result in significant sleep and sensory deprivation. Systemic absorption of topical drugs like atropine and scopolamine and the use of analgesics may also contribute.

REFERENCES

1. Ziccardi VB, Russavage J, Sotereanos GC et al: Oculocardiac reflex: Pathophysiology and case report. *Oral Surg Oral Med Oral Pathol* 71:137–138, 1991.
2. Havener WH: Autonomic drugs, in *Ocular Pharmacology*, 5th ed. St. Louis, Mosby, 1983, pp 261–417.
3. Havener WH: Secretory inhibitors, in *Ocular Pharmacology*, 5th ed. St. Louis, Mosby, 1983, pp 575–597.
4. Duncalf D, Gartner S, Carol B: Mortality in association with ophthalmic surgery. *Am J Ophthalmol* 69:610, 1970.
5. Smith B: *Ophthalmic Anesthesia*. Baltimore, University Park Press, 1983, pp 73–75.
6. Quigley HA: Mortality associated with ophthalmic surgery: A twenty-year experience at the Wilmer Institute. *Am J Ophthalmol* 77:517, 1974.
7. Petruscak J, Smith B, Breslin P: Mortality related to ophthalmological surgery. *Arch Ophthalmol* 89:106, 1973.
8. Wolf GL, Seamus L, Berlin I: Intraocular surgery with general anesthesia. *Arch Ophthalmol* 93:323, 1975.
9. Gozum ME, Turner BJ, Tipperman R: Perioperative management of the ophthalmology patient, in Merli G, Weitz H (eds): *Medical Management of the Surgical Patient*. Philadelphia, Saunders, 1992, pp 245–256.
10. Backer BA, Tinker JH, Robertson DM et al: Myocardial infarction following local anesthesia for ophthalmic surgery. *Anesth Analg* 59:257, 1980.
11. Tinker JH, Tarhan S: Discontinuing anticoagulant therapy in surgical patients with a cardiac valve prosthesis: Observation in 180 operations. *JAMA* 239:738–739, 1978.
12. Hall DL, Steen WH, Drummond JW: Anticoagulants and cataract surgery. *Annals of Ophthalmol* 12:759–760, 1980.
13. McMahan LB: Anticoagulant and cataract surgery. *J Cataract and Refractive Surg* 14:569–571, 1988.
14. Guiney SP, Robertson DM, Fay W et al: Ocular surgery of patients receiving long-term warfarin therapy. *Am J Ophthalmol* 108:142–146, 1989.
15. Hay A, Olsen KR, Nicholson DH: Bleeding complications in thrombocytopenic patients undergoing ophthalmic surgery. *Am J Ophthalmol* 109:482–483, 1990.
16. Kaplan NR, Reba RC: Pulmonary embolism as the leading cause of ophthalmologic surgery mortality. *Am J Ophthalmol* 73:159, 1972.

PROCEDURE: CATARACT SURGERY

Overview: Cataract surgery is the most frequently performed ophthalmic operation and one of the most common surgical procedures in the United States. Cataract extraction is an elective procedure and is indicated when opacification of the lens progresses to the point of functional visual impairment.

1. *Operation*
   a. Indications: Cataract formation causing visual impairment that interferes with the activities of daily living.
   b. Operative Steps: An incision is made in the superior part of the eye at the junction of the cornea and sclera. The lens is extracted by one of several techniques, and an intraocular lens implant is inserted in most cases. The wound is closed, and a subconjunctival injection of an antibiotic and steroid is given.
   c. Incision: See above.
   d. Anesthesia: The majority of cataract operations can be done under local anesthesia (retrobulbar block). General anesthesia is preferred for anxious patients, children, or patients who may not be able to lie still for 1 hour.
   e. Intraoperative Monitoring: Routine.
   f. Operative Positioning: Supine.
   g. Duration: 1 hour.
   h. EBL/Transfusions: Minimal.
   i. "Surgical Stress": Low.

2. *Expected Hospital Course/Treatment*
   a. Postoperative Monitoring
      (1) ICU Stay: Not required.
      (2) Invasive/Special Monitoring: Not required.
      (3) Parameters To Be Monitored: Routine vital signs.
   b. Positioning/Activity: Early ambulation is encouraged. No lifting more than 10 lb or bending the head below the waist.
   c. Alimentation: As tolerated.
   d. Wound Care/Drains: A patch and shield are placed over the eye which remain in place from 1 hour to several days, depending on the surgeon's preference. Rigid eye shield or protective glasses should be worn for 4 to 6 weeks after surgery.
   e. Respiratory Care: Routine.
   f. Analgesia/Postop Meds: Acetaminophen with or without codeine is appropriate.
   g. Length Of Hospital Stay: Same-day surgery.

3. *Postoperative Complications*
   a. In Hospital
      (1) Morbidity:
         i. Potential loss of vision.
         ii. Intraocular hemorrhage.
         iii. Complications of retrobulbar injection of local anesthetic such as CNS stimulation or depression, respiratory depression, hypotension, or bradycardia.
      (2) Mortality: Mortality related directly to cataract surgery is negligible.
   b. After Discharge
      (1) Increased intraocular pressure.
      (2) Endophthalmitis.
      (3) Suprachoroidal hemorrhage.

4. *Follow-up*
   a. Suggested Follow-up: Postoperative visits are scheduled at 1 day, 1 week, 4 weeks, and 6 weeks.

PROCEDURE: CORNEAL TRANSPLANT

Overview: Corneal transplant surgery is most commonly performed for corneal endothelial cell decompensation in older patients or for keratoconus in younger patients. The surgery is occasionally done on short notice due to the uncertainty of the availability of donor tissue which is usable for only 48 to 72 hours depending on the preservation medium used. Expedient medical consultation may therefore be required.

1. *Operation*
   a. Indications:
      (1) Visual impairment due to corneal disease.
      (2) Severe corneal injuries.
   b. Operative Steps: The eye is stabilized. The diseased host cornea is removed. The donor cornea is sutured in place.
   c. Incision: See above.
   d. Anesthesia: Local or general.
   e. Intraoperative Monitoring: Routine.
   f. Operative Positioning: Supine.
   g. Duration: 1 hour.
   h. EBL/Transfusions: Minimal.
   i. "Surgical Stress": Low.

2. *Expected Hospital Course/Treatment*
   a. Postoperative Monitoring
      (1) ICU Stay: Not required.
      (2) Invasive/Special Monitoring: Not required.
      (3) Parameters To Be Monitored: Routine vital signs.
   b. Positioning/Activity: No lifting more than 10 lb. No bending head below waist.
   c. Alimentation: As tolerated.
   d. Wound Care/Drains: Eye patch and shield for the first postoperative day followed by glasses or rigid eye shield for 6 weeks.
   e. Respiratory Care: Routine.
   f. Analgesia/Postop Meds: Acetaminophen with or without codeine.
   g. Length Of Hospital Stay: Same-day surgery to 1 day hospitalization.

3. *Postoperative Complications*
   a. In Hospital
      (1) Morbidity:
         i. Potential loss of vision.
         ii. Intraocular hemorrhage.
         iii. Complications of retrobulbar injection of local anesthetic such as CNS stimulation or depression, respiratory depression, hypotension, or bradycardia.
      (2) Mortality: Negligible.
   b. After Discharge
      (1) Graft rejection.
      (2) Wound leak.
      (3) Corneal ulcer.
      (4) Astigmatism.

4. *Follow-up*
   a. Suggested Follow-up: Postoperative visits are scheduled at 1 day, 1 week, 4 weeks, then monthly.

PROCEDURES: EVISCERATION, ENUCLEATION, AND EXENTERATION

Overview: This group of procedures involves removal of the contents of the eye (evisceration), removal of the entire eye (enucleation), or removal of the eye and orbital contents (exenteration). Eviscerations and enucleations are most often performed on blind painful eyes or those with intraocular tumors, infections, or trauma unresponsive to conservative therapy. Exenterations are performed when life-threatening tumors or infections invade the orbit.

1. *Operation*
    a. Indications: See above.
    b. Operative Steps: The affected tissue is removed, and a plastic or hydroxyapatite sphere implant is placed. Once the inflammation has subsided in 6 to 8 weeks, an artificial ocular prosthesis is fitted.
    c. Incision: See above.
    d. Anesthesia: General with long-acting retrobulbar anesthetic to minimize postoperative pain.
    e. Intraoperative Monitoring: Routine.
    f. Operative Positioning: Supine.
    g. Duration: 1 to 4 hours.
    h. EBL/Transfusions: Minimal.
    i. "Surgical Stress": Low.

2. *Expected Hospital Course/Treatment*
    a. Postoperative Monitoring
        (1) ICU Stay: Not required.
        (2) Invasive/Special Monitoring: Not required.
        (3) Parameters To Be Monitored: Routine vital signs.
    b. Positioning/Activity: As tolerated.
    c. Alimentation: As tolerated.
    d. Wound Care/Drains: Pressure patch for 5 to 7 days.
    e. Respiratory Care: Routine.
    f. Analgesia/Postop Meds: Parenteral narcotics are initially required.
    g. Length Of Hospital Stay: 1 to 5 days.

3. *Postoperative Complications*
    a. In Hospital
        (1) Morbidity:
            i. Orbital bleeding.
        (2) Mortality: Negligible.
    b. After Discharge
        (1) Orbital bleeding.
        (2) Infection.

4. *Follow-up*
    a. Suggested Follow-up: Postoperative visits are scheduled at 1 day, 1 week, 1 month, and 6 weeks.

PROCEDURE: GLAUCOMA SURGERY

Overview: Glaucoma filtration surgery is indicated in patients with persistently elevated intraocular pressure or progressive visual field damage from glaucoma despite maximum tolerated medical therapy and laser surgery. Since damage to the optic nerve is slowly progressive, surgery is rarely done on an emergency basis except for extremely high pressures. While most glaucomas occur in patients over age 40, congenital glaucomas do occur and require prompt surgical attention. The goal of glaucoma filtration surgery is to provide an alternate pathway for the aqueous fluid to exit the anterior chamber through a fistula between the anterior chamber and the subconjunctival space.

1. *Operation*
   a. Indications: Glaucoma refractory to medical and laser management or in patients unable to take medication.
   b. Operative Steps: A conjunctival flap is dissected in the superior portion of the eye adjacent to the cornea. A fistula is created through the sclera at the limbus connecting the area under the flap and the anterior chamber of the eye. A peripheral iridectomy is performed by excising the peripheral iris at the site of the filtration fistula. This prevents the iris from blocking the internal opening of the fistula.
   c. Incision: See above.
   d. Anesthesia: Local or general. Epinephrine is avoided in the retrobulbar block if local anesthesia is used because it may reduce blood flow to the optic nerve which can theoretically cause optic nerve damage. If general anesthesia is used, nondepolarizing relaxants are preferable to succinylcholine because they are less likely to increase intraocular pressure acutely and cause further optic nerve damage.
   e. Intraoperative Monitoring: Routine.
   f. Operative Positioning: Supine.
   g. Duration: 1 hour.
   h. EBL/Transfusions: Minimal.
   i. "Surgical Stress": Low.

2. *Expected Hospital Course/Treatment*
   a. Postoperative Monitoring
      (1) ICU Stay: Not required.
      (2) Invasive/Special Monitoring: Not required.
      (3) Parameters To Be Monitored: Routine vital signs.
   b. Positioning/Activity: Ambulation as tolerated. No lifting greater than 10 lb. No bending head below the waist.
   c. Alimentation: As tolerated.
   d. Wound Care/Drains: Eye patch and shield first postoperative day followed by glasses or rigid eye shield worn at all times for 6 weeks.
   e. Respiratory Care: Routine.
   f. Analgesia/Postop Meds: Topical steroids and cycloplegic are administered postoperatively.
   g. Length Of Hospital Stay: Same-day surgery.

3. *Postoperative Complications*
   a. In Hospital
      (1) Morbidity:
         i. Suprachoroidal hemorrhage.
         ii. Loss of vision.
      (2) Mortality: Negligible.
   b. After Discharge
      (1) Endophthalmitis.
      (2) Wound leakage.
      (3) Hypotony.

4. *Follow-up*
   a. Suggested Follow-up: Every day for the first week, every 2 to 3 days for the following week, then weekly.

PROCEDURE: STRABISMUS SURGERY

Overview: Strabismus surgery is the most frequently performed ophthalmic operation in the pediatric population. The purpose of strabismus or "squint" surgery is to reposition the extraocular muscles to restore a normal working relationship between the eyes. Although this is not always achieved, cosmetic appearance should be greatly improved. A variety of procedures are performed on the extraocular muscles, including weakening and strengthening procedures.

1. *Operation*
   a. Indications: Severe strabismus.
   b. Operative Steps: An incision is made through the outer layers of the eye near the muscle to be repositioned. A muscle hook is then passed under the muscle and the muscle is cut from the globe. The muscle is sutured to its new insertion point. Usually, two or more muscles are moved during a single operation either on one or both eyes.
   c. Incision: See above.
   d. Anesthesia: General anesthesia is preferred in children. There may be a higher risk of malignant hyperthermia in this pediatric population (see Chap. 6). Succinylcholine should be avoided in strabismus surgery because it causes tonic contraction of the extraocular muscles that may alter the forced duction test often performed at the time of surgery.
   e. Intraoperative Monitoring: Routine. ECG and blood pressure monitoring are mandatory since strabismus surgery involves placing tension on the extraocular muscles which stimulates the oculocardiac reflex.
   f. Operative Positioning: Supine.
   g. Duration: 1 hour.
   h. EBL/Transfusions: Minimal.
   i. "Surgical Stress": Low.

2. *Expected Hospital Course/Treatment*
   a. Postoperative Monitoring
      (1) ICU Stay: Not required.
      (2) Invasive/Special Monitoring: Not required.
      (3) Parameters To Be Monitored: Routine vital signs.
   b. Positioning/Activity: As tolerated.
   c. Alimentation: As tolerated.
   d. Wound Care/Drains: None.
   e. Respiratory Care: Routine.
   f. Analgesia/Postop Meds: Combination steroid and antibiotic ointment is used.
   g. Length Of Hospital Stay: Same-day surgery.

3. *Postoperative Complications*
   a. In Hospital
      (1) Morbidity: Intraoperative bradycardia due to the oculocardiac reflex.
      (2) Mortality: Negligible except for anesthetic-related risk.
   b. After Discharge
      (1) Infection.
      (2) Overcorrection or undercorrection.
      (3) Scleral perforation.

4. *Follow-up*
   a. Suggested Follow-up: Postoperative visits are scheduled at 1 day, 1 week, and 1 month.

PROCEDURE: VITREORETINAL SURGERY

Overview: Scleral buckle and vitrectomy are the two most commonly performed operations performed by vitreoretinal surgeons. The former is done for retinal detachment and the latter for a variety of indications including vitreous opacification (e.g., persistent vitreous hemorrhage), some retinal detachments, preretinal membranes, intraocular foreign body or penetrating injury, and as treatment for endophthalmitis. The goal of scleral buckle procedures is to locate the tear in the retina that caused the detachment and wall it off by creating chorioretinal adhesions around it. To reappose the retina to the underlying choroid, the subretinal fluid is drained and the choroid and sclera are invaginated by a buckle. For vitrectomy, instruments for infusion, light, cutting, and suction are placed through openings into the vitreous cavity. If the lens is too cataractous to permit adequate visualization for the procedure, a lensectomy is performed. The vitreous is then removed from the eye, and additional procedures such as membrane peeling or scleral buckle are performed. The incisions and conjunctiva are then closed. Slowly absorbing gases or silicone oil may also be injected during a vitrectomy to tamponade the retina.

1. *Operation*
    a. Indications:
        (1) Retinal detachment.
        (2) Vitreous hemorrhage.
        (3) Intraocular trauma, foreign body, or infection.
    b. Operative Steps: See description above.
    c. Incision: See above.
    d. Anesthesia: General anesthesia is preferred unless a medical contraindication exists. Gases, such as sulfur hexafluoride and perfluoropropane, may be injected intravitreally near the end of the procedure. Since these gases expand in the eye, they may cause increased intraocular pressure. Nitrous oxide should be avoided for 15 minutes before the injection of intravitreal gas and for 7 to 10 days after its injection because it can diffuse into gas-containing cavities and further elevate intraocular pressure.
    e. Intraoperative Monitoring: Routine.
    f. Operative Positioning: Supine.
    g. Duration: Scleral buckle: 2 hours. Vitrectomy: 1 to 6 hours depending upon the need to do additional retinal procedures.
    h. EBL/Transfusions: Minimal.
    i. "Surgical Stress": Low.

2. *Expected Hospital Course/Treatment*
    a. Postoperative Monitoring
        (1) ICU Stay: Not required.
        (2) Invasive/Special Monitoring: Not required.
        (3) Parameters To Be Monitored: Routine vital signs.
    b. Positioning/Activity: May require face down head position for several days if intraocular gas is used. Otherwise, no heavy lifting or bending below the waist.
    c. Alimentation: As tolerated.
    d. Wound Care/Drains: Postoperative eye patch and rigid eye shield. Glasses or rigid eye shield for 6 weeks after surgery.
    e. Respiratory Care: Routine.
    f. Analgesia/Postop Meds: Topical steroids and a cycloplegic are administered.
    g. Length Of Hospital Stay: 0 to 3 days.

3. *Postoperative Complications*
    a. In Hospital
        (1) Morbidity:
            i. Intraoperative bradycardia due to the oculocardiac reflex.
            ii. Infection.
            iii. Increased intraocular pressure.
        (2) Mortality: Negligible except for anesthetic-related risk.
    b. After Discharge: Intraocular gas takes 2 weeks (sulfur hexafluoride) to 5 weeks (perfluoropropane) to absorb. Flying should be avoided for this length of time since expansion of the bubble occurs with decreased atmospheric pressure.

4. *Follow-up*
    a. Suggested Follow-up: Postoperative visits are scheduled at 1 day, 1 week, and 4 weeks.

11 EVALUATION OF THE PATIENT UNDERGOING OTOLARYNGOLOGIC SURGERY

Jeffrey Finkelstein

Keith T. Kanel

Max Ronis

Since most minor sinus and ear procedures are now usually done in the office setting, the majority of major perioperative issues in otolaryngology arise in patients with head and neck cancer. The most common head and neck operations are total laryngectomy, partial laryngectomy, mandibulectomy, resection of the floor of the mouth, radical neck dissection, tracheostomy, panendoscopy, and tracheoesophageal puncture. Procedures for nonmalignant disease include anterior maxillary artery ligation for recurrent epistaxis, nasal polypectomy, and Caldwell-Luc sinus exploration for unremitting sinusitis. Principal inpatient otologic procedures are mastoidectomy, tympanoplasty, and resection of eighth-nerve neurilemmomas. Because of the discomfort of the above procedures and the need for control of movement, they are uniformly done under general anesthesia.

COMMON COMORBID CONDITIONS

Cardiopulmonary Disease

Many of the risk factors for head and neck cancer are common to both atherosclerotic coronary artery disease and accelerated emphysema. Patients must be screened for subclinical as well as overt disease, and careful assessment of exercise intolerance is required. Nonetheless, the overall incidence of severe cardiac complications in patients undergoing head and neck surgery is low at 2.6 percent.[1]

Postradiation Hypothyroidism

Laboratory evidence of hypothyroidism may occur as early as four months after radiotherapy for head and neck malignancies, reaching an incidence of 30 percent at two years[2] and 60 percent at three years.[3] Primary hypothyroidism is most likely the result of gland failure due to its inclusion in the radiation ports and is

characterized by rise in the serum TSH level. Coincident irradiation of the pituitary gland sometimes accompanying therapy for lesions of the cranial base and paranasal sinuses may cause secondary hypothyroidism[4] with a low serum TSH level. In such cases, a baseline thyroid panel may be useful as part of the preoperative evaluation.

Substance Abuse

Substance abuse is not uncommon in patients with painful disfiguring lesions of the head and neck. Patients should be questioned about the use of alcohol, narcotic and nonnarcotic analgesics, and benzodiazepines, and provisions should be made for preventing or controlling withdrawal symptoms. Related comorbidity should not be overlooked, including hepatitis due to alcohol or acetaminophen, gastritis from alcohol, aspirin and nonsteroidal anti-inflammatory agents, and platelet dysfunction caused by aspirin and nonsteroidal agents (see Chap. 38).

Malnutrition

Malnutrition may be significant in advanced pharyngeal lesions associated with obstructive dysphagia or odynophagia. Assessment of malnutrition and nutritional therapy are discussed in Chaps. 41 and 42.

Metastatic disease

Metastases outside the neck are uncommon in the initial presentation of most otolaryngologic tumors, and detailed staging for dissemination is usually not needed. Evaluation can usually be limited to a chest x-ray and serum liver function studies.[5] Possible metastatic lesions more often require histologic confirmation since up to 10 percent of patients with head and neck cancer may harbor a second primary tumor at the time of initial presentation. Among survivors of head and neck cancer, the risk of second malignancies rises to 20 percent after five years.

Hypercalcemia

Hypercalcemia may accompany squamous cell tumors as a paraneoplastic process. Its presence suggests significant tumor burden and should prompt a more diligent search for metastases.

Chemotherapy

Chemotherapy is occasionally used as an alternative or adjuvant modality before surgery. Surgery should be postponed until transient myelosuppression resolves. The side effects of agents used to treat otolaryngologic tumors include liver damage from methotrexate, heart failure from adriamycin, pulmonary fibrosis from bleomycin, and renal insufficiency from cisplatin.

RISK-BENEFIT ANALYSIS

There are many reasons to proceed expediently in the evaluation of patients with head and neck cancer. Delays in therapy may be associated with spread of the tumor, ongoing aspiration, worsening of nutritional status, continued pain, and the morbidity of drugs needed for pain control. Chemotherapy and radiation therapy are used as temporizing measures in medically unstable patients with aggressive tumors but are rarely curative. Many patients and surgeons are therefore willing to assume some degree of perioperative risk in moving ahead with surgery. For this reason, emphasis is placed on minimizing the risk of perioperative complications without delaying the procedure.

Medically complex patients with suspected head and neck cancer often require evaluation before panendoscopy and biopsy under general anesthesia. The need for comprehensive medical evaluation and screening for cardiac disease before this brief procedure must be weighed against delaying prompt diagnosis. In all but the most overtly high-risk patients, it is reasonable to proceed expediently with appropriate medical prophylaxis and careful monitoring. If a resectable lesion is identified, the patient can undergo a more rigorous evaluation.

The results of a medical evaluation may alter the surgical approach to a lesion. For example, a partial laryngectomy may be chosen over a total laryngectomy in patients with severe pulmonary disease. Similarly, detection of metastatic disease outside the neck may make laryngectomy for airway protection more reasonable than aggressive dissection and reconstruction.

MEDICAL IMPLICATIONS OF INDIVIDUAL OTOLARYNGOLOGIC PROCEDURES

Tracheostomy

Bypassing the glottis and thereby decreasing the physiologic end-expiratory pressure imparted by normal glottic closure increases the risk of postoperative atelectasis and pneumonia. Because effective incentive spirometry is often impossible with an uncuffed tracheostomy tube, early mobilization and pulmonary toilet and chest physical therapy are essential. Patients requiring emergency tracheostomy experience rapid decompression of a clinically obstructed airway and develop postobstructive pulmonary edema, a noncardiogenic alveolar transudate resulting from excessively high transpulmonary pressures. Some have suggested that relief of the obstruction rather than the obstruction itself causes the pulmonary edema,[6] and it most often occurs in the recovery room. Postobstructive pulmonary edema usually responds poorly to diuretics and unloading agents. Severely compromised patients may require positive-pressure ventilation.

Total Laryngectomy

Patients undergoing complete aerodigestive separation often experience an improvement in their overall medical condition with control of aspiration, enhanced nutrition, and pain relief. The incidence of serious medical complications including respiratory failure, stroke, myocardial infarction, and pulmonary embolism is low at 6.2 percent in these patients.[7] Permanent tracheostomies are required after total laryngectomy.

Partial Laryngectomy

In selected patients with limited tumors, removal of only a segment of the larynx is required. Examples of such procedures include supraglottic laryngectomy and vertical hemilaryngectomy. After a brief recovery period with a temporary tracheostomy, patients regain nearly normal phonation and swallowing. However, inevitable alteration of the deglutition mechanism may increase the risk of both short- and long-term aspiration. Up to 25 percent of patients with partial laryngectomy develop postoperative pneumonia or intolerable aspiration precluding decannulation and often require reoperation for aerodigestive separation. Larynx-sparing procedures may therefore be least suitable for patients with preexisting lung disease. Attempts to develop objective criteria such as preoperative pulmonary function parameters to predict outcome in these patients have been disappointing.[8] However, those with marked exercise intolerance, baseline hypoxemia, recurrent pulmonary infections, or intractable bronchospasm should be considered poor candidates for partial laryngectomy.

Bilateral Neck Dissection

Sacrifice of the jugular veins may result in increased intracranial pressure due to venous hypertension. Subsequent problems include headache, bradycardia, and sometimes hyponatremia. A recent study of complications associated with total laryngectomy documented stroke only among patients undergoing neck dissection, suggesting a causative role of carotid manipulation.[7] Carotid sinus hypersensitivity with cardioinhibitory, vasodepressor, or mixed responses may also develop after trauma to the carotid body.

Pharyngogastric Anastomosis and Jejunal Interposition

Gastric "pull-up" procedures or small-bowel interpositions following pharyngolaryngoesophagectomy for cancer of the hypopharynx carry the additional surgical risks of laparotomy. Intraoperative hemodynamic fluctuations during traction of the gastrointestinal tract through the mediastinum may be significant. Perioperative morbidity includes pleural effusion, cardiac arrhythmia, diarrhea, bile regurgitation, and chest infection.[9] Aggressive postoperative feeding through a small-bowel alimentation catheter is recommended since patients are often markedly malnourished.

Thyroidectomy and Parathyroidectomy

Thyroidectomy, particularly when performed as part of an extensive anterior neck dissection for tumor, may be associated with incidental complete parathyroidectomy. Affected patients may demonstrate profound symptomatic hypocalcemia within 24 hours of surgery, and serum calcium levels should be monitored expectantly. Patients exhibiting Chvostek's or Trousseau's sign or serum calcium concentrations below six mg/dl should be treated with a continuous calcium infusion. Parathyroid function may recover if the glands have been injured rather than removed and can be assessed by measuring blood levels of parathyroid hormone. Persistent hypoparathyroidism requires chronic therapy with calcium supplements and an oral vitamin D preparation. Although thyroxine replacement is not urgent, it should be instituted within the first week after surgery, provided that preoperative thyroid function was normal.

Tracheoesophageal Puncture (TEP)

This procedure permits limited phonation following total laryngectomy, but can also result in low-grade aspiration despite otherwise successful aerodigestive separation. Aspiration can usually be documented by a bedside swallowing test. TEP may therefore not be tolerated in some patients with marginal lung function.

Cranial Base Surgery

Resection of deeply seated cranial base lesions involves prolonged procedures with significant perioperative stress.[10] Dysfunction or sacrifices of structures near the base of the skull may create a variety of problems. Seizures and delirium may result from cerebral contusions incurred during brain traction, particularly when a transfrontal approach is used. Damage to the hypothalamus and neurohypophyseal tract may cause central diabetes insipidus and profound hypernatremia that should be considered during the anticipated period of postoperative diuresis. Pituitary insufficiency with secondary adrenal insufficiency and secondary hypothyroidism should be preemptively treated with hydrocortisone and L-thyroxine when the area of resection is known to encompass the gland. Cranial nerve dysfunction may be associated with vagal dysautonomia, sensory deficits, impaired swallowing, and inadequate airway protection. Surgically-induced communication between the central nervous system and the paranasal sinuses or pharynx poses the risk for intracranial infection in the form of meningitis, brain abscess, epidural abscess, or cranial base osteomyelitis. In such cases, prophylactic antibiotics are recommended, and imaging studies should be performed promptly if fever develops. Other potential complications include the syndrome of inappropriate antidiuretic hormone (SIADH), carotid compression, and respiratory failure.

Anterior Maxillary Artery Ligation for Epistaxis

Transantral arterial ligation to control refractory epistaxis is required if nonsurgical measures like temporary occlusive packing, cautery, and gel foam embolization fail. Hypertension is usually a contributing factor and should be promptly controlled. Although bleeding diatheses are often suspected, they are rarely found. Nonetheless, the platelet count, prothrombin time (PT), partial thromboplastin time (PTT), and bleeding time should be checked before surgery in all cases. The degree of blood loss is often underestimated, and blood transfusions may be required.

Nasal Polypectomy

Patients should be carefully screened for "triad asthma," consisting of nasal polyposis, recurrent sinusitis, and unremitting bronchospasm. All aspirin-containing products and nonsteroidal anti-inflammatory agents should be avoided. Glucocorticoids are often required to stabilize airway disease.

PROPHYLACTIC MEASURES

Most recommendations for perioperative prophylaxis for general surgery are applicable to otolaryngologic procedures. Because patients are mobilized early after surgery, the incidence of deep-venous thrombosis is remarkably low.[11] When recovery is less rapid, standard thromboembolism prophylaxis with low-dose heparin or intermittent pneumatic compression devices is warranted.[12] The indications for prophylaxis against gastric stress ulcer are less well-defined. However, patients with nasogastric feeding tubes are often treated with intravenous boluses or infusion of H_2-blockers or sulcrafate through the tube. The latter agent may be preferable in larynx-sparing procedures due to the increased risk of nosocomial pneumonia from aspiration of gastric bacteria when gastric acid is neutralized. Prophylaxis against seizures with phenytoin is recommended in cranial base procedures involving brain traction. Perioperative antibiotics are discussed in Chap. 44.

COMMON POSTOPERATIVE PROBLEMS

Diabetes Mellitus

Management of diabetes may be difficult in patients on postoperative tube feedings and during conversion to normal swallowing. Nasogastric feedings can also be interrupted by faulty tube function or inadvertent removal, posing the risk of hypoglycemia from previously administered insulin. Long-acting insulin preparations should be used only in select circumstances in patients undergoing swallowing retraining. Otherwise sliding scale coverage is preferable temporarily.

Chronic Obstructive Lung Disease

Metered-dose inhalers can be difficult to use for patients with tracheotomies. Few standard adapters are available for patients with tubeless stomas. In the immediate postoperative period, bronchodilators should therefore be administered by aerosolized nebulizers. Since aerosolized steroids are not available for nebulizer use, systemic steroids should be administered to steroid-dependent patients. Methylxanthines may also be useful in this setting.

Hypertension

Parenteral agents may be necessary for blood pressure control in the first few days after surgery. Sublingual agents may be unsuitable after extensive oral surgery because of swelling and poor absorption. Antihypertensive preparations in sustained release capsules work irregularly when the integrity of the capsule is violated and are therefore unsuitable for nasogastric administration.

Nutrition

Parenteral nutrition is rarely necessary. Duodenal tubes are preferable over gastric tubes to reduce the risk of aspiration and contamination of the surgical wound. Wound infection may contribute to the development of pharyngocutaneous and tracheoesophageal fistulae, a particular problem among patients with significant vasculopathy or diabetes.

REFERENCES

1. Detsky AS, Abrams HB, McLaughlin JR: Predicting cardiac complications in patients undergoing noncardiac surgery. *J Gen Intern Med* 1:211, 1986.
2. Posner MR, Ervin TJ, Fabian RL et al: Incidence of hypothyroidism following multimodality treatment for advanced squamous cell cancer of the head and neck. *Laryngoscope* 94:451–454, 1984.
3. Vrabec DP, Jeffron TJ: Hypothyroidism following treatment for head and neck cancer. *Ann Otol* 90:449–453, 1981.
4. Constine LS, Woolf PD, Cann D et al: Hypothalamic-pituitary dysfunction after radiation for brain tumors. *N Engl J Med* 328:87–94, 1993.
5. Jacobs C: The internist in the management of head and neck cancer. *Ann Intern Med* 113:771–778, 1990.
6. Kamal RS, Agha S: Acute pulmonary edema. A complication of upper airway obstruction. *Anaesthesia* 39:464–467, 1984.
7. Arriaga MA, Kanel KT, Johnson JT et al: Medical complications in total laryngectomy: Incidence and risk factors. *Ann Otol Rhinol Laryngol* 99:611–615, 1990.
8. Chow JM, Block RM, Friedman M: Preoperative evaluation for partial laryngectomy. *Head Neck Surg* 10:319–323, 1988.
9. Harrison DFN, Thompson AE: Pharyngolaryngoesophagectomy with pharyngogastric anastomosis for cancer of the hypopharynx: Review of 101 operations. *Head Neck Surg* 8:418–428, 1986.
10. Sen CN, Sekhar LN: Complications of cranial base surgery, in Post KD, Friedman E, McCormick P (eds): *Postoperative Complications in Intracranial Neurosurgery*. New York, Theme Medical, 1993, pp 111–131.
11. Spires JR, Byers RM, Sanchez ED: Pulmonary thromboembolism after head and neck surgery. *South Med J* 82:1111–1115, 1989.
12. Clagett CP, Anderson FA, Levine MN et al: Prevention of venous thromboembolism. *Chest* 102:391S–407S, 1992.

PROCEDURE: LARYNGECTOMY/RADICAL NECK DISSECTION

Overview: Procedures performed for cancer of the larynx depend on the size and location of the lesion and its classification according to the TNM staging system. Total or partial laryngectomy may be done. Partial laryngectomy may remove the portion of the larynx above the vocal cords (supraglottic) or half of the larynx (hemilaryngectomy). Other modified procedures can also be performed. Radical neck dissection includes the resection of lymphatic structures of the neck to remove metastatic or suspected metastatic lymph nodes. A classic radical neck dissection removes the submandibular gland, sternocleidomastoid muscle, tail of parotid gland, spinal accessory nerve, and internal jugular vein. Modification of this procedure may also be performed, with the most common being sparing of the spinal accessory nerve.

1. *Operation*
    a. Indications: Malignancies of the larynx.
    b. Operative Steps: The sternocleidomastoid muscle and internal jugular vein are sectioned and removed with the inferior neck lymphatics. The strap muscles of the neck are transected, and a hemithyroidectomy and isthmusectomy are performed. The paratracheal, pretracheal, and tracheoesophageal lymph nodes are removed. Tracheotomy is performed (if not previously done). The pharynx is opened prior to removal of the larynx and remaining neck dissection specimen. Cricopharyngeal myotomy and tracheoesophageal puncture with placement of a feeding tube may be performed prior to pharyngeal closure. A tracheostoma is created.
    c. Incision: A U-shaped incision generally from the mastoid tip to 1 to 2 fingerbreadths above the sternal notch. Variations will occur depending upon the extent of disease and specific procedure.
    d. Anesthesia: General with endotracheal intubation or through a tracheotomy.
    e. Intraoperative Monitoring: Routine. Arterial line with or without CVP in medically debilitated patients.
    f. Operative Positioning: Supine with neck extension.
    g. Duration: 3 to 5 hours.
    h. EBL/Transfusions: EBL is 300 to 1000 ml depending on the extent of surgery. Transfusion may be required depending on the baseline hematocrit level.
    i. "Surgical Stress": Severe.

2. *Expected Hospital Course/Treatment*
    a. Postoperative Monitoring
        (1) ICU Stay: Dictated by the patient's medical status.
        (2) Invasive/Special Monitoring: While in ICU.
        (3) Parameters To Be Monitored:
            i. Vital signs.
            ii. Urine output.
            iii. Chest x-ray 24 and 72 hours after surgery.
            iv. CBC.
            v. Electrolytes.
            vi. Drain output.
    b. Positioning/Activity: Out of bed when fully awake. May ambulate on POD 1.
    c. Alimentation: Clear liquids through a feeding tube on POD 1. Tube feedings advanced as tolerated. Oral liquids begun on POD 7 if no problems noted.
    d. Wound Care/Drains: Suction drains maintained until POD 3.
    e. Respiratory Care: Routine tracheostomy care with high-humidity tracheostomy collar.
    f. Analgesia/Postop Meds: Parenteral narcotics for 2 to 3 days, then acetaminophen with codeine through feeding tube.
    g. Length Of Hospital Stay: 1 to 2 weeks.

3. *Postoperative Complications*
    a. In Hospital
        (1) Morbidity:
            i. Pneumonia (aspiration pneumonia more common with partial laryngectomy).
            ii. Pharyngeal fistula (more common preoperative radiation therapy).
            iii. Wound infection or hematoma.
            iv. Complications associated with tracheostomy.
            v. Carotid blowout.
            vi. Chylous fistula associated with unrecognized thoracic duct transection.
            vii. Injury to mandibular, vagus, phrenic, hypoglossal, or brachial plexus nerves.
        (2) Mortality: 1%.
    b. After Discharge
        (1) Tracheal stenosis.
        (2) Pharyngeal stenosis with dysphagia.
        (3) Aphonia.
        (4) Difficulties with esophageal speech or tracheoesophageal puncture site.

4. *Follow-up*
    a. Suggested Follow-up: Patients are seen at 1 week. Prolonged cancer surveillance is necessary.

PROCEDURE: LARYNGOSCOPY

Overview: Laryngoscopy is frequently performed to diagnose and treat disorders of the larynx and hypopharynx. It allows better visualization of the larynx than flexible or mirror examinations. Laryngoscopy may be combined with microscopic visualization and/or laser treatment.

1. *Operation*

    a. Indications:

    (1) Diagnosis of acute or chronic laryngeal disease.
    (2) Removal of foreign bodies in upper aerodigestive tract.
    (3) Dilatation of a stenotic larynx.
    (4) Vocal cord injection for paralysis.
    (5) Performance of endoscopic arytenoidectomy.

    b. Operative Steps: The teeth and oral structures are protected by a mouth guard. The appropriate laryngoscope is inserted. Landmarks are exposed and examined. The instruments are removed after the appropriate procedure is performed.
    c. Incision: None or as determined by surgical procedure done in conjunction with laryngoscopy.
    d. Anesthesia: Topical or general.
    e. Intraoperative Monitoring: Routine.
    f. Operative Positioning: Supine. Both flexion and extension of the neck occur with this procedure.
    g. Duration: 30 to 60 minutes, depending upon adjunctive procedures.
    h. EBL/Transfusions: Minimal blood loss.
    i. "Surgical Stress": Moderate.

2. *Expected Hospital Course/Treatment*

    a. Postoperative Monitoring

    (1) ICU Stay: Not required.
    (2) Invasive/Special Monitoring: Not required.
    (3) Parameters To Be Monitored:

        i. Routine vital signs.
        ii. Observation for adequate air exchange after vocal cord surgery.

    b. Positioning/Activity: Elevate head initially. Advance to full activity as tolerated.
    c. Alimentation: Advance as tolerated after patient is fully awake.
    d. Wound Care/Drains: Not required.
    e. Respiratory Care: Routine with observation for adequate airway.
    f. Analgesia/Postop Meds: Oral analgesics are satisfactory.
    g. Length Of Hospital Stay: Usually outpatient depending upon associated procedures.

3. *Postoperative Complications*

    a. In Hospital

    (1) Morbidity:

        i. Tooth or oral cavity trauma.
        ii. Bleeding after biopsy.
        iii. Voice change or hoarseness.

    (2) Mortality: < 1%.

        b. After Discharge: Voice change.

4. *Follow-up*

    a. Suggested Follow-up: As determined by reason for procedure.

PROCEDURE: MASTOIDECTOMY

Overview: Mastoidectomy allows removal of disease from the temporal bone and includes resection of the mastoid bone, antrum, and middle ear. This is generally accomplished with the use of an operating microscope and high-speed drill. Mastoidectomy is reserved for patients who have failed more conservative medical management.

1. *Operation*
   a. Indications:
      (1) Acute and chronic mastoiditis unresponsive to medical treatment.
      (2) Cholesteatoma.
      (3) Otogenic brain abscess.
      (4) Petrositis.
   b. Operative Steps: After injection of local anesthetic with epinephrine, incision is made to expose the mastoid bone. Under otomicroscopy using a high-speed drill, the mastoid cortex is sequentially removed in order to expose more medial structures such as the antrum and middle ear structures. The extent of the mastoidectomy is dictated by the disease process and its location. The disease process is removed, and the wounds are closed with or without an attempt to reconstruct the hearing apparatus, depending upon the specific findings.
   c. Incision: Postauricular and transcanal.
   d. Anesthesia: General.
   e. Intraoperative Monitoring: Facial nerve monitoring is performed for unusual anatomy and some revision surgery.
   f. Operative Positioning: Supine.
   g. Duration: 2 to 4 hours.
   h. EBL/Transfusions: Minimal blood loss.
   i. "Surgical Stress": Moderate.

2. *Expected Hospital Course/Treatment*
   a. Postoperative Monitoring
      (1) ICU Stay: Dictated by the patient's medical status.
      (2) Invasive/Special Monitoring: While in ICU.
      (3) Parameters To Be Monitored:
         i. Vital signs.
         ii. Facial nerve function.
         iii. Mental status.
   b. Positioning/Activity: Elevate head of bed initially. Out of bed with assistance on day of surgery. Advance activity as tolerated. No nose-blowing. Keep ear dry.
   c. Alimentation: Advance as tolerated after any vertigo resolves.
   d. Wound Care/Drains: Drains may be used in significantly infected cases.
   e. Respiratory Care: Routine.
   f. Analgesia/Postop Meds: Oral agents are satisfactory.
   g. Length Of Hospital Stay: 1 to 2 days, depending on degree of dizziness or need for continued antibiotics.

3. *Postoperative Complications*
   a. In Hospital
      (1) Morbidity:
         i. Nausea or vertigo.
         ii. Cerebrospinal fluid leak.
         iii. Facial nerve weakness.
      (2) Mortality: < 1%.
   b. After Discharge
      (1) Persistent otorrhea.
      (2) Hearing loss.

4. *Follow-up*
   a. Suggested Follow-up: Patients are seen at 1 week.

PROCEDURE: MIDDLE EAR SURGERY

Overview: Tympanoplasty with or without ossiculoplasty involves repair and reconstruction of the middle ear hearing mechanism including the tympanic membrane and the ossicles. Stapedectomy is the surgical removal of the stapes with replacement by a prosthesis.

1. *Operation*
   a. Indications:

      Tympanoplasty with or without ossiculoplasty:

      (1) Conductive hearing loss due to ear drum perforation.
      (2) Conductive hearing loss due to ossicular destruction, disruption, or fixation.
      (3) Recurrent or chronic otitis media.
      (4) Persistent tympanic membrane perforation or hearing loss 3 months after trauma, surgery, or infection.

      Stapedectomy: Otosclerosis with significant conductive hearing loss.
   b. Operative Steps: Tympanoplasty: After injection of local anesthetic with epinephrine, a tympanomeatal flap is elevated from a transcanal or postauricular approach. The ossicular chain and middle ear are explored. The ossicular chain and tympanic membrane are then reconstructed using tissue grafts or prostheses as required. The tympanomeatal flap is replaced, and the ear canal is gently packed with absorbable packing. Stapedectomy: After exposure through a transcanal approach, the posterior-superior canal wall is trimmed to expose the incudostapedial joint. The stapes tendon is cut, the incudostapedial joint is disarticulated, the suprastructure and footplate of the stapes are removed, and a prosthesis is placed on a vein or fascial graft overlying the oval window. The prosthesis is secured to the long process of the incus, and closure is performed in the same way as tympanoplasty.
   c. Incision: Transcanal and/or postauricular.
   d. Anesthesia: Local with or without IV sedation or general, depending on the patient and extent of surgery anticipated. Stapedectomy is almost always done under local anesthesia.
   e. Intraoperative Monitoring: Routine.
   f. Operative Positioning: Supine.
   g. Duration: 1 to 3 hours (less with stapedectomy).
   h. EBL/Transfusions: Minimal blood loss.
   i. "Surgical Stress": Low.

2. *Expected Hospital Course/Treatment*
   a. Postoperative Monitoring
      (1) ICU Stay: Not required.
      (2) Invasive/Special Monitoring: Not required.
      (3) Parameters To Be Monitored:
         i. Vital signs.
         ii. Evaluate for vertigo, nystagmus, and facial palsy.
   b. Positioning/Activity: Bedrest for 24 hours. Avoid straining and nose-blowing. Keep ear dry.
   c. Alimentation: Advance as tolerated after dizziness resolves.
   d. Wound Care/Drains: Usually none.
   e. Respiratory Care: Routine.
   f. Analgesia/Postop Meds: Oral acetaminophen with codeine. Diazepam as needed for dizziness.
   g. Length Of Hospital Stay: Outpatient if no significant dizziness occurs after 2 to 4 hours of observation. Admit for continued nausea or vomiting.

3. *Postoperative Complications*
   a. In Hospital
      (1) Morbidity:
         i. Vertigo.
         ii. Nausea and/or vomiting.
         iii. Bleeding.
         iv. Facial weakness.
      (2) Mortality: < 1%.
   b. After Discharge
      (1) Persistent vertigo, nausea, or vomiting.
      (2) Facial nerve paralysis (rare).
      (3) Graft failure with persistent hearing loss.
      (4) Tinnitus.
      (5) Infection.
      (6) Loss of taste on side of tongue (usually temporary).

4. *Follow-up*
   a. Suggested Follow-up: Patients are seen at 1 week.

PROCEDURE: SINUS SURGERY

Overview: Ethmoidectomy involves removal of the septa between multiple ethmoid cells to create a large ethmoid cavity without obstruction to drainage. It is performed through an external (facial), intranasal (endoscopic), or transantral (through Caldwell-Luc) approach. The approach is determined by the degree and location of sinus disease and by the surgeon's skill and experience. A Caldwell-Luc operation allows access to the maxillary antrum to treat chronic sinus disease, biopsy pathology in the sinus, inspect or reduce fractures of the orbital floor, or retrieve fragmented root tips from extracted maxillary teeth. Access is obtained through a window created in the bony anterior sinus wall. With the advent of endoscopic sinus surgery and greater understanding of sinus pathophysiology, the Caldwell-Luc operation is less frequently performed.

1. *Operation*
   a. Indications:
      (1) Treatment of acute or chronic sinusitis unresponsive to medical therapy.
      (2) Orbital or cranial extension of maxillary or ethmoid sinusitis.
      (3) Ethmoid or maxillary polyp or tumor causing nasal obstruction.
      (4) Recurrent nasal polyps causing obstruction.
      (5) Biopsy of tumors involving respective sinuses.
      (6) Inspection and/or reduction of orbital floor and wall fractures.

   b. Operative Steps: Ethmoidectomy: In an external approach through an incision between nasal bridge and medial canthus, the anterior ethmoid artery is ligated, and the lamina papyracea and ethmoid sinuses are opened after elevation of the periosteum. Sinus surgery is performed followed by careful reapproximation of skin and subcutaneous layers. In an endoscopic approach through a lateral intranasal incision, specialized telescopes and instruments are used to open the ethmoid sinuses. A transantral approach can be performed through the opened maxillary sinus (i.e., as part of a Caldwell-Luc operation). Caldwell-Luc: An incision in the mucosa of the maxillary vestibule exposes bone in the canine fossa. A bone window is created with a chisel or drill, and the sinus is entered. The necessary procedure is performed, and the intraoral incision is closed.

   c. Incision: Ethmoidectomy: intranasal or external between nasal bridge and medial canthus. Caldwell-Luc: intraoral over area of canine fossa.
   d. Anesthesia: Local, local with IV sedation, or general.
   e. Intraoperative Monitoring: Routine.
   f. Operative Positioning: Supine with head elevated.
   g. Duration: 1 to 2 hours.
   h. EBL/Transfusions: EBL is 100 to 200 ml. Transfusions not required.
   i. "Surgical Stress": Low to moderate.

2. *Expected Hospital Course/Treatment*
   a. Postoperative Monitoring
      (1) ICU Stay: Not required.
      (2) Invasive/Special Monitoring: None.
      (3) Parameters To Be Monitored:
          i. Vital signs.
          ii. Visual fields and extraocular muscle movements.
          iii. Mental status evaluation.
          iv. Observe for facial edema.

   b. Positioning/Activity: Keep head of bed elevated. Advance activity as tolerated.
   c. Alimentation: As tolerated.
   d. Wound Care/Drains: Nasal and/or antral packing as needed. Nasal and/or external drains may be needed depending on extent of surgery.
   e. Respiratory Care: Humidified face tent especially for patients with significant nasal packing.
   f. Analgesia/Postop Meds: Acetaminophen with codeine is adequate.
   g. Length Of Hospital Stay: Outpatient or overnight stay depending on extent of surgery, type of nasal packing, or concern for postoperative complications.

3. *Postoperative Complications*
   a. In Hospital
      (1) Morbidity: Ethmoidectomy:
          i. Bleeding and eyelid ecchymosis.
          ii. Vision change (e.g., diplopia, blindness).
          iii. Facial edema.
          iv. Infection.
          v. Cerebrospinal fluid leak and meningitis.

      Caldwell-Luc:
          i. Bleeding.
          ii. Facial numbness.
          iii. Tooth numbness or damage.

      (2) Mortality: < 1%.
   b. After Discharge
      (1) Bleeding. (2) Orbital injury. (3) Recurrent sinusitis. (4) Cerebrospinal fluid leak and meningitis. (5) Oral-antral fistula.

4. *Follow-up*
   a. Suggested Follow-up: Patients are seen at 1 week.

PROCEDURE: TRACHEOTOMY

Overview: A tracheotomy is an opening made in the trachea through the neck to allow breathing when the upper airway is obstructed, narrowed, or potentially unstable. It also allows for removal of endotracheal tubes that might cause laryngotracheal irritation or damage when in place for prolonged periods of time. In general, emergency tracheotomies are associated with a higher incidence of complications.

1. *Operation*
   a. Indications:
      (1) Respiratory distress or compromise.
      (2) Prolonged intubation.
      (3) Obstructive sleep apnea with documented arterial desaturation.
      (4) Facilitation of ventilation and pulmonary toilet.
      (5) Adjunct to treatment of head and neck trauma.
   b. Operative Steps: After skin incision through the level of the platysma, the strap muscles are separated using sharp and blunt dissection. The cricoid cartilage and thyroid isthmus are exposed. Retraction or division of the thyroid isthmus is performed to expose the upper tracheal rings. A tracheal opening at the second, third, or fourth tracheal ring is created by removing an anterior window of cartilage. The trachea is suctioned. The tracheostomy tube is inserted and secured.
   c. Incision: Vertical or horizontal lower-neck incision 1 cm below the cricoid cartilage in the midline.
   d. Anesthesia: Local or general.
   e. Intraoperative Monitoring: Invasive monitors may frequently be in place in critically ill patients.
   f. Operative Positioning: Supine with neck extension.
   g. Duration: < 1 hour.
   h. EBL/Transfusions: Minimal blood loss.
   i. "Surgical Stress": Low.

2. *Expected Hospital Course/Treatment*
   a. Postoperative Monitoring
      (1) ICU Stay: Dictated by the patients medical status.
      (2) Invasive/Special Monitoring: While in ICU.
      (3) Parameters To Be Monitored:
         i. Vital signs.
         ii. Monitor for adequate ventilation and oxygenation.
         iii. Chest x-ray to evaluate tube position and exclude pneumothorax or subcutaneous emphysema.
   b. Positioning/Activity: Head elevation. Advance activity and ambulate as medical condition allows.
   c. Alimentation: Oral intake when patient is fully awake if no other limiting medical conditions.
   d. Wound Care/Drains: Initial aseptic tracheal suctioning should be done every 1 hour and as needed with cleaning and changing inner cannula every 8 to 12 hours. First tracheotomy change is performed by a qualified person at 3 to 7 days postoperatively.
   e. Respiratory Care: Tracheotomy collar with high humidification.
   f. Analgesia/Postop Meds: Mild oral analgesics as needed if patient is taking oral medications.
   g. Length Of Hospital Stay: Dependent upon original reason for tracheotomy.

3. *Postoperative Complications*
   a. In Hospital
      (1) Morbidity:
         i. Tracheotomy dislocation.
         ii. Bleeding.
         iii. Crusting and obstruction.
         iv. Pneumothorax and/or pneumomediastinum.
         v. Subcutaneous emphysema.
         vi. Local wound infection.
      (2) Mortality: 5% in elective cases, 10 to 50% in emergencies.
   b. After Discharge
      (1) Crusting and dry bleeding of mucosa.
      (2) Tube displacement.
      (3) Subglottic stenosis.
      (4) Tracheal erosion with or without vessel disruption.
      (5) Tracheocutaneous fistula after removal of tube.

4. *Follow-up*
   a. Suggested Follow-up: If the patient has the tracheotomy when leaving the hospital, follow-up is within 1 week and as needed depending on his or her ability to care for the tracheotomy. Family and patient education is very important for continued tracheotomy care at home.

PROCEDURE: UVULOPALATOPHARYNGOPLASTY (UPPP)

Overview: UPPP is a procedure used in the treatment of sleep disorders such as obstructive sleep apnea (OSA) and loud snoring. It involves removal of the tonsils (if not previously done) and redundant or excessive palatal and pharyngeal mucosa. Depending upon the severity and location of the obstruction, UPPP may be combined with septoplasty, tracheotomy, and, less frequently, partial tongue base resection. Patients with OSA presenting for this surgery are usually obese, and weight loss has been shown to improve symptoms. Severe OSA may lead to hypertension, tachycardia, and cardiac arrhythmias due to decreased O_2 saturation. UPPP is > 50% successful in treating OSA and > 80% in eliminating snoring.

1. *Operation*
   a. Indications:
      (1) Obstructive sleep apnea.
      (2) Severe snoring.
   b. Operative Steps: Tonsillectomy is performed first with mucosal incisions along the anterior tonsillar pillars. Dissection is then carried superiorly. The soft palate is incised at the uvular base with removal of palatal and tonsillar tissues. After adequate hemostasis, the anterior and posterior tonsillar pillars are sutured together and the palatal edges are sutured to themselves.
   c. Incision: Anterior and posterior tonsillar pillars. Soft palate at the uvular base level.
   d. Anesthesia: General.
   e. Intraoperative Monitoring: Routine with or without arterial line depending on severity of disease.
   f. Operative Positioning: Supine with neck extended.
   g. Duration: 2 hours.
   h. EBL/Transfusions: EBL is < 200 ml. Transfusions not required.
   i. "Surgical Stress": Moderate.

2. *Expected Hospital Course/Treatment*
   a. Postoperative Monitoring
      (1) ICU Stay: ICU monitoring for 24 hours is often necessary depending on severity of disease.
      (2) Invasive/Special Monitoring: Routine ICU care for 24 hours.
      (3) Parameters To Be Monitored:
         i. Vital signs.
         ii. Oximetry.
         iii. Cardiac rhythm.
   b. Positioning/Activity: Elevation of head of bed. Ambulate by POD 1.
   c. Alimentation: Clear liquids on POD 1. Advance to solids as tolerated.
   d. Wound Care/Drains: Oral saline rinses may be used.
   e. Respiratory Care: Careful observation for first 24 hours until acute edema has peaked.
   f. Analgesia/Postop Meds: Initially parenteral analgesics may be needed until the patient can tolerate oral acetaminophen with codeine elixir.
   g. Length Of Hospital Stay: 2 to 5 days depending upon ability to tolerate oral feedings.

3. *Postoperative Complications*
   a. In Hospital
      (1) Morbidity:
         i. Bleeding.
         ii. Exacerbation of preoperative medical problems (e.g., hypertension, cardiac arrhythmias).
         iii. Dehydration.
         iv. Postobstructive pulmonary edema.
      (2) Mortality: < 1%.
   b. After Discharge
      (1) Persistent nasal regurgitation and hypernasal speech.
      (2) Nasopharyngeal stenosis.

4. *Follow-up*
   a. Suggested Follow-up: Patients are seen at 1 week.

12 EVALUATION OF THE PATIENT UNDERGOING UROLOGIC SURGERY

David S. Macpherson

E. James Seidmon

A. Richard Kendall

Urologic surgery is commonly performed in patients of all ages and includes extensive procedures for congenital disorders in children and benign prostatic hypertrophy and cancer in older adults. Operations for prostate disease are the most common urologic procedures in the elderly. In a population-based study from Europe, 71 percent of patients undergoing surgery for benign prostatic hypertrophy were over 65 years old, and more than a third were over 75.[1] In the United States, about 20 percent of men over 60 years of age have had prostate surgery.[2] With the aging of the population, urologic surgery is likely to become even more common unless medical interventions for prostate hypertrophy prove effective and long-lasting.[3]

COMMON COMORBID CONDITIONS

Between 3 percent and 20 percent of patients seen by medical consultation services are hospitalized for urologic surgery, suggesting that comorbidity is common in urologic populations.[4-7] In those undergoing transurethral resection of the prostate, prior myocardial infarction is found in 10 percent, a history of congestive heart failure in 7 percent, angina pectoris in 15 percent, and hypertension in 31 percent.[1,8] Among noncardiac diseases, chronic obstructive pulmonary disease is present in 23 percent and diabetes in 16 percent.[1] In one study, 77 percent of patients undergoing surgery for benign prostatic hypertrophy had at least one medical disease thought to affect surgical risk.[1] In addition, long-term survival in urologic patients is strongly related to medical comorbidity and physical status.[8]

Patients with urologic disorders often present with acute urinary retention and renal insufficiency that may complicate medical management.[1] However, although renal insufficiency can be the result of obstruction to urinary flow, the prevalence of a serum creatinine over 160 μg/l in patients undergoing transurethral resec-

tion of the prostate was only 2.4 percent in one study.[8] This suggests that complete urinary outlet obstruction is usually relieved before serious renal damage occurs.

ANESTHETIC TECHNIQUES

A wide variety of anesthetic techniques are used in urologic surgery. Although more extensive procedures are usually performed under general anesthesia, transurethral resection of the prostate can be done under general, spinal, or local anesthesia.[9] The rate of perioperative complications of transurethral resection is not altered dramatically by choice of anesthesia.[10] Local anesthesia may be preferable in patients with serious medical problems but may not be an option in those who are overly anxious, those with extremely large prostates, or those in whom cancer has made the urethra rigid. Nonetheless, local anesthesia was used in one-third of cases in a series of veterans.[9]

PROPHYLACTIC ISSUES IN UROLOGIC PATIENTS

Venous Thromboembolism Prophylaxis

Venous thromboembolism is a common complication of urologic procedures and has been most extensively studied in patients undergoing transurethral resection of the prostate and open prostatectomy. The frequency of deep venous thrombosis is approximately 10 percent in those undergoing transurethral resection and 40 percent in those undergoing open procedures. For this reason, prophylaxis against thromboembolism is recommended.

Large comparative trials of prophylactic regimens are lacking in the urologic literature. However, in patients undergoing most urologic procedures, low-dose heparin appears to reduce the incidence of deep venous thrombosis (as detected by radiolabeled-fibrinogen scanning) in about 75 percent.[11] Low-dose heparin (LDH) has been shown to be effective in patients undergoing transurethral resection, but its efficacy in open prostatectomy is less certain.[12,13] External pneumatic compression devices and the combination of LDH and dihydroergotamine have proven effective in these high-risk urologic patients.[14]

Prophylaxis Against Bacterial Endocarditis

Bacteremia after urologic procedures is common and can cause endocarditis in patients with susceptible cardiac anomalies. Bacteremia following prostatectomy occurs in up to 82 percent of cases in which the urine is infected and up to 13 percent of cases in which the urine is sterile.[15] Prophylaxis against endocarditis is recommended for cystoscopy, urethral dilatation, all types of prostatic surgery, and any procedure involving the urinary tract when the urine is infected.[16] The most common bacterium implicated in endocarditis is *Enterococcus faecalis*. Gram-negative bacteremia is common but only rarely causes endocarditis in this setting. Therefore, prophylactic regimens are primarily directed against enterococcus species. Specific antibiotic regimens are discussed in Chap. 43.

Urologic Procedures in the Presence of Infected Urine

When infected urine is present at the time of instrumentation or other procedures involving the urinary tract, the risk of postoperative infection including sepsis and wound infection in patients undergoing open prostatectomy patients is probably increased.[17] However, many of the studies supporting this conclusion performed in the 1960s and 1970s were methodologically weak and were performed at a time when antibiotic choice was more limited. Nevertheless, almost all urologists attempt to sterilize infected urine before operating in the hope of preventing postoperative infection. In some patients with infected stones or indwelling catheters, sterilization of the urine may be impossible until surgery has been performed.

MEDICAL COMPLICATIONS OF SPECIFIC UROLOGIC PROCEDURES

Transurethral Resection Syndrome

Absorption of irrigating fluid during transurethral resections can lead to central nervous system and circulatory system symptoms which have been labeled the transurethral resection syndrome. Although most common during transurethral prostate resection, it has also been reported in other procedures in which irrigating solutions are used.[18] Older studies report that the frequency of this disorder is 11 to 41 percent,[19–21] but a recent prospective series of 100 patients documented no cases.[22] Changes in technique may be responsible for reducing the incidence of this complication.

Transurethral resection syndrome is caused by systemic absorption of irrigant solution through disrupted prostatic veins and extravasation of fluid through the disrupted prostatic capsule into the loose connective tissue surrounding the bladder. Irrigant solution usually contains glycine and is chosen because it is not locally toxic, can be made isoosmolar with body fluids, and is nonionic and therefore does not result in charge dispersal when electrocautery is used. Symptoms are probably related to hypervolemia and hyponatremia caused by the absorbed fluid, but direct or indirect toxicity from glycine itself may be contributory.[18] The severity of the disorder is proportional to the volume of irrigating solution absorbed and the degree of subsequent hyponatremia. The volume absorbed is related to the duration of the procedure and the pressure exerted by the solution relative to that in the prostatic veins. For this reason, transurethral resections are usually limited to one hour in duration, and the irrigating solution is placed no higher than 60 cm above the operating table. Systems to assess the amount of irrigant absorbed have been devised using low concentrations of ethanol in the irrigant that can be measured in expired air.[23] Prophylactic measures including administration of furosemide during the procedure have not been proven effective and may be harmful.[24]

Clinical manifestations of the syndrome include mild arterial hypertension during the procedure and nausea and vomiting developing within 30 to 60 minutes. In severe cases, significant hypotension supervenes at the end of the procedure and can result in anuria. Dyspnea is common and may be related to accumulation of irrigant fluid in the lungs. Neurologic symptoms include prickling or burning dysesthesias, transient visual disturbances, and even temporary complete blindness in rare cases. Apprehension and confusion can progress to coma.[23] Mild symptoms should prompt determination of the serum sodium concentration to confirm the diagnosis.

Treatment is directed toward correction of the hyponatremia and hypotension, if present. Since most absorbed irrigant fluid rapidly enters the interstitial space and the central venous pressure is low, volume expansion and vasopressor agents have been used to treat the hypotension. However, no clear remedy has been found. Optimal treatment of hyponatremia is controversial. Mild hyponatremia can be treated with loop-acting diuretics to enhance free water clearance. Hypertonic saline has been used in more severe cases. Neurologic impairment due to pontine injury can be associated with rapid correction of hyponatremia[25] but is unusual and less common when hyponatremia is of short duration.[26]

Urinary Diversion Procedures

Sections of the gastrointestinal tract have been used as an alternate route for urinary drainage for many years. Such procedures include anastamosing the ureter to the colon as in an ureterosigmoidostomy and use of segments of ileum and colon to serve as conduits for urine from the ureter or kidney to the skin or bowel. These procedures expose the gastrointestinal mucosa to urine and can result in metabolic derangement due to inappropriate absorption of electrolytes and ammonia and cause metabolic acidosis and encephalopathy.

Hyperammoniemic encephalopathy was first described in 1957 by McDermott.[27] Urinary diversion into the colon facilitates formation of increased amounts of ammonia from the urea in the urine. Serum ammonia levels rise because ammonia is absorbed more easily from the colon than the urinary tract. Because it is absorbed in ionic form,[28] inadequate hepatic clearance in patients with liver disease may produce levels high enough to cause encephalopathy. In addition, portal-systemic shunting in those with liver disease allows absorption of ammonia through hemorrhoidal veins. Urinary tract infections due to urea-splitting bacteria and situations causing prolonged contact between the colonic mucosa and urine (e.g., long ileal conduits, partially obstructed conduits, and constipation) may further increase ammonia absorption. For example, experimental obstipation produced by a rectal balloon in patients with ureterosigmoidostomies has been shown to cause hyperammoniemia and cerebral dysfunction.[29] Medical treatment of this disorder should include antibiotics for urinary tract infections, lactulose, and other laxatives. Diagnostic procedures to detect malfunctioning urinary diversions should be undertaken, and subsequent surgical correction may be necessary.

Metabolic acidosis seen in urinary diversion procedures is probably due to ammonium and concomitant passive hydrogen ion and chloride absorption through the bowel wall.[30,31] This complication occurs both in ileal conduit diversion with a frequency of 2 to 16 percent and in diversion through colonic reservoirs in 50 percent of patients.[32] Metabolic acidosis is more common with colonic reservoirs because larger surface areas of bowel are exposed to urine. Prolonged contact between urine and bowel mucosa may exacerbate metabolic derangements. Chronic acidemia can cause mobilization of buffer stores in bone and result in demineralization.[32] Treatment includes ensuring that the flow of urine is not obstructed and oral bicarbonate therapy. Experimental interventions with nicotinic acid and chlorpromazine, thought to alter intestinal electrolyte absorption through action on the cyclic AMP system, have been successful in animals and in a single patient case report.[33]

RECENT DEVELOPMENTS IN UROLOGIC SURGERY

Technical advances have enabled urologists to perform a variety of procedures with less-invasive methods. Some of these interventions are awaiting approval by the Food and Drug Administration but may be available soon. Laparoscopic surgery can be used for pelvic lymph node resection in patients requiring staging for prostate cancer, simple nephrectomy for benign disease, varicocelectomy, and bladder neck suspension. Newer techniques for prostate resection include transurethral laser-induced prostatectomy (TULIP) in which a rotating laser is inserted into the urethra and is guided by a continuous rotating ultrasonic sensor in removing glandular tissue. Transurethral balloon dilation of the prostate is being explored but thus far has proven expensive and provides only short-lived efficacy. Nerve-sparing procedures for radical prostatectomy have also been introduced. Conventional open prostatectomy results in incontinence in 20 to 30 percent of cases, and impotence is almost universal. In contrast, only 2 to 3 percent of patients undergoing nerve-sparing prostatectomy become incontinent, and sexual function is preserved in 60 to 80 percent.

Endourologic procedures and extracorporeal shock wave lithotripsy (ESWL) have almost replaced open procedures in the surgical management of renal calculi. These procedures include ureteroscopy, percutaneous nephrolithotomy, and the use of local lithotripsy devices that can be guided into the ureter and direct energy toward the calculus. ESWL has been used in millions of patients since its introduction in 1984. High-energy shock waves are used to fragment the stone into smaller pieces that pass spontaneously. The patient is placed in a water bath, and the stone is localized with varying radiology techniques. High-voltage discharges passed through an underwater spark plug lead to evaporation of a small bubble of water causing a high-pressure shock wave. The wave is reflected off an ellipsoid and is propagated to a second focal point of the ellipsoid where the stone is located. Because some energy is lost as the wave traverses the interface between the water and the skin, patients can experience pain and require anesthesia.

The frequency of perioperative complications in ESWL is low. Initially general anesthesia was required for the procedure, but more recently spinal anesthesia has been used. Logistical challenges to monitoring patients immersed in a water bath have been largely overcome.

Clinicians should be aware of contraindications to the procedure and preliminary data regarding long-term sequelae. In the past, patients with pacemakers could not undergo ESWL. However, guidelines have now been developed to allow them to proceed. In those with dual-chamber pacemakers, the device should be programmed to the VVI mode. Those with piezoelectric activity-sensing rate-responsive single-chamber pacemakers should have this feature turned off during the procedure. Those with ventricular application pacemakers require no special attention.[34]

Renal damage and hypertension are recognized complications of ESWL. Animal studies have demonstrated subcapsular and renal parenchymal hemorrhage. Perinephric hematomas that usually resolve within several weeks have been described in humans.[34] The long-term effects of ESWL on renal function are unknown. New-onset hypertension after ESWL has also been described, but it is unclear whether it develops in patients treated with ESWL more often than those with renal calculi who are not.[34]

Since renal calculi commonly recur, internists should provide recommendations in an effort to prevent recurrence. Prevention of recurrent stones depends upon the type of stone formed. Stones are composed of calcium oxalate, calcium phosphate, uric acid, struvite, and rarely cystine. Evaluation of stone disease includes measurement of 24-hour urinary excretion of calcium, magnesium, phosphorus, uric acid, creatinine, oxalate, and citrate as well as determination of pH and volume. These data together with serum concentrations of calcium, magnesium, phosphorus, uric acid, and creatinine help to define the pathogenesis of any underlying disorder. Recent comprehensive reviews can be found in the literature.[35]

REFERENCES

1. Pientka L, Van Loghem J, Hahn E et al: Comorbidities and perioperative complications among patients with surgically treated benign prostatic hyperplasia. *Urology* 38(Suppl):43–48, 1991.
2. Kiokno AC, Brown MB, Goldstein N et al: Epidemiology of bladder emptying symptoms in elderly men. *J Urol* 148:1817–1821, 1992.
3. Gormley GJ, Stoner E, Bruskewitz RC et al: The effect of finasteride in men with benign prostatic hyperplasia. *N Engl J Med* 327:1185–1191, 1992.
4. Charlson ME, Chen RE, Sears CL: General medicine consultation. *Am J Med* 75:121–128, 1983.
5. Ferguson RP, Rubenstein E: Preoperative medical consultations in a community hospital. *J Gen Intern Med* 2:89–92, 1987.
6. Golden WE, Lavender RC: Preoperative cardiac consultations in a teaching hospital. *S Medical J* 82(3):292–295, 1989.
7. Robie PW: The service and educational contributions of a general medicine consultation service. *J Gen Intern Med* 1:225–227, 1986.

8. Malenka DJ, Roos N, Fisher ES et al: Further study of the increased mortality following transurethral prostatectomy: A chart-based analysis. *J Urol* 144:224–228, 1990.

9. Sinha B, Haike G, Lange PH et al: Transurethral resection of the prostate with local anesthesia in 100 patients. *J Urol* 135:719–721, 1986.

10. McGowan SW, Smith GFN: Anaesthesia for transurethral prostatectomy. *Anaesthesia* 35:847–853, 1980.

11. Collins R, Scrimgeour A, Tusuf S et al: Reduction in fatal pulmonary embolism and venous thrombosis by perioperative administration of subcutaneous heparin: Overview of results of randomized trial in general, orthopedic and urologic surgery. *N Engl J Med* 318:1162–1172, 1988.

12. Vandendris M, Kutnowski M, Futeral B et al: Prevention of deep-vein thrombosis by low-dose heparin in open prostatectomy. *Urol Res* 8:219–221, 1980.

13. Halverstadt DB, Albert DD, Kroovand RL et al: Anticoagulation in urological surgery. *Urol* 9:617, 1977.

14. Hansberry KL, Thompson IA, Bauman J et al: A prospective comparison of thromboembolic stockings, external sequential pneumatic compression stockings and heparin sodium/dihydroergotamine mesylate for the prevention of thromboembolic complications in urologic surgery. *J Urol* 145:1205–1208, 1991.

15. Flynn N, Lawrence RM: Antimicrobial prophylaxis. *Med Clin N Am* 63:1230, 1979.

16. Dajani AD, Bisno AL, Chung KJ et al: Prevention of bacterial endocarditis. *JAMA* 264:2919–2922, 1990.

17. Richter S, Lang R, Zur F et al: Infected urine as a risk factor for postprostatectomy wound infection. *Infect Control Hosp Epidem* 12:147–149, 1991.

18. Hahn RG: The transurethral resection syndrome. *Acta Anaesth Scand* 35:557–567, 1991.

19. Logie JRC, Keengan RA, Whiting PH et al: Fluid adsorption during transurethral prostatectomy. *Br J Urol* 52:526–528, 1980.

20. Rose GA, Fitzpatrick JM, Kasidas GP: Fluid adsorption during transurethral resection. *Br Med J* 282:317, 1981.

21. Schearer RJ, Standfield NJ: Fluid adsorption during transurethral resection. *Br Med J* 282:740, 1981.

22. Goel CM, Badenoch DF, Fowler CG: Transurethral resection syndrome. *Eur Urol* 21:15–17, 1992.

23. Hahn RG: Early detection of the TUR syndrome by marking the irrigating fluid with 1% ethanol. *Acta Anaesth Scand* 33:146–151, 1989.

24. Donatucci CF, Deshon BE, Wade CE et al: Furosemide-induced disturbances of renal function in patients undergoing TURP. *Urol* 35:295–300, 1990.

25. Weissman JD, Weissman BM: Pontine myelinolysis and delayed encephalopathy following the rapid correction of acute hyponatremia. *Arch Neurol* 46:926–927, 1989.

26. Berl T: Treating hyponatremia: What is all the controversy about? *Ann Intern Med* 113:417–419, 1990.

27. McDermott WV: Diversion of urine to the intestines as a factor in ammoniagenic coma. *N Engl J Med* 256:460–462, 1957.

28. Hall MC, Koch MO, McDougal WS: Mechanism of ammonium transport by intestinal segments following urinary diversion: Evidence for ionized NH_4 transport via K-pathways. *J Urol* 148:453–457, 1992.

29. Egense J, Schwartz M: Recurrent hepatic coma following ureterosigmoidostomy. *Scand J Gastroenterol* 5(Suppl 7):149–152, 1970.

30. Boyd JD: Chronic acidosis secondary to ureteral transplantation. *Am J Dis Child* 42:366–371, 1931.

31. Koch MO, McDougal WS: The pathophysiology of hyperchloremic metabolic acidosis after urinary diversion through intestinal segments. *Surgery* 98:561–570, 1985.

32. Nurse JE, Mundy AR: Metabolic complications of cystoplasty. *Br J Urol* 63:165–170, 1989.

33. Koch MO, McDougal WS: Nicotinic acid: Treatment for the hyperchloremic acidosis following urinary diversion through intestinal segments. *J Urol* 134:162, 1985.

34. Smith LH, Drach G, Hall P et al: National high blood pressure education program (NHBPEP) review paper on complications of shock wave lithotripsy for urinary calculi. *Am J Med* 91:635–641, 1991.

35. Coe FL, Parks JH, Asplin JR: The pathogenesis and treatment of kidney stones. *N Engl J Med* 327:1141–1152, 1992.

PROCEDURE: CYSTECTOMY

Overview: Most frequently a radical cystectomy is performed for a potentially curable bladder cancer. It involves removal of the bladder, urethra, and periurethral glands (i.e., prostate and seminal vesicles) and a pelvic lymph node dissection. The ureters are then diverted into a neobladder of terminal ileum or colon. A partial cystectomy may be indicated for a small localized bladder tumor (especially adenocarcinoma), bladder diverticulum, or trauma. In a female, a total abdominal hysterectomy and urethrectomy are included as part of the operation. The male urethra is removed only if the prostatic transitional cell epithelium is positive for cancer.

1. *Operation*
   a. Indications: See description above.
   b. Operative Steps: Steps include ureteral ligation, bladder mobilization, isolation and division of the blood supply, mobilization of bladder neck and prostate off of the anterior rectum, transection of the urethra, and specimen removal. A segment of bowel (usually ileum or right colon) is taken out of circuit, bowel is reanastamosed, ureters are anastamosed to the neobladder, and a stoma is made. The transverse colon is used for diversion if the patient has had previous external beam radiation to the lower abdomen.
   c. Incision: Transverse or midline.
   d. Anesthesia: General.
   e. Intraoperative Monitoring: Arterial line and CVP.
   f. Operative Positioning: Supine. The hips may be abducted, and the hips and knees slightly flexed with the degree of flexion being determined by the need for urethrectomy.
   g. Duration: 4 to 6 hours.
   h. EBL/Transfusions: 1000 to 2000 ml.
   i. "Surgical Stress": Severe.

2. *Expected Hospital Course/Treatment*
   a. Postoperative Monitoring
      (1) ICU Stay: Generally 1 to 2 days.
      (2) Invasive/Special Monitoring: While in ICU.
      (3) Parameters To Be Monitored:
         i. Fluid intake and output, especially urine output.
         ii. CBC.
         iii. Electrolytes, BUN, creatinine.
   b. Positioning/Activity: Out of bed to chair on POD 1.
   c. Alimentation: Liquids generally started on POD 3 to 5. Usually limited by bowel anastomosis.
   d. Wound Care/Drains: Optional ureteral stents may temporarily exit stoma.
   e. Respiratory Care: Incentive spirometry encouraged.
   f. Analgesia/Postop Meds: Parenteral narcotics with transition to oral narcotics in 2 to 3 days.
   g. Length Of Hospital Stay: 10 to 14 days.

3. *Postoperative Complications*
   a. In Hospital
      (1) Morbidity:
         i. Ureteral leak at anastamotic site.
         ii. Stomal dysfunction.
         iii. Rectal injury.
         iv. Obturator nerve injury.
         v. Lymphocele formation.
         vi. Urinary tract infection.
         vii. Impotence.
      (2) Mortality: 2 to 3%.
   b. After Discharge
      (1) Stomal herniation or stenosis.
      (2) Ureteral obstruction.
      (3) Tumor recurrence.
      (4) Incisional hernia.
      (5) Bowel obstruction.

4. *Follow-up*
   a. Suggested Follow-up: Tumor surveillance and evaluation of renal function are indicated monthly for 6 months, then at intervals of every 6 months. If the urethra has been left behind, yearly swabs for cytology are indicated. Issues related to sexual dysfunction may need to be addressed.

PROCEDURE: NEPHRECTOMY

Overview: Nephrectomy includes the removal of the kidney with a variable amount of surrounding tissue. If done for malignancy (i.e., renal cell carcinoma), the encompassing Gerota's fascia, adrenal perinephric fat, regional lymph nodes, and proximal ureter are removed. If the surgery is for upper tract transitional cell carcinoma (especially within the renal pelvis), the same procedure as above is performed, but the entire ureter with a cuff of bladder is included as well. Simple nephrectomy is performed on a nonneoplastic kidney that is either obstructed, chronically infected, nonfunctioning, or traumatized when a salvage procedure is not possible. Partial nephrectomy is indicated for localized infection with calculi, congenital anomalies, trauma, or a polar tumor, either in a solitary kidney or in the presence of bilateral renal disease when it is desirable to salvage a portion of the kidney.

1. *Operation*
   a. Indications: See description above.
   b. Operative Steps: Steps include exposure of the kidney, ureteral ligation, ligation of arteries and veins, and removal of the kidney. A periaortic lymph node dissection may be added in some patients with malignancy. If a partial nephrectomy is done, the main artery is temporarily occluded with a clamp and the kidney is transected. Manual pressure is utilized to control bleeding until the vessels and calyceal system within the parenchyma can be ligated with sutures. Intravenous mannitol with saline flush may be used to protect the salvaged kidney.
   c. Incision: A simple nephrectomy may be performed through an extraperitoneal flank or subcostal incision. A radical nephrectomy requires a subcostal or chevron incision with a transperitoneal approach. Occasionally, a twelfth or eleventh rib excision may be warranted, especially in large upper-pole tumors.
   d. Anesthesia: General. Epidural anesthesia may be an adjunct for postoperative pain control.
   e. Intraoperative Monitoring: Routine except in operations for large malignancies or in medically debilitated patients in whom arterial line with or without CVP are required. Monitoring of urine output is essential.
   f. Operative Positioning: Supine or lateral decubitus.
   g. Duration: 2 to 4 hours.
   h. EBL/Transfusions: 500 to 1500 ml. EBL may be much higher in some cases of radical nephrectomy with intracaval extension. Cardiopulmonary bypass may be required if the tumor thrombus extends into the superior vena cava or heart.
   i. "Surgical Stress": Moderate to severe.

2. *Expected Hospital Course/Treatment*
   a. Postoperative Monitoring
      (1) ICU Stay: Required for medically debilitated patients or long operations with extensive blood loss or hemodynamic instability.
      (2) Invasive/Special Monitoring: While in ICU.
      (3) Parameters To Be Monitored:
         i. Fluid intake and output, especially urine output.
         ii. CBC.
         iii. Electrolytes, BUN, creatinine.
         iv. Chest x-ray to rule out ipsilateral pneumothorax.
   b. Positioning/Activity: Out of bed and ambulate on POD 1.
   c. Alimentation: After extraperitoneal approach, regular diet can frequently be resumed by POD 2 or 3; usually later for transperitoneal approach.
   d. Wound Care/Drains: Closed suction drains are optional.
   e. Respiratory Care: Incentive spirometry encouraged.
   f. Analgesia/Postop Meds: Epidural analgesia or parenteral narcotics are initially required. Oral narcotics may be substituted by POD 2 or 3.
   g. Length Of Hospital Stay: 5 to 14 days.

3. *Postoperative Complications*
   a. In Hospital
      (1) Morbidity:
         i. Inadvertent ligation of superior mesenteric artery during left radical nephrectomy.
         ii. Injury to colon, spleen, or duodenum.
         iii. Urinary retention.
         iv. Infection.
         v. Atelectasis/pneumonia.
         vi. Pulmonary embolus, especially in those patients who have tumor thrombus.
      (2) Mortality: 1%.
   b. After Discharge
      (1) Recurrent cancer.
      (2) Incisional hernia.

4. *Follow-up*
   a. Suggested Follow-up: Tumor surveillance and evaluation of renal function are performed every 3 months for the first year, then at 6-month intervals. Yearly bone scans, computed tomography, and chest x-rays are indicated for patients with renal cell carcinoma for 5 years.

PROCEDURE: RADICAL PROSTATECTOMY

Overview: This operation may be approached in two ways: (1) Extraperitoneal retropubic removal of prostate, seminal vesicles, and pelvic lymph nodes; or (2) Laparoscopic pelvic lymph node dissection followed by perineal radical prostatectomy (i.e., resection of the prostate and seminal vesicles).

1. *Operation*
   a. Indications: Radical prostatectomy is performed for localized adenocarcinoma of the prostate (stage A_2, B_1, or B_2). Radical removal of the prostate is not curative for patients with capsular penetration or invasion of the seminal vesicles (stage C) or involvement of the neurovascular bundle.
   b. Operative Steps: Steps include dissection of the anterior bladder and neck, ligation of the vas deferens, and lymph node dissection. If frozen section is negative, the surgeon proceeds with prostatectomy. The pelvic fascia and puboprostatic ligaments are divided. The membranous urethra is cut, and the prostate is dissected out. The bladder neck is opened to complete the dissection.
   c. Incision: Pfannensteil or midline incision for radical retropubic prostatectomy (RRP). Invented U-shaped incision for perineal prostatectomy (PP).
   d. Anesthesia: General. Epidural anesthesia may be performed as an adjunct for postoperative pain control.
   e. Intraoperative Monitoring: Arterial line and CVP.
   f. Operative Positioning: Supine for RRP. Exaggerated lithotomy position for PP.
   g. Duration: 3 to 4 hours.
   h. EBL/Transfusions: 500 to 1500 ml.
   i. "Surgical Stress": Moderate.

2. *Expected Hospital Course/Treatment*
   a. Postoperative Monitoring
      (1) ICU Stay: Required only for elderly or debilitated patients.
      (2) Invasive/Special Monitoring: None.
      (3) Parameters To Be Monitored:
         i. Urine output.
         ii. CBC.
         iii. Electrolytes, BUN, creatinine.
   b. Positioning/Activity: Out of bed on POD 1.
   c. Alimentation: Clear liquids started on day 1 or 2.
   d. Wound Care/Drains: Foley catheter to drain bladder and stent for urethral anastomosis. Closed suction pelvic drains for RRP. Penrose drains for PP.
   e. Respiratory Care: Incentive spirometry is encouraged.
   f. Analgesia/Postop Meds: Epidural analgesia or parenteral narcotics are initially required. Belladonna and opium suppositories are not indicated.
   g. Length Of Hospital Stay: 7 to 10 days.

3. *Postoperative Complications*
   a. In Hospital
      (1) Morbidity:
         i. Rectal injury.
         ii. Inadvertent catheter removal.
         iii. Lymphocele.
         iv. Excessive bleeding.
      (2) Mortality: 2%.
   b. After Discharge
      (1) Urinary incontinence.
      (2) Impotence.
      (3) Bladder neck contracture.

4. *Follow-up*
   a. Suggested Follow-up: Foley catheter is removed in 14 days. Assessment of voiding function, renal function, and tumor surveillance is performed monthly for 6 to 12 months, then at 6-month intervals. Prostate-specific antigen levels are checked every 6 months.

PROCEDURE: TRANSURETHRAL RESECTION OF THE PROSTATE

Overview: The portion of the prostate that is compressing the urethra and interfering with bladder emptying may usually be removed transurethrally with the aid of a resectoscope.

1. *Operation*
   a. Indications: The vast majority of enlarged prostates that are generating obstructive symptoms and are the primary cause of outflow obstruction can best be managed by endoscopic resection.
   b. Operative Steps: Cystoscopy is performed to determine if the gland is appropriate for transurethral resection. When resection is possible, pieces of prostatic tissue are removed down to the capsule with a resectoscope. The bladder is irrigated intermittently to remove chips of prostate tissue. Inspection for hemostasis is done prior to placement of a Foley catheter (2-way or 3-way irrigating catheter).
   c. Incision: None.
   d. Anesthesia: Spinal or general. Spinal is preferable in order to follow mental status changes.
   e. Intraoperative Monitoring: Routine unless medically debilitated.
   f. Operative Positioning: Modified dorsal lithotomy.
   g. Duration: 1 hour.
   h. EBL/Transfusions: EBL is difficult to estimate but may range from 500 to 1000 ml. Transfusions are rarely needed.
   i. "Surgical Stress": Low to moderate.

2. *Expected Hospital Course/Treatment*
   a. Postoperative Monitoring
      (1) ICU Stay: Only needed for complications of TUR syndrome.
      (2) Invasive/Special Monitoring: None.
      (3) Parameters To Be Monitored:
         i. Urine output.
         ii. CBC.
         iii. Electrolytes (especially sodium), BUN, creatinine.
   b. Positioning/Activity: Out of bed and ambulate on POD 1. No heavy exercise or driving a car for approximately 3 to 4 weeks postoperatively.
   c. Alimentation: As tolerated.
   d. Wound Care/Drains: A Foley catheter is placed for drainage for 1 to 3 days.
   e. Respiratory Care: Routine.
   f. Analgesia/Postop Meds: Belladonna and opium suppositories for bladder spasm.
   g. Length Of Hospital Stay: 5 days.

3. *Postoperative Complications*
   a. In Hospital
      (1) Morbidity:
         i. TUR syndrome.
         ii. Perforation of the prostatic capsule or bladder.
         iii. Excessive bleeding.
         iv. Intraoperative fracture of the sheath of the resectoscope.
      (2) Mortality: 0.1%.
   b. After Discharge
      (1) Retrograde ejaculation is common and due to resection of the bladder neck.
      (2) Incontinence.
      (3) Bladder neck contracture.
      (4) Urethral strictures.

4. *Follow-up*
   a. Suggested Follow-up: Patients are seen monthly for 3 visits, then are followed on a yearly basis. Prostate-specific antigen levels are checked yearly.

PROCEDURE: TREATMENT OF URINARY TRACT STONES

Overview: Renal calculi occur more commonly in men with a male to female ratio of 3:1. However, infected calculi are more commonly seen in women. The peak incidence of stone disease lies between the third and fifth decade. Stone formation may be influenced by genetic, environmental, diet, location, and physical/chemical factors. The composition of stones is as follows:

Calcium oxalate	33%
Calcium oxalate and phosphate	34%
Magnesium ammonium phosphate	15%
Uric acid	8%
Calcium phosphate	6%
Cystine	3%

Stone location and size usually determine the exact operation. For renal calculi < 2 cm, therapy usually involves ESWL (extracorporeal shock wave lithotripsy). For calculi > 2 cm or staghorn calculi, PCNL (percutaneous nephrolithotomy) using EHL (electrohydraulic) probes or ultrasound can destroy the calculus and leave fragments to be removed. Ureteral calculi can be treated either by ESWL therapy or ureteroscopy using stone baskets, EHL probes, or laser lithotripsy. Bladder calculi are removed by open suprapubic lithotomy, transurethral litholapaxy, ultrasonic lithotripsy, or electrohydraulic lithotripsy. Males with a bladder stone usually require transurethral resection of the prostate.

1. *Operation*
    a. Indications:
        (1) Urinary tract obstruction.
        (2) Decreasing renal function.
        (3) Systemic infection.
        (4) Renal colic.
    b. Operative Steps: See description above.
    c. Incision: ESWL, ureteroscopy, and cystoscopy: no incision. PCNL: 2-cm incision in the flank. Open suprapubic lithotomy: low transverse incision.
    d. Anesthesia: ESWL: general, epidural, or IV sedation. PCNL: general, epidural, or local with IV sedation. Ureteroscopy: general. Cystoscopy: general or spinal.
    e. Intraoperative Monitoring: Routine.
    f. Operative Positioning: ESWL: usually supine. PCNL: usually prone. Ureteroscopy and cystoscopy: usually modified dorsal lithotomy position.
    g. Duration: 1 to 3 hours.
    h. EBL/Transfusions: EBL is minimal. Transfusions are not required.
    i. "Surgical Stress": Minimal to moderate.

2. *Expected Hospital Course/Treatment*
    a. Postoperative Monitoring
        (1) ICU Stay: Rarely required.
        (2) Invasive/Special Monitoring: None.
        (3) Parameters To Be Monitored: X-ray to confirm stone destruction or removal.
    b. Positioning/Activity: As tolerated.
    c. Alimentation: Resume regular diet on POD 1.
    d. Wound Care/Drains: ESWL: no drains except when a double J catheter is inserted. PCNL and ureteroscopy: small 6F tube, usually removed on POD 1.
    e. Respiratory Care: Routine.
    f. Analgesia/Postop Meds: Oral narcotics are usually appropriate.
    g. Length Of Hospital Stay: ESWL: outpatient. PCNL: 4 days. Ureteroscopy: 2 days.

3. *Postoperative Complications*
    a. In Hospital
        (1) Morbidity:
            i. Sepsis.
            ii. Deep venous thrombosis and pulmonary embolism.
        (2) Mortality: < 0.1%.
    b. After Discharge
        (1) Retained stone fragments.
        (2) Ureteral obstruction.
        (3) Bladder perforation.
        (4) Recurrent stone formation.

4. *Follow-up*
    a. Suggested Follow-up: Patients are seen every 3 to 6 months.

13 EVALUATION OF THE PATIENT UNDERGOING NEUROSURGERY

Robert H. Rosenwasser

David F. Jimenez

Christopher C. Getch

Frank H. Brown

Neurosurgical procedures range from elective procedures like stereotactic biopsy to emergency craniotomy in unstable patients with acute head injury. Nonetheless, clinicians must be familiar with a number of situations commonly encountered in neurosurgical patients. These include coexisting medical problems, medical complications of brain injury, management of cerebral edema, and postoperative complications of specific procedures. This overview focuses primarily on patients undergoing craniotomy for intracranial hemorrhage, neoplasm, or head trauma and excludes spinal cord and peripheral nerve procedures.

COMORBID MEDICAL CONDITIONS

The prevalence of underlying medical problems in neurosurgical patients is similar to that seen in the general population. However, there are certain associations with significant perioperative implications. Intracranial aneurysms occur more commonly in patients with atherosclerotic disease, mycotic infections, and vasculitis. Aneurysmal rupture and subarachnoid hemorrhage are associated with cigarette smoking, coarctation of the aorta, fibromuscular dysplasia, polycystic kidney disease, Ehlers-Danlos syndrome, and Marfan's syndrome. Hypertension has never been established as a predisposing factor in aneurysmal rupture. However, intracerebral hematomas are commonly the result of hypertension. The incidence of alcohol and substance abuse with their attendant complications is increased in victims of head and spine trauma. Metastatic tumors requiring biopsy, shunting, or occasionally resection may be associated with risk factors such as smoking and lung disease.

In general, the risks posed by coexisting medical problems are the same as for other forms of surgery and require similar assessment and management. However, hypertension and coagulation disorders are especially important. Because of impaired autoregulation of intracranial pressure and the presence of cerebral edema, wide variations in blood pressure are poorly tolerated. Relative hypotension may result in decreased cerebral perfusion. Moreover, ischemia caused by hypotension may cause reflex vasodilation and exacerbate cerebral edema by increasing blood flow, blood volume, and intracranial pressure. Similarly, uncontrolled hypertension may increase intracranial pressure and the risk of bleeding. Because even small amounts of bleeding at the operative site can cause substantial morbidity, patients with coagulation disorders including drug-induced platelet dysfunction require careful assessment and preparation as described in Chap. 30.

MEDICAL COMPLICATIONS OF BRAIN INJURY

Depending on its location and severity, brain injury may result in a number of complications requiring medical evaluation and therapy.[1] Some of these may also occur after non-traumatic insults such as subarachnoid hemorrhage or following major neurosurgical procedures.

Cardiovascular

Severe head injury results in a marked release of catecholamines causing elevations in blood pressure, heart rate, and cardiac output. Subsequently, neurogenic hypertension, myocardial injury, and dysrhythmias may develop. Neurogenic hypertension may be due to increased intracranial pressure, brain stem compression, or medullary ischemia and may be accompanied by vagally-mediated bradycardia and changes in blood pressure, cardiac output, and systemic vascular resistance. These variations, the loss of cerebral autoregulation, and their effects on intracranial pressure and the development of cerebral edema make treatment difficult. Contributing factors like pain and hypoxia should be treated. If antihypertensives are necessary, beta-blockers or a combined alpha- and beta-blocker like labetolol are preferred. Direct vasodilators may increase intracranial pressure and should therefore be avoided.

Brain-injured patients may develop electrocardiographic changes including anterior ST-segment depression, T-wave flattening or inversion, and QT-interval prolongation. Serum levels of cardiac enzymes may be elevated, and subendocardial hemorrhage has been found in some patients at autopsy. The mechanism of myocardial injury is unclear, but it is more common in patients with the most severe head injury.

A variety of arrhythmias can be seen in brain-injured patients. Cushing's bradycardia is due to increased intracranial pressure and brain stem compression. Tachyarrhythmias are usually related to increased sympathetic tone and may be exacerbated by pain and hypoxia.

Pulmonary

The most serious respiratory complication of brain injury is neurogenic pulmonary edema, a form of the adult respiratory distress syndrome. It is characterized by tachypnea, hypoxia, decreased pulmonary compliance, and bilateral pulmonary infiltrates within the first few days of the injury. The diagnosis and treatment of ARDS is discussed in Chap. 58. Other pulmonary complications of head injury include abnormal ventilatory patterns, aspiration pneumonitis, pneumonia, pulmonary embolism, and associated pulmonary contusion.

Gastrointestinal

Decreased gastrointestinal motility is common after head injury or major neurosurgical procedures and may result in delayed feeding, increased risk of aspiration, and inability to take chronic medications. Stress-related mucosal disease is extremely common and may cause gastrointestinal hemorrhage and perforation. Prophylactic measures are detailed below.

Fluid and Electrolytes

Hyponatremia may occur in brain-injured patients and is usually due to diuretic therapy or the syndrome of inappropriate secretion of antidiuretic hormone (SIADH). Salt wasting can also be the result of excess secretion of atrial naturetic factor mediated by the hypothalamus.[2,3] SIADH is characterized by hypotonic hyponatremia and an inappropriately concentrated urine in euvolemic patients with normal renal, adrenal, and pituitary function. Serum sodium concentrations of less than 130 mmol/liter should be treated in neurosurgical patients because hypoosmolality may worsen cerebral edema and precipitate seizures. Water restriction and discontinuation of hypotonic fluids may be sufficient, but, in more severe cases, hypertonic saline is required (see Chap. 61).

Diabetes insipidus is usually attributable to trauma to the pituitary-hypothalamic axis with resultant loss of vasopressin se-

cretion or production. Awake patients may complain of polyuria and polydipsia. Urinary output may exceed 15 liters per day. The urine is dilute with a specific gravity below 1.003. Severe deficits in free water result in marked hypernatremia. Aqueous vasopressin should be administered if the rate of urine output remains at 200 to 300 ml/hr and the serum sodium continues to rise. Fluid is usually replaced with 5% glucose in water, and hyperglycemia can be treated with insulin as needed. Hypokalemia may be due to increased aldosterone secretion or the use of steroids and diuretics.

Coagulation

Approximately 40 to 70 percent of patients suffering open or closed head injuries or other severe intracranial pathology develop abnormalities in coagulation including disseminated intravascular coagulation (DIC). Coagulopathy has been attributed to the release of large quantities of brain thromboplastin into the circulation and activation of coagulation factors. The development of coagulation disorders after head injury or tumor surgery is directly proportional to the severity of the injury or the extent of the resection. In one study, the incidence of coagulation abnormalities correlated with the level of consciousness and brain stem function.[4] Almost all patients with Glasgow coma scores under 8 had abnormal coagulation tests. If DIC develops, fresh frozen plasma and platelet concentrates are given to replace clotting factors even though administration of blood components may theoretically potentiate the coagulopathy. Heparin therapy is contraindicated in most patients with acute head injury (see Chap. 65).

MEDICAL MANAGEMENT OF CEREBRAL EDEMA AND INCREASED INTRACRANIAL PRESSURE

Uncontrolled elevation of intracranial pressure (ICP) can lead to a number of complications including brain herniation, neurologic deficits, unconsciousness, and death. Marked elevation in ICP is the major cause of mortality in severely head-injured patients. Intracranial hypertension is associated with a variety of conditions affecting neurosurgical patients. One of the principal causes of increased ICP is cerebral edema. Several pathophysiologic processes affecting the central nervous system cause reactive tissue swelling. Edema can be classified as vasogenic, cytotoxic or cellular, ischemic, or interstitial.

Vasogenic edema is characterized by protein-rich exudate from plasma and is due to increased permeability in capillary endothelial cells. Albumin and other large molecules leak into the interstitial spaces with water. This type of edema is seen in patients with brain tumors, metastatic neoplasms, brain abscesses, and other conditions.

Cytotoxic or cellular edema is due to increases in intracellular volume which occur with cellular membrane energy depletion. It tends to develop immediately after a period of hypoxia and resolves with the restoration of energy substrate. With the loss of sodium-potassium ATPase function, sodium rapidly accumulates in the cells, water flows into the cell to restore the osmotic gradient and virtually all cellular components become swollen. In contrast to vasogenic edema, vascular permeability and the blood-brain barrier remain intact in patients with cellular edema. Although trauma, hypoxia, and cardiac arrest are the most common cases of cellular edema, it can also develop in acute dilutional states like SIADH. Most of these conditions are reversible with appropriate treatment of the underlying etiology.

Ischemic edema is a combination of vasogenic and cytotoxic edema but is clinically sufficiently different to be classified as a separate entity. Following an ischemic insult to the central nervous system, edema may develop in two phases. An acute initial cytotoxic phase may last 12 to 24 hours. This is followed by damage to the blood-brain barrier and subsequent vasogenic edema. The vasogenic edema lasts much longer and is associated with clinical deterioration.

Interstitial edema is most commonly seen in hydrocephalic patients with severe ventricular enlargement. Increases in intraventricular transmural pressure cause cerebrospinal fluid to move across the ependymal cells into the interstitial space.

Several factors can exacerbate intracranial hypertension.[5] Fever increases ICP by increasing cerebral blood volume and flow. The rate of cerebral metabolism is proportional to body temperature and increases 5 to 7 percent per °C. Fever should be treated with acetaminophen or cooling blankets, and all infections should be appropriately addressed. Pain and agitation also increase intracranial pressures, and adequate analgesia and sedation should be provided. Coughing or breathing against the mechanical ventilator causes elevation in central venous pressure which is in turn transmitted to the intracranial compartment. Neuromuscular paralysis may be necessary in such cases but interferes with neurologic assessment. Blood pressure control is crucial because hypotension or uncontrolled hypertension can exacerbate intracranial hypertension. Certain antihypertensives like direct vasodilators should be avoided. Seizures can also increase intracranial pressure and require strict control.

There are several therapeutic interventions available to treat intracranial hypertension.[5] Intubation and hyperventilation are often necessary. Hypocapnia with P_{CO_2} levels between 25 and 30 torr decreases cerebral blood flow (CBF), cerebral blood volume (CBV) and ICP, and increases cerebral vascular resistance. The effects of hyperventilation are immediate but transient. Mannitol decreases ICP by creating an osmotic gradient and thereby reducing total brain water. Mannitol is given at doses of 1 mg/kg and titrated to a serum osmolality of up to 310 mOsm. Complications of mannitol therapy include transient volume expansion, hypertension, and electrolyte disturbances. Loop diuretics may also be helpful, particularly when used in conjunction with mannitol, in decreasing blood volume and production of cerebrospinal fluid. Dexamethasone is the treatment of choice for vasogenic cerebral edema and produces dramatic and almost immediate results. Steroids exert their influence by stabilizing membranes and restoring the integrity of the blood-brain barrier. Hyperglycemia is the principal side effect of steroid therapy.

Barbiturate coma with pentothal can also be used to decrease ICP in patients with refractory intracranial hypertension. Pentothal is a potent vasoconstrictor which significantly decreases cerebral blood flow and metabolic rate. After an initial loading dose, pentobarbital is given by constant infusion and is titrated to burst suppression on the electroencephalogram rather than blood levels of the drug. Because barbiturate coma depresses cardiac function, a Swan-Ganz catheter and arterial line must be placed to measure pulmonary capillary wedge pressure, cardiac output, cardiac index, and systemic vascular resistance every two to four hours. The patient may require dopamine or phenylephrine to maintain blood pressure and vascular resistance at normal levels. Because coma predisposes hospitalized patients to infection, they should be closely monitored and placed on antibiotics as clinically indicated.

In addition to direct measurement of intracranial pressure, intensive care monitoring of such patients now includes measurement of the cerebral arterial-venous oxygen gradient with the help of an oxygen-sensing catheter in the jugular vein. The magnitude of the gradient is proportional to the ratio of cerebral metabolic demand to blood flow and has proven helpful in managing patients with a variety of brain insults.

MEDICAL COMPLICATIONS OF SPECIFIC PROCEDURES

Surgery for Intracranial Aneurysm

To eliminate the risk of rebleeding, surgical obliteration of intracranial aneurysms is usually performed within the first 24 to 72 hours after the initial hemorrhage. When there is evidence of vasospasm, neurologic deterioration, or coma, surgery may be delayed for more than 14 days. However, the optimal time of surgery is still controversial in such cases. If delay is necessary, the risk of rebleeding can be decreased by administering antifibrinolytic drugs like aminocaproic acid, but the use of these agents may be complicated by ischemic stroke.

Cerebral vasospasm is the most critical complication of subarachnoid hemorrhage. It is a significant cause of stroke and ischemia and accounts for 30 percent of the morbidity and mortality cited in the Cooperative Aneurysm Study.[6] It can be minimized by hypervolemic hemodilution achieved by maximizing cardiac output with fluid administration guided by Swan-Ganz catheterization. The hematocrit level is often reduced to 30 to 35 percent to improve the rheologic characteristics of the blood and increase cerebral blood flow. Hemodilution is thus accomplished by the addition of fluid rather than phlebotomy. All patients with subarachnoid bleeding due to aneurysmal rupture are given the calcium channel antagonist nimodipine for 21 days after the hemorrhage. Nimodipine causes a relative hypovolemia, a decrease in systemic vascular resistance, and possible hypotension requiring additional intravascular volume expansion.

All patients are monitored for the development of vasospasm with transcranial doppler ultrasonography (TCD) which provides an indirect measure of cerebral blood flow. Vasospasm may persist for up to two weeks, and close observation is necessary as long as TCD measurements remain elevated. Patients may require monitoring in an intensive care unit for up to three weeks if they develop vasospasm.

Infratentorial Surgery

Patients undergoing surgery in the infratentorial compartment for either tumor or vascular disease may develop lower cranial nerve dysfunction. Manipulation in the area of the infratentorial notch may cause oculomotor or trochlear nerve palsy with impairment of stereoscopic vision. Trigeminal nerve dysfunction can make chewing difficult but, more importantly, can cause anesthesia in any division of the trigeminal nerve. Involvement of the first division can also result in lid dysfunction and subsequent corneal irritation and ulceration. Special eye care with topical wetting and patching agents may prevent these complications. Corneal irritation or erythema should also prompt appropriate cultures and topical antibiotics.

Dysfunction of the facial and vestibulocochlear nerves often occurs concomitantly. Combined facial and trigeminal nerve damage causes both loss of proper eye closure and corneal sensation and often results in severe keratitis.

Glossopharyngeal and vagus nerve dysfunction causes paralysis of the vocal cords and loss of sensation in the posterior pharynx. Patients may suffer multiple aspirations and should be positioned with the intact side down to allow secretions to pool in the neurologically intact part of the pharynx. Speech pathologists may be helpful in restoring swallowing function. However, a nasogastric feeding tube or a temporary gastrostomy may be necessary until nerve function recovers. A permanent gastrostomy is needed if the nerves have been sacrificed.

PROPHYLACTIC ISSUES

Seizure Prophylaxis

Many neurosurgical patients have an increased risk of developing seizures which can contribute to perioperative morbidity. Seizures can exacerbate intracranial hypertension and increase the risk of aspiration pneumonia and pneumonitis. Many patients are therefore given prophylactic anticonvulsants. Phenytoin and phenobarbital are most often used because they can be administered parenterally. Excessively rapid intravenous administration of phenytoin can cause hypotension and arrhythmias, and parenteral phenobarbital loading can cause myocardial and respiratory depression. Other side effects of commonly used anticonvulsants are detailed in Table 13–1. Several concurrent medications influence serum concentrations of phenytoin. Those that increase serum phenytoin levels include warfarin, isoniazid, chloramphenicol, sulfonamides, disulfiram, aspirin and cimetidine. Those that decrease phenytoin levels are carbamazepine, folic acid, barbiturates, and alcohol. Metabolic abnormalities including hyponatremia and hypomagnesemia should also be corrected in an effort to prevent seizures.

TABLE 13–1. Side Effects of Commonly Used Anticonvulsants

Phenytoin
Decreased ADH release (DI)
Megaloblastic anemia
Hepatotoxicity
Blood dyscrasias
Decreased serum levels of:
warfarin
digoxin
barbiturates
Tegretol
Increased ADH release (SIADH)
Aplastic anemia
Leukopenia
Agranulocytosis
Barbiturates
Increased ADH release (SIADH)
Decreased warfarin levels

Stress-Related Mucosal Disease

Endoscopically apparent stress-related mucosal disease (SRMD) is virtually a universal finding in brain-injured patients who do not receive prophylactic therapy.[7] A multivariate analysis identified five risk factors associated with the development of postoperative gastrointestinal bleeding in neurosurgical patients.[8] These included SIADH, preoperative coma, presence of other postoperative complications, age over 60, and pyogenic infections of the central nervous system. There was no association with steroid use, sepsis or hypotension. Prophylactic therapy should be administered to patients with one or more of these factors and to any others considered to have increased risk. Antacids and H_2-blockers are effective but have been associated with bacterial overgrowth and nosocomial pneumonia. Sucralfate does not alter gastric pH and may be a better alternative (see Chap. 46).

Thromboembolism Prophylaxis

Studies have shown that the incidence of deep venous thrombosis in neurosurgical patients is 29 to 43 percent.[9] The high incidence is attributable to release of tissue thromboplastin and stasis in paretic extremities. Because of the risk of pulmonary embolism, thromboembolism prophylaxis should be considered for all patients undergoing major neurosurgical procedures. However, prophylactic options are relatively limited. Dextran is contraindicated because it can theoretically increase intracranial pressure.[9] Limited data suggest that standard low-dose heparin can be used in neurosurgical patients.[9,10] However, because of concerns about bleeding, external pneumatic compression (EPC) is considered the method of choice. A recent study found the combination of intraoperative EPC and postoperative LDH to be safe and completely effective.[11]

Nutritional Support

In the past, little attention was given to the nutritional requirements of patients with head injuries or those undergoing surgery for intracranial pathology. Although gastrointestinal function is usually intact, neurosurgical patients frequently develop an ileus due to impaired hypothalamic function. Enteral feeding is therefore often delayed for several days. Delay in feeding and fluid restriction, as practiced in the past, often complicates nutritional therapy. However, with changing trends in fluid management, parenteral hyperalimentation is now being initiated earlier.

The resting metabolic energy expenditure in patients with open or closed head injuries and in those who are extremely ill after intracranial surgery is significantly increased. Increases in caloric expenditure of 120 to 270 percent above the basal metabolic rate have been documented. The energy requirements of these patients are equivalent to those reported in patients with 30 percent burns, multiple trauma, or severe sepsis. In addition, several studies indicate that nitrogen excretion increases to as much as 25 grams per day. Early total parenteral nutrition should therefore be considered in patients with head injury and other types of intracranial pathology requiring surgery (see Chap. 42).

Parenteral nutrition is complicated by hyperglycemia and increased carbon dioxide production and oxygen consumption. In addition, preliminary experimental data indicate that hyperglycemia may potentiate cerebral ischemic injury by increasing lactic acid production. Relatively strict control of the serum glucose concentration with levels no higher than 200 mg/dl is recommended. Insulin may be added to the hyperalimentation fluid or given as a continuous infusion (see Chap. 24).

Antibiotic Prophylaxis

Neurosurgical procedures are considered clean and pose no significant risk of bacteremia. Prophylaxis against endocarditis is therefore not warranted except in the case of transphenoidal surgery. Routine antibiotic prophylaxis to prevent postoperative infection is controversial. Although definitive data cited in Chap. 44 do not support the use of prophylaxis in clean procedures, including those involving shunt placement, many neurosurgeons administer antibiotics directed against staphylococci before the procedure.

POSTOPERATIVE COMPLICATIONS

Common postoperative complications including SIADH and stress gastritis are discussed above. Postoperative fever may have infectious or noninfectious causes. So-called central fever is rare and should be viewed as a diagnosis of exclusion. Common infectious processes include aspiration pneumonia, urinary tract infection, and meningitis.

Patients with both penetrating or closed-head injury have a significant risk of bacterial meningitis. Those undergoing neurosurgical procedures for reasons other than trauma have similar risk. Fever usually develops, but other classic meningeal signs may be absent or difficult to elicit. Examination of the cerebrospinal fluid is essential, and abnormalities must be interpreted in the context of changes normally attributable to uncomplicated neurosurgery. Elevated opening pressure, increased protein concentration, and pleocytosis all occur after surgery in the absence of infection. Hypoglycorrhachia and positive gram stains are the most specific markers of infection. Postoperative meningitis is most frequently caused by staphylococci, enterococci, and gram-negative rods. Meningitis as well as shunt and ventriculostomy infections are discussed in Chap. 52.

Pulmonary embolism poses a major threat to neurosurgical patients, and anticoagulation remains the major management issue. When deep venous thrombosis or pulmonary embolism is suspected in patients with intracranial neoplasm or soon after neurosurgery, many clinicians prefer interruption of the inferior vena cava to risking bleeding with anticoagulation. However, limited data suggest that patients with primary or metastatic brain tumors can be anticoagulated without undue risk.[12] Likewise, a single study of patients who developed deep vein thrombosis after aneurysm surgery documented no complications of anticoagulation.[13]

Because these studies involved only small numbers of patients, no firm recommendations can be offered at this time.

Air embolism can occur during any neurosurgical procedure when the operative site is above the level of the heart. This was a more common complication in the past when procedures were performed in the sitting position. Significant air embolism most often presents as intraoperative hypotension. Paradoxical air embolism can also occur (see Chap. 59).

Renal insufficiency can result from renal hypoperfusion due to diuretics or hypotension. Since neurosurgical patients may undergo angiography or computerized tomography with contrast media, dye-induced acute renal failure is not uncommon.

REFERENCES

1. Kaufman HH, Timberlanke G, Woelker J et al: Medical complications of head injury. *Med Clin N Amer* 77:43–60, 1993.
2. Yamaki T, Tano-oka A, Takahashi A et al: Cerebral salt wasting syndrome distinct from the syndrome of inappropriate secretion of antidiuretic hormone (SIADH). *Acta Neurosurg* 115:156–162, 1992.
3. Lolin Y, Jackowski A: Hyponatremia in neurosurgical patients: Diagnosis using derived parameters of sodium and water homeostasis. *Br J Neurosurg* 6:457–466, 1992.
4. Olson JD, Kaufman HH, Moake J et al: The incidence and significance of hemostatic abnormalities in patients with head injuries. *Neurosurgery* 24:825, 1989.
5. Frank JI: Management of intracranial hypertension. *Med Clin N Amer* 77:61–76, 1993.
6. Locksley HB: Report on the cooperative study of intracranial aneurysms and subarachnoid hemorrhage. 1. Natural history of subarachnoid hemorrhage, intracranial aneurysms and arteriovenous malformations. *J Neurosurg* 25(Sec 5):219–239, 1966.
7. Larson G, Koch S, D'Orisio B et al: Gastric response to severe head injury. *Am J Surg* 1476:96–105, 1984.
8. Chan KH, Mann KS, Lai EC et al: Factors influencing the development of gastrointestinal complications after neurosurgery; result of multivariate analysis. *Neurosurgery* 25:378–382, 1989.
9. Powers SK, Edwards MS: Prophylaxis of thromboembolism in the neurosurgical patient: A review. *Neurosurgery* 10:509–513, 1982.
10. Cerrato D, Ariano C, Fiacchino F: Deep vein thrombosis and low-dose heparin prophylaxis in neurosurgical patients. *J Neurosurg* 49:378–381, 1978.
11. Frim DM, Barker FG, Poletti CE et al: Postoperative low-dose heparin decreases thromboembolic complications in neurosurgical patients. *Neurosurgery* 30:830–833, 1992.
12. Olin JW, Young JR, Graor RA et al: Treatment of deep vein thrombosis and pulmonary emboli in patients with primary and metastatic brain tumors. *Arch Intern Med* 147:2177–2179, 1987.
13. Tapaninaho A: Deep vein thrombosis after aneurysm surgery. *Acta Neurochir* 74:18–20, 1985.

PROCEDURE: CRANIOTOMY FOR RESECTION OF ACOUSTIC NEUROMA

Overview: Acoustic neuroma, a misnomer for a benign schwannoma involving the vestibular division of the VIII cranial nerve, is a relatively common tumor. It makes up 6 to 8% of all intracranial tumors. Approximately 2000 to 3000 new cases are diagnosed per year in the United States. It most commonly presents between the fourth and sixth decades of life as a unilateral lesion. Five percent of all acoustic neuromas are related to neurofibromatosis. Although acoustic neuromas are usually slow-growing the natural history of an untreated neuroma may be quite variable. The most common symptoms are sensory neural hearing loss, tinnitus, decreased equilibrium, and vertigo.

1. *Operation*
   a. Indications:
      (1) Presence of an acoustic neuroma.
      (2) Progressive hearing loss.
      (3) Compression of brain stem and related structures by a tumor.
   b. Operative Steps: There are three main surgical approaches: suboccipital craniotomy, translabyrinthine approach, and subtemporal craniotomy. Most operations are performed by way of the suboccipital approach described herein. Staging is rarely required.
   c. Incision: An incision is placed behind the mastoid process which may be extended far superiorly or into a modified "hockey stick" incision. The horizontal limb is located 2 cm above and parallel to the nuchal line.
   d. Anesthesia: General.
   e. Intraoperative Monitoring: Intraoperative monitoring of the facial, trigeminal, and accessory nerves is performed. The motor neurons are monitored with electromyography. Auditory brain stem responses may be monitored.
   f. Operative Positioning: Most operations for acoustic neuromas are done in the lateral or park-bench position. Few surgeons still prefer the sitting suboccipital craniectomy.
   g. Duration: 4 to 12 hours.
   h. EBL/Transfusions: EBL is minimal. Transfusions are usually not required.
   i. "Surgical Stress": Moderate to severe.

2. *Expected Hospital Course/Treatment*
   a. Postoperative Monitoring
      (1) ICU Stay: 1 to 3 days.
      (2) Invasive/Special Monitoring: None.
      (3) Parameters To Be Monitored:
         i. Neurological examination.
         ii. Blood pressure.
         iii. Hearing and lower cranial nerve function (i.e., swallowing, speech).
   b. Positioning/Activity: Supine. Head of the bed elevated to 30 degrees. Activity as tolerated.
   c. Alimentation: Assessment of vocal cord and pharyngeal musculature function should be performed prior to feeding the patient to prevent aspiration.
   d. Wound Care/Drains: Some surgeons leave subdural suboccipital drains for 24 to 48 hours. Sutures are removed at 7 days.
   e. Respiratory Care: Routine.
   f. Analgesia/Postop Meds: Parenteral narcotics are usually required initially. Diazepam is indicated if patient has cervical musculature spasm. Steroids are tapered over 1 to 2 weeks.
   g. Length Of Hospital Stay: 1 week.

3. *Postoperative Complications*
   a. In Hospital
      1. Morbidity:
         i. Facial nerve injury.
         ii. Glossopharyngeal nerve injury (e.g., dysphagia).
         iii. Vagus nerve injury (e.g., dysphagia and hoarseness).
         iv. Persistent vertigo and headaches.
      (2) Mortality: < 1%.
   b. After Discharge
      (1) Cerebrospinal fluid leaks.
      (2) Meningitis.

4. *Follow-up*
   a. Suggested Follow-up: Patients are seen regularly for 1 to 2 years.

PROCEDURE: CRANIOTOMY FOR ACUTE SUBDURAL HEMATOMA

Overview: Acute subdural hematomas (ASDH) remain a major source of morbidity and mortality (50 to 90%) in patients with severe head injury despite recent advancements in medical and surgical management. ASDH arise from bleeding that occurs over the brain surface. The bleeding may arise from torn bridging veins between the cortex and venous sinuses or contused and lacerated cortex. Rapid and aggressive management is necessary to minimize the serious complications associated with this condition. Early definitive evacuation of subdural hematomas, i.e., within 4 hours after injury, has been found to reduce the morbidity and mortality associated with these lesions significantly.

1. *Operation*
   a. Indications: ASDH of less than 5 mm in thickness rarely require surgical intervention. Clots greater than 1 cm in thickness and associated with progressive neurologic deficits, obtundation, focal or cortical distortion, and midline shifts require immediate evacuation.
   b. Operative Steps: A craniotomy flap is constructed, and the dura is exposed. The dura must be opened widely and the underlying hematoma removed with irrigation and careful suction. Bleeding is controlled, and a subdural drain is placed. The dura is closed, and the bone flap is replaced.
   c. Incision: The majority of patients require exposure of the frontotemporal and parietal lobes. However, the precise size and location of the flap are adjusted according the findings on computerized tomography. The typical trauma flap "reversed question mark" extending from midline to in front of the ear is commonly used.
   d. Anesthesia: Rapid sequence induction with general endotracheal anesthesia. Hyperventilation, osmotic agents (e.g., mannitol), and loop diuretics (e.g., furosemide) are used together to produce a slack brain.
   e. Intraoperative Monitoring: Arterial line may be indicated for unstable patients.
   f. Operative Positioning: The patient is placed supine with the head turned to the side for supratentorial hematomas. The patient is placed prone or in the lateral position for posterior fossa hematomas.
   g. Duration: 1 to 3 hours.
   h. EBL/Transfusions: 300 to 500 ml. Blood loss may be higher if a coagulopathy develops.
   i. "Surgical Stress": Minimal to moderate.

2. *Expected Hospital Course/Treatment*
   a. Postoperative Monitoring
      (1) ICU Stay: 5 to 10 days. This may be longer for patients who are initially comatose or are posturing.
      (2) Invasive/Special Monitoring: Because elevated ICP is found commonly after operation for ASDH, ICP monitor is mandatory and is inserted through a separate incision. Blood flow monitor (where available). Swan-Ganz catheter and EEG for patients who require barbiturate coma therapy.
      (3) Parameters To Be Monitored:
         i. Intracerebral pressure, cerebral perfusion pressure, and cerebral blood flow (where available).
         ii. Mental status.
         iii. Cardiovascular parameters.
         iv. PT, PTT.
   b. Positioning/Activity: The patient is supine with the head of the bed elevated at 30 degrees.
   c. Alimentation: Oral intake for awake patients. Nasogastric tube feedings for comatose patients. Parenteral nutrition for patients with an ileus.
   d. Wound Care/Drains: Subgaleal or epidural drain is left in place for 24 to 48 hours. ICP monitor remains until ICP is normal for more than 48 hours. Staples or sutures removed by POD 7.
   e. Respiratory Care: Patients are kept on mechanical ventilation and weaned as dictated by ICP, mental, and respiratory status.
   g. Analgesia/Postop Meds: With elevated ICP, deep sedation (e.g., with morphine sulfate) and muscle relaxation (e.g., with vecuronium) is mandatory. With normal ICP, codeine or acetaminophen. Dilantin or phenobarbital for seizure prophylaxis. Mannitol and furosemide when needed for ICP management.
   h. Length Of Hospital Stay: 1 to 3 weeks, longer for patients left comatose or with severe neurologic deficit.

3. *Postoperative Complications*
   a. In Hospital
      (1) Morbidity: Early detection and operation of subdural hematomas decrease morbidity significantly from 80% to 30 or 40%. Persistent coma, hemiparesis or hemiplegia, aphasia, seizures, and disseminated intravascular coagulation are common sequelae of subdural hematomas.
      (2) Mortality: 10% to 40%.
   b. After Discharge
      (1) Bone flap infections.
      (2) Subdural empyema.
      (3) Delayed neurologic deficits.

4. *Follow-up*
   a. Suggested Follow-up: 1 to 6 months, long-term for patients with seizures and neurologic deficit.

PROCEDURE: ANTERIOR CERVICAL DISCECTOMY

Overview: Although decompression may be achieved from a posterior approach (laminectomy), an anterior approach to the cervical spine is superior because it allows the surgeon the ability to deal directly with the pathology without retracting the spinal cord or roots. A herniated cervical disc (soft disc) or spondylitic osteophytes (hard disc) may be located centrally, laterally, or anterolaterally. Patients with radiculopathy may have arm, shoulder, or neck pain; occipital headaches; intrascapular pain; and sometimes chest pain. Patients with myelopathy present with progressive ataxia, lower extremity spasticity, weakness, hyperreflexia, partial Brown-Séquard syndrome, or an anterior cord syndrome. Investigation and diagnostic workup should include standard cervical spine series with flexion and extension to assess spinal stability. Originally cervical myelography was the test of choice followed by computerized tomography. Presently, a thorough MRI of the cervical spine is the test of choice.

1. *Operation*
   a. Indications:
      (1) A herniated cervical intervertebral disc with radiculopathy or myelopathy.
      (2) Degenerative disc disease associated with posterior osteophytes and radiculopathy or myelopathy.
      (3) Cervical spinal stenosis in selected cases.
      (4) Trauma of the cervical spine with anterior compressive vector forces on the spinal cord.
      (5) Dysphagia associated with cervical spondylosis.
   b. Operative Steps: The vertebral bodies are approached and exposed. The disc is completely removed along with any osteophytes. After decompression is performed, an allograft is placed in the disc space, and the fusion is allowed to take place across the affected disc space in the ensuing months.
   c. Incision: Transverse from the midline across the medial border of the sternocleidomastoid muscle. Longitudinal along the anterior border of the sternocleidomastoid muscle.
   d. Anesthesia: General.
   e. Intraoperative Monitoring: Routine. Somatosensory evoked potentials in cases of severe spinal stenosis.
   f. Operative Positioning: Supine position with moderate cervical hyperextension achieved by placing a shoulder roll and allowing the head to turn 10 degrees to the right.
   g. Duration: 2 to 3 hours.
   h. EBL/Transfusions: 100 to 300 ml. Transfusions are rarely required.
   i. "Surgical Stress": Mild to moderate.

2. *Expected Hospital Course/Treatment*
   a. Postoperative Monitoring
      (1) ICU Stay: None to 2 days.
      (2) Invasive/Special Monitoring: None.
      (3) Parameters To Be Monitored:
         i. Vital signs.
         ii. Neurological examination.
         iii. Monitor for hoarseness and dysphagia.
   b. Positioning/Activity: As tolerated with hard cervical collar.
   c. Alimentation: As tolerated.
   d. Wound Care/Drains: Some surgeons leave a drain above the anterior aspect of the spine and bring it through the lower edge of the incision. The drain is removed 12 hours after surgery.
   e. Respiratory Care: Routine.
   f. Analgesia/Postop Meds: Parenteral narcotics or acetaminophen with codeine.
   g. Length Of Hospital Stay: 2 to 4 days.

3. *Postoperative Complications*
   a. In Hospital
      (1) Morbidity: Complication rates of up to 23% have been reported. An acceptable morbidity rate is under 2%. Morbidity includes:
         i. Retractor-related injuries such as laryngeal edema.
         ii. Hoarseness.
         iii. Dysphagia.
         iv. Esophageal injury.
         v. Tracheal injury.
         vi. Cerebrovascular fluid leaks.
         vii. Vertebral artery injury.
         viii. Graft extrusion.
      (2) Mortality: < 0.1%.
   b. After Discharge
      (1) Extrusion of bone plug.
      (2) Infection.
      (3) Chronic pain.

4. *Follow-up*
   a. Suggested Follow-up: Patients are kept in a hard (Philadelphia) collar until there is radiographic evidence of bony fusion.

PROCEDURE: CRANIOTOMY FOR BRAIN TUMOR

Overview: Gliomas, or tumors arising from glial cells or astrocytes, are the most common primary brain tumor. Astrocytomas are divided into three grades: low-grade astrocytoma, anaplastic astrocytoma, and malignant astrocytoma. Glioblastoma multiforme, a malignant astrocytoma, makes up 50% of all gliomas and most commonly occurs in the fifth and sixth decades. In absolute numbers, metastatic neoplasms of the intracranial compartment are the most common intracranial malignant tumor of secondary origin. The most common benign intracranial tumor is the meningioma, constituting approximately 15% of primary brain tumors and 25% of intraspinal tumors. Typically, 60% to 70% of adult brain tumors are located in the supratentorial compartment and 30% in the infratentorial compartment. Although there are many types of tumors often requiring different approaches, this outline considers resection of supratentorial glioma as the model.

1. *Operation*
   a. Indications:
      (1) To obtain a diagnosis.
      (2) To improve, prevent, or delay neurologic symptoms.
      (3) To increase survival attributable to surgery alone.
      (4) To increase survival long enough for adjunct therapies to have an effect.
   b. Operative Steps: The goal of brain tumor surgery is to remove the entire lesion whenever possible without causing neurological deficit. This may be easily accomplished in many benign tumors but may be impossible in infiltrating malignant neoplasms. In such cases a subtotal resection is the procedure of choice.
   c. Incision: The incision and bone flap are tailored to the craniotomy site.
   d. Anesthesia: General.
   e. Intraoperative Monitoring: Arterial line and CVP monitors, EEG (for epilepsy surgery).
   f. Operative Positioning: Supratentorial tumors: supine with head turned to left or right in mild flexion or extension. Infratentorial tumors: lateral decubitus or prone. Some surgeons still prefer the sitting position.
   g. Duration: 3 to 4 hours for uncomplicated superficial tumors and approximately 9 hours for deep tumors. Large tumors may need to be staged in 2 or 3 operations.
   h. EBL/Transfusions: 300 to 700 ml. With the advent of preoperative embolization, blood loss in richly vascular tumors may be decreased by up to 75%.
   i. "Surgical Stress": Minimal for superficial small tumors (i.e., meningioma or metastasis), moderate for deep tumors, and severe for tumors invading a venous sinus or located at or near eloquent areas.

2. *Expected Hospital Course/Treatment*
   a. Postoperative Monitoring
      (1) ICU Stay: 3 to 10 days.
      (2) Invasive/Special Monitoring: In selected patients, an ICP monitor may be left in place. Other invasive monitors should remain in place while in the ICU.
      (3) Parameters To Be Monitored:
         i. Neurologic status on an hourly basis. ii. CP and cerebral perfusion pressure. iii. PT, PTT.
   b. Positioning/Activity: Supine with head of bed at 30 degrees.
   c. Alimentation: Oral as soon as possible. Comatose patients should have nasogastric tube enteral feedings started within 24 to 48 hours.
   d. Wound Care/Drains: A subgaleal drain is commonly left in place for 24 hours. Sutures or staples are removed around POD 7.
   e. Respiratory Care: Extubation is usually attempted in the operating room to improve assessment of neurologic status.
   f. Analgesia/Postop Meds: Parenteral or oral narcotics as tolerated. Steroids are tapered over 1 to 2 weeks depending on clinical and radiographic status. Anticonvulsants are continued in patients with supratentorial tumors.
   g. Length Of Hospital Stay: 7 to 14 days.

3. *Postoperative Complications*
   a. In Hospital
      (1) Morbidity:
         i. Deep venous thrombosis.   iii. Cerebrospinal fluid infection.
         ii. Hydrocephalus (immediate or delayed). iv. Difficult wound healing (affected by steroids).
      (2) Mortality: < 1%.
   b. After Discharge:
      (1) Subdural hematoma.
      (2) Recurrent tumor.
      (3) Infection.

4. *Follow-up*
   a. Suggested Follow-up: 2 weeks after surgery and then monthly thereafter as determined by the patient's clinical status. Most patients with gliomas also require radiation therapy and are followed by a radiation oncologist. For certain tumors, like medulloblastomas, chemotherapy is administered as well.

PROCEDURE: INTRACRANIAL ANEURYSM CLIPPING

Overview: Neurosurgical intervention for cerebral vascular disease is most often indicated in two conditions: aneurysmal subarachnoid hemorrhage or bleeding associated with arterial-venous malformations. Cerebral aneurysms occur in all ages but most commonly rupture in the fifth, sixth, and seventh decades. About 50% of these patients die or become permanently disabled as a result of the initial hemorrhage, and another 25% to 35% die of a later rebleed if left untreated. The present trend is to perform surgical obliteration of the aneurysm within the first 24 to 72 hours postictus. When the patient has evidence of vasospasm or neurologic deterioration or presents in coma, surgery may be delayed for 14 days or more.

1. *Operation*
   a. Indications:
      (1) Any patient with a subarachnoid hemorrhage on CT scan or significant blood on nontraumatic lumbar puncture and a documented aneurysm on cerebral angiogram is a candidate for clipping.
      (2) The development of a neurologic deficit or symptoms due to compression of adjacent neural structures by an aneurysm.
      (3) The production of emboli from an aneurysm into the distal circulation.
      (4) An asymptomatic aneurysm since it carries a risk of rupture of 3% per year.
   b. Operative Steps: The goal of surgery is the obliteration of the aneurysm by placing a metal clip along the parent vessel at the neck of the aneurysm. For some aneurysms, particularly those with a wide neck, a ligature can be used to obliterate the neck. Rarely an aneurysm may be unclippable, in which case reinforcement with muslin may be used in an effort to decrease the risk of subsequent bleeding.
   c. Incision: Straight or curved and based on the cranial flap location.
   d. Anesthesia: General anesthesia with particular emphasis on avoiding hypertension.
   e. Intraoperative Monitoring: Arterial line and CVP. EEG may be done if temporary vessel occlusion is being considered. Spinal drainage is commonly used to produce a slack easily retractable brain in order to decrease retraction injury and gain easy access to the aneurysm.
   f. Operative Positioning: Supine, lateral decubitus, park-bench, prone, or sitting position depending on the location of the aneurysm.
   g. Duration: Clipping a simple uncomplicated aneurysm may be accomplished in 2 to 3 hours whereas difficult giant aneurysms that require bypass may last as long as 12 hours or more.
   h. EBL/Transfusions: If there is no intraoperative rupture, little blood is lost. If, however, an aneurysm ruptures and the surgeon has not obtained proximal control, a patient can lose several units of blood in a few minutes.
   i. "Surgical Stress": Severe.

2. *Expected Hospital Course/Treatment*
   a. Postoperative Monitoring
      (1) ICU Stay: As long as 3 weeks if symptoms of vasospasm develop.
      (2) Invasive/Special Monitoring: Swan-Ganz catheterization to guide hypervolemic hemodilution. Transcranial doppler ultrasonography (TCD) to measure cerebral blood flow and document the development of vasospasm.
      (3) Parameters To Be Monitored:
          i. Neurological examination.   ii. Cardiovascular parameters.   iii. Cerebral blood flow.
   b. Positioning/Activity: Supine position with head of bed elevated at 30 degrees for several days. Out of bed once hemodynamic status is stable and there is no evidence of vasospasm.
   c. Alimentation: If there has been no injury to the lower cranial nerves (as in the vertebrobasilar aneurysms) and the patient is awake, an oral diet may be started on POD 1 or 2. In patients with a depressed mental status, enteral feedings are usually started as soon as normal peristalsis has resumed.
   d. Wound Care/Drains: Spinal drain is removed prior to leaving the operating room. A ventriculostomy may be placed if the patient develops hydrocephalus and is left in place until there is no clinical need for cerebrospinal fluid drainage.
   e. Respiratory Care: Extubation is attempted in the operating room to facilitate assessment of neurologic function unless airway reflexes are depressed.
   f. Analgesia/Postop Meds: Parenteral narcotics as needed. Stool softeners are routinely used.
   g. Length Of Hospital Stay: A patient with no neurologic deficits and no evidence of vasospasm may be discharged within 15 days whereas a patient with vasospasm or severe neurologic deficit may be in the hospital from 4 to 6 weeks.

3. *Postoperative Complications*
   a. In Hospital
      (1) Morbidity: Vasospasm is the most significant cause of stroke and ischemia.
      (2) Mortality: 1 to 2% for asymptomatic patients; 40 to 50% for patients presenting with stupor and coma.
   b. After Discharge:
      (1) Infection.   (4) Hemiplegia.
      (2) Memory deficit.   (5) Delayed-onset hydrocephalus.
      (3) Hypersomnolence.

4. *Follow-up*
   a. Suggested Follow-up: Two weeks after surgery, then several times during the next 6 months. Subsequent care depends on the level of neurologic function.

PROCEDURE: STEREOTACTIC SURGERY

Overview: Stereotactic surgery was originally introduced in 1908 to produce reliable and specific lesions in the cerebella of monkeys. With the use of computerized tomography and magnetic resonance imaging data, stereotactic surgery is now commonly used in modern neurosurgery to locate and treat a variety of disorders.

1. *Operation*
   a. Indications:
      (1) Diagnosis of deep-seated inaccessible lesions.
      (2) Diagnosis of lesions located in eloquent areas.
      (3) Evacuation and drainage of brain abscesses.
      (4) Treatment of certain brain and movement disorders.
   b. Operative Steps: A localization ring is placed with four skull pins under local anesthetic. A computed tomography with contrast is performed, and the lesion is localized using x and y coordinates. Coordinates are referenced with x and y coordinates of the bars of the localizer ring. In the operating room, the entry site is defined using a three-dimensional arc system, and its location is entered into the computer along with the coordinates of the lesion. The computer provides the surgeon with the appropriate trajectory and depth to reach the lesion from a defined entry point.
   c. Incision: Either burr-hole or twist-drill craniostomy is performed depending on the location of the lesion.
   d. Anesthesia: Local or general.
   e. Intraoperative Monitoring: Routine if cardiovascular status is stable.
   f. Operative Positioning: Patient is placed supine with a localizer ring and frame attached to the bed frame.
   g. Duration: 30 minutes to 2 hours.
   h. EBL/Transfusions: None.
   i. "Surgical Stress": Minimal to mild.

2. *Expected Hospital Course/Treatment*
   a. Postoperative Monitoring
      (1) ICU Stay: Overnight.
      (2) Invasive/Special Monitoring: None.
      (3) Parameters To Be Monitored:
         i. Neurologic status.
         ii. All elderly patients undergo computed tomography immediately after surgery to exclude intracranial hemorrhage.
   b. Positioning/Activity: As tolerated.
   c. Alimentation: As tolerated.
   d. Wound Care/Drains: None.
   e. Respiratory Care: Routine.
   f. Analgesia/Postop Meds: Morphine sulfate or acetaminophen with codeine as needed.
   g. Length Of Hospital Stay: 1 to 3 days.

3. *Postoperative Complications*
   a. In Hospital
      (1) Morbidity:
         i. Hemorrhage at the site of biopsy.
         ii. Infection.
         iii. Neurologic deficit.
         iv. Seizures (uncommon).
      (2) Mortality: 0.4 to 0.6%.
   b. After Discharge: Minimal to none.

4. *Follow-up*
   a. Suggested Follow-up: Follow-up depends on the results of the biopsy. If a stereotactic procedure is performed for chronic pain or movement disorder, long-term follow-up is necessary.

PROCEDURE: TRANSSPHENOIDAL SURGERY

Overview: The operating microscope, better illumination, and improved instrumentation have made the transsphenoidal approach to lesions of the sella turcica relatively easy. Preoperative testing should include prolactin, thyroid function, LH, FSH, estradiol, testosterone, and AM cortisol levels. Adjunctive studies such as a glucose tolerance test, metyrapone test, and dexamethasone suppression test may also be performed.

1. *Operation*
   a. Indications:
      (1) Sellar or suprasellar lesions such as pituitary tumors and craniopharyngiomas.
      (2) Cerebral spinal fluid leaks.
   b. Operative Steps: Sublabial gingival incision from canine to canine allows access to the pyriform opening. Submucosal tunnels are developed, and the nasal septum is reflected laterally. The floor of the sphenoid sinus is removed to allow visualization of the tumor to be resected.
   c. Incision: See above.
   d. Anesthesia: General.
   e. Intraoperative Monitoring: Arterial line with or without CVP. A spinal drain is used to allow visualization of the location of the diaphragma sella and facilitate tumor delivery.
   f. Operative Positioning: The patient is placed supine with a three-point cranial fixation. The head is turned to the right side and elevated approximately 20 degrees within the C-arm fluoroscopic unit.
   g. Duration: 4 to 6 hours.
   h. EBL/Transfusions: 200 to 300 ml.
   i. "Surgical Stress": Moderate.

2. *Expected Hospital Course/Treatment*
   a. Postoperative Monitoring
      (1) ICU Stay: 1 to 3 days. Longer if diabetes insipidus, cerebrospinal fluid leak, or visual deterioration develops.
      (2) Invasive/Special Monitoring: Invasive monitors remain in place while in the ICU.
      (3) Parameters To Be Monitored:
         i. Urinary output and specific gravity, serum and urine electrolyte levels.
         ii. Visual fields and visual acuity at frequent intervals.
   b. Positioning/Activity: Supine with head of bed at 30 to 40 degrees. Activity as tolerated.
   c. Alimentation: Clear liquids to regular diet as tolerated.
   d. Wound Care/Drains: Nasal packing is removed on POD 3. Mucosa is closed with absorbable sutures. Mouth rinse (half water and half hydrogen peroxide) for 3 to 4 days after surgery.
   e. Respiratory Care: Routine.
   f. Analgesia/Postop Meds: Mild analgesics such as codeine or acetaminophen. Postoperative medications may include DDAVP for diabetes insipidus and hormonal replacement for hypopituitarism.
   g. Length Of Hospital Stay: 6 to 8 days.

3. *Postoperative Complications*
   a. In Hospital
      (1) Morbidity:
         i. Cerebrospinal fluid leaks.
         ii. Diabetes insipidus (transient or permanent).
         iii. Visual complications from damage to the optic nerve or chiasm or postoperative hemorrhage.
      (2) Mortality: 0.5%.
   b. After Discharge:
      (1) Permanent hypopituitarism.
      (2) Permanent diabetes insipidus.

4. *Follow-up*
   a. Suggested Follow-up: Neurosurgical and endocrine follow-up as dicated by clinical status.

PROCEDURE: VENTRICULOPERITONEAL SHUNT PLACEMENT

Overview: Hydrocephalus is a common condition and is defined as a disproportionate enlargement of part of the ventricular system. It usually results from obstruction to normal cerebrospinal fluid outflow and rarely from cerebrospinal fluid overproduction. Obstruction may be due to congenital malformations (e.g., aqueductal stenosis, Dandy Walker cyst), intracranial tumors, or subarachnoid inflammation from infection or subarachnoid hemorrhage. Diagnosis is best established with computerized tomography.

1. *Operation*
    a. Indications: See above.
    b. Operative Steps: After a burr hole is made, a catheter is inserted into the lateral cerebral ventricle and is connected to a valve system. A peritoneal catheter is tunneled from the abdomen and connected to the valve system. Both wounds are closed in layers.
    c. Incision: For front shunts a curvilinear incision is placed 1 cm anterior to the coronal suture along the midpupillary line. For occipital shunt, the incision is made 2 to 3 cm lateral to the inion and 6 to 7 cm superior to this point. The peritoneal catheter is placed through a midline, paramedian or subcostal incision.
    d. Anesthesia: General.
    e. Intraoperative Monitoring: Routine with or without arterial line.
    f. Operative Positioning: Supine with head turned sharply to the side opposite the insertion site.
    g. Duration: 30 minutes to 1.5 hours.
    h. EBL/Transfusions: Minimal.
    i. "Surgical Stress": Minimal.

2. *Expected Hospital Course/Treatment*
    a. Postoperative Monitoring
        (1) ICU Stay: None.
        (2) Invasive/Special Monitoring: None.
        (3) Parameters To Be Monitored:
            i. Vitals signs.
            ii. Neurological examination.
    b. Positioning/Activity: As tolerated after recovery from anesthesia. Patients with significant ventriculomegaly may be allowed slowly out of bed over the next 24 to 48 hours.
    c. Alimentation: Patients take nothing by mouth until full peristaltic function resumes and then are advanced as tolerated to a regular diet.
    d. Wound Care/Drains: Sutures are removed between 5 and 7 days after surgery. No drains.
    e. Respiratory Care: Routine.
    f. Analgesia/Postop Meds: Codeine and acetaminophen only.
    g. Length Of Hospital Stay: 2 to 4 days.

3. *Postoperative Complications*
    a. In Hospital
        (1) Morbidity:
            i. Shunt infection.
            ii. Shunt blockade.
            iii. Subdural fluid collection.
            iv. Abdominal injury, often presenting as infection or obstruction.
        (2) Mortality: < 0.05%.
    b. After Discharge:
        (1) Shunt infection.
        (2) Shunt blockade.

4. *Follow-up*
    a. Suggested Follow-up: 2 weeks after surgery, thereafter monthly, bimonthly, semiannually, and finally annual visits. Patients with shunts should be followed long-term.

14 EVALUATION OF THE PATIENT UNDERGOING ORTHOPEDIC SURGERY

Joseph Iannotti

Kurt P. Spindler

John Kelly

Frank H. Brown

The spectrum of orthopedic surgery varies widely from arthroscopic procedures in healthy young adults to emergency fixation of unstable pelvic and long-bone fractures in patients with multiple traumatic injuries. It is therefore important for the clinician to have an overall understanding of coexisting medical problems and their implications, commonly used anesthetic and surgical techniques, postoperative complications, and various prophylactic measures needed to minimize postoperative morbidity. This chapter provides a brief overview of these issues and specific information about the most common orthopedic procedures.

COMMON COMORBID CONDITIONS

Coexisting chronic medical problems are common in patients undergoing orthopedic surgery. One study demonstrated that 71 percent of patients undergoing total hip arthroplasty had one or more preoperative medical problems.[1] The presence of major medical problems before surgery was highly correlated with the occurrence of postoperative complications and the length of hospital stay.

Advanced Age

Osteoporosis and falls are common in the geriatric population and result in an increased incidence of fractures with advancing age. Approximately 25 percent of patients admitted for orthopedic surgery are over 65. Several studies have suggested that advanced age is an independent risk factor for postoperative morbidity.[2] More importantly, the prevalence of coexisting chronic medical problems increases with age. As a result, several studies of elderly patients undergoing orthopedic procedures have shown high rates of postoperative complications. In one study of patients over 80 undergoing total hip arthroplasties, 75 percent developed complications.[3] The most common complications were excessive bleeding, postoperative confusion, urinary tract infection, and dislocation. Another study found a higher incidence of cardiovascular and gastrointestinal complications in patients over age 60.[4] A third study of elderly patients undergoing total hip replacement documented a 77 percent incidence of postoperative morbidity and a 4 percent mortality rate. Infection, adverse drug reaction, confusion, and dislocation were the most common problems adding to increased length of hospital stay.[5] Advanced age is an important independent risk factor in the development of postoperative deep-venous thrombosis and pulmonary embolism which are major causes of morbidity and mortality following orthopedic procedures.

Elderly patients with hip fractures after a fall pose special problems. In addition to assessing the overall medical condition, the clinician should evaluate the cause of the fall.[6] Although most falls are due to accidents or environmental factors, they can be due to important cardiovascular or neurologic disorders including arrhythmias, drop attacks, and orthostatic hypotension. Special consideration should also be given to alcohol and drugs as possible causes. Several studies have correlated the incidence of falls in the elderly with use of benzodiazepines, antidepressants, and diuretics. Obviously, many of these etiologies have perioperative implications, and identification of the cause may prevent future injury. Timing of surgical repair is also an important issue. Although early operative fixation is preferred, one study showed that operative delay for more than 24 hours in order to treat medical conditions did not adversely affect outcome in elderly patients.[7] A more detailed discussion of the assessment and preparation of elderly patients for surgery is presented in Chap. 39.

Cardiovascular Disease

Hypertension is the most common preoperative problem and occurs in approximately 30 percent of patients undergoing hip arthroplasty.[1] Ischemic heart disease is present in 10 percent and poses particular problems in orthopedic patients. Because the patient is often greatly limited by the underlying orthopedic condition and engages in little physical activity, assessment of anginal frequency and ischemic threshold is difficult. Preoperative assessment with adenosine-thallium or dipyridamole-thallium testing may be indicated in selected patients before major orthopedic procedures. The assessment and perioperative treatment of patients with ischemic heart disease is presented in Chap. 18.

Rheumatologic Conditions

Patients with rheumatoid arthritis undergo a variety of orthopedic procedures, ranging from hind-foot reconstruction to cervical fusion. Unfortunately, rheumatoid patients experience higher complication rates for all surgical procedures than those with osteoarthritis. Wound breakdown, infection, and loosening of implants occur more frequently in rheumatoid patients and can be attributed to poor soft-tissue envelope, compromised vascular status, and poor bone stock. Rheumatoid patients should be examined for cervical spine involvement. If present, dynamic flexion and extension radiographs should be obtained to exclude occult instability before general anesthesia is administered. A variety of other problems including anemia, pulmonary fibrosis, and pleural effusions may be present. Chronic steroid use often results in adrenal suppression, requiring perioperative administration of stress-dose steroids. Similarly, patients with systemic lupus erythematosus and other rheumatologic conditions frequently require orthopedic intervention and may pose difficult management issues that are more fully discussed in Chap. 27.

Avascular necrosis of the femoral head is a common indication for hip replacement. Although most often due to trauma, it can be associated with underlying medical problems including alcoholism, steroid use, lupus, and hemoglobinopathies.

Obesity

Obesity is a known risk factor in the development of osteoarthritis, and many patients undergoing reconstructive surgery for arthritis are overweight. Obese patients suffer higher rates of wound breakdown, thromboembolic disease, and pulmonary complications. Early patient mobilization, meticulous pulmonary toilet, and appropriate prophylaxis against deep-venous thrombosis are all necessary adjuncts to good perioperative care (see Chap. 33).

Risk of Bleeding

Orthopedic procedures may result in substantial blood loss, and excessive bleeding at the surgical site increases the chances of wound infection. Although the prevalence of underlying coagulopathies is no higher in orthopedic patients, many regularly take nonsteroidal anti-inflammatory drugs (NSAIDs) as treatment for osteoarthritis, rheumatoid arthritis, or other inflammatory conditions. Since NSAIDs are reversible inhibitors of platelet aggregation, chronic use can increase postoperative bleeding. When planning a major orthopedic procedure like total joint replacement

or spinal surgery, NSAIDs should be discontinued several days before surgery. This is usually unnecessary for minor procedures.

Malnutrition

Increasing evidence indicates that many, if not most, surgical patients are moderately to severely malnourished. The increased metabolic demand of orthopedic trauma or surgery is often not adequately met by the meager caloric consumption of some elderly patients. With inadequate caloric intake, the hypercatabolic state induced by trauma or surgery causes significant visceral and skeletal protein depletion. Malnourished patients clearly have increased rates of mortality and morbidity due to sepsis, wound complications, impaired healing, and protracted rehabilitation. While no single test conclusively demonstrates malnutrition, an array of laboratory studies and physical measurements can effectively document nutritional inadequacies. Once identified, implementation of total or peripheral parenteral nutrition should be considered. If possible, supplementation should be instituted before surgery and carefully monitored throughout the perioperative period (see Chaps. 41 and 42).

Infection

Urinary tract infections are frequently present in elderly patients undergoing orthopedic surgery. Urinary tract infections associated with bacteremia are particularly worrisome because of the possibility of bacterial seeding of metal implants. Urinary tract infection has been associated with increased risk of joint sepsis after total joint replacement, although documented cases of this are uncommon. Nonetheless, it is important to identify and treat established urinary tract infections before implant surgery. Similarly, decubitus ulcers can serve as a source of infection and bacteremia. Joint replacement performed in the presence of skin ulcers carries a higher rate of prosthetic infection.

Multiple Trauma

Many orthopedic patients are the victims of multiple traumatic injuries usually caused by motor vehicle accidents. In such cases, urgent repair of orthopedic injuries almost always takes precedence over assessment and treatment of chronic medical problems because acute stabilization of long-bone fractures dramatically reduces mortality, the incidence of adult respiratory distress syndrome, length of hospital stay, and need for mechanical ventilation. Immediate fixation of unstable pelvic and long-bone fractures limits hemorrhage, assures patient comfort, increases patient mobility, helps achieve a vertical chest, and improves pulmonary care. By allowing the patient to sit upright, such procedures facilitate oral intake. Furthermore, fracture stabilization within 24 hours reduces local inflammatory processes and reduces the overall systemic response to injury. Patients suffering multiple trauma are often in their best state of health upon admission and efforts to delay fracture stabilization are usually not in their best interest.

After surgery, it is important to recognize factors that may have caused the accident. These include alcohol and drug abuse, and unrecognized or untreated comorbid conditions such as liver disease, withdrawal syndromes, myocardial infarction, arrhythmias, seizures, and hypoglycemic agents. All of these can cause postoperative complications and may require specific diagnostic and therapeutic interventions. Medical consultants may also assist in diagnosing and treating concomitant problems such as fat embolism, pulmonary or myocardial contusion, myoglobinuric renal failure, and pancreatitis.

PROPHYLACTIC ISSUES

Thromboembolism Prophylaxis

The most important prophylactic issue in patients undergoing orthopedic surgery is the prevention of deep-venous thrombosis and pulmonary embolism. Deep-venous thrombosis develops in as many as 60 percent of patients undergoing hip surgery and total knee replacement. Hip surgery poses a particular risk because it results in proximal venous thrombi which have a high propensity to embolize. Clinically apparent pulmonary embolism occurs in approximately 20 percent of these patients.

Thromboembolism prophylaxis should therefore be considered in all patients undergoing major orthopedic procedures. Low-dose warfarin and adjusted-dose heparin have proven efficacious.[8,9] Limited data suggest that thigh-length sequential compression devices[10] and low-dose heparin-dihydroergotamine may be useful in elective hip arthroplasty.[11] Initial studies suggest that low-molecular-weight heparin may also be effective and safe in these patients.[12] Standard low-dose heparin, aspirin, and dextran have no proven benefit (see Chap. 48).

Autologous Blood Donation

Transfusion of autologous blood avoids most of the complications associated with homologous blood including transmission of disease, hemolytic transfusion reactions, and other immune phenomena. Despite existing medical problems, most patients are able to donate at least two units of autologous blood before surgery. This can enable over 90 percent of patients to avoid homologous transfusion during major orthopedic procedures. Autologous blood can normally be stored for up to 42 days; longer storage requires an expensive and complex freezing process. One unit of autologous blood can be processed from each patient every three days until three days prior to surgery, provided that the hematocrit remains at least 34 percent. Iron supplementation is recommended. Autologous transfusion and other strategies to avoid homologous transfusions are discussed in Chap. 51.

Antibiotic Prophylaxis

Prophylactic antibiotics are usually administered to patients undergoing total joint replacement because of the consequences of infected prostheses. Short courses of antibiotics are safe and effective, but longer courses have been associated with *Clostridia difficile* colitis[13] (see Chap. 44). Endocarditis prophylaxis is not warranted for clean orthopedic procedures because the risk of bacteremia is low.

ANESTHETIC TECHNIQUES

Regional anesthesia offers a number of advantages over general for patients undergoing orthopedic surgery, including less intraopera-

tive blood loss, more rapid recovery, and decreased incidence of venous thrombosis and pulmonary embolism. Blood loss may be reduced by more than 50 percent compared with that incurred under general anesthesia and may be due to associated hypotension and other independent factors. Spontaneous respiration without the increased intrathoracic pressure caused by mechanical ventilation facilitates venous return and helps maintain peripheral venous pressure at low levels. In such cases, less blood loss would be expected.

Regional anesthesia virtually eliminates the threat of postoperative nausea, and patients resume oral intake more rapidly. Patients regain full alertness faster, and pulmonary atelectasis is greatly diminished. Regional anesthesia also confers significant protection against thromboembolic phenomena in orthopedic patients. Several explanations of this phenomenon have been proposed. Blood viscosity is reduced with regional anesthetic techniques. Secondly, arterial inflow, venous capacitance, and venous emptying are enhanced by epidural anesthesia. Furthermore, epidural techniques increase fibrinolytic activity when compared to general anesthesia, and regional anesthetic agents inhibit platelet adhesion.

SURGICAL TECHNIQUES

Arthroscopic and Open Procedures

Controversies continue as to whether traditional open surgical techniques are inferior to newer arthroscopic methods. Arthroscopic procedures offer the advantages of less tissue trauma, pain, and patient inconvenience as well as improved joint visualization and faster rehabilitation. In the knee, arthroscopic procedures have almost entirely supplanted open techniques. Meniscus resection and repair, removal of loose bodies, and synovectomies all can be accomplished more effectively with arthroscopy. Ligamentous reconstructions are now largely performed with arthroscopic assistance, although entirely open reconstructions appear to cause little additional morbidity.

Arthroscopic techniques are less often used in the shoulder. Shoulder arthroscopy is invaluable as a diagnostic modality and can be particularly helpful in diagnosing certain shoulder instabilities and subtle rotator cuff tears. Furthermore, for loose body removal, glenoid labral debridement, and synovial biopsy, it is unequivocally superior. However, open procedures for repair of rotator cuff tears and treatment for shoulder instability (dislocation/subluxation) remain clearly superior to arthroscopic methods. The role of arthroscopy is less clear in the treatment of subacromial impingement in acromioclavicular joint arthritis. Equally good success rates have been reported for arthroscopic and open subacromial decompression and distal clavicle resections.

Tourniquets

Tourniquets are used to control blood loss during upper- and lower-extremity procedures. Most tourniquets are pneumatic with incorporated pressure gauges. Inappropriate tourniquet usage has been associated with both nerve and muscle damage, and tissues directly beneath and distal to the tourniquet cuff are vulnerable. Tissues directly beneath are not only subject to ischemia but also to compressive and shear forces that can result in nerve damage. To minimize this complication, the lowest pressure that will prevent capillary flow should be used. This is usually 200 mmHg for the upper extremity and 250 mmHg for the lower. The region distal to the tourniquet is subject to ischemic necrosis if tourniquet times exceed three hours. Within this time limit, local tissue metabolism is restored 20 to 40 minutes after reperfusion. In clinical practice, most clinicians do not extend tourniquet times longer than two hours. If additional time is required, the tourniquet is deflated for 10 minutes before reinflation.

Cemented Versus Noncemented Components

Total joint replacement surgery has dramatically improved over the past decade, and newer implant designs and modern materials have enabled most patients to expect at least 10 years of use from their prostheses. Joint prostheses are secured either with or without cement. Cemented prostheses use polymethylmethacrylate (PMMA) to achieve fixation between the implant and bone. Cement is applied in the operating room in a semiliquid state and hardens in about 10 minutes for immediate fixation.

Cemented components can cause a variety of problems. The cement mantle can fracture, and some patients may develop biologic intolerance to PMMA. Young patients with cemented prostheses experience a high failure rate, and revision of cemented components can present many difficulties. Cementless components have specially treated surfaces that stimulate fibers on ingrowth into the prostheses. Since ingrowth takes several weeks, the prostheses must have an initial secured "press fit" to ensure early stability. Cementless prostheses have been associated with a higher incidence of limb pain soon after the procedure. They also have been implicated in excessive release of metal ions into the systemic circulation. They are usually preferred over cemented prostheses in patients under 60 and in those undergoing surgical revision. However, while uncemented acetabular components are gaining increasing favor, cemented knee and hip components remain the standard for elderly patients.

Placement of a cemented total hip prosthesis is rarely associated with transient hypotension after compression of liquid methylmethacrylate into the femoral canal. This has been attributed to vasodilation caused by unpolymerized monomer in the cement and to fat or air embolism caused by increased pressure in the femoral canal. The hypotension usually lasts only 30 to 60 seconds and rarely results in major complications.

POSTOPERATIVE COMPLICATIONS

Anemia

Anemia is common after major orthopedic procedures like repair of hip fractures. Blood loss from the injury and surgery itself is almost always the cause. A liter of blood can be lost in the thigh without clinically apparent symptoms or signs. Blood loss and the resulting large hematoma may cause fever, reticulocytosis, indirect hyperbilirubinemia, and elevation of LDH, erroneously suggesting hemolysis.

Fever and Infection

Fever is common in the early postoperative period and is usually not due to infection. However, persistent fever, wound drainage, and continued pain at the operative site suggest infection. Most infections are due to staphylococcus species. Infection of a joint prosthesis is particularly serious and may require reoperation and removal of the infected hardware.

Pulmonary Embolism

Pulmonary embolism remains the most common cause of death after orthopedic surgery. Even in patients receiving prophylactic therapy, pulmonary embolism should be suspected in patients with unexplained tachycardia, hypoxia, chest pain, or dyspnea. The diagnosis and treatment of postoperative pulmonary embolism is discussed in Chap. 59.

Fat Embolism Syndrome

Fat embolism syndrome is a clinical symptom complex characterized by changes in mental status, fever, tachycardia, tachypnea and petechiae, usually occurring 24 to 72 hours after injury. Its incidence is particularly high in patients with open fractures, vehicular-related fractures, and fractures of several long bones. The syndrome has also been described after total joint replacement. Chest radiographs show bilateral patchy infiltrates, and blood studies reveal thrombocytopenia. The pathophysiology of fat embolism syndrome remains unclear, and treatment is largely supportive. Artificial ventilation is often necessary, and steroids may be beneficial (see Chap. 59).

Urinary Retention

Acute urinary retention occurs in up to 60 percent of patients undergoing total hip or total knee replacement. Reducing the frequency and duration of postoperative catheterization would probably decrease the risk of urinary infection. However, recent studies indicate that perioperative indwelling catheterization effectively prevents acute bladder distention and sharply diminishes both urinary retention and subsequent infection. Unfortunately, preoperative identification of patients with an increased risk of urinary retention is not consistently provided by urologic history or prostate examination.

Postoperative Delirium

Postoperative confusion is particularly common in elderly patients undergoing orthopedic surgery. Patients who develop confusion after surgery have significantly more complications and longer hospital stays. Risk factors for its development include preexisting cognitive dysfunction, depression, and concomitant use of drugs with anticholinergic effects.[14] Contributing factors may be other drugs such as narcotic analgesics and nonsteroidal anti-inflammatory agents, hypoxia, infection, and volume depletion. Alcohol withdrawal may also cause postoperative delirium (see Chaps. 38 and 70).

Compartment Syndrome

A compartment syndrome occurs when elevated pressure within a close osteofascial compartment space exceeds capillary perfusion pressure with resulting tissue ischemia. Nontraumatic etiologies include hemorrhage, closure of fascial defects, intravenous infusions, and acute exertion. Traumatic causes include blunt muscle trauma from a direct blow, fractures, burns, and crush injury. Compartment syndromes can also arise after prolonged ischemia as seen in arterial injury, revascularization procedures, lymphatic compression from lying in one position for long periods of time, or intraoperative positioning and prolonged limb elevation. Compartment syndromes commonly occur after trauma to the tibia and forearm and are less frequent in the thigh and foot.

The classical presentation of compartment syndrome is defined by the five P's—pain, pallor, pulselessness, paresthesias, and paralysis. Pain is the most consistent of these. On physical examination, the involved compartment is tense, and passive stretch of the digits or toes amplifies the patient's pain. The treatment of compartment syndrome is fasciotomy with release of the fascial coverings surrounding the involved muscle. Left untreated, compartment syndrome can lead to ischemia, necrosis, and subsequent fibrosis, leaving a contracted and compromised extremity. Measurement of compartment pressure is useful in managing compartment syndromes, although there is no universal agreement on what threshold to use to determine need for fasciotomy.

Nerve Palsies

The reported incidence of nerve palsies after total hip replacement ranges from 0.6 to 3.7 percent. The sciatic nerve and the peroneal division of the sciatic nerve are involved in 80 percent of these cases. Femoral nerve injuries occur in less than 0.5 percent, and obturator nerve injuries are rare. The possible mechanisms of nerve injury after total hip replacement include direct trauma, excessive tension, ischemia, compressive extrusion of methylmethacrylate and thermal injury from its polymerization. Prognosis for recovery is related to the degree of nerve damage.[15]

REFERENCES

1. Moran EF, Littlejohn GO: Medical problems in joint replacement patients: A retrospective study of 243 total hip arthroplasties. *Med J Aust* 152:408–413, 1990.

2. Goldman L, Caldera D, Nussbaum SR et al: Multifactorial Index of Cardiac Risk in noncardiac surgical procedures. *N Engl J Med* 297:845, 1977.

3. Boettcher WG: Total hip arthroplasties in the elderly. *Clin Orthop* 274:30–34, 1992.

4. Williams JR, Mallory TH, Danyi JJ et al: The hip replacement in the geriatric patient. *Ohio Med J* 77:671, 1981.

5. Sheppeard H, Cleak DK, Ward DJ et al: A review of early morbidity and mortality in elderly patients following Charnley total hip replacement. *Arch Orthop Trauma Surg* 97:243–248, 1980.

6. Duthie EH: Falls. *Med Clin N Am* 73:1321–1336, 1989.

7. Harries DJ, Eastwood H: Proximal femoral fractures in the elderly: Does operative delay for medical reasons affect short-term outcome? *Age and Aging* 20:41–44, 1991.

8. Mohr DN, Silverstein MD, Ilstrup DM et al: Venous thromboembolism associated with hip and knee arthroplasty: Current prophylactic practices and outcomes. *Mayo Clin Proc* 67:861–870, 1992.

9. Leyvraz PF, Richard J, Bachmann F et al: Adjusted versus fixed-dose subcutaneous heparin in the prevention of deep-vein thrombosis after total hip replacement. *N Engl J Med* 309:954, 1983.

10. Hartman JT, Pugh JL, Smith RD et al: Cyclic sequential compression of the lower limb in prevention of deep venous thrombosis. *J Bone Joint Surg* 64:1059, 1982.

11. Schondorf TH, Weber U: Heparin in orthopedic surgery. Prevention of deep-vein thrombosis in orthopedic surgery with the combination of low-dose heparin plus either dihydroergotamine or dextran. *Scan J Haematol* (Suppl) 36:126, 1986.

12. Turpie AG, Levine MN, Hirsh J et al: A randomized controlled trial of a low-molecular-weight heparin (Enoxaparin) to prevent deep-vein thrombosis in patients undergoing elective hip surgery. *N Engl J Med* 315:925–929, 1986.

13. Clarke HJ, Jinnah RH, Byank RP et al: *Clostridium difficile* infection in orthopaedic patients. *J Bone Joint Surg* 72–A:1056–1059, 1990.

14. Berggren D, Gustafson Y, Eriksson B et al: Postoperative confusion after anesthesia in elderly patients with femoral neck fractures. *Anesth Analg* 66:497–504, 1987.

15. Schmalzried TP, Amstutz HC, Dorey FJ: Nerve palsy associated with total hip replacement. *J Bone Joint Surg* 73–A;1074–1080, 1991.

PROCEDURE: ARTHROSCOPIC PROCEDURES

Overview: Arthroscopic procedures have supplanted open techniques in the treatment of meniscal tears, removal of loose bodies and soft tissue, and reconstruction of synovial joints. Many joint afflictions, however, are still best managed by traditional open techniques. Nonetheless, arthroscopic methods have greatly enriched the orthopedist's diagnostic capabilities in managing joint pathology.

1. *Operation*
   a. Indications:
      (1) Diagnostic purposes.
      (2) Removal of loose bodies.
      (3) Synovial biopsy.
      (4) Joint sepsis.
      (5) Meniscal injury.
      (6) Ligamentous reconstruction.
   b. Operative Steps: Small portals allow insertion of fiberoptic instruments for inspection of the joint. Accessory portals allow instrumentation to perform surgical procedures. Multiple portals afford excellent joint visualization and access.
   c. Incision: Only over portal sites.
   d. Anesthesia: Arthroscopy in all joints can be performed with either general, regional, or local anesthesia.
   e. Intraoperative Monitoring: Routine.
   f. Operative Positioning: Shoulder: either lateral decubitus or 60-degree beach-chair position. Knee and ankle: supine. Wrist and elbow: suspended with overhead traction.
   g. Duration: Generally 30 minutes to 2 hours.
   h. EBL/Transfusions: Negligible.
   i. "Surgical Stress": Minimal.

2. *Expected Hospital Course/Treatment*
   a. Postoperative Monitoring
      (1) ICU Stay: None required.
      (2) Invasive/Special Monitoring: None required.
      (3) Parameters To Be Monitored: Soft tissue fluid extravasation.
   b. Positioning/Activity: Compressive dressings are usually applied, and early range of motion exercises are encouraged. Weight-bearing status varies with the procedure.
   c. Alimentation: As tolerated.
   d. Wound Care/Drains: Portal sutures are usually removed in 5 to 7 days. Drains are usually not required.
   e. Respiratory Care: Routine.
   f. Analgesia/Postop Meds: Oral medications are sufficient.
   g. Length Of Hospital Stay: Outpatient surgery.

3. *Postoperative Complications*
   a. In Hospital
      (1) Morbidity:
         i. Fluid extravasation.
         ii. Neurovascular injury.
         iii. Nerve traction injury from overhead suspension for elbow, wrist, and shoulder arthroscopy.
      (2) Mortality: Negligible.
   b. After Discharge
      (1) Hemarthrosis (common).
      (2) Infection (rare).

4. *Follow-up*
   a. Suggested Follow-up: Patients are followed until full range of motion is obtained and portals are healed. Motion is usually attained by 3 weeks after surgery. Portals usually heal in 1 week.

PROCEDURE: LUMBAR LAMINECTOMY/FUSION

Overview: Low back pain is the most costly musculoskeletal ailment in the United States today. Fortunately, most lumbar spine ailments can be managed conservatively. However, a minority of patients with intractable low back pain, serious neurologic deficit, or persistent sciatica require surgery. Proper patient selection is critical in ensuring successful surgical outcomes.

1. *Operation*
   a. Indications:
      (1) Cauda equina syndrome and progressive unremitting neurologic deficit.
      (2) Lumbar radiculopathy unresponsive to conservative treatment with supportive imaging studies.
      (3) Fusion indicated only for instability associated with degenerative changes, progressive spondylolisthesis, or surgically-induced instability.
   b. Operative Steps: For laminectomy and discectomy, the lamina is either partially or wholly removed to gain access to the spinal cord. Spinal cord and nerve roots are retracted for access to disc fragments. Removal of the disc effects nerve decompression. Fusion involves decortication of bone with addition of bone graft. Metallic fixation is often employed.
   c. Incision: Straight midline posterior incision.
   d. Anesthesia: General.
   e. Intraoperative Monitoring: Spinal cord monitoring is indicated in management of difficult cases in which extensive dissection and decompression are needed.
   f. Operative Positioning: Prone with abdomen allowed to hang free to reduce intraabdominal pressure.
   g. Duration: Simple discectomy and laminectomy: 1 to 3 hours. Fusion mandates an additional 2 hours.
   h. EBL/Transfusions: Routine laminectomy and discectomy: 200 to 400 ml. Spinal fusion: 400 to 800 ml. Transfusion generally required only after fusion.
   i. "Surgical Stress": Moderate.

2. *Expected Hospital Course/Treatment*
   a. Postoperative Monitoring
      (1) ICU Stay: Uncommon and only for associated debilitating conditions.
      (2) Invasive/Special Monitoring: None.
      (3) Parameters To Be Monitored:
         i. Neurologic exam to lower extremities.
         ii. Urinary output.
   b. Positioning/Activity: After routine laminectomy and discectomy, the patient is kept supine overnight and is allowed to ambulate on the first postoperative day. Fusions may be protected by a thoracic lumbar spinal orthosis (brace). Early ambulation is still encouraged.
   c. Alimentation: Advance diet as tolerated.
   d. Wound Care/Drains: Wound is inspected on POD 2. Drains for fusion are commonly employed and are removed on POD 2 to 3. Sutures are removed 14 days after surgery.
   e. Respiratory Care: Incentive spirometry and pulmonary toilet are encouraged.
   f. Analgesia/Postop Meds: Narcotics by way of patient-controlled analgesic systems are well-tolerated. Oral agents recommended as soon as possible.
   g. Length Of Hospital Stay: Simple discectomy and laminectomy may be discharged as soon as 2 days. Complicated fusions may require up to 7 days of hospitalization.

3. *Postoperative Complications*
   a. In Hospital
      (1) Morbidity:
         i. Injury to nerve roots.
         ii. Wound infection.
      (2) Mortality: Less than 1%.
   b. After Discharge
      (1) Reherniation of disk at same level.
      (2) Inability to obtain solid fusion.
      (3) Hardware failure.

4. *Follow-up*
   a. Suggested Follow-up: The patients are seen approximately 2 weeks after surgery for wound inspection and suture removal. Radiographs are obtained to assess bone healing and guide rehabilitation. Fusions take at least 1 year to consolidate and mature.

PROCEDURE: PROCEDURES FOR RHEUMATOID ARTHRITIS

Overview: The patient with rheumatoid arthritis may have no joint spared from the deleterious effects of synovial proliferation and pannus formation. However, certain affected joints may prove especially disabling. Besides hip and knee involvement which often require total joint replacement, the rheumatoid patient may suffer from crippling hand and wrist deformities. Furthermore, foot and ankle involvement may significantly impair ambulation.

1. *Operation*
   a. Indications: Disabling joint pain or deformity unresponsive to conservative measures.
   b. Operative Steps: Hand deformities are commonly treated by joint replacement surgery. Severe wrist involvement is usually best treated with fusion. Severe foot and ankle disease is similarly best treated by fusion.
   c. Incision: Upper extremity: usually dorsal incisions over the metacarpal-phalangeal joint and wrist joint. Ankle fusions: usually anterior incisions are employed.
   d. Anesthesia: General or peripheral nerve block.
   e. Intraoperative Monitoring: Routine.
   f. Operative Positioning: Upper extremity procedures: supine with armboard. Lower extremity surgery: supine.
   g. Duration: Variable. Most arthrodeses require 1.5 to 3 hours.
   h. EBL/Transfusions: Upper extremity surgery with use of a tourniquet: minimal. Lower extremity surgery: 100 to 300 ml. Transfusion is not required.
   i. "Surgical Stress": Moderate.

2. *Expected Hospital Course/Treatment*
   a. Postoperative Monitoring
      (1) ICU Stay: None required.
      (2) Invasive/Special Monitoring: None required.
      (3) Parameters To Be Monitored: Intraoperative x-ray required.
   b. Positioning/Activity: For upper extremity surgery, the extremity is usually splinted. Motion is instituted after several days to allow for wound healing. Lower extremities are placed in a cast to allow for fusion.
   c. Alimentation: Advance as tolerated.
   d. Wound Care/Drains: Wound inspected after 2 days. Drains are optional, but are removed 24 to 48 hours postoperatively if placed.
   e. Respiratory Care: Incentive spirometry encouraged.
   f. Analgesia/Postop Meds: Parenteral narcotics generally indicated for the first 24 hours. Oral medications encouraged afterward.
   g. Length Of Hospital Stay: Upper extremity surgery patients often discharged on POD 1 to 2. Lower extremity surgery patients require 2 to 3 days of hospitalization.

3. *Postoperative Complications*
   a. In Hospital
      (1) Morbidity:
         i. Increased incidence of wound breakdown.
         ii. Infection.
      (2) Mortality: Less than 1%.
   b. After Discharge
      (1) Infection.
      (2) Delayed wound healing.
      (3) Implant failure.

4. *Follow-up*
   a. Suggested Follow-up: Variable as dictated by procedure. The patient is followed closely until fusion is successfully achieved. Hand reconstructions require protracted rehabilitation course.

PROCEDURE: REPAIR OF SCOLIOSIS

Overview: Scoliosis, or curvature of the spine, may disfigure an adolescent or cause pulmonary compromise if left untreated. School screening programs have fortunately detected many early cases, enabling prompt treatment. Bracing can prevent or lessen curve progression, but many patients ultimately require surgical correction. Newer instrumentation can restore near-normal spinal alignment in most patients if recognized early.

1. *Operation*
   a. Indications:
      (1) Adolescents with 40-degree curvatures or greater.
      (2) Adults with curvatures exceeding 50 degrees.
   b. Operative Steps: Posterior spinal laminae are exposed. Metal bars are fixed to pedicles and laminae. Compressive and tensile forces are applied to the spine to effect desired correction in three dimensions.
   c. Incision: Posterior midline.
   d. Anesthesia: General.
   e. Intraoperative Monitoring: Spinal cord monitoring essential, especially during periods of correction. Arterial line with or without CVP.
   f. Operative Positioning: Supine with the abdomen hanging freely.
   g. Duration: Variable from 2 to 7 hours.
   h. EBL/Transfusions: 1000 to 2000 ml. Transfusions are commonly required.
   i. "Surgical Stress": Moderate to severe.

2. *Expected Hospital Course/Treatment*
   a. Postoperative Monitoring
      (1) ICU Stay: One day but may be longer if respiratory status is compromised.
      (2) Invasive/Special Monitoring: Pulse oximetry or arterial blood gases to monitor oxygenation.
      (3) Parameters To Be Monitored:
          i. Neurologic exam to detect evolving deficit.
          ii. Immediate postoperative x-rays are mandatory.
          iii. CBC.
   b. Positioning/Activity: Supine. On POD 2, bed-to-chair activity is attempted. Progressive ambulation as tolerated.
   c. Alimentation: Oral intake must await return of bowel sounds which usually occurs after 48 hours.
   d. Wound Care/Drains: Hemovac drains are commonly employed and are removed 24 to 48 hours postoperatively. Wound is inspected on POD 2. Sterile dressings are applied until wound is dry.
   e. Respiratory Care: Aggressive pulmonary toilet and incentive spirometry encouraged.
   f. Analgesia/Postop Meds: Parenteral narcotics are necessary early after surgery. Patient-controlled analgesia systems are useful.
   g. Length Of Hospital Stay: 14 to 17 days.

3. *Postoperative Complications*
   a. In Hospital
      (1) Morbidity:
          i. Neurologic deficit including paralysis.
          ii. Wound infection.
          iii. Urinary retention.
      (2) Mortality: Less than 1%.
   b. After Discharge
      (1) Infection.
      (2) Failure to obtain fusion.
      (3) Implant failure.

4. *Follow-up*
   a. Suggested Follow-up: Patients are routinely examined 2 to 3 weeks after discharge. Serial radiographs are taken during the protracted recovery phase. Mature fusion may take more than 1 year to achieve.

PROCEDURE: SURGERY FOR HIP FRACTURES

Overview: The incidence of hip fractures is increasing in the United States, largely due to the growing proportion of aged patients in the population. Hip-fracture fixation is performed with either screws, screw and side plate, or rods, depending on the location of the fracture and the bone integrity of the patient. While usually enabling rapid mobilization of the patients, current operative techniques for hip fractures cannot guarantee entirely normal hip function. Many patients require ambulatory aids indefinitely. Furthermore, significant morbidity is associated with hip fractures with 3-year mortality rates approximately 50%.

1. *Operation*
   a. Indications: All fractures of the hip require operative intervention. The exception is the nonambulatory demented patient who does not have significant discomfort from the injury.
   b. Operative Steps: A fracture table and fluoroscopy are required. The lateral aspect of the proximal femur is exposed to receive the implant. Fracture reduction is obtained with longitudinal traction.
   c. Incision: Straight lateral incision centered over the proximal femur.
   d. Anesthesia: Regional or general.
   e. Intraoperative Monitoring: Foley catheter optional. Arterial line and Swan-Ganz catheter indicated if severe debilitating disease exists.
   f. Operative Positioning: Supine on fracture table.
   g. Duration: 1 to 2 hours.
   h. EBL/Transfusions: 300 to 500 ml. Transfusions necessary in approximately 50% of cases.
   i. "Surgical Stress": Moderate to severe.

2. *Expected Hospital Course/Treatment*
   a. Postoperative Monitoring
      (1) ICU Stay: Only if significant debilitating disease coexists.
      (2) Invasive/Special Monitoring: Venous ultrasonography in the operated leg should be considered in patients over 50 years of age before discharge.
      (3) Parameters To Be Monitored:

      i. Both intraoperative and postoperative x-rays required to monitor position of fixation devices.
      ii. CBC.
   b. Positioning/Activity: Patients usually supine postoperatively. Early mobilization with protected weight bearing encouraged. Unstable fracture patients may require non–weight bearing initially.
   c. Alimentation: Advance diet as tolerated. Nutritional supplementation encouraged.
   d. Wound Care/Drains: Wounds are inspected on POD 2. Drains are routinely removed 24 to 48 hours after surgery.
   e. Respiratory Care: Incentive spirometry recommended.
   f. Analgesia/Postop Meds: Parenteral narcotic analgesia required initially. After 24 to 48 hours, oral agents recommended.
   g. Length Of Hospital Stay: 5 days for uncomplicated cases. May be protracted due to delayed progress in ambulation in many elderly patients.

3. *Postoperative Complications*
   a. In Hospital
      (1) Morbidity:

      i. Deep venous thrombosis.
      ii. Fat embolism syndrome (rare).
      iii. Wound infection.

      (2) Mortality: Approximately 2% but largely dependent on patient's preexisting medical status.
   b. After Discharge
      (1) Nonunion of fracture.
      (2) Implant failure.
      (3) Avascular necrosis.

4. *Follow-up*
   a. Suggested Follow-up: Patients are seen 2 weeks after discharge for radiographs and assessment of ambulatory status. Outpatient rehabilitation is usually required.

PROCEDURE: TOTAL HIP REPLACEMENT

Overview: Total hip replacement has enabled many patients crippled with afflictions of the hip to ambulate freely. The patient's diseased hip is removed and replaced with a metal ball and polyethylene socket. Components are either fixed with cement or rely on fibrous or bony ingrowth to gain fixation. Both younger patients and those undergoing revision usually receive uncemented implants.

1. *Operation*
    a. Indications:
        (1) Hip pain failing conservative treatment in osteoarthritis, rheumatoid arthritis, posttraumatic arthritis, osteonecrosis, inflammatory arthritis, Gaucher's disease, Paget's disease, and crystal-induced arthropathy.
        (2) Failed prior prosthetic replacement.
        (3) Failed internal fixation.
    b. Operative Steps: The hip joint is exposed. The diseased femoral head is resected with an oscillating saw, and the femoral canal is reamed to accommodate the prosthetic stem. The diseased acetabulum is reamed and sized to accommodate the prosthesis. A metal-backed polyethylene socket is secured first followed by implantation of metal femoral head.
    c. Incision: For posterior approach, curved incision centered over the buttock region. For anterior approach, a curved incision beginning at the anterior pelvis and extending downward toward the proximal thigh.
    d. Anesthesia: General or regional.
    e. Intraoperative Monitoring: Foley catheterization recommended. Arterial line and Swan-Ganz catheter only if patient is medically debilitated.
    f. Operative Positioning: Either lateral decubitus or supine, depending on whether posterior or anterior approach is used. Posterior approach is more common.
    g. Duration: For primary arthroplasty, 1 to 4 hours. For revision surgery, 3 to 6 hours.
    h. EBL/Transfusions: 1000 to 1500 ml. Transfusion is usually required.
    i. "Surgical Stress": Moderate to severe.

2. *Expected Hospital Course/Treatment*
    a. Postoperative Monitoring
        (1) ICU Stay: Usually unnecessary except in patients with serious cardiopulmonary compromise.
        (2) Invasive/Special Monitoring: Venous ultrasonography of the operated leg in patients over age 50 prior to discharge.
        (3) Parameters To Be Monitored:
            i. Immediate postoperative x-ray mandatory to detect dislocation.
            ii. CBC.
            iii. Wound drainage.
            iv. Urine output.
    b. Positioning/Activity: Supine with abduction pillow to prevent dislocation. Gait training usually commences on POD 2. With cementless ingrowth implants, protected weight bearing is usually continued for 6 to 8 weeks. Cemented components allow weight bearing as tolerated.
    c. Alimentation: Diet advanced as tolerated. Nutritional supplements encouraged.
    d. Wound Care/Drains: Wounds inspected on POD 2. Drains are routinely removed between 24 and 48 hours after surgery. Sutures are removed approximately POD 14.
    e. Respiratory Care: Incentive spirometry strongly encouraged.
    f. Analgesia/Postop Meds: Parenteral narcotics usually required initially. Oral agents recommended as soon as possible.
    g. Length Of Hospital Stay: 10 to 12 days for most patients. Patients with significant debilitation, multiple joint involvement, or other limiting factors may require additional inpatient rehabilitation before discharge.

3. *Postoperative Complications*
    a. In Hospital
        (1) Morbidity:
            i. Excessive blood loss.
            ii. Femoral fracture.
            iii. Sciatic nerve injury.
            iv. Fat embolism.
            v. Hypotension secondary to use of cement.
            vi. Wound infection.
            vii. Wound hematoma.
            viii. Deep venous thrombosis and pulmonary embolism.
        (2) Mortality: Less than 1%.
    b. After Discharge
        (1) Hip dislocation, especially seen with extremes of hip flexion, adduction, and internal rotation.
        (2) Threat of infection by bacterial seeding from dental, GI, and urologic procedures.

4. *Follow-up*
    a. Suggested Follow-up: For the first 6 weeks postoperatively, patients are instructed to use elevated toilet seats and 1 to 2 pillows between the knees when lying on the unoperated side. X-rays are usually taken 6 weeks after surgery. Strengthening exercises are instituted at that time. Further follow-up visits are made at 3 months, 6 months, and 1 year with radiographs taken yearly.

PROCEDURE: TOTAL KNEE REPLACEMENT

Overview: In total knee joint replacement surgery, a diseased knee joint is replaced with a metal and plastic prosthesis that maintains joint stability and restores limb alignment. The success of total knee joint replacement has equaled, if not exceeded, that of total hip replacement in terms of patient satisfaction. Most patients report minimal or no pain with ambulation.

1. *Operation*
   a. Indications:
      (1) Osteoarthritis.
      (2) Osteonecrosis.
      (3) Rheumatoid arthritis.
      (4) Posttraumatic degenerative arthritis.
      (5) Crystal arthropathy.
      (6) Degenerative changes associated with Paget's disease.
      (7) Reconstruction following resection of tumors.
      (8) Revision of prior total knee arthroplasty.
   b. Operative Steps: The knee joint is exposed. The diseased distal femur and proximal tibia are removed with oscillating saws. Bony beds are prepared for cementing of prosthetic components. Metal femoral components and polyethylene tibial components are commonly employed. Most clinicians prefer to cement both femoral and tibial components; however, femoral components are commonly uncemented.
   c. Incision: Usually midline centered over the patella.
   d. Anesthesia: Regional or general.
   e. Intraoperative Monitoring: Foley catheter is recommended. Arterial line and the Swan-Ganz catheter only if significant debilitating conditions coexist.
   f. Operative Positioning: Supine.
   g. Duration: 1 to 3 hours. Revision surgery may require up to 5 hours.
   h. EBL/Transfusions: 250 to 1000 ml. Approximately 50% of patients require transfusion.
   i. "Surgical Stress": Moderate to severe.

2. *Expected Hospital Course/Treatment*
   a. Postoperative Monitoring
      (1) ICU Stay: Only if associated comorbid conditions exist.
      (2) Invasive/Special Monitoring: Consider venous ultrasonography of operated leg in patients over age 50 prior to discharge.
      (3) Parameters To Be Monitored:
         i. Immediate postoperative x-ray obtained to rule out dislocation.
         ii. CBC.
   b. Positioning/Activity: Immediately postoperatively, the patient is kept supine. Bed-to-chair ambulation is encouraged on POD 1. Walking with assistance is permitted as soon as tolerated. Most patients discard crutches by 6 weeks.
   c. Alimentation: Diet is advanced as tolerated. Nutritional supplements are encouraged.
   d. Wound Care/Drains: Wound is inspected at 48 hours. Hemovac drains are removed in 24 to 48 hours when drainage has abated. Sutures are removed on POD 14.
   e. Respiratory Care: Incentive spirometry encouraged.
   f. Analgesia/Postop Meds: Parenteral narcotic agents usually required for first 24 to 48 hours. Oral medications encouraged as soon as tolerated.
   g. Length Of Hospital Stay: 8 to 12 days. Additional inpatient rehabilitation may be required if multiple joint involvement, associated debilitating illness, or other limiting factors coexist.

3. *Postoperative Complications*
   a. In Hospital
      (1) Morbidity:
         i. Popliteal artery damage.
         ii. Peroneal nerve trauma.
         iii. Wound infection.
         iv. Deep venous thrombosis and pulmonary embolism.
      (2) Mortality: Less than 1%.
   b. After Discharge
      (1) Early loosening may occur in overzealous patients.
      (2) Poor return of range of motion may require manipulation under anesthesia.
      (3) Threat of infection by bacterial seeding from dental, GI, and urologic procedures.

4. *Follow-up*
   a. Suggested Follow-up: Radiographs are routinely done 6 weeks after surgery. Subsequent visits at 3, 6, and 12 months. Yearly visits are recommended to detect early signs of prosthetic loosening.

PROCEDURE: TOTAL SHOULDER REPLACEMENT

Overview: Total shoulder replacement is a highly demanding procedure reserved for a select patient population. Components are secured with or without cement, and a wide range of designs are available to accommodate different patients' needs. A total shoulder replacement, like total hip and knee replacement, affords a great deal of pain relief though by no means restores totally normal shoulder function.

1. *Operation*
   a. Indications:
      (1) Painful degenerative joint disease due to osteoarthritis, rheumatoid arthritis, osteonecrosis, crystal-induced arthropathy, or posttraumatic causes.
      (2) Tumor resection.
      (3) Selected fractures of the proximal humerus.
   b. Operative Steps: The joint is exposed, and the diseased proximal humerus is resected with an oscillating saw. The glenoid is denuded of cartilage and burred to accept the prosthesis. The medullary canal of the humerus is reamed to accept the metal prosthesis which is then inserted into the humeral canal. The shoulder is reduced, and the wound is closed in layers.
   c. Incision: Anterior incision over the deltopectoral interval.
   d. Anesthesia: General or peripheral nerve block.
   e. Intraoperative Monitoring: Routine.
   f. Operative Positioning: Supine in 30-degree beach-chair position.
   g. Duration: 2 to 4 hours.
   h. EBL/Transfusions: 400 to 500 cc.
   i. "Surgical Stress": Moderate.

2. *Expected Hospital Course/Treatment*
   a. Postoperative Monitoring
      (1) ICU Stay: Usually not necessary.
      (2) Invasive/Special Monitoring: None required.
      (3) Parameters To Be Monitored:
         i. Neurologic examination to detect brachial plexus injury.
         ii. CBC.
   b. Positioning/Activity: The patient is placed in a sling immediately after surgery. Rehabilitation is individualized according to the status of the rotator cuff. Range of motion exercises generally begin on POD 2. Active exercises should be delayed for 6 to 8 weeks.
   c. Alimentation: Diet is advanced as tolerated.
   d. Wound Care/Drains: Wound inspected on POD 2. Drains are generally used and removed 24 to 48 hours after surgery.
   e. Respiratory Care: Incentive spirometry suggested.
   f. Analgesia/Postop Meds: Parenteral narcotic analgesics usually required for first 24 to 48 hours. Oral medications recommended thereafter.
   g. Length Of Hospital Stay: 8 to 12 days.

3. *Postoperative Complications*
   a. In Hospital
      (1) Morbidity:
         i. Wound infection.
         ii. Wound hematoma.
         iii. Dislocation of prosthesis.
         iv. Injury to adjacent vascular structures.
      (2) Mortality: Less than 1%.
   b. After Discharge
      (1) Prosthetic loosening.
      (2) Joint dislocation.
      (3) Disruption of rotator cuff and deltoid repair.
      (4) Infection.

4. *Follow-up*
   a. Suggested Follow-up: Patients are seen 2 weeks after discharge, and radiographs are obtained. Intense rehabilitation is required with 12 to 18 months often necessary to reach satisfactory plateau of function.

15 EVALUATION OF THE PATIENT UNDERGOING GYNECOLOGIC SURGERY

Mark Morgan

John Mikuta

Patients undergoing gynecologic and obstetrical surgery form a diverse group, ranging from young healthy women undergoing outpatient diagnostic laparoscopy for infertility to elderly women with multiple medical conditions undergoing radical tumor debulking for advanced cancer. Procedures performed during pregnancy may involve healthy women requiring uncomplicated cesarean section for term pregnancy or acutely ill patients with severe pregnancy-induced hypertension associated with seizures, pulmonary edema, hepatic failure, and disseminated intravascular coagulation. In all cases, the physiologic changes in glucose tolerance, blood volume, respiratory function, and normal blood values observed during pregnancy should be considered in perioperative management.

This chapter briefly reviews comorbid conditions, anesthetic and surgical techniques, prophylactic issues, and postoperative complications encountered in patients undergoing gynecologic and obstetrical surgery. The second part of the chapter presents specific information about the most common gynecologic procedures.

COEXISTING MEDICAL CONDITIONS

Certain medical conditions are associated with gynecologic malignancy. For example, obesity, diabetes, and hypertension are often present in patients with endometrial carcinoma. Since cervical cancer is associated with sexual activity, patients with the disease may have a higher risk of acquiring other sexually transmitted diseases including HIV infection. Patients with common epithelial ovarian cancer typically present at an advanced stage after months of evaluation for vague abdominal complaints. Despite stable weight or increased weight due to ascites, they are often severely malnourished. Those with unusual cell types such as clear-cell carcinoma may present with hypercalcemia or otherwise unexplained thrombosis. Hydatiform moles and other forms of gestational trophoblastic neoplasms may be associated with hyperthyroidism. Trophoblastic emboli and acute respiratory distress can occur at the time of evacuation of molar tissue. All patients with gynecologic malignancies have a significantly increased risk of developing venous thrombosis.

Women undergoing surgery for nonmalignant disease are often young and healthy. However, benign disease may be associated with a variety of medical conditions. For example, renal anomalies may accompany Müllerian duct abnormalities like vaginal agenesis. Over 50 percent of women with a unicornuate uterus have an absent kidney. Women with recurrent miscarriage may have subclinical collagen-vascular disease. Those with menstrual irregularities commonly have abnormalities of thyroid function or may have an unsuspected pituitary microadenoma with hyperprolactinemia. The possibility of HIV infection should be considered in any patient with sexually transmitted disease, especially when it is unusually severe or unresponsive to conventional therapy.

PHYSIOLOGIC CHANGES IN NORMAL PREGNANCY

There are many changes in maternal physiology which should be considered when surgery is performed during pregnancy (see Chap. 40). Blood volume may increase as much as 50 percent above the nonpregnant level. Because of a relative increase in plasma volume over red blood cell mass, the hematocrit level falls slightly. Cardiac output may increase 40 percent, but a progressive drop in the systemic vascular resistance causes the baseline maternal blood pressure to decrease. Later in pregnancy, patients are susceptible to decreased cardiac output and hypotension due to compression of the inferior vena cava by the uterus when in the supine position. The electrocardiogram may show a shift in axis to the left and transient ST-segment and T-wave changes. The glomerular filtration rate increases approximately 50 percent with a subsequent decrease in the serum creatinine and uric acid levels. Urine protein concentrations of up to 300 mg in 24 hours are not considered abnormal. Ureteral dilatation and asymptomatic bacteriuria are common. The latter should be treated in view of the high risk of pyelonephritis. Pregnancy is characterized by a mild respiratory alkalosis with a mild compensatory metabolic acidosis. Although the tidal volume and vital capacity are increased, the functional residual capacity and residual volume are decreased due to elevation of the diaphragm. Glucose tolerance is impaired during pregnancy especially in the postprandial state, and it is not unusual for pregnancy to unmask diabetes in predisposed individuals. Due to an increase in serum thyroxine-binding globulin induced by increased levels of estrogen, the serum total T_4 concentration is increased, but the free thyroxine index is unchanged (see Chap. 25).

ANESTHETIC TECHNIQUES

Although general anesthesia is used in most major gynecologic surgery, the location and innervation of the pelvic organs allow many procedures to be performed with regional, spinal, or epidural anesthetic techniques. These include vaginal hysterectomy, cesarean section, dilation and curettage, cone biopsy, and various procedures involving the vulva. Although regional anesthesia can be used for abdominal hysterectomy, it is usually not suitable for oncologic surgery extending into the upper abdomen. Minor laparoscopic procedures can be performed with regional or local anesthesia, but extensive laparoscopic surgery is usually best done under general anesthesia to avoid the discomfort of pneumoperitoneum in the upper abdomen. On the other hand, regional epidural techniques are preferred for cesarean section. Because of delayed gastric emptying in pregnancy, the risk of aspiration with induction of general anesthesia is increased. In addition, many anesthesiologists feel that an epidural technique allows for optimal maternal and fetal well-being.

SURGICAL TECHNIQUES AND PATHOPHYSIOLOGY

In recent years, there has been a rapid proliferation of advanced laparoscopic and laparoscopically-assisted surgical procedures performed for gynecologic disease. Although laparoscopy has been used for many years, the advent of more sophisticated instrumentation and video capabilities allows the surgeon much more therapeutic latitude. Laparoscopic oophorectomies, laparoscopically-assisted vaginal and radical hysterectomies, and lymph node dissections are all now possible. However, the use of laparoscopy does not always improve surgical results. For example, an uncomplicated vaginal hysterectomy can be performed more quickly and with less morbidity without laparoscopic assistance. Major complications of laparoscopy include injury to vascular structures; injury to abdominal viscera; and complications of pneumoperitoneum, including hypercarbia, gas embolus, diminished venous return, and cardiac arrhythmias.

Many open procedures can be accomplished through low transverse abdominal incisions. However, other operations, particularly those for malignancy, require vertical midline incisions for adequate exposure. Low transverse incisions have less impact on pulmonary physiology than upper abdominal incisions, but pain can interfere with cough and deep breathing needed to prevent atelectasis. Postoperative ileus is common but usually short-lived, and

alimentation is not a major concern in well-nourished patients. Essential medication can be administered parenterally. If no parenteral form or substitute is available, it can be administered orally with a small amount of water.

PROPHYLACTIC ISSUES

In patients with susceptible heart disease, prophylaxis against endocarditis is recommended for most major gynecologic surgery. In the absence of infection, it is not considered necessary for dilation and curettage, therapeutic abortion, sterilization procedures, or cesarean section.[1] However, patients with high-risk valvular lesions like prosthetic valves and those with a history of endocarditis should probably receive prophylaxis for these procedures as well. Appropriate antibiotic regimens are presented in Chap. 43.

Pelvic surgery is a major risk factor in the development of postoperative deep-venous thrombosis (DVT) and pulmonary embolism. The incidence of DVT in this setting has been reported to be 20 percent. Major additional risk factors include age over 40, duration of surgery, obesity, malignancy, and a prior DVT. In addition, the use of oral contraceptives increases the risk of DVT, probably by decreasing antithrombin III.[2,3] Oral contraceptives should be discontinued at least one month prior to elective surgery after providing an alternative form of contraception.[4] Physiologic hormone replacement in postmenopausal women has not been associated with increased risk.

All women over age 40 undergoing pelvic surgery or younger women with one or more risk factors should receive prophylaxis against thrombosis. Standard low-dose heparin has been shown to be effective in most situations but has not provided adequate protection for women undergoing surgery for gynecologic malignancy.[5] External pneumatic compression devices have proven effective for these patients.[6]

COMPLICATIONS

Postoperative fever is common and is most often related to atelectasis, pelvic cellulitis, or urinary tract infection. Wound infection and pelvic abscess occur less often.[7] Injury to the gastrointestinal or urinary tract can also occur. The ureter may be injured because of its close proximity to ovarian blood vessels.[8] Gastrointestinal and genitourinary fistulae can usually be managed conservatively, but surgical repair may be necessary and is usually successful. Dysfunction of the bladder or lower bowel is also common after radical pelvic procedures. Nerve injury may occur due to positioning or the use of retractors in prolonged procedures. These may cause a sensory neuropathy in the thigh due to injury to the genitofemoral or lateral femoral cutaneous nerves, or weakness of the quadriceps muscles due to femoral nerve compression. Foot drop due to compression of the common peroneal nerve and injury to the sciatic nerve occurs infrequently. Pulmonary embolism remains a major cause of postoperative morbidity and mortality. This diagnosis should be considered in any gynecologic surgery patient with unexplained fever, tachycardia, hypoxia, dyspnea, or chest pain.

REFERENCES

1. Dajani AS, Bisno AL, Chung KJ et al: Prevention of bacterial endocarditis. *JAMA* 264:2919–2922, 1990.
2. Vesser MP, Doll R, Fanburn AS et al: Postoperative thromboembolism and the use of oral contraception. *Br Med J* 3:123, 1970.
3. Greene GR, Sarlwell PE: Oral contraceptive use in patients with thromboembolism following surgery, trauma, or infection. *Am J Public Health* 62:680, 1972.
4. DeStefano F, Peterson HB, Ory HW et al: Oral contraceptives and postoperative venous thrombosis. *Am J Obstet Gynecol* 143:227, 1982.
5. Clarke-Pearson DL, Coleman RE, Synan IS et al: Venous thromboembolism prophylaxis in gynecologic oncology: A prospective, controlled trial of low-dose heparin. *Am J Obstet Gynecol* 145:606, 1983.
6. Clarke-Pearson DL, Synan IS, Hinshaw WM et al: Prevention of postoperative venous thromboembolism by external pneumatic calf compression in patients with gynecologic malignancy. *Obstet Gynecol* 63:92–98, 1984.
7. Hemsell DL: Infections after gynecologic surgery. *Obstet Gynecol Clin of North Am* 16:381–400, 1989.
8. Neuman M, Eidelman A, Langer R et al: Iatrogenic injuries to the ureter during gynecologic and obstetric operations. *Surg Gynecol Obstet* 173:268–272, 1991.

PROCEDURE: ABDOMINAL HYSTERECTOMY FOR BENIGN DISEASE

Overview: Total abdominal hysterectomy refers to the removal of the uterus and cervix without regard to the ovaries and fallopian tubes. This is the most common procedure in the United States for benign uterine disease. Recently, some have advocated a return to the subtotal hysterectomy, which leaves the cervix, to decrease the morbidity of the procedure as well as preserve the cervix for sexual function. In general, however, there is minimal increase in risk to performing a total abdominal hysterectomy.

1. *Operation*
   a. Indications:
      (1) Dysfunctional uterine bleeding.
      (2) Benign uterine tumors (e.g., fibroids).
      (3) Preinvasive disease of the cervix or endometrium.
   b. Operative Steps: Though there are various modifications to the standard hysterectomy, the procedure has several essential steps. The pelvic peritoneum is incised, the ureters are identified, and the bladder is dissected from the lower uterine segment by either sharp or blunt dissection. The ovaries may either be preserved or removed. When preserved, the fallopian tube is usually left with the ovary to avoid compromise of the blood supply to the ovary. The uterine arteries are then clamped and ligated. The vagina is entered sharply, and the uterus and cervix are removed as one specimen. Some surgeons leave the vaginal cuff open but run a stitch around the circumference to obtain hemostasis while others close the vaginal cuff. An attempt is made to suspend the vagina to the cardinal ligament.
   c. Incision: Low transverse or vertical depending on the size of the uterus and expected associated disease.
   d. Anesthesia: General, spinal, or epidural.
   e. Intraoperative Monitoring: Routine for uncomplicated cases.
   f. Operative Positioning: Supine.
   g. Duration: 1 to 3 hours.
   h. EBL/Transfusions: If uncomplicated, < 500 ml. With complications such as pelvic inflammatory disease, extensive endometriosis, or adhesions, blood loss may exceed 1000 ml, and transfusion is sometimes necessary.
   i. "Surgical Stress": Moderate.

2. *Expected Hospital Course/Treatment*
   a. Postoperative Monitoring
      (1) ICU Stay: Not required.
      (2) Invasive/Special Monitoring: Not required.
      (3) Parameters To Be Monitored:
         i. Vital signs.
         ii. Urine output.
         iii. CBC.
   b. Positioning/Activity: Ambulate on POD 1.
   c. Alimentation: Oral feeding on POD 1 or 2, later in complicated cases.
   d. Wound Care/Drains: Drains usually not needed. Foley catheter removed on POD 1.
   e. Respiratory Care: Incentive spirometry encouraged.
   f. Analgesia/Postop Meds: Parenteral narcotics required for 1 to 3 days.
   g. Length Of Hospital Stay: 3 to 5 days.

3. *Postoperative Complications*
   a. In Hospital
      (1) Morbidity:
         i. Infection.
         ii. Hemorrhage.
         iii. Injury to the bladder or urinary tract.
      (2) Mortality: < 1%.
   b. After Discharge
      (1) Incisional hernia.
      (2) Pelvic infection.
      (3) Bowel obstruction.
      (4) Pelvic pain.

4. *Follow-up*
   a. Suggested Follow-up: Yearly Pap smears may still be indicated, especially in patients undergoing hysterectomy for preinvasive disease of the cervix. Because ovarian cancer may still arise, routine pelvic examinations are indicated.

PROCEDURE: CESAREAN SECTION

Overview: Cesarean section has been performed with increasing frequency over the last 20 years. In the United States, primary cesarean section rates of 20 to 30% are not uncommon.

1. *Operation*
    a. Indications:
        (1) When labor may be considered unsafe for the mother or fetus.
        (2) When there is significant dystocia precluding vaginal delivery.
        (3) When there is fetal distress, and imminent vaginal delivery is not anticipated.
        (4) Certain malpositions of the fetus.
        (5) Occasionally for previous uterine surgery (e.g., cornual resection).
    b. Operative Steps: Hysterotomy is usually performed through a transverse and low incision. The baby is delivered, the placenta is evacuated, and the uterus is closed. IV ergotrate or prostaglandin F_2-alpha injected into the uterus is given to produce contraction and control bleeding.
    c. Incision: Usually low transverse but occasionally vertical.
    d. Anesthesia: When time permits, a regional technique using either a spinal or epidural is preferable. General anesthesia, when used, requires rapid-sequence induction techniques because of the risk of aspiration in the pregnant patient.
    e. Intraoperative Monitoring: Routine. Arterial line, CVP, or Swan-Ganz catheter may be required in patients with pre-eclampsia.
    f. Operative Positioning: Supine with left uterine displacement to avoid compression of the inferior vena cava and aorta by the gravid uterus.
    g. Duration: 30 minutes to 2 hours.
    h. EBL/Transfusions: 700 to 1000 ml. Transfusions not required.
    i. "Surgical Stress": Moderate.

2. *Expected Hospital Course/Treatment*
    a. Postoperative Monitoring
        1. ICU Stay: Not routinely required.
        2. Invasive/Special Monitoring: None.
        3. Parameters To Be Monitored:
            i. Vital signs.
            ii. CBC.
    b. Positioning/Activity: Most patients can ambulate on POD 1.
    c. Alimentation: Most patients tolerate a regular diet on POD 1.
    d. Wound Care/Drains: Drains usually not needed.
    e. Respiratory Care: Incentive spirometry encouraged.
    f. Analgesia/Postop Meds: Parenteral narcotics for 1 to 3 days.
    g. Length Of Hospital Stay: 3 to 5 days.

3. *Postoperative Complications*
    a. In Hospital
        (1) Morbidity:
            i. Hemorrhage.
            ii. Endometritis.
            iii. Bladder injury.
            iv. Pelvic vein thrombophlebitis.
            v. Disseminated intravascular coagulation associated with placental abruption or preeclampsia.
        (2) Mortality: < 0.1%.
    b. After Discharge
        (1) Incisional hernia.
        (2) Wound infection.
        (3) Pulmonary embolus.

4. *Follow-up*
    a. Suggested Follow-up: Patients are seen at 4 to 6 weeks.

PROCEDURE: DILATION AND CURETTAGE

Overview: This procedure is intended to dilate the cervix and sample the endometrial contents. In the management of abnormal bleeding in the premenopausal period or for the diagnosis of postmenopausal bleeding, gynecologists also perform an office endometrial biopsy first. If this is not diagnostic, a formal dilation and curettage (D & C) is performed in the operating room.

1. *Operation*
   a. Indications:
      (1) Diagnosis and treatment of abnormal uterine bleeding.
      (2) Cervical stenosis.
      (3) Management of abortion (spontaneous or induced).
   b. Operative Steps: The cervix is dilated. Uterine "sounding" and curettage of endometrial cavity are then performed.
   c. Incision: None.
   d. Anesthesia: Paracervical block with sedation, regional, or general.
   e. Intraoperative Monitoring: Routine.
   f. Operative Positioning: Lithotomy.
   g. Duration: 20 to 30 minutes.
   h. EBL/Transfusions: Generally minimal.
   i. "Surgical Stress": Low.

2. *Expected Hospital Course/Treatment*
   a. Postoperative Monitoring
      (1) ICU Stay: Not required.
      (2) Invasive/Special Monitoring: Not required.
      (3) Parameters To Be Monitored: Routine vital signs.
   b. Positioning/Activity: As tolerated.
   c. Alimentation: As tolerated.
   d. Wound Care/Drains: None.
   e. Respiratory Care: Routine.
   f. Analgesia/Postop Meds: Oral codeine or nonsteroidal anti-inflammatory drugs.
   g. Length Of Hospital Stay: Same-day surgery.

3. *Postoperative Complications*
   a. In Hospital
      (1) Morbidity:
         i. Uterine perforation.
         ii. Infection.
      (2) Mortality: < 0.01%
   b. After Discharge
      (1) Recurrent bleeding.
      (2) Delayed-onset endometrial infection due to missed perforation.

4. *Follow-up*
   a. Suggested Follow-up: Patients are followed with yearly gynecologic exams.

PROCEDURE: LAPAROSCOPY

Overview: Laparoscopy is the inspection of the peritoneal cavity and pelvic organs using an endoscope. It has become the most common gynecologic procedure over the last 10 to 20 years. It is most commonly used for female sterilization, either by cauterization or ligation of the uterine tubes, but it is also indispensable in the evaluation and treatment of many disorders resulting in infertility. With the use of multiple puncture sites, it is possible to introduce grasping instruments to manipulate pelvic organs, scissors to dissect adhesions, surgical lasers for vaporization and cautery, and specially preformed suture material that permits ligation of vascular structures.

1. *Operation*
   a. Indications:
      (1) Infertility.
      (2) Undesired fertility.
      (3) Tubal pregnancy.
      (4) Pelvic masses.
      (5) Pelvic pain.
      (6) Staging of certain cancers.
   b. Operative Steps: A pneumoperitoneum is usually established by insufflating the abdominal cavity with carbon dioxide. A special sharp spring-loaded needle (Veress) is used to prevent trauma to abdominal viscera. After an adequate pneumoperitoneum is attained, the laparoscopic trocar is introduced. Pressure and volume monitoring devices are incorporated in the insufflating instruments. Separate puncture sites, usually below or around the pubic hairline, are used to introduce wands for manipulation and the surgical instruments. A probe is placed in the uterine cavity to allow manipulation of the uterus during the procedure.
   c. Incision: Either umbilical or infraumbilical.
   d. Anesthesia: General.
   e. Intraoperative Monitoring: Routine.
   f. Operative Positioning: Modified lithotomy position.
   g. Duration: Diagnostic: < 30 minutes. Therapeutic: 30 minutes to 3 hours.
   h. EBL/Transfusions: Minimal blood loss.
   i. "Surgical Stress": Low.

2. *Expected Hospital Course/Treatment*
   a. Postoperative Monitoring
      (1) ICU Stay: Not required.
      (2) Invasive/Special Monitoring: None.
      (3) Parameters To Be Monitored: Routine vital signs.
   b. Positioning/Activity: Ambulation several hours after the procedure.
   c. Alimentation: Oral intake on the evening of the procedure.
   d. Wound Care/Drains: Foley catheter intraoperatively. Special drains not required.
   e. Respiratory Care: Routine.
   f. Analgesia/Postop Meds: Oral codeine or nonsteroidal anti-inflammatory agents.
   g. Length Of Hospital Stay: Usually same-day surgery if there are no complications.

3. *Postoperative Complications*
   a. In Hospital
      (1) Morbidity:
         i. Injury to vascular structures or abdominal viscera.
         ii. Complications of pneumoperitoneum such as hypercarbia, gas embolus, cardiac arrhythmias, and subcutaneous emphysema.
      (2) Mortality: < 0.01%
   b. After Discharge
      (1) Herniation of omentum or bowel through laparoscopic incisions.
      (2) Persistence of preoperative symptoms.
      (3) Bowel obstruction.
      (4) Delayed-onset bleeding.

4. *Follow-up*
   a. Suggested Follow-up: Patients are seen 1 month after surgery.

PROCEDURE: OOPHORECTOMY FOR CANCER

Overview: Ovarian malignancies may be epithelial cancers, germ cell malignancies, or stromal tumors. Epithelial cancers are most common, have a peak incidence of 64 years of age, are metastatic at the time of diagnosis in 80% of patients, and almost always require total abdominal hysterectomy and bilateral salpingo-oophorectomy (TAH/BSO). Germ cell malignancies and stromal tumors are more likely to be localized to the ovary at the time of diagnosis, and unilateral adnexectomy is possible. Metastatic epithelial ovarian cancer frequently forms sheets of tumor over pelvic structures, and an attempt should be made to remove as much gross disease as possible. This usually involves total omentectomy and sometimes may require bowel resection or splenectomy. Many patients go into surgery with as much as 1 to 5 liters of ascites. In early ovarian cancer of any type, a thorough exploration of the abdomen and retroperitoneum is required to allow adequate staging.

1. *Operation*
    a. Indications: A TAH/BSO is performed for ovarian tumors of any type.
    b. Operative Steps: The abdoment is explored, and the uterus and ovaries are removed with pelvic peritoneum and lymph nodes. Omentectomy may be added.
    c. Incision: Thorough staging requires a vertical incision.
    d. Anesthesia: General. Epidural anesthesia may be used as an adjunct for postoperative pain control.
    e. Intraoperative Monitoring: Arterial line, CVP, and Swan-Ganz catheters are frequently needed for optimal fluid management in patients with advanced disease and concurrent medical illness.
    f. Operative Positioning: Supine.
    g. Duration: Up to 4 to 8 hours.
    h. EBL/Transfusions: Patients with extensive disease may require transfusion for blood loss of several liters.
    i. "Surgical Stress": Moderate to severe.

2. *Expected Hospital Course/Treatment*
    a. Postoperative Monitoring
        (1) ICU Stay: Patients with cardiovascular disease are usually best managed in an ICU setting.
        (2) Invasive/Special Monitoring: Invasive monitors remain in place while in ICU.
        (3) Parameters To Be Monitored:
            i. Vital signs.
            ii. Urine output.
            iii. CBC.
    b. Positioning/Activity: Ambulate on POD 1.
    c. Alimentation: Malnourished patients with advanced disease may require parenteral nutrition.
    d. Wound Care/Drains: Drains are usually not required.
    e. Respiratory Care: Incentive spirometry encouraged.
    f. Analgesia/Postop Meds: Parenteral narcotics or epidural analgesia required.
    g. Length Of Hospital Stay: 4 to 7 days. Shorter stays required for early ovarian cancer and longer if tumor debulking is necessary.

3. *Postoperative Complications*
    a. In Hospital
        (1) Morbidity:
            i. Bleeding.
            ii. Pelvic cellulitis/abscess.
            iii. Urinary tract infection.
            iv. Uretero- or vesicovaginal fistula.
            v. Genitofemoral nerve and/or obturator nerve damage.
            vi. Fluid shifts from ascites.
        (2) Mortality: 1 to 2%.
    b. After Discharge
        (1) Incisional hernia.
        (2) Adhesive bowel obstruction.
        (3) Recurrent tumor.

4. *Follow-up*
    a. Frequency of follow-up for ovarian cancer is usually dictated by subsequent therapy.

PROCEDURE: RADICAL HYSTERECTOMY

Overview: Radical hysterectomy includes a pelvic lymph node dissection and removal of most of the cardinal and uterosacral ligaments and the upper one-third of the vagina with uterine specimen. It is considered the surgical therapy of choice for stage Ib and IIa carcinoma of the cervix. Many surgeons include an evaluation of the lower paraaortic lymph nodes before proceeding with surgery. If the nodes are positive for cancer, the procedure is aborted and radiation therapy instituted. The uterus is usually left in place as a receptacle for a radiation implant.

1. *Operation*
    a. Indications: Stage Ib and IIa carcinoma of the cervix.
    b. Operative Steps: Radical hysterectomy involves exploration of the abdomen for distant disease and lymph node dissection. The ovaries are separated from the specimen if they are to be preserved. The ureters are exposed to the bladder. The uterine arteries are ligated at their origin. The bladder is raised anteriorly, and the uterosacral ligaments are clamped. The upper part of the vagina is transected, and the specimen is removed.
    c. Incision: Midline or low transverse but must allow for thorough exploration of the peritoneal cavity.
    d. Anesthesia: General. Epidural anesthesia may be used as an adjunct for postoperative pain control.
    e. Intraoperative Monitoring: Arterial line, CVP, and Swan-Ganz catheters are frequently needed for optimal fluid management.
    f. Operative Positioning: Supine.
    g. Duration: 4 to 8 hours.
    h. EBL/Transfusions: Transfusion of several units can be required in patients with extensive disease.
    i. "Surgical Stress": Severe.

2. *Expected Hospital Course/Treatment*
    a. Postoperative Monitoring
        (1) ICU Stay: Patients with cardiovascular disease are usually best monitorined in ICU setting.
        (2) Invasive/Special Monitoring: Invasive monitors remain in place while in ICU.
        (3) Parameters To Be Monitored:
            i. Vital signs.
            ii. Urine output.
            iii. CBC.
    b. Positioning/Activity: Ambulate on POD 1.
    c. Alimentation: Resuming oral intake is dependent on bowel function and may take several days. A nasogastric tube may be placed at the time of surgery.
    d. Wound Care/Drains: Most surgeons use closed suction drains in the retroperitoneal space. Bladder catheter (Foley or suprapubic) frequently needed for 3 to 5 days.
    e. Respiratory Care: Incentive spirometry encouraged.
    f. Analgesia/Postop Meds: Parenteral narcotics or epidural analgesia required.
    g. Length Of Hospital Stay: 7 to 14 days.

3. *Postoperative Complications*
    a. In Hospital
        (1) Morbidity:
            i. Bleeding.
            ii. Pelvic cellulitis/abscess.
            iii. Urinary tract infection.
            iv. Uretero- or vesicovaginal fistula.
            v. Genitofemoral nerve and/or obturatory nerve damage.
        (2) Mortality: 1 to 2%.
    b. After Discharge
        (1) Prolonged bladder and bowel dysfunction.
        (2) Ureteral stricture, especially after radiation therapy for cervical carcinoma.
        (3) Incisional hernia.
        (4) Adhesive bowel obstruction.
        (5) Recurrent tumor.

4. *Follow-up*
    a. Every 3 to 4 months for the first 2 years.

PROCEDURE: VAGINAL HYSTERECTOMY

Overview: The uterus can be removed transvaginally in some women with benign disease. In many centers, this is now being done with the aid of the laparoscope (laparoscopically-assisted vaginal hysterectomy). Vaginal hysterectomy is usually not performed in the presence of severe endometriosis or pelvic inflammatory disease because extensive adhesions may increase the risk of injury to bowel or urinary tract structures.

1. *Operation*
    a. Indications:
        (1) Uterine prolapse or pelvic relaxation.
        (2) Advanced preinvasive disease of the uterus or cervix.
        (3) Uterine leiomyomata, depending on the size of the tumors and experience of the surgeon.
    b. Operative Steps: The peritoneal cavity may be opened either posteriorly in the cul-de-sac or anteriorly after dissecting the bladder off the lower uterine segment. The uterosacral ligaments are clamped, cut, and ligated, followed by similar treatment of the cardinal ligaments and uterine vessels. The uterus is delivered through the vaginal introitus. The ovaries may be removed or preserved. The pelvic peritoneum is closed with a purse-string stitch. The uterosacral ligaments are often tied together to obliterate the cul-de-sac, and the vagina is suspended to the cardinal ligaments.
    c. Incision: Generally none, although an episiotomy is sometimes required for adequate exposure.
    d. Anesthesia: General, spinal, or epidural.
    e. Intraoperative Monitoring: Routine.
    f. Operative Positioning: Dorsal lithotomy position.
    g. Duration: 1 to 2 hours.
    h. EBL/Transfusions: If uncomplicated, < 500 ml.
    i. "Surgical Stress": Moderate.

2. *Expected Hospital Course/Treatment*
    a. Postoperative Monitoring
        (1) ICU Stay: Not required.
        (2) Invasive/Special Monitoring: None.
        (3) Parameters To Be Monitored:
            i. Vital signs.
            ii. Urine output.
            iii. CBC.
    b. Positioning/Activity: Ambulation on POD 1.
    c. Alimentation: Regular diet on POD 1.
    d. Wound Care/Drains: A Foley catheter is usually left in place for 24 hours but may remain in place longer if an anterior repair is performed.
    e. Respiratory Care: Incentive spirometry encouraged.
    f. Analgesia/Postop Meds: Parenteral narcotics for 1 to 2 days.
    g. Length Of Hospital Stay: About 3 days.

3. *Postoperative Complications*
    a. In Hospital
        (1) Morbidity:
            i. Hemorrhage.
            ii. Injury to bladder or urinary tract.
        (2) Mortality: < 0.1%.
    b. After Discharge
        (1) Vaginal prolapse.
        (2) Enterocele.
        (3) Pelvic abscess.
        (4) Bowel obstruction.

4. *Follow-up*
    a. Suggested Follow-up: Patients are seen in 4 to 6 weeks.

16 EVALUATION OF THE PATIENT UNDERGOING SURGERY FOR ENDOCRINE DISORDERS

Paul G. Curcillo II

Ernest F. Rosato

Peter J. Snyder

David R. Goldmann

This chapter discusses perioperative evaluation and management of patients with disorders of the thyroid, parathyroid, adrenal, and pituitary glands. After consideration of general principles of management pertinent to all patients undergoing endocrine surgery, preoperative evaluation and preparation and postoperative complications are discussed for procedures involving individual endocrine organ systems. Details of specific procedures are included in tabular form at the end of the chapter except for pituitary procedures which are found in Chap. 10. Discussion of less common conditions, including islet cell adenomas of the pancreas and gastrointestinal tract, multiple endocrine adenopathy syndromes, ectopic hormone production, carcinoid syndrome, and masculinizing and feminizing syndromes is excluded.

GENERAL PRINCIPLES OF MANAGEMENT

Endocrine surgery is most often performed when malignancy is suspected or glandular dysfunction cannot be adequately treated medically. Because patients requiring surgery for endocrine dysfunction do not fall into specific age groups, perioperative management must include attention to both sequelae of hormone excess or deficiency and age-related comorbid conditions. Although some endocrine surgery is performed for anatomic abnormalities of specific glands in patients without evidence of abnormal hormone production, procedures requiring management of hormone excess or deficiency demand the most care. In the case of thyroid and chromaffin tissue dysfunction, excess hormone production carries the greatest risk. In the case of adrenocortical dysfunction, hormone deficiency requires urgent attention. Both hyperfunction and hypofunction of the pituitary, parathyroids, and beta islet cells have equally important ramifications.[1]

Diagnostic certainty requires biochemical evidence of hormone excess or deficiency and accurate anatomic localization. The latter may depend upon sophisticated radiologic procedures and the former on stimulation and suppression testing of glandular function. Although a single tumor is most often the cause of hormone overproduction, it is important to exclude glandular hyperplasia, multiple tumors, or coexisting neoplasms in other endocrine organs. When possible, the goal of surgery is to remove all hypersecreting tissue while leaving behind enough normal tissue for normal function. The gross appearance of endocrine tumors may be more important than histologic examination in predicting malignant behavior. In some instances, biochemical markers provide additional evidence for malignancy.

In addition to documentation of hormonal excess or deficiency and accurate localization of suspected hormone-secreting tumors, preoperative management of patients undergoing endocrine surgery frequently includes medical therapy of hormone over- or underproduction. Because endocrine surgery is rarely urgent, there is time to reestablish relatively normal hormone levels and to treat end-organ dysfunction. Thyrotoxic patients undergoing thyroid surgery should thus be rendered euthyroid with antithyroid agents, beta-blockers, and iodide before going to the operating room. Although there is no clear-cut consensus regarding an appropriate serum calcium level in hypercalcemic patients undergoing parathyroidectomy, treatment of symptomatic hypercalcemia should be undertaken before surgery. Similarly, surgical morbidity and mortality can be significantly reduced in patients undergoing excision of a pheochromocytoma if their blood pressure is adequately stabilized with alpha- and beta-blocking agents. All patients undergoing pituitary surgery should be assured of adequate plasma levels of cortisol and thyroid hormone before the procedure.

Successful surgical treatment of endocrine disorders requires careful intraoperative management as well as comprehensive preoperative evaluation and care. Manipulation of tumors suspected of hormone production should be minimized. The function of a tumor can frequently be confirmed by sampling venous effluent for hormone, and in some cases, adequacy of excision can be confirmed by intraoperative systemic blood hormone assays or radiologic procedures. When hormone hypersecretion is due to glandular hyperplasia or unresectable metastases, a decision must be made regarding the relative benefits of removing some tissue and alternative medical treatment with chemotherapy or radiotherapy. Tissue removed for histologic examination should be carefully preserved for additional cytochemical studies when indicated.

In addition to measures included in standard postoperative care, patients undergoing surgery for hormonal over- or underproduction need continued monitoring of appropriate hormone levels after surgery. By measuring hormone levels postoperatively, the effectiveness of excision in the case of tumor hypersecretion and the need for replacement for subsequent hormone deficiency can be judged. Some patients undergoing endocrine surgery will require reoperation, additional nonsurgical therapy for definitive treatment, or palliation or hormone replacement at some point in their course. Concurrent treatment of end-organ dysfunction is often required. Examples include management of blood pressure after excision of a pheochromocytoma, hypocalcemic tetany after parathyroidectomy, and infections often seen in patients undergoing surgery for hypercortisolism. Fluid and electrolyte abnormalities accompany many endocrine disorders and require scrupulous attention.

The multiple end-organ effects of hormone excess or deficiency can complicate anesthetic management. In the case of thyroid or parathyroid surgery, positioning, airway patency, and vocal cord function are important issues. In patients with hyperthyroidism or pheochromocytoma, cyclopropane and halogenated inhalational agents may sensitize the myocardium and predispose them to arrhythmias. In such patients, thiopental is most often used for induction. Various anesthetic agents have different effects on glucocorticoid output and should be carefully chosen according to whether cortisol excess or deficiency is present. Similarly, the choice of drugs used during surgery is influenced by the hormonal milieu. For example, morphine causes release of catecholamines and may be deleterious in patients with pheochromocytoma who may have inadequate alpha-blockade.[1]

THYROID SURGERY

Thyroid surgery is performed for suspected malignancy and less frequently for thyrotoxicosis in patients who do not respond to or are not compliant with medical therapy. In the former case, fine-needle aspiration of a palpable nodule with cytologic examination in addition to standard radionuclide scintigraphy and ultrasound have improved patient selection and have decreased the need for unnecessary resection.[2] In the latter case, surgery is most frequently performed for a single functioning nodule or during pregnancy when antithyroid agents are ineffective. Thyroid surgery is also performed when glandular enlargement compromises airway patency and occasionally for cosmetic reasons.

All thyrotoxic patients undergoing thyroidectomy should be rendered euthyroid before surgery to prevent potentially dangerous cardiac arrhythmias and the development of thyroid storm with subsequent circulatory collapse. Many clinicians feel that most thyrotoxic patients can be most expeditiously prepared for surgery with beta-blockers alone.[3,4] However, others feel that patients with more severe hyperthyroidism may benefit from additional preparation with antithyroid drugs for several weeks and the use of iodine in the form of Lugol's solution a few days before surgery to shrink the gland. In both cases, beta-blockers should be continued throughout the perioperative period until the second or third postoperative day. Preparation of patients for thyroidectomy is therefore similar to that for nonthyroid surgery and is discussed in detail in Chap. 25.

Most complications of thyroid surgery occur within the first 36 to 72 hours after the procedure.[5] In addition to thyroid storm, these include hemorrhage, damage to the recurrent laryngeal nerve, hypoparathyroidism, and rarely damage to the lymphatic duct and other nerves including the cervical sympathetic trunk, phrenic nerve, and spinal accessory nerve. The treatment of thyroid storm is discussed in Chap. 25. Despite the usual presence of a drain in the neck, postoperative hematoma formation may compromise the airway and require reoperation. Laryngeal dysfunction and its duration are dependent on the extent of injury to the nerves. Serum calcium levels should be determined frequently after thyroid surgery. Asymptomatic hypocalcemia may be transient and require no therapy. However, clinical evidence of hypocalcemic tetany should be promptly treated as outlined in Chap. 61.

Even after extensive resection, replacement thyroid hormone may not be required for several weeks or months, but continued monitoring of serum thyroid function tests is mandatory. However, all patients with papillary and follicular malignancy should receive suppressive doses of thyroid hormone and periodic reevaluation for recurrence including careful physical examination, chest x-ray, serum levels of thyroglobulin, and scintigraphic scanning of the head and neck for residual tumor.[6] The indications for postoperative ablative ^{131}I therapy and management of less common thyroid neoplasms are beyond the scope of this chapter.

PARATHYROID SURGERY

Most cases of primary hyperparathyroidism are diagnosed in the course of evaluation for asymptomatic hypercalcemia.[7] Nephrolithiasis is also a common initial manifestation of hyperparathyroidism. Few patients present with all of the classic symptoms of polydipsia, bone pain, constipation, central nervous system or psychiatric dysfunction, and hypertension. Although multiple metabolic abnormalities and roentgenologic findings in the bones can be documented in patients with hyperparathyroidism, the diagnosis rests on exclusion of all other etiologies of hypercalcemia, elevation in the serum level of parathyroid hormone (or inappropriately "normal" levels in the presence of hypercalcemia), and increase in the calcium concentration in a 24-hour urine collection.[8] When hyperparathyroidism is suspected, the multiple endocrine adenopathy syndromes (types 1, 2a, and 2b) and familial hypocalciuric hypercalcemia (FHH) should be considered in carefully evaluating the family history.[9,10] The latter condition does not require surgery. About 80 percent of cases of hyperparathyroidism are due to a solitary adenoma, and 20 percent are due to hyperplasia. Less than 2 percent of tumors are malignant.[11,12] Localization efforts employing various radiologic techniques as well as venous sampling for parathyroid hormone yield variable results and more often depend upon surgical exploration. When all four glands can be identified, solitary adenomas are usually resected without further surgery. In cases of hyperplasia, a subtotal parathyroidectomy is performed.

Most agree that parathyroidectomy is indicated in patients with symptomatic primary hyperparathyroidism, but there is still controversy regarding the relative merits of medical or surgical therapy in asymptomatic cases. Although about 25 percent of asymptomatic patients eventually become symptomatic and require surgery, early operation obviates the need for expensive long-term follow-up and may initially prevent clinically inapparent sequelae.[13] It is often difficult to determine if some symptoms are due to hyperparathyroidism or other concurrent disease. In any case, severe or symptomatic hypercalcemia and associated dehydration and electrolyte disorders should be treated before surgery. This can best be accomplished with saline and furosemide. In view of the abnormalities in serum calcium levels, the electrocardiogram should be closely monitored.

Despite efforts to leave some functioning parathyroid tissue behind in the neck or forearm after subtotal parathyroidectomy, postoperative hypocalcemia is common. Serum calcium levels fall to eight to nine mg/dl between the second and seventh postoperative days. This is due to transient hypoparathyroidism resulting from excision or damage to parathyroid tissue, atrophy of remaining tissue from long-term suppression by hypercalcemia, excess calcium uptake by remineralizing bone, and occasionally pancreatitis. Excess calcium uptake by bone is seen most commonly in patients with severe osseous disease like those with chronic renal failure, renal osteodystrophy, and secondary hyperparathyroidism and can persist for several months after surgery. Persistent hypocalcemia thereafter is most often due to hypoparathyroidism with decreased levels of parathyroid hormone (PTH).

Transient postoperative hypocalcemia may facilitate return of normal PTH secretion by remaining parathyroid tissue and usually requires only monitoring. Mild symptoms of hypocalcemia can be treated with oral calcium supplements. More severe hypocalcemia requires the addition of vitamin D analogs in doses sufficient to treat symptoms but low enough to maintain the serum calcium level in the low-normal range. Severe hypocalcemia with symptomatic tetany may necessitate therapy with intravenous calcium. Resistance to therapy may be due to concomitant hypomagnesemia. The details of calcium and magnesium replacement are more fully discussed in Chap. 61. Efforts to withdraw calcium and vitamin D replacement should be made during subsequent follow-up to determine whether or not permanent hypoparathyroidism is present. Although the incidence of postoperative hypoparathyroidism soon after surgery is about 20 percent, that of persistent hypoparathyroidism is less than 3 percent.[11]

Persistent hypercalcemia, occurring in about 5 percent of patients, suggests failure to resect all abnormal parathyroid tissue and may require repeat biochemical confirmation, localization efforts, and surgical exploration.[14] Late occurrence of hypercalcemia after apparent cure usually represents regrowth of parathyroid tissue, an initially inaccurate diagnosis, or spread of parathyroid carcinoma. Recurrent disease is more common in familial forms of hyperparathyroidism.

Other complications of parathyroidectomy include those mentioned above for thyroid surgery. Hyperparathyroidism itself can predispose patientes to pancreatitis, acute pseudogout, and hyperchloremic metabolic acidosis.

ADRENAL SURGERY

Adrenal surgery is performed for cortisol- and aldosterone-secreting adenomas of the cortex, adrenal carcinoma, pheochromocytomas arising in the medulla, and tumors found incidentally on radiologic studies performed for unrelated reasons. In the latter case, algorithms have been developed to enable use of the initial hormonal evaluation and subsequent radiologic follow-up to guide management. Although hormonally active tumors and those larger than five cm are generally excised, smaller or hormonally inactive lesions should usually be carefully followed.[15]

Hypercortisolism

Hypercortisolism is most often the result of Cushing's disease in which an ACTH-producing pituitary tumor stimulates the adrenal gland to produce excess cortisol. However, autonomous cortisol-producing adenomas, nodular hyperplasia, and adrenal carcinoma, although less common, produce the same clinical syndrome. Adrenal surgery is indicated for these latter conditions and in cases of Cushing's disease when a pituitary tumor cannot be resected or pituitary ablation is unsuccessful. Adrenal carcinoma is a highly malignant disease and has usually metastasized by the time surgery is contemplated.[16] Although the classic signs and symptoms of cortisol excess are well known, the clinical manifestations of cortisol excess can be subtle.

Biochemical confirmation of hypercortisolism can usually be accomplished by documenting excessive levels of free cortisol in a 24-hour urine collection. Isolated determinations of plasma cortisol are not useful, and the one mg dexamethasone suppression test is not sufficiently specific. Higher-dose dexamethasone suppression tests and plasma ACTH levels frequently aid in differentiating Cushing's disease from hypercortisolism of adrenal origin but are occasionally unable to do so. Radiologic localization of hormone-secreting tumors depends largely on computerized tomography and magnetic resonance imaging of the head and abdomen. Scintigraphy with ^{131}I-iodomethyl-19-norcholesterol (NP–59) can also provide both anatomic and functional information about the adrenals, in some cases allowing differentiation between autonomous adenomas with contralateral nonvisualization and ACTH-dependent or independent hyperplasia with bilateral uptake.[17] In addition to diagnostic testing, preoperative management of patients with hypercortisolism requires control of blood pressure and normalization of serum glucose and electrolyte levels.

Patients suffering from hypercortisolism are prone to a variety of postoperative complications. In addition to metabolic derangements, hypercortisolism produces tissue friability resulting in excessive bleeding, poor wound healing, and increased susceptibility to infections, as detailed in Chap. 26. These patients may experience relative adrenal insufficiency when the source of excess cortisol is excised. For this reason, supraphysiologic doses of exogenous glucocorticoid should be administered during surgery and thereafter and should be tapered to appropriate physiologic doses more slowly than in other situations requiring steroid replacement. Long-term management frequently mandates careful dose adjustment.

Hyperaldosteronism (Conn's Syndrome)

Primary hyperaldosteronism due to an aldosterone-secreting adrenal tumor is usually suspected in patients with hypertension and hypokalemia that cannot be ascribed to diuretics or other causes. In about 25 percent of cases, hyperaldosteronism is due to nodular hyperplasia of the adrenals and is more often termed idiopathic. Since adrenal resection for hyperplasia cures the hypokalemia but rarely the hypertension, medical therapy with spironolactone or amilorde is the treatment of choice. On the other hand, resection of discrete aldosterone-secreting tumors improves hypertension in 50 to 70 percent of cases.[18] For these reasons, accurate preoperative documentation of hormone excess and anatomic localization are important.

Biochemical diagnosis of primary hyperaldosteronism is dependent on demonstrating autonomous aldosterone secretion.[19,20] Since hypokalemia and salt depletion normally inhibit aldosterone secretion, patients should be repleted with potassium and assured adequate sodium intake before testing. All diuretics and adrenal-blocking drugs should be discontinued for four to six weeks. Several diagnostic protocols are described in the literature, but all are designed to facilitate documentation of elevated plasma aldosterone levels after salt loading and depressed renin levels after sodium restriction, administration of a diuretic, or orthostatic maneuvers. Anatomic localization can be accomplished by computerized tomography or magnetic resonance imaging. In some institutions, NP–59 scintigraphy after giving dexamethasone has been useful in differentiating an adenoma from hyperplasia.[21] Selective measurement of aldosterone in venous effluent has been described but is not universally performed. After the diagnosis has been made, spironolactone can be given before surgery to control blood pressure, facilitate potassium repletion, and treat volume overload.

There are no significant endocrine complications of surgery for primary hyperaldosteronism except for the rare occurrence of transient hypoaldosteronism, especially in patients who have not been prepared with spironolactone. In such cases, hypotension and hyperkalemia can be treated with saline infusion and deoxycorticosterone. In those rare cases when bilateral adrenalectomy is performed, glucocorticoid replacement is necessary. Because a significant number of patients experience late recurrence of hypertension, all patients undergoing surgery for primary hyperaldosteronism require long-term follow-up.

Pheochromocytoma

The success of surgery for pheochromocytoma is largely dependent upon optimal management and anticipation of complications. Pheochromocytomas arising in the adrenal or sympathetic nerve endings are relatively rare but can present with a variety of symp-

toms and signs that often suggest other diseases. Hypermetabolic symptoms can mimic hyperthyroidism, anxiety, or psychiatric disease; polydipsia, polyuria, and elevated serum glucose levels sometimes suggest diabetes mellitus; and fever and leukocytosis are frequently taken for signs of infection. Depending upon the location of the tumor, paroxysmal attacks of hypertension and a variety of catecholamine-mediated symptoms may occur with a variety of activities or medications and manipulation or palpation of the tumor itself. Persistent hypertension is probably more common than the classic intermittent elevations in blood pressure described in the literature.[22]

Excess catecholamines from a secreting pheochromocytoma are best documented by elevated levels of metanephrines and vanillylmandelic acid (VMA) in a 24-hour urine collection. Radiologic localization can be accomplished with computerized tomography and magnetic resonance imaging. In some centers, radionuclide scanning with ^{131}I-meta-iodobenzylguanidine (^{131}I-MIBG) is used to visualize both adrenal and extraadrenal pheochromocytomas.[23]

Most patients are prepared for surgery with alpha- and beta-adrenergic blocking agents.[22] Phenoxybenzamine is preferred for long-term alpha-adrenergic blockade over the shorter-acting agent phentolamine. Phenoxybenzamine can be titrated to the blood pressure, is generally well-tolerated except for mild orthostatic hypotension, and can be continued through the morning of surgery. Although some clinicians routinely give beta-blockers, they are usually used for persistent tachycardia, cardiac arrhythmias, and angina and should only be administered after adequate alpha-blockade has been achieved. Labetolol, the combined alpha- and beta-blocker, may also be useful in this setting. Inhibitors of catecholamine synthesis like alpha-methylparatyrosine have also been used.[24] There are reports in the literature of patients who tolerate resection well with continuous infusions of nitroprusside or nicardipine without prior alpha-blockade.[22]

During surgery, the three major concerns are cardiac arrhythmias, hypertensive crises, and maintenance of a normal intravascular volume. Arrhythmias are frequently ventricular in origin and can usually be controlled with lidocaine or a short-acting beta-blocker like propranolol. Hypertensive episodes generally respond to boluses or infusions of phentolamine or infusion of nitroprusside. Hypotension usually follows removal of the tumor and responds better to fluid replacement than to pressors alone. Despite an anticipated fall in blood pressure with successful resection, the abdomen should be explored for residual or multiple tumors. Glucocorticoid replacement is indicated when substantial adrenal tissue is removed.

Postoperative care requires optimization of fluid status and control of blood pressure. Mild transient postoperative hypertension is due to relative hypervolemia and reestablishment of normal alpha-receptor sensitivity and usually responds to diuresis. Although persistent postoperative blood pressure elevation raises suspicion of residual tumor, it is often due to underlying essential hypertension and can be treated with appropriate antihypertensive agents. Repeat testing of urine catecholamine levels and adrenal cortical function should be carried out later in the follow-up period.

PITUITARY DISEASE

Pituitary adenomas comprise about 10 percent of all intracranial neoplasms. Those that secrete prolactin usually can be treated exclusively with dopamine agonists like bromocriptine.[25] Those secreting ACTH, growth hormone, or gonadotrophins, and clinically nonfunctioning adenomas usually should be treated initially by transsphenoidal surgery. The transphenoidal approach is preferable even for large adenomas exhibiting suprasellar extension.

Patients with pituitary adenomas require comprehensive neurologic and endocrine evaluation before surgery. Neurologic evaluation includes assessment of visual acuity, visual fields, and oculomotor function. Magnetic resonance imaging is necessary in evaluating the size of the tumor and in documenting the presence or absence of impingement on the optic chiasm.[26] Preoperative hormonal evaluation enables assessment of both hypersecretion and hyposecretion. In cases of hypersecretion, quantitation of specific hormone levels often determines therapy and serves as a marker by which efficacy of treatment can be judged. Detection of hyposecretion of TSH is important to document significant unsuspected secondary hypothyroidism requiring replacement before surgery. All patients should be covered with supraphysiologic doses of glucocorticoids during and after surgery.

Pituitary surgery is frequently followed by the development of diabetes insipidus with excretion of large volumes of dilute urine and is responsive to administration of fluids and aqueous vasopressin. Diabetes insipidus is usually transient after transphenoidal surgery. However, if significant symptomatic diabetes insipidus is still present five to seven days after surgery, treatment with DDAVP should be initiated.[27] Chloropropamide is contraindicated because it may produce hypoglycemia in patients with deficiencies of other anti-insulin hormones. Glucocorticoids should be tapered to a maintenance dose equivalent to 20 to 30 mg of hydrocortisone daily before the patient leaves the hospital.

A complete hormonal evaluation should be carried out four to six weeks after surgery to determine the efficacy of the procedure in eliminating hypersecretion and the need for continued supplementation of other hormones. Measuring the serum thyroxine level allows documentation of secondary hypothyroidism. If the basal morning plasma cortisol concentration is below 3 μg/dl, the determination should be repeated and, if replicated, hypocortisolism confirmed. A value above 18 μg/dl documents normal cortisol secretion. If the value is in between, ACTH reserve should be determined with a metyrapone test two or three days after exogenous glucocorticoid therapy has been discontinued.[28] Basal secretion of LH and FSH can be inferred by measuring serum estradiol levels in women under 50, but documentation of cyclical secretion must await return of menses. Serum testosterone levels can be measured in men four to six weeks after surgery, but return of adequate spermatogenesis usually requires three to six months. Screening for vasopressin deficiency can be performed by measurement of the volume of a 24-hour urine collection one or two days after DDAVP has been discontinued. If the volume is less than two liters, no further treatment is necessary. If the volume is four to five liters or more, a water deprivation test should be done to confirm continuing diabetes insipidus.[29] Levels of any hormones that were elevated before surgery and visual field examination should also be repeated as part of the postoperative assessment.

Patients undergoing pituitary therapy require long-term follow-up to monitor hormone therapy, vision, and neurologic function. Evidence of continued or recurrent hormone hypersecretion or evidence of persistence or recurrence of the adenoma on magnetic resonance imaging should prompt repeat evaluation by the internist, neurosurgeon, and neurophthalmologist to determine the need for reoperation or alternative modes of therapy such as medication or radiation.

REFERENCES

1. Proye, CAG: General concept of treatment, in Friesen SR, Thompson NW (eds): *Surgical Endocrinology, Clinical Syndromes*, 2d ed. Philadelphia, Lippincott, 1990, pp 89–94.
2. Lennquist S: The thyroid nodule: Diagnosis and surgical treatment. *Surg Clin N Am* 67(2):213–231, 1987.
3. Alderberth A, Stentstrom G, Hasselgren P: The selective B_1-blocking agent metaprolol compared with antithyroid drug and thyroxine as preoperative treatment of patients with hyperthyroidism. *Ann Surg* 205(2):182–188, 1987.
4. Lennquist S, Jortso E, Anderberg B et al: Beta-blockers compared with antithyroid drugs as preoperative treatment in hyperthyroidism: Drug tolerance, complications and postoperative thyroid function. *Surgery* 98:1141–1146, 1985.
5. Farrar WB: Complications of total thyroidectomy. *Surg Clin N Am* 63(6):1353–1361, 1983.
6. Black EG, Cassoni A, Gimlette TMD et al: Serum thyroglobulin in thyroid cancer. *Lancet* 2:443, 1981.
7. Russell C, Edis AJ: Surgical treatment of presumptive primary hyperparathyroidism: Results in 500 consecutive cases with an evaluation of the role of surgery in the asymptomatic patient. *Br J Surg* 69:244, 1982.
8. Purcell DC, Scholz DA, Smith LH: Diagnosis of primary hyperparathyroidism. *Surg Clin N Am* 57:543, 1977.
9. Marx SJ, Spiegel AM, Brown EM et al: Family studies in patients with primary parathyroid hyperplasia. *Am J Med* 62:687, 1977.
10. Marx SJ: Familial hypocalciuric hypercalcemia. *N Engl J Med* 308:810, 1980.
11. Katz AD, Hopp D: Parathyroidectomy: Review of 338 consecutive cases for histology, location and reoperation. *Am J Surg* 144:411, 1982.
12. Van Heerden JA, Weiland LH, Remind WH et al: Cancer of the parathyroid glands. *Arch Surg* 114:475, 1979.
13. Scholz DA, Purnell DC. Asymptomatic primary hyperparathyroidism; a 10-year prospective study. *Mayo Clin Proc* 56:521, 1981.
14. Roslyn JJ, Mulder DG, Gordon HE: Persistent and recurrent hyperparathyroidism. *Am J Surg* 142:21, 1981.
15. Abecassis M, McLoughlin MJ, Langer B et al: Serendipitous adrenal masses: Prevalence, significance and management. *Am J Surg* 149:783, 1985.
16. Cohn K, Brennan M: Adrencortical carcinoma. *Surgery* 100:1170, 1986.
17. Schreingart DE, Seabold JE, Gross ME et al: Iodocholesterol adrenal tissue uptake and imaging in adrenal neoplasms. *J Clin Endocrinol Metab* 52:1156, 1981.
18. Hunt TK, Roizen MF, Tyrell JB et al: Current achievement and challenges in adrenal surgery. *Br J Surg* 71:983, 1984.
19. Ferris JB, Beevers DG, Brown JJ et al: Clinical, biochemical and pathological features of low-renin ("primary") hyperaldosteronism. *Am Heart J* 95:375, 1978.
20. Weinberger NM, Grim CE, Hollifield JW et al: Primary aldosteronism; diagnosis, localization and treatment. *Ann Intern Med* 90:386, 1979.
21. Sarkar SD, Cohn ED, Bierewaltes W: A new and superior adrenal imaging agent ^{131}I-6-beta-iodomethyl-19-norcholesterol (NP–59): Evaluation in humans. *J Clin Endocrinol Metab* 45:353, 1977.
22. Bravo, EL: Pheochromocytoma: New concepts and future trends. *Kidney Int* 40(3):544–556, 1991.
23. Sisson JC, Frager MS, Valk TS et al: Scintigraphic localization of pheochromocytoma. *N Engl J Med* 305:12–17, 1981.

24. Sjoerdsma A, Engelman K, Spector S et al: Inhibition of catecholamine synthesis in man with alpha-methyl-para-tyrosine, an inhibitor of tyrosine hydroxylase. *Lancet* 2:1092, 1965.
25. Molitch ME, Elton RL, Blackwell RE et al: Bromocriptine as primary therapy for prolactin-secreting macroadenomas: Results of a prospective multicenter study. *J Clin Endocrinol Metab* 60:698–705, 1985.
26. Nabeedy MH, Haag JR, Azar-Kia B et al: MRI and CT of sellar and parasellar disorders. *Rad Clin N Am* 25:819–847, 1987.
27. Richardson DW, Robinson AG: Desmopressin. *Ann Intern Med* 103:228–239, 1985.
28. Spark RF: Simplified assessment of pituitary-adrenal reserve. Measurement of 11-deoxycortisol and cortisol after metyrapone. *Ann Intern Med* 75:717–723, 1971.
29. Miller M, Dalakos T, Moses AM et al: Recognition of partial defects in antidiuretic hormone secretion. *Ann Intern Med* 73:721–729, 1970.

PROCEDURE: ADRENALECTOMY

Overview: One or both adrenal glands may be removed to treat a variety of functional or neoplastic abnormalities of the adrenal cortex or medulla. Adrenal surgery is safer today than ever before because of (1) improved preoperative preparation and anesthetic management, (2) better preoperative localization, and (3) safer hormonal replacement therapy. The adrenal glands may be approached through a transabdominal, flank, or posterior incision. Laparoscopic adrenalectomy has been reported.

1. *Operation*
   a. Indications:
   Unilateral:
      (1) Cortical adenoma (Cushing's syndrome).
      (2) Unilateral aldosteronoma.
      (3) Pheochromocytoma.
      (4) "Incidentaloma" > 6 cm.
      (5) Adrenal carcinoma.
   Bilateral:
      (1) Pituitary hypercortisolism (Cushing's disease) failing transsphenoidal hypophysectomy, irradiation, drug therapy.
      (2) Bilateral adrenal hyperplasia.
   b. Operative Steps: Posterior approach incision is made over the twelfth rib which is excised. Gerota's fascia is opened. The adrenal veins are ligated (more dangerous on the right since the vein is short and drains directly into the vena cava). The arteries are clipped, and the gland is removed. The anterior approach is preferred for pheochromocytoma or large tumors. Left-sided lesions: The lesser sac is entered. The distal pancreas is elevated exposing the kidney, adrenal, and renal vein. Vessels are ligated, and the specimen removed. Right-sided lesions: Kocher maneuver is performed exposing the inferior vena cava. The right kidney is retracted inferiorly exposing the adrenal. Occasionally mobilization of the right hepatic lobe aids in visualization. The adrenal vein is carefully controlled and ligated, other vessels are clipped, and the specimen is removed.
   c. Incision: Posterior: twelfth rib. Flank: twelfth rib/thoracoabdominal. Anterior: midline vertical or transverse.
   d. Anesthesia: General.
   e. Intraoperative Monitoring: Arterial line is essential in pheochromocytoma surgery.
   f. Operative Positioning: Posterior approach: patient prone with bed "jackknifed." Anterior approach: supine.
   g. Duration: 2 to 4 hours.
   h. EBL/Transfusions: 500 to 2000 ml.
   i. "Surgical Stress": Moderate to severe.

2. *Expected Hospital Course/Treatment*
   a. Postoperative Monitoring
      (1) ICU Stay: Essential for pheochromocytoma patients. Preferable after longer operations with blood loss.
      (2) Invasive/Special Monitoring: Invasive monitors remain in place while in ICU.
      (3) Parameters To Be Monitored:
         i. Vital signs.
         ii. Urine output.
         iii. ECG.
         iv. CBC.
         v. Electrolytes.
         vi. Chest x-ray to exclude pneumothorax.
   b. Positioning/Activity: Out of bed in 24 to 48 hours.
   c. Alimentation: Regular diet on POD 2 to 3. May be advanced more quickly after posterior approach.
   d. Wound Care/Drains: Routine. No drains usually needed.
   e. Respiratory Care: Incentive spirometry encouraged.
   f. Analgesia/Postop Meds: Narcotics parenterally for 3 to 5 days, then orally for 1 to 2 weeks.
   g. Length Of Hospital Stay: 5 to 14 days depending upon preoperative condition.

3. *Postoperative Complications*
   a. In Hospital
      (1) Morbidity:
         i. Hemorrhage.
         ii. Wound infection.
         iii. Pancreatitis.
         iv. Electrolyte disturbance (15% of patients).
         v. Atelectasis/pneumonia.
      (2) Mortality: 1 to 2%.
   b. After Discharge
      (1) Adrenal insufficiency (after bilateral resection).
      (2) Recurrent Cushing's syndrome.
      (3) Recurrent hypertension after resection of aldosteronoma.
      (4) Incisional hernia.

4. *Follow-up*
   a. Suggested Follow-up: Patients are seen every 4 to 6 months.

PROCEDURE: PARATHYROIDECTOMY

Overview: Primary hyperparathyroidism is most often the result of benign disease. The overproduction of parathyroid hormone (PTH) is attributable to an adenoma in a single gland in 80% of cases with the remaining 20% of cases due to hyperplasia of one or all of the glands. Carcinoma of the parathyroid gland occurs in less than 1% of all reported cases. Regardless of the cause, surgical resection of the overproducing gland(s) is the only definitive treatment. Secondary hyperparathyroidism is most frequently seen in patients with chronic renal failure. Decreased phosphate excretion, impaired production of 1,25 hydroxy vitamin D, and resistance of bone to PTH result in hyperplasia of the parathyroid glands. In contrast to primary hyperparathyroidism, initial treatment of secondary hyperparathyroidism should be medical. Approximately 30% of patients become unresponsive to therapy, exhibit autonomy of their parathyroids (tertiary hyperparathyroidism), and eventually require surgical intervention.

1. *Operation*
    a. Indications:
        (1) Benign adenoma of a single gland or hyperplasia of all four glands.
        (2) Parathyroid carcinoma.
    b. Operative Steps: Exposure and evaluation of all four parathyroids is required. Identification of the superior glands is more difficult because their location is not as uniform. Finding one or two enlarged glands with the remaining glands normal in appearance allows for removal of only the enlarged glands. If three or four glands are enlarged, then hyperplasia is presumed, and a subtotal parathyroidectomy is necessary. This procedure leaves a remnant of parathyroid intact and well-vascularized. An alternative to subtotal parathyroidectomy is total parathyroidectomy with autotransplantation of the remnant into a distant site such as the forearm.
    c. Incision: Transverse collar incision.
    d. Anesthesia: General.
    e. Intraoperative Monitoring: Routine.
    f. Operative Positioning: Supine.
    g. Duration: 1 to 4 hours.
    h. EBL/Transfusions: < 200 ml.
    i. "Surgical Stress": Low to moderate.

2. *Expected Hospital Course/Treatment*
    a. Postoperative Monitoring
        (1) ICU Stay: Not required.
        (2) Invasive/Special Monitoring: None.
        (3) Parameters To Be Monitored: Serum calcium levels should be determined every 12 hours until stability is certain.
    b. Positioning/Activity: Out of bed in 24 hours.
    c. Alimentation: Regular diet by POD 2.
    d. Wound Care/Drains: Drain may be placed and removed on POD 2 or 3.
    e. Respiratory Care: Routine.
    f. Analgesia/Postop Meds: Narcotics for 2 to 3 days are usually adequate.
    g. Length Of Hospital Stay: 3 to 5 days.

3. *Postoperative Complications*
    a. In Hospital
        (1) Morbidity:
            i. Hypocalcemia.
            ii. Recurrent laryngeal nerve damage.
            iii. Hemorrhage and airway compression.
        (2) Mortality: < 1%.
    b. After Discharge:
        (1) Persistent or recurrent hypercalcemia.
        (2) Hypoparathyroidism.

4. *Follow-up*
    a. Suggested Follow-up: Periodic assessment of serum calcium, phosphate, chloride, PTH, and renal function.

PROCEDURE: THYROIDECTOMY

Overview: The extent of the procedure is dictated by both the type and extent of the disease. Many times, the decision to perform a total or near-total thyroidectomy rather than a single lobectomy is made in the operating room after visualization of the thyroid tissue and pathologic examination. Recently, total thyroidectomy has been performed with morbidity rates of less than 10%, making it a safe alternative in patients with Graves' disease and thyroid malignancy. A near-total single lobectomy is indicated in the patient with a single benign nodule and otherwise normal remaining thyroid tissue. Regardless of the procedure chosen, thyroid resection requires meticulous dissection to prevent severe hemorrhage and identify the recurrent laryngeal nerves and parathyroid glands.

1. *Operation*
   a. Indications:
      (1) Thyroid cancer.
      (2) Abnormally large goiters or thyroid nodules causing tracheal compression.
      (3) Solitary autonomous hyperfunctioning nodule.
      (4) Hyperfunctioning thyroids that have failed medical therapy.
      (5) Occasionally cosmetic reasons.
   b. Operative Steps: Exploration and dissection of the neck region require both blunt and sharp dissection. Proper mobilization of the lateral aspect of the thyroid gland allows for exposure of the parathyroid glands and laryngeal nerves. The blood supply to the thyroid is from both the external carotid and subclavian arteries. Identification and ligation of the divided arterial supply is necessary prior to removal of the gland.
   c. Incision: Transverse collar incision.
   d. Anesthesia: General.
   e. Intraoperative Monitoring: Routine.
   f. Operative Positioning: Supine.
   g. Duration: 1 to 2 hours.
   h. EBL/Transfusions: EBL usually < 200 ml but can be > 2000 ml in difficult cases involving large goiters or cancer.
   i. "Surgical Stress": Moderate.

2. *Expected Hospital Course/Treatment*
   a. Postoperative Monitoring
      (1) ICU Stay: Not required unless thyroid storm occurs.
      (2) Invasive/Special Monitoring: None.
      (3) Parameters To Be Monitored:
         i. Observe for signs of thyrotoxicosis for 24 to 72 hours.
         ii. Serum calcium levels.
   b. Positioning/Activity: Out of bed within 24 hours.
   c. Alimentation: Regular diet on POD 2.
   d. Wound Care/Drains: A drain may be left in the thyroid bed.
   e. Respiratory Care: Routine.
   f. Analgesia/Postop Meds: Narcotics generally needed for 2 to 3 days.
   g. Length Of Hospital Stay: 3 to 5 days.

3. *Postoperative Complications*
   a. In Hospital
      (1) Morbidity:
         i. Thyroid storm.
         ii. Hemorrhage and tracheal compression.
         iii. Recurrent laryngeal nerve injury.
      (2) Mortality: < 1%.
   b. After Discharge:
      (1) Hypoparathyroidism.
      (2) Hypothyroidism.

4. *Follow-up*
   a. Suggested Follow-up: Patients undergoing total thyroidectomy require life-long thyroid supplementation. Parathyroid function should be followed during the first 6 months. Patients with malignant disease require ^{131}I scanning 6 weeks after surgery to detect residual thyroid tissue.

PART

PREOPERATIVE ASSESSMENT AND MANAGEMENT OF THE SURGICAL PATIENT WITH COEXISTING DISEASE

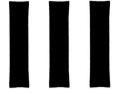

17 SURGERY IN THE HYPERTENSIVE PATIENT

Rosanne Granieri

Hypertension affects more than 58 million Americans and is a leading cause of coronary artery disease, stroke, renal disease, congestive heart failure, and retinopathy.[1] The criteria for diagnosis of hypertension in adults according to the diastolic or systolic blood pressure are listed in Table 17–1. Effective treatment of mild, moderate, and severe hypertension and isolated systolic hypertension reduces the incidence of cardiovascular and, in particular, cerebrovascular events.[2–9]

In the preoperative setting, the goals of management shift from prevention of long-term sequelae to (1) assessment of the perioperative risks of acute or chronic blood pressure elevation in itself or as a factor in underlying cardiovascular or cerebrovascular disease; (2) modification of risk to minimize primarily cardiac perioperative complications; and (3) substitution of appropriate agents for chronic oral antihypertensives in the perioperative period. Management of hypertension during and immediately after surgery is usually the responsibility of the anesthesiologist.

The finite if somewhat controversial body of knowledge on preoperative evaluation and management of patients with hypertension forms the basis of this chapter. Intraoperative and postoperative hypertension are discussed in Chap. 54.

HYPERTENSION: IS IT A RISK FACTOR FOR POSTOPERATIVE COMPLICATIONS?

Early data are conflicting regarding whether or not hypertension is associated with perioperative morbidity and mortality.[10–22] Some of these studies are retrospective, suffer from poor design, and vary in their definition of hypertension. More recent prospective studies with carefully defined outcomes assess hypertension as an independent risk factor in the development of postoperative complications rather than merely as a marker for comorbid conditions like coronary artery disease. Two important postoperative outcomes require consideration: (1) adverse cardiac outcomes such as myocardial infarctions and cardiac death; and (2) perioperative lability in blood pressure manifested as hypertension and/or hypotension.

Goldman's widely quoted study of perioperative cardiac risk demonstrated that hypertension is not an independent factor in the development of postoperative myocardial infarction, pulmonary edema, ventricular tachycardia, or cardiac death.[23,24] This finding was subsequently validated by Detsky et al. nine years later.[25]

TABLE 17–1. Classification of Hypertension in Adults

Blood Pressure	Category
Diastolic Blood Pressure (mmHg)	
< 85	Normal
85–89	High-normal
90–104	Mild hypertension
104–114	Moderate hypertension
≥ 115	Severe hypertension
Systolic Blood Pressure when Diastolic Blood Pressure < 90 mmHg	
< 140	Normal
140–159	Borderline isolated systolic hypertension
≥ 160	Isolated systolic hypertension

Source: Adapted from 1988 Joint National Committee: The 1988 report of the Joint National Committee on detection, evaluation, and treatment of high blood pressure. *Arch Intern Med* 148:1023–1038, 1988.

Goldman subsequently reexamined five groups of hypertensive patients undergoing elective noncardiac and nonneurologic surgery.[26] Group I consisted of normotensive patients on no medication (BP < 160/90). Group II consisted of normotensive patients taking diuretics for reasons other than hypertension. Group III consisted of patients with a history of hypertension (BP > 160/90) now normotensive on medication. Group IV consisted of patients who were similarly hypertensive despite treatment. Group V consisted of untreated hypertensive patients. Of those in Groups III, IV, and V, 55 percent had diastolic blood pressures between 90 and 99 mmHg, 29 percent had diastolic blood pressures over 100, and 16 percent had isolated systolic hypertension with systolic blood pressure over 160. The study specifically excluded patients undergoing cardiac and neurologic surgery, and only five patients had diastolic blood pressures over 110 mmHg. Outcome measures included pulmonary edema, myocardial infarction, ventricular tachycardia, congestive heart failure, supraventricular tachyarrhythmia, intraoperative or postoperative ischemia, cardiac death, and postoperative renal failure.

Multivariate analysis revealed that the preoperative in-hospital systolic or diastolic blood pressure did not correlate with either adverse outcome, mean nadir in intraoperative systolic blood pressure, need for intraoperative fluids or adrenergic agents, or perioperative hypertensive events (see Table 17–2). Patients with medically controlled hypertension were as likely to develop perioperative hypertension as inadequately treated or untreated hypertensive patients and were more likely to do so than normotensive patients.

The high incidence of perioperative hypertension in treated hypertensives has been confirmed by others.[27] In Goldman's early work, perioperative hypertension was also more common in those patients undergoing abdominal aortic aneurysmectomy or peripheral vascular surgery, especially carotid endarterectomy, independent of current or past blood pressure control.[24]

Although Goldman did not report higher rates of adverse outcomes resulting from perioperative hypertension, Rao et al. found that intraoperative hypertension and tachycardia were associated with a higher rate of postoperative myocardial infarction.[28] More recently, hypertension has been found to be one of several independent predictors of postoperative myocardial ischemia and in-hospital mortality in 474 male veterans. However, these data should be interpreted with caution in view of the fact that all of the patients were elderly males and had either a high risk or clear-cut evidence of preexisting coronary artery disease.[29,30]

TABLE 17–2. Multivariate Analysis of Hypertensive Surgical Patients

	Mean SBP Nadir (Intraoperative) mmHg ± SEM*	Hypertensive Episodes (%)**
Group I	94 ± 1	8
Group II	95 ± 3	6
Group III	100 ± 2	27
Group IV	97 ± 2	10
Group V	98 ± 2	15

SBP = Systolic blood pressure
* p ≤ 0.05   Group I versus Group III
** p ≤ 0.05   Group I versus Group III, IV, V
                   Group II versus Group III, IV

Source: From Goldman L, Caldera DL: Risks of general anesthesia and elective operation in the hypertensive patient. *Anesthesiology* 47:70–77, 1979.

Although it remains unclear whether perioperative hypertension independently predicts postoperative complications, Charlson found that wide swings in blood pressure correlated with postoperative renal and cardiac complications.[31,32] Goldman also found that severe reductions in intraoperative blood pressure in patients with a history of hypertension correlated with cardiac complications. Several other investigators suggest that intraoperative hypotension in turn increases the risk of postoperative cardiac and renal complications.[10,28,31,33–35]

In summary, while mild to moderate hypertension with diastolic blood pressure under 110 mmHg may not be independently associated with adverse cardiac outcomes, it may predispose the patient to develop significant intraoperative hypotension or hypertension which in turn increases the risk of postoperative cardiac and renal complications.

Cardiac Surgery and Hypertension

In a recent retrospective analysis of over 5000 patients undergoing coronary artery bypass surgery, treated hypertension was found not to be an independent predictor of postoperative mortality or morbidity, defined as myocardial infarction, need for intraaortic balloon pump support, need for mechanical ventilation for three days or more, neurological deficit, renal failure, or serious infection.[36] Systemic hypertension following revascularization is relatively common, even if blood pressure has been well controlled before surgery, and has been associated with cerebrovascular accidents and bleeding from fresh vascular suture lines.[37–39] Although data are lacking, preoperative and postoperative elevation of blood pressure in these patients should be managed in the same manner as patients undergoing noncardiac surgery.

Neurologic Surgery and Hypertension

Avoiding wide swings in blood pressure is critical in patients with chronic hypertension undergoing neurologic surgery because autoregulation of cerebral blood flow is impaired. In addition, maintenance of cerebral blood flow requires higher mean arterial blood pressures of 110 to 180 mmHg in patients with uncontrolled hypertension and 90 to 150 mmHg in those with controlled hypertension.[40,41] Hypertension and, more importantly, relative hypotension may impair cerebral perfusion and lead to cerebral ischemia as compensatory mechanisms designed to preserve optimal blood flow are blunted. Overzealous treatment of hypertension can therefore be potentially harmful. Patients with atherosclerotic cerebrovascular disease have a higher likelihood of having significant underlying coronary artery disease.[42]

Severe Hypertension

Data in the literature support the recommendation that patients with severe untreated hypertension should be treated before surgery. Prys-Roberts demonstrated that patients with diastolic blood pressure over 120 mmHg have exaggerated hypotensive responses to induction and maintenance of anesthesia and marked hypertensive responses to noxious stimuli.[43] These responses can lead to subendocardial ischemia, a risk factor in the development of adverse cardiac outcomes, especially in patients with peripheral vascular disease.[44] Another study documented an increase in postoperative mortality in patients with diastolic blood pressures over 110 mmHg undergoing abdominal surgery.[18]

PREOPERATIVE EVALUATION

Because hypertension is associated with vascular and renal disease, preoperative assessment of patients with hypertension requires a thorough history and physical examination with specific emphasis on signs and symptoms of cardiovascular and cerebrovascular disease, including congestive heart failure, valvular heart disease, recent myocardial infarction (within the last six months), angina, transient ischemic attacks, cerebrovascular accidents, and ventricular arrhythmias. Preoperative laboratory testing should include serum electrolyte levels, blood urea nitrogen (BUN), creatinine, urinalysis, chest x-ray, and electrocardiogram. A history of side effects of individual antihypertensives should be elicited. Blood pressure control should be assessed from review of available records, and clues to associated comorbid conditions, including risk factors for coronary artery disease, should be pursued. Blood pressure should be taken in both arms and in the supine and erect positions.

Primary (Essential) Versus Secondary Hypertension

Most patients with elevated blood pressure have primary or essential hypertension. The prevalence of secondary hypertension has been reported to be as high as 10 percent in a referral population[45] but is less common among unselected patients in a primary care setting.[46] Causes of secondary hypertension are listed in Table 17–3.

Suspected secondary hypertension should be evaluated before elective surgery. However, if blood pressure is controlled and se-

TABLE 17–3. Causes of Secondary Hypertension

   I. Renal Disease
      A. Parenchymal Disease
         1. Chronic Pyelonephritis
         2. Glomerulonephritis (Acute and Chronic)
         3. Nephrolithiasis
         4. Polycystic Kidney Disease
      B. Renal Artery Stenosis (Renovascular Hypertension)
      C. Renin-Producing Tumors
  II. Endocrinologic Diseases
      A. Primary Hyperaldosteronism
      B. Cushing's Syndrome or Disease
      C. Pheochromocytoma*
      D. Hyperthyroidism
      E. Congenital or Hereditary Adrenogenital Syndromes
      F. Myxedema
      G. Acromegaly
      H. Hyperparathyroidism
 III. Coarctation of the Aorta*
  IV. Substance Abuse
      A. Cocaine*
      B. Alcohol*
      C. Other Stimulants (Amphetamines)
   V. Drugs
      A. Oral Contraceptive Agents*
      B. Phenylpropanolamine, Phenylephrine
  VI. Miscellaneous
      A. Elevated Intracranial Pressure (Acute)*
      B. Fever
      C. Acute Stress or Anxiety
      D. Pregnancy*
      E. Other

*See text for further discussion.

rum electrolyte levels and renal function are within normal limits, most patients with secondary hypertension can undergo more urgent surgery and defer definitive evaluation until later. However, patients with hypertension due to pheochromocytoma, coarctation of the aorta, abuse of alcohol or cocaine, oral contraceptive use, elevated intracranial pressure, or pregnancy more often require definitive diagnosis and treatment before surgery.

Patients with unsuspected pheochromocytoma undergoing surgery have a surgical mortality rate of 50 percent. When the diagnosis is known, premedication with alpha- and beta-blockers reduces this rate significantly.[47] Patients with coarctation have an increased risk of endocarditis and require appropriate antibiotic prophylaxis before surgery. Cocaine intoxication, a recognized cause of acute hypertension,[48] has been associated with aortic dissection,[49] ventricular tachycardia,[50] pulmonary edema,[51] sudden death,[52,53] angina, and myocardial infarction.[54–56] Myocardial infarction has also been reported during cocaine withdrawal.[57] If serum or urine toxicology screens verify clinical suspicion of acute cocaine intoxication, all but the most emergent surgery should be postponed, and the patient should be carefully monitored during withdrawal. Similarly, acute alcohol intoxication or withdrawal may be associated with hypertension. Despite the paucity of data, patients in withdrawal from alcohol undergoing surgery are thought to have an increased risk of complications and should not undergo any but emergency procedures. Surgery should also be deferred in patients with hypertension due to oral contraceptives until the blood pressure returns to normal. The management of pregnant hypertensive patients is discussed in Chap. 40.[58]

Patients with elevated intracranial pressure due to a mass lesion or intracerebral hematoma may be hypertensive and require urgent surgery. Those with chronic hypertension have impaired cerebral autoregulatory responses to changes in blood pressure.[59] Aggressive treatment of blood pressure before surgery may cause significant intraoperative and postoperative hypotension, and inadequately controlled hypertension may reduce cerebral perfusion pressure.[60] If antihypertensive therapy is necessary, vasodilators should be avoided to prevent even greater increases in intracranial pressure. Resection of a mass lesion may correct systemic hypertension.

MANAGEMENT OF PREOPERATIVE HYPERTENSION

Ideally, elective surgery should be postponed in patients with acute or newly discovered moderate or severe hypertension (diastolic blood pressure above 110 mmHg) or inadequately controlled chronic hypertension until blood pressure is controlled. If urgent surgery is required, there are several effective therapeutic modalities to control blood pressure expeditiously. Patients with well-controlled hypertension on chronic therapy require careful management of their antihypertensive therapy in the perioperative period.

Acute or Inadequately Controlled Hypertension

Table 17–4 lists several therapeutic options for treating patients with newly discovered or inadequately controlled hypertension. These parenteral regimens may also be used after surgery until patients can resume oral intake. No one regimen has been proven

TABLE 17–4. Parenteral Treatment of Acute or Inadequately Controlled Hypertension or Treatment of Chronic Hypertension in Patients Unable to Take Oral Medication

Class of Drug	Dose
Vasodilators	
Sodium Nitroprusside (Nipride)	0.5–10.0 µg/kg/min, IV infusion
Nitroglycerine (Nitrostat)	5.0–400 µg/min, IV infusion
Diazoxide (Hyperstat)	1–3 mg/kg IV bolus to maximum of 150 mg q 5–15 minutes until BP acceptable
Hydralazine (Apresoline)	10–40 mg IV, repeated as necessary
Adrenergic Inhibitors	
Phentolamine HCl (Regitine)	5.0 mg IV/IM, repeated as necessary
Trimethaphan Camsylate (Arfonad)	1.0–4.0 mg/min, IV infusion
Methyldopa (Aldomet)	250–500 mg IV q 6 hours as necessary
Beta-Blockers	
Propranolol (Inderal)	a. 1–3 mg IV bolus q 4 hours as necessary b. 3 mg/hour, IV infusion
Labetalol (Normodyne, Trandate)	a. 20 mg bolus over 2 minutes, then 20–80 mg q 10 minutes until BP acceptable or 300 mg maximum b. 2 mg/min, IV infusion
Angiotensin-Enzyme Inhibitors	
Enalaprilat	0.625–1.25 mg IV q 6 hours

superior to any other. Selection should be based on individual patient needs and physician preference and experience.

Despite a paucity of data, sublingual nifedipine is often used to treat acute severe hypertension in the perioperative period.[61] Its peak effect on lowering blood pressure occurs 30 to 60 minutes after administration and lasts two to six hours.[61–63] While some studies have documented only limited side effects, there have been some recent reports of unpredictable effects including significant hypotension which is sometimes difficult to reverse.[64–66] Myocardial and cerebral ischemia have also been reported.[67,68] Even when administered sublingually, the effect of nifedipine is largely due to gastrointestinal absorption after swallowing the contents of the perforated capsule.[69] When gastrointestinal absorption is impaired in the perioperative period, whether due to ileus, inability to swallow, or nasogastric suction, other forms of antihypertensive therapy may be better. The use of sublingual nifedipine to treat hypertension has not been approved by the Food and Drug Administration.[65]

The Patient on Chronic Antihypertensive Therapy

Although it was initially thought that continuing antihypertensive therapy up to the time of surgery altered circulatory homeostasis and increased the risk of perioperative cardiovascular complications,[70–82] the bulk of more recent data would suggest otherwise. In 1971, Prys-Roberts et al. found no adverse circulatory changes in patients continuing to receive a variety of antihypertensives in the perioperative period with the possible exception of reserpine.[83] Both his group and Stone et al. confirmed that untreated hypertensives had a higher incidence of myocardial ischemia.[84] Moreover, later studies exonerated reserpine and found that it did not increase

the risk of altered circulatory reflexes or perioperative hypotension.[85] Charlson et al. found that preoperative administration of a variety of antihypertensives, including diuretics, beta-blockers, calcium channel blockers, and others did not predict either intraoperative hypotension or both hypotension and hypertension, patterns commonly associated with an increased risk of postoperative renal and cardiac complications.[31]

In fact, abrupt discontinuation of certain antihypertensive agents may be hazardous. Although the clonidine and beta-blocker withdrawal syndromes are most commonly described, withdrawal syndromes have also been reported with other agents. Rebound hypertension has been reported after withdrawal of guanethidine and bethanidine;[86] hydralazine, reserpine, and hydrochlorothiazide;[87] and methyldopa.[88–91] Many case reports of rebound hypertension involved simultaneous discontinuation of several antihypertensives, and the relative importance of individual medications may be somewhat difficult to judge. Calcium channel blockers can cause rebound vasospasm after coronary revascularization.[92] Table 17–5 lists some of the factors that predispose patients to withdrawal syndromes.

In summary, because of the relative safety of continuing antihypertensive medications in the perioperative period, the potential danger of significant rebound hypertension after abrupt discontinuation of some antihypertensives, and the potential risks of severe uncontrolled hypertension, it is recommended that antihypertensive therapy be continued up to the time of surgery. Except in the case of diuretic therapy discussed below, scheduled antihypertensives can be given on the morning of surgery with a small sip of water without adverse effect. Table 17–6 lists commonly used antihypertensives by class and outlines their suggested use in the perioperative period. A more detailed discussion of each class is presented below.

TABLE 17–5. Predisposing Factors for Acute Withdrawal Syndrome

1. Abrupt discontinuation of antihypertensive therapy
2. Centrally acting drugs
3. Beta-blockers
4. Combination of drug therapies, especially #2 with #3 above
5. High daily doses of antihypertensive therapy
6. Ischemic heart disease
7. Severe hypertension
8. Renovascular hypertension

Source: Adapted from Houston MC: Abrupt cessation of treatment in hypertension: Consideration of clinical features, mechanisms, prevention and management of the discontinuation syndrome. *Am Heart J* 102:415–430, 1981.

Diuretics

Patients on chronic diuretic therapy for hypertension undergoing surgery are prone to hypokalemia and intravascular volume depletion. Uncorrected hypokalemia may potentiate abdominal ileus, certain cardiac arrhythmias, and the effects of muscle relaxants.[93,94] Preoperative relative hypovolemia from diuretic therapy may be especially hazardous if significant blood loss or third-spacing of fluid occurs in the perioperative period. Moreover, diuretic-induced reduction in preload may be aggravated by the vasodilating effects of anesthetics and cause significant intraoperative hypotension. It is therefore recommended that diuretics be withheld for 24 to 48 hours before surgery.[93] Volume should be repleted and electrolyte abnormalities corrected preoperatively. After surgery, diuretics can be resumed based on careful daily assessment of fluid status. Parenteral furosemide or bumetanide can be used if the patient is not eating. Otherwise alternate antihypertensive agents can be used for blood pressure control if a diuretic is not advisable (see Table 17–4).

Beta-Blockers

Although there were some initial reports of intraoperative congestive heart failure and hypotension with the use of beta-blockers in the perioperative period,[79,95,96] abrupt cessation of propranolol has been associated with increasing angina, ventricular tachycardia, myocardial infarction, accelerated hypertension, and sudden death.[96–103] The risk of propranolol withdrawal is greatest four to seven days after cessation of the drug.[96] Although adverse outcomes occur mostly in patients with severe coronary artery disease, they have been reported in patients with uncomplicated hypertension.[104]

Several more recent studies actually show that continuing beta-blockers in the perioperative period carries no risk of complications,[105–107] even in patients undergoing coronary artery bypass grafting[103,108,109] or carotid endarterectomy.[110] In comparison to untreated patients, those receiving practolol before surgery developed less tachycardia and hypertension after laryngoscopy, intubation, anesthesia, and surgery and developed fewer arrhythmias and less myocardial ischemia.[111] Moreover, esmolol, an ultrashort-acting cardioselective beta-adrenergic blocker, blunts increases in heart rate and blood pressure in patients undergoing carotid endarterectomy without adverse effect.[110]

It is now recommended that beta-blockers be continued during the perioperative period, especially in patients with suspected or known coronary artery disease. The usual dose of medication can be given on the morning of surgery and resumed as soon as possible thereafter. If the patient is unable to take oral fluids for more than 24 hours, parenteral propranolol or labetolol in bolus form or continuous infusion can be used.[105,106,112,113] (See Table 17–4.) Esmolol is also effective in the perioperative period[110] but is mainly used in the treatment of supraventricular tachycardia.

Angiotensin-Converting Enzyme Inhibitors

Angiotensin-converting enzyme inhibitors (ACE inhibitors) are vasodilators that provide effective treatment of hypertension and congestive heart failure. Their half-lives are variable, and captopril has the shortest. In a controlled study of 19 patients undergoing coronary artery bypass grafting, Colson et al. reported no impairment of blood pressure regulation during anesthesia and cardiopulmonary bypass in patients receiving captopril before surgery but found that the drug failed to prevent postoperative hypertension.[114]

Pharmaceutical companies caution that the use of ACE inhibitors in patients undergoing major surgery or anesthesia with agents causing hypotension may exhibit blunted compensatory renin release and prolonged hypotension, but no clinical studies have confirmed this. Hyperkalemia may occur due to inhibition of aldosterone synthesis, and all patients should have serum potassium levels checked before surgery. It is advisable to continue ACE inhibitors up to the time of surgery and resume them thereafter. If the patient cannot tolerate oral fluids and blood pressure control is needed, intravenous enalaprilat or another parenteral agent can be used.

Centrally-Acting Sympatholytics

Centrally-acting sympatholytics include clonidine, methyldopa, and guanabenz. Abrupt withdrawal of clonidine has been associated with rebound hypertension,[86,115–123] tachycardia, headaches, agitation, sweating, palpitations, nausea, and vomiting. These symptoms may be related to an increase in arterial catecholamine levels.[118] However, a prospective study of patients with mild hypertension on various doses of clonidine during the study period failed to corroborate withdrawal phenomena.[124] Withdrawal symptoms, including overshoot hypertension, may occur less commonly than case reports suggest.[104] Patients on chronic therapy at doses above 0.8 mg/day may have a higher risk of rebound phenomena,[124] especially if other antihypertensives are withdrawn simultaneously.[104] It is therefore recommended that clonidine be given on the morning of surgery and resumed as soon as possible thereafter. If oral fluids cannot be ingested for more than 24 hours, transdermal clonidine or parenteral methyldopa are good alternative regimens.

Methyldopa should also be continued up to the time of surgery and can be given parenterally after surgery if needed (see Table 17–4). Withdrawal symptoms have been reported with abrupt discontinuation of methyldopa when used in doses ranging from 0.5 to 6 g/day.[88–94,104] Withdrawal symptoms have also been reported after discontinuation of guanabenz.[125]

Peripheral Sympatholytics

Reserpine, a peripheral sympatholytic, exerts its antihypertensive effect by depleting central and peripheral norepinephrine and decreasing sympathetic activity. Early reports in the literature warned

TABLE 17–6. Antihypertensive Medication

Strategy		Suggested Perioperative Management
I. *Diuretics*		1
Thiazides		
Chlorthalidone	(Hygroton)	
Hydrochlorothiazide	(Hydrodiuril)	
Indapamide	(Lozol)	
Metolazone	(Zaroxolyn)	
Loop-Acting		
Bumetanide	(Bumex)	
Furosemide	(Lasix)	
Potassium-Sparing		
Spironolactone	(Aldactone)	
Triamterene/HCTZ	(Dyazide, Maxzide)	
II. *Beta-Blockers*		2
Propanolol	(Inderal, Inderal LA)	
Atenolol	(Tenormin)	
Metoprolol	(Lopressor, Toprol XL)	
Timolol	(Blocarden)	
Pindolol	(Visken)	
Nadolol	(Corgard)	
Acebutolol	(Sectral)	
Labetolol*	(Trandate, Normodyne)	
* Also an Alpha-Blocker		
III. *Angiotensin-Converting Enzyme Inhibitors*		2,3
Captopril	(Capoten)	
Enalapril	(Vasotec)	
Lisinopril	(Zestril)	
Benazepril	(Lotensin)	
IV. *Central-Acting Sympatholytics*		2
Clonidine	(Catapres, Catapres TTS)	
Methyldopa	(Aldomet)	
Guanabenz	(Wytensin)	
V. *Alpha-Blockers*		3
Prazosin	(Minipres)	
Terazosin	(Hytrin)	
Doxazosin	(Cardura)	
VI. *Peripheral Sympatholytics*		3
Reserpine	(Serpasil)	
VII. *Vasodilators*		2
Hydralazine	(Apresoline)	
Minoxidil	(Loniten)	
VIII. *Calcium Channel Blockers*		3
Diltiazem	(Cardizem, Cardizem SR, Cardizem CD)	
Nifedipine	(Procardia, Adalat, Procardia XL)	
Verapamil	(Calan, Isoptin, Calan SR, Isoptin SR)	
Nicardipine	(Cardene)	
Felodipine	(Plendil)	
Isradipine	(Dynacirc)	

1 Hold 24–48 hours preoperatively. Resume postoperatively based on fluid status.
  If NPO, blood pressure control needed and diuretic clinically appropriate, IV furosemide or bumetanide.
  If NPO, blood pressure control needed and diuretic contraindicated, see Table 18–4.

2 Give usual medication the AM of surgery with sip of water.
  If NPO and blood pressure control needed, see Table 18–4 under appropriate class of drug.
    See text re: beta-blockers and clonidine.

3 Give usual medication the AM of surgery with sip of water.
  If NPO and blood pressure control needed, see Table 18–4.

that continuing this agent in the perioperative period caused hypotension during anesthesia that responded poorly to vasopressors, bradycardia, and slowed atrioventricular conduction.[93,126,127] It was recommended that reserpine be discontinued at least two weeks before nonemergent surgery to allow repletion of catecholamine stores.[127] Later studies found that patients on reserpine tolerated surgery safely[77,85,128] and had fewer episodes of hypotension than untreated hypertensive patients. Its cost-effectiveness and limited side effect profile in doses at or under 0.25 mg may lead to increased use, and clinicians should be familiar with its use in the perioperative setting.[129] Reserpine should be continued until the morning of surgery and resumed thereafter when needed. If oral fasting is prolonged, the parenteral regimens outlined in Table 17–4 can be used.

Alpha-Blockers

Prazosin, terazosin, and doxazosin are representative alpha-blockers available in the United States. No clinical data are available regarding their use in the perioperative period. It is recommended that they be continued up to the morning of surgery and resumed when possible postoperatively.

Vasodilators

Hydralazine and minoxidil directly dilate arterioles. There are no reports of adverse effects of these drugs in the perioperative period. They should be continued until surgery and resumed thereafter in the usual manner. Parenteral hydralazine is useful when oral intake is not feasible (see Table 17–4).

Calcium Channel Blockers

Calcium channel blockers are popular and effective antianginal and antihypertensive agents, and several long-acting preparations are listed in Table 17–6. Abrupt discontinuation of these drugs in the postoperative period in patients with underlying coronary artery disease can cause severe vasospasm with significant ST-segment elevation on the electrocardiogram.[92] This occurred in two of 16 patients withdrawn from diltiazem and two of 100 withdrawn from nifedipine after coronary revascularization. No adverse effects have been reported with continuation of these drugs before surgery. However, two separate reports have found them not effective against and perhaps related to a higher incidence of perioperative myocardial ischemia in patients undergoing coronary artery bypass grafting.[130,131]

It is recommended that patients continue their usual dose of medication on the morning of surgery and resume therapy thereafter as needed. If oral intake is not possible for prolonged periods, alternate antihypertensive therapy can be given. Verapamil is available in an intravenous form but is usually reserved for treatment of supraventricular arrythmias.[112] If rebound coronary artery vasospasm is a concern in patients with underlying coronary artery disease, the use of intravenous nitroglycerin may be advisable.[92]

SUMMARY

1. Diastolic blood pressure under 110 mmHg has not been definitively shown to be an independent risk factor in the development of postoperative cardiac or renal complications in patients undergoing most surgical procedures. Limited data do support preoperative treatment of diastolic blood pressures above 120 mmHg.

2. Patients with hypertension, whether controlled or uncontrolled, treated or untreated, have a higher risk of perioperative hypertension and probably hypotension as well.

3. Patients undergoing abdominal aneurysmectomy and peripheral vascular surgery, especially carotid endarterectomy, have an increased risk of developing perioperative hypertension, regardless of current or past blood pressure control.

4. Significant intraoperative hypotension appears to be associated with an increased risk of postoperative complications and may be more important than absolute blood pressure values before surgery.

5. Patients with chronic hypertension and cerebrovascular disease may have an especially high risk of adverse effects from perioperative hypotension.

6. Patients with secondary hypertension can be managed in the same way as those with essential hypertension except those with pheochromocytoma, coarctation of the aorta, alcohol and cocaine intoxication or withdrawal, oral contraceptive use, pregnancy, or increased intracranial pressure. These patients usually require diagnosis and specific therapy before surgery.

7. Ideally, elective surgery should be postponed in patients with acute or newly diagnosed hypertension until the blood pressure is controlled. In urgent cases, hypertension with diastolic blood pressure above 110 mmHg should be treated with the parenteral agents listed in Table 17–4. Sublingual nifedipine is widely used but actually requires gastrointestinal absorption and can cause significant hypotension and myocardial and cerebral ischemia. Its use is not recommended.

8. Except for diuretic therapy, chronic antihypertensive agents should be given with a sip of water on the morning of surgery and resumed as needed when the patient is able to take oral fluids. When oral fasting is prolonged because of extensive gastrointestinal surgery, ileus, or inability to take oral medication, alternative parenteral therapy as outlined in Table 17–4 is often necessary.

9. Patients previously on beta-blockers should receive parenteral propranolol or labetolol to prevent rebound hypertension and tachycardia. Those taking clonidine should be given transdermal preparations of the drug, recognizing that it will take 48 hours to achieve comparable systemic levels, or parenteral methyldopa when more rapid control is needed.

REFERENCES

1. 1988 Joint National Committee: The 1988 report of the Joint National Committee on detection, evaluation and treatment of high blood pressure. *Arch Intern Med* 148:1023–1038, 1988.
2. Veterans Administration Cooperative Study Group on Antihypertensive Agents: Effects of treatment on morbidity in hypertension: Results in patients with diastolic pressures averaging 115–129 mmHg. *JAMA* 213:1028–1034, 1970.

3. Hansson L: Current and future strategies in the treatment of hypertension. *Am J Cardiol* 61:2C–7C, 1988.
4. Veterans Administration Cooperative Study Group on Antihypertensive Agents: Effects of treatment on morbidity in hypertension: II. Results in patients with diastolic pressures averaging 90 through 114 mmHg. *JAMA* 213:1143–1152, 1970.
5. Hypertension Detection and Follow-Up Program Cooperative Group: Five-year findings of the Hypertension Detection and Follow-Up Program: I. Reduction in mortality of persons with high blood pressure, including mild hypertension. *JAMA* 242:2562–2572, 1979.
6. Management Committee of the Australian National Blood Pressure Study: The Australian therapeutic trial in mild hypertension. *Lancet* 1:1261–1267, 1980.
7. Medical Research Council Working Party: MRC trial of treatment of mild hypertension: Principal results. *Br Med J* 291:97–104, 1985.
8. SHEP Cooperative Research Group: Prevention of stroke by antihypertensive drug treatment in older persons with isolated systolic hypertension. *JAMA* 263:3255–3264, 1991.
9. MacMahon SW, Cutler JA, Furberg CD et al: The effects of drug treatment for hypertension on morbidity and mortality from cardiovascular disease: A review of randomized, controlled trials. *Prog Cardiovasc Dis* 29(Suppl):99–118, 1986.
10. Steen PA, Tinker JH, Tarhan S: Myocardial reinfarction after anesthesia and surgery. *JAMA* 239:2566–2570, 1978.
11. Driscoll AC, Haoabika JH, Steten BE et al: Clinically unrecognized myocardial infarction following surgery. *N Engl J Med* 264:633–639, 1961.
12. von Knorring J: Postoperative myocardial infarction: A prospective study in a risk group of surgical patients. *Surgery* 90:55–60, 1981.
13. Foster ED, Davis KB, Carpenter JA et al: Risk of noncardiac operation in patients with defined coronary disease: the Coronary Artery Surgery Study (CASS) registry experience. *Ann Thorac Surg* 41:42–50, 1986.
14. Tinker JH: Perioperative myocardial infarction. *Semin Anesth* 1:253, 1982.
15. Chamberlain DA, Edmonds-Seal J: Effects of surgery under general anesthesia on the electrocardiogram in ischaemic heart disease and hypertension. *Br Med J* 2:784–787, 1964.
16. Rosen M, Mushin WW, Kilpatrick GS et al: Study of myocardial ischemia in surgical patients. *Br Med J* 2:1415–1420, 1966.
17. Cooperman M, Pflug B, Martin EW et al: Cardiovascular risk factors in patients with peripheral vascular disease. *Surgery* 84:505–509, 1978.
18. Skinner JF, Pearce ML: Surgical risk in the cardiac patient. *J Chron Dis* 17:57–72, 1964.
19. Butler S, Feeney N, Levine SA: The patient with heart disease as a surgical risk. *JAMA* 95:85, 1930.
20. McQuiston JS: Relationship of arterial hypertension to surgical risk. *Proc Mayo Clin* 8:614, 1933.
21. Senturia HR: Relationship of arterial hypertension to surgical risk in breast cancer. *J Mo Med Assoc* 38:22, 1941.
22. Hamilton BE: Chronic cardiac disease as a surgical risk. *Surg Clin N Amer* 6:621, 1926.
23. Goldman L, Caldera DL, Nussbaum SR et al: Multifactorial index of cardiac risk in non-cardiac surgical patients. *N Engl J Med* 297:845–850, 1977.
24. Goldman L, Caldera DL, Southwick FS et al: Cardiac risk factors and complications in non-cardiac surgery. *Medicine* 57:357–370, 1978.
25. Detsky AL, Abrams HB, McLaughlin JR et al: Predicting cardiac complication in patients undergoing non-cardiac surgery. *J Gen Intern Med* 1:211–219, 1986.
26. Goldman L, Caldera DL: Risks of general anesthesia and elective operation in the hypertensive patient. *Anesthesiology.* 50:285–292, 1979.

27. Gal TJ, Cooperman LH: Hypertension in the immediate postoperative period. *Br J Anaesth* 47:70–74, 1975.
28. Rao TLK, Jacobs KH, El-Etr AA: Reinfarction following anesthesia in patients with myocardial infarction. *Anesthesiology* 59:499–505, 1983.
29. Browner WS, Li J, Mangano DT et al: In-hospital and long-term mortality in male veterans following noncardiac surgery. *JAMA* 268:228–232, 1992.
30. Hollenberg M, Mangano DT, Browner WS et al: Predictors of postoperative myocardial ischemia in patients undergoing noncardiac surgery. *JAMA* 268:205–210, 1992.
31. Charlson ME, MacKenzie CR, Gold JP et al: Preoperative characteristics predicting intraoperative hypotension and hypertension among hypertensives and diabetics undergoing noncardiac surgery. *Ann Surg* 212:66–81, 1990.
32. Charlson ME, MacKenzie CR, Gold JP et al: The preoperative and intraoperative hemodynamic predictors of postoperative myocardial infarction or ischemia in patients undergoing noncardiac surgery. *Ann Surg* 210:637–648, 1989.
33. Mauney FM, Ebert PA, Sabiston DC: Postoperative myocardial infarction: A study of predisposing factors, diagnosis and mortality in a high risk group of surgical patients. *Ann Surg* 172:497–503, 1970.
34. Wasserman F, Bellet S, Saichek RP: Postoperative myocardial infarction. *N Engl J Med* 252:967–974, 1955.
35. Plumlee JE, Boettner RB: Myocardial infarction during and following anesthesia and operation. *South Med J* 65:886–889, 1972.
36. Higgins TL, Estafanous FG, Loop RD et al: Stratification of morbidity and mortality outcome by preoperative risk factors in coronary artery bypass patients. *JAMA* 267:2344–2348, 1992.
37. Hoar PF, Hickey RF, Ullyot KJ: Systemic hypertension following myocardial revascularization: A method of treatment using epidural anesthesia. *J Thorac Cardiovasc Surg* 71:859–863, 1976.
38. Estafanous FG, Tarazi RC, Viljoen JF et al: Systemic hypertension following myocardial revascularization. *Am Heart J* 85:732–738, 1973.
39. Viljoen JF, Estafanous FG, Tarazi RC: Acute hypertension immediately after coronary surgery. *J Thorac Cardiovasc Surg* 71:548–550, 1976.
40. Heuser D, Gugenberger H, Fretschner R: Acute blood pressure increase during the perioperative period. *Am J Cardiol* 63:26C–31C, 1989.
41. Strandgaard S, Olesen J, Skinhoj E et al: Autoregulation of brain circulation in severe arterial hypertension. *Br Med J* 1:507–510, 1973.
42. Hertzer NR, Beven EG, Young JR et al: Coronary artery disease in peripheral vascular patients. *Ann Surg* 199:223–233, 1984.
43. Prys-Roberts C, Greene LT, Meloche R et al: Studies of anesthesia in relation to hypertension. II: Haemodynamic consequences of induction and endotracheal intubation. *Br J Anaesth* 43:531–546, 1971.
44. Raby KE, Goldman L, Creager MA: Correlation between preoperative ischemia and major cardiac events after peripheral vascular surgery. *N Engl J Med* 321:1296–1300, 1989.
45. Gifford RW: Evaluation of the hypertensive patient with emphasis on detecting curable causes. *Milbank Mem Fund Q* 47:170, 1969.
46. Rudnick KV et al: Hypertension in a family practice. *Can Med Assoc J* 17:492, 1977.
47. Apgar V, Papper EM: Pheochromocytoma; anesthetic management during surgical treatment. *Arch Surg* 62:634–648, 1951.
48. Fischman MW, Schuster CR, Resnekov L et al: Cardiovascular and subjective effects of intravenous cocaine administration in humans. *Arch Gen Psych* 33:983–989, 1976.
49. Barth CW, Bray M, Roberts WC: Rupture of the ascending aorta during cocaine intoxication. *Am J Cardiol* 57:496, 1987.
50. Nanji AA, Filipenko JD: Asystole and ventricular fibrillation associated with cocaine intoxication. *Chest* 85:132–133, 1984.

51. Allred RJ, Rwer S: Fatal pulmonary edema following intravenous "freebase" cocaine use. *Ann Emerg Med* 10:441–442, 1982.
52. Mittleman RE, Wetli CV: Death caused by recreational cocaine use. An update. *JAMA* 252:1889–1893, 1984.
53. Virmani R, Rabinowitz M, Smialek JE et al: Cardiovascular effects of cocaine: An autopsy study of 40 patients. *Am Heart J* 106:1068–1076, 1988.
54. Pasternack PF, Colvin SB, Baumann FG: Cocaine-induced angina pectoris and acute myocardial infarction in patients younger than 40 years. *Am J Cardiol* 55:847, 1985.
55. Isner JM, Ester NA, Thompson PD et al: Acute cardiac events temporally related to cocaine abuse. *N Engl J Med* 315:1438–1443, 1986.
56. Smith HW, Liberman HA, Brody et al: Acute myocardial infarction temporally related to cocaine use. Clinical, angiographic, and pathophysiologic observations. *Ann Intern Med* 107:13–18, 1987.
57. Del Aguila C, Rosman H: Myocardial infarction during cocaine withdrawal. *Ann Intern Med* 112:712, 1990.
58. Cunningham FG, Lindherimer MD: Current concepts: Hypertension in pregnancy. *N Engl J Med* 326:927–933, 1992.
59. Standgaard S, Haunso S: Why does antihypertensive treatment prevent stroke but not myocardial infarction? *Lancet* 2:658–661, 1987.
60. Heuser D, Guggenberger H, Fretschner R: Acute blood pressure increase during the perioperative period. *Am J Cardiol* 63:26C–31C, 1989.
61. Adler AG, Leahy JJ, Cressman MD: Management of perioperative hypertension using sublingual nifedipine. *Arch Intern Med* 146:1927–1930, 1986.
62. Frishman WH, Charlap S: Nifedipine in the treatment of systemic hypertension. *Arch Intern Med* 144:2335–2336, 1984.
63. Angeli P, Chiesa M, Caregaro L et al: Comparison of sublingual captopril and nifedipine in the treatment of hypertensive emergencies. A randomized single-blind clinical trial. *Arch Intern Med* 151(4):678–682, 1991.
64. Wachter RM: Symptomatic hypotension induced by nifedipine in acute treatment of severe hypertension. *Arch Intern Med* 147:556–558, 1987.
65. Opie LH: Sublingual nifedipine. *Lancet* 338:1203, 1991.
66. Kedas A, Shively M, Burres J: Nursing delivery of sublingual nifedipine. *J Cardiovasc Nurs* 3(4):31–37, 1989.
67. Nobile-Orazeo E, Sterzi R: Cerebral ischemia after nifedipine therapy. *Br Med J* 283:948, 1981.
68. Shelligar VR, Loungani R: Adverse effects of sublingual nifedipine in acute myocardial infarction. *Crit Care Med* 17:196–197, 1989.
69. van Harten J, Burggraaf K, Danhof M et al: Negligible sublingual absorption of nifedipine. *Lancet* 2:1363–1365, 1987.
70. Dingle HR: Antihypertensive drugs and anaesthesia. *Anaesthesia* 21:151, 1966.
71. Hickler RB, Vandam LD: Hypertension. *Anesthesiology* 33:214, 1970.
72. Grogono AW, Lee P: Danger lists for the anesthetist. *Anaesthesia* 25:518, 1970.
73. Smessaert AA, Hicks RG: Problems caused by rauwolfia drugs during anesthesia and surgery. *NY St J Med* 61:2399, 1961.
74. Dundee JW: Iatrogenic disease and anaesthesia. *Br Med J* 1:1433, 1958.
75. Ziegler CH, Lovette JB: Operative complications after therapy with reserpine and reserpine compounds. *JAMA* 176:916, 1961.
76. Coakley CS, Alpert S, Boling JS: Circulatory responses during anaesthesia of patients on rauwolfia therapy. *JAMA* 161:1143, 1956.
77. Ominsky AJ, Wollman H: Hazards of general anesthesia in the reserpinized patient. *Anesthesiology* 30:443, 1969.
78. Katz RL, Weintraub HD, Papper EM: Anesthesia surgery and rauwolfia. *Anesthesiology* 25:142, 1964.
79. Viljoen JF, Estafanous FG, Kellner GA: Propranolol and cardiac surgery. *J Thorac Cardiovasc Surg* 64:826–830, 1972.
80. Faulkner SL, Hopkins JT, Boerth RC et al: Time required for complete recovery from chronic propranolol therapy. *N Engl J Med* 289:607–609, 1973.
81. Coltart KJ, Mitchell NC, Stinson EB et al: Investigation of the safe withdrawal period for propranolol in patients scheduled for open heart surgery. *Br Heart J* 37:1128–1134, 1975.
82. Jones EL, Kaplin JA, Dorney EF et al: Propranolol therapy in patients undergoing myocardial revascularization. *Am J Cardiol* 38:696–670, 1976.
83. Prys-Roberts C, Meloche R, Foex P: Studies of anaesthesia in relation to hypertension. I: Cardiovascular responses of treated and untreated patients. *Br J Anaesth* 43:122–137, 1971.
84. Stone JG, Foex P, Sear JW et al: Myocardial ischemia in untreated hypertensive patients: Effect of a single small oral dose of a beta-adrenergic blocking agent. *Anesthesiology* 68:495–500, 1988.
85. Katz RL: Hazardous effects of drugs in hypertensive patients scheduled for elective surgery. *Cardiovasc Med* 3:1185–1205, 1978.
86. Goldberg AD, Raftery EB, Wilkinson P: Blood pressure and heart rate and withdrawal of antihypertensive drugs. *Br Med J* 1:1243–1246, 1977.
87. Katz JD, Croneau LH, Barash PG: Postoperative hypertension: A hazard of abrupt cessation of antihypertensive medication in the preoperative period. *Am Heart J* 92:79–80, 1976.
88. Burden AC, Alexander CPT: Rebound hypertension after acute methyldopa withdrawal. *Br Med J* 1:1056, 1976.
89. Frewin DB, Penhall RK: Rebound hypertension after sudden discontinuation of methyldopa therapy. *Med J Aust* 1:659, 1977.
90. Cannon PJ, Whitlock RT, Morris RC et al: Effect of alpha-methyldopa in severe and malignant hypertension. *JAMA* 179:673, 1963.
91. Scott JN, McDevitt DG: Rebound hypertension after acute methyldopa withdrawal. *Br Med J* 2:367, 1976.
92. Engelman RM, Hadju-Rousou I, Breyer RH et al: Rebound vasospasm after coronary revascularization in association with calcium antagonist withdrawal. *Ann Thorac Surg* 37:469–472, 1984.
93. Cygan R, Waitzkin H: Stopping and restarting medications in the perioperative period. *J Gen Intern Med* 2:270–283, 1987.
94. Hall WD: Hypertension in the surgical patient: Preoperative, intraoperative, and postoperative evaluation and management, in Lubin MF, Walter HK, Smith RB (eds): *Medical Management of the Surgical Patient.* Boston, Butterworths, 1982, p 94.
95. Edwards WT: Preanesthetic management of the hypertensive patient. *N Engl J Med* 30:158–159, 1979.
96. Goldman L: Noncardiac surgery in patients receiving propranolol. *Arch Intern Med* 141:193–196, 1981.
97. Miller RR, Olson HG, Amsterdam EA et al: Propranolol-withdrawal rebound phenomenon. Exacerbation of coronary events after abrupt cessation of antianginal therapy. *N Engl J Med* 293:416–419, 1975.
98. Alderman EL, Coltart KJ, Wettach GE et al: Coronary artery syndromes after sudden propranolol withdrawal. *Ann Intern Med* 81:625–627, 1974.
99. Mizgala HF, Counsell J: Acute coronary syndromes following abrupt cessation of oral propranolol therapy. *Circulation* 49/50(Suppl III):33, 1974.
100. Diaz RG, Somberg JC, Freeman E et al: Withdrawal of propranolol and myocardial infarction. *Lancet* 1:1068, 1973.
101. Slome R: Withdrawal of propranolol and myocardial infarction. *Lancet* 1:156, 1973.
102. Allen R, Genovese B: Propranolol withdrawal. *Ann Intern Med* 82:431, 1975.
103. Slogoff S, Keats AS, Ott E: Preoperative propranolol therapy and aortocoronary bypass operation. *JAMA* 240:1487–1490, 1978.
104. Houston MC: Abrupt cessation of treatment in hypertension: Consid-

eration of clinical features, mechanisms, prevention and management of the discontinuation syndrome. *Am Heart J* 102:415–430, 1981.

105. Smulyan H, Weinberg S, Howanitz P: Continuous propranolol infusion following abdominal surgery. *JAMA* 247:2539–2542, 1982.

106. Rotem C: Propranolol therapy in the perioperative period. *Can Med Assoc J* 114:188, 1976.

107. Magnusson J, Thulin T, Werner O et al: Haemodynamic effects of pretreatment with metoprolol in hypertensive patients undergoing surgery. *Br J Anaesth* 58:251–260, 1986.

108. Moran JM, Mulet J, Caralps JM et al: Coronary revascularization in patients receiving propranolol. *Circulation* 50(Suppl 2):116–121, 1974.

109. Kaplan JA, Dunbar RW, Bland JW et al: Propranolol and cardiac surgery: A problem for the anesthesiologist? *Anesth Analg* 54:571–578, 1975.

110. Cucchiara RF, Benefiel KJ, Matteo RS et al: Evaluation of esmolol in controlling increases in heart rate and blood pressure during endotracheal intubation in patients undergoing carotid endarterectomy. *Anesthesiology* 65:528–531, 1986.

111. Prys-Roberts C, Foex P, Biro GP et al: Studies of anaesthesia in relation to hypertension. V: Adrenergic beta-receptor blockade. *Br J Anaesth* 45:671–680, 1973.

112. *Physicians' Desk Reference*. Montvale, NJ, Medical Economics Company, 1992.

113. Leslie JB, Kalayjian RW, Sirgo MA et al: Intravenous labetolol for treatment of postoperative hypertension. *Anesthesiology* 67:413–416, 1987.

114. Colson P, Grolleau D, Chaptal PA et al: Effect of preoperative renin-angiotensin system blockade on hypertension following coronary surgery. *Chest* 93:1156–1158, 1988.

115. Bruce DL, Croley TF, Lee JS: Preoperative clonidine withdrawal syndrome. *Anesthesiology* 51:90–92, 1979.

116. Hunyor SN, Hansson L, Harrison TS et al: Effects of clonidine withdrawal: Possible mechanisms and suggestions for management. *Br Med J* 2:209–211, 1973.

117. Hansson L, Hunyor SN, Julius S et al: Blood pressure crisis following withdrawal of clonidine with special reference to arterial and urinary catecholamine levels, and suggestions for acute management. *Am Heart J* 85:605–610, 1973.

118. Bailey RR: Letter: Clonidine overshoot. *NZ Med J* 81:268–269, 1975.

119. Bailey RR, Neale TJ: Rapid clonidine withdrawal with blood pressure overshoot exaggerated by beta-blockade. *Br Med J* 1:942–943, 1976.

120. England JF: Clonidine rebound hypertension. *Med J Aust* 1:756–757, 1977.

121. Reid JL, Wing LMH, Dargie HJ et al: Clonidine withdrawal in hypertension. Changes in blood pressure and plasma and urinary noradrenaline. *Lancet* 1:71–74, 1977.

122. Strauss FG, Franklin SS, Lewin AJ et al: Withdrawal of antihypertensive therapy. Hypertensive crisis in renovascular hypertension. *JAMA* 238:1734–1776, 1977.

123. Husserl FE, deCarvalho JGR, Batson HM et al: Hypertension after clonidine withdrawal. *South Med J* 71:496–497, 1978.

124. Whitsett TL, Chrysant SG, Dillard BL: Abrupt cessation of clonidine administration: A prospective study. *Am J Cardiol* 41:1285–1290, 1978.

125. Ram CVS, Holland OB, Farichild C et al: Withdrawal syndrome following cessation of guanabenz therapy. *J Clin Pharmacol* 19:148, 1979.

126. Foster MW, Gayle RF: Dangers in combining reserpine with electroconvulsive therapy. *JAMA* 159:1520, 1955.

127. Cohen SI, Young MW, Lau SH et al: Effects of reserpine therapy on cardiac output and atrioventricular conduction during rest and controlled heart rates in patients with essential hypertension. *Circulation* 37:738–746, 1968.

128. Alper MH, Flacke W, Krayer O: Pharmacology of reserpine and its implications for anesthesia. *Anesthesiology* 24:524–542, 1963.

129. Magarian GJ: Reserpine: A relic from the past or a neglected drug of the present for achieving cost containment in treating hypertension. *J Gen Intern Med* 6:561–572, 1991.

130. Solgoff S, Keats AS: Does chronic treatment with calcium entry blocking drugs reduce perioperative myocardial ischemia? *Anesthesiology* 68:676–680, 1988.

131. Chung F, Houston PL, Cheng DCH et al: Calcium channel blockade does not offer adequate protection from perioperative myocardial ischemia. *Anesthesiology* 69:343–347, 1988.

18 THE SURGICAL PATIENT WITH CORONARY ARTERY DISEASE

Karen G. Kelly

William K. Levy

Because of the physiologic burdens imposed on the heart by surgery and anesthesia, the perioperative period may be one of instability for patients with ischemic heart disease. Perioperative myocardial infarction is a potentially serious complication with a high mortality rate. It is important to identify factors that increase cardiac risk before surgery and to follow patients with ischemic heart disease carefully. This chapter discusses the cardiac effects of anesthesia and surgery; determinants of cardiac risk; recommendations for preoperative assessment, monitoring, and postoperative care; and perioperative use of medications commonly used in patients with coronary artery disease.

CARDIAC EFFECTS OF SURGERY AND ANESTHESIA

Numerous problems can arise during surgery and anesthesia that may upset the critical balance between myocardial oxygen supply and demand in patients with ischemic heart disease. Oxygen supply can be reduced by hypoxemia, anemia, hypotension, and bradycardia induced by vagal stimulation. Oxygen supply can be increased by sympathetic stimulation, tachycardia, hypertension, laryngoscopy, and intubation. Induction of anesthesia and intubation are extremely stressful and may be associated with significant ischemia in these patients. Roy et al. documented ischemia, as indicated by ST depressions on a monitor, in 11 of 29 patients with coronary artery disease during noncardiac surgery.[1] Ischemia correlated with an increased heart rate–blood pressure product, and 73 percent of the patients who developed ischemia did so at the time of intubation. In patients undergoing coronary artery bypass surgery, up to 50 percent experience ischemia during induction and intubation as defined by ischemic ST depression or transient thallium defects.[2,3] Moreover, ischemia can occur during surgery without a documented increase in rate-pressure product and is presumably related to transient increases in coronary tone like that documented during laryngoscopy.[4] Inappropriate coronary vasodilation can also result in redistribution of the myocardial blood flow away from ischemic zones; this has been seen with isoflurane anesthesia.[5]

Mangano et al. reported intraoperative ECG changes consistent with myocardial ischemia in 27 percent of patients with known coronary artery disease or risk factors for it undergoing noncardiac surgery. Similar incidences of ischemic ST changes were seen preoperatively on ambulatory ECG monitoring in the same patients, suggesting that careful hemodynamic control may limit intraoperative ischemia to the baseline level. The highest incidence of ischemic changes occurred within the first three days after surgery, appearing in 42 percent of the patients.[6,7]

General anesthesia usually involves the use of several intravenous and inhalational agents. They have variable influence on heart rate, myocardial contractility, and afterload which variably affect hemodynamic status. Inhalational agents like halothane, enflurane, and isoflurane all depress myocardial contractility,[8] and halothane and enflurane cause significant vasodilatation. The result of these effects is a decrease in systemic blood pressure and myocardial oxygen consumption. Intravenous narcotic agents like morphine and fentanyl are often used with the inhalation agents and depress myocardial contractility less. Muscle relaxants have variable effects on heart rate; succinylcholine may cause bradycardia, and pancuronium may cause tachycardia.[9]

Spinal and epidural anesthesia do not cause direct myocardial depression. Because they produce sympathetic blockade, significant venodilation and arteriodilation may occur. This can lead to hypotension and the subsequent development of ischemia in patients with coronary artery disease. Local anesthesia has no significant hemodynamic effect, but tachycardia and hypertension may be seen if pain and anxiety are not adequately controlled.

Choice of anesthetic in patients with ischemic heart disease is the decision of the anesthesiologist. However, the medical consultant can alert the anesthesiologist to the extent of cardiac pathology and help in the details of management.

ASSESSING CARDIAC RISK

Overall perioperative cardiac risk includes the development of myocardial infarction, pulmonary edema, ventricular tachycardia, or cardiac death. In some studies, unstable angina, congestive heart failure without pulmonary edema, and other arrhythmias are included. The following section reviews factors that may be important determinants in overall cardiac risk.

Previous Myocardial Infarction

The most important cardiac risk factor is previous myocardial infarction. Numerous studies document a perioperative infarction rate of 3 to 7 percent in patients who have had a previous myocardial infarction compared to a rate of 0.13 to 0.66 percent in those with no such history.[10–13] The risk is greater when surgery is done within six months after the myocardial infarction and even higher when done within the first three months. Two studies found the incidence of perioperative reinfarction to be 27 percent and 37 percent, respectively, when major surgery was performed within three months of an infarction.[11,12] If surgery is performed four to six months after infarction, the incidences of perioperative infarction were 16 percent and 11 percent, respectively. After six months, the rate of reinfarction stabilized at 4 to 6 percent. Goldman et al.[10] reported a rate of reinfarction or cardiac death of 27 percent when surgery was performed within six months after an infarction and a rate of 4 percent when performed after the six-month period. Patients in the latter group had the same risk as those with no previous infarction.

More recently, Rao et al. have documented lower rates of perioperative myocardial infarction.[14] In an initial retrospective study between 1973 and 1976, the perioperative reinfarction rate for patients with previous myocardial infarction was 7.7 percent. In a subsequent prospective study for the period 1977 to 1982, the reinfarction rate was only 1.9 percent. Although the reinfarction

rate in both studies was higher if surgery was performed in the first three to six months after infarction, the second study documented much lower rates. In the first study, 36 percent of patients had reinfarctions when surgery was performed within three months of previous infarction, compared to 5.8 percent in the second study. For surgery within three to six months, rates were 26 percent and 2.3 percent, respectively.

The authors attributed the lower reinfarction rates in the second group to more intensive perioperative hemodynamic monitoring with arterial and pulmonary catheters in most cases. Blood pressures were not allowed to fluctuate more than 20 percent for more than five minutes. Monitoring was continued in the intensive care unit for several days after surgery in most patients.

The mortality rate of recurrent myocardial infarctions during or immediately after noncardiac surgery is reported as high as 33 to 70 percent in published studies noted in Table 18–1.[11–13,15] A high mortality rate was also documented by Rao et al. in their study of more intensively monitored patients.[14]

Angina

There is conflicting evidence whether or not stable angina increases perioperative risk. In Goldman's study, stable angina was a univariate predictor of postoperative death but not of perioperative myocardial infarction.[10] In multivariate analysis, it dropped out as a significant risk factor in the development of cardiac complications. However, Eagle et al. found that angina was both a univariate and multivariate predictor of postoperative cardiac death and myocardial infarction in a group of 200 patients undergoing vascular surgery.[16] Larsen et al., in a study of 2609 patients undergoing a variety of surgical procedures, found that patients with angina and/or infarction more than three months prior to surgery had a significantly increased risk of death or major cardiac complications including myocardial infarction, ventricular tachycardia, and cardiogenic pulmonary edema.[17] Patients with stable angina had a mortality rate of 3.5 percent as compared to 0.8 percent in the whole group and a nonfatal cardiac complication rate of 4.8 percent as compared to 1.8 percent overall.

The exact risk of noncardiac surgery in the presence of unstable or severe angina is unclear due to the small numbers of these patients in published studies. In Larsen's study, only nine patients had unstable angina, but the overall cardiac complication rate was 44 percent with one cardiac death.[17] Unstable angina should be viewed as a significant risk factor.

Congestive Heart Failure

Congestive heart failure or a depressed ejection fraction are strong predictors of perioperative cardiac complications including peri-

TABLE 18–1. Incidence of Perioperative Myocardial Infarction in Surgical Patients with Previous Infarctions

Study	Dates	No. of Patients with Previous MI	Perioperative Reinfarction Rate	Reinfarction Rate When Surgery Is Done Within 6 Months of MI	Mortality Rate of Perioperative MI
Topkins et al[13]	1959–1962	658	6.5%	55%	70%
Tarhan et al[12]	1967–1968	422	6.6%	22%	54%
Steen et al[11]	1974–1975	587	6.1%	18%	69%
Rao et al[14]	1973–1976	364	7.7%	29%	54%
Rao et al[14]	1977–1982	733	1.9%	4%	36%

TABLE 18–2. Effect of Previous Heart Failure on Postoperative Congestive Heart Failure or Pulmonary Edema

History of CHF	No. of Patients	% with Postoperative Pulmonary Edema	% with New or Worsened Post-operative CHF
Never	853	2	4
Previous, not currently	87	6	16
Persistent despite therapy	66	16	21

Source: Adapted from Goldman et al.[10]

operative pulmonary edema and cardiac death in patients with coronary artery disease.[10,17–20] The risk of postoperative pulmonary edema in Goldman's study[10] was greatest in those with overt heart failure (see Table 18–2). The overall mortality rate for patients with postoperative pulmonary edema was 57 percent with two-thirds of the deaths attributable to cardiac causes. In Larsen's study, both active congestive failure and a history of failure or pulmonary edema were strong independent predictors of cardiac complications.[17] In both studies, evidence of active congestive heart failure was the strongest risk factor for cardiac complications, quantitatively similar to a recent myocardial infarction.

In a study of 1200 patients with known ischemic heart disease followed in the Coronary Artery Surgery Study (CASS) registry, left ventricular wall-motion abnormality was the most significant independent variable relating to operative morbidity and mortality following noncardiac surgery.[18] The mortality in patients with poor left ventricular function was four times that of patients with normal function, and the nonfatal cardiac complication rate was twice as high in the group with decreased ventricular function.

Pasternac et al. studied 100 patients undergoing lower limb revascularization and found that a diminished ejection fraction was strongly associated with perioperative myocardial infarction and death.[19] (See Table 18–3.) None of the 50 patients with normal ejection fraction had a postoperative infarction despite the fact that 10 had a history of prior infarction and eight had angina. A similar trend was noted by Kazmers et al. for patients undergoing carotid surgery. In this study cardiac complication rates were significantly increased in patients with ejection fractions less than 35%.[20]

Previous Coronary Artery Bypass Surgery

Although no prospective studies have been done, most data suggest that coronary artery bypass grafting (CABG) significantly diminishes subsequent operative cardiac risk for noncardiac surgery. Low mortality rates have been seen in several studies.[21–26] Crawford et al. studied 358 patients undergoing 484 operations after CABG. The overall mortality rate was 1.1 percent, and no patient died of cardiac causes.[21] Three-quarters of the deaths and many of the medical complications occurred in patients who had

surgery within 30 days of CABG. The authors suggest delaying surgery for six weeks to three months after CABG if possible.

The CASS registry contains 1600 patients who had coronary angiograms and subsequent noncardiac surgery.[18] One group of patients had normal coronary arteries. A second group had significant coronary artery disease treated with CABG before the noncardiac surgery. A third group had coronary artery disease that was treated medically. The groups were not completely comparable because those in the second group had more advanced disease, and those in the second and third groups had more angina, left ventricular dysfunction, and more often a history of previous infarction. Nevertheless, the mortality rates for noncardiac surgery were similar for those with normal coronary arteries (0.5 percent) and for those patients after coronary artery bypass surgery (0.9 percent). The mortality rate for the patients with coronary artery disease treated medically was significantly higher (2.4 percent). The authors suggest that coronary artery bypass grafting reduces operative risk in patients with coronary artery disease to that of patients without disease. The postoperative infarction rate was not significantly different among the groups, but the numbers were small. These data do not suggest that coronary artery bypass grafting should be done solely to reduce subsequent operative risk because the mortality rate of coronary artery bypass surgery itself was 2.3 percent in the registry.[27]

These studies predominantly included patients within two to three years of CABG, although some of the patients had had the procedure as long as 12 years earlier. Graft patency declines with time, and it is unclear how long the apparent protective effect of CABG will last. Limited data are available on the risk of noncardiac surgery after angioplasty. In one nonrandomized study, Huber et al. examined the outcome of noncardiac surgery in patients who had undergone coronary angioplasty for ischemic heart disease within the prior three months, most of whom had unstable angina.[28] The cardiac mortality rate was 1.9 percent, and the perioperative mortality rate was 5.6 percent.

Abnormal Preoperative ECG

An abnormal preoperative electrocardiogram may also affect cardiac risk. In Goldman's study, electrocardiographic changes of ischemia,

TABLE 18–3. Relation Between Ejection Fraction and Perioperative MI and Death[19]

Ejection Fraction	No. of Patients	Perioperative MI	Death
> 56%	50	0	0
36–55%	42	8 (20%)	1 (2.5%)
26–35%	8	6 (75%)	1 (12.5%)

nonspecific ST–T wave changes, or conduction abnormalities were associated with an increased risk of cardiac death, although these changes were not identified by multivariate analysis as independent risk factors.[10,29] However, a cardiac rhythm other than sinus or premature atrial contractions and evidence of more than five premature ventricular contractions per minute on the electrocardiogram were independent risk factors for cardiac death.[29]

Larsen et al. also found Q waves, ST abnormalities, conduction defects, and arrhythmias on preoperative ECGs to be associated with an increased risk of cardiac complications.[17] No electrocardiographic abnormality proved to be an independent risk factor. In their study of patients undergoing vascular surgery, Eagle et al. found Q waves on the preoperative echocardiogram to be independent predictors of postoperative ischemic events including death, myocardial infarction, unstable angina, and ischemic pulmonary edema, regardless of the clinical history.[16]

NONCARDIAC FACTORS

Age

In most studies, advanced age, variously defined as over 60, 65, or 70, is independently associated with increased cardiac risk.[10,16–18] In Goldman's series, patients over 70 had an approximately tenfold increased risk of perioperative cardiac death.[10]

Among the elderly, exercise tolerance itself correlates with risk. Gerson et al. studied 100 patients over 65 years of age undergoing noncardiac surgery.[30] Inability to exercise for at least two minutes on a bicycle at a rate of 50 revolutions per minute to a heart rate greater than 99 beats per minute was a strong predictor of perioperative cardiac complications. In a study of preoperative exercise testing, five or six patients with adverse outcomes were unable to exercise to a level of 5 METS.[31] A careful history of exercise tolerance is important in identifying older patients with high risk.

Hypertension

The effect of hypertension on cardiac risk is controversial. In Goldman's study and others, neither preoperative hypertension nor a history of hypertension were predictors of cardiac risk.[10,32] However, in earlier studies[11] and in the CASS registry study[18] of patients with known coronary artery disease, hypertension was associated with significantly increased rate of postoperative complications and death. In addition, poorly controlled hypertension is associated with perioperative hemodynamic changes that may be deleterious to patients with ischemic heart disease.

Anesthetic and Surgical Factors

Both the type and timing of surgery affect cardiac risk. Patients undergoing emergency surgery are up to four times more likely to suffer postoperative myocardial infarction or cardiac death than those undergoing elective procedures.[10,17] Intraabdominal, intrathoracic, and aortic procedures are most commonly associated with increased risk of cardiac complications and cardiac death.[10–12,14–17] Other studies have also demonstrated increased risk in patients undergoing major orthopedic and carotid surgery.[33]

Anesthetic technique does not appear to affect cardiac risk. Cardiac death and perioperative myocardial infarction rates are similar in patients receiving general and spinal anesthesia.[10,11,17,34] In Goldman's study, the incidence of new or worsened congestive heart failure was greater in patients receiving general anesthesia, but overall mortality rate was the same in those getting spinal anesthesia.[10] Local anesthesia may be preferable to general anesthesia when appropriate. One study demonstrated a lower reinfarction rate for ophthalmic surgery done under local anesthesia as compared to general anesthesia in patients with a history of previous myocardial infarction.[35]

Other Factors

Poor medical condition, defined by several investigators to include a creatinine level greater than three, liver disease, hypoxia, electro-

TABLE 18–4.   Goldman's Cardiac Risk Index

Factors	Relative Point Value
History	
1. Age greater than 70 years	5
2. Recent myocardial infarction (within 6 months)	10
Cardiac Exam	
3. Signs of congestive heart failure—S$_3$ gallop or jugular vein distention	11
4. Significant aortic stenosis	3
Electrocardiogram	
5. Preoperative, rhythm other than sinus or premature atrial contractions	7
6. Documentation of 5 or more premature ventricular contractions per minute any time before surgery	7
General Medical Condition (any of the below)	3
7a. Po$_2$ < 60 or Pco$_2$ > 50	
b. Potassium < 3, bicarbonate < 20, BUN > 50, creatinine > 3	
c. Abnormal SGOT or signs of chronic liver disease	
d. Bedridden state due to noncardiac causes	
Operation	
8. Emergency	4
9. Intraperitoneal, intrathoracic, or aortic	3

TABLE 18–5. Modified Cardiac Risk Index

Factors	Relative Point Value
Coronary Artery Disease	
MI within 6 months	10
MI more than 6 months	5
Canadian Cardiovascular Society angina	
Class 3	10
Class 4	20
Unstable angina within 3 months	10
Alveolar Pulmonary Edema	
Within 1 week	10
Ever	5
Valvular Disease	
Suspected critical aortic stenosis	20
Arrhythmias	
Rhythm other than sinus or sinus plus atrial premature beats	5
Greater than 5 premature ventricular contractions	5
*Poor General Medical State**	5
Age > 70 Years	5
Emergency Surgery	10

*Defined as in Goldman's Index (see Table 18–4).

lyte abnormalities, or a requirement to be bedridden, also increases cardiac risk.[10,36] In some studies, diabetes mellitus has proven to be an independent predictor of cardiac complications in patients undergoing vascular surgery.[16,17,36]

Multivariate Indices

In an attempt to combine the many variables affecting surgical risk, Goldman et al. used the results of their multivariate analysis to assign points to various factors and developed an index to stratify overall risk (see Table 18–4).[37] The index was later modified by Detsky et al. to include more severe and unstable angina, a past history of congestive heart failure, and distant myocardial infarction (see Table 18–5).[33,38] Both indices allow overall risk to be estimated (see Table 18–6). Several groups have evaluated the original index and have validated its ability to predict cardiac risk.[39,40]

Larsen et al. developed another multivariate index using data from 2609 patients over age 40 undergoing noncardiac surgery.[17] Active congestive heart failure and recent myocardial infarction were again the most important predictors of cardiac complications.

TABLE 18–6. Cardiac Complication Rate According to Cardiac Risk Index

Type of patient	Goldman et al.	Detsky et al.[33,38]
	Unselected, age > 40 years	Preoperative medical consult requested
Overall complications*	58/1001 (6%)	27/268 (10%)
By Class:		
Class I (0–5 pts.)	5/537 (1%)	8/134 (6%)
Class II (6–12 pts.)	21/316 (7%)	6/85 (7%)
Class III (13–25 pts.)	18/130 (14%)	9/45 (20%)
Class IV (≥ 26 pts.)	14/18 (78%)	4/4 (100%)

*MI, cardiogenic pulmonary edema, ventricular tachycardia, or cardiac death.
Source: Adapted from Goldman et al.[41]

A history of more remote myocardial infarction or heart failure and angina were also independent predictors. These latter factors were included in the Detsky index but not in Goldman's (see Table 18–7).[38,41]

Vascular Surgery

Patients undergoing vascular surgery have a high prevalence of underlying coronary artery disease. Cardiac ischemic events account for more than half of the postoperative complications in these patients.[42,43] The usual measures of risk may underestimate complication rates in this population. Claudication often limits exercise, making a negative history of angina unreliable. Diabetes mellitus is common and may be associated with silent ischemia or infarction.

TABLE 18–7. Significant Predictors of Cardiac Risk

Factors	Relative Point Value
Congestive Heart Failure	
Persistent pulmonary congestion	12
No congestion but previous pulmonary edema	8
Neither of above but previous heart failure	4
Ischemic Heart Disease	
Myocardial infarction within 3 months	11
No MI within 3 months but older infarction and/or angina pectoris	3
Diabetes Mellitus	3
Elevated Serum Creatinine	2
Emergency Operation	3
Major Surgical Procedure	
Aortic operation	5
Other intraperitoneal/pleural operation	3

Source: Adapted from Larsen et al.[17]

In a study by Hertzer et al., routine preoperative coronary angiography in 1000 patients scheduled for elective vascular surgery revealed that 60 percent had significant coronary artery stenosis defined as over 70 percent occlusion of the diameter of the lumen.[42] Thirty-two percent had less severe disease, but only 8 percent had normal coronary arteries. Severe correctable disease with one or more arteries showing significant stenosis supplying an area of unimpaired myocardium was identified in 25 percent of the patients and seen more often in men. Patients with a clinical suspicion of coronary artery disease had a 78 percent incidence of significant coronary artery disease, but patients with no clinical suggestion had a 37 percent incidence of disease. Furthermore, operative mortality was increased fourfold in those with coronary artery disease.

In patients undergoing vascular surgery, a history of diabetes mellitus, congestive heart failure, prior ischemic heart disease, or myocardial infarction increased perioperative cardiac risk. In addition, Eagle et al. used multivariate analysis to show that Q waves on the ECG, diabetes mellitus, a history of angina, a history of ventricular ectopy requiring treatment, and age over 70 were independent predictors of cardiac risk after vascular surgery.[16] Moreover, reversible ischemia on dipyridamole-thallium imaging, decreased ejection fraction on radionuclide angiography, and preoperative ischemia on ambulatory ECG monitoring have also been associated with significantly increased risk in these patients.[19,44–49]

Coronary Artery Surgery

Patients undergoing coronary artery bypass surgery form a special subset with known severe coronary disease. Coronary anatomy and left ventricular function are known before surgery and the procedure is directed toward improvement in coronary artery blood flow.

Risk factors in coronary artery bypass surgery are similar to those associated with cardiac risk in patients undergoing noncardiac surgery. In the CASS registry of 8971 patients undergoing coronary bypass surgery, major determinants of operative mortality included (1) age, (2) symptoms of congestive heart failure and decreased left ventricular function, and (3) need for emergency surgery.[50] Other factors associated with high operative mortality included significant left main coronary artery disease, triple-vessel coronary artery disease, and female sex. History of prior myocardial infarction had no significant effect on operative mortality. History of unstable angina was associated but was not an independent factor in the multivariate analysis. Additional indicated cardiac procedures, especially valvular surgery and aneurysm resection, significantly increased operative risk. Overall operative mortality in this study was 2.4 percent but increased to 10.8 percent for patients undergoing emergency surgery and to 24 percent for patients undergoing both bypass surgery and mitral valve replacement.

PERIOPERATIVE MANAGEMENT

Preoperative Assessment

General recommendations for the perioperative care of patients with coronary artery disease are based on the information reviewed above. Each patient must be assessed individually in light of the extent of coronary artery disease, the presence of other risk factors, and the nature of the planned procedure. Goals of preoperative assessment include (1) identification of risk factors that can be modified before surgery to improve outcome, (2) identification of patients in whom cardiac risk outweighs the benefit of surgery, and (3) determination of whether a patient will benefit from postoperative invasive monitoring and observation in an intensive care unit.

Most cardiac risk factors can be identified with a careful history and physical examination. Details of chest pain history including precipitating factors, frequency and duration, and assessment of exercise tolerance are important in estimating risk. The severity of underlying coronary artery disease may be underestimated in elderly patients and in those limited by orthopedic injuries, neurologic disorders, or peripheral vascular disease. A history of previous myocardial infarction and congestive heart failure is clearly important. Physical examination should include special attention to signs of congestive heart failure such as an S_3 gallop, jugular venous distention, and rales. Valvular heart disease must be identified and its severity estimated. Identifying peripheral vascular disease may provide a clue to underlying coronary artery disease.

It is particularly important to identify those patients with a history of documented or suspected myocardial infarction within six months before the planned surgery. Elective or semi-elective surgery should generally be delayed until six months have passed. Emergency surgery often cannot be delayed in the patient who has had a recent myocardial infarction. However, aggressive perioperative monitoring including right-heart catheterization and close postoperative monitoring may reduce the risk of cardiac complications. In patients needing urgent but not emergent surgery, e.g., resection of a malignancy, surgery should be delayed for at least three months if possible. Exercise testing or assessment of left ventricular function may be useful in more accurately assessing cardiac risk.

Patients with stable exertional angina can safely undergo most surgical procedures. This recommendation assumes careful clinical evaluation of the severity and frequency of symptoms. In selected high-risk situations, as in major vascular surgery, further assessment with noninvasive testing or cardiac catheterization may be indicated.

Congestive heart failure, a common complication of ischemic heart disease and a potent risk factor, must be carefully identified before surgery. In many cases, surgery will have to be postponed to allow optimal treatment. Rapid overnight correction should be discouraged, especially prior to elective surgery, since it can result in electrolyte abnormalities and intravascular volume depletion that may further complicate the surgical procedure.

Electrocardiogram

An ECG is indicated in the preoperative assessment of all patients with known or suspected coronary artery disease or with significant risk factors for coronary artery disease including hypertension, diabetes mellitus, or peripheral vascular disease. It has also been recommended in men over 40 and women over 50 or 55.[5] The preoperative ECG may reveal an unrecognized recent or remote myocardial infarction or unsuspected preoperative arrhythmias. It provides a baseline for comparison should postoperative electrocardiographic abnormalities arise. Some studies indicate that an abnormal baseline ECG may also be an independent predictor of cardiac risk.

Stress Testing

The specific indications for stress testing in the preoperative setting are less clear. Routine exercise testing does not appear to add significantly to clinical evaluation in predicting cardiac risk.[31]

In certain cases exercise testing can clarify risk or select patients for coronary angiography prior to elective surgery. A patient with atypical resting chest pain scheduled for elective abdominal surgery could have unstable angina or benign noncardiac pain. Exercise testing may be useful in this setting to determine the need for preoperative cardiac catheterization. In patients with known coronary artery disease, exercise testing can be useful in determining the ischemic threshold, i.e., the heart rate and systolic blood pressure at which ischemic ST changes and chest pain occur. This information may help determine tolerable blood pressure and heart rate limits in the intraoperative and postoperative setting in order to avoid ischemia.

In general, routine exercise testing is not recommended for patients with stable ischemic heart disease scheduled for noncardiac surgery. In higher-risk patients such as those who have had a recent myocardial infarction or have significant anginal symptoms and need major abdominal, thoracic, or vascular surgery, stress testing may be useful in defining cardiac risk and selecting patients for cardiac catheterization. In patients undergoing major vascular surgery, a lower threshold for preoperative testing is required because of the high prevalence of associated coronary artery disease and greater risk of the procedure.

Investigators have sought noninvasive methods to identify those with serious coronary artery disease without having to resort to cardiac catheterization. McPhail et al. used arm ergometry or treadmill testing to study patients prior to aortic aneurysm resection or aortoiliac surgery.[52] Patients who had ischemic ST changes

and were unable to achieve 85% predicted maximum heart rate had a cardiac complication rate of 33 percent.

Because some patients, including those with peripheral vascular disease, may not tolerate exercise testing, dipyridamole-thallium scanning has been used to look for underlying ischemic heart disease.[53] This method uses dipyridamole to induce an increase in coronary blood flow in nonischemic zones and demonstrate relative decrease in thallium uptake in myocardium supplied by abnormal coronary arteries. Its sensitivity and specificity are similar to those of exercise thallium testing. Several studies demonstrate a strong association between thallium redistribution indicative of reversible ischemia and postoperative cardiac complications in patients undergoing vascular[44-47] and other noncardiac procedures.[54]

Eagle et al. combined clinical factors and results of dipyridamole-thallium scanning to identify independent clinical predictors of ischemic events after vascular surgery.[16] Q waves on the electrocardiogram, history of angina, history of ventricular arrhythmias requiring treatment, medically treated diabetes mellitus, and age over 70 all proved to be independent clinical predictors. Thallium redistribution and ischemic electrocardiographic changes during or after dipyridamole were also strong predictors. The authors suggest that dipyridamole-thallium testing is most useful in predicting risk in patients with one to two of the above clinical risk factors. In those with none, the postoperative ischemic event rate is low regardless of the thallium results. In patients with three or more risk factors, the rate is high regardless of the results of the thallium test (see Table 18–8).

Dipyridamole echocardiography and dobutamine stress thallium imaging have also been used to predict risk in patients undergoing vascular surgery.[55,56]

Ambulatory Electrocardiographic Monitoring

Ambulatory electrocardiographic monitoring can identify and quantify periods of silent myocardial ischemia. The incidence of silent

TABLE 18–8. Use of Dipyridamole-Thallium and Clinical Risk Factors to Predict Cardiac Risk in Vascular Surgery Patients

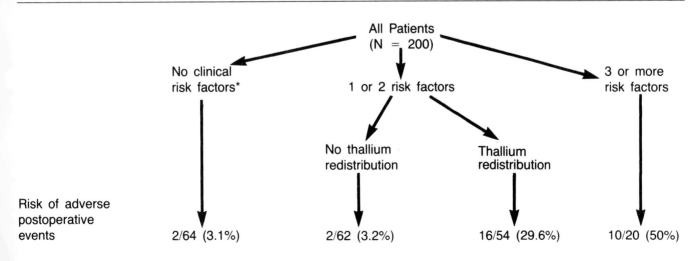

*Clinical risk factors are Q waves on ECG, age > 70, history of angina, history of PVC's requiring treatment, and diabetes requiring treatment.
Source: Adapted from Eagle et al.[47]

ischemia in preoperative patients with coronary artery disease or risk factors for it is 18 to 28 percent. Silent ischemia increases the risk of postoperative ischemic complications.[48,57,58] This testing modality has been used as an alternative to dipyridamole-thallium imaging to predict cardiac risk before vascular surgery.

Cardiac Catheterization

The indications for cardiac catheterization prior to nonemergency surgery include the usual medical indications like unstable or medically refractory angina. Catheterization is also potentially useful in patients with less severe angina and markedly positive exercise dipyridamole-thallium tests who are scheduled for high-risk procedures. In selected cases, catheterization will lead to angioplasty or coronary artery bypass surgery before noncardiac surgery if the risk of both procedures performed sequentially is acceptable. Simultaneous coronary artery bypass grafting and noncardiac surgery, like carotid endarterectomy or abdominal aortic aneurysm repair, have been performed with acceptable mortality rates when both problems require urgent correction.[59]

Perioperative Monitoring

Careful hemodynamic monitoring is essential in patients with ischemic heart disease. Hypotension, hypertension, and tachycardia are poorly tolerated in these patients. These hemodynamic changes, especially hypotension, are associated with an increased risk of intraoperative ischemia and reinfarction in patients with a history of prior myocardial infarction.[11,14] Strict control of hemodynamic variations significantly decreases the incidence of intraoperative myocardial infarction.[14]

Routine intraoperative electrocardiographic monitoring for ischemic ST changes has become common. At least two leads should be used, including lead II and lead V_5.[1] ST changes can be misleading and occur in both the presence and absence of hemodynamic changes. They have been associated with an increased incidence of perioperative myocardial infarction independent of hemodynamic changes.[2,49] Identification of such changes allows alteration in anesthetic management and/or addition of anti-ischemic agents such as intravenous nitroglycerin.

Pulmonary artery catheters allow for accurate assessment of left ventricular filling pressure, cardiac output, and systemic vascular resistance and may be useful in the hemodynamic management of high-risk cardiac patients. Need for it should be determined on an individual basis by the medical consultant, surgeon, and anesthesiologist. Appropriate candidates for this form of monitoring include patients with a history of recent myocardial infarction, those with a history of significant congestive heart failure and/or left ventricular dysfunction, and those with significant coronary artery disease scheduled for major thoracic, vascular, or intraabdominal procedures.

Postoperative Care

Sixty to eighty percent of perioperative myocardial infarctions occur postoperatively with a peak incidence on the third postoperative day.[11,12,14,15] Up to 60 percent of these are not associated with chest pain but instead present with unexplained hypotension, congestive heart failure, cardiac arrhythmias, or altered mental status.

High-risk cardiac patients should therefore be monitored in an intensive care unit for at least three days after surgery. During this period, they should have serial cardiac enzyme measurements and ECG's as well as continuous monitoring of cardiac rhythm. Volume status, vital signs, and physical examination must be followed closely and surgical pain appropriately treated.

Electrocardiographic changes may also be unreliable. Breslow et al. noted that nonspecific T-wave changes were seen in 19 percent of patients without clinical evidence of coronary artery disease or ischemia and were especially common after abdominal surgery.[60] Nondiagnostic ST-segment changes were less frequent and were therefore felt to be a more reliable indicator of cardiac ischemia.

Silent ischemic ST changes are common after surgery in patients with known coronary artery disease or those with risk factors for it.[61] In the study by Mangano et al., ischemic ST changes occurred in 41 percent of such patients and proved to be a strong predictor of adverse cardiac outcome with a ninefold increase in cardiac death, myocardial infarction, or unstable angina. New ST changes on ECG or ambulatory ECG monitoring are clinically significant and should prompt initiation of or change in the antiischemic regimen.[58]

Cardiac enzymes may be similarly difficult to interpret in the postoperative setting. Lactic dehydrogenase (LDH) and creatine phosphokinase (CK) may be elevated by the trauma of surgery. The CK-MB fraction is more specific for myocardial damage but may become negative 24 hours after a myocardial infarction. If serial electrocardiograms and CK-isoenzymes do not resolve the question of possible postoperative myocardial infarction, radionuclide imaging with technetium pyrophosphate may show diagnostic changes for one week after the event. However, false negative results are common after a small myocardial infarction.

COMMONLY USED MEDICATIONS IN THE PERIOPERATIVE PERIOD

Beta-Blockers

Nonselective and selective beta-blockers are commonly used in patients with ischemic heart disease, including those who have had a myocardial infarction and those with angina. The use of these agents in the perioperative setting was controversial in the past.[62] It was felt that the cardiac depressant effects of beta-blockers and many anesthetic agents could cause hemodynamic instability. However, the abrupt discontinuation of beta-blockers can result in hemodynamic changes such as tachycardia, hypertension, and cardiac ischemia. There may be benefit in blunting the effects of increased circulating catecholamines associated with intubation and surgical manipulation in this setting.

The safety of continuing beta-blockers before surgery has been well-documented in patients undergoing coronary artery bypass surgery.[63] Kaplan and Dunbar have also demonstrated the safety of continuing propranolol before noncardiac surgery as well.[64,65] It is therefore recommended that beta-blockers be continued up until the day of surgery with an additional dose given on the morning of surgery.

The immediate postoperative use of beta-blockers depends on the hemodynamic stability of the patient. In stable patients, a short period of cessation of beta-blockers is well-tolerated, and the agent can be restarted when the patient is able to take oral medication. Clinical effects of propranolol, one of the beta-blockers with the shortest half-life, have been documented to persist for 24 to 48 hours after discontinuation of the drug.[64] Patients who are more unstable can develop signs of beta-blocker withdrawal or angina earlier. Intravenous beta-blockers can be given as small intravenous boluses of metoprolol or propranolol, or continuous infusion of propranolol or esmolol can be titrated to the desired hemodynamic effect.[66]

Nitrates

Oral nitrates are commonly used by patients with ischemic heart disease. Intravenous nitroglycerin reduces ischemic ST changes during noncardiac surgery in patients with ischemic heart disease.[67,68] Like beta-blockers, nitrates are safe in the perioperative setting and can be beneficial. In stable patients, topical nitroglycerin can be used intraoperatively and postoperatively in place of oral nitrates. In patients with more severe disease, especially in those with unstable angina, intravenous nitroglycerin is recommended intraoperatively to allow titration of dose to blood pressure response and resolution of ischemic changes on the monitor. Intravenous nitroglycerin can also be used postoperatively in the unstable patient. Nitrate tolerance can develop after 24 to 48 hours of continuous infusion of nitroglycerin and with topical oral nitrates given without a nitrate-free period.[69] Intravenous nitroglycerin can also be useful in treating labile hypertension in the intraoperative and immediate postoperative setting in patients with coronary artery disease. Intravenous nitroprusside has the disadvantage of potentially redistributing myocardial blood flow away from ischemic zones and producing a "steal" phenomenon and subsequent increased ischemia.[70]

Calcium Channel Blockers

There is less information about the effects of calcium channel blockers in perioperative patients. Theoretically, calcium channel blockers can potentiate the myocardial depressant and vasodilatory effects of anesthetic agents, but the clinical significance of these effects is unknown. Godet et al. found that intravenous diltiazem was associated with improvement in ST-segment changes in patients with coronary artery disease undergoing vascular surgery.[71] At present, it is recommended that oral calcium channel blockers be continued in the preoperative setting without significant hemodynamic risk.[60] They can be restarted postoperatively when the patient is able to take oral medications. If they are required before bowel function returns, sublingual nifedipine or a continuous infusion of verapamil in a dose of 0.005 mg/kg/min can be used.

SUMMARY

1. Overall cardiac risk, including myocardial infarction, pulmonary edema, ventricular tachycardia, or cardiac death, is increased by previous myocardial infarction; congestive heart failure; some electrocardiographic abnormalities; age over 70; the need for major intraabdominal, intrathoracic, or vascular surgery; and poor medical condition. Stable angina and hypertension have been found to be additional risk factors in some studies. Although all types of anesthetics have cardiovascular effects, the choice of anesthetic technique, whether general or spinal/epidural, does not affect risk. The criteria developed by Goldman have been validated by other investigators and are useful in estimating risk.

2. Preoperative assessment of surgical patients should be directed at identification of risk factors on history, physical examination, and the ECG. Elective surgery in those with a history of prior myocardial infarction within six months of the procedure should be postponed.

3. Routine stress testing is not indicated before surgery, but may be useful in patients with unexplained chest pain and in those with cardiac risk factors undergoing major abdominal, thoracic, or vascular surgery who might benefit from cardiac catheterization. Patients undergoing major vascular procedures have a high prevalence of associated coronary artery disease, and the threshold for testing should therefore be lower. Dipyridamole-thallium imaging and ambulatory ECG monitoring are alternatives to exercise stress testing.

4. Continuous electrocardiographic monitoring during surgery and after surgery is indicated in all patients with known or suspected coronary artery disease. Hemodynamic monitoring is recommended in patients with severe coronary disease undergoing major abdominal, thoracic, or vascular procedures; those with a history of a recent myocardial infarction; and those with a history of congestive heart failure or left ventricular dysfunction.

5. Most perioperative myocardial infarctions occur after surgery and peak on the third postoperative day. Chest pain may be absent. ECG changes are common after surgery and may be misleading. Those representing silent ischemia are associated with an adverse outcome and should prompt initiation of or change in antianginal therapy.

6. Beta-blockers and nitrates can be safely continued until surgery and used intravenously in the perioperative period. Patients on beta-blockers who develop withdrawal tachycardia and elevated blood pressure if the drug is withheld can be effectively treated with short-acting intravenous beta-blockers like propranolol or esmolol. Since tolerance to continuous infusion of nitrates can develop, intermittent therapy with nitrate-free periods are recommended. Calcium channel blockers can also be used in the perioperative period, but data regarding their efficacy is scant.

REFERENCES

1. Roy WL, Edelist G, Gilbert B: Myocardial ischemia during noncardiac surgical procedures in patients with coronary artery disease. *Anesthesiology* 51:393, 1972.
2. Slogoff S, Keats AS: Further observations on perioperative myocardial ischemia. *Anesthesiology* 65:539, 1986.
3. Kleinman B, Henkin RE, Glisson SN et al: Qualitative evaluation of coronary flow during anesthetic induction using thallium-201 perfusion scan. *Anesthesiology* 64:157, 1986.
4. Reiz S: Myocardial ischemia associated with general anaesthesia. *Br J Anaesth* 61:68, 1988.
5. Moffitt EA, Sethna DH: The coronary circulation and myocardial oxygenation in coronary artery disease: Effects of anesthesia. *Anesth Analg* 65:395, 1986.

6. Mangano DT, Hollenberg M, Fegert G et al: Perioperative myocardial ischemia in patients undergoing noncardiac surgery: I. Incidence and severity during the four-day perioperative period. *JACC* 17:843, 1991.

7. Mangano DT, Wong MG, London MT et al: Perioperative myocardial ischemia in patients undergoing noncardiac surgery: II. Incidence and severity during the first week after surgery. *JACC* 17:851, 1991.

8. Conahan TJ: Anesthetic considerations in coronary artery disease, in Utley: *Perioperative Cardiac Dysfunction*. Baltimore, Williams & Wilkins, 1985, vol 3.

9. Well PH, Kaplan JA: Optimal management of patients with ischemic heart disease for noncardiac surgery by complementary anesthesiologist and cardiologist interaction. *Am Heart J* 102:1029, 1981.

10. Goldman L, Caldera DL, Southwick FS et al: Cardiac risk factors and complications in noncardiac surgery. *Medicine* 57:357, 1978.

11. Steen PA, Tinker JH, Tarhan S: Myocardial reinfarction after anesthesia and surgery. *JAMA* 239:2566, 1978.

12. Tarhan S, Moffitt EA, Taylor WF et al: Myocardial infarction after general anesthesia. *JAMA* 220:1451, 1972.

13. Topkins MJ, Artusio JF: Myocardial infarction and surgery. *Anesth Analg* 43:716, 1964.

14. Rao TLK, Jacobs KH, El-Etr AA: Reinfarction following anesthesia in patients with myocardial infarction. *Anesthesiology* 59:499, 1983.

15. Becker RC, Underwood DA: Myocardial infarction in patients undergoing noncardiac surgery. *Cleve Clin J Med* 54:25, 1987.

16. Eagle KA, Coley CM, Newell JB et al: Combining clinical and thallium data optimizes preoperative assessment of cardiac risk before major vascular surgery. *Ann Intern Med* 110:859, 1989.

17. Larsen SF, Olesen KH, Jacobsen E et al: Prediction of cardiac risk in noncardiac surgery. *Eur Heart J* 8:179, 1987.

18. Foster ED, Dans KB, Carpenter JA et al: Risk of noncardiac operation in patients with defined coronary disease: The coronary artery surgery study (CASS) registry experience. *Annals of Thor Surg* 41:42, 1986.

19. Pasternac PF, Imparato AM, Riles TS et al: The value of the radionuclide angiogram in the prediction of perioperative myocardial infarction in patients undergoing lower extremity revascularization procedures. *Circ* 72(Supp II):11–13, 1985.

20. Kazmers A, Cerqueira MD, Zierter RE: The role of preoperative radionuclide left ventricular ejection fraction for risk assessment in carotid surgery. *Arch Surg* 123:416, 1988.

21. Crawford ES, Moms GC, Howell JF et al: Operative risk in patients with previous coronary artery bypass. *Ann Thorac Surg* 26:215, 1978.

22. Crunchley PM, Kaplan JA, Hug CC et al: Noncardiac surgery in patients with prior myocardial revascularization. *Can Anaesth Soc J* 30:629, 1983.

23. Fudge TL, McKinnon WMP, Schoettle GP et al: Improved operative risk after myocardial revascularization. *South Med J* 74:799, 1981.

24. Mahar LT, Steen PA, Tinker JH et al: Perioperative myocardial infarction in patients with coronary artery disease with and without aorta-coronary artery bypass grafts. *J Thorac Cardiovasc Surg* 76:533, 1978.

25. McCollum CH, Garcia-Rinaldi R, Graham JM et al: Myocardial revascularization prior to subsequent major surgery in patients with coronary artery disease. *Surgery* 81:302, 1977.

26. Prorok JJ, Trostle D: Operative risk of general surgical procedures in patients with previous myocardial revascularization. *Surg Gyn Obstet* 159:214, 1984.

27. Kennedy JW, Kaiser GC, Fisher LD et al: Clinical and angiographic predictions of operative mortality from the collaborative study in coronary artery surgery (CASS). *Circulation* 63:793, 1981.

28. Huber KC, Evans MA, Bresnahan JF: Outcome of noncardiac operations with severe coronary artery disease successfully treated preoperatively with coronary angioplasty. *Mayo Clin Proc* 67:15, 1992.

29. Goldman L: Multifactorial index of cardiac risk in noncardiac surgery —a 10-year status report. *J Cardiothor Anesth* 1:237, 1987.

30. Gerson MC, Hurst JM, Hertzberg VS et al: Cardiac prognosis in noncardiac geriatric surgery. *Ann Int Med* 103:832, 1985.

31. Carliner NH, Fisher ML, Plotnick GD et al: Routine preoperative exercise testing in patients undergoing major noncardiac surgery. *Amer J Card* 56:51, 1985.

32. Cooperman M, Pflug B, Martin EW et al: Cardiovascular risk factors in patients with peripheral vascular disease. *Surgery* 84:505, 1978.

33. Detsky AS, Abrams HB, McLaughlin JR et al: Predicting cardiac complications in patients undergoing noncardiac surgery. *J Gen Int Med* 1:211, 1986.

34. Haagensen R, Steen PA: Perioperative myocardial infarction. *Br J Anaesth* 61:24, 1988.

35. Backer GL, Tinker JH, Robertson DM et al: Myocardial reinfarction following local anesthesia for ophthalmic surgery. *Anesth Analg* 59:257, 1980.

36. Browner WS, Li J, Mangano DT et al: In-hospital and long-term mortality in male veterans following noncardiac surgery. *JAMA* 268:228, 1992.

37. Goldman L, Caldera DL, Nussbaum SR et al: Multifactorial index of cardiac risk in noncardiac surgical procedures. *N Engl J Med* 297:845, 1977.

38. Detsky AS, Abrams HB, Forbath N et al: Cardiac assessment for patients undergoing noncardiac surgery. *Arch Intern Med* 146:2131, 1986.

39. Jeffrey CC, Kunsimar J, Cullen DJ et al: A preoperative evaluation of cardiac risk index. *Anesth* 58:462, 1983.

40. Zeldin RA, Math B: Assessing cardiac risk in patients who undergo noncardiac surgical procedures. *Can J Surg* 27:402, 1984.

41. Goldman L: Assessment of the patient with known or suspected ischemic heart disease for noncardiac surgery. *Br J Anaesth* 61:38, 1988.

42. Hertzer NR, Beven EG, Young JR et al: Coronary artery disease in peripheral vascular patients. *Ann Surg* 199:223, 1984.

43. Gersh BJ, Rihal CS, Rooke TW et al: Evaluation and management of patients with both peripheral vascular and coronary artery disease. *JACC* 18:203, 1991.

44. Boucher CA, Brewster DC, Darling RC et al: Determination of cardiac risk by dipyridamole-thallium imaging before peripheral vascular surgery. *N Engl J Med* 312:389, 1985.

45. Cutler BS, Leppo JA: Dipyridamole thallium-201 scintigraphy to detect coronary artery disease before abdominal aortic surgery. *J Vasc Surg* 5:91, 1987.

46. Leppo J, Plaja J, Gionet M et al: Noninvasive evaluation of cardiac risk before elective vascular surgery. *JACC* 9:269, 1987.

47. Eagle KA, Singer DE, Brewster DC et al: Dipyridamole-thallium scanning in patients undergoing vascular surgery. *JAMA* 257:2185, 1987.

48. Raby EK, Goldman L, Creager MA et al: Correlation between preoperative ischemia and major cardiac events after peripheral vascular surgery. *N Engl J Med* 321:1296, 1989.

49. Raby KE, Barry J, Creager MA et al: Detection and significance of intraoperative and postoperative myocardial ischemia in peripheral vascular surgery. *JAMA* 268:222, 1992.

50. Myers WO, Marshfield WI, Davis K et al: Surgical survival in the coronary artery surgery study (CASS) registry. *Ann Thorac Surg* 40:245, 1985.

51. Goldberger AL, O'Konski M: Utility of the routine electrocardiograph before surgery and on general hospital admission. Critical review and new guidelines. *Ann Int Med* 105:552, 1986.

52. McPhail N, Calvin JE, Shariatmadar A: The use of preoperative exercise testing to predict cardiac complications after arterial reconstruction. *J Vasc Surg* 7:60, 1988.

53. Iskandrian AS, Heo J, Askenase A et al: Dipyridamole cardiac imaging. *Am Heart J* 115:432, 1988.

54. Coley CM, Fiedl TS, Abraham SA et al: Usefulness of dipyridamole-thallium scanning for preoperative evaluation of cardiac risk for nonvascular surgery. *Amer J Card* 69:1280, 1992.

55. Elliott BM, Robinson JG, Zellner JL et al: Dobutamine-201 Tl imaging. *Circulation* 84(III):54, 1991.

56. Tischler MD, Lee TH, Hirsch AT et al: Prediction of major cardiac

events after peripheral vascular surgery using dipyridamole echocardiography. *Amer J Card* 68:593, 1991.

57. Fleisher LA, Rosenbaum SH, Nelson AH et al: The predictive value of preoperative silent ischemia for postoperative ischemic cardiac events in vascular and nonvascular surgery patients. *Amer Heart J* 122:980, 1991.

58. Mangano DT, Browner WS, Hollenberg M et al: Association of perioperative myocardiac ischemic with coronary morbidity and mortality in men undergoing noncardiac surgery. *N Engl J Med* 323:1781, 1990.

59. Reul GJ, Cooley DA, Duncan JM et al: The effect of coronary bypass in the outcome of peripheral vascular operations in 1093 patients. *J Vasc Surg* 3:788, 1986.

60. Breslow MJ, Miller CF, Parker SD et al: Changes in T wave morphology following anesthesia and surgery. A common recovery-room phenomenon. *Anesthesiology* 64:398, 1986.

61. Hollenberg M, Mangano DT, Browner WS et al: Predictors of postoperative myocardial ischemia in patients undergoing noncardiac surgery. *JAMA* 268:205, 1992.

62. Cygan R, Waitzkin H: Stopping and restarting medications in the perioperative period. *J Gen Int Med* 2:270, 1987.

63. Kopriva CJ, Brown AC, Pappas G: Hemodynamics during general anesthesia in patients receiving propranolol. *Anesthesiology* 48:28, 1978.

64. Kaplan JA, Dunbar RW: Propranolol and surgical anesthesia. *Anesth Anal* 55:1, 1976.

65. Kaplan JA, Dunbar RW, Bland JW et al: Propranolol and cardiac surgery: A problem for the anesthesiologist? *Anesth Analg* 54:571, 1975.

66. Smulyan H, Weinberg SE, Howanitz PJ: Continuous propranolol infusion following abdominal surgery. *JAMA* 247:2539, 1982.

67. Coriat P, Daloz M, Bousseau D et al: Prevention of intraoperative myocardial ischemia during noncardiac surgery with intravenous nitroglycerin. *Anesthesiology* 61:193, 1984.

68. Fusciardi J, Godet G, Bernard JM et al: Roles of fentanyl and nitroglycerin in prevention of myocardial ischemia associated with laryngoscopy and tracheal intubation in patients undergoing operations of short duration. *Anesth Analg* 65:617, 1986.

69. Thadani U, Whitsett T, Hamilton SF: Nitrate therapy for myocardial ischemic syndrome: Current perspectives including tolerance. *Curr Publ Cardiol* 11, 1988.

70. Chiariello M, Gold HK, Leinbach RC et al: Comparison between the effects of nitroprusside and nitroglycerin on ischemic injury during acute myocardial infarction. *Circulation* 54:766, 1976.

71. Godet G, Coriat P, Baron JF et al: Prevention of intraoperative myocardial ischemia during noncardiac surgery with intravenous diltiazem. *Anesthesiology* 66:241, 1987.

19 THE SURGICAL PATIENT WITH CONGESTIVE HEART FAILURE

Howard J. Eisen

Cardiomyopathy is intrinsic myocardial disease resulting from a variety of disorders including coronary artery disease, myocarditis, hypertension, valvular heart disease, and exposure to drugs and toxins like anthracyclines and alcohol. Patients with cardiomyopathy may at first be asymptomatic but ultimately develop signs and symptoms of congestive heart failure. Cardiomyopathy and congestive heart failure are the end results of a diverse group of disease processes.

CONGESTIVE HEART FAILURE AS A PERIOPERATIVE RISK FACTOR

Congestive heart failure is associated with significant mortality. Epidemiological data from the Framingham study indicate poor five-year survival in both men and women with congestive heart failure.[1] Decompensated congestive heart failure has been recognized for several years to be a risk factor in the development of significant perioperative morbidity and mortality.[2,3] Skinner and Pearce demonstrated that operative mortality correlates with severity of congestive heart failure.[4] Stratified by the New York Heart Association Functional Classification, mortality rate is 4 percent in Class I heart failure, 11 percent in Class II, 25 percent in Class III, and 67 percent in Class IV.

Goldman et al. similarly identified congestive heart failure as an important risk factor for perioperative morbidity and mortality.[3] In this study of 1001 patients over age 40 who underwent major noncardiac surgery, clinical evidence of congestive heart failure as indicated by a third heart sound or jugular venous distention was identified as the most significant risk factor. Of 35 patients with these findings, five or 14 percent had life-threatening but nonfatal cardiac complications, and seven or 20 percent suffered cardiac death. Patients without these findings had a 3.5 percent incidence of life-threatening but nonfatal cardiac complications and a 1.2 percent incidence of cardiac death. Independent risk factors more likely to occur in patients with congestive heart failure include (1) more than five premature ventricular contractions per minute documented preoperatively; (2) rhythm other than sinus or premature atrial contractions; and (3) poor general medical condition including a blood urea nitrogen level (BUN) of greater than 50, creatinine level greater than 3.0 mg/dl, and an abnormal SGOT level or other evidence of chronic liver disease.

Zeldin applied Goldman's cardiac risk index to 1140 prospectively studied patients over age 40 and verified his findings.[5] Detsky et al. prospectively studied 455 patients referred for cardiovascular evaluation before noncardiac surgery. They applied Goldman's original criteria as well as criteria from another modified multifactorial index[6,7] and found that the latter index provided additional information about risk. Both pulmonary edema within one week of surgery and a more remote history of pulmonary edema were identified as independent risk factors. Thus, several groups have identified congestive heart failure as an important risk factor in the perioperative setting.

In Goldman's study, clinical manifestations of congestive heart failure like dyspnea, orthopnea, and edema correlated with the development of intraoperative or postoperative congestive heart failure.[8] Risk ratios, defined as the relative risk of perioperative cardiac death in patients with a particular finding compared to those without these findings, were 5:1 for patients with rales on chest examination, cardiomegaly on chest x-ray, murmur of mitral regurgitation, abnormal ST segments or T waves, and congestive heart failure unresponsive to treatment; 14:1 for those with a history of pulmonary edema; and 20:1 for those with S_3 gallop, jugular venous distention, or cardiac rhythm other than normal sinus rhythm or atrial fibrillation. Not surprisingly, signs and symptoms of preoperative congestive heart failure are strongly associated with later development of pulmonary edema or exacerbation of congestive heart failure. Perioperative cardiac arrhythmias were seen in approximately 10 percent of patients with functionally significant congestive heart failure as compared to 3.9 percent in the general population.

PREDICTORS OF PERIOPERATIVE RISK FOR CARDIOVASCULAR MORBIDITY AND MORTALITY

Limitation in exercise tolerance can be obtained from the patient's history and further defined according to the New York Heart Association Functional Classification. Patients in class I have no limitation; those in class II have mild limitation with heavy exercise but are asymptomatic with daily activities; those in class III have limitation with ordinary activities such as walking three blocks or climbing one flight of stairs; and those in Class IV have dyspnea at rest.[9] This classification yields significant prognostic information about survival in patients with congestive heart failure.[10]

Goldman reviewed the correlation between preoperative heart failure and worsened postoperative heart failure.[3,8,11] A prior history of failure but none at the time of evaluation for surgery was associated with a 6 percent incidence of pulmonary edema and a 16 percent incidence of worsened heart failure. If the patient had heart failure in the past that persisted, there was a 16 percent incidence of worsened heart failure. The New York Heart Association Functional Classification also proved helpful in predicting risk of postoperative pulmonary edema and exacerbations in heart failure. Those in NYHA class I had a 3 percent incidence of pulmonary edema and a 5 percent incidence of worsened heart failure. In NYHA class II, the rates were 7 percent for both pulmonary edema and worsened congestive failure. In class III, the rates were 6 percent and 18 percent, respectively. In class IV, they were 25 percent and 31 percent, respectively. A history of pulmonary edema yields rates of 23 percent and 32 percent, respectively, and others have confirmed the importance of this historical factor.[6,7] More recently, exercise stress testing with respiratory gas analysis has been shown by Mancini et al. to be useful in predicting survival in patients with congestive heart failure.[12] However, the utility of this technique in perioperative risk assessment remains uncertain.

Three clinical signs are highly predictive of postoperative pulmonary edema and worsened heart failure. Jugular venous distention leads to a 30 percent incidence of pulmonary edema and a 35 percent incidence of worsened heart failure. Presence of a third heart sound correlates with a 35 percent incidence of pulmonary edema and a 47 percent incidence of worsened heart failure. Rales on physical exam or pulmonary infiltrates on chest x-ray yield rates of 16 percent and 26 percent, respectively. Development of pulmonary edema is an ominous event. Of those in Goldman's group who developed pulmonary edema, 57 percent died. Those who developed mild congestive heart failure postoperatively had a more benign course, with a 15 percent mortality rate but with no cardiac deaths.[3,8]

Additional risk factors in the development of postoperative congestive heart failure include age over 60, asymptomatic electrocardiographic abnormalities, and certain types of surgery. These include intrathoracic, intraperitoneal, and aortic procedures, all of which involve substantial fluid shifts. Twenty-three or 5 percent undergoing these major procedures had postoperative pulmonary edema while 11 or 2.5 percent suffered a myocardial infarction or cardiac death. In contrast, of patients undergoing less extensive procedures, only two or 0.4 percent developed pulmonary edema, seven or 1 percent had a myocardial infarction, and eight or 1 percent suffered a cardiac death. The duration of surgery had no

bearing on the development of cardiac complications.[3,8] Emergency operations always carry higher perioperative risk of cardiovascular morbidity and mortality.[3,6–8,11] In Goldman's series, a fourfold increase in mortality was noted in the emergency setting.[3]

As noted earlier, findings of preoperative congestive heart failure are associated with a higher incidence of myocardial infarction and arrhythmias. Historical factors of dyspnea and orthopnea carry an increased risk of postoperative myocardial infarction.[8] Although preoperative congestive failure is associated with higher risk of postoperative pulmonary edema, history alone does not always predict this complication. In Goldman's study, 21 of 36 patients who developed postoperative pulmonary edema did not have a prior history of heart failure. Almost all of the 21 were elderly, had abnormal electrocardiograms, and underwent major surgery.[8] Thus, prediction of postoperative congestive heart failure is limited by the lack of definite preoperative markers.

Two particular etiologies of congestive heart failure, ischemic cardiomyopathy and valvular heart disease, carry separate independent risks of morbidity and mortality above and beyond that associated with heart failure alone. Failure is a frequent result of the ischemic cardiomyopathy of coronary artery disease. The majority of these patients (64 to 85 percent) have a history of prior myocardial infarction,[13] but 10 to 15 percent do not. The risk indices of Goldman and Detsky indicate that these patients have a substantially higher risk of perioperative cardiac morbidity and mortality than patients with congestive heart failure but no prior myocardial infarction.

Patients with chronic stable exertional angina alone have a lower perioperative cardiac morbidity of 2.4 percent.[14,15] Though exact data are lacking, those with congestive heart failure and chronic stable exertional angina most likely have a higher risk of complications because of their congestive failure. Patients with angina at rest or unstable angina have a significantly greater risk of suffering a perioperative cardiac event.[11,15,16] Congestive heart failure, as an independent risk factor, no doubt contributes to this risk.

Congestive heart failure is a late result of severe valvular heart disease and is common in untreated aortic stenosis, aortic insufficiency, and mitral regurgitation. Studies reveal that 20 percent of patients with severe valvular heart disease develop new or exacerbated perioperative heart failure.[5,15] Critical or severe aortic stenosis carries an especially significant risk of perioperative morbidity and mortality in the studies of Goldman and Detsky.[3,6–8] Congestive heart failure as well as angina and syncope are considered ominous in aortic stenosis and portend an average survival of 1½ years.[17] Hemodynamically significant aortic stenosis and congestive heart failure are additive risks that dramatically increase the likelihood of perioperative cardiac morbidity and mortality.

Chronic aortic insufficiency and mitral regurgitation cause increased volume load on the left ventricle. These valvular lesions, if severe and longstanding, can also lead to congestive heart failure. Though not specifically identified as a risk factor in the literature, impairment of left ventricular function increases perioperative risk. In aortic insufficiency, the amount of valvular regurgitation is not as significant as the degree of left ventricular impairment.[15] Patients with mitral regurgitation may also have left ventricular impairment and need to be watched for the development of failure.

PREOPERATIVE EVALUATION

Patients with congestive heart failure undergoing noncardiac surgery require extensive evaluation to define the nature of their cardiac disease, the degree of their left ventricular impairment, and the extent of their functional limitations.[15-21] The history should elicit symptoms of congestive heart failure and determine the level of exercise impairment using the New York Heart Association Functional Classification as a guideline. Response to medications like diuretics, vasodilators, and oral inotropes should be documented. A history of prior myocardial infarction, especially within the last six months, is an important historical point. If the patient has angina, its pattern and the degree of exertion required to provoke it should be defined. History of valvular heart disease should be elicited including a past history of rheumatic fever.

A careful physical examination is crucial to look for the important risk factors of jugular venous distention, an S_3 gallop, and pulmonary rales. A laterally displaced diffuse point of maximal impulse is another indicator of left ventricular dysfunction. Signs of right heart failure like a right ventricular heave, palpable gallop, pedal edema, ascites, and hepatomegaly should be noted. Careful attention to the location, quality, and intensity of cardiac murmurs is essential. Evidence of aortic stenosis may be inferred from the presence of pulsus parvus et tardus or a crescendo-decrescendo murmur heard in the aortic area that radiates to the carotid arteries. The holosystolic murmur of mitral regurgitation and the decrescendo diastolic murmur of aortic insufficiency should be noted. If the nature or severity of a murmur is uncertain, echocardiography is especially useful for clarification.

The 12-lead electrocardiogram provides important information in defining perioperative risk. Past myocardial infarction as indicated by pathologic Q waves, evidence of right ventricular dysfunction implied by right ventricular hypertrophy, rhythms other than sinus, or the presence of more than five premature ventricular contractions per minute are all important factors. If significant ventricular ectopy is suspected, a 24-hour Holter monitor or telemetry can quantify overall frequency.

Hypokalemia and hypomagnesemia are frequent laboratory abnormalities in patients taking diuretics. Preoperative measurements of these electrolytes as well as digitalis and antiarrhythmic drug levels should be obtained.

Noninvasive cardiac imaging techniques play an important role in the assessment of cardiovascular disease. Multiple uptake gated acquisition (MUGA) scans, also known as radionuclide ventriculography, can define left and right ventricular ejection fractions, chamber sizes, and the presence of left ventricular wall-motion abnormalities indicative of ischemic heart disease. Left ventricular ejection fraction, as determined by MUGA scan, has been shown to be an important predictor of survival in patients with myocardial infarction[22,23] and congestive heart failure.[24] Lazor et al. retrospectively studied mortality rates of 196 patients undergoing noncardiac surgery within 60 days of obtaining a MUGA scan to determine left ventricular ejection fraction (LVEF).[25] Patients with a LVEF greater than 55% had a mortality rate of 2.2 percent. Those with a LVEF of 36 to 54% had a mortality rate of 5.4 percent. However, those with a LVEF of less than 35% had a mortality rate of 19.5 percent. More recently, the use of MUGA scans to assess left ventricular function has been evaluated prospectively by Pedersen.[26] In those patients with left ventricular

ejection fractions less than 50% or more than 70%, the cardiac complication rate was 58 percent, as compared to 12 percent in those with normal ejection fractions. Consequently, this author recommends that a noninvasive assessment of ventricular function be obtained in patients with congestive heart failure before surgery. In patients with suspicious murmurs or other findings of significant valvular disease, echocardiography is especially useful in determining the significance of valvular disease and quantitating transvalvular gradients.

The history, physical examination, and electrocardiogram are usually sufficient for estimating risk contributed by coronary artery disease. To obtain objective assessments of NYHA Functional Classification and severity of congestive heart failure, exercise stress tests with respiratory gases can be performed to measure maximal oxygen consumption.[12,27] This is helpful in patients with an ambiguous history of exercise limitation and can be combined with thallium imaging to assess regional myocardial perfusion and to look for evidence of ischemia. Routine exercise stress testing is not generally required in the majority of patients.[11,15] Cardiac catheterization should be reserved for those patients with severe angina who require delineation of their coronary artery anatomy or for those with severe valvular disease. Routine cardiac catheterization with angiography is not recommended.

In patients with severely decompensated congestive heart failure or undergoing procedures associated with large fluid shifts, it may be necessary to place a pulmonary artery catheter to measure the cardiac output, pulmonary arterial pressures, left atrial filling pressure, and pulmonary arterial oxygen saturation. This may be invaluable in guiding therapy directed at improving cardiac function and treating congestive failure.

PERIOPERATIVE MANAGEMENT

History, physical examination, electrocardiogram, laboratory tests, and noninvasive studies usually provide enough information to decide whether or not to delay or cancel surgery. Elective surgery should be cancelled or delayed in patients with clinical evidence of decompensated congestive heart failure as indicated by a third heart sound, jugular venous distention, or pulmonary rales. New atrial fibrillation, atrial fibrillation with an uncontrolled ventricular rate, atrial flutter, supraventricular tachycardia, or ventricular tachycardia as well as unstable angina, angina at rest, or hemodynamically aortic stenosis also necessitates postponement or cancellation until definitive diagnostic and therapeutic measures can be taken.[14-21]

Patients under the age of 60 with a history of chronic heart failure controlled with medical therapy who fall into NYHA functional class I or II and have minimal evidence of heart failure on physical examinations generally tolerate noncardiac surgery relatively well.[3,6-8,15-21] Medical therapy with digitalis and diuretic therapy, guided by clinical parameters, should be optimized before surgery. Patients with severe congestive heart failure as defined by NYHA functional class III or IV already have an annual mortality of at least 50 percent[28] and tolerate surgery very poorly.

The Veterans Administration Cooperative Study has demonstrated improved survival in patients with severe congestive failure using a combination of nitrates and hydralazine.[29] Others have documented benefit in survival statistics with angiotensin-converting enzyme inhibitors like captopril[30,31] and enalapril.[32] They often show dramatic improvements in exercise capacity and NYHA functional class with initiation of vasodilator therapy. No studies have evaluated the degree of reduction in perioperative risk in patients receiving such treatment preoperatively. However, the therapy can eliminate such markers of high perioperative risk as jugular venous distention, pulmonary rales, third heart sound, frequent premature ventricular contractions, and radiographic evidence of failure. Although not studied, treatment of arrhythmias should be attempted in all patients except those with chronic atrial fibrillation. Correcting these risk factors alters Goldman's cardiac risk index score substantially.

Patients with decompensated congestive heart failure should be managed in the usual manner. Digitalis preparations like digoxin can be used to enhance myocardial inotropy with care in following drug levels and avoiding hypokalemia. Digoxin is usually required long-term and may be helpful to control ventricular rate in patients with atrial arrhythmias. Some investigators believe that digoxin is most effective in patients with third heart sounds.[33] Digitalis should be continued up to and including the day of the procedure. It should not be used solely to counteract the myocardial depressant effects of anesthetic agents.

Diuretics are important in the therapy of congestive heart failure. However, aggressive preoperative therapy with diuretics can result in severe electrolyte abnormalities such as hyponatremia, hypokalemia, hypomagnesemia, or hypercarbia. Hypokalemia and hypomagnesemia can produce myocardial irritability resulting in ventricular arrhythmias and cardiac arrest.[28] They also exacerbate digitalis toxicity and lead to a variety of arrhythmias that can worsen congestive heart failure. Aggressive diuresis may cause volume depletion that is poorly tolerated in patients facing the stress of anesthesia and surgery. Diuretics may also exacerbate the vasodilatory and myocardial depressant effects of various anesthetic agents, further decrease intravascular volume from fluid shifts and blood loss, and increase the postoperative risk of thrombophlebitis. Patients with decreased left ventricular function require elevated left ventricular filling pressures to ensure adequate cardiac output, and volume depletion from diuretics can be catastrophic. Looking for orthostatic change in blood pressure and pulse is a good way to determine if the patient has been diuresed too vigorously. In euvolemic patients, diuretics usually need to be withheld only on the day of surgery.

Vasodilators have become a mainstay in the treatment of heart failure. Captopril and enalapril decrease both preload and afterload equally; nitrates decrease preload more than afterload; and hydralazine decreases only afterload. These drugs should be continued up to the time of surgery, and intravenous vasodilators like nitroprusside or nitroglycerin can be substituted when oral administration of drugs is not possible. For those with congestive heart failure and coronary artery disease, nitrates are preferable because they improve subendocardial coronary arterial blood flow and decrease left ventricular filling pressure. Enalaprilat, an intravenous angiotensin-converting enzyme inhibitor, has been used to improve hemodynamic status and cardiac output rapidly during surgery in patients with congestive heart failure and volume overload.[34]

Patients with atrial or ventricular arrhythmias who are taking antiarrhythmics should continue them up to the time of surgery. Thereafter, intravenous lidocaine or procainamide can be given to control arrhythmias until preoperative medications can be restarted. Patients with severe class IV congestive heart failure should never undergo elective surgery unless they can be improved enough to be managed on oral diuretics, digitalis, and vasodilators. Intravenous inotropic agents or even intraaortic balloon counterpulsation to maintain adequate cardiac output may be required in the urgent or emergency situation. Candidates for cardiac transplantation should be managed in this way prior to important elective noncardiac surgery. Patients who had previously undergone cardiac transplantation have successfully undergone noncardiac surgery with no significant perioperative complications at three major teaching hospitals.[35,36]

All patients undergoing surgery have continuous intraoperative electrocardiographic monitoring and frequent assessments of cuff blood pressure measurements. In patients with well-compensated congestive failure on medical therapy, such monitoring may be sufficient. If these patients are in NYHA functional classes I or II, are under age 60, have no significant electrocardiographic changes, have had no myocardial infarction within the last six months of surgery, have no significant aortic stenosis, and are not undergoing major abdominal or aortic procedures with significant blood loss, more invasive monitoring is not required. However, in patients in class I or II with additional cardiac risk factors as defined by Goldman's or Detsky's cardiac risk index, or in patients in class III or IV, more invasive monitoring should be strongly considered. This monitoring includes intraarterial measurement of systemic blood pressure and blood gases and Swan-Ganz catheterization. The lines can be inserted during the procedure and aid the anesthesiologist in rapidly responding to changes in hemodynamic status, administering intravenous fluids and blood, and initiating therapy with vasodilators and inotropic agents. Berlauk et al. have recently demonstrated the utility of preoperative optimization of hemodynamics with fluids, vasodilators, and inotropic support guided by pulmonary artery catheter measurements.[37] Cardiac morbidity and mortality was significantly lower in patients managed with the guidance of intra- and postoperative pulmonary artery monitoring than in patients who were managed solely with intraoperative arterial pressure monitoring.

Transesophageal echocardiography has recently been introduced as a noninvasive method of assessing left ventricular function and wall motion,[38,39] and can be performed intraoperatively in minutes. Although it has not been extensively evaluated in patients with congestive heart failure undergoing noncardiac surgery, it has proved successful in guiding coronary artery bypass graft surgery and valvular replacement.

There are several factors that may exacerbate heart failure in the perioperative period. Injudicious administration of intravenous fluids and blood replacement may lead to marked elevations in left ventricular end-diastolic pressure. Cooperman found that 22 of 4 episodes of pulmonary edema in patients with heart failure undergoing noncardiac surgery occurred in the first 30 minutes after anesthesia was discontinued, while 28 episodes occurred within the first hour.[40] A second peak incidence of pulmonary edema and heart failure occurred 24 to 48 hours after surgery when mobilization of intraoperative fluid occurs.[18] Excessive fluid administration has been implicated in more than half of all patients who develop heart failure postoperatively.[18] In patients with severe heart failure invasive monitoring should be continued for at least 48 hours after surgery. Postoperative volume overload can be treated effectively with diuretics.

Supraventricular tachyarrhythmias are common after surgery and are due not only to intrinsic cardiac disease but also to high levels of circulating catecholamines, infection, hypoxia, and electrolyte imbalance. These arrhythmias can exacerbate congestive heart failure by decreasing diastolic left ventricular filling time and, in some cases, by abolishing atrial systole.

As noted above, coronary artery disease is a frequent companion of congestive heart failure. Perioperative factors that precipitate myocardial ischemia and infarction include pain and volume depletion. Both increase catecholamine output and myocardial oxygen demand through changes in heart rate, afterload, and contractility. Postoperative myocardial infarctions are most likely to occur in the first five days following surgery, and 60 percent occur in the first three days.[11,14] Postoperative myocardial infarction and ischemia significantly impair an already dysfunctional left ventricle and exacerbate congestive heart failure.

Significant hypertension is likely to occur at two periods after surgery. It is seen in the first 30 to 60 minutes as the patient recovers from anesthesia and experiences pain, discomfort from the endotracheal tube, volume overload, hypothermia, and hypercarbia. It is also common between 24 and 48 hours after surgery when mobilization of intravenous fluids occurs. Increases in blood pressure and afterload can decrease cardiac output and precipitate congestive heart failure in patients with underlying left ventricular dysfunction. Intravenous vasodilators should be used to control hypertension until the patient is ready to resume oral antihypertensive medications.

Postoperative volume depletion and hypercoagulability increase the risk of thromboembolic events and are especially important in patients with congestive heart failure. Pulmonary emboli can abruptly increase pulmonary hypertension and result in acute right ventricular failure. For this reason, patients with severe congestive heart failure should receive prophylactic treatment to prevent deep-venous thrombosis. This is discussed in detail in Chap. 48.

SUMMARY

1. Patients with significant congestive heart failure and clinical findings like a third heart sound and jugular venous distention have a high perioperative risk of cardiac morbidity and mortality.

2. Congestive heart failure should be treated with digitalis derivatives, diuretics, and vasodilators prior to surgery. In most cases, arrhythmias should be treated, and excessive diuresis should be avoided.

3. Patients with a history of congestive heart failure who are in NYHA functional class I or II and have no other cardiovascular risk factors generally do not require perioperative invasive monitoring. Patients in NYHA class III or IV, or in class I or II with additional risk factors, should be monitored with systemic and pulmonary arterial catheters. Ideally, these should remain in place for 48 hours after surgery.

4. Multiple factors in the perioperative period can exacerbate congestive heart failure. These include volume overload from intravenous fluids and blood, myocardial infarction, arrhythmias, hypertension, and pulmonary emboli.

REFERENCES

1. McKee PA, Castelli WP, McNamara PA et al: The natural history of congestive heart failure: The Framingham study. *N Engl J Med* 285:1441–1446, 1971.
2. Horvat DDC: Cardiac disease, anesthesia and operation for noncardiac conditions. *Br J Anaesth* 43:288–298, 1971.
3. Goldman L, Caldera DL, Nussbaum SR et al: Multifactorial index of cardiac risk in noncardiac surgical procedures. *N Engl J Med* 297:845–850, 1977.
4. Skinner JF, Pearce ML: Surgical risk in the cardiac patient. *J Chron Dis* 17:57–72, 1964.
5. Zeldin RA: Assessing cardiac risk in patients who undergo noncardiac surgical procedures. *Can J Surg* 27:402–404, 1984.
6. Detsky AS, Abrams HB, Forbath N et al: Cardiac assessment for patients undergoing noncardiac surgery. *Arch Intern Med* 146:2131–2134, 1986.
7. Detsky AS, Abrams HB, McLaughlin JR et al: Predicting cardiac complications in patients undergoing noncardiac surgery. *J Gen Int Med* 1:211–219, 1986.
8. Goldman L, Caldera DL, Southwick FS et al: Cardiac risk factors and complications in noncardiac surgery. *Medicine* 57:357–370, 1978.
9. New York Heart Association: *Nomenclature and Criteria for Diagnosis of Diseases of the Heart and Blood Vessels.* New York Heart Association, 1953, p 359.
10. Likoff MF, Chandler SL, Kay HR: Clinical determinants of mortality in chronic congestive heart failure secondary to idiopathic dilated or to ischemic cardiomyopathy. *Am J Cardiol* 59:634, 1987.
11. Goldman L: Cardiac risks and complications of noncardiac surgery. *Ann Int Med* 98:504–513, 1983.
12. Mancini DM, Eisen H, Kussmaul W et al: Value of peak exercise oxygen consumption for optimal timing of cardiac transplantation in ambulatory patients with heart failure. *Circulation* 83:778, 1991.
13. Pantley GA, Bristow JD: Ischemic cardiomyopathy. *Prog Cardiovasc Dis* 27:95, 1984.
14. Foster E, Davis K, Carpenter J et al: Risk of noncardiac operation in patients with defined coronary artery disease: The Coronary Artery Surgery Study (CASS) Registry experience. *Ann Thor Surg* 41:42, 1986.
15. Weitz HH, Goldman L: Noncardiac surgery in the patient with heart disease, in *Medical Clinics of North America.* Philadelphia, Saunders, 1987, no 71, pp 413–432.
16. Rose SD, Corman LC, Mason DT: Cardiac risk factors in patients undergoing noncardiac surgery, in *Medical Clinics of North America.* Philadelphia, Saunders, 1987, no 63, pp 1271–1288.
17. Ross J, Braunwald E: Aortic stenosis. *Circulation* 38:V–61, 1968.
18. Wells PH, Kaplan JA: Optimal management of patients with ischemic heart disease for noncardiac surgery by complementary anesthesiologist and cardiologist interaction. *Am Heart J* 102:1029–1037, 1981.
19. Foex P: Preoperative assessment of the patient with cardiovascular disease. *Br J Anaesth* 53:731–744, 1981.
20. Silverstein DK, Karliner JS: Perioperative cardiac care. *Urol Clin NA* 10:51–63, 1983.
21. Logue RB, Kaplan JA: The cardiac patient and noncardiac surgery. *Curr Prob Cardiol* 7:1–49, 1982.
22. Serrvys PW, Simoons ML, Suryapranata H et al: Preservation of global and regional left ventricular function after early thrombolysis in acute myocardial infarction *J Am Coll Cardiol* 7:729, 1986.
23. Bigger JT, Fleiss JL, Kleiger R et al: Multicenter Post-Infarction Research Group. The relationships among ventricular arrhythmia, left ventricular dysfunction and mortality in the two years after myocardial infarction. *Circulation* 69:250, 1984.
24. Cohn JN, Ziesche SM, Archibald DG, VA Cooperative Study Group: Quantitative exercise tolerance as a predictor of mortality in congestive heart failure. The V-HeFT study. *Circulation* 74:11–447, 1986.

25. Lazor L, Russell JC, DaSilva J et al: Use of the multiple uptake gated acquisition scan for the preoperative assessment of cardiac risk. *Surg Gyn Ob* 167:234–238, 1988.

26. Pedersen T, Kelbaek H, Munck O: Cardiopulmonary complications in high-risk surgical patients. The value of preoperative radionuclide cardiography. *Acta Anesth Scand* 34:183, 1990.

27. Weber KT, Kinaesewitz GT, Janicki JS et al: Oxygen utilization and ventilation during exercise in patients with chronic cardiac failure. *Circulation* 65:1213, 1982.

28. Packer M: Sudden unexpected death in patients with congestive heart failure: A second frontier. *Circulation* 72:681, 1985.

29. Cohn JN, Archibald DG, Ziesche S et al: Effect of vasodilator therapy on mortality in chronic congestive heart failure: Results of a Veterans Administration Cooperative Study. *N Engl J Med* 314:1547, 1986.

30. Conner PJ, Powers ER, Reison D et al: A placebo-controlled trial of captopril in refractory congestive heart failure. *J Am Coll Cardiol* 2:755–763, 1983.

31. Newman TJ, Maskin CS, Dennick LG et al: Effects of captopril on survival in patients with heart failure. *Am J Med* 84(Suppl 3A):140–144, 1988.

32. CONSENSUS Trial Study Group: Effects of enalapril on mortality in serious congestive heart failure. Results of the Cooperative North Scandinavian Enalapril Survival Study (CONSENSUS). *N Engl J Med* 316:1429–1435, 1987.

33. Lee DCS, Johnson RA, Bingham JB: Heart failure in outpatients: A randomized trial of digoxin versus placebo. *N Engl J Med* 306:699, 1982.

34. Acampora GA, Melendez JA, Keefe DL et al: Intraoperative administration of the intravenous angiotensin-converting enzyme inhibitor, Enalaprilat, in a patient with congestive heart failure. *Anesth Analg* 69:833, 1989.

35. Samuels SI, Wyner J: Anaesthesia for surgery in a patient with a heart transplant (letter). *Br J Anaesth* 58:1199–1200, 1986.

36. Yee J, Petsikas D, Ricci MA et al: General surgical procedures after heart transplantation. *Can J Surg* 33:185, 1990.

37. Berlauk JA, Abrams JH, Gilmour IJ et al: Preoperative optimization of cardiovascular hemodynamics improves outcome in peripheral vascular surgery. *Ann Surg* 214:289, 1991.

38. Goldman ME, Mindich BP: Intraoperative two-dimensional echocardiography: new application of an old technique. *J Am Coll Cardiol* 7:374–382, 1986.

39. Cahalan MK, Litt L, Botvinick EH et al: Advances in noninvasive cardiovascular imaging. Implications for the anesthesiologist. *Anesthesiology* 66:356–372, 1987.

40. Cooperman LH, Price HL: Pulmonary edema in the operative and postoperative period: A review of 40 cases. *Ann Surg* 172:883–891, 1970.

20 SURGERY IN THE PATIENT WITH VALVULAR HEART DISEASE

John W. Hirshfeld, Jr.

Timothy Shapiro

Noncardiac surgery can be safely performed in virtually any patient with chronic valvular disease. However, to determine risk and plan therapy, several aspects of the patient's particular circumstances must be considered: (1) the severity and pathophysiology of the valvular lesion; (2) left ventricular contractile function; (3) the severity of any coexisting coronary artery disease; and (4) the nature of the circulatory stress imposed by the anesthesia and particular surgical procedure. Patients with valvular heart disease cannot compensate for errors in fluid replacements, drug therapy, or anesthetic management. Therefore, control of the hemodynamic and metabolic status of these patients throughout the perioperative period requires sophisticated hemodynamic and electrocardiographic monitoring.

RISK OF SURGERY IN VALVULAR HEART DISEASE

The risk of noncardiac surgery in patients with significant valvular heart disease has not been carefully studied. Much of the available information is derived from earlier studies performed before current diagnostic and monitoring procedures were available, limiting their applicability.

In 1964, Skinner and Pearce reported a mortality rate of 6 percent in patients with mitral stenosis and regurgitation undergoing noncardiac surgery.[1] Patients with aortic valve disease had an overall mortality rate of 10 percent but as high as 20 percent when only intrathoracic or intraabdominal procedures were considered. These data suggest that patients with aortic valve disease are more fragile than patients with mitral disease in the surgical setting. In Goldman's study of cardiac risk factors in noncardiac surgery, patients with a mitral regurgitant murmur of grade II or greater had a mortality rate of 7 percent, significantly higher than those

with no murmur. True aortic stenosis, with a mortality rate of 13 percent, was even more strongly associated with postoperative cardiac death and was identified as an independent risk factor. All of the major valvular abnormalities—aortic stenosis, aortic regurgitation, mitral stenosis, and mitral regurgitation—were associated with a 20 percent risk of new or worsening congestive heart failure in the postoperative period.[2]

Thus, although large studies are lacking, there is evidence that valvular heart disease can be a significant risk factor in noncardiac surgery. However, it appears that current diagnostic and therapeutic practices can reduce this risk. O'Keefe et al. reported no perioperative deaths in 48 consecutive patients with documented severe aortic stenosis undergoing noncardiac operations between 1985 and 1986.[3]

General Principles

Valvular heart disease is a heterogeneous group of disorders, each requiring a different management strategy. In addition, each disorder may vary in its hydraulic severity and associated physiologic derangement. The underlying state of left ventricular contractile function and the presence and severity of coexisting coronary artery disease are additional variables that affect operative risk and may influence management strategies. Current diagnostic techniques enable the clinician to quantify the severity of disease and to estimate risk for the individual patient. Most of the physiologic derangements produced by valvular disease are controllable if managed correctly.

The safe conduct of noncardiac surgery in a patient with valvular heart disease requires control of intravascular volume (preload), cardiac rhythm, and systemic vascular resistance (afterload). Although patients with valvular heart disease have less margin for error in fluid management, the latitude varies with the type of lesion, its severity, and left ventricular function. Problems in the management of a patient with aortic stenosis and depressed left ventricular function are entirely different from those involved in a patient with moderately severe mitral regurgitation and a normal left ventricle.

The hydraulic severity of a valvular defect can be quantitated, and severity can be correlated with the anticipated degree of circulatory embarrassment. Each defect imposes a different kind of hemodynamic burden on different chambers of the heart, and this determines the ability of the heart to respond to a particular hemodynamic stress imposed by anesthesia or surgery, like acute loss of intravascular volume or pronounced systemic arteriolar vasodilation. The quality of left ventricular function and the presence of coronary artery disease may also influence the response to stress. In addition, cardiac rhythm profoundly influences circulatory performance, and deviations from normal sinus rhythm must be corrected.

Preemptive Surgical Correction of Valvular Lesions

In most circumstances, preemptive surgical repair of a valvular defect might seem to be an excessively aggressive way to prepare a patient for a noncardiac operation. However, overall clinical status, the relative importance of the cardiac and noncardiac diseases, the possibility of short-term complications for each, and the likelihood of long-term benefit from each procedure should be considered. Certain situations are clear-cut. For example, a very elderly patient with advanced cardiac disease poorly suited to successful surgical repair and a pressing noncardiac problem should not be considered for preemptive repair of the cardiac problem because the benefits of correcting the noncardiac problem outweigh the risks of valvular repair. On the other hand, a healthy patient with a severe valvular defect who is likely to develop symptoms in the near future may present with a noncardiac problem requiring major surgery. This patient may be better served by preemptive repair of the valvular lesion prior to the noncardiac operation.

Balloon valvuloplasty has recently become available as an alternative for nonoperative palliation of valvular stenosis. It is highly effective in relieving mitral stenosis in patients with noncalcified valves.[4-6] Though it is less effective in aortic stenosis, it can reduce the severity of obstruction and may improve the patient's ability to tolerate noncardiac surgery. Several anecdotal series of preoperative balloon valvuloplasty for aortic stenosis have been reported but have not definitely shown the procedure to be a key factor in assuring successful outcome.[7-10] Nevertheless, it is reasonable to consider balloon valvuloplasty as an option in the appropriate candidate.

Stenotic Lesions

Stenotic valvular lesions are more difficult to manage than regurgitant lesions. The patient with a stenotic valve is more fragile hemodynamically and more sensitive to changes in intravascular volume, systemic vascular resistance, and cardiac rhythm. This sensitivity can be attributed to the quadratic relationship between the flow across a stenotic valve and the pressure gradient necessary to maintain flow. For flow rate across a stenotic cardiac valve to double, the pressure gradient must quadruple. A patient with aortic stenosis and a gradient of 80 mmHg at rest needs to gener-

ate a transvalvular gradient of 320 mmHg in order to double the flow rate across the valve. To maintain this acceptable arterial pressure requires a left ventricular pressure of more than 400 mmHg. Because the left ventricle cannot develop this high a pressure, the ability to increase cardiac output above resting level is greatly impaired. Patients with stenotic valves tolerate systemic vasodilation poorly because it is difficult to increase cardiac output to compensate for the decrease in systemic vascular resistance.

The pressure gradient across a stenotic valve is also influenced by the time available for flow to occur. Changes in heart rate alter this time period and therefore affect the pressure gradient independently of any change in cardiac output. Since time available for diastole decreases as heart rate increases, rapid heart rates are particularly deleterious to patients with mitral stenosis. In patients with aortic stenosis, this leads to a decrease in diastolic filling. In view of substantial left ventricular hypertrophy, relatively slow heart rates are required to insure filling of the noncompliant left ventricle and to provide adequate time for coronary artery flow to the increased muscle mass. Such hypertrophied hearts already have large metabolic requirements, and if metabolic demand increases further with rapid heart rates, a supply-demand imbalance can occur and lead to myocardial ischemia.[11]

Patients with stenotic valves are exquisitely sensitive to changes in cardiac rhythm. Rapid atrial fibrillation can be deleterious in mitral stenosis because it decreases the time available for diastolic filling. In tight aortic stenosis, it causes loss of the atrial contribution to ventricular filling. The hypertrophied left ventricle therefore loses the diastolic myocardial fiber-lengthening necessary to generate the systolic pressure needed to pump blood across the stenotic valve.

The impact of a stenotic lesion on cardiac performance is thus closely correlated with the hydraulic severity of the stenosis. The more severe the stenosis, the more likely the patient will deteriorate when subjected to hemodynamic stress. Patients with stenotic lesions are sensitive to changes in preload and poorly tolerate vasodilation and intravascular volume depletion. Careful attention must be paid to intravascular volume status and systemic vascular resistance during all phases of perioperative management.

In aortic stenosis, left ventricular contractile function is an important determinant of circulatory reserve. It is less important in patients with mitral stenosis because mitral stenosis is the only left-sided valvular lesion that does not place a direct hemodynamic burden on the left ventricle.

Regurgitant Lesions

This section discusses chronic regurgitant valvular defects and specifically excludes patients with acute valvular regurgitation. Patients with acute regurgitation often require immediate surgical correction of the valvular defect.

Patients with regurgitant defects are less difficult to manage than those with stenotic lesions. However, the determinants of systemic cardiac output are more complex in chronic regurgitation than in stenosis. Systemic cardiac output is not fixed within as narrow a range, and patients in general can adapt better to changes in intravascular volume and systemic vascular resistance. In addition, the physician can more readily influence both systemic cardiac output and left ventricular filling pressures by controlling preload, heart rate, and systemic vascular resistance.

In valvular stenosis, severity is determined principally by the degree of stenosis. However, in valvular regurgitation, the hemodynamic burden is determined not only by the severity of the valvular defect but also by hemodynamic parameters such as heart rate, systemic arterial pressure, left ventricular filling pressure, and left ventricular contractile state.[12,13] In regurgitant valvular disease, cardiovascular adaptive mechanisms are better able to handle the hemodynamic stresses of anesthesia and surgery and allow the physician greater leeway in management.

Patients with valvular regurgitation and well-preserved left ventricular function can cope with a hemodynamic change as well as patients with normal hearts. However, ability to do so decreases as left ventricular function deteriorates. Correlation between symptom status and left ventricular function is weak. Minimal symptoms do not necessarily guarantee good left ventricular function. Therefore, that function must be assessed preoperatively to guide perioperative management.

AVAILABLE DIAGNOSTIC AND MONITORING TECHNIQUES

There are several diagnostic and monitoring procedures available to aid in preoperative assessment and perioperative management of patients with valvular heart disease.

Preoperative Assessment and Management

Doppler echocardiography is an established means of detecting valvular disease and quantifying many of the variables that determine its severity and impact. A properly performed study can detect and quantify the severity of valvular stenosis and assess left ventricular contractility. A Doppler echocardiographic study should be obtained as part of the routine preoperative assessment of any patient with a significant cardiac murmur. This is particularly important in the assessment of elderly patients with systolic murmurs. A number of these patients harbor previously unrecognized significant aortic stenosis.

Gated radionuclide ventriculography (MUGA) provides an assessment of the left ventricular size and contractility in the form of a calculated left ventricular ejection fraction. This information may be redundant if a good-quality echocardiogram is available. Exercise and dipyridamole-thallium scintigraphy serve primarily to detect clinically unrecognized coronary artery disease and to assess its global severity. Cardiac catheterization and angiography are invasive procedures that provide the most accurate information in documenting the presence and severity of valvular and coronary disease and assessing left ventricular function. It should be reserved for patients in whom there is serious consideration of preemptive surgical correction of the cardiac disease before the planned noncardiac surgery.

Determination of the state of hydration is important since intravascular volume exerts a major influence on the ability to tolerate circulatory stress. There is a tendency to err on the side of hypovolemia that may be detrimental in patients with valvular heart disease. Preoperative diagnostic and preparative procedures, poor diet, and medications can exacerbate this problem. When clinical determination of the state of hydration is equivocal, invasive right-heart pressure measurement may be necessary preoperatively.

In selected patients, prophylactic use of digitalis derivatives is useful in preventing and controlling tachyarrhythmias. Its effect on the myocardial inotropic state is of no demonstrated value.

Intraoperative Monitoring Procedures

The Swan-Ganz balloon-tipped right-heart catheter is invaluable in monitoring right-heart pressures intraoperatively in patients with valvular heart disease and can be placed with minimal risk and discomfort. Although right-heart pressure monitoring is not essential in all patients with valvular heart disease, it is vital in certain subsets. It provides moment-to-moment assessment of left ventricular filling pressure, enables measurement of cardiac output and calculation of systemic vascular resistance, and allows determination of adequacy of systemic perfusion by measuring the oxygen saturation of mixed venous blood.

Monitoring systemic arterial pressure with an indwelling arterial cannula is virtually complication-free in experienced hands when maintained for less than 24 hours. It provides a continuous measurement of actual arterial pressure and is free from the ambiguities of the cuff method seen in low-output states.

AORTIC STENOSIS

Aortic stenosis is the most common valvular lesion encountered in the noncardiac surgical patient. Patients with aortic stenosis comprise the most fragile subset of patients with valvular heart disease. Failure to recognize aortic stenosis may lead to an otherwise avoidable adverse outcome. Aortic stenosis is principally a disease of the elderly, and diagnosing it among all those with omnipresent mid-systolic flow murmur is difficult in this age group. Most clinical findings consistent with aortic stenosis are related to alterations in the peripheral arterial pressure waveform caused by obstruction of the aortic valve. However, elderly patients have noncompliant great vessels that may cause the arterial waveform to appear normal and make recognition of the valvular lesion more difficult.

Any of the following clinical signs strongly suggests the presence of significant aortic stenosis. The absence of any of these clinical signs, however, does not exclude its presence.[12,13]

1. The normal arterial waveform is distorted and has a low amplitude, slow upstroke, and sometimes a palpable shudder in the carotid vessels.
2. There is palpable left ventricular hypertrophy of the pressure-overload type and a palpable fourth heart sound. This may or may not be accompanied by left ventricular hypertrophy on the electrocardiogram.
3. The systolic murmur of aortic stenosis, in contrast to the innocent systolic murmur found in the elderly, is long in duration, frequently extending almost to the pulmonic component of the second sound. The aortic component of the second sound is usually absent.
4. Calcification of the aortic valve is occasionally visible on plain x-ray. Image-intensification fluoroscopy, an easy and safe technique, provides a highly sensitive means of detection.

5. Echocardiography demonstrates a hypertrophied left ventricle and a thickened distorted aortic valve. The Doppler portion of the study can be diagnostic if a measure of aortic ejection velocity can be obtained. A technically adequate study can detect the presence of aortic stenosis, quantitate its severity, and assess left ventricular function. If a good study cannot be obtained when the diagnosis is ambiguous, cardiac catheterization should be considered.

Preoperative Preparation

Patients with aortic stenosis have limited ability to increase cardiac output in response to stress and diminished diastolic compliance. Consequently, these patients tolerate decreases in systemic vascular resistance poorly and are highly dependent on diastolic preload as determined by intravascular volume.

Particular attention must therefore be paid to the state of hydration. In this situation, it is probably better to err on the side of minimal fluid overload rather than on that of hypovolemia. Surgical patients are prone to hypovolemia from bleeding or venous pooling and are frequently subjected to perioperative stress-induced vasodilatation. Therefore, patients with aortic stenosis should go to the operating room with adequate left ventricular end-diastolic pressure. Excessive intravascular volume and pulmonary congestion can be dealt with easily in the perioperative period, but the consequence of inadequate left ventricular filling pressure can be rapid irrevocable circulatory collapse.

Operative Management

Right-heart and systemic arterial pressure monitoring are important adjuncts in operative management of patients with tight aortic stenosis. The measurements enable the anesthesiologist to regulate fluid and blood administration optimally and to interpret changes in arterial pressure accurately.

Modest changes in systemic vascular resistance can produce substantial changes in arterial pressure and coronary artery blood flow. Since increased coronary blood flow is required to satisfy increased myocardial metabolic demand, the patient is especially dependent on diastolic arterial pressure to maintain coronary artery perfusion. If the patient becomes hypotensive, coronary artery perfusion decreases, the left ventricle may become ischemic, and its systolic performance may deteriorate. This in turn can lead to a further decrease in arterial pressure, initiating a vicious cycle. It is crucial that arterial pressure be maintained.

Left ventricular stroke volume is dependent on diastolic fiber length which in the patient with aortic stenosis is sensitive to changes in cardiac rhythm. If atrial fibrillation develops, the contribution of atrial contraction to ventricular filling and myocardial fiber-lengthening is lost, and abrupt circulatory deterioration may follow, requiring emergency cardioversion. Even if the circulation appears reasonably stable with atrial fibrillation, it should be considered tenuous at best. Prompt aggressive efforts to control ventricular rate and restore sinus rhythm are indicated.

Intraoperative management should accordingly include attention to cardiac rhythm, left-heart filling pressures, and systemic vascular resistance. Spinal anesthetics should be avoided because of accompanying unpredictable vasodilatation.

Postoperative Management

Postoperative management in aortic stenosis can be difficult because of variable "third-space" fluid loss. Right-heart pressure measurements are especially useful in planning fluid therapy and blood replacement. Once again, hypovolemia may lead to circulatory collapse, and it is safer to lean toward overreplacement if renal function is normal. Excessive intravascular volume, if recognized promptly, can be easily managed with diuretics.

Atrial fibrillation should be promptly recognized and aggressively treated.[14] Moderate sinus tachycardia up to 120 is usually tolerated since it does not cause a decrease in time available for systolic ejection, but this may not be true in the presence of coronary artery disease. If sinus tachycardia is present, no effort should be made merely to slow the rate without a search for its cause and appropriate treatment. The increased basal metabolic rate that accompanies significant fever increases the demand for cardiac output, and aspirin or acetaminophen should be used to minimize temperature elevation. The value of cooling blankets for temperature reduction is debatable, but they should not be used for circulatory reasons alone.

MITRAL STENOSIS

Mitral stenosis is less common than aortic stenosis and is largely a disorder of middle-aged women, most of whom relate a history of acute rheumatic fever in childhood or adolescence. It is a more chronic insidiously progressive disease, and its symptoms, in contrast to those of aortic stenosis, correlate with the severity of the hydraulic defect. Significant mitral stenosis is thus rarely overlooked in routine preoperative evaluation. The cardiac silhouette on the chest x-ray is usually abnormal, even when the physical findings of mitral stenosis are difficult to appreciate. Difficulties in the perioperative period are directly related to the severity of obstruction.[15]

In mitral stenosis, the left ventricle is inadequately preloaded. Because of valvular obstruction, abnormally elevated left atrial pressures are needed to maintain satisfactory left ventricular end-diastolic pressures. Lowering left atrial pressure toward normal unacceptably decreases left ventricular end-diastolic pressure and may lead to a drop in cardiac output.

Patients with mitral stenosis can be divided into two groups, those with sinus rhythm and those with chronic atrial fibrillation.[14] The development of chronic atrial fibrillation is a well-recognized milestone in the natural history of mitral stenosis.

All patients with significant mitral stenosis have evidence of right ventricular enlargement and pulmonary hypertension on physical examination. Though the intensity of the murmur may vary and correlates poorly with severity, the degree of physiologic derangement can be more precisely estimated from evidence of pulmonary hypertension, tricuspid regurgitation, and low systemic cardiac output. Electrocardiographic findings are also variable and do not correlate well with severity. The chest x-ray reveals a characteristic distortion of the cardiac silhouette with enlargement of the left atrium, pulmonary artery, and right ventricle. Doppler echocardiography is highly accurate in detecting mitral stenosis and assessing its severity as well as the performance of the affected cardiac chambers.

The hemodynamic consequences of longstanding stenosis include tricuspid regurgitation and chronic right atrial hypertension. These can occasionally impair liver function that may deteriorate further with the stress of anesthesia and surgery.

Preoperative Preparation

Hydration and intravascular volume status are important determinants of a patient's ability to tolerate anesthesia and surgery. In patients with mitral stenosis, unlike those with aortic stenosis, it is preferable to aim toward hypovolemia. Although these patients can be sensitive to changes in preload, it is easier to replete volume than to treat pulmonary edema. Small increases in intravascular volume may elevate left atrial pressure to unacceptable levels. Systemic arterial hypotension is not so dangerous in patients with mitral stenosis as it is in those with aortic stenosis, and it can be easily corrected with judicious use of fluids.

When chronic atrial fibrillation is present, the ventricular response rate should be well controlled before surgery. Tachycardia can be detrimental because it reduces time available for flow across the mitral valve and can lead to the sudden development of pulmonary edema.[16] In patients with normal sinus rhythm, it may be appropriate to consider the prophylactic use of digitalis to prevent the development of rapid ventricular response should atrial fibrillation develop acutely. Many of these patients have been on chronic diuretic therapy; subsequent depletion in potassium stores may require replacement if digitalis preparations are used.

Operative Management

Clinical findings cannot reflect changes in pulmonary capillary wedge pressure in the anesthetized patient, and right-heart pressure monitoring is essential. Pulmonary capillary wedge pressure is greater than left ventricular filling pressure in patients with mitral stenosis and is usually in the range of 20 mmHg. Optimal pulmonary capillary wedge pressure varies with the severity of mitral obstruction, and a pressure of 10 to 12 mmHg in significant mitral stenosis probably indicates hypovolemia. Since the response of the pulmonary vasculature to mitral stenosis is variable, pulmonary artery diastolic pressure may not reliably reflect actual pulmonary capillary wedge pressure. Therefore, an accurate and reproducible pulmonary capillary wedge pressure is essential.

Patients with mitral stenosis are limited in their ability to increase cardiac output in response to changes in systemic vascular resistance, and vasodilating anesthetics should not be used. Since these patients also have limited capacity to handle additional intravascular volume, acute volume expansion like that seen with infusion of mannitol in neurosurgical procedures is hazardous.

The development of atrial fibrillation or sinus tachycardia requires immediate action to reestablish normal sinus rhythm or to slow ventricular response. If atrial fibrillation develops during surgery, immediate cardioversion is indicated. Sinus tachycardia should be recognized immediately and its cause sought and corrected. It may be wise to slow the ventricular response rate pharmacologically with intravenous esmolol in small increments.

Postoperative Management

Right-heart catheterization is essential to guide postoperative fluid and blood infusion rates and should be maintained until major fluid shifts have ceased. Since mild hypovolemia may be desirable preoperatively and significant postoperative "third-spacing" of fluid may be expected, there is danger of hypovolemic oliguria. Urine flow should therefore probably be maintained with diuretic administration and volume replaced in order to maintain intravascular volume.

Because of fixed obstruction to left atrial emptying, catecholamine stimulation in the hypotensive patient is usually ineffective and, if it produces tachycardia, may be counterproductive. Hypotension is not usually due to depressed left ventricular contractile function. It is more likely the result of inadequate left ventricular filling from hypovolemia, tachycardia, or some other hemodynamic change.

AORTIC REGURGITATION

Aortic regurgitation is more common than mitral stenosis but less so than aortic stenosis. Important causes of aortic regurgitation include rheumatic fever, infective endocarditis, congenital valvular abnormalities, and diseases of the ascending aorta. Since congenital defects of the aortic valve are more prevalent in men, aortic regurgitation occurs more commonly in males.[17] It is important to estimate not only the severity of regurgitation but also the quality of left ventricular function. Operative risk is influenced more strongly by the quality of left ventricular function than by the severity of regurgitation. Isolated mild aortic regurgitation is essentially a trivial disorder and does not confer additional risk.

Aortic regurgitation is recognized by its characteristic blowing decrescendo diastolic murmur heard maximally along the left sternal border. Severity is directly related to peripheral arterial findings and accompanying evidence of left ventricular volume overload. The abnormal arterial pressure-pulse contour is expressed as Quincke pulses, pistol-shot sounds heard over the femoral arteries, and low diastolic arterial pressure of 60 mmHg or less. Although peripheral signs are useful in judging severity, they may be masked in patients with enlarged ascending aortas that may act like damping chambers in decreasing the amplitude of the arterial pulse.

Severity can also be inferred from evidence of left ventricular overload as evidenced by a diffusely enlarged and displaced left ventricular impulse on physical examination, enlargement of the left ventricle on chest x-ray, and by an increase in the left ventricular end-diastolic diameter on echocardiogram. These data enable an accurate qualitative assessment of the severity of the aortic regurgitation.

Assessment of the quality of left ventricular function is a more important determinant of operative risk than regurgitation itself. Most patients with significant aortic regurgitation exhibit some electrocardiographic findings consistent with left ventricular hypertrophy. However, those with extensive repolarization changes, QRS intervals of greater than 100 ms, and abnormal P-wave vectors are more likely to have depressed left ventricular function. A greatly enlarged left ventricle on chest x-ray may also suggest depressed left ventricular function. The echocardiogram provides the best assessment of left ventricular function.[18] Left ventricular end-diastolic diameters greater than 7.5 cm and end-systolic diameters greater than 5.5 cm indicate substantially impaired left ventricular performance.

Preoperative Preparation

Patients with aortic regurgitation are not so sensitive to changes in preload as those with aortic stenosis or mitral stenosis, and precise preoperative adjustment of intravascular volume is less crucial. However, they probably tolerate the stress of anesthesia and surgery better if their intravascular volume is slightly increased.

Operative Management

Right-heart pressure and arterial pressure monitoring are important only in high-risk patients with severely impaired left ventricular function. The majority of patients can be managed effectively without such measures. Vasodilating drugs are well tolerated, and may be the most effective way to reduce left atrial pressure and treat pulmonary vascular congestion. Reduction of systemic vascular resistance decreases the degree of aortic regurgitation, leading in turn to a decrease in left ventricular end-diastolic volume and filling pressure and an increase in cardiac output. In extreme circumstances of low arterial pressure, low cardiac output, or pulmonary vascular congestion, inotropic stimulation of left ventricular contractility may be useful.

Postoperative Management

Strategy for management of aortic regurgitation in the postoperative period is similar to that detailed above. In patients with severely impaired left ventricular function, moderate hypovolemia is well tolerated. If problems with pulmonary vascular congestion develop, vasodilator therapy and/or inotropic stimulation are effective in decreasing the congestion and improving cardiac output. Vasodilator therapy should be carried out with right-heart pressure monitoring.

MITRAL REGURGITATION

Mitral regurgitation, like mitral stenosis, is more common in females and, like aortic regurgitation, has many causes. In mitral regurgitation, determinants of risk are the severity of regurgitation, its etiology, and the quality of left ventricular function.

Mitral regurgitation imposes a preload stress or volume load on the left ventricle without the afterload stress imposed by aortic regurgitation. Instead of having to eject its entire stroke volume against the relatively high impedance of the aorta, the left ventricle delivers the regurgitant fraction of mitral regurgitation into the relatively low impedance circuit of the left atrium. Afterload in mitral regurgitation is already somewhat reduced, and consequently severe left ventricular dysfunction may be masked because of the relatively low impedance against which the left ventricle pumps.[19]

The presence of mitral regurgitation is easily recognized by the detection of a blowing systolic murmur that is loudest at the left ventricular apex. However, quantitative estimation of severity is complex. Important parameters include evidence of left ventricular dilation on physical examination, chest x-ray, and echocardiogram. Patients with left ventricular dysfunction due to primary myocardial disease may develop moderate mitral regurgitation because of geometric distortion of the mitral apparatus.[19] These patients have physical signs similar to those in patients with primary mitral

regurgitation. Patients whose mitral regurgitation is caused by ischemic injury to the left ventricle or papillary muscles have a particularly high operative risk because they have, by definition, coexisting coronary artery disease and left ventricular dysfunction. Left ventricular function is best assessed through measurement of cavity dimensions and wall excursion by echocardiography.

Preoperative Preparation

Preoperative preparation of the patient with mitral regurgitation is similar to that of the patient with aortic regurgitation. Hypovolemia should be avoided, and normal or slightly increased intravascular volume is preferred. An exception to this principle is the patient with preexisting right-heart failure and resultant liver function abnormalities. In such a patient, diuresis sufficient to lower right atrial pressure to normal may better enable the liver to withstand the stress of anesthesia and surgery.

In patients with chronic atrial fibrillation, ventricular response rate should be well controlled with digoxin. Although beta blockers may be useful in controlling the ventricular response rate in mitral stenosis, they should never be used in mitral regurgitation because of their depressant effect on left ventricular function.

Operative Management

Right-heart pressure monitoring is important only for patients who have severely depressed left ventricular function and in whom appropriate pulmonary capillary wedge pressure is above 20 mmHg. Some patients with mitral regurgitation have elevated pulmonary vascular resistance, and pulmonary artery diastolic pressure may not accurately reflect wedge pressure. It is therefore necessary to obtain accurate and reproducible pulmonary capillary wedge pressure measurements.

Patients with mitral regurgitation generally withstand vasodilation well, and spinal anesthetics are well tolerated. In fact, if pulmonary vascular congestion develops, vasodilators like sodium nitroprusside are the first choice for treating inadequate systemic cardiac output and elevated pulmonary capillary wedge pressure.[20] As with aortic regurgitation, inotropic support may be necessary for the failing left ventricle.

Postoperative Management

Problems encountered in the postoperative management of patients with mitral regurgitation and the means for solving them are similar to those for patients with aortic regurgitation. However, patients with severe mitral regurgitation and right-heart failure are more likely to develop hepatic insufficiency in the postoperative period.

IDIOPATHIC HYPERTROPHIC SUBAORTIC STENOSIS

Idiopathic hypertrophic subaortic stenosis (IHSS), or asymmetric septal hypertrophy (ASH), is a hypertrophic cardiomyopathy in which there is excessive thickening of the upper portion of the intraventricular septum and distortion of the geometry of the left ventricle.[21] This causes the anterior leaflet of the mitral valve to be drawn toward the septum during left ventricular contraction in systole, thereby producing outflow obstruction.[22] In IHSS, in contrast to valvular aortic stenosis, the degree of left ventricular outflow obstruction is variable, and it changes in response to interventions that alter left ventricular size and contractility. Vasodilators which decrease left ventricular size by decreasing both venous return and arterial pressure augment the obstruction. Similarly, pharmacologic interventions like catecholamine stimulation that enhance myocardial contractility also increase obstruction.

Patients with IHSS should be approached in the same manner as those with valvular aortic stenosis. They are exquisitely sensitive to decreases in preload, both because they require adequate diastolic fiber length to maintain normal systolic performance and because reduced ventricular size increases their ventricular outflow obstruction. Consequently, the basic principles of fluid management for patients with aortic stenosis also apply to patients with IHSS. However, inotropic stimulation should never be used to treat hypotension in patients with IHSS because it aggravates the underlying left ventricular outflow obstruction that may be responsible for the hypotension. If hypotension occurs, adequate preload should be insured with volume administration, and afterload should be adjusted to produce sufficient arterial pressure. Frequently, increased afterload will improve cardiac output by decreasing the severity of left ventricular outflow obstruction.

MITRAL VALVE PROLAPSE

Mitral valve prolapse describes the ballooning of a mitral leaflet into the left atrium during ventricular systole. It is a common condition and is found in up to 28 percent of otherwise healthy young women.[23] Physical examination is notable for the presence of a nonejection midsystolic click that may be followed by a midsystolic murmur. Two-dimensional echocardiography is the most sensitive technique for detecting mitral valve prolapse and may demonstrate prolapse even when auscultatory signs are absent. Patients with mitral valve prolapse may be asymptomatic or complain of atypical chest pain, dyspnea, and palpitations. They have a slightly increased risk of developing arrhythmias, endocarditis, significant mitral regurgitation, and thromboembolism.

Preoperative management of patients with mitral valve prolapse is dependent upon the presence or absence of these complications. Arrhythmias, mitral regurgitation with congestive heart failure, or prior thromboembolism should be managed as they would in any other setting. Otherwise patients with mitral valve prolapse do not require any special preoperative preparation. However, antibiotic prophylaxis against endocarditis is appropriate even though the risk of endocarditis is extremely small.

PROSTHETIC HEART VALVES

Preoperative management of the patient with a prosthetic heart valve depends on the type of prosthesis and its location. Prosthetic valves are of two major types: tissue bioprostheses which are natural aortic valves from pigs mounted on fabric-covered metal frames; and mechanical prostheses either of the ball-and-cage type (Starr-Edwards) or of pivoting-disk design (Bjork-Shiley and St. Jude).

Clinical assessment of prosthetic valve function is difficult. Systolic murmurs are present across normally functioning aortic prostheses, and even severely stenotic mitral prostheses do not produce diastolic murmurs. Aortic periprosthetic leaks are typically accompanied by blowing diastolic murmurs, but the intensity and timing of the murmurs do not correlate with the severity of the leakage. Mitral periprosthetic leaks may be acoustically silent. In general, suspicion of prosthetic dysfunction is warranted whenever a patient is doing poorly after what appears to be a technically successful valve replacement and there are no other factors to explain the deterioration.

Within limits, Doppler echocardiography is useful in assessing the status of a prosthetic aortic valve and the underlying cardiac performance. In some circumstances technical problems limit the ability to assess the magnitude of flow-pressure gradients across prosthetic valves. However, Doppler study is very effective in detecting periprosthetic leaks.

Valve replacement never completely corrects underlying heart disease. The chamber(s) that bore the burden of the dysfunctional valve before surgery continue to be variably dysfunctional. Therefore, patients with prosthetic valves cannot be considered to have an otherwise normal heart. The extent of perioperative monitoring employed and the precautions taken should be based on careful clinical and laboratory assessment of overall cardiac function. The role of antibiotic prophylaxis in prosthetic valves is discussed in Chap. 43.

ANTICOAGULANT THERAPY

Mechanical prostheses are more prone to thrombosis and subsequent embolization than tissue prostheses, and these complications are more common with the valve in the mitral than in the aortic position.[24] Anticoagulation is most critical in patients with mechanical prostheses in the mitral position and least critical in those with bioprostheses in the aortic position. Anticoagulant management should be individualized to the particular circumstance. Considerations should include the type of surgery being conducted and the type and position of the prosthesis. It is always better to maintain anticoagulation if possible, and certain types of surgery can be performed successfully in the presence of full anticoagulation.

The recommended strategy in major operative procedures is to discontinue warfarin for three to four days before surgery.[25] For patients with mitral mechanical prostheses, this should be managed in the hospital to allow initiation of anticoagulation with heparin when the prothrombin time (PT) falls below 1.5 times the control value. For patients with aortic prostheses, preoperative heparin is not necessary, and warfarin can be safely discontinued in the outpatient setting. When the prothrombin time is less than 20 percent higher than the control value and heparin has been discontinued for six hours, the procedure can be performed with minimally increased risk of bleeding complications. After surgery, anticoagulation with heparin should be instituted as soon as the danger of bleeding has passed. If bleeding does occur, heparin can be promptly reversed with protamine.[26] Warfarin therapy should be resumed after the operation when the patient can take oral medications.

SUMMARY

1. Noncardiac surgery can be performed safely in virtually every patient with valvular heart disease. Management requires recognition of the presence and severity of the valvular defect, assessment of left ventricular contractile function, and proper control of the hemodynamic and metabolic context in which the heart functions.

2. In high-risk patients, hemodynamic monitoring, including measurement of right-heart pressure and systemic arterial pressure with indwelling catheters, is essential.

3. Patients with aortic and mitral stenosis require careful attention to intravascular volume and cardiac rhythm during and after surgery. Vasodilators are hazardous, and small changes in intravascular volume can produce profound changes in left ventricular filling pressure and cardiac output.

4. Patients with valvular regurgitation are better able to withstand perioperative stresses than are those with stenotic lesions. Their ability to respond to changes in intravascular volume, systolic vascular resistance, and cardiac rhythm is determined principally by left ventricular function.

5. Pronounced fluid shifts in the postoperative period should be anticipated. The hemodynamic monitoring employed during surgery in high-risk patients should be continued postoperatively.

6. Anticoagulation is most critical in patients with a mitral mechanical prosthesis and least critical in patients with an aortic bioprosthesis. Warfarin should be discontinued before surgery and anticoagulation maintained with heparin until six hours before the operation. Heparin followed by warfarin should be restarted postoperatively when all danger of bleeding has passed.

7. For specific recommendations regarding antibiotic prophylaxis against bacterial endocarditis in patients with valvular heart disease undergoing surgery, see Chap. 43.

REFERENCES

1. Skinner JF, Pearce ML: Surgical risk in the cardiac patient. *J Chron Dis* 17:57, 1964.
2. Goldman L, Caldera DL, Southwick FS et al: Cardiac risk factors and complications in noncardiac surgery. *Medicine* 57:357, 1978.
3. O'Keefe JH, Shub C, Rettke SR: Can patients with severe aortic stenosis safely undergo noncardiac surgery? (Abstract). *Circulation* 78(Suppl II):II–132, 1988.
4. McKay RG, Lock JE, Safian RD et al: Balloon dilation of mitral stenosis in adults: Postmortem and percutaneous mitral valvuloplasty studies. *J Am Coll Cardiol* 9:723, 1987.
5. Palacios I, Block PC, Brandi S et al: Percutaneous balloon valvuloplasty for patients with severe mitral stenosis. *Circulation* 75:778, 1987.
6. McKay CR, Kawanishi DT, Rahimtoola SH: Double catheter balloon valvuloplasty in patients with mitral stenosis. Initial experience and long-term improvement in rest and exercise hemodynamics. *Clin Res* 35:180A, 1987.
7. Hayes SN, Holmes DR Jr, Nishimura RA et al: Palliative percutaneous aortic balloon valvuloplasty before noncardiac operations and invasive diagnostic procedures. *Mayo Clin Proc* 64:753, 1989.
8. Roth RB, Palacios IF, Block PC: Percutaneous aortic balloon valvuloplasty: Its role in the management of patients with aortic stenosis requiring major noncardiac surgery. *J Am Coll Cardiol* 13:1039, 1989.
9. Levine MJ, Berman AD, Safian RD et al: Palliation of valvular aortic stenosis by balloon valvuloplasty as preoperative preparation for noncardiac surgery. *Am J Cardiol* 62:1309, 1988.
10. Schneider JF, Wilson M, Gallant TE: Percutaneous balloon aortic valvuloplasty for aortic stenosis in elderly patients at high risk for surgery. *Ann Intern Med* 106:696, 1987.
11. Marcus ML, Dott DB, Hiratzka LF et al: Decreased coronary reserve. A mechanism for angina pectoris in patients with aortic stenosis and normal coronary arteries. *New Engl J Med* 307:1362, 1982.
12. Perloff JF: Clinical recognition of aortic stenosis. The physical signs and differential diagnosis of the various signs of obstruction to left ventricular outflow. *Prog Cardiovasc Dis* 10:323, 1968.
13. Eddleman EE, Frommeyer WB, Lyle DP et al: Critical analysis of clinical factors in estimating severity of aortic valve disease. *Am J Cardiol* 31:687, 1973.
14. Mitchell JH, Shapiro W: Atrial function and the hemodynamic consequences of atrial fibrillation in man. *Am J Cardiol* 23:556, 1969.
15. Gorlin R, Gorlin G: Hydraulic formula for the calculation of area of stenotic mitral valve, other valves and central circulatory shunts. *Am Heart J* 41:1, 1951.
16. Arandi DT, Carleton RA: The deleterious role of tachycardia in mitral stenosis. *Circulation* 36:511, 1967.
17. Goldschlager N, Pfeifer J, Cohn K et al: The natural history of aortic regurgitation. A clinical and hemodynamic study. *Am J Med* 54:577, 1973.
18. Abdulla AM, Frank MJ, Canedo MI et al: Limitations of echocardiography in the assessment of left ventricular size and function in aortic regurgitation. *Circulation* 61:148, 1980.
19. Perloff JK, Roberts WC: The mitral apparatus. Functional anatomy of mitral regurgitation. *Circulation* 46:227, 1972.
20. Yoran C, Yellin EL, Becker RM et al: Mechanisms of reduction of mitral regurgitation with vasodilator therapy. *Am J Cardiol* 43:773, 1979.
21. Frank S, Braunwald E: Idiopathic hypertrophic subaortic stenosis. Clinical analysis of 126 patients with emphasis on the natural history. *Circulation* 37:759, 1968.
22. Henry WL, Clark CE, Grifith JM et al: Mechanisms of left ventricular outflow obstruction in patients with obstructive asymmetric septal hypertrophy (idiopathic hypertrophic subaortic stenosis). *Am J Cardiol* 35:337, 1975.
23. Markiewicz W, Stoner J, London E et al: Mitral valve prolapse in one hundred presumably healthy young females. *Circulation* 53:464, 1976.
24. Katholi RE, Nolan SP, McGuire LB: Living with prosthetic heart valves. Subsequent noncardiac operations and the risk of thromboembolism or hemorrhage. *Am Heart J* 92:162, 1976.
25. Tinker JH, Tarhan S: Discontinuing anticoagulant therapy in surgical patients with cardiac valve protheses. *JAMA* 239:738, 1978.
26. Chesebro JH, Adams PC, Fuster V: Antithrombotic therapy in patients with valvular heart disease and prosthetic heart valves. *J Am Coll Cardiol* 84:41B, 1986.

21 SURGERY IN THE PATIENT WITH ARRHYTHMIAS AND CONDUCTION DISTURBANCES

Francis E. Marchlinski

Improved survival in patients with heart disease has increased the patient population with greater risk of developing serious arrhythmias in the perioperative period. Moreover, advances in pharmacologic therapy and electrical devices have increased survival in those patients with life-threatening arrhythmias,[1-4] and management has become progressively more complex. This chapter reviews (1) intraoperative and postoperative factors that facilitate the development of arrhythmias, (2) preoperative clinical and electrocardiographic markers that may predict their development, (3) the value of prophylactic therapy, and (4) intraoperative and postoperative use of antiarrhythmic drugs and electrical devices.

ARRHYTHMOGENIC EFFECTS OF SURGERY AND ANESTHESIA

Continuous monitoring systems allow detailed analysis of electrocardiographic activity during surgery. Kuner et al. reviewed the electrocardiographic recordings of 154 patients undergoing surgery and found that 95 had 195 episodes of cardiac arrhythmia.[5] Most were slow supraventricular arrhythmias (in 128) including sinus bradycardia, wandering atrial pacemakers, isorhythmic atrioventricular dissociation, and junctional rhythms. Others were premature ventricular (in 28) and supraventricular premature depolarizations (in 19). Nine had supraventricular tachycardia, and five had ventricular tachycardia. Patients undergoing neurosurgical and thoracic procedures, endotracheal intubation, and operations lasting more than three hours had a higher incidence of arrhythmias. Precipitating factors included general anesthesia, hypoventilation, and intubation. Others have noted a high frequency, up to 84 percent, of transient bradyarrhythmias and premature atrial and ventricular depolarizations during surgery but a low incidence of more serious arrhythmias during surgery.[6,7]

Clinical and experimental data suggest that hypercapnea, hypoxia, hypokalemia, acidosis, and anemia increase arrhythmogenic potential, especially when they develop in association with general anesthesia.[8] Alterations in autonomic nervous system activity occurring with endotracheal intubation and central nervous system stimulation may also lead to arrhythmias. Succinylcholine, by altering potassium flux, and vasopressor agents administered with anesthetic agents have also been implicated in arrhythmogenesis.[9-11] Nitrous oxide is probably the least arrhythmogenic general anesthetic agent, but our understanding of the electrophysiologic effects of anesthetics is limited, especially in patients with severe myocardial dysfunction.

Most of the newer anesthetic agents are well tolerated unless administered in excessive concentrations. However, the effects of these agents on energy requirements for defibrillation and pacing thresholds have not been determined.[12,13] With the rapid growth of electrical devices for management of arrhythmias, documenting effects of anesthetics is important to insure optimal function in the operating room.

Electrocardiographic monitoring is now routine in the intraoperative and postoperative care of seriously ill patients. Monitoring permits prompt recognition of arrhythmias and institution of appropriate therapy. The occurrence of any rhythm disturbance should provoke a search for precipitating factors and an immediate reassessment of all ongoing therapy before additional pharmacologic intervention is undertaken.

SUPRAVENTRICULAR TACHYCARDIAS

Predictors of Intraoperative and Postoperative Events

In patients undergoing noncardiac surgery, supraventricular tachycardia occurs most frequently in those over age 70, in those with preoperative rales, and in those undergoing intraabdominal, intrathoracic, or major vascular surgery.[14] The absence of heart disease or chronic obstructive pulmonary disease does not preclude the occurrence of supraventricular tachycardia. Rogers et al. found that 21 of 50 patients who developed supraventricular tachycardia in their study had no known heart disease.[15]

A postoperative course complicated by concurrent medical problems increases the risk of developing supraventricular arrhythmias. Goldman found that of 35 patients who developed supraventricular tachycardia after noncardiac operative procedures, 22 developed atrial flutter or atrial fibrillation, three had multifocal atrial tachycardia, and six had a regular supraventricular tachycardia without discernible P waves, most likely either A-V nodal reentry or an automatic junctional (His-bundle) tachycardia.[14] Four other patients developed a rhythm disturbance that was labeled as paroxysmal atrial tachycardia. Eighteen or 52 percent of the patients developed supraventricular tachycardia by the third postoperative day. In 31 or 91 percent, factors were identified which probably contributed to the development of the arrhythmia. These factors included major infection, acute cardiac ischemia or pump dysfunction, metabolic derangements, medication effects, hypotensive events, and temperature elevation accompanying documented infection. No such factors were identified in three patients, but two of them had a history of supraventricular tachycardia. Seventeen died, but none did so as a direct consequence of arrhythmia.[14] In 14 patients, the rhythms reverted to normal without antiarrhythmic intervention. Those with arrhythmias persisting for more than six hours remained hemodynamically stable on digoxin or propranolol given for rate control.

Sometimes the nature of the surgery itself may predispose the patient to supraventricular arrhythmias. Supraventricular tachycardia, primarily atrial fibrillation or flutter, is particularly common after cardiac or thoracic surgery, with an incidence as high as 30 percent.[16] This has been attributed to pericardial and myocardial inflammation that may develop after the procedure.

Although there are clinical predictors of supraventricular tachycardia, preoperative electrocardiograms (ECG's) are of limited use. Premature atrial contractions on routine preoperative ECG's are insensitive predictors. Rogers et al. found that, of 50 patients who developed supraventricular tachycardia, only three had preoperative premature atrial depolarizations.[15] Buxton et al. reported that an increased P-wave duration was associated with an increased incidence of postoperative arrhythmias in 38 patients undergoing coronary artery bypass surgery.[17] They noted that atrial fibrillation or flutter developed only in patients with intraatrial conduction delay. Of 28 patients with a P-wave duration > 110 ms, ten developed atrial flutter or fibrillation.

Evidence of the Wolff-Parkinson-White syndrome on the routine ECG, characterized by a short PR interval and a delta wave (Fig. 21–1A), should alert the physician to the potential development of serious supraventricular arrhythmias. These patients can develop a circus-movement reentrant tachycardia with loss of the delta waves on the surface ECG and a resultant narrow QRS complex tachycardia. There is retrograde activation of the atria with the P waves following the QRS complex (Fig. 21–1C). They can also develop atrial fibrillation with very rapid conduction over the accessory pathway. This results in a wide QRS complex tachycardia with a very rapid ventricular rate (Fig. 21–1B). No prophylactic therapy is indicated in Wolff-Parkinson-White syndrome in the absence of a history of symptoms or electrocardiographic doc-

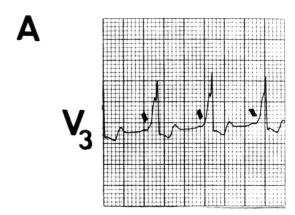

FIGURE 21–1A.   Sinus rhythm tracing in patient with Wolff-Parkinson-White syndrome. Tracing demonstrates characteristic short PR interval and delta waves seen in patients with preexcitation syndrome.

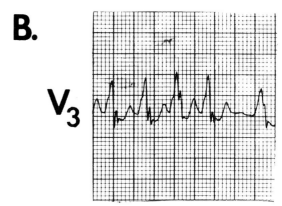

FIGURE 21–1B.   Atrial fibrillation in patient with Wolff-Parkinson-White syndrome. Tracing demonstrates rapid ventricular response and variable degrees of preexcitation characterizing this syndrome.

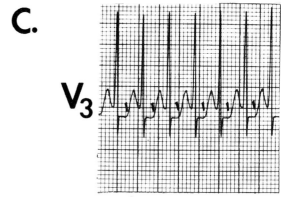

FIGURE 21–1C.   Orthodromic reentrant supraventricular tachycardia in a patient with Wolff-Parkinson-White syndrome. Tracing demonstrates narrow QRS complex with retrograde atrial activity following the QRS complex. Electrical activity proceeds over the normal A-V conduction system through ventricular muscle and returns to the atria by way of the accessory pathway.

umentation of supraventricular tachycardia. However, continuous electrocardiographic monitoring and preparation for the possible development of an arrhythmia are important.[18]

Prophylactic Therapy for Supraventricular Tachycardia

Prophylactic use of antiarrhythmic therapy for supraventricular tachycardia without a documented history of arrhythmia remains controversial. However, even in procedures associated with increased risk of supraventricular tachycardia, e.g., cardiac or thoracic surgery, prophylactic digitalis is not indicated. Juler et al. noted an increased rate of complications but no decrease in the incidence of atrial flutter or fibrillation in digitalized patients undergoing thoracotomy.[19] Tyras et al. found that prophylactic digitalization did not prevent postoperative supraventricular tachycardia in 141 consecutive patients undergoing coronary artery bypass grafting.[20] Electrolyte shifts, hypoxia, and decreased creatinine clearance can accompany major surgical procedures and predispose the patient to digitalis toxicity.[21,22] In addition, certain automatic atrial tachycardias seen after thoracotomy may mimic digitalis toxicity and confuse the issue further.

Stephenson et al. reported that small doses of propranolol (10 mg orally every six hours) significantly decreased postoperative arrhythmias in patients who had had coronary artery bypass surgery.[16] The judicious use of low-dose beta-blockers postoperatively may be considered in hemodynamically stable high-risk patients undergoing coronary artery bypass surgery if there are no known contraindications. Atrial premature contractions do not warrant specific prophylactic antiarrhythmic therapy.

History of Documented Supraventricular Tachycardia

Patients with a history of documented supraventricular tachycardia fall into three groups, each requiring distinct management strategies in the perioperative period. In the first group are those with chronic supraventricular tachycardia, typically atrial fibrillation or, less commonly atrial flutter. Preoperative use of beta-blockers, digoxin, and/or calcium channel blockers to control ventricular rate should be continued. However, excessive digitalis or beta-blockade may inappropriately blunt an expected increase in heart rate with volume loss during surgery. It may be wise to withhold these drugs on the morning of surgery and consider intraoperative hemodynamic monitoring in selected patients. Electrocardiographic evidence of a toxic drug effect should be identified preoperatively and the serum digoxin concentration measured more than six hours after the last dose.[21,22]

Supplemental rate control of atrial fibrillation or flutter during surgery and immediately thereafter can be achieved with the intravenous administration of calcium channel or beta-blockers. Esmolol, a very short-acting beta-blocker, should be used if there is concern about possible adverse effects from longer-acting agents. Supplemental digoxin therapy should be used with caution. Intraoperative and postoperative endogenous catecholamine release usually overrides the therapeutic effect of digoxin on the A-V node. Electrolyte shifts and increased autonomic nervous system activity may potentiate digoxin toxicity.

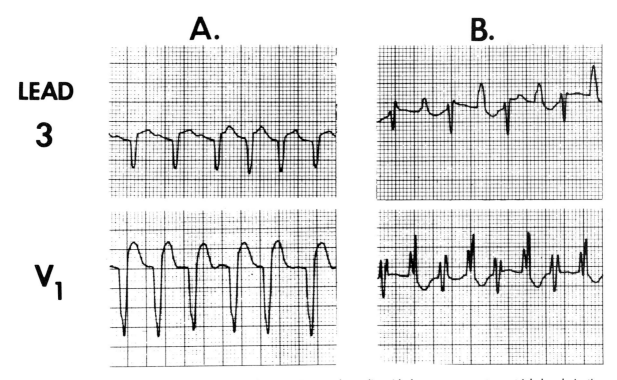

FIGURE 21–2.   A preoperative ECG rhythm strip (A) showing sinus tachycardia with frequent premature atrial depolarizations. The rhythm was misdiagnosed as atrial fibrillation, and the patient developed digoxin toxicity after receiving 2 mg of digoxin over 24 hours. The digoxin toxic rhythm (B) was a fascicular tachycardia with a characteristic narrow right bundle branch block morphology and alternating QRS axis in the frontal plane leads.

An increase in the ventricular rate in atrial fibrillation, like an increase in sinus rate, should prompt a search for other problems. Therapy may be required not only to slow A-V nodal conduction but also to reverse the abnormality causing the increased rate. Two other arrhythmias, multifocal atrial tachycardia and sinus tachycardia with atrial premature beats, are frequently misdiagnosed as atrial fibrillation. Use of digoxin therapy in these cases can have serious consequences (see Fig. 21–2).

Patients in the second group have a history of frequent paroxysms of the arrhythmia and are taking chronic drug therapy to prevent recurrence. The arrhythmia is usually atrial fibrillation or flutter, but others, including A-V nodal reentry or circus-movement tachycardias involving an accessory pathway may occur paroxysmally.[23,24] An A-V nodal blocker is often combined with a class IA agent like quinidine, procainamide, or disopyramide; a class IC drug like propafenone, flecainide, or encainide; or a class III agent like amiodarone (see Table 21–1). It is wise to look for electrocardiographic and clinical manifestations of drug toxicity and to measure serum concentrations of drugs when doses are large or toxicity is suspected.

The stress of surgery may result in supraventricular tachycardia despite preoperative drug therapy. It is important to be aware of the patient's specific arrhythmia, to review any available electrocardiographic documentation, and to understand fully the antiarrhythmic drugs being used.[25] Orally administered drugs are continued up to the time of surgery and restarted immediately thereafter. Intraoperative and postoperative management requires knowledge not only of the type of preoperative drug therapy but also of the time of administration of the antiarrhythmic agent. Supplemental A-V nodal blockade can be achieved with short-acting beta-blockers like esmolol. Alternative intravenous therapy includes calcium channel blockers like verapamil or adenosine. Intravenous procainamide is usually substituted for orally administered class IA, IC, or class III drugs in the absence of significant renal dysfunction or a past allergic reaction.

Patients in the third group have a history of rare episodes of arrhythmia that are generally well tolerated hemodynamically, and they are usually not taking antiarrhythmic drugs. The stresses of surgery may precipitate the arrhythmia and lead to hemodynamic embarrassment. Although prophylactic therapy is rarely indicated, the development of arrhythmias before and during surgery should be anticipated, and extended electrocardiographic monitoring may be necessary. Preoperative review of any available documentation of the arrhythmia and knowledge of response to prior therapy are valuable in directing therapy should the arrhythmia recur.[26]

VENTRICULAR TACHYARRHYTHMIAS

Predictors of Arrhythmia Events and Prophylactic Drug Therapy

Complex ventricular ectopy during and after surgery is common, but serious symptomatic or sustained ventricular arrhythmias are fortunately rare. Patients with a high risk of more serious arrhythmias typically have significant structural heart disease with depressed ventricular function. Those with coronary artery disease usually have (1) a history of a prior myocardial infarction often complicated by acute heart failure or heart block, (2) multivessel coronary artery disease, and (3) a left ventricular aneurysm.[27–29]

Patients with these clinical characteristics need extended periods of electrocardiographic monitoring after surgery.

Available data do not support the contention that ventricular ectopic activity is a marker for more serious ventricular arrhythmias. In one study, ventricular ectopic activity was observed in 62 percent of 283 healthy middle-aged ambulatory men monitored for six hours and is common in the general population.[31] Furthermore, ventricular premature contractions without clinical heart disease or electrocardiographic abnormalities do not significantly influence mortality.[30-32] Kennedy et al. demonstrated that only five of 25 asymptomatic patients with complex ventricular ectopy had coronary artery disease,[33] and no deaths occurred in an average follow-up period of 34 months. Ventricular ectopic activity is seen in 84 percent of patients with coronary artery disease but it does not predict ventricular tachycardia or sudden death.[34] Moss et al. reported that complex ventricular arrhythmias occurring just after infarction were associated with a high rate of cardiac death but did not specifically affect the incidence of sudden death.[35]

The importance of ventricular ectopic activity lies in its reflection of severe underlying coronary artery disease and in the degree that there is left ventricular dysfunction.[36] Goldman et al. reported that occurrence of ventricular premature depolarizations with a frequency of greater than five per minute documented any time before surgery is an independent risk factor predicting a variety of cardiac complications, if not of ventricular tachycardia itself.[37] Ventricular tachycardia occurred in only 12 of 101 patients undergoing noncardiac surgery and was not associated with ventricular ectopic activity on the routine preoperative ECG.

These data suggest that ventricular ectopic activity may be a marker for underlying cardiac disease and not a predictor of sustained ventricular arrhythmias. The potential toxicity of antiarrhythmic drugs, including initiation and aggravation of life-threatening arrhythmias has been well documented (see Table 21–1).[38–42] Caution should be exercised in the use of prophylactic antiarrhythmic drugs in situations where their efficacy has not been demonstrated. Prophylactic therapy for ventricular arrhythmias should be used only in patients who have had a myocardial infarction within 24 hours before emergency surgery.[43–46] In this setting, therapy should be instituted regardless of the degree of ventricular ectopy or the type of surgical procedure. Patients without documented sustained arrhythmias or symptoms attributable to tachyarrhythmias do not, on the basis of ventricular ectopic activity, warrant the risk of antiarrhythmic drug therapy. Careful electrocardiographic monitoring is indicated.

When required, the therapy of choice to prevent ventricular tachycardia is lidocaine as an intravenous bolus infusion of 100 to 200 mg given at a rate of 15 mg/min followed by an infusion of one to two mg/min. An alternative is procainamide as an intravenous bolus infusion of 15 mg/kg given at a rate of 40 to 50 mg/min followed by an infusion of one to four mg/min. Intravenous lidocaine and procainamide are well tolerated even in patients with significant myocardial dysfunction.[47]

History of Documented Sustained Ventricular Arrhythmia

Patients with a history of sustained ventricular arrhythmias are usually on chronic antiarrhythmic therapy. As in patients with supraventricular tachycardias on antiarrhythmics, it is crucial to review available electrocardiographic documentation of the arrhy-

TABLE 21–1. Pharmacokinetics, ECG Effects, and Major Toxicity of Antiarrhythmia Drugs

Drugs and Class	Approximate Elimination Half-Life (hr)	Primary Route of Elimination	ECG Effects and Major Toxicity
Class IA			
Quinidine	6 to 9	Hepatic	*Cardiac:* Long QT syndrome (torsade de pointes) Increased serum digoxin concentration *Noncardiac:* Gastrointestinal distress Thrombocytopenia
Procainamide	3 to 5	Renal	*Cardiac:* Long QT syndrome (torsade de pointes) *Noncardiac:* Gastrointestinal distress Neuropsychiatric, e.g., insomnia, nightmares, depression Lupus-like syndrome Agranulocytosis
Disopyramide	8 to 9	Renal	*Cardiac:* Myocardial depression Long QT syndrome *Noncardiac:* Visual blurring/closed-angle glaucoma Dry mouth Urinary retention
Class IB			
Mexiletine	10 to 17	Hepatic	*Cardiac:* None *Noncardiac:* Neurologic: ataxia, tremor, diplopia Gastrointestinal: nausea and vomiting
Tocainide	11	Hepatic	*Cardiac:* None *Noncardiac:* Hematologic: neutropenia, hypoplastic anemia, thrombocythemia Gastrointestinal: nausea and vomiting Neurologic: memory impairment, dizziness, diplopia
Class IC			
Flecainide	20	Hepatic	*Cardiac:* Myocardial depression Incessant ventricular tachycardia *Noncardiac:* Neurologic: confusion, irritability
Encainide	3 to 8	Hepatic	*Cardiac:* Myocardial depression Ventricular arrhythmias *Noncardiac:* Neurologic: dizziness, diplopia, vertigo, paresthesias
Propafenone	5 to 8	Hepatic	*Cardiac:* Myocardial depression Ventricular arrhythmias *Noncardiac:* Neurologic: dizziness
Class III			
Amiodarone	30 to 60 days	Hepatic	*Cardiac:* Marked sinus bradycardia Hypotension after surgery *Noncardiac:* Pulmonary alveolitis Hypo- and hyperthyroidism Liver enzyme elevation Neurologic: parasthesias, insomnia, muscle weakness Photosensitivity Bluish skin discoloration Corneal microdeposits Epididymitis Inhibits warafin and digoxin metabolism

thmia and the drug history of what has and has not been effective in the past (see Table 21–1). With volume loss and the vasodilatory and myocardial depressant effects of anesthetics, recurrent ventricular tachycardia that may have been tolerated preoperatively can cause hemodynamic embarrassment requiring emergent cardioversion. In addition, drug therapy well tolerated before surgery may cause significant adverse effects in the perioperative period unrelated to the development of ventricular arrhythmias. For example, patients on amiodarone may require higher-dose infusions of catecholamines to maintain adequate blood pressure and have an increased risk of developing the adult respiratory distress syndrome.[48]

Antiarrhythmic drugs are continued until surgery. If oral drugs cannot be resumed postoperatively, intravenous procainamide can be substituted at the expected time either as a continuous infusion of 0.011 mg/kg/min or every four hours at 15 mg/kg given at a rate of 25 mg/min. The dose should be adjusted if renal insufficiency is present. If renal function is severely impaired, procainamide should not be used except in a single dose for acute management of ventricular arrhythmia. Intravenous lidocaine in a dose of one to four mg/min is an alternative prophylactic drug but may be less effective. A loading dose of two mg/kg given at a rate of 15 mg/min is recommended. Serum procainamide or lidocaine levels should be monitored frequently.

Ventricular Arrhythmias Mediated or Potentiated by Catecholamines

Endogenous or exogenous catecholamines can cause most supraventricular and ventricular arrhythmias, but two particular syndromes are especially important in this regard. Although uncommon, both syndromes require recognition because of the uniqueness of their management. They occur often in young patients and in the absence of structural heart disease.

The first syndrome is repetitive monomorphic ventricular tachycardia or right ventricular outflow tract tachycardia.[49,50] It consists of repetitive runs of nonsustained ventricular tachycardia brought on by exertion or when the sinus rate is increased to a critical point. It can sometimes become sustained but has never been shown to degenerate into ventricular fibrillation. It has a left bundle branch block pattern with an inferior axis on ECG (see Fig. 21–3), and this morphology remains constant throughout the duration of the tachycardia. It is potentiated by exercise and catecholamines and usually can be prevented by beta blockers.

The second clinical entity is the congenital form of the long QT syndrome,[51–53] a neuro-cardio-electrical problem with a distinct autosomal inheritance pattern and an association with deafness. Endogenous catecholamine release brought on by emotional excitement or exercise accentuates the prolongation of the QT interval

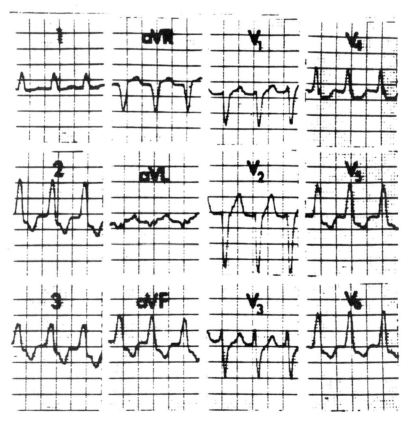

FIGURE 21–3. Characteristic ECG appearance of ventricular tachycardia that originates from the right ventricular outflow tract and occurs in the absence of structural heart disease. The tachycardia typically has a left bundle branch block morphology and an inferior axis in the frontal plane leads.

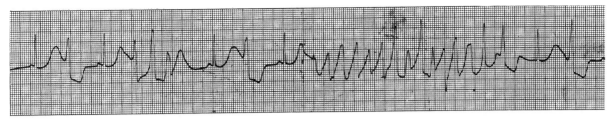

FIGURE 21–4.   Characteristic ECG appearance of prolonged QT interval noted during sinus rhythm and the polymorphic ventricular tachycardia (torsade de pointes) seen in the patient with the congenital form of the long QT syndrome.

and leads to life-threatening polymorphic ventricular arrhythmias termed torsade de pointes (see Fig. 21–4).[54] Ongoing treatment with beta-blockers, e.g., at least 160 mg of propranolol per day or the equivalent, decreases the frequency of arrhythmia recurrence and sudden death. Patients with these two uncommon arrhythmias may require supplemental beta-blockers in the perioperative period as well as extended periods of electrocardiographic monitoring. Exogenous catecholamine is contraindicated.

ANTITACHYCARDIA DEVICE THERAPY

The role of electrical devices in the management of arrhythmias is becoming increasingly important, especially in the treatment of life-threatening ventricular tachycardias.[1,3,55–57] Such devices have both cardioversion and defibrillation capabilities, and some incorporate sophisticated pacing modalities. It is important to be aware of the diagnostic and therapeutic capabilities of each device. In this regard, questions to address before surgery include:

1. What arrhythmia is being treated?
2. What kind of device (manufacturer, model number, lead number, type, and location) does the patient have?
3. How is the device activated and deactivated (e.g., by a programmer or magnet)?
4. What is the response of the device to a magnet placed over it? (Many can be at least temporarily deactivated in this way.)
5. Who is responsible for following the patient and maintaining the function of the device, and when was it last evaluated?
6. What heart rate will trigger the device?
7. Should the device remain active during surgery, or is intraoperative electrocardiographic monitoring sufficient if electrocautery may fire the device?
8. What is the response of the device should an arrythmia occur?
9. What should be done if the device fails to recognize or terminate the arrhythmia?
10. What factors influence the effectiveness of the device (e.g., drugs or extraneous electrical interference)?

If the electrical device has pacing capabilities, thresholds for pacing should be determined and the adequacy of the programmed energy output for pacing assured. Necessary equipment to permit activation and deactivation should be readily accessible. A man-

agement strategy for treating the arrhythmia should the device fail must be in place before surgery. The sophistication of these devices warrants consultation with a well-trained electrophysiologist.

BRADYARRHYTHMIAS AND CONDUCTION DISTURBANCES

Preoperative management of asymptomatic patients with sinus bradycardia or chronic bifascicular conduction disease is no longer controversial. Those with sinus bradycardia do not necessarily have sinus node dysfunction. Heart rates of less than 60 beats per minute have been observed in one-third of all males and one-sixth of all females admitted to a general medical service.[58] Resting heart rate tends to decrease with age.

Agruss et al. investigated the significance of chronic sinus bradycardia with rates of 41 to 51 beats per minute in elderly patients by assessing autonomic function and response to exercise.[59] They concluded that sinus bradycardia is not incompatible with normal cardiac performance. Josephson and Seides emphasized the role of autonomic tone in determining sinus rate and suggested that a heart rate of less than 60/min is not abnormal unless it is persistent and inappropriate in a given physiologic situation.[60]

Patients with sinus bradycardia should be questioned about palpitations followed by periods of dizziness or syncope since this is one of the most common clinical presentations of sick sinus syndrome. Those with sick sinus syndrome require insertion of a temporary pacemaker before surgery. Asymptomatic patients with persistent marked sinus bradycardia not readily explained by alterations in autonomic tone deserve further evaluation. The response to atropine (0.02 mg/kg) or exercise can predict heart rate response to the stress of surgery. Increase in heart rate to 90 or greater suggests that sinus node function is normal and that heart rate will increase appropriately during surgery. If the response is abnormal, electrophysiologic study should be considered.[61] If such study is not available, temporary pacing during surgery is indicated. Response to atropine or exercise is also useful in patients with A-V nodal dysfunction and associated bradyarrhythmias. In most cases, atropine and exercise abolish the arrhythmia and assure that the patient has a low risk of developing life-threatening bradyarrhythmias during and after surgery. Atropine should be avoided in patients with angina at rest or with minimal exercise, glaucoma, or symptoms consistent with bladder outlet obstruction.

Numerous studies confirm that preoperative prophylactic pacemakers are not needed in patients with chronic bifascicular disease but no advanced heart block or symptoms.[62–69] One of 291 patients with bifascicular block drawn from seven studies developed transient complete heart block at intubation. In addition, the presence of right bundle branch block and left posterior hemiblock, or PR-interval prolongation with an associated bifascicular conduction disturbance, do not confer additional risk.[62-69] Bellocci et al. found that, of 98 patients with chronic bifascicular block undergoing surgery of whom 51 had H-V prolongation, none developed advanced heart block in the perioperative period. However, H-V interval prolongation was associated with a higher incidence of cardiac disease and other cardiac complications.[67]

Patients with a history of syncope or dizziness and electrocardiographic evidence of bifascicular disease warrant special consideration. Placement of a prophylactic pacemaker has been recommended in these patients, but this view is not uniformly accepted.[63] Berg and Kotler suggest that patients with bifascicular disease and syncope with no previous evidence of advanced heart block be observed closely without a temporary pacemaker.[63]

Syncope, even in patients with bifascicular block, is often multifactorial. Dhingra et al. could attribute syncope to bradyarrhythmias in only six of 30 such patients. Of the 24 remaining patients, two had orthostatic hypotension, three had seizure disorders, nine had ventricular arrhythmias, one had acute blood loss, and nine had no documented etiology and no recurrent symptoms.[70] Ezri et al. noted a significant incidence of inducible sustained ventricular tachycardia in patients who experience syncope in a setting of bifascicular block and structural heart disease.[71] A complete electrophysiologic evaluation including programmed ventricular stimulation should be performed before elective surgery in patients with unexplained syncope and bifascicular block, especially in those with coronary artery disease. Criteria for placement of a temporary pacemaker at the time of surgery in patients who do not already have a permanent pacemaker in place are detailed in Table 21–2.

Before the development of the pacemaker, Vandam and McLemore found that, of 22 patients with chronic complete heart block, six suffered circulatory arrest in the operating room.[72] Although asymptomatic patients with bifascicular block generally do not go on to develop complete heart block or bradyarrhythmias and do not require prophylactic pacing, there is one important situation in which this may occur. Placement of a Swan-Ganz catheter can induce right bundle branch block in up to 5 percent of patients. Those who already have documented left bundle branch block in whom a Swan-Ganz catheter is needed should therefore first be considered for a temporary pacemaker to avoid development of complete heart block.[73,74]

Temporary pacing can usually be carried out with few complications.[62] However, Nolewajka et al. reported deep-venous thrombosis documented by venography in 37 percent of patients who had had a temporary pacing wire placed through the femoral vein.[75] The frequency of deep-venous thrombosis was even higher in a subgroup of hemodynamically compromised patients. Pacing catheters inserted through the femoral vein also have been associated with an increased risk of sepsis and pulmonary emboli. The risk of complications increases if the wire is left in place for more than 72 hours. Therefore, insertion through the brachial, internal jugular, or subclavian vein is preferred. Pacemaker function should be completely checked just prior to induction of anesthesia and at least once daily thereafter for as long as pacing is required.

Permanent Pacemakers for Bradycardia

Essential information should be acquired before surgery in all patients with bradycardia pacing systems.[62,76] This includes the manufacturer and model number, type of programmer necessary to adjust the device, response of the device to the application of a magnet, details of programmed pacing mode and rate, and indication for the device. The appropriate programming device and pacing magnet should be readily accessible during and after surgery. Normal pacing and sensing function should be documented before the procedure. If the pacemaker is functioning in the demand mode and the intrinsic heart rate exceeds the rate that triggers pacing, pacing function can be evaluated by applying a magnet to the pacemaker and activating the fixed-rate mode. The pacing threshold and status of the generator battery should be determined if more than a month has elapsed since the last evaluation or if the pacemaker generator and lead(s) were implanted within the last month.

Demand bradycardia pacemakers may be suppressed by outside electrical activity like electrocautery.[77] Maintaining the pacemaker in a fixed-rate mode or limiting the frequency and duration of electrocautery to one-second bursts separated by 10-second intervals should prevent this problem. The dispersion pad, the anode of the electrocautery device, should be placed on the patient's lower extremity away from the pacemaker generator.

SUMMARY

1. The incidence of serious arrhythmias during surgery is low but is increased by hypercapnea, hypoxia, hypokalemia, acidosis, anemia, autonomic and central nervous stimulation, and some anesthetics.

2. In patients undergoing noncardiac surgery, supraventricular tachycardia, usually atrial flutter or fibrillation, is most common in patients over 70, those with pulmonary rales, and those undergoing intraabdominal, intrathoracic, or major vascular procedures. Most of these patients have concurrent medical problems but no previous history of significant arrhythmia. The electrocardiogram is an insensitive predictor of perioperative arrhythmia except in the case of Wolff-Parkinson-White syndrome.

TABLE 21–2. Criteria for Placement of a Temporary Pacemaker Before Surgery

Symptomatic* cardioinhibitory carotid sinus hypersensitivity
Sinus node dysfunction
Sinus pauses greater than 3 sec or those resulting in symptoms
Symptomatic* sinus bradycardia
Atrioventricular nodal block
Symptomatic* second-degree heart block (Mobitz I)
Symptomatic* complete heart block
Infranodal block
New bifascicular conduction system disease (right bundle branch block and left axis deviation, right bundle branch block and left posterior hemiblock, alternating bundle branch block) associated with acute ischemia
Second-degree heart block (Mobitz II)
Complete heart block

*Symptoms include evidence of cerebral hypoperfusion, cardiac ischemia, congestive heart failure, increased ventricular irritability, and precipitation of tachyarrhythmias.

3. Prophylactic therapy with antiarrhythmic agents is generally not effective except in patients undergoing coronary bypass surgery in whom low doses of beta-blocker may decrease postoperative arrhythmias.

4. Patients on therapy for chronic supraventricular tachycardia should receive their usual medication in the perioperative period. Supplemental rate control can be achieved with calcium channel blockers, beta-blockers, or cautious use of digoxin. Those in normal sinus rhythm but on therapy for paroxysmal supraventricular tachycardia may be handled in the same manner. Knowledge of the nature of their arrhythmia facilitates therapy should it arise perioperatively. Those with a history of rarely occurring supraventricular tachycardia should be monitored expectantly.

5. Ventricular ectopic activity in those without a history of sustained arrhythmias should not be considered a marker for sudden death or serious ventricular arrhythmias in the perioperative period. However, it may reflect underlying coronary artery disease or abnormal left ventricular function. Prophylactic antiarrhythmic therapy itself carries significant risks and is not recommended except in the case of emergency surgery in patients who have suffered a myocardial infarction in the prior 24 to 48 hours.

6. Antiarrhythmic agents should be continued up to the time of surgery in those with a history of sustained ventricular arrhythmias. In the perioperative period, procainamide or lidocaine can be substituted as detailed in the text above. Drug levels should be followed carefully. Repetitive monomorphic ventricular tachycardia and congenital long QT syndrome with torsade de pointes become problematic when endogenous or exogenous catecholamine levels are increased. Patients with these syndromes require especially close monitoring and supplemental beta-blocker therapy.

7. Perioperative management of patients with antitachycardia devices requires detailed knowledge of the implanted device and warrants consultation with a cardiologist.

8. Symptomatic patients with bradyarrhythmias should be evaluated before surgery and may need a temporary pacemaker. Asymptomatic patients who respond to exercise or atropine with a heart rate above 90/min have a low risk of perioperative complications, but those who do not warrant further preoperative evaluation or temporary pacing.

9. Patients with chronic bifascicular block with no evidence of advanced heart block or symptoms do not require preoperative prophylactic placement of a pacemaker. Electrophysiologic study should be considered in patients with bifascicular block and a history of syncope or dizziness. Although only some develop bradyarrhythmias, they may have underlying structural heart disease and be subject to sustained ventricular tachycardia during surgery. Indications for perioperative temporary pacing are outlined in Table 21-2.

10. Management of patients with permanent bradycardia pacemakers also requires detailed knowledge of their particular devices. Pacemaker function should be fully evaluated before surgery, and an appropriate programming device and pacing magnet should be available at all times. Suppression of pacemaker activity by electrocautery devices can be avoided by maintaining the pacemaker in a fixed-rate mode or limiting the frequency and duration of electrocautery.

REFERENCES

1. Marchlinski FE, Flores BT, Buxton AE et al: The automatic implantable cardioverter-defibrillator: Efficacy, complications, and device failures. *Ann Intern Med* 104:481–488, 1986.
2. Miller JM, Kienzle MG, Harken AH et al: Subendocardial resection for ventricular tachycardia: Predictors of surgical success. *Circulation* 70:624–631, 1984.
3. Marchlinski FE, Buxton AE, Flores BF: The automatic implantable cardioverter defibrillator: Follow-up and complications, in El-Sherif N, Samet P (eds): *Cardiac Pacing and Electrophysiology* Orlando, Grune & Stratton, 1990, pp 756–777.
4. Wilber DJ, Garan H, Finkelstein D et al: Out-of-hospital cardiac arrest. Use of electrophysiologic testing in the prediction of long-term outcome. *N Engl J Med* 318:19–24, 1986.
5. Kuner J, Enescu V, Utsu F et al: Cardiac arrhythmias during anesthesia. *Dis Chest* 52:580, 1967.
6. Bertrand CA, Steiner NV, Jameson AG et al: Disturbances of cardiac rhythm during anesthesia and surgery. *JAMA* 216:1615, 1971.
7. Vanik PE, Davis HS: Cardiac arrhythmia during halothane anesthesia. *Anesth Analg* 47–299, 1968.
8. Katz RL, Bigger JT: Cardiac arrhythmias during anesthesia and operation. *Anesthesiology* 33:193, 1970.
9. Walker DE, Barry JM, Hodges CV: Succinylcholine-induced ventricular fibrillation in the paralyzed urology patient. *Urol* 113:111, 1975.
10. Gronest GA, Theye RA: Pathophysiology of hyperkalemia induced by succinylcholine. *Anesthesiology* 43:89, 1975.
11. Katz RL, Epstine RA: The interaction of anesthetic agents and adrenergic drugs to produce cardiac arrhythmias. *Anesthesiology* 29:763, 1968.
12. Mendoza IG, Kleinman RB, Marchlinski FE: Electrophysiologic effects of the anesthetic propofol at postoperative defibrillator testing. *J Am Coll Cardiol* 19(3):221A, 1992.
13. Hook BG, Perlman RL, Callans DJ et al: Acute and chronic cycle length dependent increase in ventricular pacing threshold. *PACE* 15:1437, 1992.
14. Goldman L: Supraventricular tachyarrhythmias in hospitalized adults after surgery. *Chest* 73:4, 1978.
15. Rogers WR, Wrobleski F, LaDue JS: Supraventricular tachycardia complicating surgical procedures. *Circulation* 7:192, 1952.
16. Stephenson LW, MacVaugh H, Tomasello D et al: Propranolol for the prevention of postoperative cardiac arrhythmias. A randomized study. *Ann Thorac Surg* 29:113, 1980.
17. Buxton AE, Kastor JA, Josephson ME: Role of P wave duration as a predictor of postoperative atrial arrhythmias. *Chest* 80:68–73, 1981.
18. Packer DL, Prystowsky EN: Wolff-Parkinson-White Syndrome: Further progress in evaluation and treatment, in Zipes DP, Rowlands DJ (eds): *Progress in Cardiology*. Philadelphia, Lea & Febiger, 1988, pp 231–253.
19. Juler GL, Stemmer EA, Connelly JE: Complications of prophylactic digitalization in thoracic surgical patients. *J Thorac Cardiovasc Surg* 58:352, 1969.
20. Tyras DH, Stothert JC, Kaiser GC et al: Supraventricular tachyarrhythmias after myocardial revascularization: A randomized trial of prophylactic digitalization. *J Thorac Cardiovasc Surg* 77:310, 1979.
21. Fisch C, Knoebel SB: Digitalis cardiotoxicity. *J Am Coll Cardiol* 5:91A–98A, 1985.
22. Smith TW: Pharmacokinetics, bioavailability and serum levels of cardiac glycosides. *J Am Coll Cardiol* 5:43A–50A, 1985.
23. Calkins H, Langberg J, Sousa J et al: Radiofrequency catheter ablation of accessory atrioventricular connections in 250 patients: Abbreviated therapeutic approach to Wolff-Parkinson-White syndrome. *Circulation* 85:1337–1346, 1992.
24. Jazayeri MR, Hempe SL, Sra JS et al: Selective transcatheter ablation of the fast and slow pathway using radiofrequency energy in patients

with atrioventricular nodal reentrant tachycardia. *Circulation* 85:1318–1328, 1992.

25. Koblin DD, Romanoff ME, Martin DE et al: Anesthetic management of the parturient receiving amiodarone. *Anesthesiology* 66:551–553, 1987.

26. Kay GN, Pressley JC, Packer DL et al: Value of the 12-lead electrocardiogram in discriminating atrioventricular nodal reciprocating tachycardia from circus movement atrioventricular tachycardia utilizing a retrograde accessory pathway. *Am J Cardiol* 59:296, 1987.

27. Marchlinski FE: Ventricular tachycardia associated with coronary artery disease, in Zipes DP, Rowlands DJ (eds): *Progress in Cardiology* Philadelphia, Lea & Febiger, 231–253, 1988.

28. Marchlinski FE, Waxman HL, Buxton AE et al: Sustained ventricular tachyarrhythmias during the early postinfarction period: Electrophysiologic findings and prognosis for survival. *J Am Coll Cardiol* 2:240–250, 1983.

29. Marchlinski FE: Ventricular tachycardia soon after myocardial infarction: Risk and management. *Int J Cardiol* 5:761–766, 1984.

30. Desai DC, Hershberg PI, Alexander S: Clinical significance of ventricular premature beats in an outpatient population. *Chest* 4:564, 1973.

31. Hinkle LE, Carver ST, Stevens M: The frequency of asymptomatic disturbances of cardiac rhythm and conduction in middle-aged men. *Am J Cardiol* 24:629, 1969.

32. Rodstein M, Wolloch L, Gubner RS: Mortality study of the significance of extrasystole in an insured population. *Chest* 64:564, 1973.

33. Kennedy HL, Pescarmona JE, Bouchard RJ et al: Coronary artery status of apparently healthy subjects with frequent and complex ventricular ectopy. *Ann Intern Med* 92:179, 1980.

34. Kotler MN, Tabtznik B, Mower NM et al: Prognostic significance of ventricular ectopic beats with respect to sudden death in the late postinfarction period. *Circulation* 47:959, 1973.

35. Moss AJ, Davis HT, Decamille J et al: Ventricular ectopic beats and their relation to sudden and non-sudden cardiac death after myocardial infarction. *Circulation* 60:998, 1979.

36. Schulze RA, Rouleau J, Rigo P et al: Ventricular arrhythmias in the late hospital phase of acute myocardial infarction: Relation of left ventricular function detected by gated blood pool scanning. *Circulation* 52:1006, 1975.

37. Goldman L, Caldera DL, Southwick FS et al: Multifactorial index of cardiac risk in noncardiac surgical procedures. *N Engl J Med* 297:845, 1977.

38. Koster RW, Wellens HJ: Quinidine-induced ventricular flutter and fibrillation without digitalis therapy. *Am J Cardiol* 38:519, 1976.

39. Meltzer RS, Robert EW, McMorrow M et al: Atypical ventricular tachycardias: A manifestation of disopyramide toxicity. *Am J Cardiol* 42:1049, 1978.

40. Nicholson WJ, Martin CE, Gracey JG et al: Disopyramide-induced ventricular fibrillation. *Am J Cardiol* 43:1053, 1979.

41. Cohen IS, Jick H, Cohen SI: Adverse reactions to quinidine in hospitalized patients: Findings based on data from the Boston Collaborative Drug Surveillance Program. *Prog Cardiovasc Dis* 20:151, 1977.

42. Horowitz LN: Drugs and proarrhythmia, in Zipes DP, Rowlands DJ (eds): *Progress in Cardiology*. Philadelphia, Lea & Febiger, 1988, pp 109–125.

43. Lie KI, Wellens HJ, VanCapelle FJ et al: Lidocaine in the prevention of primary ventricular fibrillation. *N Engl J Med* 291:1324, 1974.

44. Noneman JW, Rogers JF: Lidocaine prophylaxis in acute myocardial infarction. *Medicine* 57:501, 1978.

45. Harrison DC: Should lidocaine be administered routinely to all patients after acute myocardial infarction? *Circulation* 58:581, 1978.

46. Lie KI, Wellens HJ, Downar E et al: Observations on patients with primary ventricular fibrillation complicating acute myocardial infarction. *Circulation* 52:755, 1975.

47. Burton JR, Matthew MJ, Armstrong PW: Comparative effects of lidocaine and procainamide on acute impaired hemodynamics. *Am J Cardiol* 43:98, 1979.

48. Greenspon AJ, Kidwell GA, Hurley W et al: Amiodarone-related postoperative adult respiratory distress syndrome. *Circulation* 84(Suppl 5):407–415, 1991.

49. Buxton AE, Waxman HL, Marchlinski FE et al: Right ventricular tachycardia: Clinical and electrophysiologic characteristics. *Circulation* 68:917–927, 1983.

50. Coumel P, Leciercq JF, Slama R: Repetitive monomorphic idiopathic ventricular tachycardia, in Zipes DP, Jalife J (eds): *Cardiac Electrophysiology and Arrhythmias*. Orlando, Grune & Stratton, 1985, pp 455–466.

51. Callaghan AC, Normandale JP, Morgan M: The prolonged Q-T syndrome: A review with anaesthetic implications and a report of two cases. *Anaesth Intens Care* 10:50–55, 1982.

52. Wig J, Bali IM, Singh RG et al: Prolonged Q-T interval syndrome. Sudden cardiac arrest during anaesthesia. *Anaesthesia* 34:37–40, 1979.

53. Moss AJ, Schwartz PJ, Crampton RS et al: The long QT syndrome: A prospective international study. *Circulation* 71:17–21, 1985.

54. Schwartz PJ: Idiopathic long QT syndrome: Progress and questions. *Am Heart J* 109:399–410, 1985.

55. Troup PJ: Implantable cardioverters and defibrillators, in O'Rourke RA, Crawford MH (eds): *Current Problems in Cardiology* New York, Year Book Med Pub, 1989, pp 675–843.

56. Gaba DM, Wyner J, Fish KJ: Anesthesia and the automatic implantable cardioverter/defibrillator. *Anesthesiology* 62:786–792, 1985.

57. Carr CM, Whiteley SM: The automatic implantable cardioverter/defibrillator. Implications for anesthetists. *Anesthesia* 46(9):737–740, 1991.

58. Kirk JE, Kvorning SA: Sinus bradycardia: A clinical study of 515 consecutive cases. *Acta Med Scand* (Suppl) 266:625, 1952.

59. Agruss NS, Rosen EV, Adolph RJ et al: Significance of chronic sinus bradycardia in elderly people. *Circulation* 46:924, 1972.

60. Josephson ME: *Clinical Cardiac Electrophysiology: Techniques and Interpretations*. Philadelphia, Lea & Febiger, 1993, pp 71–166.

61. Gann D, Tolentino R, Samet P: Electrophysiologic evaluation of elderly patients with sinus bradycardia. *Ann Intern Med* 90:24, 1979.

62. O'Neill MJ, Davis D: Pacemakers in noncardiac surgery. *Surg Clin N Am* 63:1103–1112, 1983.

63. Berg GR, Kotler MN: The significance of bilateral bundle branch block in the preoperative patient. *Chest* 59:62, 1971.

64. Kundstadt D, Punga M, Cagin N et al: Bifascicular block: A clinical and electrophysiologic study. *Am Heart J* 86:173, 1983.

65. Venkataraman K, Madias JE, Hood WB: Indications for prophylactic preoperative insertion of pacemakers in patients with right bundle branch block and left anterior hemiblock. *Chest* 86:501, 1975.

66. Pastore J, Yurchak PM, Janis KM et al: The risk of advanced heart block in surgical patients with right bundle branch block and left axis deviation. *Circulation* 57:677, 1978.

67. Bellocci F, Santanelli P, DiGennano M et al: The risk of cardiac complication in surgical patients with bifascicular block: A clinical and electrophysiologic study in 98 patients. *Chest* 77:343, 1980.

68. Rooney SM, Goldiner PL, Muss E: Relationship of right bundle branch block and marked left axis deviation to complete heart block during anesthesia. *Anesthesiology* 44:65, 1976.

69. Goldman L, Caldera DL, Southwick FS et al: Cardiac risk factors and complications in noncardiac surgery. *Medicine* 57:357, 1978.

70. Dhingra RC, Denes P, Wu D et al: Syncope in patients with chronic bifascicular block. *Ann Intern Med* 81:302, 1974.

71. Ezri MD, Lerman BB, Marchlinski FE et al: Electrophysiologic evaluation of syncope in patients with bifascicular block. *Am Heart J* 106:693–697, 1983.

72. Vandam LD, McLemore GA: Circulatory arrest in patients with complete heart block during anesthesia and surgery. *Ann Intern Med* 47:518, 1957.

73. Thomson IR, Dalton BC, Lappos DG et al: Right bundle branch block and complete heart block caused by the Swan-Ganz catheter. *Anesthesiology* 31:359, 1979.

74. Campo I, Garfield G, Escher DJ et al: Complications of pacing by pervenous subclavian semi-float electrodes including two extraluminal insertions. *Am J Cardiol* 26:627, 1970.

75. Nolewajka AJ, Goddard MP, Brown TC: Temporary transvenous pacing and femoral vein thrombosis. *Circulation* 62:646, 1980.

76. Simon AB: Perioperative management of the pacemaker patient. *Anesthesiology* 46:127, 1977.

77. Lerner SM: Suppression of a demand pacemaker by transurethral electrocautery. *Anesth Analg* 52:703, 1973.

22 PREOPERATIVE EVALUATION AND PREPARATION OF PATIENTS WITH PULMONARY DISEASE

Horace M. DeLisser

Michael A. Grippi

Significant alterations in pulmonary function occur during and after surgery in patients with normal and diseased lungs and are usually well tolerated (see Table 22–1). However, patients with underlying lung disease have a higher risk of postoperative pulmonary complications. This chapter focuses on preoperative evaluation and preparation of these patients. First, expected changes in pulmonary function are reviewed, pulmonary complications of surgery are outlined, and general and respiratory-specific risk factors are discussed. Next, preoperative clinical and laboratory assessment of the patient is considered including that of patients undergoing lung resection. Finally, recommendations regarding preoperative therapy and postoperative management are made.

CHANGES IN PULMONARY FUNCTION WITH SURGERY

Many postoperative complications can be considered an exaggeration of the usual postoperative changes in pulmonary function arising from surgical, anesthetic, or pharmacologic interventions.

TABLE 22–1. Changes in Pulmonary Function with Surgery

Reduction in lung volumes (restrictive defect)
Diaphragm dysfunction
Impaired gas exchange, including hypoxemia
Respiratory depression due to residual effects of anesthesia or postoperative narcotics
Impaired cough and mucociliary clearance

Knowledge of normal pulmonary physiology is essential for understanding many postoperative problems. Five areas are considered: (1) lung volumes; (2) diaphragmatic function; (3) gas exchange; (4) control of breathing; and (5) lung defense mechanisms.[1–3] In addition, effects of specific anesthetics and the nature of the surgery must be addressed.

Lung Volumes

Following thoracic and abdominal surgery, restrictive changes occur in lung function, characterized by moderate to severe reductions in vital capacity (VC) and smaller, but more important reductions in functional residual capacity (FRC) (see Fig. 22–1).[1–6] Impairment is similar in upper-abdominal and thoracic surgery, but smaller changes in VC and FRC are seen in lower-abdominal procedures.[4] Surgery involving the extremities is usually not associated with changes.[3,4] During the first 24 hours after upper-abdominal surgery, VC and FRC may be reduced by more than 70% and 50%, respectively, and may remain depressed for more than a week.[1,4–6] It is therefore not surprising that pulmonary complications are more common in thoracic and upper-abdominal surgery than in other procedures.[3]

Other lung volumes, including total lung capacity (TLC), inspiratory capacity (IC), expiratory reserve volume (ERV), and residual volume (RV) are also reduced.[3,6] While the forced expiratory volume in one second (FEV_1) is decreased, the ratio of FEV_1 to the forced vital capacity (FEV_1/FVC) remains unchanged, indicating that major airway obstruction does not occur.[6]

Surgery in other areas of the body does not result in major changes in lung volumes, and in many patients FRC in the early postoperative period may remain unchanged.[4,7–9] Alternatively, re-

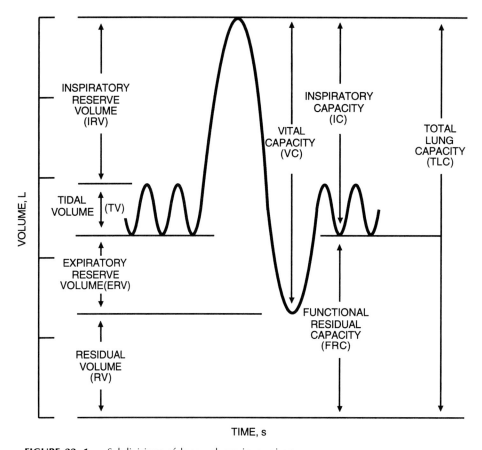

FIGURE 22–1. Subdivisions of lung volume in a spirogram.
Source: From Fishman AP (ed): *Pulmonary Disease and Disorders.* New York, McGraw-Hill, 1988, with permission.

duction in FRC may be the result of impaired lung mechanics due to pain and muscle splinting. However, since effective pain control using epidural anesthesia or intercostal nerve block fails to restore VC or FRC to preoperative levels,[10–13] other mechanisms must be operative. Diaphragmatic dysfunction may be an important contributing factor.

Reduced FRC is of major physiologic significance because of its relationship to closing capacity (CC). FRC is the lung volume at the end of a normal tidal expiration. CC is the lung volume at which small airways in the lung bases begin to close during expiration (see Fig. 22–2). In a normal lung, FRC is always greater than CC, and airways remain open throughout a tidal breath. However, when CC is greater than FRC, lung volume fails to increase sufficiently during tidal breathing to open all of the airways. Consequently, some alveolar units remain closed and constitute areas of atelectasis. If CC exceeds lung volume for part of the time during each tidal breath, airways open for only a portion of the respiratory cycle, thereby creating areas of low ventilation relative to perfusion. In summary, any situation that decreases FRC below CC or that increases CC above FRC produces regions of reduced ventilation and atelectasis. Table 22–2 outlines some of the conditions that may alter this relationship.

Diaphragm Function

Dysfunction of the diaphragm contributes to postoperative reduction in lung volumes.[8,9,13–16] In a study of patients undergoing

TABLE 22–2. Conditions that Alter the Relationship Between Functional Residual Capacity (FRC) and Closing Capacity (CC)

Decrease FRC	Increase CC
Supine position	Advanced age
Obesity	Smoking
Pregnancy	COPD
General anesthesia	Pulmonary edema
Abdominal pain	

cholecystectomy, the contribution of the diaphragm to quiet tidal breathing after surgery was shown to be significantly reduced.[14] Pain does not account for the impairment.[13] Measurements of transdiaphragmatic pressure during maximal phrenic nerve stimulation after upper-abdominal surgery indicate decreased central nervous system output to the phrenic nerves. This may be the result of inhibitory reflexes arising from sympathetic, vagal, or splanchnic receptors.[8]

Gas Exchange

Postoperative arterial hypoxemia is common and occurs in two phases.[17–23] In the first several hours after surgery,[1,20] it is related largely to residual effects of anesthesia. These include ventilation-

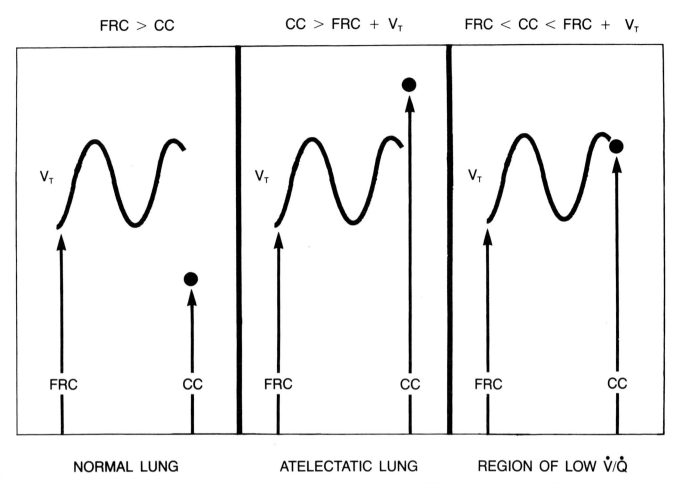

FIGURE 22–2.   The relationship between functional residual capacity (FRC) and closing capacity (CC).

perfusion mismatch, anesthetic-induced inhibition of hypoxic pulmonary vasoconstriction, right-to-left shunting, alveolar hypoventilation, depressed cardiac output, and increased oxygen consumption by peripheral muscle. This phase resolves within 24 hours.

After thoracic or upper-abdominal surgery, hypoxemia may persist for several days or weeks.[6,18,19,22,24] This second phase correlates with reductions in FRC and, more specifically, with changes in the FRC-CC relationship. Other processes contributing to late postoperative hypoxemia include alveolar hypoventilation; increased dead space ventilation due to rapid shallow breathing; and decreased mixed venous oxygen tension due to increased oxygen consumption, impaired cardiac output, and reduced oxygen-carrying capacity.[1,2]

Control of Breathing

Two factors are responsible for postoperative respiratory depression. First, residual effects of anesthetics inhibit respiratory drive and reduce the ventilatory response to hypercapnia, hypoxia, and acidemia.[25–28] Second, narcotics given for postoperative analgesia depress both hypoxic and hypercapnic ventilatory drives, resulting in decreased tidal volume, reduced minute ventilation, and increased Pa_{CO_2}.[29] Narcotics also alter the pattern of breathing, reducing the frequency of sighs or eliminating them entirely.[25] In addition, sleep apnea may develop in patients treated with narcotic analgesics.[30]

Lung Defense Mechanisms

A number of mechanisms protect the lung from environmental and infectious agents.[31] Two of the most important, cough and mucociliary transport, are impaired postoperatively, contributing to an increased risk of pulmonary infection.[32] Coughing is inhibited as a result of postoperative pain or excessive use of narcotics. Furthermore, alterations in lung mechanics result in reduced expulsive force generated with each cough.[2] Mucociliary clearance is decreased for up to six days following upper-abdominal surgery[33] and is related to ciliary damage from inhalation of dry gases,[34] endotracheal intubation,[35] and use of hyperoxic gas mixtures.[36] Other factors include reduction in tracheal mucus velocity from the endotracheal tube,[2] inhibition of mucociliary transport from anesthetic agents,[31] and reduced clearance of lower tract secretions from atelectasis.[3]

Effects of Type of Anesthesia

The pulmonary effects of general anesthesia have been reviewed extensively.[37–39] Impairment of oxygenation and carbon dioxide elimination are two of the most important. These effects are due to anesthetic-induced changes in the shape and motion of the chest wall and diaphragm that in turn lead to increases in alveolar dead space, shunt fraction, and ventilation-perfusion mismatch. These alterations may contribute to subsequent pulmonary morbidity and mortality.

The use of regional anesthesia should be considered in patients with underlying pulmonary disease. Epidural anesthesia to a T4 sensory level does not alter FRC, VC, FEV_1, the alveolar-arterial oxygen gradient, shunt fraction, or cardiac output.[8] However, with the exception of several reports documenting a reduced risk of postoperative thromboembolism with epidural anesthesia,[40-44] there are no good studies indicating that regional anesthesia results in a lower incidence of other postoperative pulmonary complications.[45] Although one study suggests that, in patients with COPD, spinal anesthesia is associated with lower postoperative mortality,[46] other studies fail to demonstrate this advantage with other forms of regional anesthesia.[47,48]

Effects of Surgical Site

The anatomic site of operation is a significant factor in the development of postoperative pulmonary complications.[3] The complication rate in upper- and lower-abdominal operations is about 10 percent compared with a 0.6 percent rate for procedures that do not involve abdomen or thorax.[49] For upper-abdominal surgery the complication rate ranges from 7 to 76 percent,[6,48-53] while for lower-abdominal procedures it is 0 to 5 percent.[48,50,53] In lung resection, the complication rate is dependent on other factors, including the presence of underlying lung disease, the amount of functional lung removed, and the extent to which the "bellows" function of the lung is impaired.[3]

PULMONARY COMPLICATIONS

Criteria for defining postoperative respiratory morbidity and mortality vary considerably. However, there are several major categories of complications:[6,49,51,54-60] (1) atelectasis; (2) infection, including acute tracheobronchitis and pneumonia; (3) exacerbation of underlying chronic lung disease; and (4) prolonged mechanical ventilation and respiratory failure. Two additional problems with significant postoperative morbidity and mortality,[2,61] venous thromboembolism and permeability pulmonary edema, have been excluded in many studies addressing postoperative pulmonary complications. In thoracic surgery, several additional unique pulmonary complications may occur and are summarized in Table 22–3.[52,53,62-72]

Because of the marked variability in defining postoperative pulmonary complications, an overall incidence ranging from 5 to 90 percent has been reported in the literature. Although a young healthy nonsmoker of normal weight has a very low risk of postoperative pulmonary complications (approximately one percent[3]), the presence of preexisting lung disease and a number of other "general" factors increase the risk of developing complications. These general risk factors for postoperative pulmonary complications include: (1) age, (2) obesity, (3) smoking history, (4) nutritional status, (5) antecedent respiratory tract infection, (6) type of surgical incision, (7) duration of anesthesia, and (8) general state of health.

Age

Data from both older retrospective and some more recent prospective studies suggest that advanced age is a major risk factor in the development of postoperative pulmonary complications.[3,51,55] However, other prospective analyses fail to confirm this when other confounding variables are excluded.[6,49,73-76] In a large study of 520 patients undergoing elective thoracic or abdominal surgery, no association between age and postoperative pneumonia was noted.[74] Similar results were noted in another study of 200 consecutive patients admitted for a variety of elective surgical procedures.[76]

Correlation between age and complication rate is also not seen in patients undergoing lung resection.[77-80] In a study of patients undergoing thoracotomy for lung cancer, 30-day postoperative mortality was somewhat higher in patients over 70, but the incidences of postoperative pulmonary complications, hospital stay, and survival were not statistically different.[80] Advanced age alone should not be considered a contraindication to surgery.

Obesity

Several changes in respiratory mechanics and pulmonary function test parameters occur in obese patients.[81-83] Accumulation of fat in the chest wall, diaphragm, and abdomen may reduce total respiratory compliance by more than 60%, a change that is amplified

TABLE 22–3. Pulmonary Complications Associated with Thoracic Surgery

Procedure	Complication	Incidence	References
Coronary artery bypass grafting	Phrenic nerve damage	10%	[60]
	Late pleural effusions*	—**	[61, 62]
Thoracotomy with lung resection	Bronchopleural fistula and/or empyema	5–20%***	[63–67]
Median sternotomy	Sternal wound infection (mediastinitis and/or osteomyelitis)	1–2%	[68–70]
Esophagectomy and/or gastrectomy	Anastamotic leak	3–6%	[71, 72]

*Pleural effusions arising after discharge from hospital.
**Incidence not noted in published reports.
***Higher for patients with sarcoidosis and aspergilloma.

when the patient is supine. Reduced compliance in turn increases the work of breathing. Minute ventilation, oxygen consumption, and carbon dioxide production are further increased above levels that are already elevated as a result of the increased metabolic demands imposed by the obese state.[82]

Spirometry in obese patients reveals no evidence of airways obstruction, but a reduction in expiratory reserve volume (ERV) is found consistently. The magnitude of reduction correlates with the degree of obesity,[83] and areas of low ventilation relative to perfusion and atelectasis result.[84] In addition to these mechanical changes, obese patients have larger gastric volume and lower pH and may be predisposed to aspiration.[85]

Data on the incidence of postoperative pulmonary complications in obese patients are conflicting. In a review of 10 large series of obese patients undergoing gastric bypass, Pasulka et al. found a 3.9 percent incidence of pneumonia and atelectasis and a one percent incidence of pulmonary embolism and thrombophlebitis. These frequencies are similar to those seen in the general population.[81] Another retrospective review of 48 obese patients undergoing cholecystectomy demonstrated no increase in the rate of postoperative pneumonitis or atelectasis compared with nonobese.[86]

Few prospective studies have been conducted on the subject.[6,49,74] Small numbers of patients have been studied,[6,52] nonuniform definitions of obesity have been employed,[6,49] and height has not been routinely considered.[74] In one series, no significant difference in the incidence of pulmonary complications was documented when patients of normal weight and those 5% above ideal weight were compared.[49] However, in another study in which obesity was defined as a body weight greater than 10% above ideal, investigators noted an association between obesity and postoperative pulmonary problems, particularly atelectasis, in 18 of 19 obese patients.[6] While it appears that obesity may increase the risk of postoperative pulmonary complications, the magnitude and significance of this risk are unknown.

Smoking History

Smoking increases the risk of postoperative respiratory complications independent of its association with chronic obstructive lung disease.[48,74,76,87] Adverse changes in respiratory epithelium and pulmonary function correlate well with the amount of tobacco use.[88-92] In patients undergoing coronary artery bypass graft surgery, the risk is significant when tobacco use exceeds 20 pack-years.[87] A statistically significant reduction in complications occurs only when patients stop smoking for at least eight weeks before surgery. This finding is consistent with previous reports showing that pulmonary function abnormalities may take weeks to months to reverse after smoking cessation.[89,90]

Nutritional Status

Malnutrition and severe starvation have significant effects on the respiratory system, including diminished ventilatory response to hypoxia, decreased diaphragmatic muscle function, impaired cell-mediated and humoral immunity, and alterations in the elastic properties of the lung with development of "emphysema-like" changes.[93-96] While many hospitalized patients show some signs of malnutrition,[97,98] it is unclear whether it produces clinically significant changes in pulmonary function or an increased incidence of

postoperative pulmonary complications.[54,93] Although aggressive preoperative nutritional support does improve biochemical parameters,[99,100] its effect in decreasing postsurgical pulmonary morbidity is unknown.[101]

Antecedent Respiratory Tract Infection

Viral respiratory tract infections may cause enhanced airway reactivity and increased airway resistance. The increased resistance may persist for several weeks following resolution of acute symptoms.[102] Viral infections have also been associated with diaphragmatic dysfunction.[103] While no studies have addressed whether concomitant viral infection increases the risk of postoperative pulmonary complications, it seems prudent to avoid elective surgery in this setting.

Type of Surgical Incision

In abdominal procedures, vertical laparotomy incisions carry a higher incidence of postoperative complications than do horizontal incisions.[104,105] In one prospective study of 100 patients undergoing biliary tract surgery, those who had vertical incisions experienced a 20 percent rate of pulmonary complications compared with a 2 percent rate in those who had transverse incisions.[104]

Duration of Anesthesia

The incidence of pulmonary complications increases significantly in procedures lasting longer than three to four hours.[6,55,58,74,75] The risk of postoperative pneumonia may be five times higher in procedures lasting four or more hours compared with those lasting less than two.[74]

General State of Health

Overall clinical status, as categorized by the American Society of Anesthesiologists' (ASA) classification shown in Table 22–4, correlates with the likelihood of developing postoperative pulmonary complications.[51,54] In patients undergoing abdominal surgery, the ASA classification is a powerful predictor of risk.[51]

RISKS ASSOCIATED WITH CHRONIC LUNG DISEASE

Operative risk is considered in patients with three common categories of chronic lung disease: (1) chronic obstructive pulmonary

TABLE 22–4. American Society of Anesthesiologists' (ASA) Clinical Classification

ASA I	Otherwise healthy patient who is undergoing elective surgery
ASA II	Patient with single system or well-controlled disease which does not affect daily life
ASA III	Patient with multisystem or well-controlled major system disease which limits daily activity
ASA IV	Patient with severe, incapacitating disease which is poorly controlled or end-stage
ASA V	Patient who is in imminent danger of death and is not expected to survive 24 hours

disease; (2) restrictive lung diseases; and (3) pulmonary vascular diseases. Operative risk in patients with asthma is discussed in Chapter 23.

Chronic Obstructive Pulmonary Disease

Since chronic obstructive pulmonary disease (COPD) is the most common chronic pulmonary disorder, most studies addressing the impact of preexisting lung disease on surgical risk have focused on it. The reported incidence of postoperative pulmonary complications in patients with COPD varies from 25 percent to 100 percent. The type of surgery, the magnitude of preexisting respiratory impairment, and the criteria used to define a complication influence the statistics.[106]

In a large prospective study in which the presence of COPD was determined on the basis of clinical findings and chest x-ray without the use of pulmonary function tests, 26 percent of patients with COPD developed a complication compared with 8 percent of those without preexisting disease.[49] When preoperative pulmonary function testing is considered, an association between airflow obstruction and subsequent postoperative pulmonary morbidity has been demonstrated.[106] In one study, a postoperative pulmonary complication rate of 60 percent was found in patients who had abnormal preoperative pulmonary function tests but no preoperative preparation.[49] In another study, pulmonary complications developed in all patients who had a preoperative FEV_1 less than 65% and an FVC less than 70% of the predicted normal value.[6]

In patients with severe disease, the issue of "prohibitive" pulmonary function tests commonly arises. Is there a cutoff of pulmonary function below which the risk of developing a major life-threatening pulmonary complication is so high that it precludes anesthesia and surgery? In the 1950s Miller et al. proposed such a cutoff,[107] but their work has not been validated in an appropriate population of patients. Other studies have suggested that the concept of an absolute "prohibitive" level of lung function is obsolete.[108,109] Although patients with hypercapnic COPD have an increased risk of postoperative pulmonary morbidity,[109,110] data do not otherwise support the Miller hypothesis. In a study of 16 patients with severe COPD with "prohibitive" pulmonary function tests as defined by Miller's criteria, only three of 16 or 19 percent developed major pulmonary complications, and one patient died. The three complications occurred after pulmonary resection, and the one fatality was not the result of pulmonary problems.[108] Other investigators have found that patients with an FEV_1 as low as 450 ml can safely tolerate surgery.[109] Hence, patients should not be denied necessary surgery solely on the basis of poor pulmonary function. The importance of the operative procedure must be weighed against the risk.

The increased incidence of postoperative pulmonary complications in patients with COPD is due to an increase in the closing capacity, favoring the development of areas of low ventilation-to-perfusion ratios and atelectasis. In addition, in patients who continue to smoke, impaired ciliary function and chronic tracheobronchitis may be contributing factors.[88-92]

Restrictive Lung Diseases

Restrictive lung disease (RLD) refers to a heterogeneous group of conditions that includes interstitial lung disease, structural abnormalities of the chest wall like kyphoscoliosis, and neuromuscular disorders. These diseases are classified in the "restrictive" category on the basis of a common pattern on pulmonary function tests.[111]

The risk of pulmonary complications in patients with RLD undergoing surgery is unknown. While there is some reported experience with patients undergoing thoracic and orthopedic surgery, there are few data regarding risk in abdominal and other procedures. A higher incidence of postoperative respiratory complications might be expected because FRC is reduced, favoring the formation of areas of poor ventilation and atelectasis, and coughing and the ability to clear respiratory secretions are impaired.

Experience with postoperative pulmonary complications in patients with RLD has been reported in three situations: (1) corrective surgery for kyphoscoliosis; (2) myasthenia gravis with associated thymoma; and (3) sarcoidosis complicated by aspergilloma and hemoptysis. Patients with kyphoscoliosis may undergo corrective surgery for a variety of reasons, including deterioration of pulmonary function.[112] In one large retrospective study, an overall postoperative complication rate of 17 percent was noted.[113] Risk factors included the presence of nonidiopathic scoliosis, anterior spinal fusion procedures, age over 20, mental retardation, preoperative hypoxemia, and obstructive pulmonary function tests. Complications involving the pleural space, such as pneumothorax, pleural effusion, bronchopleural fistula, and empyema, appear to be especially significant in this population.[113,114]

Thymectomy is commonly performed in patients with myasthenia gravis.[115] Prolonged ventilatory support for more than three days is required in up to 30 percent of patients.[116-118] Factors that correlate with the need for prolonged mechanical ventilation are myasthenic symptoms for more than six years, a history of associated respiratory disease, a preoperative pyridostigmine dose requirement of more than 750 mg/day, and a preoperative vital capacity of less than 2.9 liters.[119] However, other data suggest that maximal static expiratory pressure may be the best predictor of need for prolonged ventilatory support. The clinical severity of the disease is only marginally predictive, and preoperative measurements of vital capacity are not helpful.[116]

Virtually all patients with myasthenia gravis are managed with anticholinesterases. These agents are sometimes stopped prior to surgery to minimize tracheobronchial secretions. However, there is no consensus on when to restart the medication.[120] Some authorities advocate withholding anticholinesterases for at least 24 hours following thymectomy to avoid cholinergic crisis, but others argue for restarting the drug as soon as possible.[117] The value of preoperative plasmapheresis in preventing postthymectomy pulmonary complications is uncertain.[121]

Some patients with sarcoidosis develop diffuse interstitial fibrosis and cavitary changes, primarily involving the upper lobes. These cavities are prone to infection with aspergillus species and formation of aspergillomas or "fungus balls." Aspergillomas may be the source of recurrent and at times life-threatening hemoptysis.[68,69] Such patients have very poor lung function, and conservative medical management rather than surgery is usually chosen. However, patients may require thoracotomy and lung resection which is often complicated by the development of a bronchopleural fistula or empyema.[68]

Pulmonary Vascular Diseases

The risk of postoperative pulmonary complications in patients with underlying pulmonary vascular disease and normal lung mechanic is unknown. One might anticipate an exaggeration or prolongation of postoperative hypoxemia. In addition, pulmonary reserve in these patients is usually reduced, and additional insults are poorly tolerated.

EVALUATION OF THE PATIENT

Four components of the preoperative evaluation are considered: (1) history and physical examination; (2) chest x-ray; (3) arterial blood gas analysis; and (4) pulmonary function tests. (See Fig. 22–3.)

History and Physical Examination

A comprehensive history is a vital part of the preoperative evaluation. The physician should review the patient's smoking history; pertinent history of respiratory symptoms like cough, chest pain, and dyspnea; the extent of preexisting lung disease; and any history of recent respiratory tract infection. The physical examination is rarely helpful in identifying pulmonary risk factors. When the history is negative, the physical examination is usually unremarkable. The initial examination does, however, provide a baseline for future comparison.

Chest X-Ray

The preoperative chest x-ray is rarely of benefit when risk factors and abnormal physical findings are absent.[122,123] In patients with known cardiopulmonary disease, an admission or screening chest radiograph is more likely to show an abnormality but usually reconfirms previously known abnormalities and only rarely alters management.[122–124] A preoperative chest x-ray is therefore indicated when there are new or unexplained symptoms or signs, when there is a history of underlying lung disease and no recent chest x-ray available, or when thoracic surgery is planned.

Arterial Blood Gas Analysis

Since CO_2 retention is associated with an increased incidence of postoperative pulmonary morbidity, an arterial blood gas analysis should be obtained before surgery in all patients with significant chronic lung disease.[109,110] It may also be wise to draw one from a patient who has new or unexplained pulmonary signs or symptoms. Data do not support the use of arterial blood gas analysis as a routine preoperative screening test.[125]

Pulmonary Function Tests

An increased risk of respiratory complications has been demonstrated only in patients with obstructive pulmonary disorders.[106] Although there are theoretical reasons to expect a higher incidence of postoperative problems in patients with restrictive lung diseases, there are no data correlating the degree of restriction as assessed by lung volumes with subsequent pulmonary morbidity. While a complete battery of pulmonary function tests may be useful in quantitating restriction, spirometry to evaluate for airway obstruction is all that is required in patients with increased risk.

Pulmonary function testing should be performed in patients with a history of chronic lung disease,[6,48,106,126] in those with a cigarette smoking history of more than 20 pack-years,[89,90,93,126] in those with cough (especially if productive) or unexplained dyspnea,[49,76] and in those undergoing lung resection. Although some consider advanced age an indication for pulmonary function testing,[3] data to support this recommendation are lacking. Pulmonary function testing is of unproved value merely as a routine test before abdominal procedures.[126,127] It is of questionable use in evaluating obese patients[83,126] and is of unknown value in the assessment of those who have had a recent respiratory tract infection. Normal pulmonary function tests do not guarantee a postoperative course free of complications and do not lessen the need for diligent and attentive care.

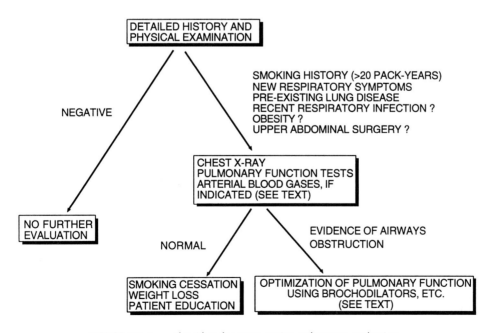

FIGURE 22–3. Algorithm for preoperative pulmonary evaluation.

EVALUATION FOR LUNG RESECTION

In evaluating patients for lung resection, the clinician must consider two questions: What is the surgical morbidity and mortality due to the patient's underlying chronic lung disease? Will postoperative lung function be adequate? To address these questions several diagnostic studies, including pulmonary function tests, lung scans, and arterial blood gas analyses, have been used routinely. Others have been utilized less commonly.

Pulmonary Function Tests, Lung Scans, and Arterial Blood Gas Analyses

Studies from the 1950s indicate that the risk of postoperative pulmonary complications following lung resection, especially pneumonectomy, increases significantly when the FEV_1 is less than 2 liters or when the FVC or maximal voluntary ventilation (MVV) is less than 50% of the predicted value.[63,106,128–132] In such "high-risk" patients, a number of additional tests have been used to predict postoperative pulmonary function.[106] Quantitative radionuclide perfusion and ventilation lung scans have been found to be the most helpful.[133–141] These scans estimate the relative blood flow or ventilation to one lung or lung region and enable prediction of postoperative FEV_1 and determination of the likelihood of postoperative respiratory disability. Ventilation and perfusion scintigraphy are equally accurate in calculating the postoperative FEV_1,[139,141] although perfusion scanning is more commonly used because it is technically easier to perform.[135]

For pneumonectomy, the predicted postoperative FEV_1 may be calculated as:

$$\text{Predicted postoperative } FEV_1 = \text{Preoperative } FEV_1 \times \text{\% perfusion to remaining lung}$$

For lobectomy, regional quantitative perfusion scans may be used.[139,141] Alternatively, the postoperative FEV_1 may be predicted with comparable accuracy using the following equation:[139–141]

$$\text{Predicted postoperative } FEV_1 = \text{Preoperative } FEV_1 \times \frac{\text{Number of lung segments remaining after resection}}{\text{Total number of segments in both lungs}}$$

A predicted postoperative FEV_1 of 800 ml has been used as a cutoff for withholding resection because below that level many patients are disabled and develop CO_2 retention.[106,134] Studies in which this criterion is met report "acceptable" surgical and postoperative morbidity and mortality,[130,132,133,135] but no prospective studies have confirmed the significance of this value.[134] Furthermore, an FEV_1 of 800 ml depends upon a number of factors, including the patient's body size. An FEV_1 of 800 ml may be adequate in meeting the respiratory needs of a small person but not those of someone with a larger body size. Another criterion—using a predicted postoperative FEV_1 of more than 40% of a predicted normal value—has been proposed.[141] In any case, calculation of predicted FEV_1 may therefore be of greater value in determining operability than in predicting postoperative function.[106] Most patients undergoing lung resection have lung cancer, and it is therefore important to exercise caution in applying arbitrary exclusionary criteria.

As noted above, hypercarbia in the setting of chronic lung disease is associated with a higher incidence of postoperative respiratory morbidity.[109,110] However, hypoxemia is not a good predictor of subsequent pulmonary morbidity. In fact, resection of areas of the lung with significant ventilation-perfusion mismatch may improve the level of oxygenation.[133] A preoperative arterial blood gas analysis should be obtained in all patients with preexisting lung disease undergoing lung resection. Although supportive data are lacking, it is common practice to obtain one even in patients without significant underlying lung disease. It frequently serves as a basis for comparison when later measurements are obtained.

Other Tests for Evaluating Patients for Lung Resection

Several other studies, including exercise testing, measurement of diffusing capacity, bronchospirometry, the lateral position test, and unilateral pulmonary artery occlusion have been advocated in the preoperative evaluation of candidates for lung resection. The role of exercise testing in preoperative assessment is not yet clarified. Some have found measurement of maximal oxygen consumption ($\dot{V}O_2$ max) to be useful in predicting postoperative morbidity and mortality.[106,141–145] A value of less than one l/min[144] or 20 ml/kg/min[142,143] is associated with an increased incidence of postoperative complications. In addition, exercise-induced arterial oxygen desaturation with a decline of more than two percent may predict postoperative complications, including death and respiratory failure.[141]

Measurement of the diffusing capacity (D_LCO) previously has proved helpful in assessing operative risk.[129,146,147] However, in a recent report, determination of the predicted postoperative D_LCO using a formula similar to the one used for predicting postoperative FEV_1 has also been shown to be of value. A predicted postoperative D_LCO of less than 40% of the predicted value is associated with high operative morbidity and mortality.[141] Bronchospirometry, in which oxygen uptake is measured individually in each lung,[148] the so-called "lateral position test,"[149–151] and measurement of pulmonary artery pressure during temporary unilateral pulmonary artery occlusion[106,134] are techniques that have been utilized in the past to assess the risk of thoracotomy in borderline patients. These tests are not currently used because of technical problems and concerns over reproducibility of results.[106]

Recommended Approach

In evaluating patients for lung resection, we recommend a modified version of the approach outlined by Markos et al.:[141]

1. Operability for full pneumonectomy is determined in the event it becomes necessary to remove the tumor completely or because of an intraoperative complication. If the preoperative FEV_1 is two liters or greater, or at least 80% of the predicted normal value, pneumonectomy can be performed and no further testing is required. If the preoperative FEV_1 falls below these values, the predicted postoperative FEV_1 should be calculated. Pneumonectomy may proceed if the predicted postoperative FEV_1 is at least 40% of the predicted normal value. The patient is considered borderline if this value is between 30 and 40% of the predicted value and is considered a poor candidate if the value is less than 30%.

2. In borderline patients or in those with significant dyspnea or disability despite an "operable" FEV_1 or predicted postoperative FEV_1, the predicted postoperative D_LCO should be determined. The patient can undergo pneumonectomy if this value is at least 40% of the predicted normal value.

3. If confirmatory evidence of operability is required, an exercise test can be performed. The patient can pneumonectomy if the $\dot{V}O_2$ max is at least 20 ml/kg/min and arterial oxygen saturation declines less than two percent.

4. If these criteria cannot be met, but the patient appears to be a good candidate for lobectomy, steps 1 and 2 should be followed to calculate the predicted postlobectomy FEV_1 and D_LCO.

When respiratory insufficiency occurs as a result of pulmonary resection, it does so within the first several weeks after surgery. After three months, the development of respiratory insufficiency attributable to the surgery itself is rare.[130,137]

PREOPERATIVE PREPARATION

Surprisingly, data supporting the notion that aggressive preoperative pulmonary preparation decreases postoperative pulmonary morbidity and mortality are limited. In one study, "high-risk" patients, as defined by pulmonary function tests, were randomly assigned to a "no-treatment" group or to a group that received a standard respiratory therapy regimen including a smoking-cessation program, antibiotics when indicated, preoperative and postoperative bronchodilator treatments, inhalation of humidified gases, and chest physiotherapy. Therapy for the "no-treatment" group was left to the discretion of the patients' physicians. In the treated group, five of 23 patients or 22 percent experienced a pulmonary complication compared with 15 of 25 or 60 percent in the control group. While none of the treated patients undergoing thoracic surgery suffered a fatal complication, four of 17 or 22.6 percent in the "no-treatment" group died.[56]

Using historical controls, another group of investigators examined the postoperative complication rate in 157 patients with COPD who received a preoperative regimen of nebulized isoproterenol, inhalation of humidified air, chest physiotherapy, oral hydration, theophylline, and smoking cessation. The preoperative interventions decreased the incidence of postoperative complica-

tions by more than 50 percent, but mortality was unaffected.[48] In another large retrospective study, patients with COPD who received preoperative prophylactic therapy were shown to have a greater than 50 percent reduction in postoperative respiratory complications compared with a similar group who received no preoperative preparation.[46] While data on preoperative preparation are limited, it appears that, at least for patients with significant obstructive airways disease, intensive preoperative respiratory therapy is beneficial as outlined in Table 22–5.[46,48,51,81,87] Efforts to optimize pulmonary function should begin at least 48 to 72 hours before surgery. For elective procedures, when there is a reasonable chance of patient compliance with a weight-loss program or smoking cessation, surgery should be postponed accordingly.

POSTOPERATIVE PROPHYLACTIC MEASURES

Several postoperative measures designed to prevent respiratory complications are listed in Table 22–6 and deserve comment. Since FRC decreases by 500 to 1000 ml in the supine position and predisposes the patient to atelectasis,[39] early patient mobilization may reduce the incidence of this complication. Deep breathing and incentive spirometry are equally effective measures to inflate the lungs and maintain FRC.[56,152,153] Intermittent positive pressure breathing (IPPB) is ineffective.[152] In studies supporting its use, complication rates and costs have been higher than with other techniques.[58] Recent reports of intermittent continuous positive airway pressure (CPAP) applied by face mask indicate that it is at least equivalent to deep breathing exercises and incentive spirometry in preventing and treating atelectasis.[153-155] However, while CPAP may be useful in the patient who cannot cooperate with inspiratory maneuvers, its role in the management of patients capable of taking deep breaths is unclear.[156] Several other postoperative interventions have been shown to be ineffective, including the use of "blow bottles,"[152] carbon dioxide–induced hyperventilation,[152] chest physiotherapy in the absence of excessive secretions or sputum production,[157] and routine application of positive end-expiratory pressure in mechanically ventilated patients.[158]

Effective pain control is vital in the early postoperative period since pain inhibits coughing and deep breathing and discourages early mobilization, factors that contribute to an increased risk of pulmonary complications. Parenteral narcotics have been used for postoperative analgesia despite the risk of respiratory depression, and concerns over adverse respiratory effects may lead to inadequate dosing and inadequate pain relief. To overcome this, alterna-

TABLE 22–5. Preoperative Prophylactic Measures in Patients with Pulmonary Risk Factors

Smoking cessation (ideally a minimum of 8 weeks prior to surgery)
Optimization of airway function in patients with obstructive lung disease:
  Bronchodilators
  Corticosteroids if indicated
  Antibiotics if infection suspected
  Chest physiotherapy
Weight reduction for obese patients
Patient education on:
  Postoperative deep-breathing exercises
  Importance of coughing
  Use of incentive spirometry

TABLE 22–6. Postoperative Measures for the Prevention of Respiratory Complications

Early patient mobililzation and ambulation
Prophylactic lung expansion maneuvers:
  Incentive spirometry
  Deep-breathing exercises
  Continuous positive airway pressure (CPAP)
Provision of adequate analgesia:
  Narcotics as necessary
  Regional anesthesia (e.g., epidural anesthesia, intercostal nerve blocks)
Prophylaxis against thromboembolism

tive approaches including use of epidural analgesia and intercostal nerve blocks have been studied.[45,159-165] While they provide equivalent or superior analgesia to parenteral narcotics, data are still accumulating as to whether they decrease the incidence of postoperative pulmonary complications.

SUMMARY

1. Surgery and anesthesia affect lung volumes, diaphragmatic performance, gas exchange, control of breathing, and lung defense mechanisms.

2. Factors that may contribute to the development of postoperative pulmonary morbidity include overall clinical status, chronic lung disease (particularly chronic obstructive pulmonary disease), increased age, obesity, cigarette smoking, poor nutritional status, antecedent respiratory tract infection, type and duration of anesthesia, surgical site, and type of incision.

3. Preoperative evaluation should include a comprehensive history and careful physical examination. A chest x-ray is indicated if there are new or unexplained symptoms or signs, in patients with underlying lung disease who have not had a recent film, or when thoracic surgery is planned. Arterial blood gas measurement should be reserved for those with a significant new pulmonary process and should not be performed routinely. Pulmonary function tests should be performed in patients with a history of chronic lung disease or a smoking history of more than 20 pack-years, in those with cough or unexplained dyspnea, and in those requiring lung resection.

4. Patients undergoing lung resection who have a history of smoking, respiratory symptoms, preexisting lung disease, or abnormal physical findings in the lung should be more extensively evaluated, and postoperative respiratory function should be estimated before surgery.

5. Patients with symptomatic chronic obstructive pulmonary disease should receive intensive preoperative therapy that may include antibiotics, bronchodilators, steroids, and chest physiotherapy. Weight reduction in obese patients, smoking cessation, and patient education should be initiated several weeks before elective surgery.

6. In an effort to prevent postoperative respiratory complications, early mobilization, lung expansion maneuvers, adequate analgesia, prophylaxis against thromboembolism, and careful monitoring should be provided to all patients.

REFERENCES

1. Craig DB: Postoperative recovery of pulmonary function. *Anesth Analg* 60:46–52, 1981.
2. Fairshter RD, Williams JH: Pulmonary physiology in the postoperative period. *Crit Care Clin* 3:287–306, 1987.
3. Tisi GM: Preoperative evaluation of pulmonary function. Validity, indications and benefits. *Am Rev Respir Dis* 119:293–310, 1979.
4. Ali J, Weisel RD, Layug AB et al: Consequences of postoperative alterations in respiratory mechanics. *Am J Surg* 128:376–382, 1974.
5. Meyers JR, Lembeck L, O'Kane H et al: Changes in functional residual capacity of the lung after operation. *Arch Surg* 110:576–583, 1975.
6. Latimer RG, Dickman M, Day WC et al: Ventilatory patterns and pulmonary complications after upper abdominal surgery determined by preoperative and postoperative computerized spirometry and blood gas analysis. *Am J Surg* 122:622–632, 1971.
7. Colgan FJ, Mahoney PD: The effects of major surgery on cardiac output and shunting. *Anesthesiology* 31:213–221, 1969.
8. Dureuil B, Vires N, Cantineau JP et al: Diaphragmatic contractility after upper abdominal surgery. *J Appl Physiol* 61:1775–1780, 1986.
9. Dureuil B, Cantineau JP, Desmonts JM: Effects of upper or lower abdominal surgery on diaphragmatic function. *Br J Anaesth* 59:1230–1235, 1987.
10. Wahba WM, Craig DB, Don HF et al: The cardio-respiratory effects of thoracic epidural anesthesia. *Can Anaesth Soc J* 19:8–19, 1972.
11. Wahba WM, Don HF, Craig DB: Postoperative epidural analgesia: Effects on lung volumes. *Can Anaesth Soc J* 22:519–527, 1975.
12. Woltering EA, Flye MW, Huntley S et al: Evaluation of bupivacaine nerve blocks in the modification of pain and pulmonary function changes after thoracotomy. *Ann Thorac Surg* 30:122–127, 1980.
13. Simonneau G, Vivien A, Sartene R et al: Diaphragm dysfunction induced by upper abdominal pain. Role of postoperative pain. *Am Rev Respir Dis* 128:899–903, 1983.
14. Ford GT, Whitelaw WA, Rosenal TW et al: Diaphragm function after upper abdominal surgery in humans. *Am Rev Respir Dis* 127:431–436, 1983.
15. Ford GT, Guenter CA: Toward prevention of postoperative pulmonary complications. *Am Rev Respir Dis* 130:4–5, 1984.
16. Dureuil B, Desmonts JM, Mankikan B et al: Effects of aminophylline on diaphragmatic dysfunction after upper abdominal surgery. *Anesthesiology* 62:242–246, 1985.
17. Alexander JI, Spence AA, Parikh RK et al: The role of airway closure in postoperative hypoxaemia. *Br J Anaesth* 45:34–40, 1973.
18. Diament ML, Palmer KN: Postoperative changes in gas tensions of arterial blood and in ventilatory function. *Lancet* 2:180–182, 1966.
19. Knudsen J: Duration of hypoxaemia after uncomplicated upper abdominal and thoraco-abdominal operations. *Anaesthesia* 25:372–377, 1970.
20. Marshall BE, Wyche MQ: Hypoxemia during and after anesthesia. *Anesthesiology* 37:178–209, 1972.
21. Parfrey PS, Harte PJ, Quinlan JP et al: Pulmonary function in the early postoperative period. *Br J Surg* 64:384–389, 1977.
22. Parfrey PS, Harte PJ, Quinlan JP et al: Postoperative hypoxaemia and oxygen therapy. *Br J Surg* 64:390–393, 1977.
23. Kitamura H, Sawa T, Ikenzono E: Postoperative hypoxemia: The contribution of age to the maldistribution of ventilation. *Anesthesiology* 36:244–252, 1972.
24. Aldren CP, Barr LC, Leach RD: Hypoxaemia and postoperative pulmonary complications. *Br J Surg* 78:1307–1308, 1991.
25. Kafer ER, Marsh HM: The effect of anesthetic drugs and disease on the chemical regulation of ventilation. *Int Anesthesiol Clin* 15:1–38, 1977.
26. Knill RL, Gelb AW: Ventilatory responses to hypoxia and hypercapnia during halothane sedation and anesthesia in man. *Anesthesiology* 49:244–251, 1978.
27. Knill R, Chung D, Baskerville J: Ventilatory response to acute "Iso P_{CO_2}" acidosis in awake and anesthetized man (abstract). *Clin Res* 26:379A, 1978.
28. Knill RL, Manninen PH, Clement JL: Ventilation and chemoreflexes during enflurane sedation and anesthesia in man. *Can Anaesth Soc J* 26:353–360, 1979.
29. Weil JV, McCullough RE, Kline JS et al: Diminished ventilatory response to hypoxia and hypercapnia after morphine in normal man. *N Engl J Med* 292:1103–1106, 1975.
30. Catley DM: Postoperative analgesia and respiratory control. *Int Anesthesiol Clin* 22:95–111, 1984.

31. Brain JD: Anesthesia and respiratory defense mechanisms. *Int Anesthesiol Clin* 15:169–198, 1977.

32. Sugimachi K, Ueo H, Natsuda Y et al: Cough dynamics in oesophageal cancer: Prevention of postoperative pulmonary complications. *Br J Surg* 69:734–736, 1982.

33. Gamsu G, Singer MM, Vincent HH et al: Postoperative impairment of mucus transport in the lung. *Am Rev Respir Dis* 114:673–679, 1976.

34. Chalon J, Ali M, Ramanathan S et al: The humidification of anaesthetic gases: Its importance and control. *Can Anaesth Soc J* 26:361–366, 1979.

35. Klainer AS, Turnsdorf H, Wu WA et al: Surface alterations due to endotracheal intubation. *Am J Med* 58:674–683, 1975.

36. Laurenzi GA, Yin S, Guarneri JJ: Adverse effect of oxygen on tracheal mucus flow. *N Engl J Med* 279:333–339, 1968.

37. Rehder K, Sessler AD, Marsh HM: General anesthesia and the lung. *Am Rev Respir Dis* 112:541–563, 1975.

38. Rehder K: Anaesthesia and the respiratory system. *Can Anaesth Soc J* 26:451–462, 1979.

39. Foltz BD, Benumof JL: Mechanisms of hypoxemia and hypercapnia in the perioperative period. *Crit Care Clin* 3:269–286, 1987.

40. Modig J, Hjelmstedt A, Sahlstedt B et al: Comparative influences of epidural and general anaesthesia on deep venous thrombosis and pulmonary embolism after total hip replacement. *Acta Chir Scand* 147:125–130, 1981.

41. Modig J, Borg T, Karlstrom G et al: Thromboembolism after total hip replacement: Role of epidural and general anesthesia. *Anesth Analg* 62:174–180, 1983.

42. Davis FM, Laurenson VG: Spinal anaesthesia or general anaesthesia for emergency hip surgery in elderly patients. *Anaesth Intens Care* 9:352–358, 1981.

43. McKenzie PJ, Wishart HY, Gray I et al: Effects of anaesthetic technique on deep vein thrombosis. A comparison of subarachnoid and general anaesthesia. *Br J Anaesth* 57:853–857, 1985.

44. Hendolin H, Mattila MA, Poikolainen E: The effect of lumbar epidural analgesia on the development of deep vein thrombosis of the legs after open prostatectomy. *Acta Chir Scand* 147:425–429, 1981.

45. Scott NB, Kehlet H: Regional anaesthesia and surgical morbidity. *Br J Surg* 75:299–304, 1988.

46. Tarhan S, Moffitt EA, Sessler AD et al: Risk of anesthesia and surgery in patients with chronic bronchitis and chronic obstructive pulmonary disease. *Surgery* 74:720–726, 1973.

47. Ravin MB: Comparison of spinal and general anesthesia for lower abdominal surgery in patients with chronic obstructive pulmonary disease. *Anesthesiology* 3:319–322, 1971.

48. Gracey DR, Diverte MB, Didier EP: Preoperative pulmonary preparation of patients with chronic obstructive pulmonary disease. A prospective study. *Chest* 76:123–129, 1979.

49. Wightman JA: A prospective survey of the incidence of postoperative pulmonary complications. *Br J Surg* 55:85–91, 1968.

50. Forthman HJ, Shephard A: Postoperative pulmonary complications. *South Med J* 62:1198–1200, 1969.

51. Hall JC, Tarala RA, Hall JL et al: A multivariate analysis of the risk of pulmonary complications after laparotomy. *Chest* 99:923–927, 1991.

52. Ellis FH, Gibb SP, Watkins E: Overview of the current management of carcinoma of the esophagus and cardia. *Can J Surg* 28:493–496, 1985.

53. Nishi M, Hiramatsu Y, Hioki K et al: Risk factors in relation to postoperative complications in patients undergoing esophagectomy or gastrectomy for cancer. *Ann Surg* 207:148–154, 1988.

54. Velanovich V: The value of routine preoperative laboratory testing in predicting postoperative complications; a multivariate analysis. *Surgery* 109:236–243, 1991.

55. Pederson T, Eliasen K, Henriksen E: A prospective study of risk factors and cardiopulmonary complications associated with anesthesia and surgery: Risk indications of pulmonary morbidity. *Acta Anaesthesiol Scand* 34:144–145, 1990.

56. Stein M, Cassara EL: Preoperative pulmonary evaluation and therapy for surgery patients. *JAMA* 211:787–790, 1970.

57. Bartlett RH, Brennan ML, Gazzaniga AB et al: Studies on the pathogenesis and prevention of postoperative pulmonary complications. *Surg Gyn Ob* 137:925–933, 1973.

58. Celli BR, Rodriquez KS, Snider GL: A controlled trial of intermittent positive pressure breathing, incentive spirometry, and deep breathing exercises in preventing pulmonary complications after abdominal surgery. *Am Rev Respir Dis* 130:12–15, 1984.

59. Fogh J, Willie-Jorgensen P, Brynjolf I et al: The predictive value of preoperative perfusion/ventilation scintigraphy, spirometry and x-ray of the lungs on postoperative complications. A prospective study. *Acta Anaesthesiol Scand* 31:717–721, 1987.

60. Roukema JA, Carol EJ, Prins JG: The prevention of pulmonary complications after upper abdominal surgery in patients with noncompromised pulmonary status. *Arch Surg* 123:30–34, 1988.

61. Reasbeck PG, Guerrini S, Harper J et al: Incidence of deep vein thrombosis after major abdominal surgery in Brisbane. *Br J Surg* 75:440–443, 1988.

62. Delisser HM, Grippi MA: Phrenic nerve injury following cardiac surgery, with emphasis on the role of topical hypothermia. *J Intensive Care Med* 6:295–301, 1991.

63. Kollef MH, Peller T, Knodel A et al: Delayed pleuropulmonary complications following coronary artery revascularization with the internal mammary artery. *Chest* 94:68–71, 1988.

64. Stelzner TJ, King TE, Anton VB et al: The pleuropulmonary manifestations of the postcardiac injury syndrome. *Chest* 84:383–387, 1983.

65. Lockwood P: The relationship between pre-operative lung function tests results and post-operative complications in carcinoma of the bronchus. *Respiration* 30:105–116, 1973.

66. Nagasaki F, Flehinger BJ, Martini N: Complications of surgery in the treatment of carcinoma of the lung. *Chest* 82:25–29, 1982.

67. McGovern EM, Trastek VF, Pairolero PC et al: Completion pneumonectomy: Indications, complications and results. *Ann Thorac Surg* 46:144–146, 1988.

68. Israel HL, Lenchner GS, Atkinson GW: Sarcoidosis and aspergilloma. The role of surgery. *Chest* 82:430–432, 1982.

69. Glimp RA, Bayer AS: Pulmonary aspergilloma. Diagnostic and therapeutic considerations. *Arch Intern Med* 143:303–308, 1983.

70. Lovich SF, Iverson LIG, Young JN et al: Omental pedical grafting in the treatment of postcardiotomy sternotomy infection. *Arch Surg* 124:1192–1194, 1989.

71. Loop FD, Lytle BW, Cosgrove DM et al: Sternal wound complications after isolated coronary artery bypass grafting: Early and late mortality, morbidity and cost of care. *Ann Thorac Surg* 49:179–187, 1990.

72. Ottino G, DePauls R, Pansini S et al: Major sternal wound infection after open-heart surgery; a multivariate analysis of risk factors in 2579 consecutive operative procedures. *Ann Thorac Surg* 44:173–179, 1987.

73. Jezek V, Ourednik A, Lichtenberg J et al: Cardiopulmonary function in lung resection performed for bronchogenic cancer in patients above 65 years of age. *Respiration* 27:42–50, 1970.

74. Garibaldi RA, Britt MR, Coleman ML et al: Risk factors for postoperative pneumonia. *Am J Med* 70:677–680, 1981.

75. Hansen G, Drablos PA, Steiner TR: Pulmonary complications, ventilation and blood gases after upper abdominal surgery. *Acta Anaesth Scand* 21:211–215, 1977.

76. Mitchell C, Garrahy P, Peake P: Postoperative respiratory morbidity: Identification and risk factors. *Aust NZ J Surg* 52:203–209, 1982.

77. Yellin A, Benfield JR: Surgery for bronchogenic carcinoma in the elderly. *Am Rev Respir Dis* 131:197, 1985.

78. Breyer RH, Zippe C, Pharr WF et al: Thoracotomy in patients over

age seventy years. *J Thorac Cardiovasc Surg* 81:187–193, 1981.

79. Ginsberg RJ, Hill LD, Eagan RT et al: Modern thirty-day operative mortality for surgical resections in lung cancer. *J Thorac Cardiovasc Surg* 86:654–658, 1983.

80. Sherman S, Guidot CE: The feasibility of thoracotomy for lung cancer in the elderly. *JAMA* 258:927–930, 1987.

81. Pasulka PS, Bistrian BR, Benotti PN et al: The risk of surgery in obese patients. *Ann Intern Med* 104:540–546, 1986.

82. Luce JM: Respiratory complications of obesity. *Chest* 78:626–631, 1980.

83. Ray CS, Sue DY, Bray G et al: Effects of obesity on respiratory function. *Am Rev Respir Dis* 128:501–506, 1983.

84. Barrera F, Hillyer P, Ascanio G et al: The distribution of ventilation diffusion and blood flow in obese patients with normal and abnormal blood gases. *Am Rev Respir Dis* 108:819–830, 1973.

85. Vaughan RW, Bauer S, Wise L: Volume and pH of gastric juice in obese patients. *Anesthesiology* 43:636–639, 1975.

86. Pemberton LB, Manax WG: Relationship of obesity to postoperative complication after cholecystectomy. *Am J Surg* 121:87–90, 1971.

87. Warner MA, Divertie MB, Tinker JH: Preoperative cessation of smoking and pulmonary complications in coronary artery bypass patients. *Anesthesiology* 60:380–383, 1984.

88. Ide G, Suntzeff V, Cowdry EV: A comparison of the histopathology of tracheal and bronchial epithelium of smokers and nonsmokers. *Cancer* 12:473–484, 1959.

89. Buist AS, Sexton GJ, Nagy JM et al: The effect of smoking cessation and modification on lung function. *Am Rev Respir Dis* 114:115–122, 1976.

90. Bode FR, Dosman J, Martin RR et al: Reversibility of pulmonary function abnormalities in smokers. A prospective study of early diagnostic tests of small airways disease. *Am J Med* 59:43–52, 1975.

91. Chalon J, Tayyab MA, Ramanathan S: Cytology of respiratory epithelium as a predictor of respiratory complications after operation. *Chest* 67:32–35, 1975.

92. Chang SC: Microscopic properties of whole mounts and sections of human bronchial epithelium of smokers and nonsmokers. *Cancer* 6:1246–1262, 1957.

93. Martin TR: The relationship between malnutrition and lung infections. *Clin Chest Med* 8:359–373, 1987.

94. Pingleton SK: Nutritional support in the mechanically ventilated patient. *Clin Chest Med* 9:101–112, 1988.

95. Wilson DO, Rogers RM, Hoffman RM: Nutrition and chronic lung disease. *Am Rev Respir Dis* 132:1347–1365, 1985.

96. Rochester DR, Esau SA: Malnutrition and the respiratory system. *Chest* 85:411–415, 1984.

97. Bistrian BR, Blackburn GL, Hallowell E et al: Protein status of general surgical patients. *JAMA* 230:858–860, 1974.

98. Bistrian BR, Blackburn GL, Vitale J et al: Prevalence of malnutrition in general medical patients. *JAMA* 235:1567–1570, 1976.

99. Dempsey DT, Mullen JL, Buzby GP: The link between nutritional status and clinical outcome: Can nutritional intervention modify it? *Am J Clin Nutr* 47:352–356, 1988.

100. Buzby GP, Williford WD, Peterson OL et al: A randomized clinical trial of total parenteral nutrition in malnourished surgical patients: The rationale and impact of previous clinical trials and pilot study on protocol design. *Am J Clin Nutr* 47:357–365, 1988.

101. The Veterans Affairs Total Parenteral Nutrition Cooperative Study Group: Perioperative total parenteral nutrition in surgical patients. *N Engl J Med* 325:525–532, 1991.

102. Hall WJ, Hall CB, Speers DM: Respiratory syncytial virus infection in adults. Clinical, virologic, and serial pulmonary function studies. *Ann Intern Med* 88:203–205, 1978.

103. Mier-Jedrzejowicz A, Brophy C, Green M: Respiratory muscle weakness during upper respiratory tract infection. *Am Rev Respir Dis* 138:5–7, 1988.

104. Halasz NA: Vertical vs. horizontal laparotomies. *Arch Surg* 88:911–914, 1964.

105. Vaughan RW, Wise L: Choice of abdominal operative incision in the obese patient: A study using blood gas measurements. *Ann Surg* 181:829–835, 1975.

106. Gass GD, Olsen GN: Preoperative pulmonary function testing to predict postoperative morbidity and mortality. *Chest* 89:127–135, 1986.

107. Miller WF, Wu N, Johnson RL: Convenient method of evaluating pulmonary ventilatory function with a single breath test. *Anesthesiology* 17:480–493, 1956.

108. Williams CD, Brenowitz JB: "Prohibitive" lung function and major surgical procedures. *Am J Surg* 132:763–766, 1976.

109. Milledge JS, Nunn JF: Criteria of fitness for anaesthesia in patients with chronic obstructive lung disease. *Br Med J* 3:670–673, 1975.

110. Stein M, Koota GM, Somon M et al: Pulmonary evaluation of surgical patients. *JAMA* 181:765–770, 1962.

111. Grippi MA, Metzger LF, Krupinski AV et al: Pulmonary function testing, in Fishman AP (ed): *Pulmonary Diseases and Disorders*. New York, McGraw-Hill, 1988, pp 2469–2523.

112. Bradford DS: Adult scoliosis. Current concepts of treatment. *Clin Ortho* 229:70–87, 1988.

113. Anderson PR, Puno MR, Lovell SL et al: Postoperative respiratory complications in nonidiopathic scoliosis. *Acta Anaesthesiol Scand* 29:186–192, 1985.

114. Westfall SH, Akbarnia BA, Merenda JT et al: Exposure of the anterior spine. Technique, complications and results in 85 patients. *Am J Surg* 154:700–704, 1987.

115. Seybold ME: Myasthenia gravis. A clinical and basic science review. *JAMA* 250:2516–2521, 1983.

116. Younger DS, Braun NM, Jenetzki A et al: Myasthenia gravis: Determinants for independent ventilation after transsternal thymectomy. *Neurology* 34:336–340, 1984.

117. Sivak ED, Mehta A, Hanson M et al: Postoperative ventilatory dependency following thymectomy for myasthenia gravis. *Cleve Clin Q* 51:585–589, 1984.

118. Gracey DR, Divertie MB, Howard FM et al: Postoperative respiratory care after transsternal thymectomy in myasthenia gravis. A three-year experience in 53 patients. *Chest* 86:67–71, 1984.

119. Leventhal S, Orkin F, Hirsch R: Prediction of the need for postoperative mechanical ventilation in myasthenia gravis. *Anesthesiology* 53:26–30, 1980.

120. Spence PA, Morin JE, Katz M: Role of plasmapheresis in preparing myasthenic patients for thymectomy: Initial results. *Can J Surg* 27:303–305, 1984.

121. Gorty SR: Recovery room care after thoracic surgery. *Int Anesthesiol Clin* 21:173–184, 1983.

122. Tape TG, Mushlin AI: The utility of routine chest radiographs. *Ann Intern Med* 104:663–670, 1986.

123. Rucker L, Frye EB, Staten MA: Usefulness of screening chest roentgenograms in preoperative patients. *JAMA* 250:3209–3211, 1983.

124. Hubbell FA, Greenfield S, Tyler JL et al: The impact of routine admission chest x-ray films on patient care. *N Engl J Med* 312:209–213, 1985.

125. Raffin TA: Indications for arterial blood gas analysis. *Ann Intern Med* 105:390–395, 1986.

126. Zibrack JD, O'Donnell CR, Marton K: Indications for pulmonary function testing. *Ann Intern Med* 1122:703–771, 1990.

127. Lawrence VA, Page CP, Harris GD: Preoperative spirometry before abdominal operations. A critical appraisal of its predictive value. *Arch Intern Med* 149:280–285, 1989.

128. Gaensler EA, Cugell DW, Lindgren I et al: The role of pulmonary insufficiency in mortality and invalidism following surgery for pulmonary tuberculosis. *J Thorac Surg* 29:163–187, 1955.

129. Mittman C: Assessment of operative risk in thoracic surgery. *Am Rev Respir Dis* 84:197–207, 1961.

130. Boushy SF, Billig DM, North LB et al: Clinical course related to preoperative and postoperative pulmonary function in patients with bronchogenic carcinoma. *Chest* 59:383–391, 1971.

131. Boysen PG, Block AJ, Moulder PV: Relationship between preoperative pulmonary function tests and complications after thoracotomy. *Surg Gyn Ob* 152:813–815, 1981.

132. Miller JI, Grossman GD, Hatcher CR: Pulmonary function test criteria for operability and pulmonary resection. *Surg Gyn Ob* 153:893–895, 1981.

133. Kristersson S, Lindell S, Svanberg L: Prediction of pulmonary function loss due to pneumonectomy using ^{133}Xe-radiospirometry. *Chest* 62:694–698, 1972.

134. Olsen GN, Block AJ, Swenson EW et al: Pulmonary function evaluation of the lung resection candidate: A prospective study. *Am Rev Respir Dis* 111:379–387, 1975.

135. Olsen GN, Block AJ, Tobias JA: Prediction of postpneumonectomy pulmonary function using quantitative macroaggregate lung scanning. *Chest* 66:13–16, 1974.

136. Boysen PG, Block J, Olsen GN et al: Prospective evaluation for pneumonectomy using the 99m technetium quantitative perfusion lung scan. *Chest* 72:422–425, 1977.

137. Boysen PG, Harris JO, Block AJ et al: Prospective evaluation for pneumonectomy using perfusion scanning follow-up beyond one year. *Chest* 80:163–166, 1981.

138. Ali MK, Mountain CF, Ewer MS et al: Predicting loss of pulmonary function after pulmonary resection for bronchogenic carcinoma. *Chest* 77:337–342, 1980.

139. Wernly JA, DeMeester TR, Kirchmer PT et al: Clinical value of quantitative ventilation-perfusion lung scans in the surgical management of bronchogenic carcinoma. *J Thorac Cardiovasc Surg* 80:535–543, 1980.

140. Veneskoski T, Sovijarvi AR: Prediction of ventilatory function after subtotal lung resection using preoperative dynamic spirometry and radiospirometry. *Eur J Respir Dis* 68:167–172, 1986.

141. Markos J, Mullan BP, Hillman DR et al: Preoperative assessment as a predictor of mortality and morbidity after lung resection. *Am Rev Respir Dis* 139:902–910, 1989.

142. Smith TP, Kinasewitz GT, Tucker WY et al: Exercise capacity as a predictor of post-thoracotomy morbidity. *Am Rev Respir Dis* 129:730–734, 1984.

143. Bechard D, Wetstein L: Assessment of exercise oxygen consumption as preoperative criterion for lung resection. *Ann Thorac Surg* 44:344–349, 1987.

144. Eugene J, Brown SE, Light RW et al: Maximum oxygen consumption: A physiologic guide to pulmonary function. *Surg Forum* 33:260–262, 1982.

145. Miyoshi S, Nakahara K, Ohno K et al: Exercise tolerance test in lung cancer patients: The relationship between exercise capacity and post-thoracotomy hospital mortality. *Ann Thorac Surg* 44:487–490, 1987.

146. Reichal J: Assessment of operative risk of pneumonectomy. *Chest* 62:570–576, 1972.

147. Legge JS, Palmer KN: Pulmonary function in bronchial carcinoma. *Thorax* 28:588–591, 1973.

148. Neuhaus H, Cherniack NS: A bronchospirometric method of estimating the effect of pneumonectomy on the maximum breathing capacity. *J Thorac Cardiovasc Surg* 55:144–148, 1968.

149. Marion JM, Alderson PO, Lefrak SS et al: Unilateral lung function. Comparison of the lateral position test with radionuclide ventilation-perfusion studies. *Chest* 69:5–9, 1976.

150. Jay SJ, Stonehill RB, Kilbawi SO et al: Variability of the lateral position test in normal subjects. *Am Rev Respir Dis* 121:165–167, 1980.

151. Schoonover GA, Olsen GN, McLain WC et al: Lateral position test and quantitative lung scanning in the preoperative evaluation for lung resection. *Chest* 86:854–859, 1984.

152. Bartlett RH, Gazzaniga AB, Geraghty TR: Respiratory maneuvers to prevent postoperative pulmonary complications. A critical review. *JAMA* 224:1017–1021, 1973.

153. Stock MC, Downs JB, Gauer PK et al: Prevention of postoperative pulmonary complications with CPAP, incentive spirometry and conservative therapy. *Chest* 87:151–157, 1985.

154. Ricksten S, Bengtsson A, Soderberg C et al: Effects of periodic positive airway pressure by mask on postoperative pulmonary function. *Chest* 89:774–781, 1986.

155. Williamson DC, Modell JH: Intermittent continuous positive airway pressure by mask: Its use in the treatment of atelectasis. *Arch Surg* 117:970–972, 1982.

156. O'Donohue WJ: Prevention and treatment of postoperative atelectasis. Can it and will it be adequately studied? *Chest* 87:1–2, 1985.

157. Kirilloff LH, Owens GR, Rogers RM et al: Does chest physical therapy work? *Chest* 88:436–444, 1985.

158. Good JT, Wolz JF, Anderson JT et al: The routine use of positive end-expiratory pressure after open heart surgery. *Chest* 76:397–400, 1979.

159. Baxter AD, Jennings FO, Harris RS et al: Continuous intercostal blockade after cardiac surgery. *Br J Anaesth* 59:162–166, 1987.

160. Yeager MP, Glass DD, Neff RK et al: Epidural anesthesia and analgesia in high-risk surgical patients. *Anesthesiology* 66:729–736, 1987.

161. Rosenberg PH, Heino A, Scheinin B: Comparisons of intramuscular analgesia, intercostal block, epidural morphine and on-demand IV fentanyl in the control of pain after upper abdominal surgery. *Acta Anaesth Scand* 28:603–607, 1984.

162. Cushieri RJ, Morran CG, Howie JC et al: Postoperative pain and pulmonary complications: Comparison of three analgesic regimens. *Br J Surg* 72:495–498, 1985.

163. Hjortso NC, Neuman P, Frosig F et al: A controlled study on the effect of epidural analgesia with local anaesthetics and morphine on morbidity after abdominal surgery. *Acta Anaesth Scand* 29:790–796, 1985.

164. Engberg G, Wiklund L: Pulmonary complications after upper abdominal surgery: Their prevention with intercostal blocks. *Acta Anaesth Scand* 32:1–9, 1988.

165. Sabanathan S, Smith PJ, Pradhan GN et al: Continuous intercostal nerve block for pain relief after thoracotomy. *Ann Thorac Surg* 46:425–426, 1988.

23 SURGERY IN THE PATIENT WITH ASTHMA

Gregg J. Fromell

Asthma is a chronic lung disease that affects over 10 million Americans, and the prevalence of the disease appears to be steadily increasing. Between 1979 and 1987, the proportion of the population with asthma increased by about one-third.[1] A major problem in studying asthma is the difficulty of defining it. In 1962, the American Thoracic Society proposed the following definition:

> Asthma is a disease characterized by an increased responsiveness of the trachea and bronchi to various stimuli and manifested by a widespread narrowing of the airways that changes in severity either spontaneously or as a result of therapy. The term "asthma" is not appropriate for the bronchial narrowing which results solely from widespread pulmonary emphysema or from cardiovascular disorders.

Since then, a number of attempts to refine this definition have been made, but none has been universally accepted.[2] Most recently, the National Asthma Education Program has compiled an executive summary of the Guidelines for the Diagnosis and Management of Asthma.[3] Its proposed definition states that asthma is a lung disease characterized by "obstruction that is reversible (but not completely so in some patients) either spontaneously or with treatments, airway inflammation and airway hyperresponsiveness to a variety of stimuli." Most would agree that asthma involves bronchial hyperreactivity resulting in variable obstruction to airflow and hyperinflation of the lungs, and many accept that this is usually associated with mucus secretion and some mucosal thickening. Problems in definition confound the study of surgical risk in the asthmatic patient. It is accepted that asthmatic patients have a higher risk of pulmonary complications after surgery,[4] though the statistical risk and exact likelihood of specific complications are not precisely known.

The incidence of postoperative wheezing is significantly higher in patients with mild preoperative wheezes than those without them.[5] Therefore, asthmatic patients should be free of wheezes before surgery. When the disease is so severe that baseline wheezing is present when the patient is asymptomatic, one must weigh the necessity of the surgery against the increased risk of postoperative pulmonary complications.

SURGICAL CONSIDERATIONS

Operative risks in the asthmatic patient can be divided into those attributable to the disease itself and those attributable to extrinsic factors such as the nature of the procedure, tracheal intubation, and specific anesthetic agents. Upper-abdominal surgery is frequently associated with elevation of the diaphragm and lower-lobe atelectasis leading to a marked reduction in lung volumes.[6-8] These abnormalities are not seen in lower-abdominal surgery which carries a comparatively lower risk of pulmonary complications.[9] For unclear reasons, a raised left hemidiaphragm frequently develops in patients undergoing coronary bypass surgery, resulting in postoperative reductions in lung volumes.[10] Similarly, thoracic surgery involving resection of lung tissue increases risk in asthmatic patients. Even those asthmatics undergoing dental surgery require careful management to avoid complications.[11] The duration of surgery is also related to the likelihood of developing pulmonary complications.[12] Management of asthmatic patients under these conditions involves maximizing medical therapy before surgery, providing aggressive postoperative pulmonary toilet thereafter, and daily monitoring for exacerbation of asthma.

ANESTHETIC CONSIDERATIONS

Though choice of anesthetic agent is left to the anesthesiologist, it is important that the clinician understand the effects of these agents on the patient's underlying disease. Inhaled anesthetic agents themselves have been used to control severe asthma.[13,14] Until recently, halothane was considered the agent of choice for the asthmatic patient undergoing surgery because of its role in treating refractory status asthmaticus in intubated patients who do not respond to usual medical treatment.[15-17] However, because of possible adverse reactions to halothane in patients with asthma (discussed below), enflurane and isoflurane have been shown to have several advantages over halothane and may be used as first-line anesthetics.

The mechanisms by which halothane and other inhaled anesthetic agents cause bronchial smooth-muscle relaxation is unclear.

Clinically used concentrations of halothane have no apparent direct effect on relaxing bronchial smooth muscle in vitro,[18] and there is no effect on histamine release after its administration.[19] However, although halothane does not affect bronchial muscle relaxation directly, it decreases the ability of the bronchial smooth muscle to contract and depresses parasympathetic-mediated reflexes that control airway smooth muscle.[18]

Halothane is not without potential adverse effects. It is associated with increased cardiac irritability that can result in ventricular dysrhythmias and cardiac arrest.[16,20,21] Barton reports dysrhythmias ranging from supraventricular tachycardia to bigeminal and multifocal premature ventricular contractions in patients receiving aminophylline and halothane.[5] Aminophylline stimulates synthesis and release of endogenous catecholamines,[18] and halothane sensitizes the myocardium to their effects,[22] providing a possible explanation for the proarrhythmic effects of the combination. Withdrawing theophylline preparations prior to surgery decreases the arrhythmogenic effects but may increase the risk of perioperative bronchospasm.[5] Richards suggests attempting to maintain theophylline levels in a low therapeutic range (e.g., 10 μg/ml) to help reduce the incidence of cardiac arrhythmias induced by the combination of these drugs. However, even at reduced levels of theophylline, the incidence of arrhythmias is as high as 33 percent in experimental animals.[20]

Enflurane and isoflurane do not sensitize the myocardium to the effects of catecholamines.[16,20] In addition, isoflurane depresses the myocardium less than the other agents, making it a favorable choice in the asthmatic patient. Ketamine, an intravenous agent, is another alternative because of its sympathomimetic bronchodilating properties, but its use is limited because of unpleasant side effects on emerging from anesthesia including alterations in mood, extracorporeal or floating sensations, vivid dreams, and delirium.[23] Another option is the use of intravenous lidocaine, administered as a bolus followed by a continuous infusion, because it reduces the concentration of inhaled agent required to prevent reflex bronchospasm and may therefore decrease the risk of cardiac depression by inhaled agents like halothane.[16]

The route of administration of anesthesia may affect underlying asthma. Regional anesthesia carries lower pulmonary risk and should remain a first choice.[15,16] Local anesthesia is not without risk since certain local anesthetics of the ester type have been associated with allergic phenomena (see Chap. 49). Also, preparations in multi-use vials may contain metabisulfites as stabilizing agents, and many contain the preservative methylparaben. Use of local anesthetic agents containing these substances has rarely been associated with allergic reactions including bronchospasm.[24,25] In addition, there are case reports of bronchospasm after spinal anesthesia,[26,27] but their significance is unclear.

In the past, it was common to avoid intubation when general anesthesia was required in asthmatics in an effort to reduce the incidence of so-called intubation-induced bronchospasm. It is now thought that intubation allows better control of the airway and that intubation-stimulated bronchospasm is the result of inadequate depth of anesthesia.[15]

There are no controlled studies of the use of preoperative medications in asthmatic patients. However, the administration of narcotics and benzodiazepines is appropriate but not in such large doses that may lead to unnecessary respiratory depression. Antihistamines, because of their theoretical advantage as H_1 antagonists, may also be used as sedatives, although their role in decreasing exacerbation of asthma in surgical patients has been disappointing.

Succinylcholine can stimulate histamine release in vitro but in practice does not appear to increase the incidence of bronchospasm.[28,29] Concentrations of thiopental required to stimulate histamine are higher than those needed to induce clinical anesthesia.[18]

EVALUATION OF THE PATIENT

The history and physical examination provide important information about the activity of the patient's disease and other associated processes that may increase the risk of surgery. Table 23–1 summarizes important points of the history that are helpful in determining risk. Although the physical examination can be helpful in assessing the activity of the disease, normal findings can be misleading because asymptomatic asthmatics may still have abnormal lung functions studies.[30] Pratter et al. have pointed out that wheezes do not always indicate asthma. Using methacholine provocation of bronchospasm as a diagnostic gold standard, they found that pulmonologists diagnosing asthma clinically were correct only 54 percent of the time. They suggest combining clinical evaluation with either a methacholine bronchoprovocation challenge or spirometry before and after administration of a bronchodilator if baseline spirometry shows more than a minimal decrease in flow rates.[31] However, it is often impractical for the consultant to use these methods to confirm the diagnosis of asthma in every patient. Confirmatory testing can be reserved for those patients with a confusing presentation or other associated disease processes that might confuse diagnosis. When spirometry with bronchodilator testing is performed, reversible airway disease is considered present when there is an increase of 200 ml or 10% or more increase in the FEV_1[32] or an improvement in $FEV_{25-75\%}$ of 45 percent with bronchodilators.[33]

It is important to identify subsets of patients who may have an even greater risk of complications than the average asthmatic. Interestingly, patients with frequent exacerbations of asthma have increased endurance of their respiratory muscles.[34] In one group, there was measurable hypertrophy of the sternocleidomastoid muscles.[35] Although patients with recurrent episodes may be more likely to experience a perioperative exacerbation, they may be better equipped to withstand it than an asthmatic with less respiratory muscle training. On the other hand, frequent or chronic use of corticosteroids may lead to respiratory muscle weakening and decreased ability to handle a perioperative exacerbation of their asthma.[36]

TABLE 23–1. Important Points in the History of the Asthmatic Patient

History of hospitalization for asthma
History of intubation during an asthmatic exacerbation
Frequency of asthmatic exacerbations
Use of single versus multiple classes of bronchodilator medications
History and frequency of steroid use (systemic versus inhaled)
Previous peak flow or pulmonary function values
History of cardiac dysrhythmias
Other associated cardiac or pulmonary diseases

Pulmonary Function Testing

Since there are no large studies correlating preoperative pulmonary function tests with surgical risk, it is unclear which pulmonary function parameters predict risk the best and which patients should have preoperative pulmonary function tests. Single-breath spirographic studies are useful in assessing impairment of pulmonary function that may not be clinically apparent. A simple spirogram is therefore often informative and relatively inexpensive and should be obtained before surgery in patients with asthma. Preoperative values provide a baseline for comparison should a subsequent exacerbation occur. If spirometry is normal, patients can be spared routine perioperative use of intravenous aminophylline and steroids.

Although the $FEV_{25-75\%}$ may be a better indicator of small airway disease,[33] the FEV_1 is an adequate measure. Most agree that the FEV_1, FVC, and FEV_1/FVC are the most important parameters.[37] Peak expiratory flow rate can be measured with a simple hand-held meter at the bedside and, when done properly, correlates well with the FEV_1 measured by spirometry.[38] Nowak has shown that marked decreases in FEV_1 and peak flow to less than one liter and 200 ml, respectively, can predict hypercarbia and hypoxemia in patients with acute exacerbations.[39] Simple tests like FEV_1 or peak flow can therefore be useful in assessing asthmatic disease and following improvement during treatment. Before surgery, these values are more meaningful if there are previous baseline studies with which to compare.

There have been attempts to classify the severity of asthma according to abnormalities in spirographic studies and peak flow measurements (see Tables 23–2 and 23–3). However, moderate-to-severe disease should be apparent clinically, and no classification of asthma has been validated as a predictor of surgical risk. There are studies of pulmonary function tests as predictors of pulmonary complications in general but none specifically for asthma. In these studies, an FEV_1 of less than one liter is associated with increased surgical risk.[40] Cebul has suggested that an FEV_1 of less than 75% of the predicted normal value is associated with significantly increased risk of postoperative pulmonary complications.[41]

Chest X-ray

The chest x-ray is not a useful routine preoperative screening test in patients with asthma. Asymptomatic asthmatics commonly exhibit hyperaeration, increased lung markings, peribronchial thickening, and subsegmental atelectasis on chest x-ray,[42] and these findings do not provide information that will alter management of

TABLE 23–2. Severity of Asthmatic Disease Correlated with Spirographic Measurement

Clinical Classification	% of Predicted FEV_1, FVC
Normal	80–100
Mild	75–79
Moderate	50–74
Severe	35–49
Status Asthmaticus	< 35

Source: Adapted from Kingston et al[16] and Atkins.[63]

TABLE 23–3. Severity of Asthmatic Disease Correlated with Peak Flow Measurements

Clinical Classification	% of Predicted Peak Flow
Normal	80–100*
Mild to Moderate	50–79†
Severe	< 50††

*Measurements of 80–100% predicted are within normal range.

†Measurements of 50–80% predicted suggest that either acute exacerbation is present or that overall asthma is not under sufficient control.

††Measurements of less than 50% signal medical alert for acute treatment.

Source: Adapted from National Asthma Education Program.[3]

the patient. The chest x-ray should be reserved for those with complicating factors associated with their asthma such as congestive heart failure, pneumonia, or irreversible chronic obstructive pulmonary disease.

Electrocardiogram

There are several abnormalities seen on the electrocardiogram during an acute exacerbation of asthma including right bundle branch block, ventricular premature beats, and acute increase in right atrial size.[43] In status asthmaticus, p-pulmonale is the most common electrocardiographic abnormality seen and is thought to be indicative of hypercapnia and more severe obstruction. ST-segment and T-wave abnormalities suggesting myocardial ischemia are found in approximately 10 percent of patients.[37] These temporary changes resolve with resolution of the bronchospasm. The decision to obtain a preoperative electrocardiogram should be based on an appropriate cardiac history or factors other than the patient's asthma.

The Arterial Blood Gas

Asthma is a reversible ventilation problem. The arterial blood gas determination (ABG) is therefore of little value as a preoperative screening test in the asymptomatic patient. The ABG is valuable in managing the patient with an acute attack, especially if the patient is showing signs of fatigue.

PRETREATMENT OF THE ASTHMATIC SURGICAL PATIENT

General approaches to managing preoperative patients with asthma have evolved over the years, although rigorous study of specific approaches has never been undertaken. In the United States, asthmatics are often started on intravenous aminophylline the day before surgery and receive inhaled beta-agonists through a pressurized nebulizer on a regular basis. In the United Kingdom, asthmatics generally receive less rigorous preoperative preparation.[4] Grouping asthmatic patients according to level of severity has been advocated in order to design specific treatment to prevent complications. The following classification of asthmatic patients is a synthesis of suggestions culled from the literature and is put forth in an effort to temper the tendency to treat all asthmatic patients with preoperative bronchodilators. Elective surgery should be postponed for patients in any group who are wheezing until they are free of wheezes and spirograms either are only minimally abnormal or approach baseline.

Group 1

Patients in this group have a history of asthma but do not take bronchodilators and have not had an episode in several years. The physical examination and spirographic studies or peak flow rates are usually normal. These patients can usually be managed without bronchodilators. An appropriate anesthetic agent should be chosen to avoid bronchospasm. Confirmatory testing with a pre- and postbronchodilator or bronchoprovocation testing prior to surgery need only be done if there is diagnostic uncertainty.

Group 2

Patients in this group have mild episodes of wheezing that are easily managed with an inhaled bronchodilator and do not require prophylactic theophylline or cromolyn sodium. If their physical examinations and spirometry or peak flows are normal, they can be managed with an inhaled bronchodilator given every four to six hours before surgery and postoperatively as needed. The beta-agonist can be administered in a hand-held metered-dose inhaler with a spacer device. An appropriate anesthetic agent should be chosen.

Group 3

Patients in this group have frequent attacks and may or may not use theophylline preparations. They either have more severe disease or may not be receiving optimal therapy. If they are wheeze-free and spirograms show an FEV_1 of greater than 75% of the predicted normal value, they can receive intravenous aminophylline on the day of surgery. Therapeutic theophylline levels should be documented prior to the procedure. Inhaled bronchodilators may be added as necessary. If spirometry shows more than mild abnormalities and there are no baseline values for comparison, intravenous aminophylline and inhaled bronchodilators should be started the day before surgery. Moderate-to-severe spirometric abnormalities are usually associated with wheezing on examination. In these cases, surgery should be postponed until these abnormalities have resolved.

Group 4

Patients in this group take steroids, give a history of recent or chronic steroid use, or have a history of severe asthmatic attacks sometimes requiring intubation. These patients may exhibit more abnormal baseline spirometry values. They must be monitored closely and should receive intravenous aminophylline, inhaled beta-agonist, and steroids at least 24 hours prior to surgery. Dosing for intravenous steroids is outlined below. Patients who have taken supraphysiologic doses of steroids for more than a week or two in the year before surgery require stress doses of steroids in the perioperative period.[44]

MEDICAL TREATMENT

Inhaled Beta-Agonists

Patients in group 1 or 2 are likely to be easily managed with inhaled bronchodilators. It was previously thought that an acute exacerbation was better treated with beta-agonist delivered with an air- or oxygen-driven pressurized small-volume nebulizer than with a metered-dose inhaler. However, with a spacer device to simplify use, a metered-dose inhaler provides equal therapeutic benefit.[45] Spacer devices obviate the need for timed inspiration and allow for better delivery of the medication when proper coordination of regular hand-held inhalers is in question.[46] The usual dosing interval is every four to six hours. The administration of bronchodilators need not be interrupted by surgery since there are various means of administering bronchodilators in the anesthesia circuit.[47,48]

Theophylline

Patients taking oral theophylline preparations should receive intravenous aminophylline for greater reliability in maintaining therapeutic theophylline levels. Patients admitted for "same-day surgery" should not take their regular morning dose and then receive maintenance intravenous aminophylline with appropriate supplemental boluses as dictated by the serum theophylline level. If they have already taken theophylline before surgery, a maintenance intravenous aminophylline drip should be started and supplemented as needed. Theophylline levels should be closely monitored.

Patients who have not been taking theophylline or who have undetectable levels can be managed with an initial loading dose of aminophylline of 5.6 mg/kg followed by a continuous intravenous infusion of 0.9 mg/kg/hr.[49] Most agree on this loading dose,[50,51] but some believe that this fixed maintenance dose is too high for many adults. Kelly et al. have summarized data from several sources and have developed maintenance dosing recommendations that more reliably yield a therapeutic level (see Table 23–4).[65]

The loading dose of aminophylline should be calculated using total body weight in kilograms and administered as a bolus over 20 to 30 minutes. The maintenance dose should be calculated using ideal body weight because theophylline clearance is reduced in obese patients and therefore less drug is required.[52,53] The serum theophylline level should not be determined until one to two hours after completion of the infusion.[64] In the determination of an

TABLE 23–4. Aminophylline Maintenance Dose

Category	Initial Clearance (ml/kg/hr)	IV Dose (mg/kg/hr)
Uncomplicated		
nonsmoking	40 ± 12	0.5
smoking	70 ± 28	0.8
Critically ill, all varieties (Westerfield et al.64)	43 ± 16	0.5
Congestive heart failure or severe pneumonia (Powell et al.52)	25 ± 12	0.2

Source: Adapted from *Drug Therapy for Asthma.*[65]

appropriate supplemental bolus dose for patients with measurable but subtherapeutic levels, it can be assumed that the serum theophylline level will increase approximately two $\mu g/ml$ for every mg/kg aminophylline given.

Certain drugs such as phenobarbital, phenytoin, rifampin, and intravenous isoproterenol cause more rapid metabolism of theophylline. Conversely, erythromycin, cimetidine (but not other H_2 blockers), allopurinol, and oral contraceptive steroids reduce clearance of theophylline. Close monitoring of theophylline levels and appropriate adjustments in dosing should be made in patients taking these drugs.

Corticosteroids

Steroids should be given to patients in group 4 to avoid the complications of possible adrenal axis suppression resulting from chronic or frequent steroid use. Steroids are effective in the treatment of asthma, but the exact doses required remain uncertain.[54,55] During an exacerbation, hydrocortisone 250 mg intravenously every six hours or methylprednisolone 40 mg intravenously every six hours should be given. If the patient is not wheezing, steroids can be given twice daily. Oral steroids are well absorbed and equally effective, but the intravenous form is preferred in patients who may not be able to eat. Hydrocortisone has more mineralocorticoid effect than methylprednisolone; the latter may therefore be preferable in patients with a history of congestive heart failure.

Oxygen

During surgery and immediately thereafter, oxygen therapy is managed by the anesthesiologist. Oxygen should otherwise be reserved for treatment of the symptomatic asthmatic. Oxygen improves hypoxemia resulting from impaired ventilation during bronchospasm. In addition, it prevents transient worsening of hypoxemia that can sometimes be seen during clinical improvement in bronchospasm.[39,56] This initial fall in arterial oxygen concentration is thought to be the result of improved ventilation of previously underventilated areas that may still be underperfused because of a lag in resolution of reflex vasoconstriction in the pulmonary vasculature serving those areas.

Anticholinergics

Anticholinergic agents are generally reserved for treatment of severe exacerbations of asthma and have no role in the medical management of asymptomatic asthmatics going to surgery.

Beta-Blockers

Beta-blockers are generally contraindicated in asthmatics. However, there are instances such as in thyrotoxic patients when they may be quite useful. Case reports show that selective beta-adrenergic receptor blockers can be used safely with careful monitoring of the underlying asthma.[57]

Other Medications

Calcium channel blockers like verapamil and nifedipine have been shown to have bronchodilating properties in asthmatics,[58–60] but their role in managing asthma in or outside the surgical setting remains unclear. The beneficial effect of calcium channel blockers may be a consideration in selecting an antihypertensive agent in asthmatic patients with hypertension.

Theoretically, H_2 blockers may affect control of asthma through their effect on histamine release but do not appear to worsen asthma clinically.[61,62] A more important effect is the increase in theophylline levels that has been documented with cimetidine.

SUMMARY

1. There are no controlled studies estimating surgical risk in asthmatic patients apart from those with chronic obstructive pulmonary disease. However, pulmonary complications are more common in thoracic and upper-abdominal procedures. Different anesthesia and drug combinations may also increase risk and lead to exacerbation of bronchospasm.

2. Classification of asthmatics by history, physical examination, and simple pulmonary function tests is useful in determining appropriate management. Patients should be free of wheezing and have an FEV_1 of 75% of the predicted normal value before elective surgery.

3. Inhaled beta-agonists, intravenous aminophylline, and parenteral steroids are used in various combinations depending on the severity of the underlying asthma.

4. All patients who are taking or have taken supraphysiologic doses of steroids for more than two weeks during the past year require adrenal coverage with the equivalent of 200 to 300 mg of hydrocortisone intravenously per day in the perioperative period.

REFERENCES

1. National Heart, Lung, and Blood Institute: *Data Fact Sheet—Asthma Statistics*. Bethesda, NHLBI Education Programs, 1989.
2. Gross NJ: What is this thing called love? Or defining asthma. *Am Rev Resp Dis* 121:203–204, 1980.
3. National Heart, Lung, and Blood Institute: *Executive Summary: Guidelines for the Diagnosis and Management of Asthma*. Publication No. 91-3042A. Bethesda, NHLBI Education Programs, 1991.
4. Morgan C, Gillbe C: Anesthetizing the asthmatic. *Br J Hosp Med* 34:326–330, 1985.
5. Barton DM: Anesthetic problems with aspirin-intolerant patients. *Anesth Analg* 54(3):376–380, 1975.
6. Dureuil B, Viires N, Cantineau JP et al: Diaphragmatic contractility after upper abdominal surgery. *J Appl Phys* 61:1775–1780, 1986.
7. Ford GT, Whitelaw WA, Rosenal TW et al: Diaphragm function after upper abdominal surgery in humans. *Am Rev Resp Dis* 127:431–436, 1983.
8. Simonneau G, Vivien A, Sartene R et al: Diaphragm dysfunction induced by upper abdominal surgery. *Am Rev Resp Dis* 128:899–903, 1983.
9. Tobin MJ: Respiratory muscles in disease. *Clin Chest Med* 5:669–683, 1984.
10. Large S, Heywood LJ, Flower CD et al: Incidence and etiology of a raised hemidiaphragm after cardiopulmonary bypass. *Thorax* 40:444–447, 1985.
11. Geist ET, Diaz JH: Management of the asthmatic patient undergoing dental surgery. *J Am Dent Assoc* 105:65–69, 1982.
12. Dripps RD, Deming M: Postoperative atelectasis and pneumonia. *Ann Surg* 124:94–109, 1946.

13. Fuchs AM: The interruption of the asthmatic crisis by tribromethanol (avertin). *J Allergy* 8:340–346, 1937.

14. Maytum CK: Bronchial asthma: Relief of prolonged attack by colonic administration of ether. *Med Clin N Am* 15:201, 1931.

15. Schwiesow J: Anesthesia for the asthmatic patient. *Am Assoc Nurse Anesth* 47:407–411, 1979.

16. Kingston HG, Hirshman CA: Perioperative management of the patient with asthma. *Anesth Analg* 63:844–855, 1984.

17. Schwartz SH: Treatment of status asthmaticus with halothane. *JAMA* 251:2688–2689, 1984.

18. Hirshman CA, Edelstein G, Peetz S et al: Mechanism of action of inhalational anesthesia on airways. *Anesthesiology* 56:107–111, 1982.

19. Hermens JM, Edelstein G, Hanifin JM et al: Inhalational anesthesia and histamine release during bronchospasm. *Anesthesiology* 61:69–72, 1984.

20. Richards W, Thompson J, Lewis G et al: Cardiac arrest associated with halothane anesthesia in a patient receiving theophylline. *Ann Allergy* 61:83–84, 1988.

21. Roizen MF, Stevens WC: Multiform ventricular tachycardia due to the interaction of aminophylline and halothane. *Anesth Analg* 57:738–741, 1978.

22. Hall AD, Norris FH: Fluothane sensitization of the dog heart to the action of epinephrine. *Anesthesiology* 19:631–641, 1958.

23. Rock MJ, Reyes De La Rocha S, L'Hommedieu CS et al: Use of ketamine in asthmatic children to treat respiratory failure refractory to conventional therapy. *Crit Care Med* 14:514–516, 1986.

24. Blackmore JW: Local anesthetics and sulphite sensitivity. *J Can Dent Assoc* 54:349–352, 1988.

25. Schwartz HF, Gilbert IA, Lenner KA et al: Metabisulfite sensitivity and local dental anesthesia. *Ann Allergy* 62:83–86, 1989.

26. Eldor J, Frankel DZ: Acute bronchospasm during epidural anesthesia in asthmatic patients. *J Asthma* 26(1):15–16, 1989.

27. Mallampati SR: Bronchospasm during spinal anesthesia. *Anesth Analg* 60(11):839–840, 1981.

28. Adriani J, Rosenstine EA: The effect of anesthetic drugs upon bronchi and bronchioles of exised lung tissue. *Anesthesiology* 4:253–262, 1943.

29. Crago RR, Bryan AC, Laws AK et al: Respiratory flow resistance after curare and pancuronium measured by forced oscillation. *J Can Anaesth Soc* 19:607–614, 1972.

30. McFadden ER, Kiser R, deGroot WJ: Acute bronchial asthma: Relations between clinical and physiological manifestations. *N Engl J Med* 288:221–225, 1973.

31. Pratter MR, Hingston DM, Irwin RS: Diagnosis of bronchial asthma by clinical evaluation—an unreliable method. *Chest* 84:43–45, 1983.

32. Conrad SA: *Pulmonary Function Testing; Principles and Practice*. New York, Churchill Livingstone, 1984, p 216.

33. McFadden ER, Linden DA: A reduction in maximum mid-expiratory flow rate. A spirographic manifestation of small airway disease. *Am J Med* 52:725–737, 1972.

34. McKenzie DK, Gandevia SC: Strength and endurance of inspiratory, expiratory, and limb muscles in asthma. *Am Rev Resp Dis* 134:999–1004, 1986.

35. Lavietes MH, Reichman L (eds): *Diagnostic Aspects and Management of Asthma*. New York, Purdue, 1982, pp 27–38.

36. Melzer E, Souhrada JF: Decrease of respiratory muscle strength and static lung volumes in obese asthmatics. *Am Rev Resp Dis* 121:17–22, 1980.

37. Gershwin ME (ed): *Bronchial Asthma, Principles of Diagnosis and Treatment*. Orlando, Grune & Stratton, 1986, p 473.

38. Nowak RM, Pensler MI, Parker DD: Comparison of peak expiratory flow and FEV_1: Admission criteria for acute asthma. *Ann Emerg Med* 11:64–69, 1982.

39. Nowak RM, Tomlanovich MC, Sarkar DD et al: Arterial blood gases and pulmonary function testing in acute bronchial asthma—predicting outcomes. *JAMA* 249:2043–2046, 1983.

40. Hodgkin JE: Preoperative evaluation of pulmonary function. *Am J Surg* 138:355–360, 1979.

41. Cebul RD, Williams SV, Kussmaul WG et al: Predicting postoperative pulmonary complication after elective thoracic surgery. Presented at the Second Annual Meeting of the Society for Medical Decision Making. Washington DC, September 1980.

42. Gershel JC, Goldman HS, Stein REK et al: The usefulness of chest radiographs in first asthma attacks. *N Engl J Med* 11:336–339, 1983.

43. Weiss EB, Segal MS (eds): *Bronchial Asthma, Mechanisms and Therapeutics*. Boston, Little Brown, 1975, p 279.

44. Morgan C, Gillbe C: Anaesthetising the asthmatic. *Br J Hosp Med* 34(6):326–330, 1985.

45. Yao FSF, Artusio JF: Asthma-COPD, in *Anesthesiology, Problem-Oriented Patient Management*. Philadelphia, Lippincott, 1988, pp 3–25.

46. Morley TF, Marozsan E, Zappasodi S et al: Comparison of beta-adrenergic agents delivered by nebulizer versus metered dose inhaler with inspirease in hospitalized asthmatic patients. *Chest* 94:1205–1210, 1988.

47. Konig P: Spacer devices with metered-dose inhalers: Breakthrough or gimmick. *Chest* 88(2):276–284, 1985.

48. Diamond MJ: Delivering bronchodilators into the anesthesia circuit. *Anesthesiology* 64:531, 1986.

49. Newell R, Schulman MS: The administration of bronchodilators into the anesthesia circuit. *Anesthesiology* 66:716–717, 1987.

50. Mitenko PA, Ogilvie RI: Rational intravenous doses of theophylline. *N Engl J Med* 289:600–603, 1973.

51. Kordash TR, Van Dellen RG, McCall JT: Theophylline concentrations in asthmatic patients after administration of aminophylline. *JAMA* 238:139–141, 1977.

52. Powell JR, Vozeh S, Hopewell P et al: Theophylline disposition in acutely ill hospitalized patients. The effect of smoking, heart failure, severe airway obstruction and pneumonia. *Am Rev Respir Dis* 118:229–238, 1978.

53. Gal P, Jusko WJ, Yurchak AM et al: Theophylline disposition in obesity. *Clin Pharmacol Ther* 23:438–444, 1978.

54. Hendeles L, Weinberger M, Johnson G: Monitoring serum theophylline levels. *Clin Pharmacokinet* 3:294, 1978.

55. Fanta CH, Tossing TH, McFadden ER: Glucocorticoids in acute asthma. A critical controlled trial. *Am J Med* 74:845–851, 1983.

56. Haskell RJ, Wong BM, Hansen JE: A double-blind, randomized clinical trial of methylprednisolone in status asthmaticus. *Arch Int Med* 143:1324–1327, 1983.

57. Tai E, Read J: Response of blood gas tensions to aminophylline and isoprenaline in patients with asthma. *Thorax* 22:543–549, 1967.

58. Dial P, Hastings PR: The use of a selective beta-adrenergic receptor blocker for the preoperative preparation of the thyrotoxic patient. *Ann Surg* 196:633–635, 1982.

59. Henderson AF, Heaton RW, Dunlop LS et al: Effects of nifedipine on antigen-induced bronchoconstriction. *Am Rev Resp Dis* 127:549–553, 1983.

60. Schwartzstein RS, Fanta CH: Orally administered nifedipine in chronic stable asthma. *Am Rev Resp Dis* 134:262–265, 1986.

61. Solway J, Fanta CH: Differential inhibition of bronchoconstriction by the calcium channel blockers, verapamil and nifedipine. *Am Rev Resp Dis* 132:666–670, 1985.

62. Lichtenstein LM, Gillespie E: Inhibition of histamine release by histamine controlled by H_2 receptors. *Nature* 244:287–288, 1973.

63. Atkins PC: The risks of surgery in patients with asthma, in Goldmann DR, Brown FH, Levy WB et al (eds): *Medical Care of the Surgical Patient*. Philadelphia, Lippincott, 1982, pp 422–426.

64. Westerfield BT, Carder AJ, Light RW: The relationship between arterial blood gases and serum theophylline clearance in critically ill patients. *Am Rev Resp Dis* 124:17–20, 1981.

65. Kelly WH, Murphy S, Jenne JW: *Drug Therapy for Asthma*. New York, Marcel Dekker, 1987, p 1038.

24 THE SURGICAL PATIENT WITH DIABETES MELLITUS

Alicia M. Conill

David A. Horowitz

Seth Braunstein

Diabetes mellitus is common in the general population. In 1985, Reynolds reported that there were 10 million Americans, or approximately five percent of the population, with diabetes mellitus of whom half would require surgery at some point in life.[1] In 1988, Dunnet et al. reported that diabetes affects 5 to 10 percent of the population between the ages of 60 and 80 and one to two percent of the population as a whole.[2] Wetterhall et al. reported that in 1987 there were 6.82 million people in the United States with known diabetes and perhaps an equal number with the disease but no knowledge of it. They estimated that the number had increased by more than one million in the previous eight-year period.[3] The incidence of diabetes increases with age, and the prevalence of the disease between the ages of 65 and 74 is 18 percent in whites, 25 percent in blacks, and 33 percent in Hispanics.[4,5] Hospitalization rates for patients with some of the major complications of diabetes mellitus are rising proportionately. In addition to hospitalizations for stroke, diabetic ketoacidosis, cardiovascular disease, and end-stage renal disease,[3,6] diabetics undergo a wide array of procedures, including vitrectomy, cataract extraction, kidney transplantation, penile prosthesis implantation, ulcer debridement, vascular repairs, amputations, and coronary artery bypass surgery.[7]

In the early 1960s, Galloway and Shuman reported that the mortality rate was 3.6 percent and the morbidity rate was 17.2 percent in diabetic patients undergoing surgery.[8] In the late 1970s and early 1980s these numbers were corroborated by other investigators.[9,10] As recently as 1992, Milaskiewicz and Hall reported that the mortality rate in diabetics after surgery is 1.5 times that in the general population.[11]

Diabetes has been shown to be a risk factor in patients undergoing a variety of procedures. A retrospective study of patients undergoing biliary surgery suggests increased morbidity among diabetics in 1500 consecutive cases requiring both emergency and elective procedures.[12] Of the 12.6 percent of patients with diabetes, those undergoing emergency surgery had a mortality rate of 3.1 percent compared to 1.1 percent mortality in the nondiabetic group. Septic complications, especially wound infections, were more common in the diabetic group. Larsen et al. developed a prospective model for the prediction of perioperative cardiac risk from multivariate regression analysis of risk factors in 2609 noncardiac major operative procedures.[13] Although diabetes mellitus proved to be an independent risk factor, five other factors proved significant: congestive heart failure, ischemic cardiac disease, a serum creatinine level above 130 μmol/l, the need for emergency surgery, and the type of surgery. Three of these risk factors are known complications of diabetes mellitus. In a more recent study, Hollenberg et al. noted that diabetics in a population of male veterans with significant known coronary artery disease experienced a greater incidence of postoperative myocardial ischemia than a similar group of nondiabetics.[14]

Several studies suggest that diabetes itself may not be an independent risk factor predicting morbidity and mortality and that preexisting cardiac, renal, vascular, and neurological abnormalities, more common in diabetics, are responsible for surgical complications.[15–18] In comparing surgical outcome in diabetic patients and nondiabetic controls, Hjortrup et al. found that diabetes in itself does not increase the risk of complications after surgery for hip fracture or major abdominal or vascular procedures.[15] MacKenzie et al. found that in a cohort of diabetic patients, serious cardiac morbidity and death were best predicted by preexisting cardiac disease including congestive heart failure and valvular heart disease.[16] The same study suggests that infection, renal insufficiency, and cerebral ischemic events were more likely in diabetics with preoperative end-organ dysfunction. In diabetics without underlying nephropathy, neuropathy, or retinopathy, complications were rare. There are few data correlating surgical outcome measures with the type of diabetes, duration of disease, severity of complications, specifics of glucose control, or management strategies.

However, descriptive reports, some animal data, and knowledge of the natural history of diabetes and its complications allow identification of areas of concern in the preoperative assessment and perioperative management of patients with diabetes.

As suggested above, atherosclerotic cardiovascular disease is the most important concern in evaluating diabetic patients before surgery. Coronary artery disease occurs four times more often in diabetics as in age-matched patients without diabetes and accounts for an increased incidence of perioperative ischemia and myocardial infarction.[14] Congestive heart failure is also more frequent among diabetics and may be related to diabetic cardiomyopathy or subclinical ischemia. Cerebrovascular disease is probably more common in diabetics, potentiating the threat of cerebral ischemia and thrombotic and embolic stroke following episodes of hypotension, hypertension, or hypoxia. Dysfunction of other organs can lead to a variety of perioperative complications. Diabetic autonomic neuropathy, sometimes manifested by a lack of variation in cardiac rate and postural hypotension, can cause unpredictable autonomic nervous system responses to surgical stress.[17,18] Peripheral sensory neuropathy predisposes bedridden patients to pressure ulcers and skin necrosis. Underlying diabetic nephropathy can make fluid and electrolyte balance a difficult and complex management problem.[19] Delayed wound healing due to hyperglycemia has been demonstrated in many experimental studies.[20–22] Abnormalities in leukocyte phagocytosis and antibody response to staphylococcal antigen have been documented when blood glucose levels exceed 200 to 250 mg/dl and predispose patients to postoperative infections including those caused by gram-negative bacteria.[23,24]

In summary, although it is still not entirely clear whether diabetes mellitus independently predicts perioperative morbidity and mortality, it appears certain that patients with diabetic-related end-organ dysfunction do have an increased risk of complications during and after surgery. Therefore, it is crucial that the preoperative evaluation be thorough in defining the nature and extent of end-organ disease and that perioperative management be especially careful as it relates to myocardial ischemia and infection.

CARBOHYDRATE METABOLISM AND SURGERY

An understanding of the physiology of normal carbohydrate metabolism facilitates perioperative management of patients with diabetes mellitus.[25–29] Appreciation of the differences between the fed and fasting states and the effects of the stress of surgery upon these states allows the clinician to anticipate and prevent perturbations in glucose homeostasis. The liver plays a central role in the utilization of ingested carbohydrate, protein, and fat. Insulin, the chief anabolic hormone, is most active in the fed state and stimulates hepatic glycogenesis and lipogenesis. It also stimulates glucose uptake into fat and muscle tissue and promotes protein anabolism. Insulin-deficiency or insulin-resistance mimics the fasting state. In the absence of insulin, the effects of counterregulatory hormones go unchecked, and stored glycogen, fat, and protein are catabolized to maintain substrate levels adequate for energy production. Glucagon promotes gluconeogenesis and glycogenolysis in the liver. Cortisol facilitates protein breakdown in peripheral tissues to create substrate for hepatic gluconeogenesis. Catecholamines promote lipolysis and glycogenolysis. Energy homeostasis is thus maintained at the expense of body stores of carbohydrate, fat, and protein. Prolonged fasting leads to starvation in which alternate substrates are utilized to produce energy. Catabolism of fatty acids ultimately leads to formation of ketone bodies. In diabetic patients, insulinopenia can thus lead to hyperglycemia, hyperosmolarity, dehydration, electrolyte abnormalities, and, in extreme cases, diabetic ketoacidosis (DKA) or hyperosmolar hyperglycemic nonketotic coma (HHNC).

The stresses of surgery and anesthesia exert major effects on glucose homeostasis. Reactive hyperglycemia develops during and after surgery even in patients without diabetes. The "stress" of surgery causes an outpouring of catecholamines and cortisol that increase insulin resistance and hyperglycemia. In diabetic patients, underlying insulin resistance and deficiency are exacerbated by these effects. In addition, general anesthesia itself suppresses endogenous insulin secretion.[30] Vasoactive substances used in the operating room can exert or potentiate anti-insulin effects. For example, epinephrine has been reported to promote insulin resistance in noninsulin-dependent diabetics undergoing open-heart surgery.[31]

PREOPERATIVE EVALUATION AND MANAGEMENT

Preoperative evaluation of patients with diabetes, whether or not they are insulin-dependent, requires correction of metabolic, fluid, and electrolyte disturbances as well as assessment of underlying complicating disease. The latter requires particular attention to cardiovascular, cerebrovascular, renal, and neurological function as well as evaluation of independent contributing risk factors to end-organ damage such as hyperlipidemia, smoking, obesity, and family history of disease. In addition to a good history and physical examination, every patient should have blood electrolyte, blood urea nitrogen, and creatinine levels measured; a complete blood count; and a urinalysis. A glycohemoglobin level may be helpful to estimate the degree of control in the preceding eight to 10 weeks, but is not essential. The preoperative electrocardiogram may be useful in identifying conduction abnormalities and evidence of old myocardial infarction or ongoing ischemia. Stress testing, even with thallium imaging, is not specific enough to use as a screening tool to identify silent ischemia in patients with or without diabetes,[32] and there is still controversy regarding its prognostic value in many surgical settings.[33–36] However, stress testing may be useful in patients with symptoms suggestive of coronary artery disease such as breathlessness or fatigue with modest activity or in those with ECG changes suggesting ongoing ischemia.

Careful assessment of volume status and renal function is an important element of the preoperative evaluation. In patients with insulin-dependent diabetes mellitus (IDDM), the presence of more than 30 mg/dl of protein in a dipstick-positive spot urine specimen generally implies significant impairment of renal function and a reduction in glomerular filtration rate that may not yet be reflected in the serum creatinine level. Proteinuria in patients with noninsulin-dependent diabetes mellitus (NIDDM) may not be associated with as ominous a prognosis as it would in those with IDDM, but some studies suggest that even a small amount of proteinuria may be a marker for increased cardiovascular morbidity and mortality in these patients.[37,38]

All diabetics and especially those with nephropathy are more sensitive to intravenous contrast agents. Hydration before and during the procedure, administration of mannitol, and use of nonionic contrast agents reduce the risk of contrast-induced renal failure.[39] Contrast-induced nephropathy is discussed in detail in Chap. 45.

Preoperative evaluation of glucose control is essential in managing patients with both IDDM and NIDDM. Serum glucose, fluid, and electrolyte management will be easier in the perioperative period if glucose control is optimal before surgery. Patients who are poorly controlled with diet or with diet and oral hypoglycemic agents may benefit from treatment with insulin for several days or weeks before elective surgery if time allows.[40]

Home glucose monitoring before and after meals affords the best measure of therapeutic effectiveness. Patients already on insulin may need adjustments in their dosages. Ideal goals include a fasting plasma glucose level under 140 mg/dl and premeal levels of about 180 mg/dl, but these may need to be tempered by the individual patient's risk of hypoglycemia, his or her willingness and ability to comply with therapeutic recommendations, and the time available before the procedure. Obviously, urgent or emergency procedures do not allow the luxury of time, but even patients in these settings benefit from some attempt to bring the serum glucose level under control.

The benefits of better preoperative glucose management include:

1. Normalization of fluid and electrolyte abnormalities and intracellular and extracellular volume;
2. Reduced tissue resistance to insulin allowing easier perioperative management of the blood sugar;[41]
3. Enhanced endogenous beta-cell responsiveness with increased insulin secretion in those with NIDDM;[41]
4. Decreased hepatic gluconeogenesis;[41] and
5. Improved leukocyte function and wound healing.[20–22]

Diabetic patients can generally be divided into two groups—those with noninsulin-dependent diabetes (NIDDM) and those with insulin-dependent diabetes (IDDM). Patients with NIDDM may use diet, oral hypoglycemic agents, or insulin (or any combination of the three) to control hyperglycemia. The use of insulin does not necessarily mean that a patient is definitely insulin-dependent. Patients with NIDDM tend to develop their disease after the age of 40, are more often overweight, and have a strong family history of diabetes. They generally do not develop ketoacidosis in the absence of insulin but can do so when stressed by trauma, surgery, or infection. Patients with IDDM are absolutely dependent on exogenous insulin. They have no residual beta-cell activity and do not respond to oral hypoglycemic agents. In the absence of insulin they can become ketoacidotic, and stress can potentiate the rapidity of its onset and severity. Patients usually develop IDDM before the age of 30, but there are many patients who develop ketosis-prone diabetes later in life.

It is often impossible to determine which patients taking insulin have NIDDM and which have IDDM and are therefore prone to develop ketosis. For this reason, it is safer to treat all such patients as if they were insulin-dependent and to use insulin before and after surgery. While patients with IDDM are thought to have a greater tendency to develop diabetic complications than those with NIDDM, nephropathy, retinopathy, neuropathy, and cardiovascular involvement commonly occur in those with NIDDM. Since the population of patients with NIDDM is so much larger, the number with complications is as great or greater than that in the population of those with IDDM.

Assuming that glucose control is already good, preoperative management of patients with NIDDM and IDDM is usually dictated by their previous specific regimens. For those with NIDDM controlled with oral hypoglycemic agents, the drugs should be stopped the night before surgery. Patients on agents like chlorpropamide (with a half-life of 36 hours and potential continuing activity up to 60 hours) and glyburide (with activity up to 24 hours) may require intravenous glucose when fasting before surgery and during the procedure.

The patient controlled with diet alone, shorter-acting oral hypoglycemic drugs, or both can usually be maintained without food or intravenous glucose before and during surgery with no ill effects. In these patients, the blood glucose level may rise somewhat during the procedure, but frequent monitoring will allow corrective administration of small quantities of regular insulin if needed.

Patients with NIDDM who are under reasonable control with insulin before surgery can be given insulin up to the morning of surgery. In those who take an evening dose of insulin, it is important to remember that the effect of intermediate-acting NPH or Lente insulin may persist past the usual morning meal. If food is withheld, this may lead to hypoglycemia by midmorning. Therefore, if the fasting glucose level is usually well controlled below 120 to 140 mg/dl, the evening dose of intermediate insulin can be reduced by 20% or an intravenous glucose infusion can be started in the morning. In such cases, careful glucose monitoring by finger-stick technique at 7 AM and every two to three hours while waiting for surgery is recommended. A progressive reduction in the serum glucose level indicates a need for glucose infusion.

If it can be determined with some confidence that a patient with NIDDM taking insulin is really not insulin-dependent and the serum glucose level on the morning of surgery is less than 180 mg/dl, insulin can be withheld if no glucose infusion is initiated. If it is unclear whether or not a patient is insulin-dependent, insulin and glucose should be administered before surgery. Although a variety of regimens are detailed in the literature,[42–46] one-half the usual total morning dose, given as NPH, is typically used when surgery is scheduled early in the morning. If the patient is to undergo surgery later in the day or as an outpatient, it is best to withhold insulin, monitor the serum glucose level, and administer small doses of regular insulin if the glucose concentrations rise while waiting for the procedure.

The preoperative management of patients with IDDM is often more complex. Although intraoperative stress stimulates counter-regulatory hormones like cortisol and epinephrine in all patients, those with IDDM are solely dependent on exogenous insulin to counteract their effects. Circulating insulin must be present in adequate amounts to prevent excessive gluconeogenesis, lipolysis, and consequent hyperglycemia and ketoacidosis. Many patients with IDDM are still treated with twice-daily injections of intermediate-acting insulin with or without supplementary shorter-acting insulin. These patients can be given one-half of their usual morning dose as intermediate-acting insulin and an infusion of 5% glucose at a rate of 80 to 100 ml/hour. The serum glucose level should be checked during the procedure, and more regular insulin can be administered if necessary. Patients taking regular insulin before meals and intermediate- or long-acting insulin at bedtime can receive a slightly smaller-than-usual dose of regular insulin every six hours with a glucose infusion beginning on the morning of surgery. It is important not to withhold a dose of insulin during surgery because, in the absence of intermediate-acting insulin, serum and tissue levels of insulin can fall and precipitate ketosis. During a long procedure, if serum glucose levels are low six hours after a dose, one can delay giving insulin and check the levels hourly. Insulin should then be administered as soon as the blood glucose concentration starts to rise without waiting until the beginning of the next six-hour interval.

In patients with subcutaneous insulin pumps, the device should be turned off and removed on the morning of surgery. Glucose control can be achieved with regular subcutaneous insulin as described above. However, insulin pumps can be continued if the patient is awake during surgery and can therefore participate in management.

Glucose control with continuous intravenous insulin has been well detailed in the literature and is especially popular in Great Britain for managing insulin-dependent diabetics before, during, and after major surgery.[47,48] The goal is to achieve as near-to-steady-state plasma glucose levels as possible. Alberti and Thomas developed a method using infusions containing fixed proportions of glucose, insulin, and potassium known as the GIK regimen.[47] In most cases, five units of regular insulin are added to 500 ml of 10% dextrose containing 7.4 meq of potassium chloride and infused at a rate of 100 ml/hr beginning one-half hour before the operation. Taitelman's modification of the method is more flexible because glucose and insulin can be infused separately and can be varied independently.[48] He initially recommends giving 500 ml of 5% dextrose over the first hour followed by 125 ml/hr of dextrose and two units per hour of regular insulin. The basal level of insulin in the infusion can be adjusted by using an algorithm that depends on the patient's maintenance dose of subcutaneous insulin and intraoperative measurements of serum glucose.[49] These regimens require frequent determinations of the serum glucose concentration during surgery and increase the risk of hypoglycemia. Although continuous intravenous insulin is less popular in the United States, it is often used in pregnant patients undergoing surgery in whom optimal glucose control is required to prevent fetal morbidity. Occasionally, some patients already receiving continuous intravenous insulin, such as those with diabetic ketoacidosis, require surgery. In such cases, the regimen can be continued during the procedure with careful monitoring.

In the past decade, the use of subcutaneous insulin has been compared to that of intravenous insulin in the perioperative period. Pezzarossa et al. found that intravenous insulin yielded better glucose control during the procedure but offered no advantage in glucose control in the pre- and postoperative periods.[49] Evaluating the two modalities in minor surgery, Christiansen et al. found that intravenous insulin resulted in lower intra- and postoperative serum glucose measurements but no difference in levels of lactate, 3-hydroxybutyrate, glycerol, alanine, glucagon, insulin, and growth hormone when compared to subcutaneous regimens.[50] Further studies comparing the effects of different regimens on patient outcome are clearly needed.

If a choice is available, local or regional anesthesia is favored over general in diabetics because the patients are more likely to be able to report symptoms of hypoglycemia during and immediately after surgery and to take food postoperatively.

POSTOPERATIVE MANAGEMENT

Upon arrival in the recovery room or intensive care unit, the patient's serum glucose level should be immediately determined. If the patient received no insulin or glucose preoperatively and the initial postoperative serum glucose concentration is under 200 mg/dl, the level can be monitored every four to six hours. A glucose infusion is usually started until it is clear if the patient will tolerate food, and in many cases the serum glucose will rise, especially in those with IDDM and those with NIDDM who were taking insulin before surgery. Insulin should be administered if the serum glucose level is persistently elevated above 220 mg/dl. Even patients who were controlled on diet or oral agents preoperatively may require insulin therapy in the postoperative period. They should be carefully monitored every six hours while not eating and then before meals and at bedtime. Regular insulin can then be administered subcutaneously at these latter times. Within the first 24 hours after surgery, it is often possible to predict if a patient will need insulin, and it is more desirable to anticipate the insulin requirements rather than to act after the fact with a predetermined "sliding scale." Patients with NIDDM treated with insulin before surgery generally require insulin postoperatively, especially if they are given a glucose infusion. Those with IDDM definitely require insulin. The major exception to this rule is the mother with IDDM in the immediate postpartum period when insulin may not be required for up to 24 or 36 hours.

The common sliding-scale method of insulin administration in which insulin requirements and dosage are determined by monitoring the finger-stick or serum glucose level every four to six hours is not physiological and often leaves the patient poorly controlled. Since orders are often written to give no insulin below a certain glucose level and the glucose is not checked again for four to six hours, insulin is frequently withheld just at the time it is needed as the effect of the previous dose of insulin is beginning to wane. This results in elevation of the serum glucose concentration over the ensuing four- to six-hour interval. Moreover, the next time the glucose level is checked, a large bolus of insulin is often required, increasing the risk of subsequent hypoglycemia. The patient's glucose level thus continues to rise and fall with poor overall control. In patients with IDDM, withholding insulin for six hours after surgery may lead to ketogenesis and in some cases to frank ketoacidosis. In patients with NIDDM, high serum glucose levels suppress endogenous insulin production by the pancreas and decrease tissue responsiveness to insulin, thereby increasing the requirement for exogenous insulin.[41]

Adequate control of the serum glucose level requires anticipation of the patient's needs. The goal is to maintain the serum glucose level between 150 and 200 mg/dl after surgery. Insulin requirements usually increase in the first 24 to 48 hours after surgery in both patients with IDDM and NIDDM previously treated with insulin. Patients require at least their usual total daily dose given in four divided doses of regular insulin. If the patient is eating, these doses can be given before meals and at midnight or simply every six hours if the patient is receiving intravenous glucose. Bedside capillary blood glucose monitoring is most often used to determine the effectiveness of a dose of subcutaneous insulin given six hours previously. If the level is too high or too low, the subsequent dose should be adjusted appropriately. In this way, a reasonable steady-state level can be achieved over a 24-hour period.

In the early postoperative period, many patients with NIDDM previously controlled by diet or medication require some regular insulin almost every six hours whether they are eating or not. If the blood glucose level is low-normal, it is appropriate to wait and retest at hourly intervals and administer insulin as soon as the glucose level begins to rise even if it is still within the desired range. If testing is delayed another full six hours, the glucose level will definitely be elevated. These management principles are also frequently applicable to patients with NIDDM previously treated with insulin. In all cases, stresses related to surgery and concomitant conditions may cause the serum glucose level to change rapidly in either direction and should be considered when planning insulin doses.

Patients with IDDM and those with NIDDM who are particularly stressed by infection, stroke, or myocardial infarction or who are receiving steroids, epinephrine, or total parenteral nutrition may require continuous intravenous insulin after surgery. Those with IDDM frequently require a baseline dose of only 0.7 to 1.2 units of insulin per hour to maintain glucose homeostasis but may need more when subjected to one or more of the above stresses. Those with NIDDM are often obese and resistant to insulin and may require four to 10 units per hour to maintain acceptable serum glucose levels. When continuous intravenous insulin is used, it is easier to bring high glucose levels into acceptable ranges with hourly bolus intravenous insulin in doses of five to ten units and to rely on the continuous insulin infusion for maintenance. Merely increasing the infusion rate to correct elevated glucose levels often acutely results in hypoglycemia or the same erratic pattern obtained when subcutaneous insulin is given based on a rigid sliding scale. When using intravenous insulin in bolus form, it is important to remember that peak activity lasts about one hour. Bolus intravenous insulin repeated every two to four hours without continuous infusion only leads to poor control.

Nutritional supplementation administered by intravenous hyperalimentation or enterostomy tube often greatly increases insulin requirements in patients with IDDM and those with NIDDM previously treated with insulin and even in previously diet-controlled patients with NIDDM. Insulin added to intravenous hyperalimentation fluid often produces good glucose control and may be supplemented with subcutaneous or intravenous bolus insulin until the optimal dose of intravenous insulin in the hyperalimentation fluid is determined. In patients receiving enterostomy feedings, regular insulin can be initially administered subcutaneously every six hours or given in a continuous intravenous infusion. As the feeding cycle is established and the patient becomes less stressed, combinations of NPH and regular insulin once or twice daily can often be used to achieve glucose control, depending on the length of the feeding cycle. In patients with NIDDM, no insulin may be necessary at the end of enterostomy feeding. In this case, insulin may be best administered only at the start and perhaps eight or ten hours into the tube feeding. Only short-acting regular insulin may be necessary for the second dose if the tube feeding is scheduled to end in another four or six hours. For longer feedings, combinations of NPH and regular insulin may be preferable for the second dose as well.

Once the patient is transferred to the surgical floor, all measures of optimal postoperative care, including prophylaxis against deep venous thrombosis, early ambulation, incentive spirometry, and prompt evaluation and treatment of postoperative fever should be initiated. Frequent glucose monitoring should continue until the patient is tolerating a full diet and a daily regimen of an oral agent or insulin is resumed. Postoperative insulin requirements should decrease toward preoperative levels over time. If they do not, reasons for insulin resistance like occult infection or interference by concomitant medications should be promptly elucidated. In view of the increased prevalence of coronary artery disease in patients with diabetes, current standard of practice calls for repeating an electrocardiogram postoperatively. Many clinicians do so just after surgery and 48 to 72 hours later when postoperative myocardial ischemia is statistically most likely to occur.

SPECIAL CONSIDERATIONS

Mention must be made of the difficult management problems encountered when a patient in diabetic ketoacidosis (DKA) requires surgical intervention. These problems are compounded by the fact that DKA alone may often cause abdominal pain mimicking an acute abdomen, nausea, vomiting, ileus, and even hyperamylasemia, all of which resolve with treatment of ketoacidosis. Moreover, surgical conditions requiring emergent intervention such as trauma or severe infection often trigger development of DKA in diabetic patients. Surgical mortality is dramatically increased in patients with DKA,[8] and surgery should be postponed as long as possible in an attempt to correct associated metabolic abnormalities. However, in some cases, the surgery itself may be essential for resolution of DKA, as in the case of a gangrenous extremity requiring amputation. Clearly, elective procedures must be postponed in a diabetic patient in DKA. An in-depth discussion of the diagnosis and management of DKA is beyond the scope of this chapter. However, intravenous hydration and insulin by continuous infusion should be instituted and guided by frequent monitoring of arterial pH, glucose concentration, and potassium levels. Bicarbonate therapy is controversial but may be beneficial in extreme cases when the arterial pH falls below 7.1. When infection is suspected, broad-spectrum antibiotics should be given after appropriate cultures are obtained. It must be remembered that DKA does occur in IDDM patients without excessive elevations in blood glucose. In one series, 17 percent of patients with DKA have plasma glucose levels less than 300 mg/dl, and DKA has been reported in patients with plasma glucose levels as low as 100 mg/dl.[51,52]

Hyperglycemic hyperosmolar nonketotic coma (HHNC) presents similar management problems in diabetic patients undergoing surgery. It is characterized by extreme hyperglycemia with glucose levels usually in the range of 700 to 2000 mg/dl without ketoacidosis. Fluid replacement therapy before surgery is essential because anesthesia in these usually elderly volume-depleted individuals may exacerbate hypotension and lead to decreased organ perfusion, myocardial ischemia, or renal failure. HHNC is often accompanied by lactic acidosis due to poor tissue perfusion. It can usually be corrected by adequate fluid repletion and small doses of insulin.

Diabetic patients undergoing open-heart surgery involving cardiopulmonary bypass have especially high insulin requirements. Unusually high serum glucose levels may be due to the large amounts of glucose infused,[53] insulin resistance associated with hypothermia,[54] and the hyperglycemic effects of commonly used adrenergic drugs.[55] Management includes limiting glucose infusions, increasing insulin doses, and monitoring serum glucose levels every 15 to 30 minutes. In other situations, surgery causes a rapid fall in insulin requirements. These include removal of an infected organ, drainage of an abscess, removal of a pheochromocytoma with rebound hyperinsulinism, and delivery of the placenta after pregnancy.[1]

Patients may develop acute or subacute unilateral pain syndromes due to truncal neuropathy, mimicking acute cholecystitis, appendicitis, myocardial infarction, and diverticulitis. A distinguishing feature of these pain syndromes is the usual presence of a zone of hypesthesia or anesthesia over the dermatome supplied by the involved nerve root. Pain usually subsides spontaneously in several weeks to months. The Charcot joint, also known as diabetic osteoarthropathy, can also pose diagnostic problems. Presenting with a warm erythematous and swollen foot, ankle, or lower leg with little or no pain, it is often confused with cellulitis, deep-venous thrombosis, or acute gout. If ulceration is present, osteomyelitis may be suspected. Radiographic changes may be absent initially, but subsequent bony changes caused by osteoarthropathy may mimic osteomyelitis and prompt unnecessary debridement and even amputation. Although the early phase of standard triple-phase scintigraphy may be positive, indium scans are negative in cases of diabetic osteoarthropathy if no ulcers are present. Magnetic resonance imaging cannot differentiate osteoarthropathy from osteomyelitis well enough to be useful.

COMPLICATIONS

Poor wound healing and a higher frequency of wound infections have been confirmed in many experimental studies.[20–24] The incidence of wound infections is 10.4 to 10.7 percent in diabetics compared with 4.8 to 7.4 percent in nondiabetics.[20] Age and obesity may be important cocontributing factors.

Simple epithelial repair is not influenced by hyperglycemia. However, repair of deeper wounds requiring collagen formation is adversely affected. The impaired wound healing and increased risk of infection in hyperglycemic diabetics is attributable to diminished phagocytic activity, chemotaxis and adherence of granulocytes, and impaired synthesis of protocollagen and collagen.

Some aspects of experimental wound healing improve with insulin administration alone while others require that enough insulin be administered to lower the serum glucose to levels below 250 mg/dl. For this reason, it is recommended that serum glucose levels in diabetics be maintained below 250 mg/dl after surgery to enhance wound healing and decrease the risk of infection.[20–22] Experimental studies suggest that defects in wound healing may also be partially corrected by the administration of zinc or large amounts of vitamin A, but clinical data on their efficacy in the surgical setting are lacking.[24]

Other postoperative complications in patients with diabetes have already been discussed in the first part of this chapter. Cardiovascular complications, most often associated with tissue ischemia and necrosis, frequently account for much of the observed morbidity and mortality in diabetics undergoing surgery. Myocardial infarction, cerebrovascular accidents, and systemic emboli are not infrequent. Other infectious complications follow in frequency and significance and require careful surveillance and prompt therapy.

Postoperative DKA and HHNC are uncommon if not present preoperatively. They usually reflect inadequate intraoperative glucose monitoring and control or a major intraoperative event such as myocardial infarction or stroke. Diabetic gastroparesis should always be considered in patients with protracted postoperative nausea and vomiting, and metaclopramide may be useful in such cases.

SUMMARY

1. Diabetes mellitus is common in the general population. Recent data suggest that perioperative mortality rates in diabetic patients are about 1.5 times those of nondiabetics. Postoperative morbidity and mortality are related to diabetic-related end-organ dysfunction. Myocardial ischemia and infection remain the two most significant complications.

2. Insulin-deficient patients suffer exaggerated metabolic responses to the stress of surgery and anesthesia. Significant hyperglycemia is the result of insulin lack or resistance and the release of anti-insulin hormones.

3. Preoperative evaluation of diabetic patients must include a thorough and accurate assessment of metabolic status, including glucose control, fluid status, and electrolyte balance as well as cardiovascular, renal, and neurological function. In addition to a thorough history and physical examination, all patients should undergo laboratory evaluation of electrolytes, BUN, creatinine and glucose levels, urinalysis, and ECG. Preoperative cardiac stress testing with thallium imaging should be considered in clinically selected high-risk patients. Diagnostic studies involving the use of contrast dye agents should be avoided.

4. Patients with NIDDM controlled by diet alone usually do not require insulin or glucose infusion before or during surgery but should be carefully monitored.

5. Patients with NIDDM taking oral hypoglycemic agents should discontinue them on the day before surgery. Long-acting agents should be discontinued two days prior to the procedure. These patients can usually be managed like those controlled with diet alone. Postoperative hyperglycemia can be controlled with supplemental regular insulin guided by finger-stick blood glucose measurements.

6. Preoperative management of patients with NIDDM taking insulin preoperatively and those with IDDM is dictated by the specifics of their insulin regimens. In general, they should receive half of their usual morning dose of intermediate-acting insulin with a glucose infusion on the morning of surgery and then monitored carefully. Continuous intraoperative intravenous insulin and glucose infusion is most often used in pregnant women undergoing surgery, patients undergoing cardiopulmonary bypass, and those already on continuous infusions for the treatment of DKA. In most other cases, continuous insulin infusion offers no advantage and may cause hypoglycemia.

7. Postoperative management should be guided by the individual patient's anticipated needs and not by rigid adherence to a fixed sliding-scale regimen of insulin. In general, most diabetics require regular insulin in the first 24 to 48 hours after surgery. Appropriate monitoring will allow optimal timing of insulin therapy to achieve smooth glucose control. The goal of therapy is maintenance of a serum glucose level of 150 to 200 mg/dl in the first few days after surgery.

8. Elective surgery should be postponed in diabetic patients with DKA or HHNC. In emergency situations, a delay of one or two hours to correct metabolic abnormalities can decrease surgical mortality.

9. Postoperative stresses including infection, stroke, and myocardial infarction and the administration of steroids, adrenergic agents, and total parenteral nutrition can worsen hyperglycemia and in some cases may require continuous intravenous insulin therapy.

10. Because diabetics often have cardiovascular, renal, and neurologic dysfunction and increased susceptibility to infection, they require scrupulous and expectant postoperative care in addition to management of their diabetes. This should include repeating the ECG following the procedure and again 48 to 72 hours later to exclude silent myocardial ischemia. Patients with known significant coronary artery disease may benefit from postoperative continuous electrocardiographic monitoring.

11. Administration of insulin and correction of hyperglycemia decreases the incidence of defective wound healing and susceptibility to infection in patients with diabetes mellitus.

REFERENCES

1. Reynolds C: Management of the diabetic surgical patient. *Postgrad Med* 77:265–279, 1985.
2. Dunnet JN, Holman RR, Turner RC et al: Diabetes mellitus and anesthesia. *Anesthesia* 43:538–542, 1988.
3. Wetterhall SF, Olson DR, DeStefano F et al: Trends in diabetes and diabetic complications, 1980–1987. *Diab Care* 15(8):960–967, 1992.
4. Harris MI, Hadden WC, Knowler WC et al: Prevalence of diabetes and impaired glucose tolerance and plasma glucose levels in U.S. population aged 20–74 years. *Diabetes* 36:523–524, 1987.
5. Harris MI: Epidemiological correlates of NIDDM in Hispanics, whites and blacks in the U.S. population. *Diab Care* 14(Suppl 3):639, 1991.
6. Macleod CA, Murchison LE, Russel EM et al: Measuring outcome of diabetes: A retrospective survey. *Diab Med* 6(1):59–63, 1989.
7. Hirsch IB, McGill JB, Cryer PE et al: Perioperative management of surgical patients with diabetes mellitus. *Anesthesiology* 74(2):346–359, 1991.
8. Galloway JA, Shuman CR: Diabetes and surgery: A study of 667 cases. *Am J Med* 34:177–191, 1963.
9. Byyny R: Management of diabetics during surgery. *Postgrad Med* 68:191–202, 1980.
10. Molitch M, Reichlin S: The care of the diabetic patient during emergency surgery and postoperatively. *Ortho Clin N Am* 9:811–824, 1978.
11. Milaskiewicz RM, Hall GM: Diabetes and anesthesia: The past decade. *Brit J Anesth* 68(2):198–206, 1992.
12. Reiss R, Deutsch AA, Nudelmann J: Biliary surgery in diabetic patients; statistical analyses of 189 patients. *Dig Surg* 4:37, 1987.
13. Larsen SF, Olesen KH, Jacobsen E et al: Prediction of cardiac risk in noncardiac surgery. *Eur Heart J* 8:179, 1987.
14. Hollenberg M, Mangano DT, Browner WS et al: Predictors of postoperative myocardial ischemia in patients undergoing noncardiac surgery. The Study of Perioperative Ischemia Research Group. *JAMA* 268(2):205–209, 1992.
15. Hjortrup A, Sorensen C, Dyremose E et al: Influence of diabetes mellitus on operative risk. *Br J Surg* 72:783–785, 1985.
16. MacKenzie R, Charlson M: Assessment of perioperative risk in the patient with diabetes mellitus. *Surg Gyn Obstet* 167:293–299, 1988.
17. Charlson, ME, MacKenzie CR, Gold JP et al: Preoperative characteristics predicting intraoperative hypotension and hypertension among hypertensives and diabetics undergoing noncardiac surgery. *Ann Surg* 212(1):66–81, 1990.
18. Burgos LG, Ebert TJ, Asiddao C et al: Increased intraoperative cardiovascular morbidity in diabetics with autonomic neuropathy. *Anesthesiology* 70(4):591–597, 1989.
19. Charlson, ME, MacKenzie CR, Gold JP et al: Postoperative renal dysfunction can be predicted. *Surg Gyn Obstet* 169(4):303–309, 1989.
20. McMurry J: Wound healing with diabetes mellitus. *Surg Clin N Am* 64:769–778, 1984.
21. Terranova A: The effects of diabetes mellitus on wound healing. *Plast Surg Nurs* 11(1):20–25, 1991.
22. Rosenberg CS: Wound healing in the patient with diabetes mellitus. *Nurs Clin N Am* 25(1):247–261, 1990.
23. Nolan CM, Beaty HN, Bagdade JD et al: Further characterization of the impaired bactericidal function of granulocytes in patients with poorly controlled diabetes. *Diabetes* 27:889–894, 1978.
24. Mowat AG, Baum J: Chemotaxis of polymorphonuclear leukocytes from patients with diabetes mellitus. *N Eng J Med* 284:621–627, 1971.
25. Daykin AP: Anesthetic and surgical stress in the diabetic patient: Carbohydrate homeostasis. *Int Anesth Clin* 26(3):206–212, 1988.
26. Gavin LA: Perioperative management of the diabetic patient. *Endocrin Metab Clin N Am* 21(2):457–475, 1992.
27. Trevisan R, Marassotti C, Avogero A et al: Effects of different insulin administrations on plasma amino acid profile of insulin-dependent diabetic patients. *Diab Res* 12(2):57–62, 1989.
28. Bak JF, Jacobsen VK, Jorgneson FS et al: Insulin receptor function and glycogen synthetase activity in skeletal muscle biopsies from patients with insulin-dependent diabetes mellitus: Effects of physical training. *J Clin Endocrin Metab* 69(1):158–164, 1989.
29. Hirsch IB, Herter CD: Intensive insulin therapy. Part I: Basic principles. *Am Fam Phys* 45(5):2141–2147, 1992.
30. Hirsch IB, McGill JB: Role of insulin in the management of surgical patients with diabetes mellitus. *Diab Care* 13(9):980–991, 1990.
31. Caruso M, Orszulak TA, Miles JM et al: Lactic acidosis and insulin resistance associated with epinephrine administration in a patient with non-insulin-dependent diabetes mellitus. *Arch Intern Med* 147(8):1422–1424, 1987.
32. Kotler TS, Diamond GA: Exercise thallium-201 scintigraphy in the diagnosis and prognosis of coronary artery disease. *Ann Intern Med* 113(9):684–702, 1990.
33. Camp AD, Garvin PJ, Hoff J et al: Prognostic value of intravenous dipyridamole thallium imaging in patients with diabetes mellitus considered for renal transplantation. *Am J Cardiol* 65(22):1459–1463, 1990.
34. Holley JL, Fenton RA, Arthur RS et al: Thallium stress testing does not predict cardiovascular risk in diabetic patients with end-stage renal disease undergoing cadaveric renal transplantation. *Am J Med* 90(5):563–570, 1991.
35. Clement R, Rovsov JA, Engleman RM et al: Perioperative morbidity in diabetics requiring coronary artery bypass surgery. *Ann Thorac Surg* 46(3):321–323, 1988.
36. Bhan A, Das B, Wasir HS et al: Profile of coronary artery disease in diabetic patients undergoing coronary arterial bypass grafting. *Int J Cardiol* 31(2):155–159, 1991.
37. Mattock MB, Morrish NJ, Viberti G et al: Prospective study of microalbuminuria as predictor of mortality in NIDDM. *Diabetes* 41:736, 1992.
38. Dumsgaard EM, Froland A, Jorgensen OD: Eight to nine year mortality in known non-insulin dependent diabetics and controls. *Kidney Int* 41:731–735, 1992.
39. Hamburger S: Medical management of the surgical patient with diabetes mellitus. *JAMA* 34:155–167, 1979.

40. Walts L, Miller J, Davidson MB et al: Perioperative management of diabetes mellitus. *Anesthesiology* 55:104–109, 1981.

41. Rossetti L, Giaccari A, DeFronzo RA: Glucose toxicity. *Diab Care* 13(6):610–630, 1990.

42. Steinke J: Management of diabetes mellitus and surgery. *New Eng J Med* 282:1472, 1970.

43. Marble A, Steinke J: Physiology and pharmacology in diabetes mellitus; guiding the diabetic patients through the surgical patient. *Anesthesiology* 24:442–447, 1963.

44. Forsham PH: Management of diabetes during stress and surgery, in Williams RH (ed): *Diabetes*. New York, Harper & Row, 1965, pp 511–515.

45. Shipp, JC: Diabetes mellitus, anesthesia, and surgery. *Int Anesth Clin* 6:189–209, 1968.

46. Stanley VF, Giesecke AM, Selzer HS: Anesthesia for the diabetic patient. *Clin Anesth* 3:263–274, 1968.

47. Alberti KG, Thomas DJB: The management of diabetes during surgery. *Br J Anaesth* 51:693–708, 1979.

48. Taitelman U, Reece EA, Bessman AN: Insulin and the management of the diabetic surgical patient. Continuous intravenous infusion versus subcutaneous administration. *JAMA* 237:658–660, 1977.

49. Pezzarossa A, Taddei F, Cimicchi MG et al: Perioperative management of diabetic subjects. *Diab Care* 11:52–57, 1988.

50. Christiansen CL, Schurizek BA, Malling B et al: Insulin treatment of the insulin-dependent diabetic patient undergoing minor surgery. Continuous intravenous infusion compared with subcutaneous administration. *Anesthesia* 43(7):533–537, 1988.

51. Monro JF, Campbell IW, McCuish AG et al: Euglycemic diabetic ketoacidosis. *Br Med J* 2:578, 1973.

52. Bradley RF: Diabetic ketoacidosis and coma, in Marble A, White P, Krall L, et al (eds): *Joslin's Diabetes Mellitus*, 2d ed. Philadelphia, Lea & Febiger, 1971, pp 361–416.

53. Crock PA, Ley CJ, Martin IK et al: Hormonal changes during hypothermic coronary artery bypass surgery in diabetic and nondiabetic subjects. *Diab Med* 5(1):47–52, 1988.

54. Gill GV, Sherif IH, Alberti KG: Management of diabetes during open heart surgery. *Br J Surg* 68:171–172, 1982.

55. Clutter WE, Rizza RA, Gerich JA et al: Regulation of glucose metabolism by sympathochromaffin catecholamines. *Diab Metab Rev* 4:1–15, 1988.

25 THE SURGICAL PATIENT WITH THYROID DISEASE

Margaret L. Lancefield

Anatomic and functional abnormalities of the thyroid gland are common in surgical patients. The prevalence of goiter on physical examination is reported to be as high as four to nine percent in the general population, and autopsy surveys report an even higher incidence of nodular thyroid disease. The annual incidence of Graves' disease and thyroiditis is estimated to be 0.2 to 0.8 per 1000. Although spontaneous myxedema is uncommon, occurring in only 0.01 to 0.08 percent of all persons admitted to the hospital, the incidence of ^{131}I and drug-induced hypothyroidism is rising. A variety of illnesses affect the interpretation of thyroid function tests and can disguise the signs and symptoms of thyroid dysfunction. In one study of seriously ill hospitalized patients, more than 17 percent had some abnormality in their thyroid function tests. Fewer than half were ultimately found to have significant thyroid disease.[1]

Thyroid physiology in euthyroid surgical patients is discussed in the first section of this chapter. Particular attention is given to assessment of thyroid function and the effects of anesthesia, surgery, and both acute and chronic illness on thyroid hormone metabolism and commonly used thyroid function studies. The following section covers estimation of surgical risk in patients with hyperthyroidism and overall assessment and management in both elective and emergency procedures. Emphasis is placed on prevention and treatment of thyroid storm. The final section deals with the same issues in patients with hypothyroidism and myxedema coma.

THYROID PHYSIOLOGY IN THE SURGICAL PATIENT

The anterior pituitary hormone thyrotropin or thyroid-stimulating hormone (TSH) is the primary stimulus of synthesis and secretion of thyroid hormone. TSH release is in turn initiated by thyrotropin-releasing hormone (TRH) from the ventro-median hypothalamus. Thyroxine (T_4) and 3,5,3'-triiodothyronine (T_3) are the principal biologically active hormones. The thyroid gland is the sole source of T_4, but up to 90 percent of circulating T_3 is derived from peripheral conversion of T_4 to T_3 mediated by the enzyme 5'-deiodinase present in muscle, liver, heart, and kidney. Another enzyme converts T_4 to 3,3',5'-T_3 or reverse T_3 (rT_3), which is biologically inactive.

About 70 percent of circulating T_4 is bound to thyroxine-binding globulin (TBG), and most of the remainder is bound to thyroxine-binding prealbumin (TBPA) and albumin. Only about 40 percent of T_3 is bound to TBG and most of the rest to albumin. Only free unbound T_4 and T_3 are biologically active. T_3 is three to four times more potent than T_4. Binding of thyroid hormones by plasma proteins can be affected by surgery, medications, and acute and chronic illness.

Normal thyroid function requires an average daily intake of 100 μg of iodine. Dietary iodine is concentrated in thyroid follicular cells and combines with tyrosine residues on thyroglobulin to produce monoiodotyrosine and diiodotyrosine. Oxidative coupling of monoiodotyrosine and diiodotyrosine produce T_3 and T_4 that are bound to thyroglobulin and stored extracellularly in the lumen of the thyroid follicle. T_4 and T_3 are secreted as free hormones after hydrolysis from thyroglobulin in follicular cell lysosomes. The thyroid gland normally contains 5000 to 7000 μg of organic iodine mostly bound to thyroglobulin. This pool serves as a buffer to counter fluctuations in thyroid hormone synthesis. Even after complete suppression of thyroid hormone synthesis for one or two weeks, there is no change in plasma TSH level or the normal secretion of T_4 and T_3.

Biochemical estimates of thyroid status are usually based on measured levels of total T_4 and TSH and calculated levels of free T_4 (the free thyroxine index or FTI) based on measurements of T_3-resin uptake (T_3RU). T_3RU varies inversely with total TBG concentration and with the number of unoccupied hormone binding sites on the TBG molecule. If the concentration of TBG is constant, a low T_3RU implies more free sites available on the TBG molecules, as seen in hypothyroidism. Likewise, if the concentration of TBG increases with no change in overall thyroid status, T_3RU will fall. FTI is the calculated product of total T_4 and T_3RU.

Serum total T_3 levels can also be measured but are rarely useful in routine evaluation. Serum T_3 concentration is affected by nonthyroidal illness such as malnutrition, cirrhosis, neoplasm, chronic renal failure, and toxemia of pregnancy, and reduced levels are due to a decreased peripheral conversion of T_4 to T_3. Reduced T_3 levels have been noted in as many as 70 percent of hospitalized patients. It has been suggested this reduction of T_3 levels serves to conserve energy and maintain metabolic homeostasis during periods of illness.[2-4]

A new test for TSH that is about ten times more sensitive than previous assays is now widely available. With rare exceptions, high serum T_4 concentrations suppress TSH secretion by the pituitary. In otherwise healthy patients, TSH determination can usually distinguish between the euthyroid state and thyrotoxicosis, in which TSH levels fall below 0.1 μIU/nl. This information may obviate the need for a TRH stimulation test in cases of questionable thyrotoxicosis.[5-7] This test requires the intravenous injection of 400 μg of TRH and defines hyperthyroidism if there is a minimal or no rise in serum TSH levels over 30 to 60 minutes. In those rare situations in which hypothyroidism is caused by pituitary or hypothalamic failure, TSH will be low and will not be stimulated by TRH. In the majority of ambulatory patients, a careful history, physical examination, and measurement of T_4, T_3RU, FTI, and TSH levels are sufficient to assess thyroid status.

Thyroid physiology is altered by anesthesia, surgery, chronic illness, medications, fasting, and infection. T_4 and free T_4 concentrations are not significantly altered by general anesthesia or epidural block. However, many studies document an immediate and prolonged fall in T_3 levels with elective and emergency nonthyroid surgery independent of the type of anesthesia.[8,9]

Acute illness may be associated with a slight increase in serum T_4 and T_3RU levels and a decrease in serum T_3 concentrations because of decreased peripheral conversion. Reverse T_3 (rT_3) levels rise. TSH levels remain normal and rise appropriately after TRH stimulation. As the illness continues, T_4 and T_3RU levels fall to normal, and T_3 concentration may decrease further to as low as 25% of normal. Absolute free T_4 levels rise commonly as a result of interaction of TBG with plasma proteins and subsequent decrease in binding of T_4 to TBG. In severe chronic illness, serum T_4, T_3RU and T_3 levels may all be low. Lack of response to TRH is common in severe chronic illness and suggests depressed pituitary function. The effects of chronic starvation or malnutrition are similar to those of chronic illness.[10-12]

Chronic liver disease may cause confusing changes in thyroid function tests in clinically euthyroid patients. In cirrhosis, TBG and TBPA levels are usually decreased with the expected elevation in T_3RU. Total T_4 concentration is also decreased resulting in a normal or slightly decreased FTI. Because much of the peripheral conversion of T_4 to T_3 occurs in the liver, T_3 levels are reduced in proportion to the severity of liver damage. Patients with chronic liver disease may have mildly increased TSH levels which may rise in response to TRH stimulation, suggesting true hypothyroidism. In contrast, TBG levels are markedly elevated in acute hepatitis. T_4 concentration is increased, and T_3 production is normal. T_3RU is low because of the elevation in TBG levels, and the calculated FTI is therefore near normal.

Total T_4, FTI, and T_3 levels may all be decreased in severe chronic renal failure. These patients are clinically euthyroid and do not require exogenous thyroid hormone. Infection or fever may increase T_4 and T_3 turnover as much as fourfold by activating hepatic enzymes. This increase in T_4 turnover may explain precipitation of myxedema coma by infection that can occur in hypothyroid patients.

THYROTOXICOSIS

Clinical Manifestations

Separation of the signs and symptoms of hyperthyroidism into adrenergic and metabolic categories is clinically useful. Metabolic effects due to excess thyroid hormone develop over weeks and months and take longer to reverse than adrenergic effects.

Adrenergic Effects

Adrenergic effects place hyperthyroid patients at greatest risk during surgery. The striking similarities between the effects of excessive thyroid hormone and enhanced sympathetic activity have long been recognized. Palpitations, tremors, increased sweating, heat intolerance, and anxiety are common in both states. Nevertheless, recent investigations have failed to demonstrate adrenergic hypersensitivity or excess circulating catecholamines in hyperthyroid states.[13] There have been reports of increased beta-adrenergic receptors in the hearts of hyperthyroid animals, and T_3 and T_4 exert direct inotropic and chronotropic effects on cardiac muscle. Cardiac hypertrophy is common in hyperthyroidism, and there is reversible cardiomyopathy in which left ventricular ejection falls with exercise. Atrial fibrillation occurs in 10 to 15 percent of thyrotoxic patients. Arrhythmias are difficult to control until hyperthyroidism is treated. Basal increase in output in hyperthyroidism significantly limits cardiac reserve during surgery.[13]

Metabolic Effects

Although both synthesis and breakdown of protein increase in thyrotoxicosis, catabolism predominates and results in negative nitrogen balance. Increased basal oxygen consumption, atrial fibrillation, underlying heart disease, mild anemia, or vitamin B_6 deficiency due to increased coenzyme requirements may contribute to cardiac decompensation. Response to digoxin is often inadequate and may reflect increased drug metabolism.

Dyspnea without congestive heart failure is common in hyperthyroidism and is probably due to weakened respiratory muscles. Pulmonary function tests show decreased vital capacity and pulmonary compliance and increased basal minute ventilation. Bulbar muscle dysfunction, present in a small percentage of patients, may complicate postoperative respiratory management in the untreated thyrotoxic patient.

Most thyrotoxic patients are malnourished despite increased food intake. Preparation for surgery may therefore require sufficient time for nutritional supplementation. Hypoalbuminemia reflects generalized protein wasting. Insulin metabolism is increased, glucose tolerance may be abnormal, and net lipid degradation may produce ketosis, especially when the patient is fasting.

Gastrointestinal signs and symptoms may be atypical and confusing. Intestinal hypermotility and mucosal edema may complicate the evaluation of patients with abdominal pain. Hepatomegaly and splenomegaly accompanied by lymphadenopathy may be present. Paradoxically, anorexia occurs in as many as 30 percent, and constipation is seen in 25 percent, of elderly hyperthyroid patients. The insidious onset of hyperthyroidism in patients over 60 and its often nonspecific presentation place elderly patients at greatest risk for misdiagnosis.

A variety of other laboratory abnormalities may be found in

hyperthyroid patients. The serum alkaline phosphatase level may be elevated and the prothrombin time prolonged. Anemia and neutropenia with relative lymphocytosis in not unusual. Thrombocytopenia may be critical. Several patients with presumed idiopathic thrombocytopenic purpura (ITP) have been found to be thyrotoxic.[14] Serum T_4 and T_3RU levels should be checked in all patients with ITP before splenectomy to exclude occult hyperthyroidism.

Aspects Unique to Graves' Disease

Certain signs and symptoms of hyperthyroidism are unique to Graves' disease and appear unrelated to elevations in thyroid hormone. Thyroid-stimulating immunoglobulins (TSIG) are a group of antibodies found in the serum of such patients, and those with infiltrative ophthalmopathy and pretibial myxedema usually have detectable levels. Autoimmune diseases such as myasthenia gravis and pernicious anemia are associated with both Graves' disease and Hashimoto's thyroiditis and may complicate perioperative management.

Diagnosis

When hyperthyroidism is suspected by history and physical examination, measurements of T_4, T_3RU and FTI levels are usually sufficient for confirmation. Measuring serum T_4 concentration alone may be misleading, because increased TBG levels often cause elevation in the T_4 level in euthyroid patients. If this is so, T_3RU is decreased, and the calculated FTI is normal. Elevation of TBG can occur in pregnancy and as a result of increased estrogen levels from exogenous hormone or from estrogen-producing tumors. It can also be seen in familial disorders of protein binding, some liver diseases, and as a result of drugs like fluorouracil, heroin, and methadone. TBG is decreased in cirrhosis, nephrotic syndrome, acromegaly, and Cushing's syndrome or with use of androgens, anabolic steroids, or glucocorticoids.[15] In these situations, thyroid status can be clarified by measurement of T_3RU and calculation of FTI from the product of total T_4 and T_3RU.

Occasionally a normal FTI can be seen in early hyperthyroidism. In such cases, an elevated serum T_3 concentration or very low TSH level renders the diagnosis evident. A TRH stimulation test is rarely necessary. In hyperthyroidism, there is virtually no rise in TSH after administration of TRH.

The radioactive iodine uptake may be misleading in diagnosing hyperthyroidism. Hyperthyroid patients exposed to iodine in food, topical iodine agents, or contrast dye may have a normal or low uptake. In contrast, euthyroid patients from iodine-deficient environments may have a high uptake.

Measurement of T_4, T_3RU, and FTI may falsely lead to a diagnosis of hyperthyroidism. Drugs such as propranolol and amiodarone, certain radiopaque dyes (e.g., Oragrafin or Telopaque), and amphetamines promote hyperthyroxinemia by blocking peripheral conversion of T_4 to T_3. However, TSH secretion is not decreased in these situations and therefore clarifies the situation. Marked transient hyperthyroxinemia may also occur in acute or chronic psychiatric illness, hyperemesis gravidarum, and symptomatic hyponatremia. In these situations, TSH secretion may actually be suppressed and raise the question of thyrotoxicosis. A serum T_3 level and TRH stimulation may be warranted.[3,15]

Risk of Surgery

The greatest risk confronting surgical patients with untreated thyrotoxicosis is thyroid storm. An early study of more than 2000 patients collected over a 25-year period prior to 1950 documented 36 cases of thyroid storm. Twenty-five developed after surgery, and 16 patients died.[16] The use of antithyroid agents and adrenergic antagonists over the last 40 years has decreased the risk of thyroid storm. However, in those who develop storm, the mortality rate can still be as high as 40 percent.

Any thyrotoxic patient undergoing surgery has a higher-than-normal risk of developing thyroid storm. Case reports of cardiac arrest or storm after minor procedures in patients with unrecognized thyrotoxicosis illustrate the importance of preoperative recognition and prompt treatment. Reports of storm in surgical patients on seemingly adequate medical regimens for hyperthyroidism emphasize the need for close perioperative monitoring.[17]

There are no published studies on the risks of surgery in patients with mild hyperthyroidism due to causes other than Graves' disease, including multinodular goiter, thyroiditis, or excess doses of thyroid hormone. The lack of such data suggests that the risk of serious complications or death during surgery in these patients is probably low and that elective surgery can safely proceed with perioperative use of beta-blockers, as discussed below.[18] If beta-blockers are contraindicated because of asthma or significant congestive heart failure, elective surgery should be delayed even in mildly hyperthyroid patients until they are rendered euthyroid.

The morbidity of surgery in hyperthyroid patients other than that due to thyroid storm is related to the adrenergic and metabolic effects of excess thyroid hormone and includes arrhythmias like atrial fibrillation and cardiac ischemia and decompensation.[13] Increased basal oxygen consumption, relative malnutrition, and respiratory muscle weakness may all contribute to prolonged intubation. Glucose regulation may be difficult, and patients with Type I diabetes mellitus more often develop ketoacidosis. Neutropenia, anemia, and thrombocytopenia may increase the risk of infection and bleeding.

Perioperative Management

Once the diagnosis of hyperthyroidism has been made, definitive treatment may vary depending on the etiology of the disease. If clinical findings clearly suggest thyrotoxicosis, treatment may need to be started even before laboratory results are available. Elective surgery should be postponed and treatment started immediately. In emergency situations, the goal in all thyrotoxic patients, regardless of etiology, is prevention of thyroid storm.

Perioperative screening for cardiopulmonary disease is essential in all hyperthyroid patients. Measurement of arterial blood gases, forced expiratory volume, minute ventilation, and maximum breathing capacity are recommended. Congestive heart failure should be treated before surgery and all patients should be monitored continuously for arrhythmias. If significant cardiopulmonary disease is present, an arterial line and Swan-Ganz catheter should be inserted preoperatively. Cooling blankets should be used during surgery if hyperthermia develops.[19]

Antithyroid Agents

If surgery can be delayed for several months, hyperthyroid patients should be treated with an antithyroid agent of the thionamide class. Propylthiouracil (PTU) and methimazole (MMI) are those most commonly used, and they act by inhibiting the oxidation and organification of iodide and the coupling of iodotyrosines. In high doses, PTU also inhibits the peripheral conversion of T_4 to T_3. Because these drugs decrease synthesis but not release of thyroid hormone, hyperthyroidism persists until hormone stores are depleted. Clinical improvement can be seen within two weeks, and normal serum hormone levels may return to normal within six weeks. However, if the patient has received large quantities of iodine before treatment, it may take months for stores of hormone in the thyroid to be depleted. Larger doses of antithyroid agent may help shorten this latency period.[20]

Dosage depends on the patient's clinical status. The usual initial dose of PTU is 100 mg orally every six to eight hours. Those with severe thyrotoxicosis or large goiters may require much higher doses. It is often helpful to increase the daily dosage and shorten the dosing interval to every four hours. Once the patient is euthyroid, the dose can usually be decreased by as much as one-third. Although PTU is often recommended over methimazole because of its ability to block peripheral conversion of T_4 to T_3, it has a shorter serum half-life than methimazole. Using a single daily dose of the latter may significantly increase patient compliance.

Patients undergoing emergency surgery should be given a loading dose of 1000 mg of PTU orally to block organification of iodide and peripheral conversion of T_4 to T_3. Propranolol should be started immediately to block catecholamine effects if there are no contraindications to its use. Sodium iodide should follow one hour after the PTU for reasons discussed below. There are no parenteral preparations of PTU or MMI.

Adverse reactions to thionamides are reported in 3 to 12 percent of patients. Most are mild hypersensitivity reactions like skin rash or fever that usually occur early in treatment with high doses and resolve when the drug is discontinued. If one thionamide causes such a reaction, the other may be tried. More serious reactions including agranulocytosis or serum sickness reactions are reported in less than 0.5 percent of patients. These may occur at any time but are more common early in treatment. A case of severe perioperative bleeding has been reported in a patient on PTU and may have been related to thrombocytopenia. Patients should discontinue the drug immediately if fever, pharyngitis, stomatitis, proctitis, or bleeding develops. As many as 10 percent of hyperthyroid patients have baseline white blood cell counts below 4000, and thionamide-induced neutropenia may be mistakenly attributed to underlying thyroid disease. Marrow recovery occurs in virtually all patients after discontinuation of the drug.

Thyrotoxic patients with known intolerance or prior adverse reactions to PTU or methimazole can be prepared for urgent or emergent surgery with sodium ipodate. This oral cholecystographic agent blocks conversion of T_4 to T_3, inhibits hormone secretion from the thyroid, and may reduce hormone uptake in tissues. Sodium ipodate contains large amounts of iodine that are released during its metabolism. Excess iodine transiently inhibits the organification and release of hormone from the thyroid. The optimal dose of sodium ipodate is 500 mg daily for five days orally if surgery can be safely postponed. Even one dose can be of some benefit in emergency situations.[21,22] There are reports of recurrence of hyperthyroidism in some patients treated for more than two weeks with sodium ipodate, and it is not recommended for long-term suppression of Graves' disease.[23]

Iodine

Iodine is rarely used alone in the treatment of hyperthyroidism. More often a thionamide is administered for several weeks, and iodine is added seven to 10 days before surgery. Iodine is especially important in managing hyperthyroid patients facing emergency surgery and those with thyroid storm. Iodine acutely inhibits the release of T_4 and transiently inhibits organification (Wolff-Chaikoff effect). Some patients escape from the initial effectiveness of iodine, and exacerbation of thyrotoxicosis may occur when iodine is withdrawn. If iodine is used and fails, radioiodine ablation and antithyroid agents are ineffective for several weeks or months because they cannot be taken up by an iodine-replenished gland.

When emergency surgery is necessary, the recommended dose of iodine is five drops of saturated solution of potassium iodide (SSKI) orally three times daily used in conjunction with PTU, propranolol, and corticosteroids. The first dose of iodine should be given one hour after the loading dose of PTU to allow time for the PTU to block organification. Iodine should be discontinued after seven to 14 days. Adverse reactions are uncommon when recommended doses are used. However, in larger doses, symptoms of iodism may occur, including headache, mucosal edema, skin rash, fever, and sialadenitis. These resolve with discontinuation of iodine. Sodium iodide is available in intravenous form and can be given in doses of one gram every eight to 12 hours.

Adrenergic Antagonists

In recent years propranolol has become the drug of choice for patients with symptomatic thyrotoxicosis and impending or actual thyroid storm. Doses of 10 to 40 mg orally every six hours usually control the symptoms of catecholamine excess, although occasionally larger doses are required. Other longer-acting nonselective or $beta_1$ selective beta-blockers have been used successfully and avoid breakthrough of adrenergic symptoms.[24] During surgery, intravenous propranolol in small doses of one mg/min is used to control tachycardia, hypertension, fever, and arrhythmias.

The very short-acting cardioselective intravenous beta-blocker esmolol has recently been used successfully in a hyperthyroid patient undergoing emergency appendectomy after conventional therapy with rectal PTU, intravenous propranolol, and corticosteroids had failed.[25] Esmolol is usually given in a loading dose of 500 μg/kg over one minute and gradually titrated from 25 μg/kg/min to as high as 300 μg/kg/min until tachycardia and hypertension are controlled.

Beta-blockers are contraindicated in patients with asthma and should be avoided in patients with significant congestive heart failure or brittle insulin-dependent diabetes. In those with cardiac dysfunction due to hyperthyroidism, beta-blockers may be cautiously administered, but thionamides and iodine remain the drugs of choice.

Corticosteroids

If time or patient tolerance does not allow adequate preoperative treatment with antithyroid agents, corticosteroids are often added to propranolol and iodine. They protect against adrenal insufficiency and decrease serum levels of T_4 and TSH. Thyrotoxicosis may be associated with increased degradation of corticosteroids and compensatory hyperplasia of the adrenal cortex. Although the adrenal response to acute stress is usually normal in thyrotoxicosis, adrenal reserve as measured after two days of stimulation with ACTH is often subnormal.

Anesthesia

Heavy preoperative sedation is not adequate prophylaxis against thyroid storm. The anesthesiologist often avoids the use of atropine that may stimulate adrenergic activity. Short-acting barbiturates or diazepam may be used as premedications. The anesthetic of choice is often a balanced technique of intravenous narcotics or barbiturates and inhalational agents that blunt the sympathetic response to surgical stimulation. Epidural blockade may be used when applicable.[26]

Thyroid Storm

The risk of thyrotoxic crisis is greatest during surgery and in the first 18 hours after the procedure. Thyroid storm usually occurs in patients undergoing emergency surgery or in those undergoing even minor elective surgery in whom hyperthyroidism was not recognized beforehand. Thyroid storm is nearly always abrupt in onset. In one series, all 22 patients studied had fever, diaphoresis, and tachycardia. Most had sinus tachycardia, but a significant proportion had other arrhythmias. Eleven developed congestive heart failure, and two became hypotensive. Patients exhibited a variety of changes in mental status, including agitation, somnolence, psychosis, and coma. Half experienced diarrhea or hyperdefection, but jaundice, tender hepatomegaly, and abdominal pain were less frequent.[27] The differential diagnosis of thyroid storm includes malignant hyperthermia, neuroleptic malignant syndrome, sepsis, delirium tremens, pheochromocytoma, acute drug intoxication with agents like amphetamines and cocaine, and even acute psychiatric illness.[28,29] A case of thyroid storm has been misdiagnosed as hyperemesis gravidarum.[30] Thyroid storm is fatal if untreated. Stupor or coma develop within 24 hours, rapidly followed by pulmonary edema, circulatory collapse, and death. With treatment, improvement can be seen within 12 hours, and the crisis may resolve in an average of three days.

There are no laboratory markers for thyroid storm. Thyroid function studies do not differ from those seen in stable thyrotoxicosis. Hyperglycemia occurs in 50 percent of patients because thyroid hormone causes impaired insulin secretion, insulin resistance, and increased glycogenolysis. Plasma cortisol levels may be below 12 μg/dl, suggesting decreased adrenal reserve. Leukocytosis of 10,000 to 20,000 is present in about half of the patients and raises the question of concomitant infection.

Treatment must begin as soon as the diagnosis is considered, even before laboratory results are known. It may be lifesaving and is unlikely to harm those who are not actually in storm. PTU in a dose of 1000 mg is immediately given orally or through a nasogastric tube to block organification of iodine and is followed by 200 mg every six hours until the patient is euthyroid. Hydrocortisone should be given immediately in a dose of 300 mg intravenously, followed by 100 mg daily until the crisis resolves.

Propranolol is given intravenously at a rate of one mg/min to a maximum of 10 mg, acts within minutes, and may be repeated as necessary every three hours. Oral propranolol in a dose of 20 mg to 80 mg every six hours takes one hour to work but lasts up to eight hours. The benefit of propranolol in patients with congestive

heart failure due to thyroid storm probably outweighs the risk. However, digoxin should be given before propranolol to compensate for depression of myocardial contractility. Propranolol should not be used in patients with asthma. Iodine should be given one hour after the first dose of PTU in the same doses outlined above. Intravenous esmolol may be used instead of propranolol.

Aggressive supportive care with cooling blankets, intravenous fluid, glucose, and oxygen is essential. Aspirin may displace T_4 from its carrier protein and should not be used to lower temperature. Serum electrolytes, glucose, and calcium levels and arterial blood gas measurements should be followed closely. Congestive heart failure should be treated with diuretics and digoxin. Supplementary vitamins, particularly B-complex, are often recommended. Precipitating factors causing thyroid storm must be identified and treated promptly. Infection or sepsis may be precipitants and should be aggressively treated. However, antibiotics need not be used prophylactically. Plasmapheresis and peritoneal dialysis have been used in thyroid storm to remove excess T_4 but are not necessary if other measures are taken.

HYPOTHYROIDISM

Clinical Manifestations

The manifestations of hypothyroidism can be protean. Clinical features can include dry skin, constipation, fatigue, cold intolerance, hoarseness, menorrhagia, anemia, easy bruising, and impaired mentation, as well as periorbital edema, lateral thinning of the eyebrows, dry brittle hair, goiter, bradycardia, hypo- or hypertension, and delayed relaxation phase of the deep-tendon reflexes. The symptoms of early hypothyroidism due to glandular hypofunction may be insidious and nonspecific. However, development of the full clinical picture is rapid in patients who either discontinue their exogenous hormone or from whom replacement is withheld after thyroidectomy. Symptoms appear within three weeks and become flagrant within three months.

The term myxedema is derived from the puffy edematous appearance of patients with severe hypothyroidism. Hyaluronic acid accumulates in all tissues, binds water, and produces mucinous edema. The skin becomes pale, cool, and dry, and bruising is common from increased capillary fragility. Surgical wounds heal slowly because of the slow growth rate of tissues. Macroglossia, cardiomegaly, pleural and pericardial effusions, and ascites are seen in some patients.

Hemodynamic Abnormalities

In myxedema heart, histologic examination reveals diffuse interstitial vacuolations in the myocardium containing mucopolysaccharide and proteinaceous deposits. These materials also account for the pericardial effusions found in as many as 60 percent of overtly hypothyroid patients. Accumulation is gradual, and tamponade is rare. Myocardial function is abnormal due to prolonged preejection time, decreased heart rate, and reduced stroke volume, which can lower cardiac output by as much as 40 percent. Pulse pressure is often narrowed. The electrocardiogram may show sinus bradycardia, decreased voltage, and flattening or inversion of the T wave in lead II. Peripheral vascular resistance is increased and blood volume decreased. These changes coupled with baroreceptor dysfunction may contribute to the tendency of hypothyroid patients to become hypotensive in response to a variety of anesthetic agents. Minimal blood loss may precipitate hypotension while rapid transfusion can result in congestive heart failure. Fluid replacement must be closely monitored, and arterial lines and Swan-Ganz catheters are recommended during surgery in overtly hypothyroid patients.

Angina from occult coronary artery disease may develop with thyroid replacement, especially if the replacement is rapid or the patient is stressed. The serum concentrations of cardiac enzymes in hypothyroidism can be high without apparent cardiac disease, making the diagnosis of myocardial infarction difficult. Hypothyroid patients who have angina before hormone replacement usually have severe coronary artery disease.

Pulmonary Abnormalities

Hypothyroid patients may have decreased maximal breathing capacity and diminished diffusing capacity (DL_{CO}). However, lung volumes, minute ventilation, P_{O_2}, and P_{CO_2} are usually normal. Both hypoxic and hypercapnic ventilatory drive may be markedly depressed. Pleural effusions may be present, and there may be myxedematous infiltration of the respiratory muscles. The reduced DL_{CO} is believed to be due to thickening of capillary membranes or a decreased pulmonary capillary bed. Respiratory failure can occur following the administration of respiratory depressants. Pandya et al. described three ventilator-dependent patients who were successfully extubated once their hypothyroidism was corrected.[31]

Gastrointestinal Abnormalities

Decreased peristalsis with distention and constipation is common in myxedema and may complicate diagnosis in the surgical patient. Hypomotility may progress to atony and, if accompanied by pain and vomiting, may resemble mechanical obstruction. Myxedematous ascites is high in protein and mucopolysaccharides. Autoimmune diseases involving the gastrointestinal tract are associated with hypothyroidism, although malabsorption is uncommon. Among patients with primary hypothyroidism, half have achlorhydria, one-third have circulating parietal cell antibodies, and 10 percent have pernicious anemia.[32] Gastrointestinal hemorrhage has been reported in hypothyroidism and is probably due to both increased capillary fragility and reductions in coagulation factors.

Hematologic Abnormalities

There are a variety of hemostatic abnormalities in hypothyroidism in addition to a nonspecific normocytic normochromic anemia. Edson et al. studied the hemostatic profiles of 16 hypothyroid patients. Most exhibited decreased platelet adhesiveness, and many had decreased levels of at least one clotting factor (VII, VIII, IX, or XI).[33] These abnormalities disappeared after replacement with thyroid hormone.

Close monitoring for bleeding is essential in hypothyroid patients undergoing surgery. If there are no known clotting abnormalities, special preoperative testing or preparation is not necessary. If bleeding develops in the setting of a prolonged prothrombin time or partial thromboplastin time, fresh frozen plasma should be used.

Fluid and Electrolytes

Hyponatremia is well-recognized in hypothyroidism but is of uncertain etiology. Abnormal free-water excretion is reported in 75 percent of patients and can be corrected with replacement of thyroid hormone. In this setting, superimposed secretion of antidiuretic hormone precipitated by postoperative pain may lead to life-threatening hyponatremia. Serum electrolytes and intravenous fluid replacement should therefore be followed closely.

Adrenal Function

Patients with primary hypothyroidism due to Hashimoto's thyroiditis have a higher incidence of concurrent Addison's disease. Patients with secondary hypothyroidism from pituitary disease often have associated adrenal insufficiency. Hypothyroid patients may have decreased adrenal reserve when stressed or when receiving rapid replacement of thyroid hormone. Such patients should receive supplemental glucocorticoid in the perioperative period.

Central Nervous System Abnormalities

Cerebral blood flow is reduced in hypothyroidism without a concomitant decrease in cerebral oxygen consumption, increasing the chances of cerebral hypoxia during anesthesia. Extreme sensitivity to central nervous system depressants mandates careful use of tranquilizers, narcotics, and hypnotics.[34]

Diagnosis

The clinical signs and symptoms of hypothyroidism are especially nonspecific in ill hospitalized patients. The only physical findings that may be reliable are delayed ankle reflexes, a husky voice, and dry skin. Total serum T_4, T_3RU, and FTI are all decreased in hypothyroidism. Serum T_3 levels may be normal or decreased and therefore do not help in confirming the diagnosis. Measurement of TSH differentiates primary hypothyroidism due to thyroid failure from secondary hypothyroidism due to pituitary failure. TSH is elevated in the former and normal or absent in the latter. If a patient has been taking thyroid hormone, it should be discontinued for four to six weeks before the diagnosis can be confirmed with a TSH level.

There is a continuous spectrum of laboratory abnormalities in hypothyroidism. Patients may be asymptomatic with FTI's in the normal range and mild elevations in TSH levels. Mildly symptomatic patients may have similar FTI's with higher elevations in TSH levels (above 10). Moderately symptomatic patients have lower FTI's with TSH levels above 10. Those with severe hypothyroidism have FTI's less than one and TSH levels above 20. There is generally a good correlation between clinical severity and degree of elevation in the TSH level.

Of the 0.5 to 0.8 percent of the adult population who are hypothyroid, most are those who have had surgery or received radioactive iodine for thyrotoxicosis and are inadequately replaced with thyroid hormone. A good medication history is therefore essential. Several drugs can induce hypothyroidism, such as lithium carbonate, cholestyramine, and prolonged nitroprusside infusion. Amiodarone, phenobarbital, and phenytoin may not affect normal patients but may render those with subclinical thyroid insufficiency frankly hypothyroid.

Severely ill patients hospitalized for prolonged periods of time often have abnormal thyroid function tests. T_4, FTI, and TSH may all be low and represent the "euthyroid sick" condition. This reflects reduced metabolic rate in response to prolonged illness.[4] Thyroid hormone replacement is not indicated in such cases. However, it is crucial to distinguish this state from secondary pituitary hypothyroidism, in which adrenal and gonadal dysfunction may also be present.

Risk of Surgery

Because of the various physiologic and metabolic derangements seen in hypothyroidism, it has long been felt that hypothyroidism is an absolute contraindication to any but the most emergency surgery. However, more recent data suggest that the risk of surgery in patients with mild-to-moderate hypothyroidism has been overestimated. Weinberg et al. reviewed surgical outcomes in 59 patients with mild to moderate untreated hypothyroidism. They were similar to controls in lowest temperatures and blood pressures recorded during surgery, need for postoperative respiratory assistance, use of vasopressors, incidence of bleeding complications and fluid and electrolyte imbalances, need for steroid support, time to extubation, frequency of arrhythmias, incidence of myocardial infarctions, and time to discharge from the hospital.[35]

Similarly, Ladenson et al. studied 40 patients undergoing elective or semi-elective procedures including cardiac surgery, most of whom had mild-to-moderate partially treated hypothyroidism. No differences were noted in blood loss, duration of hospitalization, pulmonary complications, or death or in the incidence of perioperative arrhythmias, hypothermia, hyponatremia, delayed extubation, or impaired wound healing when compared to control patients. Intraoperative hypotension and congestive heart failure were, however, more common in the hypothyroid group. The hypothyroid patients more often failed to mount fevers and had more gastrointestinal and neuropsychiatric complications after surgery.[36]

In both of these studies there were too few profoundly hypothyroid patients to draw any conclusions. Elective surgery should still be avoided in these patients until thyroid hormone is replaced. Even one week of replacement may be of some benefit. Hypothyroid patients undergoing coronary artery bypass surgery deserve specific comment. In each case, the risk of surgery without hormone replacement must be balanced against the possibility of worsening cardiac ischemia with preoperative hormone replacement.[37]

Perioperative Management

When the diagnosis of hypothyroidism has been established, replacement with L-thyroxine should be instituted. Although young patients usually tolerate rapid replacement, gradual therapy is recommended in adults who may have occult coronary artery disease. An initial oral dose of 25 to 50 μg of L-thyroxine daily can be increased by 25 μg every two weeks until full replacement doses of 100 to 200 μg daily are reached. In the early stages of therapy, hormone levels should be checked every four weeks. The TSH level returns to normal about four to six weeks after optimal replacement has been achieved.

Hypothyroid patients with angina may not tolerate thyroid hormone replacement. However, angina is not an absolute contraindication to replacement if the patient has symptomatic hypothyroidism, and in some patients angina improves with replacement. The initial dose of L-thyroxine in such cases should be 15 μg daily orally with increases of 15 μg every two weeks. If angina worsens and is unresponsive to antianginal medications, the dose of thyroid hormone should be decreased and coronary artery bypass surgery or angioplasty considered.

Patients with mild-to-moderate hypothyroidism should preferably begin oral replacement before surgery or alternatively with the resumption of oral intake thereafter. Patients with adequately treated hypothyroidism may omit their dose on the day of surgery. T_4 has a half-life of more than seven days and can be restarted when the patient is eating. T_4 is also available in intravenous form if oral replacement is impossible for a prolonged period of time.

Profoundly hypothyroid patients tolerate emergency surgery and trauma poorly. In such cases, a slow intravenous infusion of 300 to 500 μg of L-thyroxine has been shown to increase the basal metabolic rate and correct electrocardiographic abnormalities within six hours, and should be given preoperatively.[38] Hydrocortisone in a dose of 300 mg intravenously should also be given before surgery and continued in a dose of 100 mg intravenously daily for several days to avoid exhausting limited adrenal reserve by an acute increase in basal metabolic rate. Swan-Ganz catheters and arterial lines should be used to monitor hemodynamic status. Smaller daily doses of thyroid hormone can be given intravenously or through a nasogastric tube. There is no indication for the use of T_3 instead of T_4.

Fluid and electrolyte status should be monitored closely. Since hypothyroid patients may not mount adequate fevers, vigilance for potential infection is important. Prolonged constipation and ileus as well as neuropsychiatric complications require careful differential diagnosis and appropriate treatment.

MYXEDEMA COMA

Myxedema coma is a medical emergency with a mortality rate of 50 percent even after aggressive treatment. It is usually precipitated by infection, cold exposure, central nervous system depressants, or trauma. Over half of reported cases occur after hospital admission in patients with unrecognized hypothyroidism. Grand mal seizures occur in 25 percent, cerebellar signs are common, and frank psychosis may precede coma. The electroencephalogram is usually markedly abnormal but correlates poorly with prognosis. Recovery has been reported in patients with flat electroencephalograms.[39] Although hypotension is present at presentation in 50 percent of patients, hypertension has also been reported.

Mechanisms of coma in myxedema include hypothermia, hypercapnia, and hyponatremia. Hypothermia is present in over 80 percent of patients with myxedema coma. Heat loss should be prevented and intravenous fluids warmed to body temperature, but external warming may worsen hypotension and is therefore contraindicated. Hypoventilation and CO_2 retention may contribute to the development of coma. Airway obstruction may precipitate acute respiratory failure. If breathing is spontaneous, an oral airway should be inserted to prevent obstruction by the tongue. Arterial blood gas measurements should be done every few hours. Oxygen should be carefully administered to prevent further CO_2 retention. Intubation may be necessary.

Hyponatremia occurs in 50 percent of patients and is also implicated in the development of coma. Free-water restriction is generally sufficient treatment. However, if hyponatremia is severe with serum sodium concentrations under 115 meq/liter, normal or hypertonic saline may be cautiously administered. If the patient is hypotensive, fluids should be given before pressors. Response to pressors is poor in hypothyroidism. Simultaneous administration of thyroid hormone and pressors may precipitate life-threatening arrhythmias.

In one study, hypoglycemia was reported in four of 23 severely myxedematous patients, and three of the four died.[40] Glucose-containing solutions should therefore be given along with corticosteroids to prevent adrenocortical insufficiency.

Administration of thyroid hormone is critical in the treatment of myxedema coma. Because of severe hypometabolism and variable gastrointestinal absorption, intravenous L-thyroxine is recommended. A single dose of 500 μg replaces the extrathyroidal pool and need not be repeated for several days. When the patient is conscious, oral L-thyroxine should be administered daily as described above. Stress doses of intravenous hydrocortisone are also recommended.

SUMMARY

1. The serum concentrations of T_4, T_3, and T_3RU may be affected by surgery, anesthesia, and a variety of illnesses. Diagnosing hyperthyroidism or hypothyroidism may therefore be difficult.

2. Thyrotoxic patients have a higher risk of complications and death in the perioperative period. Elective surgery should be delayed and PTU should be administered daily for several weeks until the patient is euthyroid.

3. If surgery cannot be delayed, patients with mild hyperthyroidism may safely undergo surgery after premedication with a beta-blocker. Those with more severe hyperthyroidism should receive PTU in a dose of 1000 mg orally and hydrocortisone in a dose of 300 mg intravenously, followed by SSKI in a dose of five drops orally three times daily or sodium iodide in a dose of one gram intravenously three times daily. Propranolol in a dose of one mg/min intravenously or 20 to 40 mg every six hours orally can be used to control tachycardia, hypertension and arrhythmias. The very short-acting intravenous cardioselective beta-blocker esmolol can also be useful in this setting. Thyroid storm is a medical emergency requiring immediate treatment with the same regimen.

4. Urgent surgery can be performed in patients with mild-to-moderate hypothyroidism with no increased risk. L-thyroxine in a dose of 25 μg daily should be started before or after surgery and the dose increased 25 μg every two weeks. Slower replacement with 15 μg of L-thyroxine daily and increasing increments of 15 μg every two weeks is suggested for elderly patients or patients with angina. Elective surgery should be delayed in patients who are markedly hypothyroid until they are clinically and chemically euthyroid.

5. If surgery in severely hypothyroid patients cannot be delayed, L-thyroxine in a dose of 300 to 500 μg intravenously and hydrocortisone in a dose of 300 mg intravenously should be administered preoperatively. Hydrocortisone in a dose of 100 mg

daily should be continued for at least one week. L-thyroxine in a daily oral dose of 25 μg can be instituted several days postoperatively and increased in an incremental fashion. Myxedema coma is a medical emergency requiring immediate treatment with L-thyroxine and hydrocortisone in the same manner.

REFERENCES

1. Spencer C, Elgen A, Shen D et al: Specificity of sensitive assays of thyrotropin used to screen for thyroid disease in hospitalized patients. *Clin Chem* 33:1391–1396, 1987.
2. Hay ID, Klee CG: Thyroid dysfunction. *Endoc Metab Clin North Am* 473–509, 1988.
3. Borst GC, Eil C, Burman KD: Euthyroid hyperthyroxinemia. *Ann Intern Med* 98:366–378, 1983.
4. Wortofsky L, Burman KP: Alterations in thyroid function in patients with systemic illness. The "euthyroid sick syndrome." *Endoc Rev* 3(2):164–217, 1982.
5. Simons RJ, Simon JM, Demers LM et al: Thyroid dysfunction in elderly hospitalized patients. *Arch Intern Med* 150:1249–1253, 1990.
6. Watts NB: Use of a sensitive thyrotropin assay for monitoring treatment with Levothyroxine. *Arch Intern Med* 144:309–312, 1989.
7. Ehrmann DA, Weinberg M, Sarine DH: Limitations to the use of a sensitive assay for serum thyrotropin in the assessment of thyroid status. *Arch Intern Med* 149:367–372, 1989.
8. de Los Santos ET, Stauch GH, Mazzaferri EL: Sensitivity, specificity, and cost-effectiveness of the sensitive thyrotropin assay in the diagnosis of thyroid disease in ambulatory patients. *Arch Intern Med* 149:526–532, 1989.
9. Surks MI, Chopra IJ, Mariash CN et al: American Thyroid Association guidelines for use of laboratory tests in thyroid disorders. *JAMA* 263:1529–1532, 1990.
10. Rutberg H, Anderberg B, Håkanson E et al: Influence of extradural blockade on serum thyroid hormone concentrations after surgery. *Acta Chir Scand* 151:97–103, 1985.
11. Noreng MF, Jensen P, Tjellden NU: Pre- and postoperative changes in the concentration of serum thyrotropin under general anaesthesia, compared to general anaesthesia with epidural analgesia. *Acta Anaesth Scand* 31:292–294, 1987.
12. Vinik AI, Kalk WJ, McLaren H et al: Fasting blunts the TSH response to synthetic thyrotropin-releasing hormone (TRH). *J Clin Endoc Metab* 40:509, 1975.
13. Woeber KA: Thyrotoxicosis and the heart. *N Engl J Med* 327:94–97, 1992.
14. Herman J: Thrombocytopenic purpura and thyroid disease. *Ann Intern Med* 93:934, 1980.
15. Gavin LA: The diagnostic dilemmas of hyperthyroxinemia and hypothyroxinemia. *Adv Intern Med* 33:185–203, 1988.
16. McArthur JW, Rawson RW, Means JH et al: Thyrotoxic crisis. *JAMA* 134:868, 1947.
17. Strube PJ: Thyroid storm during beta-blockade. *Anaesthesia* 39:343–346, 1984.
18. Alderbeith A, Stenstrom G, Hasslegren PO: The selective beta blocking agent metoprolol compared with antithyroid drugs as preoperative treatment of patients with hyperthyroidism. Results from a preoperative randomized study. *Ann Surg* 205:182–188, 1987.
19. Wartofsky L: Emergency thyrotoxic storm. *Hosp Prac* 28:123–142 1992.
20. Cooper DS: Antithyroid drugs. *N Engl J Med* 321:1353–1362, 1984
21. Berghout A, Wiersinga WA, Brummelkamp WH: Sodium ipodate in the preparation of Graves' hyperthyroid patients for thyroidectomy *Horm Res* 31:256–260, 1989.
22. Martino E, Balgano S, Bartelana L et al: Therapy of Graves' disease

with sodium ipodate is associated with a high recurrence rate of hyper-thyroidism. *J Endoc Invest* 14:847–851, 1991.

23. Caldwell G, Errington M, Toft AD: Resistant hyperthyroidism induced by sodium ipodate used as treatment for Graves' disease. *Acta Endo-crinol* 120:215–216, 1989.

24. Geffner DL, Hershman JM: Beta-adrenergic blockade for the treatment of hyperthyroidism. *Am J Med* 93:61–68, 1992.

25. Isley WL, Dahl S, Gibbs H: Use of esmolol in managing a thyrotoxic patient needing emergency surgery. *Am J Med* 89:122–123, 1990.

26. Bendixen HH, Ngai SH: Anesthesia in thyroid surgery, in Werner SC, Ingbar SH (eds): *The Thyroid*, 4th ed. Hagerstown, Harper & Row, 1978, p 584.

27. Mazzaferri EL, Skillman TG: Thyroid storm: A review of 22 episodes with special emphasis on the use of guanethidine. *Arch Intern Med* 124:684, 1969.

28. Peters KR, Nance P, Wingard DW: Malignant hyperthyroidism or ma-lignant hyperthermia? *Anesth Analg* 60:613–615, 1981.

29. Rosenberg MR, Green M: Neuroleptic malignant syndrome. *Arch In-tern Med* 149:1927–1931, 1989.

30. Dozeman R, Kaiser FE, Case O et al: Hyperthyroidism appearing as hyperemesis gravidarum. *Arch Intern Med* 143:2202–2203, 1983.

31. Pandya K, Lal C, Scheinhorn D et al: Hypothyroidism and ventilatory dependency. *Arch Intern Med* 149:2115–2116, 1989.

32. Tudhope GR, Wilson GM: Deficiency of vitamin B_{12} in hypothyroid-ism. *Lancet* 1:703, 1962.

33. Edson JR, Fecher DR, Doe RP: Low platelet adhesiveness and other hemostatic abnormalities in hypothyroidism. *Ann Intern Med* 82:342, 1975.

34. Murkin JM: Anesthesia and hypothyroidism: A review of thyroxine physiology, pharmacology, and anesthetic implication. *Anesth Analg* 61:371–382, 1982.

35. Weinberg AD, Brennan MD, Gorman CA et al: Outcome of anesthesia and surgery in hypothyroid patients. *Arch Intern Med* 143:893–897, 1983.

36. Ladenson PN, Levin AA, Ridgway EC, Daniels GH: Complications of surgery in hypothyroid patients. *Am J Med* 77:261–266, 1984.

37. Levine HD: Compromise therapy in the patient with angina pectoris: A clinical assessment. *Am J Med* 69:411–418, 1980.

38. Holvey DN, Goodner CJ, Nicoloff JT et al: Treatment of myxedema coma with intravenous thyroxine. *Arch Intern Med* 113:89, 1964.

39. Urbanic RC, Mazzaferri EL: Thyrotoxic crisis and myxedema coma. *Heart Lung* 7:435, 1978.

40. Nickerson JF, Hill SR Jr, McNeill JH et al: Fatal myxedema, with and without coma. *Ann Intern Med* 53:475, 1960.

26 THE SURGICAL PATIENT ON STEROIDS

David R. Goldmann

Ever since the initial case reports of intraoperative cardiovascular collapse in patients taking exogenous glucocorticoids, the literature has reflected continuing concern about the potential risk of this serious complication.[1-8] The use of steroids for the treatment of a variety of diseases is widespread. Through their effect on the hypothalamic-pituitary-adrenal (HPA) axis, they are the most common cause of unsuspected adrenal suppression. Adrenocortical insufficiency induced by withdrawal of steroids can remain clinically inapparent until the stress of surgery supervenes. In addition, steroids affect both wound healing and host defenses against infection, two important concerns in the perioperative period.

Although severe adrenal insufficiency and endogenously or exogenously induced Cushing's syndrome are usually readily recognized, preoperative patients who have taken or are taking steroids can be difficult to identify. When steroids are discontinued, resulting adrenal insufficiency can be subtle in its presentation with few, if any, clearly defined signs and symptoms. Both adrenal insufficiency and the so-called steroid withdrawal syndrome can cause anorexia, weight loss, malaise, myalgias, arthralgias, emotional lability, and even low-grade fever, but in the latter baseline and stimulated cortisol levels are normal.[9,10] Exogenous steroids can produce some of the same manifestations as endogenous Cushing's syndrome but can also cause others not seen in the native disease.[11,12] Obesity, edema, poor wound healing, and psychiatric symptoms are common to both situations, but benign intracranial hypertension, glaucoma, posterior subcapsular cataracts, pancreatitis, panniculitis, and aseptic necrosis of bone are peculiar to patients taking exogenous steroids. Hypertension, acne, menstrual irregularities, hirsutism, striae, purpura, and plethora are more commonly seen in those with endogenous Cushing's syndrome. Equivalent doses of steroids administered over a given period of time may produce more side effects in some patients than in others. For these reasons, a detailed history of steroid use is often more helpful than physical examination or routine laboratory testing for electrolyte abnormalities.

This chapter reviews the physiology of the HPA axis, the biochemistry and pharmacology of commonly used steroids, and the effects of steroids on the HPA axis, wound healing, and host defenses against infection.

STEROID PHYSIOLOGY, BIOCHEMISTRY, AND PHARMACOLOGY

The production of cortisol by the adrenal cortex is controlled by adrenocorticotropic hormone (ACTH) from the anterior pituitary gland. The secretion of both hormones is episodic and exhibits diurnal variation with peak secretion in the early morning and significantly less in the evening. The secretion of ACTH is in turn controlled by corticotrophin-releasing hormone (CRH) from the hypothalamus. Neural stimuli from higher centers stimulate the secretion of CRH. There is a clearly defined negative-feedback mechanism in which cortisol from the adrenal cortex suppresses the secretion of ACTH. This same inhibition of ACTH production and secretion is produced by exogenous steroids.

Pharmacologically active steroids are all variants of cortisol or hydrocortisone with 21 carbon atoms arranged in the characteristic four-ringed compound common to all steroid hormones. Variations in the saturation of the rings and the presence of various side-chains determine the half-lives and potencies of these agents. Table 26–1 lists some of the most commonly used steroids grouped according to their durations of action and relative potencies in suppressing ACTH secretion.[13,14] Equivalent doses of short-acting steroids produce ACTH suppression for 24 to 36 hours, intermediate-acting compounds for 24 to 48 hours, and long-acting agents for more than 48 hours.

The duration and potency of these compounds in suppressing ACTH secretion do not correlate strictly with serum half-life or duration of biologic effect. Though the serum half-life of prednisolone is about twice that of hydrocortisone, in equivalent doses they are both short-acting in their suppression of ACTH. Since steroids must enter the cell nucleus to exert their biologic effects, neither serum half-life nor potency in suppressing ACTH correlates with

TABLE 26–1. Commonly Used Glucocorticoids

Steroids	Glucocorticoid Potency*	Equivalent Glucocorticoid Dose (mg)
Short-acting		
Cortisol (hydrocortisone)	1	20
Cortisone	0.8	25
Prednisone	4	5
Prednisolone	4	5
Methylprednisolone	5	4
Intermediate-acting		
Triamcinolone	5	4
Long-acting		
Betamethasone	25	0.60
Dexamethasone	30	0.75

*The values given for glucocorticoid potency are relative. Coritsol is arbitrarily assigned a value of 1.

duration of action in various target tissues. Moreover, the duration of one biologic effect exerted by a particular dose of steroid may differ from that of another effect. For example, although several different pulmonary function tests are useful in monitoring the effect of steroids in patients with asthma, the duration of improvement in one parameter may differ from that in another.[15]

The effects of surgical stress on the HPA axis have been well studied. In normal subjects, the plasma concentration of cortisol rises to a peak of five to 10 times normal approximately six hours after surgery and, unless stress continues, falls to normal levels within 24 hours.[16–18] A similar rise is seen after a dose of exogenous ACTH.[19] Epidural anesthesia delays but does not prevent this response.[20] Cortisol secretion remains episodic during stress, but the number of episodes per unit of time and the amount of cortisol secreted during each are greater than under normal conditions.[21] A rise in ACTH occurs before a rise in cortisol and in one study was found to begin 15 to 45 minutes after skin incision.[22] There are minor and probably clinically unimportant changes in the hepatic conjugation and renal excretion patterns of steroid metabolites after surgery.[23] Though a temporal relationship between the rise in plasma concentration of adenosine 3',5'-cyclic phosphate (cyclic AMP) and cortisol has been documented, the exact mechanism of HPA activation, whether neural or humoral, remains undefined.[24–27] The adrenal response to the stress of surgery remains essentially intact in the elderly.[28]

Several tests have been used to evaluate the effect of exogenous steroids on one or more components of the HPA axis. Although administration of pyrogen or production of hypoglycemia with insulin simulates stress, these methods are impractical and potentially dangerous. The two best standardized and clinically most useful tests to measure adrenal reserve and the integrity of the HPA axis are, respectively, the ACTH test and the metyrapone test.[29,30] Adrenal reserve is tested by measurement of the plasma cortisol concentration before and 30 to 60 minutes after a parenteral dose of 250 µg of synthetic ACTH (cosyntropin).[21–24] From a basal plasma level of six µg/dl to 25 µg/dl, a rise to greater than 20 µg/dl or an incremental increase of more than seven µg/dl in plasma cortisol concentration is considered normal. Although there are several variations of the metyrapone test, all involve inhibition of the final 11-hydroxylation step in the production of cortisol (compound F) from 11-deoxycortisol (compound S). After administration of metyrapone, plasma concentration of cortisol falls,

ACTH secretion increases, and production of 11-deoxycortisol rises. An increase in plasma 11-deoxycortisol levels to above 10.5 µg/dl with a simultaneous plasma cortisol concentration of 8 µg/dl or less assures the integrity of both the pituitary and the adrenal components of the HPA axis.

SUPPRESSION OF THE HYPOTHALAMIC-PITUITARY-ADRENAL AXIS AND ITS IMPLICATIONS FOR THE SURGICAL PATIENT

It is thought that adrenal suppression by exogenous glucocorticoids is dangerous during periods of stress because lack of acutely required cortisol can lead to hypotension, cardiovascular collapse, and even death. Since the early 1950s, numerous case reports have documented such complications during surgery in patients taking steroids for a number of inflammatory diseases.[1–8] Some provide histologic evidence of adrenal atrophy at autopsy, but only a few supply biochemical evidence of low plasma concentrations of cortisol or one of its metabolites at the time of these complications.[1–3,31–33] It is important to know what type of steroid given at what dose and frequency produces suppression, what is the best way to define and measure suppression, how long the suppression lasts, and how much time is required for recovery of the HPA axis. Even more important is the question of whether abnormalities in the HPA axis adversely alter surgical outcome.

Studies of HPA axis suppression by exogenous steroids fall into two major groups.[12,14] Some only document suppression by abnormalities in one or more biochemical tests, while others attempt to correlate suppression with clinical outcome in the surgical setting. Though the latter are more relevant to questions posed in this chapter, both groups suffer from lack of uniform methodology and together reach no definitive conclusions. They evaluate heterogeneous groups of patients with different underlying diseases on a variety of different steroid regimens and employ different biochemical tests to define suppression.

Clinical studies of surgical outcome in patients taking exogenous steroids provide the most relevant data. Danowski et al studied 117 patients on various steroid regimens approximating replacement doses undergoing 80 different stresses, including surgery, pregnancy, diagnostic procedures, and acute illness. None developed signs or symptoms of adrenal insufficiency.[34] Another group of 13 men underwent 15 major or minor surgical procedures three to 24 months after interrupting replacement doses of steroid and similarly experienced no mishap. Although no biochemical testing of the HPA axis was performed, this clinical study provides firm evidence that patients taking replacement doses of steroid at the time of surgery or at any time within the preceding two years tolerate stress and surgery well and therefore require no perioperative steroid coverage.

Patients taking supraphysiologic doses of steroids greater than the equivalent of about 7.5 mg/day of prednisone present a more difficult problem. The best early study is probably that of Sampson et al.[32] They studied 35 patients with ulcerative colitis undergoing elective surgery, 17 of whom had never received steroids and 18 of whom had been on various regimens within two years of surgery. Two days after steroid was stopped, ACTH tests were performed in all patients, and plasma cortisol concentrations were determined hourly during surgery. In all patients but three of those who had taken steroids before surgery, the ACTH test and intra-operative plasma cortisol levels were normal. Of the three with abnormal ACTH tests, one underwent surgery with steroid coverage and two did so without. Both of the latter had subnormal intraoperative plasma cortisol determinations and suffered unexplained hypotension that responded to intravenous hydrocortisone. Despite the small number of patients, the authors concluded not only that larger doses of exogenous steroids can produce HPA axis suppression and increase the risk of perioperative collapse but also that a preoperative ACTH test predicts both lack of adrenal response to stress and subsequent surgical complications.

This work has been confirmed and extended by others. Jasani et al. showed that plasma 11-hydroxycorticosteroid levels rise appropriately in response to synovectomy of the knee in 16 of 21 steroid-treated patients with rheumatoid arthritis with normal preoperative ACTH stimulation tests.[31] Levels were clearly subnormal in patients with abnormal tests and intermediate in those with a normal response to ACTH but subnormal response to one or more of three other tests of the HPA axis. There was only one case of severe intraoperative hypotension in a patient on low-dose steroids with an abnormal ACTH test. The authors concluded that the results of the ACTH test correlate best with the adrenal response to the stress of surgery and may be useful in predicting intraoperative complications and the need for steroid coverage. The conclusions of this work were reaffirmed by Kehlet and Binder with the caveats that abnormalities in any stimulation test do not always correlate with intraoperative outcome and that intraoperative hypotension may occur for a variety of reasons unrelated to HPA axis function.[19]

Other studies supply limited information about the time course of suppression and recovery of HPA axis function during and after a course of exogenous steroids. These data allow the physician to decide what length of steroid course at what time before surgery will likely produce clinically significant HPA axis suppression, especially when surgery cannot await the results of an ACTH stimulation test. Graber et al. studied the time course of recovery of each component of the HPA axis after discontinuation of supraphysiologic doses of exogenous steroids given for one to 10 years or after surgical removal of an adrenocortical tumor causing Cushing's syndrome.[35] Through measurements of plasma ACTH and basal and ACTH-stimulated 17-hydroxycorticosteroid levels, they defined four phases of HPA axis recovery. During the first month, ACTH and 17-hydroxycorticosteroid levels are low, and the ACTH stimulation test is abnormal. In the second through the fifth months, ACTH levels rise to normal or supranormal levels while basal and stimulated 17-hydroxycorticosteroids remain low. In the sixth through ninth months, 17-hydroxycorticosteroid levels return to normal, but adrenal responsiveness remains abnormal. Only after nine months do all parameters return to normal. Graber concluded that recovery of adrenocortical function lags behind that of the pituitary and may not occur for up to a year or more after discontinuation of exogenous steroids.

Livanou et al. studied the recovery of HPA axis function by measuring plasma levels of 11-hydroxycorticosteroids before and after insulin-induced hypoglycemia in control subjects and patients who were either still taking steroids or had discontinued them for periods ranging from 24 hours to more than a year.[36] Although basal 11-hydroxycorticosteroid levels returned to normal after about one month, stimulated levels did not normalize in all patients for a year or more. Basal levels of 11-hydroxycorticosteroids

normalized more quickly if exogenous steroid doses were equivalent to 7.5 mg/day daily or less of prednisone. In this low-dose group, stimulated levels returned to normal more quickly if the duration of therapy had been less than 18 months. These authors emphasized the importance of considering both variables of dosage and duration of therapy in predicting response to stress.

Data on the steroid dosage and duration of therapy necessary to produce HPA axis suppression are conflicting, but Streck and Lockwood demonstrated that high-dose short-term steroid therapy given twice daily for only five days can affect HPA axis function.[37] They measured cortisol response to both ACTH and insulin-induced hypoglycemia two and five days after discontinuation of therapy in 10 normal men and found both to be impaired after two days with the response to ACTH remaining subnormal after five days. Unfortunately, testing was not carried out for more than five days after steroids had been stopped.

Steroid regimens involving other than systemic routes of administration and various dosage frequencies affect HPA axis function differently. Although infrequent and usually mild, adrenal suppression has been documented in patients receiving large quantities of topical or intranasal steroids.[38–41] The effect of dosage frequency on the HPA axis can be more significant. Harter et al. documented that alternate-day prednisone therapy not only produced significantly fewer side effects than daily therapy but also preserved normal adrenal response to ACTH.[42] Ackerman and Nolan found that alternate-day high-dose prednisone lowered basal plasma 17-hydroxycorticosteroid levels but had no effect on response to insulin-induced hypoglycemia.[43] Others have extended this work to other steroids and intermittent dosage regimens.[44] Alternate-day administration of the long-acting steroid dexamethasone produces profound adrenal suppression, and HPA axis dysfunction cannot be avoided by regimens in which it is given on three consecutive days each week.[45–47] Triamcinolone given once daily in the morning produces less HPA axis suppression than divided or even single doses given later in the day.[48,49] Administration of ACTH does not produce significant HPA axis suppression.[14,50]

In summary, although the available data are far from consistent, HPA axis suppression can be expected from supraphysiologic doses of exogenous steroids given for as few as five days. Full recovery may require up to a year and cannot be easily predicted from information on dosage and duration of treatment. Suppression of the HPA axis can be minimized by using the lowest possible single daily morning dose of a short-acting agent only as long as necessary. Alternate-day therapy is most desirable because it produces virtually no HPA suppression if long-acting potent agents like dexamethasone are avoided. In addition, alternate-day therapy is effective in controlling most chronic disease except for temporal arteritis.

A careful history is important in preparing patients taking steroids for surgery. Precise information regarding the dosage, its duration and frequency, and the interval between the last dose and the operative procedure allows the clinician to predict the possibility of adrenal insufficiency under stress and determine the need for steroid coverage in the perioperative period. When time permits before surgery, especially if an accurate history cannot be obtained, an ACTH stimulation test provides the most reliable index of adrenocortical response to stress. Patients with a normal test can undergo surgery without coverage and thereby avoid potential problems with wound healing and increased susceptibility to infection that may result from steroid use. Those with an abnormal or equivocal test should receive appropriate coverage. In an emergency situation, it is reasonable to provide preoperative steroid coverage when the patient has taken supraphysiologic doses of steroid for more than a week in the year preceding surgery or when the history is unclear. If immediate coverage and measurement of adrenal reserve are desired, dexamethasone can be used since it does not interfere with standard plasma cortisol assays required in ACTH testing.

The nature of the underlying disease may be a determinant of risk in predicting steroid-related perioperative complications. In one recent study, the incidence of such complications was higher in patients with chronic pulmonary disease.[51] The authors also demonstrated a rough correlation between steroid dose and duration of therapy and the development of complications. However, until these findings are confirmed in larger numbers, all patients who meet the above historical and biochemical criteria for coverage should receive appropriate doses of steroids in the perioperative period.

There are many steroid coverage regimens outlined in the literature, all of which are largely empirical but theoretically based on matching the normal output of about 250 mg of cortisol from the adrenal under stressful conditions.[52–54] For major surgery, hydrocortisone hemisuccinate in a dose of 100 mg can be given intravenously the evening before surgery, at the beginning of the procedure, and every eight hours until the end of the period of stress. Adequate salt- and glucose-containing fluid should be provided with careful monitoring of blood pressure and serum electrolyte and glucose concentrations. H_2-antagonists should be administered to avoid steroid-induced gastrointestinal bleeding. Some investigators have been successful using doses smaller than 100 mg in patients undergoing elective procedures and increasing the dose if complications arise.[55] However, until such data are widely confirmed, the above doses are recommended. Equivalent doses of other steroids can be substituted as long as they are administered intravenously. Intramuscular cortisone acetate should be avoided because of its uncertain absorption and the need for hepatic reduction to active cortisol. For minor surgical procedures, the same regimen can be used for 24 hours, and, for stressful diagnostic procedures, a simple intravenous dose of 100 mg of hydrocortisone just before the operation should suffice.

Many different steroid tapering schedules are described in the literature,[54] but none has been rigorously evaluated. In uncomplicated minor or elective surgery requiring coverage for no more than a few days or for diagnostic procedures, steroids can usually be discontinued without tapering. In more complicated cases requiring prolonged coverage, steroids should be tapered over a longer period. This can usually be accomplished by halving the dose of hydrocortisone each day until the patient is receiving 25 mg intravenously every eight hours. After one day on this dose, the drug can be given in a dose of 25 mg twice daily for one day, then 25 mg once daily for one day, and then discontinued. Patients undergoing adrenalectomy or hypophysectomy for Cushing's syndrome have been accustomed to hypercortisolism for a long time and may require even slower tapering. If a maintenance dose of steroid for an underlying disease is required, it can be resumed at an appropriate point in the tapering schedule and given orally when the patient is eating.

STEROID THERAPY AND WOUND HEALING

Clinicians have long recognized thinning of skin, easy bruisability, and delayed wound healing in patients with endogenous or exogenous hypercortisolism. However, the literature on surgical wound healing in patients taking steroids is scant. Much must be inferred from series of patients with Cushing's syndrome undergoing adrenalectomy or pituitary surgery, animal work dealing with the physics of wound healing, and in vitro studies of collagen biochemistry. Given the number of patients on long-term steroid therapy undergoing surgery and those requiring perioperative steroid coverage for suspected HPA axis suppression, it is important that the effect of these agents on the normal process of wound healing be assessed.

Solem and Lund reviewed their experience with 449 steroid-treated patients undergoing surgery with high-dose cortisone coverage over a 10-year period.[56] They found that steroids rarely interfere with healing unless doses are unduly high for long periods of time and protein intake is inadequate. In a later series of 44 patients undergoing bilateral adrenalectomy for Cushing's disease, only one patient who could not be easily weaned from replacement cortisone experienced delayed wound healing.[57]

On the other hand, steroids have been found to affect wound healing in animal studies. Baker and Whitaker inflicted standardized wounds in the skin of rats before and after local application of cortisone and studied the gross and histologic morphology of the healing process.[58] They found that cortisone delayed formation of granulation tissue and wound closure and caused thinning of the dermis, atrophy of collagen fibers, and a decrease in fibroblast and new blood vessel proliferation. Howes et al. found that subcutaneous cortisone affected granulation tissue formation in rabbits and rats in a dose-dependent fashion and significantly decreased the tensile strength of sutured wounds.[59]

Data on the effects of different steroid doses and the temporal relationship between drug administration and wounding are conflicting. Several investigators have found that moderate-to-large doses of steroids exert most of their morphologic effects on healing within three days of injury. They postulate that inhibition of the early inflammatory process after wounding is responsible for delayed healing.[60,61] In these studies, vitamin A protected against delayed healing, presumably because of its effect on stabilizing lysosomes. However, other investigators have found that smaller doses of steroid have variable effects.[62,63] Moreover, the effects of different doses of steroid on the proliferation of fibroblasts, production of collagen, and uptake of nucleic and amino acids in tissue cultures from humans remain unclear.

Later work relies on techniques to measure several different physical and biochemical parameters of connective tissue. In one study, rats given long-term moderate doses of cortisol were wounded, and tissue from the wound and a distant site were tested both biochemically for collagen content and mechanically for tensile strength, stress-strain relationships, failure energy, extensibility, and elastic stiffness.[64] Although the investigators found that steroids only slightly impaired the mechanical properties of healing, they documented a systemic effect of wounding itself independent of steroid treatment on skin distant from the wound. The distant skin revealed increased collagen content and decreased stiffness.

Despite the inconclusiveness of the data, clinical experience suggests that steroid treatment may have a deleterious effect o wound healing. For this reason, meticulous care of wounds in patients on glucocorticoids is recommended.

STEROID THERAPY AND INFECTION

Increased susceptibility to infection is another generally accepted complication of steroid therapy relevant to the surgical setting. However, satisfactory data on which to base an assessment of risk are difficult to find. Conclusions must be drawn from clinical studies of infection in steroid-treated nonsurgical patients and from in vitro studies examining the effects of glucocorticoids on cellular processes of host defense.

Winstone and Brooke documented four cases of septicemia among 18 surgical patients on steroids given steroid coverage but none in 17 others on steroids not given coverage.[65] In a controlled retrospective study of 100 patients on steroids undergoing major and minor surgical procedures with appropriate coverage, there were 11 wound infections in the steroid-treated group and only one among the controls.[66] Though patients and controls were matched for age and sex, they were not matched for underlying disease. In contrast, Kaalund-Jensen and Elb observed no increase in the incidence of wound or other infections in an uncontrolled series of 419 patients undergoing surgery with steroid coverage.[67] Oh and Patterson found only one minor suture abscess among a group of 17 steroid-dependent asthmatics undergoing 21 surgical procedures.[68] In four series of patients with Cushing's disease undergoing adrenalectomy, rates of wound infection ranged from 2.3 percent to 21 percent.[57,69–71] In a more recent meta-analysis of 71 studies, there was a two-fold increase in relative risk of infection in over 2000 patients in a variety of clinical settings.[72] Though the data are conflicting, largely uncontrolled, and drawn from patients with serious underlying diseases, there is some evidence that long-term steroid use and perhaps steroid coverage itself may predispose some surgical patients to postoperative wound infection.

Other clinical data to support the contention that steroids may predispose to infection can be drawn from the nonsurgical literature.[73–75] Soon after their introduction into clinical practice, steroids were found to worsen infection despite their effects in reducing fever and toxicity. Patients treated with steroids have a higher-than-usual incidence of infection with gram-negative bacteria and other more unusual opportunistic organisms. In addition, there is some evidence to suggest that steroid therapy may predispose patients with systemic lupus erythematosus and patients undergoing renal transplantation to serious complications and death from infection.[76,77] There are also data to suggest that alternate-day steroid therapy may decrease this risk in patients with a variety of chronic diseases.[74,78]

The accumulation of experimental data on the effects of steroids on host defenses and cellular immunity provides a theoretical basis for clinical observation.[74] Steroids exert multiple effects on the kinetics, distribution pattern, and function of granulocytes and mononuclear cells. Though glucocorticoids cause a brisk neutrophilic leukocytosis, they suppress accumulation of granulocytes at the inflammatory site, probably by altering their surface and preventing adherence to and egress from the vascular epithelium. Steroid-induced lymphocytopenia is probably due to redistribution of circulating lymphocytes, particularly T lymphocytes, out of the intravascular space through as yet undefined mechanisms. Steroids also antagonize macrophage interaction with the soluble products of activated lymphocytes.[79] The same mechanisms that allow glucocorticoids to exert their beneficial anti-inflammatory and immunosuppressive effects in many disease states may be responsible for increasing host susceptibility to infection.

In summary, the incidence of postoperative infection, particularly of the surgical wound, may be increased in steroid-treated patients. For this reason, steroids should be used perioperatively only when required to treat an underlying disease or when adrenal suppression is suspected. Meticulous wound care is essential to prevent infection, but prophylactic antibiotics are not indicated.

SUMMARY

1. Decreased adrenal reserve due to suppression of the HPA axis by exogenous steroids should be suspected in any patient who has taken supraphysiologic doses of glucocorticoids (more than the equivalent of 7.5 mg/day of prednisone) for more than a week in the year preceding surgery.

2. If the history is unclear, an ACTH stimulation test provides an adequate measure of the ability of the adrenal glands to meet the stress of surgery. When emergency surgery is required and time does not permit testing, steroid coverage should be given.

3. Appropriate steroid coverage for major surgery consists of hydrocortisone hemisuccinate in a dose of 100 mg intravenously the evening before surgery, another dose at the beginning of the procedure, and 100 mg every eight hours thereafter until the stress of the postoperative period has passed. The same regimen can be used for 24 hours for minor procedures. One dose of 100 mg of hydrocortisone should be given just before stressful diagnostic procedures. Intramuscular cortisone acetate should be avoided because of its uneven absorption. Adequate glucose- and salt-containing fluid and H$_2$-antagonists should be given. Blood pressure and serum electrolyte and glucose concentrations should be followed.

4. Tapering of the steroid dose is required only if coverage is required for ongoing postoperative stress for more than a few days. Patients who require maintenance glucocorticoid for their underlying diseases should be continued on parenteral therapy until they can restart their usual oral dose.

5. Steroids may delay wound healing and predispose patients to wound infection. They should therefore be used only when indicated in the perioperative period. However, they should never be withheld if adrenal suppression is suspected. Meticulous wound care and surveillance for infection are essential.

REFERENCES

1. Fraser CG, Preuss FS, Bigford WD: Adrenal atrophy and irreversible shock associated with cortisone therapy. *JAMA* 149:1542, 1952.
2. Lewis L, Robinson RF, Yee J: Fatal adrenal cortical insufficiency precipitated by surgery during prolonged continuous cortisone treatment. *Ann Intern Med* 39:116, 1953.
3. Salassa RM, Bennett WA, Keating FR: Postoperative adrenal cortical insufficiency: Occurrence in a patient previously treated with cortisone. *JAMA* 152:1509, 1953.
4. Slaney G, Brooke BN: Postoperative collapse due to adrenal insufficiency following cortisone therapy. *Lancet* 1:1167, 1957.

5. Hayes MA, Kushlan SD: Influence of hormonal treatment for ulcerative colitis upon the course of surgical treatment. *Gastroenterology* 30:75, 1956.

6. Harmagel EE, Kramer WG: Severe adrenocortical insufficiency following joint manipulation. *JAMA* 158:1518, 1955.

7. Robert JG: Operative collapse after corticosteroid therapy—a survey. *Surg Clin N Am* 50:363, 1970.

8. Cope CL: The adrenal cortex in internal medicine. *Br Med J* 2:847, 1966.

9. Armatruda TT Jr, Hollingsworth DR, D'Esopo ND et al: A study of the mechanism of the steroid withdrawal syndrome. Evidence for integrity of the hypothalamic-pituitary-adrenal system. *J Clin Endoc Metab* 20:239, 1960.

10. Armatruda TT Jr, Hurst MM, D'Esopo ND: Certain endocrine and metabolic facets of the steroid withdrawal syndrome. *J Clin Endoc Metab* 25:1207, 1965.

11. Ragan C: Corticotropin, cortisone, and related steroids in clinical medicine: Practical consideration. *Bull NY Acad Med* 61:1, 1964.

12. Christy NP: Iatrogenic Cushing's syndrome in the human adrenal cortex, in Christy NP (ed): *The Human Adrenal Cortex.* New York, Harper & Row, 1971, p 395.

13. Harter JG: Corticosteroids: Their physiologic use in allergic disease. *NY State J Med* 66:827, 1966.

14. Axelrod L: Glucocorticoid therapy. *Medicine* 55:39, 1976.

15. Ellul-Micallef R, Borthuricle RC, McHardy GJR: The time-course of response to prednisolone in chronic bronchial asthma. *Clin Sci* 47:105, 1974.

16. Thoren L: General metabolic response to trauma including pain influence. *Acta Anaesth Scand* 55(suppl):9, 1974.

17. Haugen HN, Brinde-Johnsen T: The adrenal response to surgical trauma. *Acta Chir Scand* 357(suppl):100, 1966.

18. Plumpton FS, Besser GU: The adrenocortical response to surgery and insulin-induced hypoglycemia in corticosteroid-treated and normal subjects. *Br J Surg* 55:857, 1968.

19. Kehlet H, Binder C: Value of an ACTH test in assessing hypothalamic-pituitary-adrenocortical function in glucocorticoid-treated patients. *Br Med J* 1:147, 1973.

20. Lush D, Thorpe NN, Richardson DJ et al: The effect of epidural analgesia on the adrenocortical response to surgery. *Br J Anaesth* 44:1169, 1972.

21. Wise L, Margraf HW, Ballinger WF: A new concept on the pre- and postoperative regulation of cortisol secretion. *Surgery* 72:290, 1972.

22. Ichikawa Y, Kawagoe M, Nishikai M et al: Plasma corticotropin (ACTH), growth hormone (GH), and 11-OHCS (hydroxycorticosteroid) response to surgery. *J Lab Clin Med* 78:882, 1971.

23. Wise L, Margraf H, Ballinger WF: The effect of surgical trauma on the excretion and conjugation pattern of 17-ketosteroids. *Surgery* 71:625, 1972.

24. Gill GV, Prudhoe K, Cook DB et al: Effect of surgical trauma on plasma concentrations of cyclic AMP and cortisol. *Br J Surg* 62:441, 1975.

25. Hime DH, Bell CC, Barker F: Direct measurement of adrenal secretion during operative trauma and convalescence. *Surgery* 52:174, 1962.

26. Greer MA, Allen CF, Gibbs FB et al: Pathways at the hypothalamic levels through which traumatic stress activates ACTH secretion. *Endocrinology* 86:1404, 1970.

27. Witorsch RN, Brodish A: Evidence for acute ACTH release by extrahypothalamic mechanisms. *Endocrinology* 90:1160, 1972.

28. Blichert-Toft M, Hippe E, Kaalund-Jensen H: Adrenal cortical function as reflected by the plasma hydrocortisone and urinary 17-ketogenic steroids in relation to surgery in elderly patients. *Acta Chir Scand* 133:591, 1967.

29. Speckart PF, Nicoloff JT, Bethune JE: Screening for adrenocortical insufficiency with cosyntropin (synthetic ACTH). *Arch Intern Med* 128:761, 1971.

30. Spark RF: Simplified assessment of pituitary-adrenal reserve: Measurement of serum 11-deoxycortisol and cortisol after metyrapone. *Ann Intern Med* 75:717, 1971.

31. Jasani MK, Freeman PA, Boyle JA et al: Studies of the rise in plasma 11-hydroxycorticosteroids (11-OHCS) in corticosteroid-treated patients with rheumatoid arthritis during surgery: Correlations with the functional integrity of the hypothalamo-pituitary-adrenal axis. *Q J Med* 37:407, 1968.

32. Sampson PA, Brooke BN, Winstone NE: Biochemical confirmation of collapse due to adrenal failure. *Lancet* 1:1377, 1961.

33. Sampson PA, Winstone NE, Brooke BN: Adrenal function in surgical patients after steroid therapy. *Lancet* 2:322, 1962.

34. Danowski TS, Bonessi JV, Sabeh A et al: Probabilities of pituitary adrenal responsiveness after steroid therapy. *Ann Intern Med* 61:11, 1964.

35. Graber AL, Ney RI, Nicholson WE et al: Natural history of pituitary-adrenal recovery following long-term suppression with corticosteroids. *J Clin Endoc Metab* 25:11, 1965.

36. Livanou T, Ferriman D, James VHT: Recovery of hypothalamo-pituitary-adrenal function after corticosteroid therapy. *Lancet* 2:856, 1957.

37. Streck W, Lockwood DH: Pituitary-adrenal recovery following short-term suppression with corticosteroids. *Am J Med* 66:910, 1979.

38. Munro DD, Feiwel M, James VHT: The influence of topical corticosteroids on hypothalamic-pituitary-adrenal function, in Jadassohn W, Schirren CF (eds): *XII Conpressus Internationalis Dermatologiae.* Berlin, Springer Verlag, 1967, p 94.

39. Scoggins RB, Kliman B: Percutaneous absorption of corticosteroids: Systemic effects. *N Engl J Med* 273:832, 1965.

40. Feiwel M, James VHT, Barnett ES: Effect of potent topical steroids on plasma-cortisol levels of infants and children with eczema. *Lancet* 2:485, 1969.

41. Czarny D, Brostoff J: Effect of intranasal beta-methesone-17-valerate on perennial rhinitis and adrenal function. *Lancet* 1:189, 1968.

42. Harter JG, Reddy WJ, Thorn GW: Studies on an intermittent corticosteroid dosage regimen. *N Engl J Med* 269:591, 1963.

43. Ackerman GL, Nolan CM: Adrenocortical responsiveness after alternate-day corticosteroid therapy. *N Engl J Med* 278:405, 1968.

44. Jasani MK, Boyle JA, Dick WC et al: Corticosteroid-induced hypothalamo-pituitary-adrenal axis suppression: Prospective study using two regimens of corticosteroid therapy. *Ann Rheum Dis* 27:352, 1968.

45. Rabhan NB: Pituitary-adrenal suppression and Cushing's syndrome after intermittent dexamethasone therapy. *Ann Intern Med* 69:1141, 1968.

46. Martin MM, Gaboardi F, Podolsky S et al: Intermittent steroid therapy. *N Engl J Med* 279:273, 1968.

47. Malone DN, Brant IWV, Percy-Robb IW: Hypothalamus-pituitary-adrenal function in asthmatic patients receiving long-term corticosteroid therapy. *Lancet* 1:733, 1970.

48. Grant SP, Forsham PH, DiRaimondo VC: Suppression of 17-hydroxycorticosteroids in plasma and urine by single and divided doses of triamcinolone. *N Engl J Med* 273:1115, 1965.

49. Nichols T, Nugent CA, Tyler FH: Diurnal variation in suppression of adrenal function by glucocorticoids. *J Clin Endoc Metab* 25:343, 1965.

50. Carter ME, James VHT: Pituitary-adrenal response to surgical stress in patients receiving corticotrophin treatment. *Lancet* 2:328, 1970.

51. Reding R: Surgery in patients on long-term steroid therapy: A tentative model for risk assessment. *Br J Surg* 77:1175, 1990.

52. Paris J: Pituitary-adrenal suppression after protracted administration of adrenal cortical hormones. *Proc Mayo Clin* 36:305, 1961.

53. Olin R: When should you consider a cortisone prep? *Med Time* 100:64, 1972.

54. Byyny RL: Preventing adrenal insufficiency during surgery. *Postgrad Med* 67:219, 1980.

55. Symreng T et al: Physiological cortisol substitution of long-term steroid-treated patients undergoing major surgery. *Br J Anaesth* 53:949, 1981.

56. Solem JH, Lund I: Surgery in patients treated with cortisone or cortisone-like steroids: A 10-year study. *J Oslo City Hosp* 19:3, 1969.

57. Ernest I, Ekman H: Adrenalectomy in Cushing's disease; a long-term follow-up. *Acta Endocrinol* 160(suppl):3, 1972.

58. Baker BL, Whitaker WL: Interference with wound healing by the local action of adrenocortical steroids. Endocrinology. 46:544, 1950.

59. Howes EL, Plotz CM, Blunt JW et al: Retardation of wound healing by cortisone. *Surgery* 28:177, 1950.

60. Ehrlich HP, Hunt TK: Effects of cortisone and vitamin A on wound healing. *Ann Surg* 167:324, 1968.

61. Sandberg N: Time relationship between administration of cortisone and wound healing in rats. *Acta Chir Scand* 27:446, 1964.

62. Stern SF, Shuman A: The effect of locally administered corticosteroids (soluble and insoluble) on the healing times of surgically induced wounds in guinea pigs. *J Am Pod Assoc* 63:374, 1973.

63. Vogel HG: Tensile strength of skin wounds in rats after treatment with corticosteroids. *Acta Endocrinol* 64:295, 1970.

64. Oxlund H, Fogdestam I, Viidik A: The influence of cortisol on wound healing of the skin and distant connective tissue response. *Surg Gynecol Obstet* 148:876, 1979.

65. Winstone NE, Brooke BN: Effects of steroid treatment on patients undergoing operation. *Lancet* 1:973, 1961.

66. Engquist A, Backer OG, Jarnum S: Incidence of postoperative complications in patients subjected to surgery under steroid cover. *Acta Chir Scand* 140:343, 1974.

67. Kaalund-Jensen J, Elb S: Pre- og postoperative komplikationer hos kortikosteroid-behandlede patienter. *Nord Med* 76:975, 1966.

68. Oh SH, Patterson S: Surgery in corticosteroid-dependent asthmatics. *J Allergy Clin Immunol* 53:345, 1974.

69. Walbourn RB, Montgomery DAD, Kennedy TL: The natural history of treated Cushing's syndrome. *Br J Surg* 58:1, 1971.

70. Bennett AH, Cain JP, Dluhy RC et al: Surgical treatment of adrenocortical hypoplasia: 20-year experience. *J Urol* 109:321, 1973.

71. Hradec E: Surgical treatment of hyperadrenocorticalism (Cushing's syndrome). *J Urol* 109:533, 1973.

72. Stuck AE, Minder CE, Frey FJ: Risk of infections complications in patients taking glucocorticosteroids. *Rev Inf Dis* 11:954-963, 1989.

73. David DS, Grieco MH, Cushman P: Adrenal glucocorticoids after twenty years: A review of their clinically relevant consequences. *J Chronic Dis* 22:637, 1970.

74. Fauci AS, Dale DC, Balow JF: Glucocorticoid therapy: Mechanisms of action and clinical considerations. *Ann Intern Med* 84:304, 1976.

75. Dale DC, Petersdorf RG: Corticosteroids and infectious diseases. *Med Clin North Am* 57:1277, 1973.

76. Staples PJ, Gerding DN, Decker JL et al: Incidence of infection in systemic lupus erythematosis. *Arthritis Rheum* 17:1, 1974.

77. Myerowitz RC, Mederios AA, O'Brien TF: Bacterial infection in renal homotransplant recipients: A study of 53 bacteremic episodes. *Am J Med* 53:3081, 1972.

78. Dale DC, Fauci AS, Wolff SM: Alternate-day prednisone: Leukocyte kinetics and susceptibility to infections. *N Engl J Med* 291:1154, 1974.

79. Boumpas DT, Chrousos GP, Wilder RL et al: Glucocorticoid therapy of immune related diseases: Basic and clinical correlates. *Ann Intern Med*, in press.

27 SURGERY IN THE PATIENT WITH RHEUMATOLOGIC DISEASE

Brian F. Mandell

There have been no systematic studies of preoperative assessment or postoperative complications in patients with rheumatic disorders. Management of these patients before and after elective or emergency surgery must therefore be based on largely anecdotal reports of surgical complications and internists' experiences. This chapter focuses on potential perioperative problems of rheumatic patients but excludes discussion of orthopedic surgery itself, prophylaxis against thromboembolic disease, and adrenal insufficiency from long-term steroid therapy, which are covered in other parts of this book.

Specific surgical risks and complications in patients with rheumatic disorders depend upon the underlying disease. For example, older patients with osteoarthritis undergoing surgery are comparable to similar age-matched controls unless their arthritis causes mechanical impingement on the spinal cord, nerve roots, or vascular structures. Patients with inactive systemic lupus erythematosus may have an elevated sedimentation rate or mild pancytopenia but may flare with a sudden change in their hematologic profile and require immunosuppressive treatment. On the other hand, patients with scleroderma do not characteristically exhibit these hematologic abnormalities as part of their underlying disease. Therefore, postoperative leukopenia or thrombocytopenia in these patients may more likely indicate sepsis with disseminated intravascular coagulation. A complete history of a patient's autoimmune disorder may be invaluable in the perioperative setting.

CHRONIC NONCRYSTALLINE POLYARTHRITIS

The most common inflammatory noncrystal arthropathy is rheumatoid arthritis (RA), and a large number of patients with this disorder undergo surgery each year. These patients may require joint reconstruction or tendon repair to improve functional capability or may develop cutaneous, vascular, or visceral problems that demand surgical intervention. In addition, drug therapy with nonsteroidal anti-inflammatory drugs (NSAIDs) can also create potential surgical problems due to gastrointestinal bleeding. Many of the perioperative issues in patients with ankylosing spondylitis (AS), juvenile rheumatoid arthritis (JRA), and the seronegative spondyloarthropathies with inflammatory skin or gastrointestinal disease are similar to those of patients with RA. (See Table 27–1.)

RA is a systemic disease characterized by chronic polyarthritis, predominantly of the small joints. A positive assay for rheumatoid factor in the blood or nodules on physical examination need not be present. Crystalline joint diseases should be excluded by synovial fluid analysis in patients with atypical features of the disease, including occurrence in men, asymmetric joint involvement, and seronegativity. Disease activity should be assessed before elective surgery by evaluating symptoms of joint stiffness, swelling, and fatigue. Those with mild disease activity benefit most from postoperative physical and occupational therapy. It may be helpful to use short courses of prednisone in doses of 7.5 mg per day or less to assure this. Steroid therapy is not usually otherwise required in most emergency surgery unless active visceral vasculitis is present or the patient's adrenal axis has been suppressed by past steroid use. Those with active vasculitis may also require immunosuppressive agents.

Joint-Related Issues

The cervical spine is commonly involved in RA and AS, and neck manipulation required in intubation may pose a risk in these patients. Some have recommended that all patients with RA have preoperative cervical spine x-rays, but there are no studies that assess the medical value or cost-effectiveness of obtaining them. Depending on the article cited, the cervical spine is involved with RA in 25 to 90 percent of patients.[1] Clinical and standard radiographic assessment may not always correlate, but x-rays are probably more sensitive. Newer imaging modalities like magnetic resonance imaging may increase sensitivity. Intubation may be especially difficult in patients with AS who have ankylosis on examination and x-ray.[2] In JRA radiographic findings may be present early in the course of the disease, but in RA clinically apparent cervical disease with x-ray abnormalities may not appear for years,

TABLE 27–1. Issues in Preoperative Assessment: Chronic Polyarthritis

Overall Medical Condition
   Cardiopulmonary risk in the inactive patient
Activity of Disease
   Medication changes
Intubation
   Mandibular joints
   Larynx
   Cervical spine
Pulmonary
   Fibrosis
   Risk for thromboembolism
Skin
   Nodules/fragility
   Raynaud's
   Leg ulcers
Hematologic
   Cytopenias
   Lupus anticoagulant
   Felty's syndrome
Prosthetic Joints
   Antibiotic prophylaxis
Medications
   Adrenal suppression
   Bleeding/platelet dysfunction
   Pain control while not eating
   Flare in disease
   Renal insufficiency

and then usually only in patients with seropositive joint-deforming disease.[1,3]

Surgical treatment of rheumatoid cervical disease is controversial, but is rarely necessary unless neurological signs of severe subluxation are present. Five-year postoperative survival in patients undergoing cervical spine surgery has been reported to be only 54 percent,[4] and even lower with coexistent rheumatoid lung disease. RA also involves tendons and ligaments, and cervical spine instability may be the result of ligamentous laxity resulting from inflammation. Subsequent vertebral body translocation can result in various cord, nerve root, or vascular syndromes and in atlantoaxial joint dislocation. Mild dislocation can produce neck pain and headache; severe translocation can result in central cord lesions following acute flexion or extension injury or transsection. Cervical collars do not prevent anterior subluxation of the atlas in maximal flexion.[5] Subaxial subluxation and superior migration of the odontoid process may also occur. Patients with AS and JRA often have proliferative bone growth in response to inflammation. Ligamentous calcification, apophyseal joint fusion, and ankylosis may result in an inflexible fragile spine. Neurologic syndromes that may occur include occiput and neck pain from C_2 root irritation; fluctuating paresthesias and weakness in the extremities from intermittent stretching of roots; evidence of cord compression with long tract signs, posterior column findings, and sphincter dysfunction; and decreased sensation in the first branch of the trigeminal nerve.

Since significant cervical disease in RA is not common at the outset of disease, newly diagnosed neurologically asymptomatic patients do not need preoperative spine films. It is useful to maintain all patients in a soft collar during transportation in the hospital to act as a reminder for caution, but a collar is no substitute for careful handling of the neck. Patients with peripherally destructive arthritis, neurologic symptoms, or limited neck motion should have cervical films including lateral views in gentle extension and flexion. Magnetic resonance imaging studies may provide further information but will probably not alter management.

Patients with neurologic symptoms or unstable spines on x-ray require meticulous care during induction of anesthesia. Spinal anesthesia or awake intubation may be required. Elective surgery may need to be postponed until fixation of the unstable spine is performed. The physician should be certain that a thorough preoperative neurological examination is recorded in the chart, and neurosurgical consultation may be helpful. RA patients may have neurologic deficits from nerve entrapment (e.g., median or ulnar neuropathy or tarsal tunnel syndrome) that should be identified preoperatively to avoid confusion later with myelopathy or other operative complications.

The cricoarytenoid joints uncommonly become inflamed and can cause vocal cord adduction. Symptoms include hoarseness, dysphagia, or even stridor. Traumatic intubation can exacerbate mild inflammation, and emergency tracheostomy may be needed. Symptomatic patients should be evaluated by an experienced otorhinolaryngologist before surgery,[6] especially in the setting of active articular disease. Locally injected or topical steroids may be helpful.

Temporomandibular (TM) joint dysfunction is especially common in JRA, but may also be seen in other forms of polyarthritis. This may limit mouth opening and may mandate nasotracheal intubation. Patients with amyloidosis may develop macroglossia that can interfere with intubation. Although patients with RA do not usually have lumbar spine disease, those with AS develop bony proliferation that can affect positioning for spinal anesthesia.

Pain control is important in the perioperative management of patients with rheumatoid joint disease. When aggressive physical therapy is required after joint reconstruction, inflammation and pain may slow progress. Preoperative intraarticular injections of corticosteroid into one or two active joints can avoid this problem. Narcotics ease mechanical pain but do little for the stiffness of inflammation. They may be less effective in those who are already taking them for chronic pain. NSAID's should be reinstituted early, and low-dose oral corticosteroids added to keep the patients from developing stiffness. Joints like the wrist may need splinting to avoid positioning injuries during transportation. Range-of-motion exercise should be an integral part of postoperative care even in those with minimally active polyarthritis. Passive range of motion and active joint movement using soft clay or sponges for hand gripping also decrease stiffness. Paraffin soaks may also be helpful.

Cardiopulmonary Concerns

Patients with RA or other chronic arthritides may have clinically apparent or occult pulmonary fibrosis. This usually involves the lung bases in RA, but in AS it may be apical. Nodules and cavities can occur, but isolated nodules should not be assumed to be rheumatoid without appropriate evaluation. In patients undergoing intrathoracic surgery or procedures with a high risk of pulmonary embolism, preoperative pulmonary function tests and arterial blood gas measurements may be helpful, but the criteria for ordering these tests are generally the same as for those without rheumatic disease.[7] Pleural disease is common but not usually significant. Patients with AS may have kyphosis and limitation of chest-wall expansion which mimics restrictive lung disease. These patients require postoperative incentive spirometry and breathing exercises. Those with Sjogren's syndrome may have chronic cough that can exacerbate perioperative pain. Cough suppressants, lozenges, and humidified air may be helpful.

Myocardial involvement in both RA and AS is well-documented and can occasionally cause conduction system disease and aortitis with aortic insufficiency. Requirements for antibiotic prophylaxis are the same as in other patients with valvular heart disease. Heart block is more common in patients with the HLA-B27 antigen and is may be first recognized on the preoperative electrocardiogram. Pericardial effusions on echocardiogram may be present in 40 percent of patients with RA, but these rarely cause symptoms or hemodynamic problems. Costochondritis is quite common in the chronic arthritides and SLE and may cause chest pain mimicking acute cardiac or pulmonary disease. Tenderness of the costochondral joints is present, but swelling or warmth is rare. On the other hand, costochondral disease can be dramatically exacerbated by any acute pulmonary event requiring increased ventilatory effort. Treatment of costochondritis includes narcotics, NSAID's, or local instillation of anesthetic with or without steroids. In patients bedridden with severe RA, it may be impossible to assess cardiopulmonary risk by history. Formal cardiac or pulmonary testing may be required.

Hematologic Problems

A mild anemia of chronic disease is common in rheumatologic disease. Microcytosis should prompt evaluation for iron deficiency,[8] which should not be assumed to be due to NSAID use. Thrombocytosis is common in patients with active rheumatologic disease. Profound neutropenia is seen in patients with Felty's syndrome. These patients may have recurrent leg ulcers, splenomegaly, and are prone to infection. Treatment with splenectomy is controversial, but neutropenia may respond to gold or cyclophosphamide.

Lupus anticoagulants may be present in the serum and are most often recognized when the partial thromboplastin time is prolonged. Their presence does not correlate with clinical bleeding but may be associated with thrombosis. No specific treatment is required in the absence of a history of thrombosis.

Other Disease-Related Issues

Patients with RA, JRA, and AS may run low-grade fevers with flares of their underlying disease, but, except in systemic pattern JRA or adult Still's disease, significant fever is uncommon. Fever must therefore be carefully evaluated before ascribing its presence to the underlying illness.

Despite the lack of conclusive studies, patients with prosthetic joints should receive antibiotics according to the recommendations of the American Heart Association for endocarditis prophylaxis.[9] Postoperative flares in arthritis, especially if monoarticular, may represent septic arthritis and require evaluation. Patients with RA, and especially those on immunosuppressive therapy, have an increased risk of septic arthritis.[10]

Patients with chronic inflammatory arthritis frequently undergo elective joint reconstruction, synovectomy, or semielective tendon repair following rupture due to inflammation. Emergency surgery is rarely required for complications of the underlying disease itself.

Exceptions include laparotomy for intestinal ischemia from rheumatoid or Sjogren's vasculitis and severe gastrointestinal bleeding due to NSAID therapy. Since most surgery can be planned in advance, decisions regarding postoperative anticoagulation, physical therapy, and use of NSAID's can be made preoperatively.

Perioperative Management of Medications

Most patients with rheumatoid disease require ongoing therapy with NSAID's. These cause some degree of gastric irritation, but even parenteral or rectal administration can lead to gastric erosion,[11] presumably because of systemic inhibition of gastric prostaglandin synthesis. All NSAID's except nonacetylated salicylate interfere with platelet function and may prolong the bleeding time. Aspirin irreversibly acetylates cyclo-oxygenase, but NSAID inhibition is reversible.

Limited studies have not documented a dramatically increased risk of surgical bleeding with these agents.[12] However, it is not unreasonable to withhold NSAID's for several days and aspirin for at least a week before surgery, especially in intraocular, neurosurgical, or some vascular procedures. There are isolated reports of unexpected bleeding in patients on NSAID's, and increased bloody drainage after coronary artery bypass surgery has been seen in patients treated with aspirin.[13-16] NSAID's can be restarted as soon as the patient is eating. If this is not possible, low-dose parenteral steroid equivalent to 7.5 mg or less of prednisone daily or rectal acetaminophen can be used. It is unclear whether or not noncemented joint prostheses bleed more frequently if the patient is taking NSAID's.

NSAID's can also cause renal insufficiency by altering renal blood flow and glomerular filtration rate or by producing allergic nephritis and glomerulonephritis. The former is more common in patients with compromised renal perfusion or underlying renal disease. NSAID's can also produce or exacerbate hyperkalemia by causing a type IV renal tubular acidosis.

Often patients with chronic diseases like RA, especially if treated with corticosteroids, will experience poor wound healing and skin breakdown. Those patients with longstanding RA who have fragile skin may benefit from external padding over prominent bones or nodules that may otherwise be traumatized and superinfected. Heels, occiput, sacrum, and olecranons should be carefully examined. However, in a controlled study of 100 RA patients undergoing orthopedic procedures, there was only a minimal increase in failure of surgical wound healing by primary intention and no significant difference in infection rate or time required for healing.[17] Patients treated with corticosteroids for more than three years, regardless of daily dose, had only slightly more difficulty with healing. The use of "stress" dose steroids in such patients is fully discussed in Chapter 26.

New therapy for underlying disease should not be started in the perioperative period except for occasional use of low-dose steroids for flares of inflammation. Patients on stable doses of weekly or monthly gold injections can receive their regular dose on schedule. Increasing the dose in the perioperative period and risking a complication is unwise. Hydroxychloroquine can be given as long as the patient is eating, and missing several doses usually does not cause problems. Some feel that penicillamine should be withheld for about a week before and after surgery to prevent effects of the drug on collagen synthesis and wound healing. Unless necessary to treat life-threatening systemic vasculitis, azathioprine, cyclophosphamide, and methotrexate should probably be withheld after surgery to avoid accumulation of toxic metabolites in the setting of acute renal failure. Methotrexate has also been associated with an increased risk of perioperative infections,[18] but this has not been confirmed.

CRYSTALLINE ARTHROPATHY

Attacks of urate and calcium pyrophosphate crystalline arthritis commonly occur in the perioperative period. Gouty arthritis can be precipitated by acute changes either up or down in serum uric acid levels. Many factors affect uric acid levels during hospitalization (see Table 27–2).[19] Patients with recent attacks are more prone to recurrence because of variation in these levels induced by often unavoidable changes in hypouricemic therapy and volume status after surgery.

Drugs commonly used for prophylaxis include NSAID's, allopurinol, and colchicine. These can be withheld before surgery and resumed when the patient is eating. Acute attacks in those with new onset gout or in those who have not had a recent attack can be treated with oral agents or intravenous colchicine. Patients with recent or polyarticular attacks should receive ongoing prophylactic therapy with intravenous colchicine in the perioperative period.

Intravenous colchicine requires a carefully inserted peripheral catheter to avoid irritation to soft tissues. Given parenterally, it causes no diarrhea, is not ulcerogenic, and has no adverse effects on platelets. In patients with renal or liver dysfunction, toxic intracellular levels can cause marrow suppression and even multiorgan failure without warning.[20] Intravenous prophylactic doses should not exceed 0.5 mg daily for a short time if renal and hepatic function are normal. In the presence of hepatic or renal dysfunction, it is safer to withhold prophylactic therapy and treat an acute attack if it occurs. Use of intravenous therapy following chronic oral therapy may be dangerous.

For acute gout or pseudogout, an initial intravenous dose of two mg can be given followed by another one mg in 8 to 12 hours. No more than four mg, including both oral and intravenous forms, should be given in any 48-hour period, and frequent boluses should be avoided. Colchicine, although not a general antipyretic, will treat the fever of crystalline arthritis.[21] If the patient does not respond, it is unlikely that additional doses will be successful.

Other treatment options include narcotics for pain relief and corticosteroids. Steroids can be administered systemically for several days to treat polyarticular attacks or may be injected into the joint in monoarticular attacks, if infection has been excluded.

TABLE 27–2. Perioperative Factors Influencing Serum Uric Acid Levels

Volume Status
Renal Failure
Organic Acids
Intravenous Dye Studies
Drugs (Addition or withdrawal)
Allopurinol
Parenteral nitroglycerin
Salicylates
Diuretics (except aldactone)
Alcohol
Cyclosporine

Hypouricemic therapy should not be started in the setting of acute gouty arthritis, but patients on chronic allopurinol should resume the drug as soon as possible. Sometimes arthrocentesis alone is sufficient to relieve symptoms of acute crystal-induced arthritis. When diagnostic arthrocentesis is performed, the joint should be drained as much as possible. Rectal suppositories of indomethacin can be used, but the risk of gastric erosion is not eliminated.[11] There are few data on the use of the parenteral NSAID ketorolac in this setting.

OSTEOARTHRITIS

Osteoarthritis (OA) is a disease of older patients. Younger patients without a history of trauma who have clinical and radiologic features of the disease should be screened for superimposed crystal disease and other disorders like hemochromatosis, avascular necrosis, Paget's disease, Wilson's disease, and hemoglobinopathies. Some patients require reconstructive joint surgery, but most patients with OA undergo surgery for unrelated reasons. Postoperative flares are usually manifested by back pain after prolonged immobility. Pain can usually be managed with acetaminophen and local measures, including heating pads, mattress cushions, and collars or back corsets.

OA can affect the entire spine, but radiographic findings are more common than clinical symptoms. OA of the spine can lead to nerve root entrapment and spinal stenosis. The latter can cause pseudoclaudication that may be confused with vascular insufficiency. New-onset severe back pain in elderly patients should be viewed with concern for malignancy or infection even if radiographic findings suggest OA or vertebral compression from osteoporosis. These issues should be considered prior to performing elective surgery.

NSAID's can be withheld in the perioperative period. Systemic corticosteroid therapy should not be used for increased postoperative pain in patients with OA. Localized pain may be due to periarticular causes like anserine bursitis. This can be treated with local extraarticular anesthetic and corticosteroid injection.

SJOGREN'S SYNDROME

Sjogren's syndrome with the sicca complex of xerophthalmia and xerostomia can occur alone or in association with underlying rheumatic illness. Patients may have multiple drug allergies, dry skin, purpura, and parotitis that may be acute and asymmetric. Sjogren's can rarely be associated with arteritis, renal tubular acidosis, pulmonary fibrosis, and pseudo- or B-cell lymphoma. Cough due to bronchial dryness and ciliary dysfunction is common and may lead to postoperative respiratory problems. Hard candy or lozenges may be helpful as oral lubricants. Anticholinergic drugs should be avoided. In patients with severe xerophthalmia, eye lubricants should be used during prolonged surgery to avoid corneal drying and abrasions.

SYSTEMIC LUPUS ERYTHEMATOSUS

Systemic lupus erythematosus (SLE) is a multisystem disorder with some complications that may require surgery. SLE itself and treatment with steroids are associated with avascular necrosis that may require joint reconstruction. Splenectomy or laparotomy to diagnose and treat intestinal infarction may rarely be required. Patients with SLE may undergo surgery because some disease manifestations such as peritonitis, pancreatitis, mesenteric ischemia, renal vein thrombosis, lupoid panniculitis, and severe Raynaud's phenomenon may mimic or represent true surgical emergencies. Elective surgery should not be performed in patients with clinically active disease and perhaps in those with acutely worsening serologic studies.

Assessment of disease activity should include questioning about fevers, fatigue, change in menses, weight loss, dysphagia, rashes, alopecia, muscular weakness, neurologic symptoms, abdominal pains, and Raynaud's phenomenon. Physical examination should include looking for asymptomatic oral and nasal ulcerations, hypertension, tachycardia, adenopathy, skin lesions, focal neurologic lesions, retinal lesions, and myopathy. Laboratory examination should include a complete blood count, protime (PT), partial thromboplastin time (PTT), platelet count, reticulocyte count (if hemolysis is suspected), urinalysis, CPK level, liver function tests, and serologies, including anti-DNA, C3 and C4 levels.

Patients may have a history of venous or arterial thrombosis due to the presence of a lupus anticoagulant with a normal or elevated PTT.[22] Such patients should be screened for antiphospholipid antibodies, and, if present, prophylactic anticoagulation measures should be taken. More commonly, a prolonged PTT prompts a search for a coagulation factor deficiency. The presence of a lupus anticoagulant, an antibody that reacts with the prothrombin activator complex, causes prolongation of the PTT. Occasionally, it will only prolong the prothrombin time (PT) or have no effect on either test.

The lupus anticoagulant has also been associated with thrombocytopenia, pulmonary artery hypertension, frequent miscarriages, and thrombotic stroke. It is virtually never associated with bleeding unless profound thrombocytopenia or an antifactor antibody is also present. Prolongation of coagulation tests mandates demonstration of the lupus anticoagulant and exclusion of a factor deficiency. The presence of a lupus anticoagulant should not interfere with surgery.[23]

Abnormal liver function tests may not always reflect liver disease. Myositis can cause elevations in ALT, AST, LDH, and aldolase levels. Measurement of CPK, while not specific for myositis, helps to distinguish muscle involvement from subclinical hepatitis.

Patients with severe active SLE should be cared for by physicians experienced with the disease, but a few guidelines may be helpful to the generalist. "Stress dose" hydrocortisone 100 mg intravenously preceding and every eight hours after surgery may be needed to avoid effects of decreased adrenal reserve. Some clinicians believe that the stress of surgery may trigger a flare of SLE and will increase the baseline dosage of corticosteroids for several weeks after surgery. Although this has not been formally studied in this setting, pregnant SLE patients managed this way had no documented increase in postpartum flares.[24]

Patients may have chronic, stable, and asymptomatic laboratory abnormalities. Leukopenia, anemia, and mild thrombocytopenia may not reflect disease activity. Mild thrombocytopenia usually does not cause bleeding, but antiplatelet drugs or overzealous anticoagulation should be avoided. Platelets should be available if needed for more serious thrombocytopenia with bleeding, but their half-life in the circulation may be reduced. If bleeding occurs with thrombocytopenia, high-dose steroids, intravenous gamma-globu-

lin, and/or danazol treatment should be considered. Aside from splenectomy, corticosteroids and immunoglobulin probably work most rapidly.

Rashes are common and need no specific preoperative attention other than to provide local care to avoid breakdown and secondary infection of vasculitic lesions. Nasal ulcers and large asymptomatic perforations should be documented before nasal intubation. Raynaud's phenomenon can be triggered by the stress of surgery and cool operating room temperatures, and care should be taken to keep the extremities warm. Raynaud's can be significant even in the absence of systemic disease activity.

Renal involvement with SLE can be asymptomatic or marked by edema from nephrosis, hypertension from nephritis, or depressed glomerular filtration. Tubular-interstitial disease may predominate, causing occult or apparent renal tubular acidosis with either low or elevated serum potassium levels. A normal creatinine level may not reflect an entirely normal glomerular filtration rate, and measuring a creatinine clearance may be useful as a baseline. Nephrotoxic drugs should be used with caution.

Cardiopulmonary disease most commonly occurs from serosal involvement with SLE. Patients with longstanding disease may have restrictive lung disease, diaphragmatic dysfunction[25] or pulmonary hypertension. Pleuritic chest pain may be due to pleuritis, pericarditis, costochondritis, or even pulmonary embolism, a concern in patients with a lupus anticoagulant. Cardiac involvement is common but often subclinical.[26] Libman-Sachs vegetative valvular disease may predispose to bacterial endocarditis. The use of antibiotic prophylaxis has not been formally studied but should be considered in view of the increased risk of developing bacterial endocarditis.[27] Heart murmurs do not correlate with the presence of lupus valvular disease.

The most common neurologic manifestations of SLE are subtle personality changes and neuropsychiatric disorders. Strokes may occur and are usually related to vascular thrombosis. Cerebral arteritis is rare. Seizures or other central nervous system events can occur abruptly, even in the absence of clinical or laboratory evidence of active disease. In cases of central nervous system flare, the cerebrospinal fluid is usually normal with occasional mild pleocytosis or protein elevation. Oligoclonal immunoglobulins may be found.

Abdominal pain occurring in patients with SLE may be due to lupoid peritonitis, pancreatitis, mesenteric ischemia, or renal vein thrombosis. Differentiation of these syndromes from other causes of severe abdominal pain may require laparotomy. The distinction is even more difficult when the patient is receiving corticosteroid therapy, which may increase the peripheral white blood cell count and blunt physical findings. Early treatment with high-dose corticosteroids has been advocated when ischemic bowel is suspected.[28] However, lack of a prompt and continued response should warrant consideration of laparoscopy or laparotomy. Salmonellosis has been reported to occur more commonly in lupus patients hospitalized in a city hospital setting and can mimic many aspects of lupus flare.[29]

Management of preoperative medications is usually straightforward. Hydroxychloroquine used to control skin and joint disease and NSAID's can be withheld until the patient can eat. Narcotics or acetaminophen can be used for control of pain. Immunosuppressives such as cyclophosphamide and azathioprine can be similarly withheld, but cyclophosphamide can be given in a monthly intravenous bolus. Corticosteroids management is discussed above. If severe visceral flares occur, steroid dose can be increased and given parenterally in a dose equivalent to one mg/kg of prednisone or higher. NSAID's have been rarely reported to cause reversible hepatitis when given to those with active flares.[30] Aseptic meningitis and a severe systemic syndrome of fever and hypotension has been described in patients with SLE taking NSAID's like ibuprofen.[31]

MYOSITIS

Patients with polymyositis (PM) rarely require surgery for disease-related problems. However, dermatomyositis in adults may be associated with a malignancy requiring surgery. Juvenile dermatomyositis commonly results in muscular calcification called myositis ossificans which occasionally requires surgical treatment. Most patients with primary myositis or myositis associated with other collagen vascular diseases undergo the same procedures as age-matched patients with these same underlying diseases without myositis. Other reasons for myositis and an elevated CPK, including hypothyroidism, drugs (e.g., lovastatin, clofibrate, and alcohol), and intramuscular injection, should be considered.

Patients with PM may develop pulmonary fibrosis or myocardial involvement reflected in conduction system disease or congestive failure, but most of their surgical risk is related to muscle disease. Patients with severe disease can have respiratory muscle compromise. They should have preoperative pulmonary function tests including arterial blood gas, maximal inspiratory force, and maximal ventilatory measurements. Pharyngeal involvement can cause dysphagia and contribute to aspiration.

Although there are no data showing that patients with active disease have a worse surgical outcome, elective surgery should probably be postponed. Muscle enzyme abnormalities may return to baseline rapidly with drug therapy, but true disease control allowing drug withdrawal without subsequent flare takes considerably longer to achieve. The MB fraction of CPK can be elevated in the serum without clinical cardiomyopathy, representing either myocarditis or inflammation of rapidly regenerating skeletal muscle. Immunosuppressive drugs like methotrexate, azathioprine, and cyclophosphamide should be withheld until renal and hematologic parameters are stable.

Steroid-treated patients should be treated with stress doses as discussed above. Steroid myopathy is a complication of long-term corticosteroid therapy. It is characterized by normal serum muscle enzymes but clinical proximal weakness indistinguishable from PM except for the fact that respiratory muscle involvement is not characteristic of steroid myopathy. Myopathy poses a difficult problem in patients undergoing joint replacement who will require postoperative physical therapy. Rehabilitation potential and formal strength testing should be evaluated before the procedure.

SCLERODERMA (SYSTEMIC SCLEROSIS)

Scleroderma (SS) is a rare disorder marked by variably progressive fibrosis of skin and lung, severe Raynaud's phenomenon, conduction system disease, pulmonary hypertension, intestinal and esophageal dysmotility, malabsorption, reflux esophagitis and aspiration, and telangiectasias of the skin and gastrointestinal tract. Life-

threatening hypertensive renal crises can develop. There are few of the inflammatory features seen in SLE.

Fibrosis of the skin can make venous access difficult. Chest-wall involvement may cause restrictive ventilatory dysfunction. Mouth opening may be limited enough to make oral intubation impossible. Raynaud's phenomenon may cause tissue necrosis, and radial artery cannulation should be avoided to prevent vascular compromise. Some have described a "visceral Raynaud's" in which exposure of the extremities to cold causes a marked rise in pulmonary artery pressure and alterations in intrarenal blood flow.[32] If pulmonary fibrosis is severe, pulmonary function tests and arterial blood gas measurement should be performed before elective surgery. Lung fibrosis may be exacerbated by repetitive gastric aspiration caused by esophageal dysmotility and lower esophageal sphincter incompetence. The head of the bed should be elevated as much as possible. Pulmonary artery hypertension may not become obvious until volume is replenished. Cardiac involvement may cause pericardial effusions, conduction system disease, pseudoinfarction patterns on electrocardiogram, and sudden death. Syncope or presyncope should be thoroughly evaluated.

Intestinal dysmotility can result in pseudoobstruction and pose a diagnostic dilemma that may require laparotomy. Decreased motility favors bacterial overgrowth and results in malabsorption. Oral medications may not be fully absorbed. Gastric or intestinal telangiectasias may cause significant bleeding.

Renal crisis in scleroderma is marked by acute hypertension and rapid development of fulminant renal failure. The urine sediment is generally benign. Aggressive control of the hypertension must be achieved rapidly.[33] Angiotensin-converting enzyme inhibitors are commonly used, but any potent antihypertensive agent may suffice. Marrow suppression from captopril may develop in renal failure. Anemia, thrombocytopenia, leukopenia, and an elevated sedimentation rate are otherwise not characteristic laboratory findings in SS, but most patients have a positive antinuclear antibody test.

Although there is no proven therapy for SS, many patients are treated with penicillamine for skin and lung disease. This drug can be withheld in the perioperative period if the patient is not eating. Calcium channel blockers are used to control Raynaud's phenomenon and hypertension, and H_2 antagonists to limit acid reflux. These drugs should be continued in parenteral form throughout the perioperative period. Potent vasodilators should be used with caution in the presence of pulmonary hypertension, and parenteral alpha-agonist or beta-antagonist use should be limited in Raynaud's phenomenon.

PAGET'S DISEASE

Patients with Paget's disease frequently require orthopedic procedures for fracture fixation or joint replacement or modification. Diphosphonate therapy should be avoided in the setting of new fractures. Since pagetic bone is extremely vascular, elective joint surgery should be preceded, if possible, by several weeks of therapy with calcitonin or diphosphonates to limit blood loss and the risk of hypercalcemia and overly vigorous bone growth. A full medical, neurologic, and physical therapy evaluation should precede surgery.

ACUTE ARTHRITIS IN THE POSTOPERATIVE PERIOD

Acute arthritis may occur in the postoperative setting. It may be clinically apparent or present as unexplained fever or immobility in intubated or otherwise uncommunicative patients (see Fig. 27–1). Few nonorthopedic procedures predispose patients to arthritis, although jejunoileal bypass for morbid obesity is associated with a sterile immune complex–mediated arthritis.[34] Parathyroidectomy may precipitate pseudogout and, as discussed above, any surgery may spark an attack of acute gout. Septic arthritis can develop after bacteremias from any source. Acute oligo- or polyarticular arthritis is more likely to be crystal-induced than infectious, but clear-cut diagnosis is essential.[35] The presence or absence of leukocytosis or fever does not distinguish crystalline disease from septic arthritis.[36] Septic arthritis requires prompt and often repetitive joint drainage[37] as well as systemic antibiotics to avoid loss of function. Radiographic studies are useless in diagnosing acute septic arthritis.

The presence of an acute joint effusion mandates arthrocentesis and fluid examination for cell count, crystal analysis, and culture. Cultures may be affected by preoperative antibiotics and should be allowed to incubate for a longer period of time. Gram stains are sometimes positive[36] and can be diagnostic. If the fluid contains more than 5000 white blood cells and 85% neutrophils with no crystals, parenteral antibiotics that cover staphylococcus should be considered. Gram-negative coverage is necessary if the genitourinary or gastrointestinal tract has been manipulated, if the patient is on hemodialysis, or if a central line is in place. Methicillin-resistant staphylococcus requires vancomycin. Intra-articular antibiotics are not needed. If crystals are seen, treatment for crystalline disease as described above is sufficient, even in the presence of fever or leukocytosis. Measurement of serum uric acid levels or erythrocyte sedimentation rate does not distinguish between septic and crystalline arthritis. Other less common forms of arthritis in the perioperative setting are shown in Fig. 27–1. Septic arthritis should be excluded in all patients with a monoarticular flare in the postoperative period.

Infections in prosthetic joints can lead to loss of the prosthesis and joint function and result in chronic osteomyelitis. Approximately 50 percent of such infections occur within one year of joint replacement. The most common bacterial agent in both early and late infection is *S. epidermidis*,[38] suggesting contamination at the time of surgery. Reoperations on prosthetic joints can introduce infection more often in the knees than the hips. Septic arthritis of native or prosthetic joints can present with pain without fever, leukocytosis, or abnormal radiographic and nuclear imaging studies. Arthrocentesis and appropriate cultures should be performed whenever infection is suspected. Arthroscopy can be followed by an acute inflammatory, noninflammatory, or hemorrhagic synovial reaction characterized by pain and effusion that can confuse diagnosis.

SUMMARY

1. Patients with chronic noncrystalline polyarthritis undergoing surgery require careful evaluation to assess activity of their joint disease, specific systemic manifestations related to other organ systems, and medication-related problems.

2. Such patients may require low doses of steroids to control disease activity or larger stress doses if they have been on significant doses of steroids in the year preceding surgery. NSAID's should be avoided in the perioperative period to minimize gastrointestinal, hematologic, and renal side effects. New therapy for underlying polyarthritis should not be instituted in the perioperative period. Those already on immunosuppressive agents deserve careful surveillance for infection.

3. Acute gout is common in the perioperative period and can be precipitated by a variety of factors listed in Table 27–2. It should be confirmed by arthrocentesis and synovial fluid analysis and treated with intravenous colchicine or steroids if oral therapy is not possible.

4. Perioperative flares of osteoarthritis are usually manifested by back pain after prolonged immobility. After excluding other causes, osteoarthritic flares can be managed with analgesics and local measures.

5. In patients with Sjogren's disease, xerostomia and cough due to bronchial dryness can be eased with lozenges. Xerophthalmia should be treated with eye lubricants. Anticholinergic use should be limited.

6. Systemic lupus erythematosus (SLE), polymyositis, and scleroderma are multisystem disorders with manifestations that may require surgery, mimic surgical conditions, or complicate the surgical course. Patients with complicated disease are best managed in conjunction with rheumatologic consultants.

7. Patients with active Paget's disease should be treated with calcitonin or diphosphonates for several weeks before joint surgery to reduce the vascularity of the bone and limit blood loss, hypercalcemia, and overly vigorous bony regrowth. Diphosphonates should be avoided in patients with acute fractures.

8. The development of acute arthritis in the perioperative period mandates arthrocentesis and analysis of the synovial fluid. Crystalline arthritis is most common, but septic arthritis must be

FIGURE 27–1. Evaluation of New-Onset Arthritis in the Postoperative Patient

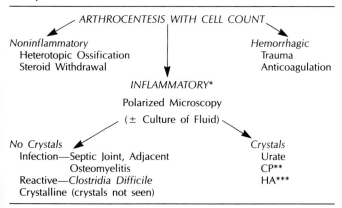

ARTHROCENTESIS WITH CELL COUNT

Noninflammatory
Heterotopic Ossification
Steroid Withdrawal

Hemorrhagic
Trauma
Anticoagulation

INFLAMMATORY*
Polarized Microscopy
(± Culture of Fluid)

No Crystals
Infection—Septic Joint, Adjacent
            Osteomyelitis
Reactive—*Clostridia Difficile*
Crystalline (crystals not seen)

Crystals
Urate
CP**
HA***

*> 85% PMNs; All may be associated with fever
**CP: Calcium pyrophosphate
***HA: Hydroxyapatite

excluded with appropriate cultures, especially in patients with prosthetic joints and in those on immunosuppressive therapy.

REFERENCES

1. Bland JH: Rheumatoid arthritis of the cervical spine. *J Rheumatol* 3:319–341, 1974.
2. Sinclair JR, Mason RA: Ankylosing spondylitis: The case for awake intubation. *Anesthesia* 39:3–10, 1984.
3. Winfield J, Cooke D, Brook AS et al: A prospective study of the radiological changes in the cervical spine in early rheumatoid disease. *Ann Rheum Dis* 40:109–114, 1981.
4. Saway PA, Blackburn WD, Halla JT et al: Clinical characteristics affecting survival in patients with rheumatoid arthritis undergoing cervical spine surgery: A controlled study. *J Rheumatol* 16:890–896, 1989.
5. Althoff BO, Goldie IF: Cervical collars in rheumatoid atlanto-axial subluxation: A radiographic comparison. *Ann Rheum Dis* 39:485–489, 1980.
6. Bridger MWM, Jahn AF, Nostrand AWP: Laryngeal rheumatoid arthritis. Laryngoscope 90:296–303, 1980.
7. Zibrak JD, O'Donnell CR, Marton K: Indications for pulmonary function testing. *Ann Int Med* 112:763–771, 1990.
8. Mandell BF: Laboratory findings in rheumatoid arthritis, in Schumacher HR, Gall EP (Eds): *Rheumatoid Arthritis*. Philadelphia, Lippincott, 1988, pp 2.1–2.12.
9. Blackburn WD, Alarcon GS: Prosthetic joint infections. A role for prophylaxis. *Arth Rheum* 34:110–117, 1991.
10. Goldenberg DL: Infectious arthritis complicating rheumatoid arthritis and other chronic rheumatic disorders. *Arth Rheum* 32:496–502, 1989.
11. Hansen TM, Matzen P, Madsen P: Endoscopic evaluation of the effect of indomethacin capsules and suppositories on the gastric mucosa in rheumatic patients. *J Rheumatol* 11:484–487, 1984.
12. Amrein PC, Ellman L, Harris WH: Aspirin-induced prolongation of bleeding time and perioperative blood loss. *JAMA* 245:1825–1828, 1981.
13. Paris GL, Waltuch GF: Salicylate-induced bleeding problem in ophthalmic plastic surgery. *Ophthalmic Surg* 13:627–629, 1982.
14. Stage J, Jensen JH, Bonding P: Posttonsillectomy hemorrhage and analgesics. *Clin Otolaryngol* 13:201–204, 1988.
15. Ferraris VA, Ferraris SP, Lough FC et al: Preoperative aspirin ingestion increases operative blood loss after coronary artery bypass grafting. *Ann Thorac Surg* 45:71–74, 1988.
16. Merriman E, Bell W, Long DH: Surgical postoperative bleeding associated with aspirin ingestion. *J Neurosurg* 50:682–684, 1979.
17. Garner RW, Mowat AG, Hazleman BL: Wound healing after operations on patients with rheumatoid arthritis. *J Bone Joint Surg* 55B:134–144, 1973.
18. Bridges SL, Lopez-Mendez A, Han KH et al: Should methotrexate be discontinued before elective orthopedic surgery in patients with rheumatoid arthritis? *J Rheumatol* 18:984–988, 1991.
19. Beck LH: Clinical disorders of uric acid metabolism. *Med Clin N Am* 65:401–411, 1981.
20. Wallace SL, Singer JZ: Review: Systemic toxicity associated with the intravenous administration of colchicine—guidelines for use. *J Rheumatol* 15:495–499, 1988.
21. Berger RG, Levitin PM: Febrile presentation of calcium pyrophosphate dihydrate deposition disease. *J Rheumatol* 15:642–643, 1988.
22. Gastineau DA, Kazmier FJ, Nichols WL et al: Lupus anticoagulant: An analysis of the clinical and laboratory features of 219 cases. *Am J Hematol* 19:265–275, 1985.
23. Kelly JP, Thomas L, Moulder PV et al: Coronary bypass surgery in patients with circulating lupus anticoagulant. *Ann Thorac Surg* 40:261–263, 1985.
24. Lockshin MD: Pregnancy does not cause systemic lupus erythematosus to worsen. *Arth Rheum* 32:665–670, 1989.
25. Thompson PJ, Dhillon DP, Ledingham J et al: Shrinking lungs, diaphragmatic dysfunction, and systemic lupus erythematosus. *Am Rev Resp Dis* 132:926–928, 1985.
26. Mandell BF: Cardiovascular involvement in systemic lupus erythematosus. *Sem Arth Rheum* 10:655–658, 1987.
27. Lehman TJA, Palmeri ST, Hastings C et al: Bacterial endocarditis complicating systemic lupus erythematosus. *J Rheumatol* 10:655–658, 1983.
28. Zizic TM, Classen JN, Stevens MB: Acute abdominal complications of systemic lupus erythematosus and polyarteritis nodosa. *Am J Med* 73:525–531, 1982.
29. Abramson S, Kramer SB, Radin A et al: Salmonella bacteremia in systemic lupus erythematosus. *Arth Rheum* 28:75–79, 1985.
30. Seaman WE, Ishak KG, Plotz PH: Aspirin-induced hepatotoxicity in patients with systemic lupus erythematosus. *Ann Int Med* 80:1–8, 1974.
31. Mandell BF, Raps EC: Severe systemic hypersensitivity reaction to ibuprofen occurring after prolonged therapy. *Am J Med* 82:817–820, 1987.
32. Fahey P, Utell M, Condemi J et al: Raynaud's phenomenon of the lung. *Am J Med* 76:263–269, 1984.
33. Traub YM, Shapiro AP, Rodnan GP et al: Hypertension and renal failure in progressive systemic sclerosis. *Medicine* 62:335–352, 1983.
34. Clegg DO, Samuelson CO, Williams HJ et al: Articular complications of jejunoileal bypass surgery. *J Rheumatol* 7:65–70, 1980.
35. Epstein JH, Zimmerman B, Ho G: Polyarticular septic arthritis. *J Rheumatol* 13:1105–1107, 1986.
36. Goldenberg DL, Cohen AS: Acute infectious arthritis. A review of patients with nongonococcal joint infections. *Am J Med* 60:369–377, 1976.
37. Broy SB, Schmid FR: A comparison of medical drainage (needle aspiration) and surgical drainage (arthrotomy or arthroscopy) in the initial treatment of infected joints. *Clin Rheum Dis* 12:501–522, 1986.
38. Inman RD, Gallegos KV, Brause BD et al: Clinical and microbial features of prosthetic joint infection. *Am J Med* 77:47–53, 1984.

28 SURGERY IN THE PATIENT WITH HEMATOLOGIC DISEASE

Bonnie J. Goldmann

Marc J. Kahn

Patients with blood disorders commonly have superimposed illnesses requiring surgery. This chapter reviews the available data on the surgical risk and management of patients with underlying blood disorders and outlines an approach to patients with anemia, polycythemia, leukemia, leukopenia, and platelet disorders in the surgical setting. Problems of hemostasis are covered in Chapter 30.

RED BLOOD CELL DISORDERS

Anemia

It has long been accepted that anemia increases the risk of surgery and anesthesia. A survey of over 1200 hospitals in the United States revealed that 88.1 percent required patients to have a hemoglobin level of greater than 9 g/dl before elective surgery.[1] However, the hypothesis that anemia increases risk by compromising the oxygen-carrying capacity of blood is poorly supported by conflicting data in the literature. Lunn and Elwood, in a retrospective review of the association between preoperative hemoglobin levels and postoperative complications, found that men but not women with low hemoglobin levels were hospitalized longer and had more postoperative complications than average.[2] Mortality was higher in both men and women with anemia. Although the authors show a relationship between preoperative anemia and postoperative complications, they do not establish causality because anemia may be indicative of more severe underlying disease. In contrast, Rawstron found that anemia was not associated with an increased number of postoperative complications.[3] More recently, in a case-control study of 125 surgical patients refusing blood transfusion for religious reasons, preoperative hemoglobin level was a clear-cut predictor of postoperative mortality independent of other confounding variables.[4] Operative mortality was found to be inversely related to these levels. Mortality rates were also related to blood loss during the surgical procedure.

It is also thought that severe anemia reduces tolerance to anes-

thesia. Rawstron found that a 45 percent reduction in hemoglobin was required to decrease tolerance to halothane anesthesia in mice.[5] However, Cullen and Eger found that in animals a fall in hematocrit to 10 percent of normal over a period of several days did not significantly alter anesthetic requirements.[6] The applicability of these studies to humans is unknown.

Finally, anemia has been thought to adversely affect wound healing. In one prospective study, however, Heughen et al. clearly showed that mild normovolemic anemia did not compromise healing.[7] This has also been documented in iron-deficiency anemia.[8]

Despite this controversy, most physicians accept that anemia increases overall surgical risk.[9,10] However, there is less agreement regarding the lowest acceptable preoperative hemoglobin level at which risk begins to increase. A hemoglobin of 10 g/dl provides more oxygen to tissue than is needed for normal metabolic requirements.[9] Ventricular function decreases with levels of hematocrit between 24% and 31% but remains stable at levels between 32% and 42%, and coronary blood flow is maximal at a hematocrit of 32%.[11] At hemoglobin levels of 5 to 10 g/dl, blood flow to the left ventricle is evenly distributed, but at lower levels it is shunted away from the subendocardium with resultant ischemia.[12] There is some tentative evidence in dogs that anemia influences the amount of myocardium liable to necrosis.[13] Cardiac reserve is excellent when the hemoglobin level is 10 g/dl or more, but increases in cardiac output are inconsistent as hemoglobin decreases to seven g/dl.[9]

It is therefore difficult to establish clear-cut preoperative hemoglobin requirements for surgery and to determine when preoperative transfusion is necessary. The standard practice before elective surgery is to define the anemia and if possible to correct it, proceeding only when the hemoglobin concentration is 9 to 10 g/dl or higher. Possible exceptions to this rule are sickle-cell disease and anemia associated with chronic renal disease in which hemoglobin levels as low as 4 g/dl have been accepted in the perioperative setting.[9]

Although anesthesiologists[14,15] and surgeons[15,16] generally believe that a hemoglobin of less than 10 g/dl or a hematocrit of less than 30 percent requires preoperative transfusion, more emphasis is now placed on evaluating the individual patient[15,17] in order to balance benefits and risks of giving blood. In the case-control study cited above,[4] although surgical mortality was found to be related to preoperative hemoglobin concentration, the "break point" level was determined to be 8 g/dl. A patient was 16.2 times more likely to die if his preoperative hemoglobin level was less than 8 g/dl than if it was greater. Intraoperative blood loss was significantly and independently related to postoperative mortality. The authors suggested that the usually accepted requirement of 10 g/dl be reexamined and that both preoperative hemoglobin level and anticipated surgical blood loss be considered in determining the need for transfusion.[4] Alternatives to transfusion should be considered where appropriate. Pharmacologic alternatives include the use of recombinant human erythropoietin (r-HuEPO) several weeks prior to surgery to stimulate erythropoiesis for autologous donation. In addition, intraoperative blood salvage has been used to decrease the need for transfusion during and after surgery.[18]

Once the decision to transfuse has been made, it is recommended that it be done at least 24 hours before surgery. It is easier to manage fluid status and avoid volume overload at that time than immediately before or during surgery. In addition, levels of 2,3-DPG in transfused blood are low. This causes a shift to the left in the oxygen dissociation curve and decreases oxygen delivery to the tissues. More than 24 hours are necessary to replete red cell 2,3-DPG levels after significant transfusion.[19,20]

Anemia Related to Hemoglobinopathies

Sickle-cell anemia is associated with high surgical morbidity and mortality.[21] Patients with hemoglobin SS, hemoglobin SC, and hemoglobin S/beta-thalassemia have the highest risk. Those who have sickle-cell disease with persistent fetal hemoglobin or sickle trait do not share this risk, although those with sickle trait may develop symptoms when they become severely hypoxic.[22,23] Conditions that precipitate sickle-cell crisis include hypoxia, hypothermia, infarction, acidosis, and dehydration. Administration of oxygen for at least 24 to 48 hours before surgery has been recommended by some authors,[24] but others argue that it decreases erythropoietin production and reticulocytosis and may worsen the anemia.[25]

Controversy surrounds the issue of perioperative transfusion in patients with hemoglobinopathies. Although Browne recommends that elective surgery be postponed until the hemoglobin level is 8 g/dl,[26] others suggest that transfusions be avoided until it falls to 5 to 7 g/dl.[27,28] Recent reports are conflicting and suggest hemoglobin levels of 9,[29] 10,[30] or more than 11 g/dl[31,32] as appropriate.

It is still unclear what hemoglobin S concentration predicts sickling. Preoperative transfusion or partial exchange transfusion to reduce the concentration of hemoglobin S, even in patients with sickle-cell trait, is essential in open-heart, major thoracic, neurosurgical, and vascular procedures.[24,26,27] In such cases, hemoglobin S concentration should be reduced to less than 30 percent.[31,32] The logic behind this recommendation is based on the experimental work of Lessin[33] in which optimal blood flow was seen in the range of 30 to 40 percent. Vasoocclusive crises only occurred when the hemoglobin S concentration was greater than 50 percent.

Therefore, despite the finding of one study that the complication rate was higher in transfused patients,[22] perhaps because they were more seriously ill, most recommend that preoperative transfu-

sions be given to patients with sickle cell anemia before major surgery.[31,32,34] The type of transfusion—simple, serial, or partial exchange—remains controversial. Janik and Seeler reported no mortality or morbidity in a series of 35 children with sickle hemoglobinopathies undergoing 46 operative procedures who were transfused preoperatively to a hematocrit of 36 percent.[32] In another series, there was no advantage to partial exchange over simple transfusions.[31] Some suggest that transfusion or exchange transfusion be continued after surgery to maintain a hemoglobin concentration of 10 g/dl or more for about 10 weeks.

Surgical risk is not increased in patients with glucose-6-phosphate dehydrogenase (G6PD) deficiency so long as various drugs like antimalarials, sulfonamides, para-aminosalicylic acid, chloramphenicol, nitrofurantoin, prilocaine, and sodium nitroprusside are avoided.[35]

Polycythemia

Surgical patients with uncontrolled polycythemia vera have a higher risk of hemorrhage or thrombosis.[36] Wasserman and Gilbert reviewed the courses of 68 patients with polycythemia vera undergoing 81 procedures[37] and documented an increased overall complication rate of 46 percent and a mortality rate of 16 percent. Patients with hematocrit levels less than 52 percent prior to surgery experienced a morbidity rate of 28 percent and a mortality rate of five percent compared to those with uncontrolled disease in whom the rates were 79 percent and 36 percent, respectively. Patients in whom levels of hemoglobin had been controlled for four months or more before surgery did better than those in whom control had been achieved for less than four.[38]

The perioperative risk of hemorrhage or thrombosis in patients is uncertain. Since risk may vary depending on whether polycythemia is primary or secondary, it is necessary to establish a clear-cut diagnosis of polycythemia vera, secondary erythrocytosis (physiologically appropriate or inappropriate), or relative erythrocytosis. Patients with a hematocrit over 50% all have some form of polycythemia,[17] but only a hematocrit above 60% reliably predicts an abnormally high red blood cell mass.[39] Those with a hematocrit below 60% may have a normal or even low red blood cell mass. Therefore, it is important to measure the red cell mass with ^{51}Cr-labeled red blood cells to help differentiate among polycythemia vera, secondary polycythemia and relative erythrocytosis.

Polycythemia vera is a myeloproliferative disorder characterized by an increase in red blood cell mass and may be associated with thrombocytosis, leukocytosis, and splenomegaly. The increased red blood cell mass results in hypervolemia and increased blood viscosity. Increased blood viscosity leads to decreased cardiac output and peripheral blood flow, stasis and tissue hypoxia, decreased coronary blood flow, and increased coronary and peripheral resistance.[40] The increased blood viscosity predisposes patients to both thrombosis and hemorrhage.[37] Thrombocytosis is common and may exert an anticoagulant effect.[37,41] Some patients also exhibit qualitative platelet abnormalities that can lead to postoperative hemorrhage.[37]

The hematocrit should be reduced in patients with polycythemia vera before surgery. Most investigators recommend a target hematocrit below 45%.[17,42,43] In elective cases, the hematocrit can be reduced over time by phlebotomy alone.[17,43] Some believe that both phlebotomy and myelosuppressive agents should be used to control the hemoglobin level for several months before surgery.[44] In emergency surgery, phlebotomy should be performed preoperatively, and volume loss should be replaced with plasma or plasma expanders.[17,42,43] Intraoperative hemodilution may also help to lower the hematocrit.[43]

The issues of risk and perioperative management are not straightforward in patients with secondary polycythemia. Many studies have shown extensive bleeding in patients with secondary polycythemia. Both thrombosis and hemorrhage are associated with the severe secondary polycythemia seen in those with congenital heart disease.[37] However, in mild or moderate secondary polycythemia, there is no evidence of increased operative risk or need for phlebotomy.

Secondary polycythemia can be physiologically appropriate or inappropriate. In the latter case, the erythrocytosis is due to erythroid-stimulating substances elaborated by tumors (e.g., ovarian or renal cell), hypersecretion of adrenocorticoids, or kidney disease like hydronephrosis or renal cysts. In preparing such patients for elective surgery, it has been variously recommended that the hematocrit be reduced to 42 to 46%[39] or 45 to 50%[17] before surgery. In any case, the hematocrit should definitely be under 60% to prevent decreases in arterial blood flow and decrease the risk of thromboembolic complications.

In physiologically appropriate secondary polycythemia, erythrocytosis is a response to a decrease in tissue oxygenation. This is seen at high altitudes and in patients with congenital cyanotic heart disease, pulmonary disease, or hemoglobinopathies in which the hemoglobin molecule has a high affinity for oxygen. Whether or not to reduce the hematocrit in these patients is more controversial. Doing so alters the compensatory mechanism for decreased tissue oxygenation.[39] However, animal data suggest that oxygen delivery becomes impaired when the hematocrit rises above 60% because of the resulting increase in blood viscosity.[39] Management of these patients must therefore be empiric and individualized. Hematocrit levels somewhere between 50% and 60% are probably appropriate. If phlebotomy is performed, attention to volume replacement is essential.[39,43]

The perioperative management of patients with relative polycythemia is even more controversial. Patients with relative polycythemia have an elevated hematocrit that does not reflect a true increase in red blood cell mass. They may have either a high-normal red blood cell mass with a low-normal plasma volume or a normal red blood cell mass with a low plasma volume.[39] Patients with relative polycythemia have an increased risk of thromboembolic disease with a prevalence approaching 30 percent. Patients with low plasma volumes have the highest risk of these complications. The role of phlebotomy in these patients in general or in the perioperative setting is unclear.

Various reports indicate that elevated hematocrit levels, regardless of the volume of the red cell mass, predict a higher rate of surgical complications including wound healing.[16] Some of the risk may be related to abnormalities in plasma volume both before and after phlebotomy. It is therefore important that sufficient fluid replacement with colloid be given if phlebotomy is performed.[16,43]

WHITE BLOOD CELL DISORDERS

Leukemia and Leukopenia

With the advent of sophisticated supportive measures such as broad-spectrum antibiotics, platelet and granulocyte transfusions, and colony-stimulating factors, surgery has become possible in leukemic patients.[45] Such patients now live longer and experience complications of their disease and therapy that require more frequent surgery.[46] In one report of nine patients with acute myelocytic leukemia undergoing 10 major abdominal or thoracic procedures, six or 66 percent survived for more than one month.[45] In another study, 8 of 11 patients survived.[46]

Successful surgical outcome is no longer dependent on hematologic remission.[46] In a recently reported retrospective review of 23 leukemic patients undergoing elective or emergency intraabdominal procedures, the authors conclude that close observation and early surgical intervention are often required despite thrombocytopenia, granulocytopenia, or ongoing chemotherapy.[47] The overall operative mortality rate in this series was 29 percent. In chronic leukemia it was 17 percent, and in acute leukemia it was 42 percent. Although the numbers of patients were small, mortality did not correlate with hematologic diagnosis, status of the disease, or presence of thrombocytopenia or granulocytopenia. A more recent review suggests that nonemergent procedures be delayed in patients with reversible granulocytopenia until it resolves.[17]

Perioperative management of leukemic patients includes administration of specific antibiotics when infection is suspected, platelet transfusions if counts are under 50,000/mm[3] even without evidence of bleeding, and careful monitoring and correction of coagulation abnormalities.[45] The role of granulocyte transfusions is not well-defined, but they may reduce the risk of surgery in leukopenic patients. Unless below 500/mm[3], low granulocyte counts probably do not significantly affect wound healing or increase the risk of infection.[22] Bodey et al. have demonstrated a quantitative relationship between the number of circulating white blood cells and the prevalence of infection.[48] The rate of infection increases somewhat when the absolute neutrophil count falls below 1000/mm[3] but rises markedly with counts under 500/mm[3]. Granulocyte transfusions are most effective in granulocytopenic patients who do not respond to antibiotics alone.[49] Some recommend that if the marrow is hypoplastic and the granulocyte count is less than 200/mm[3], granulocyte transfusions should be given for 10 days after surgery. If the marrow is not hypoplastic, transfusions should be withheld unless complications arise.[22]

Colony-stimulating factors influence the survival, proliferation, differentiation, and functional activation of myeloid hematopoietic cells.[50] The two forms commercially available in the United States are granulocyte colony-stimulating factor (G-CSF) and granulocyte-macrophage colony stimulating factor (GM-CSF). Their primary role is to accelerate neutrophil recovery after cytotoxic chemotherapy, but they may also have a role in increasing granulocyte counts in disease states like cyclic neutropenia,[51] myelodysplastic syndromes,[52] and aplastic anemia.[53] The use of colony stimulating factors in surgical patients has not been specifically studied, but they may provide an alternative to granulocyte transfusions in the perioperative period.

Because a granulocytopenic patient may not form pus, the only manifestation of infection may be fever. A significant fever of 101°F or higher should be thoroughly evaluated and treated. If no source can be found, the patient should be treated with an appropriate antibiotic combination designed to be effective against a broad spectrum of bacteria including pseudomonas.

PLATELET DISORDERS

Thrombocytopenia

Bleeding may occur with thrombocytopenia or essential thrombocytosis or when platelets are dysfunctional as in dysproteinemias, scurvy, or collagen vascular disease. Surgical bleeding is rarely a problem when the platelet count exceeds 50,000/mm³, and spontaneous bleeding usually does not occur until the count falls below 10,000/mm³. However, the risk of bleeding at a particular count may be greater in patients with sepsis or in those taking certain antibiotics that affect platelet function.[54] These include the penicillins, especially those that are semisynthetic.

The etiology of thrombocytopenia dictates management. In the patient with nonimmune-mediated thrombocytopenia requiring surgery, platelet transfusions with platelets that are not matched for HLA antigens can be administered preoperatively to maintain a platelet count of 50,000/mm³. For central nervous system or cardiac procedures, it is desirable to have platelet counts higher than 100,000/mm³.[17] Multiple transfusions both during and after surgery may be required.[55] In elective procedures, transfusions should be given 24 hours before surgery, the bleeding time checked, and the platelet count maintained by small frequent transfusions.[22] For every desired increment of 10,000/mm³ in the platelet count, the patient requires the number of units equal to his weight in kilograms divided by 70. Transfused platelets survive approximately four days. Transplant candidates or those sensitized to random donors should receive single-donor HLA-matched platelets.[56,57]

Although often used as a predictor of bleeding in surgical patients with thrombocytopenia, the bleeding time or clotting time does not identify which patients will actually experience excessive hemorrhage during surgery.[58] Recently, data from 23 studies in the literature were compared to look for a correlation between the degree of thrombocytopenia and the bleeding time.[59] With the exception of one study,[60] the published data relating platelet count and bleeding time were broadly scattered. The authors concluded that in the individual patient it is impossible to use one of these parameters to make a precise prediction about the other.[59]

In immune-mediated thrombocytopenia, transfused platelets are destroyed rapidly and are generally ineffective in raising the platelet count or decreasing bleeding. Although not extensively studied in the surgical setting, administration of intravenous gamma globulin often results in a rapid although unsustained increase in the platelet count sufficient to decrease the risk of bleeding during invasive procedures.[61-63] If splenectomy is required in patients with this disorder, platelets need not be given preoperatively unless the count is less than 10,000/mm³. If needed, they should be given immediately before surgery and again after the splenic pedicle is clamped.[22,24] In those who require both a splenectomy and other emergency surgery, the splenectomy should be done first and platelet transfusions given thereafter before the second procedure is performed. Intravenous gamma-globulin has also been used in preparing patients for splenectomy, but the ideal temporal relation between its administration and splenectomy requires further elucidation. It is unclear whether gamma-globulin is more useful in patients who have not responded to steroids and are about to undergo splenectomy or whether it is of greater benefit after splenectomy in those without a satisfactory response.

Thrombocytosis

Platelet counts of greater than 1,000,000/mm³ are usually due to myeloproliferative disorders such as polycythemia vera, chronic myelogenous leukemia, myeloid metaplasia, or essential thrombocythemia and are associated with an increased risk of hemorrhagic and thromboembolic events. The temporary thrombocytosis seen after splenectomy, trauma, or infection is not usually associated with bleeding[64] except in myeloproliferative disorders in which postoperative thrombocytosis can lead to either hemorrhagic or thrombotic complications.[65] In the latter case, preoperative reduction in the platelet count is advisable.

It has recently been recommended that this be done only in high-risk patients, especially older patients with a history of previous bleeding, thrombotic complications, or known vascular disease.[17] In elective surgery, the platelet count can be lowered with myelosuppressive agents. In emergency situations, plateletpheresis has been successfully used to achieve levels below 1,000,000/mm³ before surgery and may be performed postoperatively for maintenance.[66]

Qualitative Platelet Disorders

Qualitative platelet disorders may or may not accompany a variety of systemic illnesses like dysproteinemias, leukemia, and uremia. They may also be caused by drugs, and aspirin, other anti-inflammatory agents, and high-dose penicillin are the most common offenders. If a platelet abnormality is suspected, a bleeding time measurement should be performed. The bleeding time can be affected by thrombocytopenia and is inversely related to the number of circulating platelets below 100,000/mm³.[67] Only rarely are more sophisticated tests of platelet function indicated. When platelet dysfunction is recognized, contributing underlying processes should be identified and treated. Platelet transfusions should be administered preoperatively and the bleeding time repeated to check for correction.[24]

Platelet transfusions are not useful in dysproteinemias or uremia. If the bleeding time is prolonged in uremia, dialysis prior to surgery has been suggested to minimize bleeding[24]. Alternatively, cryoprecipitate,[68] conjugated estrogens,[69] and 1-deamino-8-D-arginine vasopressin (DDAVP)[70] all decrease the bleeding time in uremic patients. However, only cryoprecipitate and DDAVP have been shown to decrease clinical bleeding in patients with renal failure.[68,70] The role of conjugated estrogens in the management of clinical bleeding due to uremic platelet dysfunction remains to be determined.

A single 650 mg dose of aspirin can significantly prolong the bleeding time in normal patients for as long as seven days.[24,71] Even 150 mg of acetylsalicylic acid inhibits platelet aggregation for a similar period of time.[72] However, it is unknown whether the use of acetylsalicylic acid in surgical patients constitutes a major risk for bleeding.[73] One study of platelet function in normal patients on no medications undergoing surgery documented progressive, although slight, inhibition of aggregation. The authors suggested that drugs known to cause platelet dysfunction be avoided because of their additive effect.[74]

In patients with preexisting hemostatic abnormalities like hemophilia and von Willebrand's disease, the effect of aspirin on platelets is potentiated.[75] Carbenicillin and other penicillins in high doses induce abnormal platelet aggregation lasting two to four days after the drug has been discontinued and have been associated with bleeding complications.[76] It seems prudent to avoid these agents, to monitor the bleeding time, and to postpone surgery if necessary. In emergency surgery, platelet transfusions should control perioperative bleeding.

SUMMARY

1. Anemic patients generally do not require hemoglobin levels above 10 g/dl to undergo surgery safely. The decision to transfuse anemic patients must be individualized and should include consideration of preexisting illness, the type of surgery, anticipated blood loss, and the preoperative hemoglobin level.

2. Patients with hemoglobin SS, SC, and sickle-cell beta-thalassemia have increased operative risk. Hemoglobin S concentration should be reduced to less than 30% before major surgery. During anesthesia, inhaled gas should contain at least 50% oxygen.

3. Patients with G6PD deficiency do not have increased operative risk, but drugs known to increase hemolysis should be avoided.

4. Patients with polycythemia vera are prone to thrombosis and hemorrhage. Elective surgery should be delayed until the hematocrit is less than 45% and the platelet count is less than 500,000/mm³ for several months. Before emergency surgery, the hematocrit should be reduced to 52% by phlebotomy.

5. Patients with mild or moderate secondary polycythemia do not share the risk of those with polycythemia vera.

6. Surgery should not be withheld in leukemic patients. Antibiotics, platelet transfusions, and granulocyte transfusions may be required. The role of granulocyte colony stimulating factor is not clearly established in the perioperative setting, but it may be useful in facilitating recovery of the white blood cell count and avoiding granulocyte transfusions.

7. In patients with thrombocytopenia, random-donor platelets should be administered before surgery to maintain the platelet count above 50,000/mm³. Intravenous gamma-globulin may be useful in preparing patients with immune thrombocytopenia for elective surgery or splenectomy. In the case of splenectomy, if the platelet count is less than 10,000/mm³, platelets should be given immediately before surgery and again after the splenic pedicle is clamped.

8. The bleeding time does not correlate well with decreases in the platelet count and cannot be used reliably to guide platelet transfusion therapy. However, it may be usefull in detecting a qualitative platelet disorder.

9. Patients with myeloproliferative disorders and platelet counts in excess of 1,000,000/mm³ are prone to bleeding and thrombosis. Myelosuppressive therapy should be used before elective surgery and plateletpheresis before emergency procedures.

10. Aspirin prolongs the bleeding time and should be avoided if possible in the seven to ten days before surgery.

REFERENCES

1. Kowalshyn TJ, Prager D, Young J: A review of the present status of preoperative hemoglobin requirements. *Anesth Analg* 51:75, 1972.
2. Lunn JN, Elwood PC: Anaemia and surgery. *Br Med J* 3:71, 1970.
3. Rawstron RE: Anaemia and surgery: A retrospective clinical study. *Aust NZ J Surg* 39:425, 1970.
4. Carson JL, Spence RK, Poses RM et al: Severity of anemia and operative mortality and morbidity. *Lancet* 1:727, 1988.
5. Rawstron RE: Oxygen and anemia. Their effects in mice on induction time and survival time. *Br J Anaesth* 40:214, 1968.
6. Cullen DJ, Eger EL: The effects of hypoxia and isovolemic anemia on the halothane requirements (MAC) of dogs. III: The effects of acute isovolemic anemia. *Anesthesiology* 32:46, 1970.
7. Heughen C, Grislis G, Hunt TK: The effect of anemia on wound healing. *Ann Surg* 179:163, 1974.
8. Macon WL, Aries WJ: The effect of iron deficiency anemia on wound healing. *Surgery* 69:792, 1971.
9. Rawstron RE: Preoperative hemoglobin levels. *Anaesth Intens Care* 4:179, 1976.
10. Moore F: Transcapillary refill, the unrepaired anemia and clinical hemodilution. *Surg Gynecol Obstet* 139:245, 1974.
11. Case RB, Berglund E, Sarnoff SJ: Ventricular function. VII: Changes in coronary resistance and ventricular function resulting from acutely induced anemia and the effects thereof on coronary stenosis. *Am J Med* 18:397, 1955.
12. Brazier J, Cooper N, Maloney JV et al: Acute normovolemic anemia. Effects on the adequacy and distribution of coronary blood flow. *Surg Forum* 24:203, 1973.
13. Hoffman M, Schaper W: Infarct size manipulation by alteration of hematocrit (abstract). *Am J Cardiol* 45:484, 1980.
14. Barrera M, Miletich J, Albrecht RF et al: Hemodynamic consequences of halothane anesthesia during chronic anemia. *Anesthesiology* 61:36-42, 1984.
15. Summary of National Institutes of Health Consensus Development Statement on Perioperative Red Cell Transfusion.
16. Messmer KFW: Acceptable hematocrit levels in surgical patients. *World J Surg* 11:41, 1987.
17. Fellin F, Murphy S: Hematologic problems in the preoperative patient. *Med Clin N Am* 71:477, 1987.
18. Goodnough LT, Shuck JM: Risks, options and informed consent for blood transfusion in elective surgery. *Am J Surg* 159:602–609, 1990.
19. Valtis DJ, Kennedy AL: Defective gas transport function of stored red blood cells. *Lancet* 1:119, 1954.
20. Beutler E, Wood L: The in vivo regeneration of red cell 2,3-diphosphoglycemic acid (DPG) after transfusion of stored blood. *J Lab Clin Med* 74:300, 1969.
21. Spigelman A, Warden J: Surgery in patients with sickle cell disease. *Arch Surg* 104:761, 1972.
22. Watson-Williams EJ: Hematologic and hemostatic considerations before surgery. *Med Clin N Am* 63:1178, 1978.
23. Szentpetery S, Robertson L, Lower RR: Complete repair of tetralogy associated with sickle cell anemia and G6PD deficiency. *J Thorac Cardiovasc Surg* 72:279, 1976.
24. Cooper BS, Churchill WH: Hematology, in Vandam L (ed): *To Make the Patient Ready for Anesthesia.* Reading MA, Addison-Wesley, 1980.
25. Embury SH, Garcia JF, Mohandas R et al: Effects of O_2 inhalation on endogenous erythropoietin kinetics, erythropoiesis, and properties of blood cells in sickle-cell anemia. *N Engl J Med* 311:291–295, 1984.

26. Browne RA: Anesthesia in patients with sickle cell anemia. *Brit J Anaesth* 37:181, 1965.

27. Holzman L, Finn H, Lichtman HS et al: Anesthesia in patients with sickle cell disease. *Anesth Analg Curr Res* 48:566, 1969.

28. Scarle JE: Anaesthesics in sickle cell states: A review. *Anesthesia* 28:48, 1973.

29. Warner CE: Surgical management in sicklemia. *J Nat Med Assoc* 71:457, 1979.

30. Coker NJ, Milner PF: Elective surgery in patients with sickle cell anemia. *Arch Otolaryngol* 108:574, 1982.

31. Fullerton MW, Philippart AI, Sarnaik S et al: Preoperative exchange transfusion in sickle cell anemia. *J Ped Surg* 16:297, 1987.

32. Janik J, Seeler RA: Perioperative management of children with sickle hemoglobinopathy. *J Ped Surg* 15:117, 1980.

33. Lessin LS, Kurantsin-Mills J, Klug PP et al: Determination of rheologically optimal mixtures of AS and SS erythrocytes for transfusion, in Kruckeberg WC, Eaton JW, Brewer GJ (eds): *Erythrocyte Membranes: Recent Clinical and Experimental Advances.* New York, Liss, 1978.

34. Esseltine DW, Baxter MRN, Bevan JC: Sickle cell states and the anaesthetist. *Can J Anaesth* 35:385, 1988.

35. Smith CL, Snowden SL: Anesthesia and glucose-6-phosphate dehydrogenase deficiency. A case report and review of the literature. *Anaesthesia* 42:281, 1987.

36. Barabas AP: Surgical problems associated with polycythaemia. *Br J Hosp Med* 23:289, 1980.

37. Wasserman LR, Gilbert HS: Surgical bleeding in polycythemia vera. *Ann NY Acad Sci.* 115:125, 1964.

38. Cole WH: Operability in the young and aged. *Ann Surg* 138:145, 1953.

39. Golde DW, Hocking WG, Koeffer HP et al: Polycythemia: Mechanism and management. *Ann Int Med* 95:71, 1987.

40. Kemble JVH, Hickman JA: Postoperative changes in blood viscosity and the influence of hematocrit and plasma fibrinogen. *Br J Surg* 59:629, 1972.

41. Spaet TH, Bulleic S, Melamed S: Hemorrhagic thrombocythemia: A blood coagulation disorder. *Arch Intern Med* 98:377, 1956.

42. Berkman SA: Hematologic care of the surgical patient. *Hosp Prac* 21:124DD, 1986.

43. Cundy J: Aspects of anaesthetics: The perioperative management of patients with polycythemia. *Ann Roy Coll Surg Engl* 62:470, 1980.

44. Wasserman LR, Gilbert HS: The treatment of polycythemia vera. *Semin Hematol* 13:57, 1976.

45. Bjornsson S, Yates JW, Mittelman A et al: Major surgery in acute leukemia. *Cancer* 34:1275, 1974.

46. Seligman BR, Rosmer F, Ritz ND: Major surgery in patients with acute leukemia. *Am J Surg* 124:632, 1972.

47. Vaughn EA, Key CR, Sterling WA: Intraabdominal operations in patients with leukemia. *Am J Surg* 156:51, 1988.

48. Bodey GP, Buckley M, Sathe YS et al: Quantitative relationship between circulating leukocytes and infection in patients with acute leukemia. *Ann Intern Med* 64:328, 1966.

49. Alavi JB, Root R, Djerassi I et al: A randomized clinical trial of granulocyte transfusion for infection in acute leukemia. *N Engl J Med* 296:706, 1977.

50. Lieschke GJ, Burgess AW: Granulocyte colony stimulation factor and granulocyte-macrophage colony stimulating factor. *N Engl J Med* 322:28–35, 1992.

51. Hammond WP, Price TH, Souza LM et al: Treatment of cyclic neutropenia with granulocyte-macrophage colony stimulating factor. *N Engl J Med* 320:1306–1311, 1989.

52. Negrin RS, Haeuber DH, Nagler A et al: Maintenance treatment of patients with myelodysplastic syndromes using recombinant human granulocyte colony stimulating factor. *Blood* 76:36–43, 0000.

53. Vadhan-Raj S, Beuscher S, Broxmeyer HE et al: Stimulation of myelopoiesis in patients with aplastic anemia by recombinant human granulocyte-macrophage colony stimulating factor. *N Engl J Med* 319:1628–1634, 1988.

54. Kelton JG, Ali AM: Platelet transfusions—a critical appraisal. *Clin Oncol* 2:549, 1983.

55. Bergin JJ, Zuck TF, Miller RE: Compelling splenectomy in medically compromised patients. *Ann Surg* 178:761, 1973.

56. Kahan BD, Green D, Ruder A et al: Single donor, HLA-matched platelet transfusions for thrombocytopenic patients undergoing surgery. *Surgery* 77:247, 1975.

57. McCredie KB: Platelet and granulocyte transfusion therapy. *Postgrad Med* 62:150, 1977.

58. Lind SE: The bleeding time does not predict surgical bleeding. *Blood* 77:2547–2552, 1991.

59. Rodgers RPC, Levin J: A critical reappraisal of the bleeding time. *Sem Thromb Hemost* 16(1):1–20, 1990.

60. Harker LA, Slichter SJ: The bleeding time as a screening test for evaluation of platelet function. *N Engl J Med* 287:155–159, 1972.

61. Newland AC, Minchinton RM, Treleaven JG et al: High-dose intravenous IgG in adults with autoimmune thrombocytopenia. *Lancet* 1:84, 1983.

62. Carroll CR, Noyes WD, Rossi WF et al: Intravenous immunoglobulin administration in the treatment of severe chronic and immune thrombocytopenic purpura. *Am J Med* 76:181, 1984.

63. Oral A, Nusbacher J, Hill JB et al: Intravenous gamma globulin in the treatment of chronic idiopathic thrombocytopenic purpura in adults. *Am J Med* 76:187, 1984.

64. Silver D, McGregor FH Jr: Nonmechanical causes of surgical bleeding. *Cur Probl Surg* 1:000, 1970.

65. Murphy S: Thrombocytosis and thrombocythaemia clinic. *Haemotology* 12:89, 1983.

66. Panlilio AL, Russ RF: Therapeutic plateletpheresis in thrombocythemia. *Transfusion* 19:147, 1979.

67. Harken LA, Stichter SJ: The bleeding time as a screen test for evaluation of platelet function. *N Engl J Med* 287:155, 1972.

68. Janson PA, Jubelirer SJ, Weinstein MJ et al: Treatment of the bleeding tendency in uremia with cryoprecipitate. *N Engl JK Med* 303:1318–1322, 1980.

69. Livio M, Mannucci M. Vigano G et al: Conjugated estrogens for the management of bleeding associated with renal failure. *N Engl J Med* 315:731–735, 1986.

70. Mannucci PM, Remuzzi G, Pusineri F et al: Deamino-8-D-arginine vasopressin shortens the bleeding time in uremia. *N Engl J Med* 308:8, 1983.

71. Cohen LS: Clinical pharmacology and acetylsalicylic acid. *Semin Thrombo Hemostas* 2:146, 1976.

72. O'Brien JR: Effects of salicylates on human platelets. *Lancet* 1:779, 1968.

73. Meriman E, Bell W, Conlin M, et al: Surgical postoperative bleeding associated with aspirin ingestion. Report of two cases. *J Neurosurg* 50:682, 1979.

74. Kokores JA, Economopoulos TC, Alexopoulos C et al: Platelet function test during major operation for gastrointestinal carcinoma. *Br J Surg* 64:149, 1977.

75. O'Brien JR: Aspirin haemostasis and thrombosis. *Br J Haematol* 29:524, 1975.

76. Brown CH, Natelson EH, Bradshaw M et al: The hemostatic defect produced by carbenicillin. *N Engl J Med* 291:265, 1974.

29 SURGERY IN THE PATIENT WITH CANCER

Kevin R. Fox

Although an improved understanding of the biology and natural history of cancer has modified the nature of cancer surgery, allowing for less radical procedures in many cases, about 90 percent of all cancer patients will undergo surgery at some time for cure or palliation. Approximately 75 percent of cancer patients depend upon surgical resection for cure.[1] Nearly one million new cases of cancer are diagnosed yearly in the United States, excluding non-melanomatous skin cancer and noninvasive cervical cancers. The physician therefore faces many potential problems in cancer patients undergoing surgery.

Uncomplicated cancer patients respond to operative stress in a manner no different from those without cancer.[2] The principles of general operative and anesthetic risk set forth by Dripps et al.[3,4] can be applied to the cancer population. The majority fall within ASA classes I and II with a mortality of approximately 0.01 to 0.03 percent. True operative mortality, however, varies with the type of surgery and is more difficult to predict on the basis of physical status alone. The physician must identify distant and systemic effects of cancer that affect overall functional status in order to minimize risk.

SYSTEMIC EFFECTS OF CANCER

This section discusses the variety of generalized metabolic, nutritional, and other systemic effects associated with cancer and its treatment. In each case, these effects are considered in the context of their bearing upon operative risk and perioperative management of cancer patients.

Nutritional Effects of Cancer

As many as one-third of newly hospitalized cancer patients suffer from nutritional problems severe enough to warrant preoperative intervention.[4] The incidence of malnutrition varies widely with the type of primary tumor and may exceed 80 percent in the case of pancreatic and gastric cancer.[5] This protein-calorie malnutrition has

many causes, including decreased oral intake from structural impairment, anorexia, depression, fistula formation, increased gastrointestinal losses from malabsorption, and increased nutritional requirements from increased host metabolism or host-tumor competition for nutrients.

Nutritional assessment and therapy of the cancer patient is covered more fully in Chapter 41. Although the value of parenteral nutritional support in cancer patients is unclear,[6] its use in the perioperative setting appears to be beneficial. Abundant data suggest that an intensive seven-day preoperative course of parenteral nutrition followed by continued parenteral support until adequate oral intake is possible may reduce operative mortality and morbidity and the incidence of postoperative wound infection in those with moderate-to-severe nutritional deficiency.[7,8]

Metabolic and Endocrine Effects of Cancer

Disturbances in host metabolism, endocrine function, and electrolyte homeostasis are well-recognized complications in newly diagnosed untreated cancer patients. These disturbances are paraneoplastic phenomena and can be attributed to the production of a variety of hormonal substances by the cancer (see Table 29–1). Less commonly, infiltration of an endocrine organ by tumor may cause alterations in hormone production. These phenomena may usually be documented through a careful history, physical examination, and routine laboratory screening tests. Those with relevance to the perioperative setting will be discussed.

Ectopic production of ACTH with resulting Cushing's syndrome is seen in up to 2 percent of all patients with lung cancer and up to 5.5 percent of those with small-cell lung cancer.[9,10] Less frequently, ACTH is produced by carcinoids, neural crest tumors, pheochromocytomas, and thymomas.[11] Although the syndrome is best treated by surgical extirpation of the tumor or by systemic chemotherapy, the physician is often challenged by its attendant manifestations of hypokalemia, hyperglycemia, and hypertension requiring electrolyte replacement, insulin, and antihypertensives.

Delayed wound healing or infection in the patient from cortico-

TABLE 29–1. Humoral Substances Secreted by Cancers

ACTH	Calcitonin
Vasopressin	Prolactin
Somatomedins	Somatostatin
Parathyroid hormone	Erythropoietin
Growth hormone	Pituitary hormone releasing factors
Glucagon	Prostaglandins

steroid excess is a more difficult problem. Preoperative use of inhibitors of cortisol production like mitotane or aminoglutethimide to prevent these complications is unwise, and the risk of postoperative adrenal suppression is considerable. However, meticulous attention to wound care and appropriate treatment of postoperation infections are crucial.

Hyponatremia due to inappropriate secretion of vasopressin is an uncommon manifestation of malignancy found almost exclusively in patients with small-cell carcinoma of the lung. The physician must therefore exclude other causes of hyponatremia in patients with cancer. In patients with small-cell carcinoma, central nervous system manifestations may be due to hyponatremia or metastatic disease in the brain. Focal neurological findings have been documented in patients with hyponatremia in the absence of brain metastases.[12]

Serum sodium levels may be corrected by fluid restriction in mild cases. The rate of response may be slower than in hyponatremia from other causes. Saline and diuretic therapy with furosemide can be administered in more severe cases, and hypertonic saline may be used in those who are clearly symptomatic. Demeclocycline should be reserved for cases in which the aforementioned measures are inappropriate or ineffective.[13] Chemotherapeutic treatment of the underlying malignant small-cell cancer should be undertaken before surgery is performed.

There is no absolutely safe level of serum sodium at which surgery can be performed in patients with hyponatremia due to inappropriate vasopressin secretion. However, isolated hyponatremia is not associated with increased perioperative risk if uncorrected provided that volume status is near normal.[14] In elective cases, it is prudent to aim for a serum sodium level above 135 mg/liter to ensure optimal outcome.

Hypercalcemia is more common in cancer patients and occurs in about 10 percent, of whom 15 percent have no bone metastases.[15,16] Breast cancer, nonsmall-cell lung cancer, and myeloma account for the majority of cases, but squamous-cell cancers of the head, neck, and esophagus as well as renal carcinoma can result in hypercalcemia as well. The surgical and anesthetic risks of hypercalcemia itself are unclear. However, perioperative management of hypercalcemia should include normalization of volume status with saline hydration and correction of the serum calcium level. A search for intracranial metastases should be considered in patients with neurological disturbances, particularly with breast and lung carcinomas. Dietary calcium restriction is of little value. The addition of furosemide to lower the serum calcium level is questionable and can be dangerous but may be of value in preventing or controlling fluid overload and maintaining diuresis.

Further reduction in the serum calcium level may be achieved with a variety of agents, including calcitonin (4 to 8 units/kg intramuscularly every six to eight hours), mithramycin (25 µg/kg intravenously every two days), etidronate, pamidronate, gallium

nitrate, or, in the case of myeloma, prednisone (40 to 100 mg/day). With the exception of mithramycin, which can cause myelosuppression and thrombocytopenia seven or more days after administration, these agents carry little toxicity. An optimum serum calcium level for elective surgery in cancer patients has not been defined. However, no anesthetic or postoperative risk should be expected if the corrected level is maintained below 11.5 to 12.0 mg/dl in euvolemic patients.[17,18]

Hyperuricemia may be seen in hematologic malignancies both before and after treatment and, when severe, may lead to renal insufficiency. Drugs that cause hyperuricemia should be discontinued, and adequate hydration with diuresis should be maintained. Alkalinization of the urine with oral or intravenous bicarbonate is recommended. Allopurinol should be given in doses of 300 to 900 mg/day. When hyperuricemia is accompanied by acute oliguria, ultrasonographic evaluation to look for ureteral obstruction is warranted. Hemodialysis is reserved for renal failure that cannot otherwise be reversed.

Hyperuricemia due to malignancy that is treated before surgery should be carefully monitored thereafter. Allopurinol should be reinstituted as soon as possible, and adequate intravascular volume and urine output should be maintained. The dynamics of tumor-induced hyperuricemia may cause elevation of urate levels again in a matter of days, resulting in postoperative renal failure or acute gout.[19]

Hypoglycemia is a rare complication of islet-cell tumors of the pancreas, hepatomas, and bulky sarcomas. In the perioperative setting, intravenous glucose infusions provide sensible short-term symptom control while definitive antitumor therapy is undertaken.

Adrenal insufficiency due to destruction of the gland by tumor infiltration is uncommon. Symptoms of adrenal insufficiency such as nausea, fatigue, and anorexia are nonspecific but common in cancer patients. However, these symptoms, when accompanied by orthostatic hypotension, electrolyte disturbances, and adrenal enlargement on computerized axial tomography, may indicate adrenal insufficiency requiring replacement therapy before any planned surgery.[20,21]

Hematologic Disorders in Cancer Patients

Many hematologic problems encountered in cancer patients are related to treatment. However, the untreated patient may display a variety of derangements of hematopoiesis or coagulation. Although the mainstay of urgent perioperative management is red cell transfusion, the clinician should perform a rudimentary evaluation of the anemia including the blood count, reticulocyte, test for occult blood in the stool, and examination of the peripheral blood smear.

Anemia is seen in most cancer patients at some time during their clinical course and is most commonly due to chronic disease. The anemia is usually characterized as normochromic and normocytic but can be hypochromic and microcytic in up to one-half of cases. Serum iron and transferrin levels are decreased, marrow iron stores are normal, and serum ferritin levels may be normal or elevated.

This anemia must be distinguished from iron-deficiency anemia, in which microcytosis is more pronounced, transferrin levels are elevated, and ferritin levels and marrow iron stores are decreased. Ten to fifteen percent of all cases of iron-deficiency anemia caused by blood loss are due to gastrointestinal cancer.[22] Oral iron replacement therapy is of value only in documented cases of iron deficiency. Iron will act to restore preoperative hemoglobin levels over weeks to months depending upon the severity of anemia and the degree of ongoing blood loss.

Myelophthisis due to replacement of the marrow by tumor with resulting anemia and other cytopenias causes anemia in patients with a variety of malignancies, particularly breast, lung, and prostate carcinoma. Hematologic neoplasms often involve the marrow, but the frequency of involvement is variable and the correlation with anemia is difficult to predict.[23] True myelophthisic anemia is characterized by leukoerythroblastosis, i.e., the appearance of immature white and red blood cell forms on the peripheral blood smear. In the perioperative setting, these anemias are best managed by packed red blood cell transfusion to maintain a hemoglobin of 10 g/dl or greater.

Hemolytic anemias occur occasionally in untreated cancer patients. Microangiopathic hemolysis with or without disseminated intravascular coagulation is seen most frequently in gastric and other mucin-secreting cancers. Immune hemolysis is most common in chronic lymphocytic leukemia, lymphoma, myeloma, and thymoma[24] and is rare in carcinoma. Hypersplenism as a cause of anemia is found most often in hematologic neoplasms. Pure red cell aplasia is associated with thymoma in up to 7 percent of cases.

Thrombocytopenia in the untreated patient may be caused by hypersplenism, myelophthisis, disseminated intravascular coagulation, drug effects, or immune thrombocytopenia. The latter is most commonly associated with chronic lymphocytic leukemia. Although the platelet count alone may be an inadequate predictor of hemorrhagic risk, most major surgical procedures can be performed at platelet counts of 50,000/μl or greater. When required, transfusion of six to eight units of donor platelets can be expected to raise the count by 10,000/μl per unit within one hour of transfusion. If the patient is alloimmunized or peripheral platelet destruction is ongoing, platelet transfusion will be of little value. Spontaneous hemorrhage does not usually occur until the platelet count falls below 20,000/μl. Nonemergent surgical procedures should be avoided until levels of 50,000/μl can be maintained consistently.

Thrombocytosis is a common accompaniment of many solid tumors,[25] and counts occasionally exceed 1,000,000/μl. Platelet dysfunction with counts in this range is not well understood, but preoperative measures to normalize the platelet count are not indicated routinely. However, the reactive thrombocytosis associated with malignancy must be differentiated from thrombocytosis due to chronic myeloproliferative disorders. In essential thrombocytosis, polycythemia vera, myeloid metaplasia, and chronic myelogenous leukemia, dramatic elevations in the platelet count may be associated with an intrinsic platelet defect and an increased risk of hemorrhage.

Unfortunately, the absolute level of the platelet count and the bleeding time correlate poorly with risk of hemorrhage.[26] Therefore, dramatic measures to correct either parameter rapidly before elective surgery are unwarranted in patients without a definite history of abnormal bleeding. In those with a bleeding history, thrombocytosis can be corrected with hydroxyurea, radioactive phosphorus, or alkylating agents. Those who suffer hemorrhagic complications after surgery can be managed with transfusions of normal platelets, DDAVP,[27] or plateletpheresis, although none of these measures has been systematically evaluated in the postoperative setting.

Leukocyte abnormalities become relevant in the perioperative setting when the granulocyte count is depressed by the primary disease process. This is seen in the setting of all types of hematologic neoplasms but almost never in that of solid tumors.[28] Management of the granulocytopenic patient is discussed further below.

Coagulation abnormalities, both hemorrhagic and thrombotic, are well-recognized in cancer patients. Some authors recommend routine perioperative use of prophylactic subcutaneous heparin in all patients with malignancy who have no contraindication to anticoagulation.[29] However, disseminated intravascular coagulation and subsequent bleeding may be seen in promyelocytic leukemia and prostate carcinoma. Although heparin therapy may be effective in controlling the coagulation defect in these cases, surgery should be avoided until the underlying disease is treated. Dysproteinemias in myeloma and macroglobulinemia are associated with bleeding for a variety of reasons.[30] Bleeding correlates poorly with abnormalities in prothrombin time, partial thromboplastin time, platelet count, and bleeding time. It may be a manifestation of the hyperviscosity syndrome, and signs of accompanying central nervous system, ocular, and cardiovascular disturbances may also be present. Plasmapheresis remains the mainstay of treatment for this condition if surgery is contemplated.[31]

The many hematologic abnormalities seen in the cancer patient may raise the question of the necessity of performing a bone marrow examination. A list of indications for this procedure is included in Table 29–2.

Neurological Disorders in Cancer Patients

Neurological problems may be seen in 17 percent of hospitalized cancer patients.[32] They may be due to direct structural involvement by the tumor itself in the form of brain metastases, epidural spinal cord compression, or carcinomatous meningitis. Cancer patients with symptoms or signs of neurological disease deserve neurologic evaluation because structural complications often carry a grave prognosis and may increase surgical and anesthetic risk. In some patients surgical resection of a solitary brain metastasis may be beneficial.[33] In others, surgical decompression of a spinal cord metastasis, when other therapy has failed or when a diagnosis depends upon surgical intervention, can be carried out successfully with a minimum of operative and anesthetic risk.[34,35] However, success is less likely in those with greater preoperative neurological deficit,[36] and preoperative use of corticosteroids should be considered to minimize the deficit. In patients with neurological deficits but no structural lesions, metabolic abnormalities such as hypercalcemia, hyponatremia, and hepatic encephalopathy are a common cause of neurological symptoms and signs and are usually easily detectable.

Paraneoplastic phenomena may account for unexplained neurological deficits.[37] Conditions most important in the perioperative setting are those most likely to affect neuromuscular function and

TABLE 29–2. Indications for Bone Marrow Examination

Pancytopenia
Presence of nucleated red cells in the peripheral blood
Presence of immature leukocyte forms in the peripheral blood
Areticulocytosis
Paraproteins
Unexplained anemia (including evaluation of iron stores)
Unexplained isolated leukopenia or thrombocytopenia

thereby compromise pulmonary toilet. Myasthenia gravis occurs in up to 50 percent of patients with thymoma. The Lambert-Eaton syndrome has been described in up to 6 percent of patients with small-cell lung carcinoma.[38] Dermatomyositis and polymyositis are strongly associated with cancer, particularly in men over age 50.

Patients with known malignancy exhibiting signs and symptoms of neuromuscular weakness should be evaluated preoperatively with pulmonary function testing, electromyography, and measurement of muscle enzymes. Pulmonary function can often be improved in myasthenic patients with cholinergic and immunosuppressive agents, steroids, plasmapheresis, or treatment of an accompanying thymoma. Patients with polymyositis or dermatomyositis can remit dramatically with treatment of the underlying cancer, and those with Lambert-Eaton syndrome occasionally improve with successful cancer treatment. Because of their respiratory problems, these patients should be monitored in an intensive care unit.

The interval between surgery and extubation or transfer from the intensive care unit is highly variable in patients with neuromuscular weakness due to malignancy. Measurement of inspiratory force is helpful in deciding upon extubation, and determination of vital capacity is often used to look for signs of ventilatory deterioration.[39] Sometimes patients with no known malignancy who fail to recover from the effects of neuromuscular blocking agents in a timely fashion are diagnosed with Lambert-Eaton syndrome and may develop their malignancy thereafter.[40,41]

Infectious Problems in Cancer Patients

Aggressive use of cytotoxic chemotherapy and radiation predisposes cancer patients to a broad array of infectious complications. However, those in whom a diagnosis of cancer has not been made or to whom no treatment has been given also have an increased risk of infection for a variety of reasons. These patients, when febrile, should have the same thorough fever evaluation as those without cancer. However, the physician should be aware of those situations unique to these patients.

Fever and infection may be direct local effects of tumor. Primary skin carcinomas may ulcerate and become infected with skin flora. Oropharyngeal carcinomas may do the same but are affected by a broader array of aerobic and anaerobic organisms. Obstruction of the paranasal sinuses by the tumor may result in sinusitis, otitis, or meningitis. Bronchial obstruction is common in newly diagnosed lung cancer,[42] and, when accompanied by postobstructive infection, requires urgent radiotherapy or urgent chemotherapy in the case of small-cell lung carcinoma. Antibiotic management of postobstructive pneumonia should include anaerobic coverage. Similarly, obstruction of the ureters and intestinal perforation must be considered in patients with abdominal and pelvic malignancies with unexplained fever.

The bacterial flora in untreated cancer patients with infection do not differ greatly from that of other patients. However, certain malignancies carry a risk of particular immunological defects and thus predispose to unique infections. The association between Hodgkin's disease and defects in cell-mediated immunity is well established.[43] Although other opportunistic infections are rare, these patients have a higher risk of herpes zoster. Defects in B-lymphocyte function and humoral immunity are usually present in patients with multiple myeloma and chronic lymphocytic leukemia, and predispose to infections with encapsulated organisms such as *S. pneumonia*, *H. influenza*, and *N. meningitidis*.

The management of febrile patients with neutropenia unrelated to treatment is difficult because recommendations are based largely on clinical data in patients with treatment-induced neutropenia. However, when febrile, they should be assumed to be infected until proven otherwise and managed in the same way as neutropenic patients discussed below.

Cardiopulmonary Disease in the Cancer Patient

Both the patient in whom surgery is contemplated for diagnosis of an intrathoracic mass and the patient with known cancer involvement of the heart, pleura, and mediastinum in whom surgery is planned pose difficult management issues. The patient with an undiagnosed mediastinal mass with or without superior vena caval obstruction requires careful preoperative evaluation. The fundamental question is whether or not surgery requiring endotracheal intubation actually needs to be performed. Life-threatening bronchial or tracheal obstruction or compression of a major vascular structure may arise during any phase of anesthesia and may be fatal.[44] Although asymptomatic patients share this risk, a thorough history and physical examination are essential in this situation. Symptoms of dyspnea, wheezing, or cough, particularly postural symptoms, suggest involvement of critical structures.[45] Physical signs as innocent as a systolic murmur may imply pulmonary artery obstruction, and those of facial edema and venous dilatation in the head, face, thorax, and arms suggest obstruction of the superior vena cava. A finding of increased pulsus paradoxus may point to pericardial involvement. Contrast-enhanced computerized tomography of the chest should be obtained in all patients with undiagnosed mediastinal abnormalities.[46] Flow-volume loops and echocardiography may also be helpful.

Evaluation should be directed toward seeking alternative means of diagnosis. Cervical, supraclavicular, or axillary nodes may accompany mediastinal masses in Hodgkin's disease, non-Hodgkin's lymphoma, or bronchogenic carcinoma, in which cases node biopsy under local anesthesia may confirm the diagnosis. Examination of the bone marrow by both aspiration and biopsy may disclose the presence of lymphoblastic lymphoma or, less frequently, small-cell lung carcinoma and other types of non-Hodgkin's lymphoma. Evaluation of the blood for elevated serum levels of alpha-fetoprotein and beta-human chorionic gonadotrophin aids in the diagnosis of the germ-cell cancers in the mediastinum. Thoracentesis of a pleural effusion may be a reliable means of diagnosis particularly in bronchogenic carcinoma, and sputum cytology will occasionally confirm this malignancy.[47,48] Bronchoscopy is clearly recommended in cases of suspected bronchogenic carcinoma when these less-invasive measures are unsuccessful or not feasible.

When a decision must be made between performing diagnostic mediastinoscopy or thoracotomy, or initiating emergent therapy without histologic diagnosis, the following guidelines should be considered:

1. The patency of the trachea and large airways should be evaluated with computerized tomography, plain radiographs of the trachea, and flow-volume loops.[49] The presence of airway obstruction should be considered a relative contraindication to general anesthesia.[44,50]

2. In the absence of airway obstruction, superior vena cava syndrome may not be a contraindication to surgery,[51] and in

experienced hands, mediastinoscopy can be performed with low morbidity.[52] However, the quantity of tissue obtainable by mediastinoscopy may be inadequate to diagnose Hodgkin's disease or certain non-Hodgkin's lymphomas.

3. Symptoms of airway obstruction may be relieved by corticosteroids which may reduce edema or, in the case of lymphoblastic lymphoma, exert a direct cytolytic effect on the tumor. Symptom relief from steroids alone has not been systemically studied with respect to subsequent operative risk.

4. If the institution of radiotherapy without histologic confirmation is the only recourse, subsequent biopsy of a treated tumor mass will still yield a diagnosis in many cases.[53,54]

Pericardial effusion with or without tamponade is a well-known complication of cancer and cancer therapy. However, as many as half of patients with known cancer have pericardial disease that is not malignant,[55,56] such as radiation-induced or idiopathic pericarditis. The symptoms and signs of pericardial disease in cancer patients are reviewed elsewhere[55-57] and are rarely overlooked on history and physical examination. Chest x-ray is abnormal in only 50 percent of patients, and electrocardiography is unreliable in making the diagnosis.[58] Carcinomas of the lung and breast as well as lymphoma, leukemia, and melanoma account for most cases of malignant pericardial disease. Pericardial effusion with or without tamponade is an extraordinarily uncommon presenting sign of malignancy.[59] Two-dimensional echocardiography remains the mainstay of diagnosis in pericardial disease[60] and should be performed whenever signs, symptoms, or radiographic abnormalities suggest the presence of disease.

The presence of malignant pericardial effusion is a relative contraindication to surgery and general anesthesia. Establishing a diagnosis of pericardial disease and instituting definitive management should be done in an intensive care unit. Diagnosis and treatment may range from emergency pericardiocentesis to pericardiectomy. Relief of tamponade can almost always be accomplished by pericardiocentesis or subxiphoid placement of a pericardial window, often requiring no general anesthesia and offering significant symptom relief with low morbidity.[61] Survival is poor in patients with a known cancer and malignant effusion.[55] Radical surgery, such as complete pericardiectomy, is associated with high morbidity and should be reserved for cases of radiation-induced pericardial constriction. Definitive management of pericardial disease and relief of tamponade should precede all unrelated surgery when possible.

Thoracentesis remains the mainstay of diagnosis and short-term therapy in cancer patients with pleural effusion, although reaccumulation often occurs within days.[62] Definitive therapy is best accomplished with placement of a thoracic drainage tube followed by pleurodesis or sclerosis with irritants like tetracycline. Occasional patients with breast cancer may respond to chemotherapy or hormonal therapy. Those with lymphomas frequently respond to chemotherapy or radiation to the mediastinum. Radiation is most effective in nonmalignant effusions caused by lymphatic obstruction from mediastinal disease. Surgical intervention with pleurectomy is associated with high mortality[63] and is rarely required.

Preoperative treatment of malignant pleural effusions is not always necessary, and preoperative pulmonary function tests do not necessarily predict operative risk. However, simple spirometry and blood gas measurements are recommended for patients with malignant effusions undergoing elective surgery. Those who are sympto-matic from their effusion or who fail to meet the preoperative pulmonary criteria outlined by Tisi[64] should probably undergo thoracentesis. Postoperative chest x-rays are helpful in monitoring reaccumulation and determining the need for repeat thoracentesis.

SYSTEMIC EFFECTS OF CANCER THERAPY

The cancer patient may require surgery after treatment with chemotherapy and/or radiation therapy has been administered. In some cases, indications for surgery are unrelated to the patient's cancer, while in others "neoadjuvant" chemotherapy or radiation therapy or both are given to reduce tumor bulk and to improve operability. This is seen in locally advanced cancers of the head and neck, breast, and bladder. Resection of residual disease is performed in some types of metastatic disease, as in the cases of testicular cancer and "second look" laparotomy for ovarian cancer.

The physician needs a working knowledge of chemotherapeutic agents used in cancer treatment including their acute and chronic toxicities. A detailed history of the type of drug, dosage, cumulative dose, and schedule of treatment is imperative in the patient undergoing surgery. A list of such agents appears in Table 29–3.

Chemotherapy and Anesthesia

Chemotherapy can increase anesthetic and surgical risk through its effects on immune, cardiac, pulmonary, and metabolic function.[65-67] Several chemotherapeutic agents are associated with hepatic dysfunction that is usually apparent on routine preoperative laboratory evaluation. Methotrexate can commonly cause acute transient elevations in serum transaminases that may be of no clinical significance, but daily administration over several months may lead to frank hepatic fibrosis.[68] Percutaneous liver biopsy may be required for accurate assessment of the degree of fibrosis. 6-mercaptopurine may also cause transaminase elevation and hepatocellular necrosis after months of continuous use that resolves with cessation of therapy. Streptozotocin, L-asparaginase, and cytosine arabinoside may raise serum transaminase levels. High doses of mithramycin can cause biochemical abnormalities and acute liver dysfunction. Although most cases of hepatotoxicity caused by chemotherapeutic agents are transient, patients with suspected or confirmed liver dysfunction are best treated with anesthetic agents that are not metabolized in the liver. If such drugs are needed, reduced doses should be used. Direct hepatotoxins should be avoided.[65-67]

Chemotherapeutic agents have several other noteworthy effects. Cyclophosphamide and thiotepa have been associated with decreases in serum cholinesterase activity, and prolonged apnea after the use of succinylcholine has been reported.[69] The recovery period of cholinesterase activity may be variable, and succinylcholine should therefore be used only in a properly monitored setting. Procarbazine inhibits monoamine oxidase in animals and may also do so in humans. Indirect-acting sympathomimetic drugs and tricyclic antidepressants should therefore be avoided. In addition, procarbazine may act synergistically with barbiturates and narcotics. The effects of vincristine and cis-platinum on peripheral nerve function and those of procarbazine, 5-FU, and L-asparaginase on the central nervous system demand careful preoperative evaluation. Postoperative neurological deficits might otherwise be incor-

TABLE 29–3. Chemotherapeutic Agents

Type of Drug	Generic Name	Toxicities
Alkylating agents	Cytoxan	Marrow, GI, bladder, heart
	Melphalan	Marrow, GI
	Chlorambucil	Marrow, GI
	Nitrogen mustard	Marrow, GI
	Thiotepa	Marrow, GI
	Busulfan	Marrow, GI, lung
	BCNU (carmustine)	Marrow, GI, pulmonary
	CCNU (lomustine)	
	Methyl-CCNU	
	Streptozotocin	Marrow, GI
	Dacarbazine (DTIC)	Marrow, GI, liver
Antimetabolics	Methotrexate	Marrow, GI, renal
	5-Fluorouracil	Marrow, GI, CNS
	FUDR	Marrow, GI, hepatic
	Cytarabine (Ara-C)	Marrow, hepatic, GI
	Mercaptopurine	Marrow, GI, hepatic
	Thioguanine	Marrow, GI, hepatic
Vinca alkaloids	Vincristine	Neurological, GI
	Vinblastine	Marrow, neurological
Antibiotics	Dactinomycin	Marrow, GI
	Daunorubicin	Marrow, cardiac
	Doxorubicin (Adriamycin)	Marrow, cardiac
	Bleomycin	Pulmonary, skin, fever
	Mithramycin	Hepatic, GI, marrow
	Mitomycin-C	Marrow, renal, cardiac
Miscellaneous	Procarbazine	Marrow, GI
	cis-Platinum	Renal, GI, otologic, neurologic, marrow
	Hydroxyurea	Marrow, GI
	Asparaginase	GI, fever
	Etoposide (VP-16)	Marrow, GI
Hormones	Tamoxifen	GI
	Diethylstilbestrol	GI, coagulation
	Megestrol acetate	Skin, coagulation
	Fluoxymesterone	Skin
	Prednisone	GI, skin, metabolic, CNS
	Dexamethasone	GI, skin, metabolic, CNS

rectly attributed to anesthesia or intraoperative central nervous system events.

Cancer Therapy and Wound Healing

Although some retrospective studies find no increased risk of infectious complications in previously irradiated patients undergoing abdominal surgery,[70] there are no data from controlled studies to refute the long-accepted tenet that high doses of radiation may increase operative morbidity. Surgery should therefore be delayed for five weeks or more after radiation therapy in doses above 4000 rads to avoid poor wound healing. When urgent or emergency surgery is required in a radiated field, meticulous attention to intraoperative aseptic technique, wound care, and treatment of wound infections is mandatory.

The risk of operative morbidity in patients treated with chemotherapy is more difficult to assess. Several animal studies demonstrate retarded wound and anastomotic healing in rats and mice treated perioperatively with agents like 5-FU and adriamycin.[71–73] However, data in humans is conflicting.[74,75] One retrospective study over a 10-year period in patients receiving chemotherapy within three weeks of surgery suggests that the risk of operative morbidity and mortality is not excessively high.[76] In another large

series of patients undergoing limb-salvage for bone sarcoma, the perioperative complication rate was increased when chemotherapy was given before rather than after surgery.[77] These data imply that recent chemotherapy is not necessarily a contraindication to elective surgery.

In emergency situations, the clinician should be aware of the potential hematologic toxicity of chemotherapy given before the procedure. Although such toxicity is usually transient and resolves within days to weeks, granulocytopenic patients may develop fever after surgery and should receive broad-spectrum antibiotics with expanded gram-negative coverage.

Pulmonary Toxicity

Radiation injury is dose- and field-dependent, and acute and intermediate radiation changes occurring up to nine months after treatment often resolve spontaneously. More severe injury may lead to chronic changes that appear nine months or more after therapy.[78] A minority of patients develop acute radiation pneumonitis, characterized by dyspnea, cough, and occasionally hemoptysis or fever. Most patients recover completely, but some are left with an element of chronic lung injury that stabilizes after about two years.

Preoperative evaluation of patients with a history of radiotherapy to the lung or mediastinum should include pulmonary function tests and arterial blood gases. Decreased lung volumes, impaired diffusing capacity, and decreased compliance may be present.[79,80] Surgical and anesthetic risk should be extrapolated from data on nonirradiated patients with similar defects (see Chap. 22).

Some chemotherapeutic agents cause significant pulmonary toxicity. Busulfan may cause severe alveolar and interstitial infiltration and a syndrome of cough, dyspnea, and fever months to years after therapy. Hypoxemia, restrictive lung volumes, loss of diffusing capacity, and progression to death can occur. Bleomycin lung toxicity occurs during therapy or within months of completion of treatment. Dry cough, tachypnea, and dyspnea are the earliest symptoms. Chest x-ray shows a diffuse or occasionally patchy interstitial infiltrate. Pulmonary function tests and blood gas measurements show hypoxemia, a decrease in diffusion capacity, and restrictive lung volumes. Bleomycin toxicity can occur at low cumulative doses, but risk increases substantially after cumulative doses of 450 mg have been reached, with a 10 percent incidence of death.[79] Bleomycin toxicity is more likely to occur in patients over age 60 or in those with a previous history of lung irradiation or subsequent oxygen therapy.

Increased perioperative mortality has been reported in patients treated with bleomycin and has been attributed to high concentrations of inspired oxygen or to excessive replacement of crystalloid and colloid, causing irreversible interstitial edema.[80,81] Although not all investigators support these findings,[82–86] it is recommended that inspired oxygen concentrations not exceed 30% and that a Swan-Ganz catheter be used to maintain perfusion with minimal crystalloid or colloid replacement.

Other chemotherapeutic agents, including cytoxan, nitrosoureas, methotrexate, ara-C, and procarbazine have been implicated in acute and chronic lung toxicity. Enhancement of toxicity by high concentrations of inspired oxygen has not been unequivocally demonstrated with these drugs. However, if the history, physical examination, chest x-ray, and pulmonary function tests suggest drug-induced lung toxicity, intraoperative oxygen supplementation and fluid replacement should be guided by careful monitoring.[87]

Cardiac Complications

Radiation therapy to the mediastinum may injure the pericardium and myocardium. The best-understood complication of mediastinal radiation is pericarditis. This phenomenon is dose-dependent and occurs in 5 percent of patients who have received at least 4000 rads to more than 50 percent of their heart volume.[88] Acute pericarditis typically appears within a year of therapy and may result in tamponade. Chronic pericarditis usually causes an asymptomatic pericardial effusion presenting several years after therapy. Chronic pericarditis may resolve spontaneously or may progress to constrictive pericarditis.[89]

Radiation injury to the myocardium can cause premature coronary artery disease. The overall incidence is low, but risk increases with higher doses, particularly with those delivered to an anterior field.[90] Modern radiation techniques, utilizing postero-anterior fields, probably reduce this risk.

The perioperative implications of mediastinal irradiation and its relation to heart disease are unknown. Patients with a history suggestive of myocardial ischemia who have received mediastinal irradiation should be carefully evaluated regardless of age. It may be well more than ten years before coronary artery disease appears. The electrocardiogram may be abnormal in many patients[91] but may not predict coronary or pericardial disease.

Many chemotherapeutic agents have been implicated in pericardial and myocardial toxicity, but anthracycline cardiomyopathy is the most common. The anthracyclines doxorubicin and daunorubicin cause a dose-dependent cardiomyopathy that presents as biventricular failure. Although it can occur at any cumulative dose, the incidence rises steadily with increasing cumulative doses, reaching approximately 7 percent at 550 mg/m² [92] and increasing abruptly thereafter. Congestive heart failure can develop a few weeks to several months after treatment but can also occur during therapy or years thereafter.[93] Radionuclide assessment of the left ventricular ejection fraction may show a higher incidence of cardiac dysfunction but may not predict clinical congestive failure.[94] Mediastinal irradiation, age, hypertension, and preexisting heart disease increase the risk.

The risk of anesthesia and surgery in patients who have received anthracyclines is unclear. One retrospective series documented an incidence of perioperative complications of 6.3 percent but found no correlation between complications and age, total anthracycline dose, or time interval from the last dose of anthracycline.[95] Most of the patients who experienced complications had a history of congestive heart failure or were symptomatic with congestive failure at the time of surgery.

The preoperative evaluation of patients who have received anthracyclines should include a calculation and confirmation of cumulative dose received and determination of additional cardiac risk factors. Radionuclide estimation of ejection fraction can be done but does not predict operative risk. Patients with a history of congestive failure or active failure at the time of evaluation should be treated medically with digitalis, diuretics, and/or vasodilators to improve cardiac performance.[96] These patients are candidates for intraoperative monitoring of pulmonary arterial and radial artery blood pressures.

Hematologic Effects of Cancer Therapy

Most of the chemotherapeutic agents listed in Table 29–3 cause some degree of hematologic toxicity. The depth and duration of the resulting decreases in white blood cell count, platelet count, and hematocrit are dependent on dose and dosage schedule. Most drug regimens given in cyclic combination produce predictable and reversible reductions in the granulocyte and platelet count that occur within 7 to 14 days of therapy and resolve within several days. The most intensive regimens like those used in treating acute leukemia will produce more sustained and severe suppressions of the blood counts lasting several weeks. Chronic therapy with low doses of drugs like cytoxan, melphalan, chlorambucil, busulfan, hydroxyurea, 6-mercaptopurine, or 6-thioguanine produces chronic suppression of blood counts that resolves only upon withdrawal of the drug. Several agents carry unique hematologic toxicities and require separate consideration. Mitomycin-C and nitrosoureas may produce a delayed suppression of granulocyte and platelet counts four to six weeks after therapy, and mitomycin-C has been associated with a syndrome of microangiopathic hemolytic anemia and acute renal failure. Busulfan may cause permanent bone marrow aplasia in excessive doses.

The perioperative management of drug-induced anemia or thrombocytopenia is straightforward and is covered elsewhere in this book (see Chap. 28). Granulocytopenia induced by chemotherapy rarely requires granulocyte transfusions, and such therapy should be reserved for patients with documented infections who do not respond to appropriate antimicrobial therapy, and only if spontaneous recovery in the white blood cell count is not expected to occur within a week.[97]

Although the administration of granulocyte colony stimulating factors (G-CSF) may shorten the duration of granulocytopenia in patients treated with chemotherapy, their benefit has only been clearly demonstrated when they are given before the expected drop in the white cell count.[98] The use of these factors in the perioperative setting has not been evaluated. They need not be used before elective procedures, when waiting three to four weeks after chemotherapy (or six to eight weeks in the case of nitrosoureas or mitomycin) is all that is required. When emergency surgery must be performed in patients who are significantly granulocytopenic, colony-stimulating factors may be useful in hastening white cell recovery. In this case, they should be given daily in accordance with accepted guidelines[98] until the granulocyte count recovers.

Renal, Metabolic, and Endocrine Effects

Renal toxicity is a common and usually transient effect of several chemotherapeutic agents. Cis-platinum causes dose-dependent direct toxicity to the distal tubular epithelium. This occurs from several days to two weeks after therapy and is usually reversible. Asymptomatic hypomagnesemia is common, but symptomatic tetany may occur. Careful perioperative monitoring of renal function as well as electrolytes and magnesium levels with appropriate replacement therapy is mandatory. The nitrosourea streptozotocin can cause renal tubular damage that may progress to Fanconi's syndrome.[99] High-dose methotrexate, mitomycin-C, mithramycin, and the other nitrosoureas may also cause variable degrees of renal toxicity.

Electrolyte disturbances in the absence of renal damage are seen in many treated cancer patients because of drug-induced nausea and vomiting, mucositis resulting in poor oral intake, and diarrhea or anorexic effects of systemic malignancy. High-dose cyclophosphamide may cause hyponatremia and inappropriate urinary concentration mimicking the syndrome of inappropriate antidiuretic hormone secretion.[100] Most of these disturbances will have little impact on perioperative morbidity if detected and corrected preoperatively.

Frank disruption of normal endocrine function is uncommon in cancer therapy. Patients who have received mantle radiation therapy for Hodgkin's disease will have a 10 to 20 percent incidence of hypothyroidism, and as many as half of these patients will have elevations of serum thyroid-stimulating hormone levels.[101] Patients who have received radiation therapy to the neck for treatment of squamous cancers may also have an increased risk of hypothyroidism. These abnormalities may occur many months to years after therapy, and thyroid function should be evaluated in all of these patients. Elective surgery should be postponed until appropriate replacement therapy has been given. When surgery is urgently or emergently indicated, replacement therapy with intravenous thyroxine may be given according to the guidelines in Chapter 25.

Adrenal insufficiency may result from the use of mitotane in adrenal carcinoma and aminoglutethimide in adrenal, prostate, and breast carcinoma. A cortrosyn stimulation test should be performed in patients who have received these agents to evaluate adrenal reserve and determine the need for appropriate "stress" doses of steroids in the perioperative period.

Infectious Complications of Cancer Treatment

Treated cancer patients who become febrile pose complex problems. They are susceptible to many pathogens because of the immunosuppressive effects of cancer therapy. Though fever can be due to chemotherapeutic or antimicrobial drugs, tumor necrosis, blood products, or the tumor itself, it is infectious in origin in more than 50 percent of cases.[102]

Susceptibility to infection is enhanced by granulocytopenia, defined as fewer than 500 granulocytes/mm^3, counting both polymorphonuclear leukocytes and band forms. A first step in the evaluation of a febrile cancer patient should be determination of the granulocyte count. The general evaluation is otherwise the same as in any sick hospitalized patient. However, broad-spectrum antibiotics should be given at the first sign of fever in the granulocytopenic patient after appropriate cultures are obtained.

Physical examination fails to demonstrate a cause of infection in most cases.[103] The inflammatory response is impaired in the granulocytopenic state, and subtle indications like pain, tenderness, or erythema may be the only signs of infection. Two sets of blood cultures, urine culture, chest x-ray, and cultures of any suspected sites of infection should be obtained. Special attention should be paid to the perirectal area and sites of intravenous and other indwelling catheters.

Immediate broad-spectrum antibiotic therapy is mandatory and generally includes a third-generation cephalosporin or antipseudomonas penicillin plus an aminoglycoside to maximize gram-negative bacterial coverage. Some investigators have demonstrated equivalent efficiency of single-antibiotic therapy with a third-generation cephalosporin,[103] while others have recommended the inclusion of vancomycin to cover coagulase-negative staphylococci.[104] These recommendations remain controversial, and the physician should follow institutional guidelines based on infection patterns and predominant bacterial flora in the particular hospital. Granulocytopenic patients who undergo emergency surgery may require additional coverage against gram-positive skin flora and anaerobes indigenous to the mouth and gastrointestinal tract.

In patients who defervesce with no source of infection, antibiotic therapy can be discontinued after the neutropenia has resolved. If an infectious source and pathogen are identified, a longer course of narrowed coverage is appropriate if the duration of neutropenia is short.[105] In patients with longer periods of granulocytopenia, continuation of antibiotic therapy for 14 days is recommended. A significant minority of these patients become febrile again and in most cases respond to the reinstitution of the original antibiotic.[105,106]

Granulocytopenic patients who remain febrile or who experience recurrent fever despite antibiotic therapy pose a more difficult problem. In this case, antibiotics should be continued since septic complications are frequent. Empiric antifungal therapy is recommended after four to seven days of persistent fever. More than 30 percent of these patients develop invasive fungal disease.[105] Amphoterocin B in doses of at least 0.4 mg/kg/day remains the drug of choice in these situations.

Neutropenic patients who develop pulmonary infiltrates may have localized infection due to bacteria, mycobacteria, fungi, and viruses including herpes and cytomegalovirus. More diffuse or interstitial infiltrates may be caused by legionella, mycoplasma, chlamydia, pneumocystis, toxoplasmosis, and a variety of other fungi, bacteria, and viruses. If the patient fails to respond to antibacterial and antifungal therapy or becomes clinically unstable, bronchoscopy or open-lung biopsy may be necessary.

Elective surgical procedures should be postponed in patients with granulocytopenia until it resolves. However, situations that may require emergency surgery in neutropenic patients include necrotizing enterocolitis or typhlitis, an inflammatory lesion of the cecum caused by resistant gram-negative organisms.[107] Its presentation may mimic pseudomembranous colitis caused by *C. difficile*, requiring assay of stools for bacterial toxin and therapy with oral vancomycin or metronidazole.

Sometimes patients receiving ongoing cancer therapy without neutropenia require evaluation of fever. These patients develop infections similar to those of the general population. Patients receiving corticosteroid therapy have a higher risk of pulmonary infections with mycobacteria. Those receiving steroids or aggressive combination chemotherapy may get *Pneumocystis carinii* pneumonia. Cytomegalovirus pneumonia is occasionally seen in such patients after allogenic bone marrow transplantation.

Fever in the absence of infection is a well-described paraneoplastic phenomenon. "Tumor fever" occurs in as many as 5 percent of cancer patients at some time in their clinical course. It is always a diagnosis of exclusion and should never obviate the need for thorough evaluation whether or not the cancer has been treated. Fever due to underlying malignancy should resolve after successful treatment with surgery, radiotherapy, or chemotherapy. If the tumor is uncontrolled or end-stage and no appropriate therapy is available, fever may be palliated by standard doses of nonsteroidal anti-inflammatory agents.[108,109]

ETHICAL AND PRACTICAL CONSIDERATIONS

The physician faces one fundamental question in the cancer patient facing surgery: Is the procedure curative or palliative? An operation intended to cure might be considered always appropriate, while a palliative procedure for symptom relief might be questioned. However, situations may arise that may run counter to this thinking. Resection of an asymptomatic nonobstructing colon carcinoma may not be appropriate in a patient with crippling cardiomyopathy or end-stage liver disease. Similarly, elective cholecystectomy for minimally symptomatic cholelithiasis in a patient with rapidly progressive metastatic sarcoma who has failed chemotherapy might seem foolhardy. Conversely, coronary artery bypass surgery to relieve incapacitating angina unresponsive to medical therapy may be appropriate in a patient with metastatic prostate carcinoma who is functionally intact. However, hemipelvectomy for pain relief in a patient with metastatic osteosarcoma may be excessive if adequate doses of narcotics have not been tried.

When considering the appropriateness of surgery in patients with metastatic cancer, the physician should not rely on crude five-year survival statistics because the natural history of malignant disease may be quite different in individual patients with a similar tumor type. Each case must be assessed individually, and the goals of surgery, whether curative or palliative, must be discussed fully

beforehand. A thorough understanding of the natural history of the patient's own cancer and objective assessment of the tumor burden and rate of growth are necessary to provide a sound basis for advice. Consideration of alternative therapies such as chemotherapy, radiation, or narcotic analgesia should be reviewed and input from oncology consultants should be ingredients in the decision-making process.

Physicians should recognize situations in which surgical resection of metastatic lesions with curative intent is appropriate. Patients with metastatic testicular tumors may have residual disease in the lymph nodes or retroperitoneum after chemotherapy that requires surgery. Resection of solitary lung metastases is curative in a small number of patients and may improve survival in others with a wide variety of malignancies, particularly in the case of sarcomas. Similarly, resection of solitary liver metastases may be curative in some patients with colon carcinoma. Surgery in such cases should only be considered if (1) the primary tumor is amenable to cure, (2) an exhaustive search for metastatic disease elsewhere is unrevealing, and (3) resection can be performed without jeopardizing remaining organ function.

SUMMARY

1. Malignancy may cause nutritional compromise, metabolic alterations, endocrine disturbances, hematologic abnormalities, neurologic disorders, cardiopulmonary disease, and immune dysfunction. These phenomena are due to direct tumor invasion of essential structure or to distant paraneoplastic phenomena and affect operative and anesthetic risk in predictable ways.

2. Organ dysfunction in patients with cancer is managed in the same way as in it is in those without malignancy.

3. The toxic effects of cancer therapy can also cause organ dysfunction. A working knowledge of the toxicities induced by chemotherapy and radiotherapy is necessary to predict operative risk and manage patients with cancer undergoing surgery.

REFERENCES

1. Daly JM, Decosse JJ: Principles of surgical oncology, in Calabrese P, Schein PS, Rosenberg SA (eds): *Medical Oncology*. Toronto, Macmillan, 1985, p 261.
2. Brennan MF: Metabolic response to surgery in the cancer patient. *Cancer* 43:2053, 1979.
3. Dripps RD, Lamont A, Eckenkoff JE: *Introduction to Anesthesia*. Philadelphia, Saunders, 1977.
4. Mullen J, Buzby G, Matthew D: Reduction of operative morbidity and mortality by combined preoperative and postoperative nutritional support. *Ann Surg* 192:604, 1980.
5. Dewys WD, Begg C, Lavin PT: Prognostic effect of weight loss prior to chemotherapy in cancer patients. *Am J Med* 69:491, 1980.
6. Williams R, Heatley R, Lewis M: Preoperative parenteral nutrition in patients with stomach cancer, in *Clinical Parenteral Nutrition*. Chester, England, Geistlich Education, 1977, p 25.
7. Muller JM, Dienst C, Brenner V: Preoperative parenteral feeding in patients with gastrointestinal carcinoma. *Lancet* 1:68, 1982.
8. McGeer A, Dersky A, O'Rourke K: Parenteral nutrition in patients receiving cancer chemotherapy. *Ann Int Med* 9:734, 1989.

9. Rassam JW, Anderson G: Incidence of paramalignant disorders in bronchogenic carcinoma. *Thorax* 30:86, 1975.
10. Lokich JJ: The frequency and clinical biology of the ectopic hormone syndromes of small cell carcinoma. *Cancer* 50:2111, 1982.
11. Lees LH: The biosynthesis of hormones by nonendocrine tumors—a review. *J Endocrinol* 67:143, 1975.
12. Trump DL, Baylin SB: Ectopic hormone syndromes, in Abeloff, MD (ed): *Complications of Cancer: Diagnosis and Management*. Baltimore, JHU Press, 1979, p 211.
13. Cohen MH, Bunn PA, Ihde DC: Chemotherapy rather than demeclocycline for inappropriate secretion of antidiuretic hormone. *N Eng J Med* 298:1423, 1978.
14. Sendak M: Monitoring and management of perioperative fluid and electrolytic therapy, in Rogers, MC, Tinker JH, Covino BG (eds): *Principles and Practice of Anesthesiology*. St. Louis, Mosby, 1992, p 863.
15. Myers WPL: Differential diagnosis of hypercalcemia and cancer. *Cancer* 27:258, 1977.
16. Mundy GR, Martin TJ: The hypercalcemia of malignancy: Pathogenesis and management. *Metabolism* 1:1247, 1982.
17. Gurst MA, Drop LJ: Chronic hypercalcemia secondary to hyperparathyroidism; a risk factor for anesthesia? *Br J Anaesth* 52:507, 1980.
18. Sieber FE: Evaluation of the patient with endocrine disease and diabetes mellitus, in Rogers MC, Tinker JH, Covino BG (eds): *Principles and Practice of Anesthesiology*. St. Louis, Mosby, 1992, p 285.
19. Kjellstrand CM, Campbell DC, Von Hortitzsch B: Hyperuricemic acute renal failure. *Arch Int Med* 133:349, 1974.
20. Seidenwurm DJ, Lerner EB, Kaplan LM: Metastases to the adrenal glands and the development of Addison's disease. *Cancer* 54:552, 1984.
21. Redman BG, Pazdur R, Zingas AP: Prospective evaluation of adrenal insufficiency in patients with adrenal metastases. *Cancer* 60:103, 1987.
22. Fry J: Clinical patterns and course of anemias in general practice. *Br Med J* 2:1732, 1961.
23. Devita VT, Jaffe ES, Mauch P: Lymphocytic lymphomas, in Devita VT, Hellman S, Rosenberg SA (eds): *Cancer—Principles and Practice of Oncology*. Philadelphia, Lippincott, 1989, p 1766.
24. Pirofsky B: Clinical aspects of autoimmune hemolytic anemia. *Semin Hematol* 13:251, 1976.
25. Levin J, Conley CL: Thrombocytosis associated with malignant disease. *Arch Int Med* 114:497, 1964.
26. Schafer AI: Bleeding and thrombosis in the myeloproliferative disorders. *Blood* 64:1, 1984.
27. Richardson DW, Robinson AG: Desmopressin. *Ann Int Med* 103:228, 1985.
28. McCarthy JH, Sullivan JR, Ungar B: Two cases of carcinoma of the lung characterized by a bone marrow agar pattern resembling acute myeloid leukemia. *Blood* 54:530, 1979.
29. McClay MD, Bellet RE: Preoperative evaluation of the oncology patient. *Med Clin N Amer* 71(3):529, 1987.
30. Lackner H: Hemostatic abnormalities associated with dysproteinemia. *Semin Hematol* 10:125, 1973.
31. Beck JR, Quinn BM, Meier FA: Hyperviscosity syndrome in paraproteinemia. *Transfusion* 22:51, 1982.
32. Allen JC, Deck MD, Foley FM: *Neuro-oncology: II*. New York, Sloan-Kettering, 1979, p 47.
33. Galicich JH, Sundaresan N, Arbit E: Surgical treatment of single brain metastasis: Factors associated with survival. *Cancer* 45:381, 1980.
34. Tindal S: Anesthesia for spinal decompression for metastatic disease. *Anesth Analg* 66:894, 1987.
35. Siegal T: Surgical decompression of anterior and posterior malignant epidural tumors compressing the spinal cord: A prospective study. *Neurosurgery* 17:424, 1985.
36. Gilbert RW, Kim JH, Posner JB: Spinal cord compression from metastatic tumor: Diagnosis and treatment. *Ann Neurol* 3:40, 1978.
37. Bunn PA, Ridgwa EC: Paraneoplastic syndromes, in Devita VT,

Hellman S, Rosenberg SA (eds): *Cancer—Principles and Practice of Oncology*. Philadelphia, Lippincott, 1989, p 1896.
38. Lambert EH, Eaton LM, Rooke ED: Defect of neuromuscular conduction associated with malignant neoplasms. *Am J Physiol* 187:612, 1956.
39. Olanow CW, Wechsler AS: The surgical management of myasthenia gravis, in Sabiston D (ed): *Textbook of Surgery*. Philadelphia, Lippincott, 1986, p 2119.
40. MacDonnell RA, Rich JM, Cros D: The Lambert-Eaton myasthenic syndrome: A cause of delayed recovery from general anesthesia. *Arch Phys Med Rehab* 73:98, 1992.
41. Small S, Ali HH, Lennon VA: Anesthesia for an unsuspected Lambert-Eaton myasthenic syndrome with autoantibodies and occult small cell lung cancer. *Anesthesiology* 76:142, 1992.
42. Miller WE: Roentgenographic manifestations of lung cancer, in Straus W (ed): *Lung Cancer: Clinical Diagnosis and Treatment*. New York, Grune & Stratton, 1977, p 175.
43. Brown RS, Haynes HA, Foley HJ: Hodgkin's disease. Immunological, clinical, and histologic features of 50 untreated patients. *Ann Intern Med* 67:291, 1967.
44. Mackie AM, Watson CB: Anesthesia and mediastinal masses: A case report and review of the literature. *Anaesthesia* 39:899, 1984.
45. Tonnesen AS, Davis FG: Superior vena caval obstruction during anesthesia. *Anesthesiology* 45:91, 1976.
46. Baron RL, Lee JK, Sagel SS: Computed tomography evaluation of mediastinal widening. *Radiology* 138:107, 1981.
47. Perez CA, Presant CA, VanAmburg AL: Management of superior vena cava syndrome. *Semin Oncol* 5:124, 1978.
48. Schranfinagel DE, Hill R, Leech JA: Superior vena caval obstruction: Is it a medical emergency? *Am J Med* 70:1169, 1981.
49. Neuman GG, Weingarten AE, Abramowitz RM: The anesthetic management of the patient with an anterior mediastinal mass. *Anesthesiology* 60:144, 1984.
50. Halpern S, Chatten J, Meadows A: Anterior mediastinal masses: Anesthesia hazards and other problems. *J Pediatrics* 102:407, 1983.
51. Ahmann FR: A reassessment of the clinical implications of the superior vena caval syndrome. *J Clin Oncol* 2:961, 1984.
52. Lewis RJ, Sisler GE, Mackenzie JW: Mediastinoscopy in advanced superior vena cava obstruction. *Ann Thor Surg* 32:458, 1981.
53. Davenport D, Ferree C, Blake D: Radiation therapy in the treatment of superior vena caval obstruction. *Cancer* 42:2600, 1978.
54. Loeffler JA, Leopold KA, Recht A: Emergency prebiopsy radiation for mediastinal masses: Impact on subsequent pathologic diagnosis and outcome. *J Clin Oncol* 4:716, 1986.
55. Posner MA, Cohen GI, Skarin AT: Pericardial disease in patients with cancer. *Am J Med* 71:407, 1981.
56. Adenle AD, Edwards JE: Clinical and pathological features of metastatic neoplasms of the pericardium. *Chest* 81:166, 1982.
57. Hancock WE: Pericardial disease in patients with neoplasm, in Reddy PS (ed): *Pericardial Disease*. New York, Raven Press, 1982, p 325.
58. Glover DJ, Glick JH: Oncologic emergencies and special complications, in Calabrese P, Schein PS, Rosenberg SA (eds): *Medical Oncology*. Toronto, Macmillan, 1985, p 1261.
59. Sulkes A, Weshler Z, Kopolovic Y: Pericardial effusion as first evidence of malignancy in bronchogenic carcinoma. *J Surg Oncol* 20:71, 1982.
60. Morris AL: Echo evaluation of tamponade. *Circulation* 53:746, 1976.
61. Hankins JR, Scatterfield JR, Aisner J: Pericardial window for malignant pericardial effusion. *Ann Thorac Surg* 30:465, 1980.
62. Anderson CB, Philpott GW, Ferguson TB: The treatment of malignant pleural effusions. *Cancer* 33:916, 1974.
63. Jensik R, Cagle JE, Milloy F: Pleurectomy in the treatment of pleural effusion due to metastatic malignancy. *J Thorac Cardiovasc Surg* 46:322, 1963.
64. Tisi GN: *Pulmonary Physiology in Clinical Medicine*. Baltimore, Williams & Wilkins, 1980, p 143.

65. Selvin BL: Cancer chemotherapy: Implications for the anesthesiologist. *Anesth Analg* 60:425, 1981.
66. Chung F: Cancer, chemotherapy, and anesthesia. *Can Anesth Soc J* 29:364, 1982.
67. Ciresi SA: The anesthetic implications of chemotherapy. *JAANA* 51:26, 1983.
68. Dahl MG, Gregoing MM, Suheuer PJ: Methotrexate hepatotoxicity in psoriasis: Comparison of different dose regimens. *Br Med J* 1:654, 1972.
69. Gurman GM: Prolonged apnea after succinylcholine in a case treated with cytostatics for cancer. *Anesth Analg* 51:761, 1972.
70. Donato D, Angelides A, Irani H: Infectious complications after gastrointestinal surgery in patients with ovarian carcinoma and malignant ascites. *Gynecol Oncol* 44:40, 1992.
71. Cohen SC, Gabelnick HL, Johnson RK: Effects of antineoplastic agents on wound healing in mice. *Surgery* 78:238, 1975.
72. Deveraux DF, Thibault L, Bonetas J: The quantitative and qualitative impairment of wound healing by adriamycin. *Cancer* 43:932, 1979.
73. Morris T: Retardation of healing of large-bowel anastomoses by 5-fluorouracil. *NZ J Surg* 9:743, 1979.
74. Cohn I, Slack NH, Fisher B: Complications and toxic manifestations of surgical adjuvant chemotherapy for breast cancer. *Surg Gyn Ob* 127:1201, 1968.
75. Finney R: Adjuvant chemotherapy in the radical treatment of carcinoma of the breast. *Am J Roent Rad Ther Nuc Med* 111:137, 1971.
76. Finn D, Steele G, Osteen RT: Morbidity and mortality after surgery in patients with disseminated or locally advanced cancer receiving systemic chemotherapy. *J Surg Oncol* 13:237, 1980.
77. McDonald DJ, Capanna R, Gherlinzoni F: Influence of chemotherapy on perioperative complications in limb salvage surgery for bone tumors. *Cancer* 65:1509, 1990.
78. Rosenaw EC: The spectrum of drug-induced pulmonary disease. *Ann Int Med* 77:977, 1972.
79. Blum RH, Carter SK, Agre K: A clinical review of bleomycin—a new antineoplastic agent. *Cancer* 31:903, 1973.
80. Goldiner PL, Schweizer O: The hazards of anesthesia and surgery in bleomycin-treated patients. *Sem Oncol* 6:121, 1978.
81. Goldiner PL, Carlon GC, Cuitkovic E: Factors influencing postoperative morbidity and mortality in patients treated with bleomycin. *Br Med J* 1:1664, 1978.
82. Allen SC, Riddell GS, Butchart GC: Bleomycin therapy and anesthesia. *Anaesthesia* 36:60, 1981.
83. Douglas MJ, Coppin CM: Bleomycin and subsequent anesthesia: A retrospective study at Vancouver General Hospital. *Can Anaesth Soc J* 27:449, 1980.
84. Hulbert JC, Grossman JE, Cummings KB: Risk factors of anesthesia and surgery in bleomycin-treated patients. *J Urol* 130:163, 1983.
85. Kochansky SW: Anesthetic management of the surgical patient on bleomycin sulfate. *JAANA* 51:146, 1983.
86. LaMantia KR, Glick JH, Marshall BE: Supplemental oxygen does not cause respiratory failure in bleomycin-treated surgical patients. *Anesthesiology* 60:65, 1984.
87. Klein DS, Wilds PR: Pulmonary toxicity of antineoplastic agents: Anaesthetic and postoperative implications. *Can Anaesth Soc J* 30:399, 1983.
88. Stewart JR, Fajardo LF: Radiation-induced heart disease: Clinical and experimental aspects. *Rad Clin N Am* 9:511, 1971.
89. Morton DL, Kagan AR, Roberts WC: Pericardiectomy for radiation-induced pericarditis with effusion. *Ann Thorac Surg* 8:195, 1969.
90. Brosius FC, Waller BF, Roberts WC: Radiation heart disease: Analysis of 16 young (aged 15 to 33 years) necroscopy patients who received over 3500 rads to the heart. *Am Med* 70:519, 1981.
91. Perrault DJ, Gilbert BW, Levy MD: Long-term effects of upper mantle radiation on the heart in patients with lymphoma. *Proc ASCO* 21:349, 1980.
92. VonHoff DD, Layard MW, Basa P: Risk factors for doxorubicin-induced congestive heart failure. *Ann Int Med* 91:70, 1979.
93. Buzdar AU, Marcus C, Smith TL: Early and delayed clinical cardiotoxicity of doxorubicin. *Cancer* 55:2761, 1985.
94. Dresdale A, Bonow RO, Wesley R: Prospective evaluation of doxorubicin-induced cardiomyopathy resulting from postsurgical adjuvant treatment of patients with soft tissue sarcomas. *Cancer* 52:51, 1983.
95. Burrows FA, Hickey PR, Colan S: Perioperative complications in patients with anthracycline chemotherapeutic agents. *Can Anaesth Soc J* 32:149, 1985.
96. Saini J, Rich MW, Lyss AP: Reversibility of severe left ventricular dysfunction due to doxorubicin cardiotoxicity. *Ann Int Med* 106:814, 1987.
97. Deisserath A, Wallerstein R: Use of blood and blood products, in Devita VT, Hellman S, Rosenberg SA (eds): *Cancer—Principles and Practice of Oncology*. Philadelphia, Lippincott, 1989, p 2045.
98. Lieschke GJ, Burgess AW: Granulocyte colony stimulating factor and granulocyte-macrophage colony stimulating factor. *N Eng J Med* 327:2899, 1992.
99. Schein PS, O'Connell MJ, Blom J: Clinical antitumor activity and toxicity of streptozotocin. *Cancer* 34:993, 1974.
100. DeFronzo RA, Brainc H, Calvin OM: Water intoxication in man after cyclophosphamide therapy. *Ann Int Med* 78:861, 1973.
101. Glatstein E, McMardy-Young S, Brast N: Alterations in serum thyrotropin (TSH) and thyroid function following radiotherapy in patients with malignant lymphoma. *J Clin Endocrinol Metab* 32:833, 1971.
102. Browder AA, Hoff JA, Petersdorf RE: The significance of fever in neoplastic disease. *Ann Int Med* 55:932, 1961.
103. Pizzo PA, Hathorn JW, Hiemenz JW: A randomized trial comparing ceflazidime alone with combination antibiotic therapy in cancer patients with fever and neutropenia. *N Eng J Med* 315:552, 1986.
104. Karp JE, Dick JD, Angelopoulos C: Empiric use of vancomycin in prolonged treatment-induced granulocytopenia. Randomized, double-blind, placebo-controlled clinical trial in patients with acute leukemia. *Am J Med* 81:237, 1986.
105. Pizzo PA, Meyers JA: Infections in the cancer patient, in Devita VT, Hellman S, Rosenberg SA (eds): *Cancer—Principles and Practice of Oncology*. Philadelphia, Lippincott, 1989, p 2008.
106. Pizzo PA, Robichaud KJ, Gill FA: Duration of empiric antibiotic therapy in granulocytopenic cancer patients. *Am J Med* 67:194, 1979.
107. Skibber JM, Matler GJ, Lotke MT: Right lower quadrant complications in young patients with leukemia: A surgical prospective. *Ann Surg* 206:711, 1987.
108. Bodel P: Tumors and fever. *Ann NY Acad Sci* 230:6, 1974.
109. Petersdorf RG: Fever and cancer. *Hosp Med* 1:2, 1965.

30 SURGERY IN THE PATIENT WITH CLOTTING ABNORMALITIES

David H. Henry

Bleeding is a major concern in surgical patients. Most intraoperative and postoperative bleeding is the result of compromise in the structural integrity of a vessel resulting from the surgery itself. However, an underlying bleeding disorder requires clarification before the procedure to avoid bleeding complications. This chapter discusses the evaluation of the patient with a known or suspected bleeding diathesis and the management of specific clotting abnormalities before surgery.

PREOPERATIVE EVALUATION

Patients with bleeding disorders come to surgery either already diagnosed and requiring specific preoperative therapy or with a suspected problem that needs definition. In the latter case, the history is the most important element in the process.[1] Isolated laboratory studies may underestimate or overestimate a bleeding problem. The patient should be questioned about previous stresses to his own clotting system and those of family members and about the adequacy of the response.

Patients with platelet abnormalities usually have a history of easy bruising, heavy menses, or ecchymoses, while those with clotting-factor disorders more often experience bleeding into muscles, joints, or the retroperitoneum. Prolonged bleeding after dental extraction can be seen in either group. Platelet disorders are characterized by continuous oozing for more than 24 hours, while clotting-factor abnormalities result in delayed recurrence of bleeding after initial hemostasis. In the latter case, a platelet plug stops initial bleeding, but the fibrin meshwork necessary for complete clotting never properly forms.

The value of a careful history has been demonstrated many times. Liver disease, use of anticoagulants, hemophilia, or malabsorption of vitamin K can often be readily diagnosed from the patient's history.[2-4] In one survey of 97 preoperative patients with prolongation of the activated partial thromboplastin time (aPTT),

37 were taking anticoagulants, 27 had known liver disease, four had hemophilia, four had undergone intestinal bypass surgery, and one had malabsorption due to cystic fibrosis. In 10 patients, the abnormal PTT was the result of laboratory error. The remaining 14 patients had unexplained prolongation of the PTT by less than 10 seconds above the control value, but none had bleeding complications during surgery.[2] The usefulness of a routine admission protime determination (PT) as a screening test for bleeding has also been studied.[3] In 97 percent, a prolonged PT could have been predicted by history alone. Of additional note is the fact that screening coagulation tests may be normal in patients with a clear-cut history of bleeding.[4,5]

When the history and physical examination suggest a hemostatic abnormality, a platelet count, bleeding time, prothrombin time (PT), and activated partial thromboplastin time (aPTT) should be performed. One or more of these four tests will be abnormal in over 95 percent of patients with clinically significant coagulation problems when they are actually bleeding. However, coagulation tests may all be normal in patients with significant bleeding disorders who have not as yet been stressed by surgery (see Fig. 30–1). Only 25% of the normal level of each factor is required to produce a normal PT or aPTT. A patient with 35% factor XI deficiency may have a normal aPTT preoperatively but suffer significant bleeding at surgery after much of the factor XI has been consumed. Repeated intraoperatively, the aPTT would become prolonged as the factor level falls below 25%. In all cases, an abnormal preoperative clotting study should be repeated for verification.

The PT, aPTT, platelet count, and bleeding time may suggest specific defects in the clotting system.[6] The PT tests the integrity of the extrinsic coagulation pathway, and the aPTT tests the intrinsic coagulation sequence. If the aPTT is prolonged and the PT is normal, the defect lies in one or more of the factors in the intrinsic pathway. Hemophilia A and B are sex-linked congenital deficiencies of factors VIII and IX, respectively. Factor VIII deficiency can also occur in von Willebrand's disease. Factor XI defi-

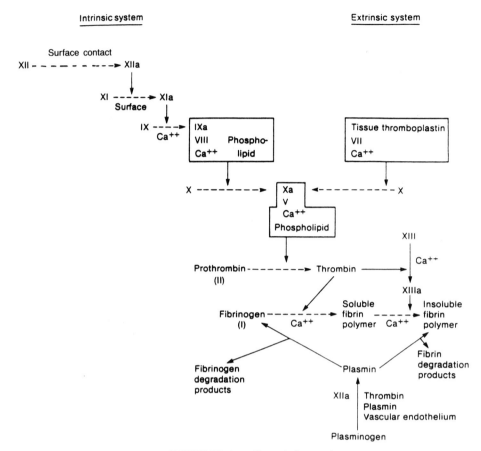

FIGURE 30–1. Coagulation pathway.

ciency has an autosomal recessive inheritance pattern and is seen most commonly in Jews of northern European extraction. Factor XII deficiency does not result in clinical bleeding.

A prolonged aPTT with a normal PT can also suggest the presence of a lupus anticoagulant, an antibody that exerts its effect at the beginning of the final common pathway. The lupus anticoagulant binds lipid in the PT and aPTT assays. Large quantities of lipid are used in the PT assay and overwhelm the effect of the lupus anticoagulant, thereby resulting in a normal test result. However, little lipid is used in the aPTT assay, and the lupus anticoagulant affects the test in such a way as to prolong the result. The lupus anticoagulant does not result in bleeding in vivo because excess lipid is always present.

If the PT is prolonged and the aPTT is normal, the coagulation defect lies in factor VII. Factor VII deficiency is rarely responsible for clinical bleeding. If both tests are abnormal, many factors may be deficient, but more often there is a major defect in the final common pathway involving factors X, V, II (prothrombin), or I (fibrinogen). Liver disease, vitamin K deficiency, and disseminated intravascular coagulation (DIC) commonly affect factors in both pathways.

A platelet count and bleeding time are useful in evaluating the integrity of the other arm of the coagulation system involved in the formation of the initial platelet plug. If the platelets are decreased in number, the tendency to bleed is roughly inversely proportional to the decrement in the count below $100,000/\mu l$.

However, even if the platelet count is normal, platelet function may be abnormal and may cause significant bleeding. A standard Ivy bleeding time provides a measure of platelet function and vascular integrity. According to large population studies, a bleeding time of less than 10 minutes assures that the platelet count, platelet function, and blood vessel integrity are all normal. However, a normal or prolonged bleeding time in an individual patient has not been shown to correlate with the risk of bleeding across a wide range of clinical situations, including coronary artery bypass graft surgery, orthopedic procedures, and uremia.[7] Consequently, a single normal or abnormal bleeding time should be interpreted with caution in light of the clinical setting. The bleeding time is predictably abnormal when the platelet count is low and need not be performed. Aspirin, von Willebrand's disease, and uremia all prolong the bleeding time through their effects on platelet function; and scurvy, amyloid, and the aging process can alter vascular integrity.

PREOPERATIVE MANAGEMENT

When the history and laboratory evaluation provide evidence of an unsuspected bleeding disorder or confirm one already known, specific prophylactic therapy may be needed to minimize the risk of bleeding. Several common conditions requiring special attention are detailed below.

Bleeding Due to Aspirin and Other Drugs

Aspirin causes an irreversible defect in platelet aggregation for the remainder of the seven- to ten-day life of the platelet. Aspirin acetylates the enzyme cyclo-oxygenase, inhibiting the release of adenosine diphosphate (ADP) and preventing aggregation. Aspirin does not always prolong the bleeding time but may still cause increased bleeding during or after surgery. Many other drugs also Von Willebrand's disease is an autosomal dominant disorder in which platelet adhesion and factor VIII are abnormal. The aPTT and bleeding time may not be prolonged preoperatively but may ever, their residual effects on platelet function usually dissipate within hours after discontinuance. Clinical bleeding due to platelet malfunction may also occur following the administration of high-dose intravenous penicillins. Semisynthetic penicillins like carbenicillin and ticarcillin are the most frequent offenders since they are given in large doses. Their effects can last 24 to 48 hours after they are discontinued.

Correction of a prolonged bleeding time due to drug-induced platelet malfunction requires stopping the drug. If rapid correction of a prolonged bleeding time is necessary for urgent surgery, platelet transfusion is required. Desmopressin (DDAVP) may help reverse aspirin-induced platelet malfunction for unclear reasons.[9]

Von Willebrand's Disease

Von Willebrand's disease is an autosomal dominant disorder in which platelet adhesion and factor VIII are abnormal. The aPTT and bleeding time may not be prolonged preoperatively but may become so during or after surgery. Therapy consists of increasing the factor VIII coagulant activity and von Willebrand factor protein. In most patients, DDAVP in a dose of 0.3 to 0.4 µg/kg intravenously over 15 to 20 minutes every 8 to 12 hours will accomplish this. The peak effect is almost immediate but may fatigue after 24 hours of repeated dosing.[9] Therefore, for major procedures the addition of cryoprecipitate may be necessary in a dose of 0.1 to 0.2 bags/kg every 12 hours.[10,11] Therapeutic effect should be monitored both before and after surgery. The bleeding time and ristocetin aggregation tests should both normalize with appropriate therapy, and then the bleeding time alone will suffice if it correlates well with the ristocetin aggregation test. Factor VIII levels of above 25% are required for proper hemostasis.

Uremia

Uremic patients commonly have a prolonged bleeding time due to a dialyzable factor that impairs platelet function. If dialysis is not feasible or does not correct the abnormality, therapy with cryoprecipitate or DDAVP is usually effective.[12] Correction with DDAVP is prompt but short-lived. If immediate correction is not essential, two other therapeutic options are available. Conjugated estrogens in a dose of 0.6 mg/kg intravenously daily for 4 to 5 days will slowly correct the bleeding time. The effect lasts for an additional five days after the estrogens are stopped.[13] Recombinant human erythropoietin (r-HuEPO) is also useful in correcting the bleeding time in uremia and in reversing the associated anemia. By raising the hematocrit above 30% with r-HuEPO, the bleeding time can be progressively shortened. The hematocrit rises slowly over several weeks.[14]

Hemophilia

Hemophilia A (factor VIII deficiency) and hemophilia B (factor IX deficiency) are the most common inherited clotting-factor abnormalities. Hemophilia C (factor XI deficiency) is less common but is becoming increasingly recognized. Hemophilias A and B are sex-linked recessive disorders, and hemophilia C is autosomal recessive and more common in northern European Jews. In all of these disorders, the bleeding time is normal, but the aPTT is usually prolonged. However, if the plasma level of the deficient factor is greater than 25%, the aPTT may also be normal. Bleeding problems during surgery are associated with plasma levels significantly below 25%.

Treatment consists of factor replacement before and after surgery. In hemophilia A, the necessary quantity of cryoprecipitate or antihemophilic factor required to raise the factor VIII level to 80% of normal should be infused one hour before surgery (40 to 50 units/kg). Half of the loading dose should be given every 12 hours for 10 to 14 days following major surgery. A shorter postoperative course can be given after minor surgery. The factor VIII level should be maintained above 30% during and after major procedures, but levels of 20% to 30% are adequate for minor surgery. Therapy can be monitored by measuring factor VIII levels or the aPTT.[10,15] In some minor procedures like dental surgery, epsilonaminocaproic acid (EACA) can be used alone in a dose of one to two grams every four hours orally for several days.[16] If a factor VIII inhibitor is detected before surgery, the same principle of treatment can be applied, but plasmapheresis or immunoadsorptive measures will usually be necessary to keep the inhibitor low.

In hemophilia B, factor IX levels of 50% are required for major surgery. An initial dose of 50 units/kg followed by half this dose every 12 to 24 hours for 7 to 10 days after surgery provides adequate hemostasis. In hemophilia C, patients with factor XI levels below 20% should be treated with fresh frozen plasma before surgery.[17] A dose of 15 to 20 ml/kg followed by 3 to 6 ml/kg every 12 hours is recommended and should be continued for at least several days.

Bleeding Due to Acquired Anticoagulants

Factor VIII Inhibitor. Acquired antibodies to factor VIII may occur spontaneously in nonhemophiliac individuals and cause clinical bleeding. Factor VIII antibodies are seen in the postpartum state, autoimmune disease, lymphoid malignancies, certain skin disorders, and with drugs like penicillin and ampicillin or may occur without underlying cause. In one-third of cases, they disappear spontaneously. If therapy is necessary, steroids and immunosuppressive agents have been shown to be effective.[18,19]

Lupus Anticoagulant. The lupus anticoagulant (LA) can be associated with systemic lupus erythematosus but more commonly occurs without underlying cause. It prolongs the aPTT by interfering with the assay and does not affect clotting or lead to clinical bleeding. Some lupus anticoagulants may actually cause thrombosis because of their inflammatory interaction with lipid on the surface of vascular endothelial cells.[20]

Like anticardiolipin antibodies, the LA belongs to a family of antiphospholipid antibodies consisting of IgG, IgM, or both molecules. While usually idiopathic, it can be induced by medications.

Phenothiazines are most often implicated, but hydralazine, procainamide, and quinidine have also been reported to induce it.[21] Systemic lupus erythematosus (SLE), chronic inflammatory states, and chronic infections like HIV have been associated with the LA.

Although the LA does not cause clinical bleeding, it can induce thrombosis.[20] It may irritate endothelial cells or inhibit prostacyclin synthesis in these cells, but the actual molecular basis of action remains unknown.[22,23] The LA may induce thrombocytopenia by activating platelets and thereby increasing their consumption.[24]

Patients with thromboses due to the LA usually require prolonged therapy. Warfarin is most effective in treating recurrent venous thrombosis. Prednisone, aspirin, or immunosuppressive therapy are less effective and are associated with a variety of side effects. When the LA is associated with an autoimmune disease, treatment of the underlying process with immunosuppressive therapy will often decrease thrombosis. Arterial thrombosis is more difficult to treat, but low-dose aspirin may be the best choice. Thrombocytopenia associated with the LA is best treated with corticosteroids.

Other Clotting Abnormalities

Malnutrition, malabsorption, and bowel sterilization can all lead to a deficiency of vitamin K, resulting in decreased hepatic activation of factors II, VII, IX, and X. A patient who is receiving intravenous antibiotics and not eating may become vitamin K–deficient with subsequent prolongation of the PT and aPTT after only one week. Vitamin K in a dose of 10 mg subcutaneously corrects the deficiency and can normalize the clotting parameters within 8 to 12 hours. Immediate correction to control bleeding requires fresh frozen plasma.

Acquired coagulation abnormalities associated with liver disease and decreased factor production are quite variable. Vitamin K can be given but may be only marginally effective. Patients with minimal clotting abnormalities who do not require invasive procedures require no therapy. Those with a prolonged PT of more than three seconds above the control value should be tested for an inhibitor with a 1:1 mix test. If no inhibitor is present, vitamin K should be administered. If the PT and aPTT are still significantly prolonged, fresh frozen plasma should be given in large volumes. Quantities approximating 25% of plasma volume (5% of total body dry weight) are initially required followed by half that amount every six hours. If the fibrinogen level is less than 100 mg/dl, cryoprecipitate in a dose of 5 to 10 units, alone or in addition to fresh frozen plasma, may significantly shorten clotting times. Thrombocytopenia with counts under 20,000/μl or platelet dysfunction accompanying liver disease should also be treated if bleeding occurs or invasive procedures are planned. Desmopressin (DDAVP) in a dose of 0.3 mg/kg intravenously is useful in correcting platelet dysfunction.[9]

Low plasma fibrinogen levels can also be seen in patients with disseminated intravascular coagulation (DIC) or inherited dysfibrinogenemias and can be associated with impaired hemostasis and wound healing. DIC is induced by either extensive injury to vascular endothelial cells, extensive tissue damage, or both. In patients with shock, burns, sepsis, or obstetrical emergencies, clotting and anticlotting factors are systemically activated and consumed, upsetting the balance between the two and leading to bleeding, thrombosis, or both. Correction of the underlying disease process is the cornerstone of treatment and should be attempted before surgery is undertaken.

Emergency surgery may be necessary to treat the underlying cause of DIC (e.g., abruptio placenta or perforated viscus with sepsis). If clotting is severely impaired with a PT above 15 seconds, fibrinogen level below 100 mg/dl, and platelet count under 20,000/μl, simultaneous treatment with low-dose heparin in a dose of 5 to 10 units/kg/hr, clotting factors, and platelets may be required. Heparin presumably slows down factor consumption but must be administered with extreme care. Cryoprecipitate should be used initially to increase the fibrinogen level above 100 mg/dl, changing to fresh frozen plasma if the PT remains prolonged above 15 seconds.

Factor X deficiency, reported in patients with systemic amyloidosis, may cause severe bleeding and requires fresh frozen plasma. Finally, deficiency of factor XIII, although rare, may lead to significant bleeding. Factor XIII deficiency may be congenital or acquired and can be associated with isoniazid therapy. This diagnosis should be considered when the PT, aPTT, platelet count, and bleeding time are all normal but when bleeding continues in the absence of a demonstrable structural defect. Factor XIII crosslinks soluble fibrin at a point in the coagulation process after that measured by the PT and PTT. Diagnosis of factor XIII deficiency depends on a clot solubility test, and therapy requires fresh frozen plasma or cryoprecipitate.

Hypercoagulable States

Hypercoagulable states can be inherited or acquired. Inherited defects include antithrombin III, protein C, and protein S deficiencies. Acquired hypercoagulability can arise after surgery or can be seen in patients with malignancy, hyperviscosity, and polycythemia and in those who are elderly or taking estrogen.[25] Whenever possible, the underlying condition should be treated to decrease the risk of clotting. Otherwise, patients with acquired hypercoagulable states should receive appropriate prophylaxis against thromboembolism as described in Chap. 48.

Inherited hypercoagulable states require specific treatment.[26] Antithrombin III deficiency can be treated with antithrombin III factor concentrate. This factor has a half-life of 48 hours and can be given in an initial dose of 50 units/kg followed by 60% of the original dose 24 hours later to maintain factor levels above 80%. Most patients with protein C deficiency are heterozygotes and have plasma levels under 55%. Since the half-life of protein C is six hours, fresh frozen plasma or protein C concentrate must be given frequently to maintain levels above 70%. Most patients require chronic warfarin or heparin therapy.

Patients on Anticoagulants

Patients who are taking anticoagulants and undergoing surgery fall into two categories: (1) those already on heparin or coumadin-like anticoagulants for a prior or concurrent condition; and (2) those placed on prophylactic low-dose heparin or coumadin for the prevention of postoperative venous thrombosis and thromboembolism. When low-dose heparin or coumadin regimens are used, the clotting times need not be followed since they are usually not prolonged. When adjusted-dose heparin or therapeutic doses of coumadin are used, clotting times should be checked and therapy interrupted in the perioperative period. Reversal of clotting times to completely normal levels is usually not necessary.

Patients taking anticoagulants for prior or concurrent thrombosis are usually fully anticoagulated with either coumadin-like agents or heparin. If the indication for anticoagulation is tenuous or the patient has had nearly a full course of the therapy, anticoagulation should be stopped or reversed. However, patients who have suffered prior thromboembolic events have a high risk of recurrent episodes. In this case, prophylaxis with low-dose heparin is indicated in the perioperative period. Some authors advocate full therapeutic doses.

In patients requiring continuous full therapeutic anticoagulation, most major surgical procedures can be safely performed with brief interruption in anticoagulation. However, those undergoing eye, central nervous system, or liver procedures require complete normalization of their clotting parameters before surgery.[27,28] The aPTT usually normalizes about 12 hours after heparin is discontinued. If more rapid correction is required, anticoagulation can be reversed with protamine sulfate in a dose of one mg for every 100 units of heparin still in the circulation. Full heparin anticoagulation can usually be resumed three days after major surgery and one to two days after minor procedures. Patients with aortic heart valves have had heparin therapy interrupted for as long as one to three days without thromboembolic complications.[29,30]

In patients on chronic warfarin therapy undergoing surgery, the dose should be lowered to achieve a PT less than 15 seconds for minor procedures.[31,32] Warfarin should be discontinued to allow the PT to reach normal levels before major elective surgery. When surgery is more urgent, fresh frozen plasma or vitamin K can be given before the procedure. If there is delay between normalization of the PT and surgery, heparin can be used to achieve needed anticoagulation and interrupted 6 to 12 hours before the procedure.

SUMMARY

1. A personal or family history of bleeding is often more important than laboratory studies in identifying patients with increased risk of hemorrhage in the perioperative period.

2. When the history or examination suggests a hemostatic abnormality, a PT, aPTT, platelet count, and bleeding time should be obtained. At least one of the four will be abnormal in 95 percent of patients who are bleeding at the time of the testing, but all may be normal in the absence of bleeding.

3. When abnormal, coagulation tests are useful in characterizing the nature of the hemostatic abnormality. An abnormal aPTT suggests either a clotting-factor deficiency or the presence of the lupus anticoagulant. Abnormalities in both the PT and aPTT suggest liver disease, vitamin K deficiency, or DIC. The bleeding time can be abnormal in patients with thrombocytopenia or in those with qualitative platelet disorders. The risk of bleeding due to thrombocytopenia correlates with how far the platelet count is below 100,000/μl.

4. Aspirin, von Willebrand's disease, and uremia affect platelet function and prolong the bleeding time. Platelet dysfunction due to aspirin can last 7 to 10 days after discontinuation of the drug but may respond to DDAVP. Patients with von Willebrand's disease may respond to DDAVP initially, but prolonged therapy may require treatment with cryoprecipitate. Platelet dysfunction induced by uremia can be treated with DDAVP or cryoprecipitate but also improves with conjugated estrogens and recombinant human erythropoietin (r-HuEPO).

5. Patients with inherited clotting-factor deficiencies can be treated with specific factor concentrates or fresh frozen plasma before surgery.

6. Acquired anticoagulants include factor VIII inhibitor and the lupus anticoagulant. Factor VIII inhibitor is associated with the postpartum state, autoimmune disease, certain drugs, lymphoid malignancies, and skin disorders and can be treated with steroids and immunosuppressive agents if necessary. The lupus anticoagulant does not cause clinical bleeding but may cause thrombosis. It is associated with SLE, certain drugs, and other chronic inflammatory states and infections. Treatment should be aimed at the underlying disease. Venous thrombosis can be treated with coumadin; arterial thrombosis may be prevented with aspirin.

7. Malnutrition, bowel sterilization, and antibiotic therapy associated with surgery may lead to vitamin K deficiency or hemostatic abnormalities that respond to parenteral vitamin K. Chronic liver disease can be associated with factor deficiency, decreased fibrinogen levels, and thrombocytopenia or platelet dysfunction. Therapy includes fresh frozen plasma, cryoprecipitate to replace fibrinogen, and platelet transfusions as needed.

8. The thrombocytopenia and abnormal PT and aPTT seen in DIC respond to treatment of the underlying disease but may also require platelets, clotting factors, and, rarely, judicious use of heparin.

9. Patients with inherited hypercoagulable states can now be treated with specific antithrombin III or protein C concentrates. Acquired hypercoagulability is best managed by treating the underlying disease and using standard anticoagulants as needed.

10. Patients on full-dose anticoagulants can safely undergo most surgical procedures with brief interruption in anticoagulation therapy. However, anticoagulation should be completely reversed in those undergoing eye, central nervous system, or liver surgery. In elective cases, discontinuing warfarin usually allows the PT to normalize in about three days, but fresh frozen plasma or vitamin K can be given in more urgent situations. Discontinuing heparin allows the aPTT to normalize in about 12 hours. The anticoagulant effect of heparin can be reversed immediately with protamine.

REFERENCES

1. Myers AM: Evaluation of the hemorrhage-prone patient. *Postgrad Med* 67:161–170, 1980.
2. Robbins JA, Rose SD: PTT as a screening test. *Ann Intern Med* 90:796, 1979.
3. Eisenberg JM, Goldfarb S: Clinical usefulness of measuring prothrombin time as a routine admission test. *Clin Chem* 22:1644, 1976.
4. Bowie EJW, Owen CA: Clinical and laboratory diagnosis of bleeding disorders, in *Disorders of Hemostasis.* Philadelphia, Saunders, 1991, vol 3, pp 48–75.
5. Aggeler PM, Haag MS, Wallerstein RO et al: The mild hemophilias: Occult deficiencies of AHF, PTC and PTA frequently responsible for unexpected surgical bleeding. *Am J Med* 30:84, 1961.

6. Bowie EJW, Owen CA: The significance of abnormal preoperative hemostatic tests. *Prog Hemostas Thromb* 5:179–209, 1980.

7. Rodgers RPC, Levin J: A critical reappraisal of the bleeding time. *Sem Thromb Hemostas* 16:1, 1990.

8. Malpass TW, Harker LA: Acquired disorders of platelet function. *Semin Hematol* 17:242–258, 1980.

9. Manucci PM: Desmopressin: A nontransfusional form of treatment for congenital and acquired bleeding disorders. *Blood* 72:1449–1455, 1988.

10. Fellin F, Murphy S: Hematologic problems in the preoperative patient. *Med Clin N Am* 71:477–487, 1987.

11. Blomback M, Johansson G, Johnson M et al: Surgery in patients with von Willebrand's disease. *Br J Surg* 76(4):392–400, 1989.

12. Manucci PM, Remuzzi G, Pusineri F et al: DDAVP shortens the bleeding time in uremia. *N Eng J Med* 308:8, 1983.

13. Livio M, Mannucci PM, Vigano G et al: Conjugated estrogens for the management of bleeding associated with renal failure. *N Engl J Med* 315:731, 1986.

14. Moia M, Mannucci PM, Vizzotto L et al: Improvement in the hemostatic defect of uremia after treatment with recombinant human erythropoietin. *Lancet* 2:1227, 1987.

15. Kitchens CS: Surgery in hemophilia and related disorders. *Medicine* 65:34–45, 1986.

16. Caughman WF, McCoy BP, Sisk AL et al: When a patient with a bleeding disorder needs dental work. How you can work with the dentist to prevent a crisis. *Postgrad Med* 88(6):175–182, 1990.

17. Asakai R, Chung DW, Davie EW et al: Factor XI deficiency in Ashkenazi Jews in Israel. *N Engl J Med* 325(3):153–158, 1991.

18. Green D, Lachner K: A survey of 215 nonhemophiliac patients with inhibitors to factor VIII. *Thromb Haemost* 45:200–203, 1981.

19. Shapiro SS: Antibodies to blood coagulation factors. *Clin Haematol* 8:207–214, 1979.

20. Creagh MD, Greaves M: Lupus anticoagulant. *Blood Rev* 5(3):162–167, 1991.

21. Zarrabi MH, Zucker S, Miller F et al: Immunologic and coagulation disorders in chlorpromazine-treated patients. *Ann Int Med* 91:194, 1979.

22. Cines DB, Lyss AP, Reeber M et al: Presence of complement-fixing antiendothelial cell antibodies in systemic lupus erythematosus. *J Clin Invest* 73:611, 1984.

23. Carreras LO, Defrey NG, Machin SJ et al: Arterial thrombosis, intrauterine death and "lupus" anticoagulant: Detection of immunoglobulin interfering with prostacyclin formation. *Lancet* 1:244, 1981.

24. Harris EN, Asherson RA, Gharavi AE et al: Thrombocytopenia in SLE and related autoimmune disorders: Association with anticardiolipin antibody. *Br J Haematol* 59:227, 1985.

25. Schafer, AI: The hypercoagulable states. *Ann Int Med* 102:814, 1985.

26. Eason JD, Mills JL, Beckeett WC: Hypercoagulable states in arterial thromboembolism. *Surg Gynecol Obstet* 174(3):211–215, 1992.

27. Ellison N, Ominsky AJ: Clinical considerations for the anesthesiologist whose patient is on anticoagulant therapy. *Anesthesiology* 39:328, 1973.

28. Vander Woude JC, Milam JD et al: Cardiovascular surgery in patients with congenital plasma coagulopathies. *Ann Thorac Surg* 46(3):283–288, 1988.

29. Katholi RE, Nolan SP, McGuire LB: The management of anticoagulation during noncardiac operations in patients with prosthetic heart valves: A prospective study. *Am Heart J* 96:163–165, 1978.

30. Tinker JH, Tarhan S: Discontinuing anticoagulant therapy in surgical patients with cardiac valve prostheses: Observations in 180 operations. *JAMA* 239:738–739, 1978.

31. Wieberdink J: Safe preoperative anticoagulation. *Thorax* 22:567, 1967.

32. Kloster FE, Briwtow JD, Seaman A: Cardiac catheterization during anticoagulant therapy. *Am J Cardiol* 28:67, 1971.

31 SURGERY IN THE PATIENT WITH HIV INFECTION

Susan C. Hunt

Matthew N. Klain

The number of individuals with human immunodeficiency virus (HIV) infection and acquired immunodeficiency syndrome (AIDS) continues to increase worldwide. The World Health Organization (WHO) predicts that between 30 to 40 million people will be infected with HIV by the year 2000.[1] The incidence of HIV infection and AIDS is increasing among women, minorities, parenteral drug users, and infants.[2]

Since the introduction of the antiviral agent zidovudine in 1986, the natural history of AIDS has changed dramatically.[3,4] As a result of early therapy with zidovudine and the newer antiviral agents ddI and ddC, patients with HIV infection are living longer with fewer symptoms before developing AIDS-defining illness.[5] Patients with AIDS treated with antivirals may suffer fewer and less severe opportunistic infections and may have increased survival time.[6,7] Ongoing research and clinical trials of new antiviral medications increase the likelihood of a better quality of life, a delay in the onset of symptoms, and increasingly prolonged survival for patients with HIV infection and AIDS. The development of prophylactic therapy for opportunistic infections has significantly decreased morbidity for infected patients.

SURGERY IN HIV-INFECTED PATIENTS

Current data on surgical interventions in AIDS patients are limited to retrospective uncontrolled case reports. These studies often fail to classify patients by HIV-related symptoms, CD4+ lymphocyte counts, or nutritional status parameters. Only more recent studies have stratified HIV-infected patients undergoing surgery.

Most postoperative complications, including bacterial sepsis, wound infection, and delayed healing occur in AIDS patients who suffer from poor nutrition.[8–11] In one retrospective study of patients with HIV infection and AIDS undergoing surgery,[10] the rate of postoperative complications was 20 percent. There was no difference in rate between HIV-infected and AIDS patients except for the more frequent occurrence of bacterial sepsis among those with AIDS. Wound infection and delayed healing correlated with a decreased number of circulating neutrophils.

Studies in noninfected patients underline the importance of nutritional and immune status in determining outcome,[12–14] but few similar studies have been done in HIV-infected or AIDS populations. In one such study, the combination of hypoalbuminemia with serum albumin levels below 2.5 g/liter and a history of opportunistic infection was associated with decreased survival after surgery.[11] In noninfected patients, anesthesia, surgery itself, and postoperative recovery depress killer-cell activity, lymphocyte proliferation, and blastogenic function,[15,16] but these changes are transient and rarely contribute to surgical morbidity.

Poor outcome in HIV-infected and AIDS patients undergoing surgery is more likely due to complications of AIDS than to complications of surgery. Several studies document few surgical complications but find that mortality is influenced by the progression of opportunistic infections and malignancies.[17,18] In two such studies of AIDS patients, the 39-day postoperative mortality rate approached 22 percent.[19,20] In another study of both HIV-infected and AIDS patients, the 30-day rate was 19 percent after emergency surgery and 9 percent after elective procedures. No increase in the number of wound infections has been reported among asymptomatic HIV-infected patients.[10] Procedures associated with an especially low rate of complications include biopsies of the skin, lymph nodes, and brain; placement of central venous catheters; splenectomy; and appendectomy.[18,19]

Elective and emergency surgical procedures can thus be performed in HIV-infected and AIDS patients with acceptable rates of postoperative complications and mortality.[11] Recommendations in the early literature calling for restricting surgery in these patients[9,20,21] were based on methodologically flawed studies involving small numbers of patients and are now outdated.

PREOPERATIVE EVALUATION OF THE HIV-INFECTED SURGICAL PATIENT

A complete history and physical examination is required to determine the clinical stage of HIV infection and to identify potential complications. Many patients are well informed about their disease while others have just been informed of the diagnosis. The history should include inquiries about the most recent CD4 lymphocyte count, previous or ongoing therapy with antiviral or prophylactic agents, medications, allergies, and occurrence of AIDS-defining opportunistic infections or malignancy. Progressive immunodeficiency should be assessed by eliciting a history of weight loss, skin rash, diarrhea, oral thrush, and bacterial infections. Coinfections such as hepatitis, sexually transmitted diseases, herpes simplex or zoster, vaginal or anorectal disease, and tuberculosis (including active disease, exposure, and PPD status) should also be documented. A careful review of systems is important in uncovering AIDS-associated end-organ dysfunction that might affect surgical risk, and should include quantification of drug or alcohol use. Patients should be asked about advance medical directives and a durable power of attorney for health care. This is especially important if an HIV-infected patient wishes to designate a surrogate who is not a legal spouse or family member.

Physical examination requires particular attention to the skin, oropharynx, lymph nodes, and perirectal area and should include assessment of mental status and neurologic function. In addition to routine preoperative laboratory tests, CD4+ lymphocyte count, RPR, and serum albumin and transferrin levels should be measured, and, if appropriate, a one-hour ACTH stimulation test should be performed. A PPD and anergy panel should be placed unless the PPD is known to be reactive. A nutritional consultation is also recommended.

Hematologic Abnormalities

All hematopoietic elements are affected by HIV infection, and these effects increase with advancing disease. In one study, anemia, granulocytopenia, and thrombocytopenia were found in 17 percent, 8 percent, and 13 percent, respectively, of asymptomatic HIV-infected patients and in 70 percent, 65 percent, and 43 percent, respectively, of patients with AIDS.[22] The lupus anticoagulant has also been isolated from the sera of those with AIDS.[23–25]

The incidence of anemia is 70 to 90 percent in AIDS patients, 15 percent in symptomatic HIV-infected patients, and 8 percent in asymptomatic HIV-infected patients.[22,26–28] The causes of anemia are multiple and include ineffective erythropoiesis, medication effects, nutritional deficiencies, and infiltrative disease of the bone marrow. Anemia due to ineffective erythropoiesis in HIV-infected or AIDS patients is usually normochromic and normocytic. Serum iron studies are most often consistent with the anemia of chronic disease,[29] and the reticulocyte count is low.[30] Zidovudine causes anemia by suppressing the bone marrow only rarely in asymptomatic HIV-infected patients[31] but does so in up to 40 percent of AIDS patients.[32] Chronic use of human recombinant erythropoietin (r-HuEPO) can be effective in treating zidovudine-induced anemia.[33] Macrocytosis develops in a majority of patients after two weeks of antiviral treatment.[34] Although positive direct antiglobulin tests and autoantibodies have been found in the sera of AIDS patients, clinically significant hemolytic anemia is rare.[32] HIV-infected and AIDS patients undergoing surgery may require trans-fusions, and there is recent evidence that transfusion of leukocyte-containing blood products may accelerate the dissemination of HIV and progression of disease. Therefore, leukocyte-depleted packed red blood cells should be used.[35,36]

Leukopenia occurs with about the same frequency as anemia. The majority of patients with AIDS and about 15 percent of asymptomatic HIV-infected patients are leukopenic.[30,22] Leukopenia may present as granulocytopenia, lymphopenia, or both. It results from an ineffective bone marrow[30] or can be induced by medication. Trimethoprim-sulfamethoxazole and zidovudine can exacerbate leukopenia,[34] but many other medications used in treating HIV-infected patients are associated with its development.

As long as HIV-infected patients are not severely neutropenic, leukopenia is generally well tolerated. Even a mild neutropenia with counts of 500 to 1000/mm^3 usually has no clinical sequelae in HIV-infected and AIDS patients without active bacterial infections.[37] The role of prophylactic antibiotics or colony-stimulating factors in preventing bacterial infections in severely neutropenic HIV-infected and AIDS patients has not yet been clarified.

Thrombocytopenia in the absence of anemia or leukopenia has been reported in up to 13 percent of asymptomatic patients[38] and is usually the result of immunologically-mediated destruction of platelets. Circulating immune complexes, platelet-bound immunoglobulins and serum IgG with antiplatelet activity all have been found in patients presenting with HIV-associated thrombocytopenia.[38–40] Examination of the bone marrow reveals a normal to increased number of megakaryocytes.

Clinical bleeding is less common in HIV-associated thrombocytopenia than in patients with chronic immune thrombocytopenic purpura.[41,42] Some investigators have reported spontaneous improvement without therapy.[43,44] However, hemophiliacs with HIV-associated thrombocytopenia appear to have an increased risk of bleeding, especially in the central venous system.[45]

Treatment of HIV-related thrombocytopenia has included corticosteroids, intravenous gamma globulin, zidovudine, danazol, and splenectomy. Oksenhendler et al. found that 58 percent of patients with HIV-associated thrombocytopenia and clinical bleeding responded to one mg/kg/day of prednisone after four weeks, but only 23 percent had continued response after steroid therapy was tapered.[39] Walsh et al. also found that, although most thrombocytopenic patients responded to steroids, the majority relapsed when the drug was withdrawn.[43] The use of high-dose corticosteroid therapy in these patients may cause reactivation of latent infections or hasten development of opportunistic infections.[39,43,46]

Intravenous gamma globulin has also been used successfully in these patients. In one study of 17 patients, 71 percent responded to a two to five consecutive day infusion.[39] No patient achieved a sustained remission but none suffered side effects from the therapy. Bussel et al. also reported successful treatment with intravenous gamma globulin.[46] Responses were better in asymptomatic HIV-infected patients than in those with AIDS. Tertian et al. reported a 75 percent response rate following a single dose of intravenous gamma globulin. Platelet counts rose to a maximum within four days and lasted 11 to 60 days.[47] Although the mechanism of its action on the immune system has not been elucidated, intravenous gamma globulin has not been shown to cause clinically significant immunosuppression.

Zidovudine appears to be effective in increasing platelet counts in patients with HIV-related thrombocytopenia and is most often used in outpatients. Oksenhendler et al. documented twofold increases or more in platelet counts and a reduction in mild clinical bleeding in 15 of 34 patients when zidovudine was given for 12 weeks.[50] Improvement in platelet counts have been noted after eight days of therapy.[51] With the exception of one case report,[52] danazol has not been found effective in treating HIV-associated thrombocytopenia.[39,53,54]

Thrombocytopenia in HIV-infected and AIDS patients may also result from bone marrow suppression, infiltration, or medication toxicity. All medications that may contribute to thrombocytopenia should be discontinued. Examination of the bone marrow is indicated when the cause of thrombocytopenia remains uncertain.

Splenectomy is an appropriate treatment for patients with severe sustained thrombocytopenia resistant to medical therapy who require surgery. Response is excellent in most patients,[43] and postoperative complications are minimal.[39,42,43] Relapses after splenectomy have been reported.[39,42] Antipneumococcal vaccination before and long-term penicillin prophylaxis after splenectomy are recommended.[39] There is some concern that splenectomy may increase the risk of progression to AIDS.[42,43,47–49]

In summary, patients with HIV-associated immune thrombocytopenia undergoing surgery may require high-dose intravenous steroids or intravenous gamma globulin before the procedure. Because splenectomy may contribute to the progression of HIV disease, it is reserved for life-threatening situations. In those with thrombocytopenia due to bone marrow suppression, platelet transfusions can be given before surgery. Recent data suggest that leukocyte-depleted platelets should be used.[35,36] For elective procedures, zidovudine may be effective and is often concurrently indicated for progressive disease.[50] Therapy should be closely monitored for toxicity.

The presence of the lupus anticoagulant, an IgG or IgM immunoglobulin capable of prolonging lipid-dependent coagulation tests, has been reported in AIDS patients but has not been associated with thrombotic complications.[23,25,55] In one study, several patients with the lupus anticoagulant had coincident factor deficiency, thrombocytopenia, or a qualitative platelet disorder and an increased risk of bleeding.[23] There may be an association between the appearance of the lupus anticoagulant and the onset of an opportunistic infection, and between the subsequent disappearance of the anticoagulant and resolution of the infection.[23,25] However, the lupus anticoagulant has also been documented in patients with asymptomatic and symptomatic HIV infection and in those with AIDS who have not experienced opportunistic infections.[53] A prolonged PTT due to the lupus anticoagulant does not increase the risk of bleeding and requires no treatment.

Immunologic Abnormalities

HIV infection should be viewed as a spectrum of disease ranging from those who are asymptomatic to those who are critically ill with AIDS. The Centers for Disease Control classification for HIV-associated disease[56] and the Walter Reed staging classification of HIV infection[57] categorize patients on the basis of degree of immunodeficiency. Although the timing of progression from asymptomatic infection to symptomatic infection (sometimes known as AIDS-related complex or ARC) and finally to AIDS is not predictable in a given individual, there are clinical and immunologic markers that allow some determination of the risk of developing AIDS over time. The terms AIDS-related complex (ARC), persistent generalized lymphadenopathy (PGL), and lym-

phadenopathy syndrome (LAS) have all been applied to patients at different points in the spectrum between asymptomatic HIV infection and AIDS. Unfortunately, these terms have not been applied uniformly and have attempted to create a homogeneous category for a heterogeneous group of patients.

HIV-infection results in progressive loss of CD4+ lymphocytes and worsening immunodeficiency. The CD4+ lymphocyte count in noninfected healthy individuals is approximately 1000 cells/mm^3. The average drop in the number of CD4+ lymphocytes in the first year after seroconversion is 200 to 300 cells/mm^3,[58] followed by an average loss of about 85 cells/mm^3 per year thereafter[59] and a more precipitous fall just before the development of an opportunistic infection.[60] Ten years after seroconversion, almost all patients have less than 200 CD4+ lymphocytes/mm^3.[61]

Persistent generalized lymphadenopathy alone in an HIV-infected individual is not predictive of a low CD4+ lymphocyte count or imminent development of AIDS.[62,63] Kaslow et al., in a cohort of gay and bisexual HIV-infected men, found that thrush, fever, low hematocrit, and low neutrophil count each correlated independently with a mean CD4+ lymphocyte count of less than 250 cells/mm^3.[62] However, it is important to remember that each of these clinical findings can have other causes. Most AIDS-defining opportunistic infections and malignancies occur in patients with CD4+ lymphocyte counts under 200 cells/mm^3. Infections with *Toxoplasma gondii*, *Cryptococcus neoformans*, cytomegalovirus (CMV), and *Mycobacterium avium intracellulare* (MAI) usually develop in patients with counts under 100 cells/mm^3.

The number of circulating CD4+ lymphocytes is a sensitive but nonspecific surrogate marker for the development of AIDS. Although most patients with AIDS have a CD4+ cell count of less than 200 cells/mm^3, only 25 to 30 percent with counts under 200 cells/mm^3 develop AIDS within two years.[61] If a low CD4+ is accompanied by the presence of p24 antigen, the risk of developing AIDS in one study increased to 50 percent within one year and 67 percent within two.[61] Moss et al. found that, among HIV-infected patients who had normal absolute number and percentage of CD4+ lymphocytes, normal serum beta$_2$ microglobulin levels, normal packed-cell volume, and negative serum p24 antigen tests, the risk of developing AIDS within three years was only 7 percent.[59] Among patients with two or more abnormal parameters, the risk was 57 percent over three years.

Once a patient develops AIDS, estimating survival time is difficult. In one large study of AIDS patients diagnosed between 1981 and 1985, the cumulative probability of survival was about 48 percent at one year and 15 percent at five years.[64] Because of better medical management of AIDS, therapy with antiviral drugs, and prophylaxis for *Pneumocystis carinii* pneumonia, most published survival data are now outdated.

Antiviral therapy may be briefly interrupted in the immediate perioperative period. If possible, medications for prophylaxis of opportunistic infections, particularly those for *P. carinii* pneumonia, should be continued.

Endocrine Abnormalities

Endocrine dysfunction in patients with AIDS can be the result of opportunistic infection, malignancy, or drug therapy. Recognition of endocrine disorders, particularly adrenal insufficiency, is important in the surgical patient. Much that is known about adrenal involvement in AIDS is derived from autopsy studies. Adrenal necrosis is commonly seen at autopsy in patients with localized or disseminated cytomegalovirus (CMV) infection at the time of death. In a study by Tapper et al., all but one patient with evidence of a CMV infection elsewhere had adrenal involvement at autopsy.[65] Adrenal insufficiency was neither suspected nor investigated before death in any of the patients. In an autopsy series of 41 patients reported by Glasgow et al., lipid depletion of the adrenal gland was present in 100 percent of the cases. CMV infection was seen in more than half of the cases and was more extensive in the medulla than the cortex.[66] *Mycobacterium avium intracellulare*, *Cryptococcus neoformans*, and Kaposi's sarcoma were found in others. Necrosis never involved more than 70 percent of the gland and was less than that normally seen in adrenal insufficiency. Of the 32 patients with clinical data, only two were suspected of adrenal insufficiency. However, 75 percent had hypoglycemia, 34 percent had hypotension, and most had a variety of nonspecific symptoms. Adrenal infiltration with *P. carinii* has been reported in a patient with disseminated pneumocystosis.[67]

Several investigators have studied adrenal function in patients with AIDS. Dobs et al. found normal cortisol responses to adrenocorticotrophin (ACTH) stimulation in 92 percent of ambulatory patients.[68] Greene et al. screened 20 patients with symptoms and signs of adrenal insufficiency and found abnormal ACTH stimulation tests in 20 percent.[69] In a study of 75 severely ill hospitalized patients, Membreno et al. documented that more than half had a subnormal one-hour response to ACTH, suggesting marginal adrenal function.[70] Of the four patients with adrenal insufficiency, none had hyperpigmentation, and ACTH levels were not elevated.

Anorexia, weight loss, fatigue, and hypotension are common in patients with AIDS and in those with adrenal insufficiency. It is therefore not unusual to overlook the possibility of adrenal insufficiency in those with AIDS. Laboratory data can be atypical. Baseline cortisol levels in sick patients with AIDS have been reported to be normal or high.[69,70] Hyponatremia or an elevated ACTH level need not be present. Patients with CMV or MAI infections or with metastatic Kaposi's sarcoma may have a higher risk of developing adrenal insufficiency.[69,70] Adrenal insufficiency has also been reported after therapy with ketoconazole[71,72] and rifampin.[73,74] It is recommended that, if time permits, all severely ill patients with HIV infection or AIDS undergo a one-hour ACTH stimulation test prior to surgery. If adrenal insufficiency is suspected, patients should be treated with stress-dose steroids in the perioperative period until test results are known.

Thyroid abnormalities in hospitalized patients with AIDS are for the most part similar to those observed in patients with severe nonthyroidal illnesses and require no treatment.[75-77] Distinctly unusual alterations in thyroid function have been observed in HIV-infected patients and include increased serum T_4 and thyroxine-binding globulin, as well as decreased rT_3 and normal serum T_3 levels in the context of worsening illness.[78] At autopsy, involvement of the thyroid by CMV, *Cryptococcus neoformans*, Kaposi's sarcoma, and *P. carinii* have been reported.[79,80] Ketoconazole, rifampin, and interferon have been implicated in the development of hypothyroidism in patients who do not have AIDS.[81]

Hypoglycemia can be a complication of pentamidine therapy in patients with AIDS. Stahl-Bayliss et al. reported hypoglycemia in 27 percent of 37 patients receiving pentamidine for *P. carinii* pneumonia.[82] The hypoglycemia was associated with drug-induced nephrotoxicity and developed during or shortly after pentamidine

therapy was given. Serum glucose and creatinine concentrations should be checked daily in patients receiving pentamidine therapy, and glucose levels should be monitored for several days after the completion of therapy. The syndrome of inappropriate ADH secretion (SIADH) and hypocalcemia have also been reported as rare complications of pentamidine therapy.[83] Drug-induced pancreatitis can be a complication of therapy with ddI and ddC.

Nutritional Considerations

HIV infection is often complicated by severe weight loss and nutritional deficiency. Numerous studies have documented the negative impact of nutritional depletion on immune function.[84] Malnutrition may compound the immunodeficiency of AIDS. The multiple opportunistic infections and atypical neoplasms in AIDS have been compared to the illnesses seen in children suffering from severe protein calorie malnutrition.[85]

Several studies have shown that preoperative nutritional repletion reduces surgical morbidity and mortality.[86-88] However, there are no studies clearly demonstrating an improved surgical outcome in patients with AIDS. Extrapolating data from the former studies suggests that optimal nutritional status in patients with AIDS improves surgical outcome, contributes to the quality of life, and may prevent additional impairment of the immune system. Preoperative and ongoing nutritional assessment by a trained consultant is an important part of the management of these patients. Reviews in the literature and Chap. 41 of this book detail methods of preoperative nutritional assessment.[87,89] Many malnourished patients can be identified by a serum albumin concentration under 3 gm/dl and a serum transferrin level under 200 mg/dl.[89]

Patients with AIDS who are not undergoing surgery have nutritional requirements comparable to those of other metabolically stressed patients. General recommendations for nutritional repletion of these patients are available.[90,91] They require 2.0 to 2.5 g/kg/day of protein (normal 0.8 to 1.5 g/kg/day) to maintain lean body weight. Their total daily caloric requirements are also greater at 35 to 40 kcal/kg/day (normal 25 to 30 kcal/kg/day). Because bowel function is often compromised, the ideal diet should have low osmolality and high caloric content. It should be low in fat with high concentrations of glutamine and branched-chain amino acids, the preferred energy source of the small intestine. It should contain no lactose and provide adequate minerals, vitamins, and trace elements.

Nutritional supplementation can be complicated by diarrhea. Diarrhea should be aggressively evaluated to exclude infectious causes. Step-wise treatment involves the use of antidiarrheal agents and BRAT diet consisting of bananas, rice, apples, and tea.[90,92,93]

Institution of total parenteral nutrition (TPN) is indicated in cases of severe dehydration, electrolyte imbalance, intolerance to enteral feedings, or intraabdominal pathology resulting in intermittent or continuous mechanical bowel obstruction.[90] Before starting TPN, specific goals of therapy and prognosis must be carefully assessed. TPN regimens used in patients with AIDS are comparable to those used in others and should be based on total caloric and protein requirements. Complications of TPN include mechanical and infectious complications due to indwelling central venous catheters and metabolic derangements.[89] These can be minimized by meticulous care of the catheter and diligent monitoring of metabolic parameters.

POSTOPERATIVE MANAGEMENT

The management of postoperative complications in HIV-infected and AIDS patients is similar to that in noninfected patients. However, aggressive management and a high clinical suspicion are especially important in those with HIV disease. Although prolonged unexplained fever after surgery with spontaneous defervescence on or about the fourth postoperative day has been reported,[35] infection should be considered as the etiology until proven otherwise. HIV-infected patients with postoperative fever require a complete physical examination with attention to the sinuses, oral mucosa, skin, perirectal area, and sites of surgical intervention and catheter placement.

In addition to impaired cell-mediated immunity, patients with HIV infection have abnormal B-cell antibody response to encapsulated organisms and impaired neutrophil function, particularly late in the disease.[94] Bacterial infections are more frequent and have atypical presentations.[95-98] Frequent prior hospitalizations and therapy with broad-spectrum antibiotics make HIV-infected and AIDS patients vulnerable to nosocomial infections.

Pneumonia in the Perioperative HIV-Infected Patient

The presence of a pulmonary infiltrate before or after surgery in an HIV-infected patient requires careful evaluation. The differential diagnosis must include not only opportunistic infections resulting from T-cell immunodeficiency but also bacterial pneumonias. Nosocomial pneumonias frequently have a severe clinical course, often requiring mechanical ventilation, and are associated with a higher mortality rate than community-acquired pneumonias.[97]

The radiographic presentation of bacterial pneumonia in AIDS may be typical or atypical. *Streptococcus pneumoniae* pneumonia may cause the expected segmental or lobar consolidation on chest x-ray,[99] but may also cause multilobar involvement.[100] A diffuse interstitial infiltrate on chest film, indistinguishable from that of *P. carinii* pneumonia, has been reported in *Hemophilus influenzae* infections.[96] Bacterial infections may coexist with opportunistic infections, and chest x-rays may be difficult to interpret in the setting of preexisting pulmonary malignancies or scarring from previous *P. carinii* pneumonia.

The majority of nosocomial bacterial pneumonias in patients with AIDS are due to gram-negative organisms, usually *Pseudomonas aeruginosa*, *Klebsiella pneumoniae*, and *Enterobacter aerogenes*.[97] Pneumonia due to *P. aeruginosa* is more common in neutropenic patients or as a complication of bacteremia from indwelling central venous catheters.[97,101] Gram-positive organisms also frequently cause nosocomial infections.[98,101] *Staphylococcus aureus* pneumonia has become increasingly more common in patients with AIDS, either as a complication of bacteremia or as a result of primary lung infection.[101] *S. aureus* pneumonia can also occur in conjunction with *P. carinii* pneumonia and Kaposi's sarcoma in the lung.[101]

Nosocomial pneumonia requires empiric coverage for both gram-negative and gram-positive organisms, including methicillin-resistant *S. aureus*. Fiberoptic bronchoscopy with bronchoalveolar lavage is required in postoperative patients in whom no pathogen is identified by laboratory tests of sputum and blood and in those who fail to improve clinically on antimicrobial therapy.[98]

Bacteremia in the Perioperative HIV-Infected Patient

The diagnostic evaluation of the febrile perioperative patient with AIDS must include consideration of bacteremia due to a wide variety of organisms. A study by Kumholz et al. underscores the need for a high level of suspicion of bacteremia in patients with AIDS.[102] Only about half of bacteremic patients became febrile or tachycardic, and about 25 percent had totally vital signs. Abnormalities in temperature, heart rate, respiratory rate, and blood pressure are not sensitive indicators of bacteremia in AIDS patients.

Nosocomial bacteremia in AIDS can be caused by common bacterial pathogens. Both gram-positive and gram-negative organisms must be considered. Whimby et al. found that bacteremias in hospitalized patients with AIDS were most frequently due to *S. pneumoniae* and *H. influenzae* as complications of pneumonias. *S. aureus* was most often a complication of pneumonia or soft-tissue infection.[101] *Pseudomonas aeruginosa*, *S. epidermidis*, and *S. fecalis* bacteremias were reported most often in neutropenic patients. An indwelling venous catheter was associated with bacteremias caused by *P. aeruginosa*, *S. aureus*, *S. epidermidis*, and *Candida albicans*. *Clostridium perfringens* and *Streptococcus bovis* bacteremias have been reported in association with gastrointestinal Kaposi's sarcoma.[102,103] In another study, the rate of indwelling central venous catheter infections was 35 percent in AIDS patients and only 8 percent in noninfected patients.[104]

Because of the T-cell defect in AIDS, other organisms to consider include *Salmonella* species, *Listeria monocytogenes*, *Cryptococcus neoformans*, and *Histoplasma capsulatum*.[101] *Salmonella* bacteremia has a high rate of recurrence in these patients despite antibiotic therapy and is difficult to eradicate.[105] Fungemias and bacteremias due to *Coccidioides immitis*, *Nocardia asteroides*, *Aspergillus*, and *Mycobacterium tuberculosis* have been reported.[106-108] *Mycobacterium avium intracellulare* (MAI) is a common cause of bacteremia in patients with AIDS.[109-111] Despite the common finding of oropharyngeal and esophageal candidiasis in AIDS patients, *Candida albicans* fungemia is rare and is usually associated with neutropenia, prolonged hospitalization, the use of indwelling central venous catheters, and administration of broad-spectrum antibiotics.[101-112]

SUMMARY

1. Increasing numbers of HIV-infected and AIDS patients will require elective and emergency surgery as the dramatic increase in HIV infection continues in the United States and worldwide.

2. Surgery can be performed in HIV-infected and AIDS patients with acceptable complication rates. Most studies have been retrospective and uncontrolled, and there are no data to support any contraindication to surgery in these patients. In determining risk, each patient should be evaluated on an individual basis.

3. Because of improved expertise in managing patients with HIV infection, including therapy with antiviral agents and prophylaxis against opportunistic infections, HIV-infected patients live a longer and better life before developing AIDS. Early ongoing care is critical and should be facilitated both during and after hospitalization.

4. A complete history and physical examination allows assessment of risk of potential surgical complications. Medical directives and durable power of attorney for heath care should be discussed with all patients.

5. Hematologic abnormalities are common in patients with HIV disease. Leukopenia without severe neutropenia is generally well tolerated in HIV-infected and AIDS patients without active infections. The role of prophylactic antibiotics to prevent bacterial infections in neutropenic HIV-infected patients is not established.

6. Thrombocytopenia in HIV-infected patients can be the result of immune-mediated platelet destruction or may be due to marrow failure. In the former case, intravenous corticosteroids or gamma globulin can be used before urgent surgery. Platelet transfusions are given when thrombocytopenia is due to marrow failure. Splenectomy is reserved for patients who are unresponsive to medical therapy or in life-threatening situations. Zidovudine can be used in clinically stable patients undergoing elective procedures.

7. Clinical and immunological parameters are helpful in assessing the severity of immunodeficiency and the risk of developing AIDS in HIV-infected patients. One surrogate immunologic marker is the CD4+ lymphocyte count. Most opportunistic infections occur in patients with counts under 200 cells/mm³.

8. HIV-infected patients have an increased risk of infection with *Mycobacterium tuberculosis* that often precedes the diagnosis of AIDS.[113–117] The number of cases of multidrug-resistant tuberculosis in HIV-infected patients is rapidly increasing. All HIV-infected patients, except those with a known prior positive test, should be skin-tested for tuberculosis and cutaneous anergy. Those who are positive should be screened for active infection and treated with preventive therapy if active infection is not present. A negative skin test may reflect HIV-induced cutaneous anergy and does not exclude infection.[57,114]

9. Adrenal insufficiency is not uncommon in patients with HIV infection and, because of its nonspecific symptoms and signs, can be easily overlooked. All severely ill HIV-infected and AIDS patients undergoing major surgery should have a one-hour ACTH stimulation test. If adrenal insufficiency is clinically suspected, patients should be treated with stress-dose steroids in the perioperative period pending test results.

10. A preoperative nutritional assessment is an important component in the management of HIV-infected and AIDS patients. Protein and calorie requirements are high. The diet should be lactose-free and low in osmolality and should provide adequate vitamins, minerals, and trace elements. Diarrhea can severely compromise nutritional status and should be aggressively evaluated to exclude infection and then treated with a step-wise approach.

11. Postoperative management should include vigilance for infection. Both gram-positive and gram-negative organisms can cause nosocomial bacterial infections in HIV-infected and AIDS patients. Central venous catheter infections are particularly common.

REFERENCES

1. Anonymous: *Global Program on AIDS*. Geneva, World Health Organization, 1991.

2. Berkelman RL, Heyward WL, Stehr-Green JK et al: Epidemiology of human immunodeficiency virus infection and acquired immunodeficiency syndrome. *Am J Med* 86:761–770, 1989.

3. Fischl MA, Richman DD, Grieco MH et al: The efficacy of azidothymidine (AZT) in the treatment of patients with AIDS and AIDS-related complex. *N Engl J Med* 317(4):185–191, 1987.

4. Yarchoan R, Mitsuya H, Broder S: AIDS therapies. *Sci Am* 259(4):110–119, 1988.

5. Marx JL: Wider use of AIDS drugs advocated. *News and Comments* 245:811, 1989.

6. Graham NMH, Zeger SL, Park PL et al: The effect on survival of early treatment of HIV infection. *N Engl J Med* 326:1037–1042, 1992.

7. Hamilton JD, Hartigan PM, Simberkoff MS et al: A controlled trial of early versus late treatment with zidovudine in symptomatic HIV. *N Engl J Med* 325:437–443, 1992.

8. Burack JH, Mandel MS, Bizer LS: Emergency abdominal operations in the patients with acquired immunodeficiency syndrome. *Arch Surg* 124:285–286, 1989.

9. Wexner SD, Smithy WB, Milson JW et al: The surgical management of anorectal diseases in AIDS and pre-AIDS patients. *Dis Colon Rectum* 29:719–723, 1986.

10. Vipond MN, Ralph DJ, Stotter AT: Surgery in HIV-positive and AIDS patients: Indications and outcome. *J R Coll Surg Edinb* 36:254–258, 1991.

11. Diettrich NA, Cacioppo JC, Kaplan G et al: A growing spectrum of surgical disease in patients with HIV/AIDS. *Arch Surg* 126:860–866, 1991.

12. Brown R, Bancewicz J, Hamid J: Failure of delayed hypersensitivity skin testing to predict postoperative sepsis and mortality. *Br Med J* 284:851–857, 1982.

13. Law KK, Dudrick SH, Abdov NI: Immunocompetence of patients with protein-calorie malnutrition. *Ann Int Med* 79:545–549, 1973.

14. Mullen JL, Buzby GP, Matthews DC: Nutritional predictors of surgical outcome. *Ann Surg* 604–610, 1980.

15. Scannel KA: Surgery and human immunodeficiency virus disease. *J Acquired Immuno Synd* 2(1):43–53, 1989.

16. Jubert A, Lee ET, Hirsch EM: Effects of surgery, anesthesia, and intraoperative blood loss on immunocompetence. *J Surg Res* 15:399–403, 1973.

17. Nugent P, O'Connell TX: The surgeon's role in treating acquired immunodeficiency syndrome. *Arch Surg* 121:1117–1120, 1986.

18. Robinson G, Wilson SE, Williams RA: Surgery in patients with acquired immunodeficiency syndrome. *Arch Surg* 122:170–175, 1987.

19. LaRaja RD, Rothenberg RE, Odom JW et al: The incidence of intraabdominal surgery in the acquired immunodeficiency syndrome: A statistical review of 904 patients. *Surgery* 5(2,1):175–179, 1986.

20. Ferguson CM: Surgical complications of human immunodeficiency virus infection. *Am Surg* 54(1):4–9, 1988.

21. Miller JI: The thoracic surgical spectrum of acquired immune deficiency syndrome. *J Thorac Cardiovasc Surg* 92:977–980, 1986.

22. Zon LI, Arkin C, Groopman JE: Haematologic manifestations of the human immune deficiency virus (HIV). *Br J Haematol* 66:251, 1987.

23. Cohen AJ, Philips TM, Kessler CM: Circulating coagulation inhibitors in the acquired immunodeficiency syndrome. *Ann Int Med* 104:175–180, 1986.

24. Bloom EJ, Abrams DI, Rodgers GM: Lupus anticoagulant in the acquired immunodeficiency syndrome. *JAMA* 256:491, 1986.

25. Gold JE, Haubenstock A, Zalusky R: Lupus anticoagulant and AIDS. *N Engl J Med* 314:1252, 1986.

26. Frontiera M, Myers AM: Peripheral blood and bone marrow abnormalities in the acquired immunodeficiency syndrome. *West J Med* 147:157, 1987.

27. Namiki TS, Boone DC, Meyer PR: A comparison of bone marrow findings in patients with acquired immunodeficiency syndrome (AIDS) and AIDS-related conditions. *Hematol Oncol* 5:99, 1987.

28. Weber JN, Walker D, Engelkins H et al: The value of hematological

screening for AIDS in an at-risk population. *Genitourin Med* 61:325, 1985.

29. Castella A, Croxson TS, Mildvan D et al: The bone marrow in AIDS: A histologic, hematologic and microbiologic study. *Am J Clin Pathol* 84:425, 1985.

30. Perkocha LA, Rodgers GM: Hematologic aspects of human immunodeficiency virus infection: Laboratory and clinical considerations. *Am J Hematol* 29:94–105, 1988.

31. Volberding PA, Lagakos SW, Koch MA et al: Zidovudine in asymptomatic HIV. *N Engl J Med* 322:941–949, 1990.

32. Zon LI, Groopman JE: Hematologic manifestations of the human immune deficiency virus (HIV). *Sem Hematol* 25(3):208–218, 1988.

33. Fischl M, Galpin JE, Levine JD et al: Recombinant human erythropoietin therapy for AIDS patients treated with zidovudine: A double-blind, placebo-controlled clinical study. *N Engl J Med* 322(21):1488–1493, 1990.

34. Richman DD, Fischl MA, Grieco MH et al: The toxicity of azidothymidine (AZT) in the treatment of patients with AIDS and AIDS-related complex: A double-blind, placebo-controlled trial. *N Engl J Med* 317(4):192–197, 1987.

35. Bosch MP, Tzong HL, Heitman J: Allogenic leukocytes but not therapeutic blood elements induce reactivation and dissemination of latent HIV Type I infection: Implications for transfusion support of infected patients. *Blood* 80(8):2128–2135, 1992.

36. Klein HG: Wolf in wolf's clothing: Is it time to raise the bounty on the passenger leukocyte? (editorial) *Blood* 80(8):1885–1888, 1992.

37. Shaunak S, Bartlett JA: Zidovudine-induced neutropenia: Are we too cautious? *Lancet* 2:91–92, 1989.

38. Walsh CM, Nardi MA, Karpatkin S: On the mechanism of thrombocytopenic purpura in sexually active homosexual men. *N Engl J Med* 311:635, 1984.

39. Oksenhendler E, Bierling P, Farcet J et al: Response to therapy in 37 patients with HIV-related thrombocytopenic purpura. *Br J Haematol* 66:491–495, 1987.

40. Stricker RB, Abrams DI, Corash L et al: Target platelet antigen in homosexual men with immune thrombocytopenia. *N Engl J Med* 313:1375, 1985.

41. Walsh C, Krigel R, Lannetta E et al: Thrombocytopenia in homosexual patients. *Ann Int Med* 103:542–545, 1985.

42. Abrams DI, Kiprov DD, Goedert JJ et al: Antibodies to human T-lymphotropic virus type III and development of the acquired immunodeficiency syndrome in homosexual men presenting with immune thrombocytopenia. *Ann Int Med* 104:47, 1986.

43. Walsh C, Krigel R, Lannetta E et al: Thrombocytopenia in homosexual patients. *Ann Int Med* 103:542–545, 1985.

44. Goldsweig HG, Grossman R, William D: Thrombocytopenia in homosexual men. *Am J Hematol* 21:243, 1986.

45. Ragni MV, Bontempo FA, Myers DJ et al: Hemorrhagic sequelae of immune thrombocytopenic purpura (ITP) in HIV-infected hemophiliacs. *Blood* 75:1267–1272, 1990.

46. Bussel JB, Haimi JS: Isolated thrombocytopenia in patients infected with HIV: Treatment with intravenous gamma globulin. *Am J Hematol* 28:79–84, 1988.

47. Tertian G, Risler N, Le Bras P et al: Intravenous gamma globulin treatment for thrombocytopenic purpura in patients with human immunodeficiency virus (HIV) infection. *Eur J Haematol*. 39:180–181, 1987.

48. Morris L, Distenfeld A, Amorosi E et al: Autoimmune thrombocytopenic purpura in homosexual men. *Ann Int Med* 96:714–717, 1982.

49. Ravikman TS, Allen JD, Bothe A et al: Splenectomy: The treatment of choice for human immunodeficiency virus–related immune thrombocytopenia. *Arch Surg* 124:625–628, 1989.

50. Oksenhendler E, Bierling P, Ferchal F et al: Zidovudine for thrombocytopenic purpura related to human immunodeficiency virus (HIV) infection. *Ann Int Med* 110:365–368, 1989.

51. The Swiss Group for Clinical Studies on the Acquired Immunodeficiency Syndrome (AIDS): Zidovudine for the treatment of thrombocytopenia associated with human immunodeficiency virus (HIV): A prospective study. *Ann Int Med* 109:718–721, 1988.

52. Anonymous: One case report (letter). *Ann Int Med* 104(6):583, 1986.

53. Costello C, Treacy M, Lai L: Treatment of immune thrombocytopenic purpura in homosexual men. *Scand J Haematol* 36:507–510, 1986.

54. Lynch EC, Huston DP: Immune thrombocytopenia in homosexual men. *Ann Int Med* 104:583–584, 1986.

55. Bloom EJ, Abrams DI, Rogers GM: Lupus anticoagulant in the acquired immunodeficiency syndrome. *Blood* 64:93A, 1984.

56. Centers for Disease Control: Classification system for human T-lymphotropic virus III/lymphadenopathy-associated virus infections. *Ann Int Med* 105:234–237, 1986.

57. Redfield RR, Wright DC, Tramont EC: The Walter Reed staging classification for HILV-III LAV infection. *N Engl J Med* 314(2):131–132, 1986.

58. Bartlett JG: *A Guide to HIV Care from the AIDS Care Program of the Johns Hopkins Medical Institutions*, 2d ed. Baltimore, Johns Hopkins, 1992.

59. Moss AR, Bacchetti P, Osmond D et al: Seropositivity for HIV and the development of AIDS or AIDS-related condition: Three-year follow-up of the San Francisco General Hospital cohort. *Br Med J* 296:745–750, 1988.

60. Eyster ME, Gail MH, Ballard JO et al: Natural history of human immunodeficiency virus infections in hemophiliacs: Effects of T-cell subsets, platelet counts, and age. *Ann Int Med* 107(1):1–6, 1987.

61. Eyster ME, Ballard JO, Gail MH et al: Predictive markers for the acquired immunodeficiency syndrome (AIDS) in hemophiliacs: Persistance of p24 antigen and low T4 cell count. *Ann Int Med* 110:963–969, 1989.

62. Kaslow RA, Phair JP, Friedman HB et al: Infection with the human immunodeficiency virus: Clinical manifestations and their relationship to immune deficiency. *Ann Int Med* 107:474–480, 1987.

63. Goedert JJ, Biggar RJ, Melbye M et al: Effect of T4 count and cofactors on the incidence of AIDS in homosexual men infected with human immunodeficiency virus. *JAMA* 257(3):331–334, 1987.

64. Rothenberg R, Woelfel M, Stoneburner R et al: Survival with the acquired immunodeficiency syndrome. *N Engl J Med* 317:1297–1302, 1987.

65. Tapper ML, Rotterdam HZ, Lerner CW et al: Adrenal necrosis in the acquired immunodeficiency syndrome. *Ann Int Med* 120(2):239–241, 1984.

66. Glasgow BJ, Steinsapir KD, Anders K et al: Adrenal pathology in the acquired immune deficiency syndrome. *Am J Clin Pathol* 84:594–597, 1985.

67. Unger PD, Rosenblum M, Krown SE: Disseminated *Pneumocystis carinii* infection in a patient with acquired immunodeficiency syndrome. *Human Path* 19(1):113–116, 1988.

68. Dobs AS, Dempsey MA, Ladenson PW et al: Endocrine disorders in men infected with human immunodeficiency virus. *Am J Med* 84:611–616, 1988.

69. Greene LW, Cole W, Greene JB et al: Adrenal insufficiency as a complication of the acquired immunodeficiency syndrome. *Ann Int Med* 101(4):447–448, 1984.

70. Membreno L, Irony I, Dere W et al: Adrenocortical function in acquired immunodeficiency syndrome. *J Clin Endoc Metab* 65:482–487, 1987.

71. Best TR, Jenkins JK, Murphy FY et al: Persistent adrenal insufficiency secondary to low-dose ketoconazole therapy. *Am J Med* 82:676–680, 1987.

72. Tucker WS Jr, Snell BB, Island DP et al: Reversible adrenal insufficiency induced by ketoconazole. *JAMA* 253:2413–2414, 1985.

73. Kyriazopoulou V, Parparousi O, Vagenaskis AG: Rifampicin-induced adrenal crisis in Addisonian patients receiving corticosteroid replacement therapy. *J Clin Endoc Metab* 59:1204–1206, 1984.

74. Hey AA, Coaglen JV, Espiner EA: Rifampicin-induced adrenal crisis. *NZ Med J* 96:988–989, 1983.

75. Frank TS, LiVolsi VA, Connor AM: Cytomegalovirus infection of the thyroid in immunocompromised adults. *Yale J Biol Med* 60:1–8, 1987.

76. Tibaldi JM, Surks MI: Effects of nonthyroidal illness on thyroid function. *Med Clin N Am* 69:899–911, 1985.

77. Chopra IJ, Hershman JM, Padrige MD et al: Thyroid function in nonthyroidal illness. *Ann Intern Med* 98:946–957, 1983.

78. LoPresti JS, Fried JC, Spencer CA et al: Unique alterations of thyroid hormone indices in the acquired immunodeficiency syndrome (AIDS). *Ann Int Med* 110:970–975, 1989.

79. Welch K, Finkbeiner W, Alpers CE et al: Autopsy findings in the acquired immune deficiency syndrome. *JAMA* 252:1152–1159, 1984.

80. Machac J, Nejatheim M, Goldsmith SJ: Gallium-67 critrate uptake in cryptococcal thyroiditis in a homosexual male. *J Nucl Med Allied Sci* 29:283–285, 1985.

81. Yarchoan R, Mitsuya H, Broder S: Clinical and basic advances in the antiretroviral therapy of human immunodeficiency virus infection. *Am J Med* 87:191–200, 1989.

82. Stahl-Bayliss CM, Kalman CM, Laski OL: Pentamidine-induced hypoglycemia in patients with the acquired immune deficiency syndrome. *Clin Pharmacol Ther* 39:271–275, 1986.

83. Andersen R, Boedicker M, Ma M et al: Adverse reactions associated with pentamidine isethionate in AIDS patients: Recommendations for monitoring therapy. *Drug Intell Clin Pharm* 20:862–868, 1986.

84. Chandra RK: Nutrition, immunity and infection. *Lancet* 1:688–691, 1983.

85. Gray RH: Similarities between AIDS and protein caloric malnutrition. *Am J Pub Health* 73(11):1332, 1988.

86. Meakins JL, Rietch JB, Bubenick O: Delayed hypersensitivity: Indicator of acquired failure of host deficiencies in sepsis and trauma. *Ann Surg* 186:241–250, 1977.

87. Buzby GP, Mullen JL, Mathews DC: Prognostic nutritional index in gastrointestinal surgery. *Am J Surg* 139:160–167, 1980.

88. Mullen JL, Gertner MH, Buzby GP: Implications of malnutrition in the surgical patient. *Arch Surg* 114:121–125, 1979.

89. Buzby GP, Mullen JL. Nutrition and surgical patient, in Goldmann DR, Brown FH, Levy WK et al (eds): *Medical Care of the Surgical Patient*. Philadelphia, Lippincott, 1982, pp 188–200.

90. Hickey MS, Weaver KE: Nutritional management of patients with ARC and AIDS in gastroenterology. *Clin N Am* 17(3):545–561, 1988.

91. Task Force on Nutrition Support in AIDS: Guidelines for nutrition support in AIDS. *Nutrition* 5(1):39–46, 1989.

92. Gedlin JS, Shike M, Alcock W: Malabsorption and mucosal abnormalities of the small intestine in acquired immunodeficiency syndrome. *Ann Int Med* 102:619–622, 1985.

93. Kottler DP: Nutritional considerations in AIDS. *Res and Staff Phys* 33(10):30–41, 1987.

94. Nichols L, Balogh K, Silverman M et al: Bacterial infections in AIDS. *Am J Clin Pathol* 92:787–790, 1990.

95. Simberkoff MS, Sadr WE, Schiffman GS et al: *Streptococcus pneumoniae* infections and bacteremia in patients with acquired immune deficiency syndrome, with report of a pneumococcal vaccine failure. *Am Rev Resp Dis* 130:1174–1176, 1984.

96. Polsky B, Gold JWM, Whimbey E et al: Bacterial pneumonia in patients with the acquired immunodeficiency syndrome. *Ann Int Med* 104:38–41, 1986.

97. Witt DJ, Craven DE, McCabe WR: Bacterial infections in adult patients with the acquired immune deficiency syndrome (AIDS) and AIDS-related complex. *Am J Med* 82:900–906, 1987.

98. Fells AOS: Bacterial and fungal pneumonias. *Clin Chest Med* 9(3):449–457, 1988.

99. Stover DA, White DE, Romano PA et al: Spectrum of pulmonary diseases associated with the acquired immune deficiency syndrome. *Am J Med* 78:429, 1985.

100. Murata GH, Ault MJ, Meyers RD: Community-acquired bacterial pneumonias in homosexual men: Presumptive evidence for a defect in host resistance. *AIDS Res* 1:379, 1984/1985.

101. Whimbey E, Gold JWM, Polsky B et al: Bacteremia and fungemia in patients with the acquired immunodeficiency syndrome. *Ann Int Med* 104:511, 1986.

102. Kumholz HM, Sande MA, Lo B: Community-acquired bacteremia in patients with acquired immunodeficiency syndrome: Clinical presentation, bacteriology, and outcome. *Am J Med* 86:776–779, 1989.

103. Glaser JB, Landesman SH: *Streptococcus bovis* bacteremia and acquired immunodeficiency syndrome (letter). *Ann Int Med* 99(6):878, 1983.

104. Raviglione MC, Battan R, Pablos-Mendez A et al: Infections associated with Hickman catheters in patients with AIDS. *Am J Med* 86:780–786, 1989.

105. Fischl MA, Dickinson GM, Sinave C et al: *Salmonella* bacteremia as manifestation of acquired immunodeficiency syndrome. *Arch Int Med* 146:113–115, 1986.

106. Abrams DI, Robia M, Blumenfeld W et al: Disseminated coccidioidomycosis in AIDS (letter). *N Engl J Med* 310:986–987, 1984.

107. Holtz HA, Lavery DP, Kapila R: *Actinomycetales* infection in the acquired immunodeficiency syndrome. *Ann Int Med* 102:203–205, 1985.

108. Mess TP, Hadley WK, Wofsy CB: Bacteremia due to *Mycobacterium tuberculosis* (MTB) and *Mycobacterium avium* intracellulare (MAI) in homosexual males, in *Abstracts from the Internal Conference on Acquired Immunodeficiency Syndrome, 14–17 April 1985, Atlanta, Georgia*. Philadelphia, American College of Physicians, 1985, p 47.

109. Macher AM, Kovacs JA, Gill V et al: Bacteremia due to *Mycobacterium avium intracellulare* in the acquired immunodeficiency syndrome. *Ann Int Med* 99:782–785, 1983.

110. Pierce PF, DeYoung DR, Roberts SG: Mycobacteremia and the new blood culture systems. *Ann Int Med* 99:786–789, 1983.

111. Wong B, Edwards FF, Kiehn TE et al: Continuous high-grade *Mycobacterium avium intracellulare* bacteremia in patients with the acquired immune deficiency syndrome. *Am J Med* 78:35–40, 1985.

112. Armstrong D: Fungal infections in the compromised host, in Rubin RH, Young LS (eds): *Clinical Approach to Infection in the Compromised Host*. New York, Plenum, 1981, pp 195–228.

113. Rieder HL, Cauthem GM, Bloch AB et al: Tuberculosis and acquired immunodeficiency syndrome—Florida. *Arch Int Med* 149:1268–1273, 1989.

114. Centers for Disease Control: Tuberculosis and human immunodeficiency virus infection: Recommendations of the advisory committee for the elimination of tuberculosis (ACET). *MMWR* 38(14):236–242, 1989.

115. Selwyn PA, Hartel D, Lewis VA et al: A prospective study of the risk of tuberculosis among intravenous drug users with human immunodeficiency virus infection. *N Engl J Med* 320(9):545–550, 1989.

116. Chaisson RE, Schector GF, Theuer CP et al: Tuberculosis in patients with the acquired immunodeficiency syndrome: Clinical features, response to therapy, and survival. *Am Rev Resp Dis* 136:570–574, 1987.

117. American Thoracic Society: Mycobacterioses and the acquired immunodeficiency syndrome. *Am Rev Resp Dis* 136:492–496, 1987.

32 SURGERY IN THE PATIENT WITH CHRONIC RENAL FAILURE

Neil Shusterman

More than 122,000 patients with end-stage renal disease (ESRD) are currently maintained on dialysis in the United States, and many times this number of people have milder degrees of renal insufficiency.[1] Most surgical conditions develop at least as frequently in patients with chronic renal failure (CRF) as in those with normal renal function. Some procedures like parathyroidectomy are required more commonly in those with CRF, and others like vascular access surgery or renal transplantation are performed exclusively in such patients. Preexisting renal insufficiency increases the risk of complications in the perioperative period.[2] However, surgery can be performed in patients with CRF with an acceptably low rate of complications if careful preoperative evaluation and treatment are carried out.[3,4]

SURGICAL RISK OF CHRONIC RENAL FAILURE

Excretion of intracellular constituents released into the extracellular fluid (ECF) during surgery and changing sodium excretion in response to surgically induced shifts in the volume of ECF are renal functions essential to homeostasis.[5] As renal function decreases, much of the adaptive ability of the remaining viable kidney is used to maintain ECF homeostasis in the steady state, and very little is available to defend against the acute stresses of the perioperative period. In addition, CRF is often complicated by other systemic abnormalities like hypertension, anemia, and coagulopathy. Dysfunction of other organs caused by CRF or by diseases responsible for the renal failure may further increase risk of surgery.

The incidence of systemic complications in the perioperative period increases with the severity of the renal failure. If the glomerular filtration rate (GFR) is above 50 ml/min, surgery is usually well tolerated, and no specific precautions are necessary. Renal function is most commonly assessed by measuring serum creatinine levels. Though a better marker of GFR than blood urea nitrogen concentration (BUN), it has several limitations. With age,

glomerular filtration rate declines. If creatinine production remained constant, the serum creatinine level would rise. However, creatinine production is directly proportional to muscle mass. As mass declines with aging, serum creatinine concentration remains "normal" even though GFR has decreased substantially.[6] A serum creatinine level of 1.0 mg/dl in a 25-year-old probably reflects a glomerular filtration rate of 120 to 130 ml/min, while the same serum creatinine level in a 75-year-old represents a GFR of 60 to 70 ml/min. This is particularly important when administering medications which are excreted by the kidney. Creatinine clearance is therefore a better measure of renal function than the serum creatinine level. This can be determined either by measuring creatinine in a 24-hour urine collection and obtaining a simultaneous serum creatinine or by estimating it from the following equation:[7]

$$\text{Creatinine Clearance} = \frac{(140 - \text{Age}) \times \text{Weight in kg}}{\text{Serum Creatinine} \times 72}$$

For women the value obtained should be multiplied by a factor of 0.85.

If the GFR is below 20 ml/min, perioperative complications are more likely to occur unless specific preventive steps are taken. The type of underlying renal disease may influence the risk of perioperative complications but is less important than the level of azotemia. For example, patients with chronic interstitial renal diseases or diabetes mellitus are more likely to develop complications like hyperkalemia and metabolic acidosis because of abnormal tubular function. However, these complications can occur in any type of renal disease.

COMPLICATIONS OF DECREASED RENAL FUNCTION

Extracellular Fluid (ECF) Volume

CRF limits the ability of the kidney to respond to situations requiring either maximum sodium excretion or conservation.[8] Homeostatic changes that do occur do so more slowly and less completely than in patients with normal renal function. The administration of large quantities of intravenous fluids can easily lead to ECF volume expansion and overload, particularly when the GFR has dropped below 10 ml/min. In patients with only mild or moderate renal failure, a sodium load can be excreted by the kidneys, and volume overload does not occur unless other conditions that independently inhibit sodium excretion—congestive heart failure, cirrhosis, or nephrotic syndrome—are present. Maximum sodium excretion is nonetheless decreased even in patients with only moderately advanced azotemia, and extremely large sodium loads given quickly can cause significant volume expansion.

If ECF volume expansion is present preoperatively, it should be treated with sodium restriction and either diuretics or, in patients with ESRD, dialysis.[9] Potent parenteral diuretics like furosemide or bumetanide are usually required in large doses. The addition of a modest dose of metolazone may significantly increase the diuresis.

ECF volume depletion is even more common in patients with mild or moderately advanced renal failure. CRF causes enhanced fractional excretion of sodium as remaining nephrons adapt to meet demand for sodium excretion. Decreased sodium intake or increased loss from an extrarenal source in patients with fever, diarrhea, nasogastric suction, fistulous tracts, or vomiting can cause further ECF volume depletion. Volume depletion in patients with CRF commonly goes unrecognized until serious complications develop. Careful monitoring of the ECF volume may require the use of central venous pressure monitoring. In patients with significantly impaired left ventricular function, consideration should be given to the placement of a flow-directed pulmonary artery catheter for accurate measurement of left-heart filling pressures.

Tonicity and Serum Sodium Concentration

In CRF the ability to conserve or excrete free water is limited.[10] Because of ongoing osmotic diuresis in each nephron, urinary dilution and concentration are limited. Dilutional ability is maintained longer than concentrating function. Maximum urinary concentrating ability is lost when the GFR drops below 60 ml/min. Despite these abnormalities, ECF tonicity remains normal because water intake is adjusted by the thirst mechanism. However, if enough free water is given in the perioperative period, the ability of the kidneys to excrete it is exceeded, and hyponatremia develops.[10] This is exacerbated by elevated levels of antidiuretic hormone due to pain, nausea, or use of narcotics. Conversely, if free-water intake is inappropriately restricted, hypernatremia may develop. The clinical consequences and the treatment of these ECF abnormalities are discussed in Chap. 60.

Acidosis

Chronic metabolic acidosis is usually present in patients with moderately advanced CRF.[11] The serum bicarbonate concentration begins to decrease when the GFR falls below 20 to 30 ml/min. The acidosis of CRF is usually well compensated by respiratory hyperventilation, and blood pH is maintained at a level only slightly below normal.

Patients with CRF can develop severe acidemia with a sudden increase of hydrogen ions in the ECF. The serum bicarbonate concentration should be 18 meq/liter or higher before surgery,[9] and enough oral or intravenous bicarbonate should be given to reach that level. The sodium load given with the bicarbonate is tolerated by most patients.[12] In patients on chronic dialysis, the bicarbonate concentration is generally above 18 meq/liter between dialysis treatments, making supplemental bicarbonate unnecessary.

It is important to obtain preoperative arterial blood gas measurements when the bicarbonate concentration is less than 18 meq/liter and when the serum creatinine level is above 6 mg/dl regardless of serum bicarbonate concentration. In the latter case, a normal serum bicarbonate level may be the result of a mixed acid-base disorder. Winters' formula ($Pco_2 = 1.5[HCO_3^-] + 8 \pm 1$) allows assessment of respiratory compensation for metabolic acidosis.[13] If the Pco_2 is higher than the expected calculated value, compensation is inadequate, and immediate evaluation of pulmonary function before surgery becomes crucial.

During and after surgery, hydrogen ions are released from ischemic cells into the ECF. Cellular ischemia occurs at the operative site and elsewhere due to changes in blood pressure, regional blood flow, and systemic oxygenation. The release of hydrogen ions causes an added acid load requiring buffering. In CRF, the patient is already hyperventilating to compensate for a chronic metabolic acidosis. If hyperventilation cannot be maintained, Pco_2 will rise, and pH will fall.[14] Even an increase in Pco_2 to normal will result in a significant fall in blood pH.

Hyperkalemia

Hyperkalemia does not appear in most patients with CRF until end-stage disease develops.[15] Though they can usually maintain a normal steady-state serum potassium concentration, they do not tolerate sudden shifts of potassium ions into the ECF.[16] Hyperkalemia is therefore a common complication of surgery in such patients.[17,18] The risk of hyperkalemia increases with the severity of renal failure. Intraoperative hyperkalemia is more likely to occur at a given level of renal insufficiency in patients with chronic interstitial disease or diabetes mellitus than in patients with other types of renal failure. The risk of hyperkalemia during surgery correlates with the preoperative serum potassium concentration and, in patients undergoing chronic dialysis, with the predialysis potassium concentration. The serum potassium level should be below 5 meq/liter immediately before surgery.

Any reversible factor interfering with potassium excretion should be addressed. Volume depletion and increased sodium reabsorption occur in heart failure, cirrhosis, and the nephrotic syndrome. There is increased sodium reabsorption in the proximal tubule and decreased delivery of sodium to distal tubular sites where sodium reabsorption is necessary for potassium secretion. Careful fluid repletion in patients who are volume-depleted or taking diuretics should be undertaken. If more than 50 to 60 meq/day of sodium are excreted in the urine, distal sodium delivery can be considered adequate to permit distal tubular potassium secretion.

Various drugs can interfere with potassium excretion. Those that inhibit the action of aldosterone, such as spironolactone, triamterene, or amiloride, should be discontinued. Nonsteroidal anti-inflammatory agents can cause hyperkalemia by inhibiting prostaglandin production and should be discontinued if hyperkalemia is present.[19] Heparin inhibits the production of aldosterone and may rarely contribute to hyperkalemia.[20] Beta-adrenergic antagonists may predispose the patient to intraoperative hyperkalemia by decreasing cellular uptake of potassium.[21] Angiotensin-converting enzyme inhibitors have also been associated with hyperkalemia in patients with CRF, presumably because of their tendency to reduce aldosterone levels.[22]

If preoperative hyperkalemia is not reversible, the serum potassium level must be lowered by other means. Kayexalate (sodium polystyrene sulfonate) is the treatment of choice and is equally as or more effective than dialysis in removing potassium. It should be given in a dose of 30 to 50 grams every two to three hours orally in sufficient sorbitol to promote its elimination. Though less effective, it may be administered as a rectal retention enema. If Kayexalate proves ineffective or cannot be used because of gastrointestinal disease, dialysis should be performed.

During and after surgery, the load of potassium introduced into the ECF increases significantly. Causes of this increase include acidemia, cellular ischemia, and release of potassium ions from muscle cells exposed to succinylcholine. Potassium ions may also be introduced in transfused blood or as cations in a variety of drugs including antibiotics.

The principle risk of hyperkalemia is cardiac irritability.[23] In one large series of patients with ESRD undergoing renal transplantation, the incidence of intraoperative cardiac arrhythmias was approximately 10 percent and that of serious rhythm disturbances 3 percent.[18] Postoperative hyperkalemia in patients with CRF is the major indication for emergency dialysis in the 24 hours following surgery, a time when dialysis is most likely to increase the risk of postoperative bleeding. Efforts to control the serum potassium concentration are therefore important to reduce the need for emergency dialysis.

Calcium and Phosphate

Disorders of calcium and phosphate homeostasis in patients with CRF are not exacerbated by surgery and do not generally cause postoperative complications. Marked hypocalcemia increases the cardiovascular risk of general anesthesia and should be treated preoperatively, but it is seldom severe enough to constitute a risk factor. Treatment of severe hypocalcemia should begin with control of the serum phosphate level. If this level is greater than 6 mg/dl in a patient with severe hypocalcemia, oral phosphate binders or, in an emergency situation, dialysis should be used to lower it. Decreasing the serum phosphate concentration to 5.5 mg/dl or less may cause a slight increase in the serum calcium level and allow safe administration of calcium. If time permits, hypocalcemia can be treated over several days with oral calcium supplements in doses of at least one gram per day of elemental calcium and the rapidly acting vitamin D derivative 1,25-dihydroxycholecalciferol in a dose of 0.50 to 0.75 μg/day. If more rapid therapy is needed, intravenous calcium can be given.

Symptomatic hypocalcemia may also develop in the postoperative period. If a large amount of intracellular phosphate is released into the ECF during surgery, the serum phosphate level may rise dramatically. Because renal phosphate excretion is limited in CRF, the serum calcium level may fall. Serum phosphate levels should be controlled before direct efforts to increase serum calcium concentrations are made. Intravenous calcium should be considered only if definite signs and symptoms of hypocalcemia are present.

SYSTEMIC COMPLICATIONS OF CHRONIC RENAL FAILURE

Hypertension

Hypertension is seen commonly in patients with CRF, particularly in those with advanced azotemia. The operative risks of inadequately treated hypertension are the same for patients with CRF as for normals. However, some important treatment considerations should be reviewed. In patients with renal failure, hypertension is often due to ECF volume expansion,[24] and potent diuretics or dialysis will reduce ECF volume and thereby lower blood pressure. However, even in ESRD hypertension may not be volume-dependent, and in such cases depletion of ECF volume is not effective. In addition, the use of nitroprusside to control severe or malignant hypertension in patients with CRF leads to accumulation of thiocyanate, which is largely dependent on glomerular filtration for elimination.[25] However, complications generally occur only if the infusion is continued for more than a few days. Dialysis may be necessary to lower extremely high thiocyanate levels. Other parenteral agents like labetolol or trimethaphan can be used in this setting. For those unable to take oral medications who do not require parenteral therapy, the clonidine patch is a useful alternative. Its transcutaneous absorption system provides for steady-state drug levels over a seven-day period. The dose can be titrated as needed, and central nervous system side effects are less marked than with the oral preparation.

Anemia

Anemia is an almost universal feature of advanced CRF. Although anemia theoretically increases perioperative risk, most patients with CRF do not develop complications because of it.[9] Anemia in CRF is chronic and remarkably well tolerated. Even patients with ESRD who have hematocrit levels of 20% to 24% tolerate major surgery without prior transfusion in most cases. More recently, the use of recombinant erythropoietin in anemic patients with CRF, before dialysis is needed and once it has begun, allows maintenance of hematocrit levels above 30% and obviates the need for transfusion.[26,27]

Although transfusions are usually not required before surgery, they are occasionally necessary for acute blood loss. The risks associated with transfusion in patients with CRF include hepatitis, iron overload, transfusion reactions, transmission of retrovirus infection, and volume overload. Patients with hematocrit levels above 25% do not require red cells before surgery, but those with levels below 20% probably should be transfused. Decreased postoperative wound healing, a feared consequence of anemia, is not a major factor in patients with CRF, although it is in those with acute renal failure. If transfusions are required, washed red cells are necessary only if a patient has had a previous transfusion reaction due to sensitization to white blood cell antigens.

Coagulation Defects

Though patients with CRF have normal clotting factor levels, they have an increased tendency to bleed excessively because of defective platelet aggregation. This abnormality is multifactorial in cause. Retained uremic toxins, abnormal platelet arachadonate metabolism, excess vascular prostacyclin production, and abnormal von Willebrand factor generation have all been implicated in the pathogenesis of the uremic platelet disorder.[28] Reduced hematocrit levels may contribute to bleeding by increasing the distance between platelets and the vessel wall. The use of recombinant erythropoietin to increase levels above 30% lowers the bleeding time in patients with CRF and improves platelet adhesion to the subendothelium in vitro.[29]

Although a number of in vitro tests demonstrate platelet abnormalities in uremic patients, the only test that correlates with clinical bleeding is the bleeding time.[30] The bleeding time is often prolonged by 1.5 to 2 times normal. Most patients with CRF tolerate even major surgery without hemorrhagic complications, but it is worthwhile to obtain a bleeding time in any patient with CRF who has a past history of excessive bleeding.

If the bleeding time is prolonged, several options are available. If the patient is already receiving dialysis and there is time before surgery, more intensive dialysis may shorten the bleeding time.[31] If surgery is more urgent, intravenous desmopressin can be used in a dose of 0.4 µg/kg immediately before the procedure.[32] The drug has a rapid onset of action and is effective for approximately six to eight hours. Additional doses should not be given in less than 24 hours because of the development of tachyphylaxis. If longer duration of action is required, oral or intravenous estrogens can be administered.[33] Onset of action is slower, but therapeutic effect persists significantly longer than that of desmopressin. Cryoprecipitate has been shown to improve the bleeding time and reduce hemorrhagic complications, but as a pooled blood product it carries an increased risk of transmitting viral infections.[34]

Routine hemodialysis also increases the risk of perioperative bleeding if it is performed less than six hours before surgery or in the first 24 hours thereafter.[34] However, if dialysis is absolutely necessary during these periods, it can be performed without heparin.[36,37] Advances in technique allow this to be done with a surprisingly low incidence of clotting in the extracorporeal dialyzer circuit. An alternative to "no-heparin" dialysis is regional citrate anticoagulation.[38] Sodium citrate is administered before the dialyzer, and calcium is administered after the dialyzer to chelate the citrate and reverse its effects. After the first 24 hours following surgery, standard "low-dose" heparin techniques can be used.[39] This is continued for about one week to reduce the incidence of bleeding from the wound.

Nutritional Status

It is not unusual for patients with severe renal failure to be malnourished.[40] As a result of decreased protein intake and uremia itself, many develop both somatic and visceral protein depletion. Malnutrition may contribute to poor wound healing and infectious complications. In a recent review of surgery and nutritional support in patients with CRF, patients receiving enteral or parenteral nutrition had a markedly improved survival rate compared to patients with inadequate nutrition.[41] All patients with CRF undergoing major surgery should be considered for nutritional support if they are unable to resume oral nutritional intake within several days after surgery. The enteral route is preferable because it allows a natural route of absorption and a lower rate of complications. However, parenteral nutrition should not be avoided if it is the only practical method of hyperalimentation.

It is difficult to administer standard parenteral nutrition solutions to patients with advanced renal failure not undergoing dialy-sis without worsening azotemia or fluid overload. In this case, administration of essential amino acids with concentrated carbohydrate solutions containing 70% dextrose and lipids provides good nutrition and minimizes nitrogenous waste and fluid excess. Standard nutrition solutions may be used in those receiving dialysis. In all of these patients, it is important to monitor potassium, magnesium, and phosphorus levels frequently and to adjust their concentrations in hyperalimentation fluids appropriately. Because patients may have difficulty eliminating free water, it is often necessary to add sodium, often up to 140 meq/liter, to prevent hyponatremia. Sodium acetate prevents hyponatremia and combats metabolic acidosis as well.

Infections

Infectious complications are neither more frequent in the perioperative period nor more difficult to treat in patients with CRF or ESRD. Except for necessary changes in antibiotic dosages, indications for prophylactic antibiotics and treatment of established infections are the same for patients with renal failure as those with normal renal function.

Atherosclerotic Cardiovascular Disease

Atherosclerotic cardiovascular disease is common in patients with renal failure and is more often a consequence of other underlying conditions.[42] The perioperative risks associated with atherosclerotic cardiovascular disease and its treatment are discussed in Chap. 18.

PERIOPERATIVE PRESERVATION OF RENAL FUNCTION

The preservation of renal function in the perioperative period is crucial in patients with CRF who have not progressed to ESRD. Preexisting renal insufficiency is one of the most important risk factors in the development of postoperative acute renal failure. A substantial number of patients with CRF suffer an acute decrease in renal function with surgery. Moreover, a postoperative decrement in renal function in a patient with CRF is seldom fully reversible. It is therefore imperative that all other situations that increase the risk of acute renal failure be avoided or minimized (see Chap. 63).

Volume depletion is common in patients with CRF in the perioperative period. In the event of postoperative oliguria or a rising serum creatinine level, intravascular volume should be assessed promptly. If the assessment is equivocal, a volume challenge of 500 ml of normal saline is recommended.

The use of nonsteroidal anti-inflammatory drugs in the immediate preoperative period, although unproven, may increase the risk of acute renal failure in these patients by inhibiting protaglandin synthesis.[43] Patients with CRF may be dependent on renal prostaglandin production for maintenance of maximum renal function.

Other risk factors include intravenous and intraarterial radiocontrast agents and aminoglycoside antibiotics.[44] Ultrasound or magnetic resonance imaging should be used to avoid radiocontrast dye whenever possible. When radiocontrast studies are unavoidable, gentle diuresis should be initiated with one-half normal saline solution started one to two hours before the study and continued for four to six hours thereafter. A loop-acting diuretic like furosemide or bumetanide may be necessary to initiate the diuresis.

Aminoglycoside antibiotics accumulate in the renal cortex where they cause tubular damage.[45] Given the availability of antibiotics with broad gram-negative bacterial coverage such as aztreonam and ceftazidime, it should be possible in many cases to avoid aminoglycoside antibiotics in patients with CRF. If they must be given, tobramycin and netilmicin should be considered because they are less nephrotoxic than gentamicin.[45] Careful attention to proper dosing with frequent monitoring of plasma levels and serum creatinine is important.

Anesthetic Concerns

Preoperative sedation with any of the commonly used agents is safe in patients with CRF. Although the metabolism of some may be altered by a decreased GFR, one or two doses will not cause complications. General anesthesia of any type causes a reduction in renal blood flow that is proportional to the depth of anesthesia.[46] Spinal anesthesia is associated with only minimal alterations in renal hemodynamics, but hypotension due to sympathetic blockade must be avoided.[46] Despite the theoretical advantages of spinal anesthesia, no study comparing it to general anesthesia has been done in patients with CRF. The requirements of the procedure rather than the presence of CRF should dictate the choice of anesthesia. Local or regional anesthesia may also be used in CRF patients without alteration of dose or technique.

The choice of general anesthetic is of some concern. Methoxyflurane is a potential nephrotoxin and can produce a clinical picture akin to diabetes insipidus through metabolic production of fluoride.[47] Although the incidence of renal failure following methoxyflurane anesthesia is low in patients with normal renal function, it should not be used in patients with preexisting renal failure who are not on dialysis. Enflurane is also metabolized to fluoride and has been associated with acute renal failure in patients with CRF.[48] However, fluoride levels are elevated only after prolonged exposure, and short exposures may be safe for patients with CRF. Isoflurane, because it is not extensively metabolized and does not release inorganic fluoride, is the most widely used inhalational agent in patients with CRF.[49]

Muscle relaxants should be carefully chosen. Succinylcholine is generally well tolerated. However, it causes a rise in serum potassium level in both normal patients and in those with CRF. Although the increase is similar in both groups, it may be deleterious in patients with CRF who have previously been hyperkalemic or require repeated doses of the drug. Gallamine should be avoided in patients with decreased renal function because it depends primarily on glomerular filtration for elimination and can produce prolonged paralysis in patients with CRF.[46] Although the half-life of D-tubocurarine is increased by 30 to 70 minutes in patients with CRF, it can be used safely. Cases of prolonged or recurrent paralysis after successful reversal by neostigmine have been reported in patients with renal failure, but such cases are uncommon and easily managed if accurately diagnosed.[50] Pancuronium is eliminated by the kidneys, and multiple doses can result in an unpredictably long duration of action. Vecuronium and atracurium are probably the muscle relaxants of choice in renal failure. Vecuronium is appropriate for rapid intubations, but cumulative effects may be seen with repeated doses. Atracurium is not affected by renal or hepatic dysfunction and does not accumulate in patients with CRF, making it the ideal muscle relaxant in this setting.

Modification of Drug Doses

Alterations in the doses of some drugs are necessary in CRF because either the drugs or their active or toxic metabolites are eliminated by the kidneys. Doses of such agents must be decreased to maintain safe concentrations in the body. Changes in doses of other drugs are necessary because of alterations in protein binding or volume of distribution induced by azotemia. Recent studies have noted that patients with CRF are very sensitive to narcotic analgesics.[51,52] Some have reported that morphine metabolism is diminished in renal failure, causing a marked increase in the plasma half-life of the drug.[51] Other studies have instead documented retention of morphine metabolites that may reach levels high enough to be biologically active.[52] Morphine is an appropriate analgesic in these patients, but doses must be reduced to avoid excessive sedation and respiratory depression. Administration of meperidine in repeated doses should be avoided because it may lead to seizures in patients with CRF.[53] Its main metabolite, normeperidine, is epileptogenic and accumulates in toxic levels. Other investigators have noted that codeine metabolism is also abnormal and suggest lower doses in those with compromised renal function.[54] A detailed discussion of dosage modifications for other drugs is found in a review by Bennett et al.[55]

DIALYSIS AND SURGERY

Most patients with CRF who are not already on chronic dialysis do not require dialysis immediately before surgery. Electrolyte and volume disturbances can generally be corrected without dialysis. Patients occasionally require their initial dialysis and surgery at the same time. If one or more complications of uremia requires dialysis in these patients, surgery should be postponed until a minimum of four or five hemodialysis treatments have been performed, or until at least 48 to 72 hours of peritoneal dialysis have been completed. If surgery must be performed urgently, three or four hours of hemodialysis should be performed with an anticoagulation protocol designed to minimize postdialysis bleeding.[36,37] Two to three hours should elapse between the completion of dialysis and the beginning of surgery. If absolutely necessary, dialysis can be continued throughout the operative procedure.

Published reports do not support the impression that patients established on dialysis are poor surgical candidates. They have an acceptably low postoperative mortality rate, ranging in a number of case series from 0 to 3.5 percent.[56] In the most recent series, a two percent mortality rate was documented in patients undergoing major procedures.[56] All of the deaths were among those requiring urgent or emergency surgery. The most frequent postoperative complication occurring in the first day or two after surgery was hyperkalemia in 19 percent of these patients. Hypotension was seen early in seven percent and was related to volume shifts, autonomic dysfunction, and depressed left ventricular function. Later in the postoperative period at five to seven days after surgery, wound complications assumed greater importance in up to five percent of cases.

Particular attention must be paid to preserving the vascular access of patients on hemodialysis in the perioperative period. Pressure on the access should be avoided by proper positioning of the limb, protection of the site during surgery, and frequent examination for detection of decreased function. If possible, hypotension should be avoided during and after the procedure. Intravenous catheter placement, blood drawing, and blood pressure measurement should not be performed in the extremity with the access. Alteration in access function should prompt evaluation by a vascular surgeon. Despite these precautions, thrombosis occurs in 3 percent of cases.[56] Vascular access can become infected during surgery if bacteremia occurs. Infection is more likely to develop in synthetic grafts but is also seen in autologous arteriovenous fistulas. All patients on hemodialysis should receive antibiotic prophylaxis before any procedure that may cause bacteremia. The guidelines of the American Heart Association for prophylaxis against endocarditis are appropriate for patients on hemodialysis (see Chap. 43).[57]

Patients on a regular treatment program should receive their last treatment between 4 and 30 hours before surgery. If it is done more than 30 hours before surgery, chances of intraoperative hyperkalemia are greater. If it is performed less than four hours before the operation, the possibility of intraoperative bleeding is increased. After surgery, dialysis should be delayed for at least 24 hours. The approach to preoperative and postoperative anticoagulation has already been discussed.

Cardiac Surgery

Cardiac surgery in the patient on dialysis presents special demands. Though one report has indicated a high mortality rate, particularly in older patients,[58] several others document no greater mortality than in those without renal failure.[59,60] Patients on dialysis did have a greater incidence of complications, including longer duration of mechanical ventilation and vasopressor support and longer intensive care unit and hospital stays.[60] Nonetheless, these data suggest that cardiac surgery can be performed successfully in this population. Because coronary disease is so prevalent in dialyzed patients, these findings have wide applicability.

Control of intravascular volume and serum potassium levels are important during open-heart surgery. Intraoperative hemodialysis or arteriovenous hemofiltration may be needed to achieve this. Intraoperative hemodialysis is easy to perform and has been shown to delay the need for postoperative dialysis and provide better control of potassium levels than standard dialysis regimens.[61] After surgery, continuous arteriovenous hemofiltration (CAVH)[62] and continuous arteriovenous hemodialysis[63] provide dialytic support to hemodynamically unstable patients. These techniques utilize highly permeable filters to allow solute and fluid removal with the patient's own blood pressure providing the force to circulate the blood through the extracorporeal circuit.

Peritoneal Dialysis Patients and Surgery

Today there are more than 15,000 patients alive on chronic peritoneal dialysis in the United States.[1] Although the preceding comments generally apply to those on peritoneal dialysis, specific issues should be addressed. If a patient on peritoneal dialysis is to receive general anesthesia, the abdomen should be drained of peritoneal fluid just before the procedure and the peritoneal catheter filled with a heparin-containing solution and capped. This reduces

intraabdominal pressure, facilitates ventilation of the patient, and reduces the chances of aspiration during induction. In addition, extubation of the patient at the end of the procedure is more easily accomplished.

Peritoneal dialysis can be resumed any time after a nonabdominal procedure. However, after abdominal surgery, peritoneal dialysis may be associated with anastomotic leaks, poor wound healing, and late incisional hernia formation. An alternative technique like hemodialysis or continuous arteriovenous hemodialysis is recommended. The peritoneal catheter should be flushed weekly with a heparin-containing saline solution, and standard exit-site care should be performed daily. If possible, peritoneal dialysis should not be resumed for at least four to six weeks. When dialysis is resumed, small intraperitoneal volumes should be used initially to reduce the chances of leakage or patient discomfort. If peritoneal dialysis must be started sooner, only small volumes of 500 to 1000 ml in frequent exchanges should be used.

Peritoneal dialysis patients chronically lose albumin in the peritoneal fluid and serum albumin levels are slightly lower than in hemodialysis patients. Some investigators have demonstrated impaired delayed hypersensitivity responses in these patients[64] and have suggested that early nutritional support is important if oral feedings cannot be resumed within several days of surgery.[65]

Wounds need to be carefully closed to achieve water-tightness in order to prevent dehiscence, leaks, and late hernia formation. Skin sutures are generally left in place longer than in other patients because of slow healing. Drains need to be removed before dialysis is resumed. The formation of an ostomy generally precludes further peritoneal dialysis because of the high risk of peritonitis. In such cases, the patient must be transferred to hemodialysis.[65]

THE RENAL TRANSPLANT PATIENT AND SURGERY

Renal transplantation is an accepted modality in the treatment of ESRD. More than 40,000 patients in the United States are alive with a functioning transplant.[1] Though most of these patients are cared for at specialized transplant centers, the chances that such patients will receive care in other medical settings increase as more transplants are performed. In general, most transplant patients can be treated like other patients, depending on their level of renal function. For patients with a creatinine clearance of greater than 50 ml/min, no special precautions are necessary. However, because many transplant patients have reduced renal function due to chronic graft rejection or recurrent disease, they need to be treated similarly to other patients with CRF.

All transplant patients do, however, differ from others by virtue of the immunosuppressive medications they receive. These medications include prednisone, azathioprine, and cyclosporine. Because of adrenal suppression, transplant patients undergoing surgery require increased doses of corticosteroids in the perioperative period. In patients taking azathioprine, a myelosuppressive drug, the absence of an elevated white blood cell count may not exclude an inflammatory or infectious process. Azathioprine can be administered intravenously in the same doses taken before surgery. Note that allopurinol inhibits the metabolism of azathioprine, thereby increasing the frequency of toxicity. If the two drugs must be used

TABLE 32–1. Major Cyclosporine Drug Interactions

Drugs That Increase Cyclosporine Levels (increasing risk of nephrotoxicity)	Drugs That Decrease Cyclosporine Levels (increasing risk of rejection)
Ketoconazole	Carbamazepine
Erythromycin	Phenobarbital
Diltiazem	Phenytoin
Nicardipine	Sulfamethoxazole/Trimethoprim (IV)
Cimetidine	Isoniazid
Oral Contraceptives	Rifampin

together, the azathioprine dose should be decreased to two-thirds or three-quarters of the previous dose.[66]

The immunosuppressive agent cyclosporine has greatly improved the outcome of allograft transplantation. It does not cause bone marrow suppression like azathioprine, but it can cause acute and chronic renal damage.[67] Acute renal toxicity is often associated with elevated blood levels of the drug and responds to dose reduction. Renal vasoconstriction may mediate this form of toxicity. Chronic toxicity is less likely to respond to dose reduction or discontinuation of the drug, and interstitial fibrosis is found on renal biopsy.

Hypertension occurs frequently in patients treated with cyclosporine[68] and can be managed in the usual manner. Cyclosporine can also interfere with tubular secretion of potassium and cause hyperkalemia. Hyperkalemia rarely reaches critical levels, but, if additional demands are placed on renal potassium excretion (e.g., increased potassium release from surgically traumatized tissue), it may require treatment. Serum potassium levels should be monitored in all patients receiving cyclosporine after transplant. When a patient is unable to take oral cyclosporine, it can be administered intravenously in one-third the oral dose. Cyclosporine blood levels are altered by the concomitant administration of a number of medications as shown in Table 32–1. When these medications are required, cyclosporine levels should be followed closely.[69]

Other than the need for careful dosing of immunosuppressive medications, postoperative care of renal transplant patients is not much different from that of other patients.[70] There is, however, a higher incidence of urinary tract infections in transplant patients.

SUMMARY

1. Patients with CRF can undergo surgery safely with proper care in the perioperative period.

2. Volume overload and depletion should be avoided with judicious use of diuretics or dialysis for the former and saline replacement for the latter.

3. Serum electrolyte levels should be measured regularly in the perioperative period. Serum sodium concentration should be maintained between 130 and 150 meq/liter by avoiding unnecessary free-water administration or replacing excessive water losses as needed.

4. Hyperkalemia is a continuous threat to patients with CRF and requires careful monitoring to maintain serum potassium levels below 5 meq/liter. Drugs like NSAID's, beta-blockers, and heparin that impair potassium handling should be avoided. Kayexalate and dialysis are effective in removing excess potassium from the body.

5. Abnormalities of calcium and phosphorus metabolism are usually not problematic in the perioperative period. However, serum calcium levels below 7.5 mg/dl should be treated with calcium replacement before surgery, but only after elevations of serum phosphate concentration have been corrected.

6. Most patients with CRF have a mild metabolic acidosis. Arterial blood gas measurements should be obtained before surgery in those with serum bicarbonate concentrations under 18 meq/liter or serum creatinine levels above 6 mg/dl. Serum bicarbonate levels should be maintained above 18 meq/liter and P_{CO_2} levels should be kept low to avoid mixed metabolic and respiratory acidoses.

7. Hypertension in patients with CRF can be treated with currently available medications and control of volume overload. If nitroprusside is needed for more than one or two days, thiocyanate levels should be monitored to avoid toxicity.

8. The anemia and coagulopathy of CRF can be treated with recombinant erythropoietin, and transfusion is usually necessary only when the hematocrit level is below 20%. Patients with prolonged bleeding times despite an adequate hematocrit level can be treated with estrogens or desmopressin. Anticoagulation with heparin should be avoided in the period four hours before and 24 hours after the procedure and kept to a minimum in the first week after surgery.

9. Nutritional assessment should be performed frequently in patients with CRF, and oral or parenteral nutritional support should be insititued if protein or calorie deficits are detected.

10. Infections do not occur more commonly in patients with CRF, but dosage of antibiotics may require adjustment for the reduction in renal function.

12. Patients with CRF have a high risk of developing further deterioration in renal function in the postoperative period. Efforts should be made to prevent volume depletion; avoid nephrotoxic drugs such as aminoglycosides, radiocontrast agents, and NSAID's and nephrotoxic anesthetics like methoxyflurane. Dosages of narcotics should be reduced. The muscle relaxants of choice in patients with CRF are vecuronium and atracurium.

13. Patients on dialysis generally tolerate major surgery without increased morbidity and mortality. Dialysis should be performed 4 to 30 hours before the procedure. Postoperative dialysis should be performed with an anticoagulation regimen designed to minimize bleeding at least 24 hours thereafter. Patients on peritoneal dialysis require backup hemodialysis after abdominal procedures and should not resume peritoneal dialysis for four to six weeks.

14. Hyperkalemia, hypotension, and wound complications are the most frequent postoperative problems in patients with CRF. Vascular access should be carefully protected during and after surgery to prevent thrombosis.

15. Patients with a renal transplant should be treated according to their level of renal function. Those with a creatinine clearance above 50 ml/min require no special precautions, and those with

clearances below this should be treated like other patients with CRF.

16. Immunosuppressive agents should be continued in the perioperative period, and stress doses of steroids may be needed. Azathioprine and cyclosporine can be administered intravenously with reduction in the dose of the latter by two-thirds. Drug interactions should be kept in mind at all times.

REFERENCES

1. Executive summary, excerpts from United States renal data system. 1991 annual data report. *Am J Kid Dis* 18(Supp 2):9–16, 1991.
2. Brenowitz JB, Williams CD, Edwards WS: Major surgery in patients with chronic renal failure. *Am J Surg* 134:765, 1977.
3. Hampers CL, Bailey GL, Hager EB et al: Major surgery in patients on maintenance hemodialysis. *Am J Surg* 115:747, 1968.
4. Lissos I, Goldberg B, Van Blerk PJP et al: Surgical procedures on patients in end-stage renal failure. *Br J Urol* 45:359, 1973.
5. Harris RC, Meyer TW, Brenner BM: Nephron adaptation to renal injury, in Brenner BM, Rector FC (eds): *The Kidney*, 3d ed. Philadelphia, Saunders, 1986, pp 1553–1585.
6. Rose BD: *Pathophysiology of Renal Disease*, 2d ed. New York, McGraw-Hill, 1987, pp 6–10.
7. Cockcroft DW, Gault MH: Prediction of creatinine clearance from serum creatinine. *Nephron* 16:13, 1976.
8. Depner TA, Gulyassy PF: Chronic renal failure, in Earley LE, Gottshalk CW (eds): *Straus and Welt's Diseases of the Kidney*. Boston, Little, Brown, 1979, p 211.
9. Blythe WB: The management of intercurrent medical and surgical problems in the patient with chronic renal failure, in Earley LE, Gottshalk CW (eds): *Straus and Welt's Diseases of the Kidney*. Boston, Little, Brown, 1979, p 517.
10. Kleeman CR, Adams OA, Maxwell MH: An evaluation of maximal water diuresis in chronic renal disease. I: Normal solute intake. *J Lab Clin Med* 58:169, 1961.
11. Sebastian A, McSherry E, Morns RC: Metabolic acidosis with special reference to the renal acidosis, in Brenner BM, Rector FD (eds): *The Kidney*. Philadelphia, Saunders, 1987, p 165.
12. Husted FC, Nolph KD, Moher JF: $NaHCO_3$ and NaCl tolerance in chronic renal failure. *J Clin Invest* 56:414, 1975.
13. Albert MD, Dell RB, Winters RW: Quantitative displacement of acid-base equilibrium in metabolic acidosis. *Ann Intern Med* 66:312, 1967.
14. Goggin MJ, Joeskes AM: Gas exchange in renal failure. I: Dangers of hyperkalemia during anesthesia. *Br Med J* 2:244, 1971.
15. Gonick HC, Kleeman CR, Rubin ME et al: Functional impairment in chronic renal disease. III: Studies of potassium excretion. *Am J Med* 261:281, 1971.
16. Keith NM, Osterberg AE: The tolerance for potassium in severe renal insufficiency: A study of ten cases. *J Clin Invest* 26:773, 1947.
17. Takacs FJ: Surgery with impaired renal function. *Surg Clin N Am* 50:719, 1970.
18. Aldrete JA, O'Higgins JW, Starzl DTE: Changes in serum potassium during renal homotransplantation. *Arch Surg* 101:82, 1970.
19. Tan SY, Shapiro R, Franco R et al: Indomethacin-induced prostaglandin inhibition with hyperkalemia. A reversible cause of hyporeninemic hypoaldosteronism. *Ann Intern Med* 9G:783, 1979.
20. Phelps KR, Oh MS, Carroll HJ: Heparin-induced hyperkalemia. Report of a case. *Nephron* 25:209, 1980.
21. Rosa RM, Silva P, Young JB et al: Adrenergic modulation of extrarenal potassium disposal. *N Engl J Med* 302:401, 1980.
22. Textor SG, Bravo EL, Fouad F et al: Hyperkalemia in azotemic patients during angiotensin-converting enzyme inhibition and aldosterone reduction with captopril. *Am J Med* 73:719, 1982.
23. Korde M, Ward BE: Serum potassium concentrations after succinylcholine in patients with renal failure. *Anesthesiology* 36:142, 1972.
24. Vertes V, Cangiano J, Berman L et al: Hypertension in endstage renal disease. *N Engl J Med* 280:978, 1969.
25. Cohn JN, Burke LP: Nitroprusside. *Ann Intern Med* 91:752, 1979.
26. Eschbach JW, Kelly MR, Haley NR et al: Treatment of the anemia of progressive renal failure with recombinant human erythropoietin. *N Engl J Med* 321:158–163, 1989.
27. Eschbach JW, Egrie JC, Downing MR et al: Correction of the anemia of end-stage renal disease with recombinant human erythropoietin: Results of a combined phase I and II clinical trial. *N Engl J Med* 316:73–78, 1987.
28. Llulo M, Benigni A, Remuzzi G: Coagulation abnormalities in uremia. *Sem Neph* 5:82, 1985.
29. Moia M, Vizzotto L, Cattaneo M et al: Improvement in the hemostatic defect of uremia after treatment with recombinant human erythropoietin. *Lancet* 2:1227–1229, 1987.
30. Steiner R, Coggins C, Carvalho A: Bleeding time in uremia: A useful test to assess clinical bleeding. *Am J Hematol* 7:107, 1979.
31. Stewart JH, Castaldi PA: Uremic bleeding: A reversible platelet defect corrected by dialysis. *QJ Med* 36:409, 1967.
32. Mannucci PM, Remuzzi G, Pusineri F et al: Deamino-8-*d*-argininine vasopressin shortens the bleeding time in uremia. *N Engl J Med* 303:1318, 1983.
33. Livio M, Mannucci P, Vigano G et al: Conjugated estrogens for the management of bleeding associated with renal failure. *N Engl J Med* 315:731, 1986.
34. Janson PA, Jubeliere SJ, Weinstein MJ et al: Treatment of the bleeding tendency in uremia with cryoprecipitate. *N Engl J Med* 303:1318, 1980.
35. Kjellstrand CM, Buselmeier TJ: A simple method of anticoagulation during pre- and postoperative hemodialysis avoiding rebound phenomenon. *Surgery* 72:630, 1972.
36. Schwab SJ, Onorato JJ, Sharer LR et al: Hemodialysis without anticoagulation; one-year prospective trial in hospitalized patients at risk for bleeding. *Am J Med* 83:405, 1987.
37. Carvana RJ, Raja RM, Bush JV et al: Heparin-free dialysis: Comparative data and results in high-risk patients. *Kidney Int* 31:1351, 1987.
38. Pinneik RV, Wiegmann TB, Diederich DA: Regional citrate anticoagulation for hemodialysis in the patient at high risk for bleeding. *N Engl J Med* 308:258, 1983.
39. Swartz RD, Port FK: Preventing hemorrhage in high-risk hemodialysis: Regional versus low-dose heparin. *Kidney Int* 16:5–13, 1979.
40. Kopple JD: Causes of catabolism and wasting in acute or chronic renal failure. *Proc Int Congr Nephrol* 9:1498, 1984.
41. Giacchino JL, Geis WP, Wittenstein BH et al: Surgery, nutritional support, and survival in patients with end-stage renal disease. *Arch Surg* 116:634, 1981.
42. Rostand SG, Greles JC, Kirk KA et al: Ischemic heart disease in patients with uremia undergoing maintenance hemodialysis. *Kidney Int* 16:600, 1979.
43. Torres VE, Strong CG, Romero JC: Indomethacin enhancement of glycerol-induced acute renal failure in rabbits. *Kidney Int* 7:170, 1975.
44. Shusterman NH, Strom BL, Murray TG et al: Risk factors and outcome of hospital-acquired acute renal failure. Clinical epidemiologic study. *Am J Med* 83:65, 1987.
45. Humes HD: Aminoglycoside nephrotoxicity. *Kidney Int* 33:900, 1988.
46. Muller M: Anesthesia for the patient with renal dysfunction, in Priebe HJ (ed): *The Kidney in Anesthesia*. International Anesthesiology Clinics, vol 22. Boston, Little, Brown, 1984, pp 169–188.
47. Churchill D, Knaack J, Chirito E et al: Persisting renal insufficiency after methoxyflurane anesthesia. Report of two cases and review of literature. *Am J Med* 56:575, 1974.
48. Cousins MS, Fulton A, Haynes WD et al: Enflurane nephrotoxicity and preexisting renal dysfunction. *Anaesth Intens Care* 6:277, 1972.

49. Graybar GB, Work J, Barber WH: Anesthetic considerations for the dialysis patient. *Sem Dial* 2:108, 1989.

50. Miller RD, Cullen DJ: Renal failure and postoperative respiratory failure. Recurarization. *Br J Anaesth* 48:253, 1976.

51. Ball M, McQuay HJ, Moore RA et al: Renal failure and the use of morphine in intensive care. *Lancet* 1:784, 1985.

52. Chauvin M, Sandook P, Scherrmann JM et al: Morphine pharmacokinetics in renal failure. *Anesthesiology* 66:327, 1987.

53. Szeto HH, Inturrisi CE, Houde R et al: Accumulation of normeperidine, an active metabolite of meperidine, in patients with renal failure or cancer. *Ann Intern Med* 86:738, 1977.

54. Barnes JN, Williams AJ, Toseland PA et al: Opioid drugs and renal failure. *Lancet* 2:748, 1984.

55. Bennett NM, Aronoff GR, Golper TA et al: *Drug Prescribing in Renal Failure: Dosing Guidelines for Adults*. Philadelphia, American College of Physicians, 1988.

56. Pinson CW, Schuman ES, Gross GF et al: Surgery in long-term dialysis patients. Experience with more than 300 cases. *Am J Surg* 151:567, 1986.

57. Dajani AS, Biksno AL, Chung KJ et al: Prevention of bacterial endocarditis. *JAMA* 264:2919, 1990.

58. Rostand SG, Rutsky EA: Ischemic heart disease in chronic renal failure: Management considerations. *Sem Dial* 2:98, 1989.

59. Zamora JL, Burdine JT, Karlberg H et al: Cardiac surgery in patients with end-stage renal disease. *Ann Thorac Surg* 42:113, 1986.

60. Deutsch E, Bernstein RC, Addonizio VP et al: Coronary artery bypass surgery in patients on chronic hemodialysis: A case-control study. *Ann Intern Med* 110:369, 1989.

61. Ilson B, Bland P, Jorkasky D et al: Intraoperative versus routine hemodialysis in ESRD patients undergoing open heart surgery (abstract). *Kidney Int* 35:249, 1989.

62. Golper T: Continuous arteriovenous hemofiltration in acute renal failure. *Am J Kid Dis* 6:373, 1985.

63. Sigler M, Teehan B, Van Valkenburgh D: Solute transport in continuous hemodialysis. A new treatment for acute renal failure. *Kidney Int* 32:562, 1987.

64. Newberry WM, Sanford JP: Detective cellular immunity in renal failure: Depression of reactivity of lymphocytes to phytohemagglutinin by renal failure serum. *J Clin Invest* 50:1262, 1971.

65. Moffat F, Deitel M, Thompson D: Abdominal surgery in patients undergoing long-term peritoneal dialysis. *Surgery* 92:598, 1982.

66. Zimm S, Collins JM, O'Neill D et al: Inhibition of first pass metabolism in cancer chemotherapy; interaction of 6-mercaptopurine and allopurinal. *Clin Pharmacol Ther* 43:810, 1983.

67. Mihatsch M, Thiel G, Ryffel DB: Cyclosporine nephropathy. A tubulinterstitial and vascular disease, in Bertanit, Remuzzi G (eds): *Drugs and the Kidney*. New York, Raven Press, 1986, pp 153–169.

68. Bennett WM, Porter GA: Cyclosporine-associated hypertension. *Am J Med* 85:131–133, 1988.

69. Lake KD: Cyclosporine drug interactions: A review. *Card Surg* 2:617, 1988.

70. Halasz N: Surgery in the patient with a functioning renal transplant, in Love J (ed): *Cardiac Surgery in Patients with Chronic Renal Disease*. Mount Kisco, NY, Futura, 1982, p 105.

33 PERIOPERATIVE MANAGEMENT OF THE OVERWEIGHT PATIENT

Sankey V. Williams

A significant portion of the population is overweight. Many of these patients suffer from a number of related medical disorders and carry a higher risk of surgical complications. This chapter describes the natural history and the medical consequences of being overweight. It concludes with a discussion of common surgical complications in overweight patients.

THE DEFINITION OF OBESITY

Measurements of simple body weight do not account for height or separate differences in body size from differences in body composition. Because most experts believe that body fat is more important than body size, investigators have developed indices which combine height and weight to measure body fat indirectly. Two of the most popular indices are the body-mass index, also called the Quetelet index, and the relative weight, sometimes called the desirable or ideal weight.[1-4] The body-mass index equals the weight in kilograms divided by the square of the height in meters. The relative weight equals the actual weight divided by the mid-point of desirable weight for medium-frame persons in the 1959 or 1983 Metropolitan Life Insurance Company tables. Reading reports about the health of overweight persons is difficult, because different investigators use different indices. However, these measures are closely correlated, and few if any of the important conclusions drawn from the literature would be different if the alternative index were used.[5]

Regardless of measure, distinguishing normal-weight people from those who are overweight remains a problem. In 1985 a consensus-development conference sponsored by the National Institutes of Health concluded that body weight 20% or more above relative weight constitutes a health hazard.[6] Applying this definition to the United States in the period 1971 to 1974, 14 percent of men and 24 percent of women between the ages of 20 and 74 were overweight.[7]

Weight may vary but is stable over long periods of time. When 5209 residents of Framingham, Massachusetts, were weighed every other year for 18 years, the mean difference between the highest and lowest weights was 21 pounds.[8] For most people, however, weight at one age was closely related to weight later in life. Average weight increased until age 54, remained stable until age 62, and then declined.

MEDICAL COMPLICATIONS OF OBESITY

Longevity

Between 1903 and 1979, five large studies based on life insurance records have examined the relationship between weight and longevity, and all found increased weight to be associated with a shorter lifespan.[8] Five additional prospective studies not restricted to holders of life insurance policies reached the same conclusion.[9-14] Deaths attributed mostly to coronary artery disease and diabetes mellitus but also to gallbladder disease, cerebrovascular disease, and cancer account for much of the excess mortality.[11] As weight increases, mortality increases. Compared to average-weight persons, those 20 to 30% heavier have a 30 percent higher mortality rate which increases to 90 percent for persons who are at least 40% heavier than average.[11] Weights slightly lower than average are associated with longer life, but those 20% or more below average have a 25 percent increase in mortality.[5,11,13,15]

Characteristics other than simple weight affect longevity. Becoming overweight at a younger age increases risk.[12] Distribution of fat is also an important factor.[16-18] People with fat distributed predominantly in the upper body and abdomen have higher mortality rates than those with fat distributed mainly in the hips and thighs. Age of onset and distribution of fat may also modulate the effect of weight on other medical complications.

There is some evidence that weight loss decreases mortality.[19] One study describes 2300 overweight subjects required to pay a higher premium on life insurance because of their weight. Those

319

who subsequently lost enough weight to pay a lower premium had a lower mortality rate than those who did not lose weight but still had a higher rate than people of normal weight.

Hypertension

The association between hypertension and obesity is supported by convincing epidemiologic data.[20–26] Between one-fifth and one-third of adults with hypertension are overweight. In the Framingham study, there was a moderately strong correlation between blood pressure and body weight.[8,21] Correlations were better for diastolic than for systolic blood pressure and were slightly more evident in women and in younger people. Depending on age and sex, between 20 to 50 percent of the most overweight patients had hypertension.

Universal acceptance of the relationship between hypertension and body weight has been delayed by conflicting answers to two questions: (1) Does obesity artificially increase blood pressure measurements obtained with a cuff? (2) Does weight loss without sodium restriction decrease blood pressure? Several studies show that mean blood pressure determinations in groups are approximately the same with adequate cuff or intraarterial measurements.[20,27–29] There is still controversy about the effect of weight loss on blood pressure, although many[23–25] but not all[30] reviewers believe that weight loss alone will reduce blood pressure. A loss of 10 pounds produces a decrease in mean blood pressure of about 20 torr.

Lipid Abnormalities

Body weight correlates with blood lipid levels, and changes in weight produce alterations in these levels. In the Framingham study, relative weight was directly correlated with blood levels of triglycerides, total cholesterol, low-density (LDL) cholesterol, and very low-density (VLDL) cholesterol.[31,32] There was an even stronger inverse correlation between relative weight and high-density (HDL) cholesterol. These associations were strongest in men and young people, except for those with HDL cholesterol, where there were no age or sex differences.

A large study conducted by the Lipid Research Clinics confirmed the inverse correlation between weight and HDL cholesterol.[33,34] The difference in mean HDL-cholesterol levels between those in the tenth and ninetieth percentiles for body weight was 6 to 7 mg/dl, enough to affect cardiovascular mortality rates. These relationships persisted when the effects of other factors affecting lipid levels were discounted. When all variables were considered simultaneously, body weight, cigarette smoking, and alcohol use were most strongly and consistently associated with HDL-cholesterol levels.[34]

There is also a strong relationship between changes in body weight and changes in lipid levels. In one study, for each 10 percent change in relative weight in men, there was a change of 11.3 mg/dl in total cholesterol levels. In women, the corresponding change was 6.3 mg/dl.[32] Other studies describe similar variations in total cholesterol levels with weight loss and gain.[32,34–36]

Atherosclerotic Vascular Disease

The overweight state is associated with the development of cardiovascular disease but is also associated with known risk factors for heart disease itself. These include hypercholesterolemia, hypertension, and diabetes mellitus. Most short-term studies asking if being overweight is an independent predictor of cardiovascular disease have found that weight exerts its effect by influencing other risk factors.[8,37–39] More recently, however, long-term results from the Framingham study show that being overweight predicts the development of cardiovascular disease independently when adjusted for the effects of age, systolic blood pressure, serum cholesterol level, cigarette smoking, glucose intolerance, and left ventricular hypertrophy on electrocardiogram.[40] Being 20% over desirable weight at the beginning of the study was associated with a 20 percent increase in the relative risk of developing cardiovascular disease during the 26-year follow-up period in both men and women. More recent studies support the idea that being overweight should be considered both an independent risk factor for cardiovascular disease and a marker for other risk factors.[41,42]

The relationship between body weight and cerebrovascular disease is less clear. Most studies have found no independent effect and have concluded that being overweight only appears to increase the incidence of stroke because it raises blood pressure.[8,43,44] However, in the Framingham study and a large study of London civil servants, being overweight independently predicted the development of thrombotic stroke.[40,42,45]

Some studies have unexpectedly documented an inverse relationship between weight and peripheral vascular disease,[8,43] but others have found no consistent correlation.[40] One suggested explanation is that overweight people are limited in their ability to exercise and avoid stress that would otherwise lead to symptoms.[40,43]

Other Cardiopulmonary Abnormalities

As body weight increases, the cardiovascular system responds with comparable increases in blood volume, resting cardiac output, and heart size.[46–48] Increased heart size is the result of myocardial hypertrophy and not fatty infiltration.[49] Increase in cardiac output with exercise is normal, but pulmonary artery pressure and left ventricular end-diastolic filling pressure rise above normal with exercise in most overweight subjects. With increasing weight, there is an increase in cardiac work that can be disproportionate to the degree of obesity.

The respiratory system responds to moderate increases in body weight by increasing minute ventilation, resulting in normal arterial PO_2 and normal or reduced PCO_2 levels despite increased resting oxygen consumption and carbon dioxide production.[50] Increased work of breathing is explained by the fact that respiratory muscles must work against abnormal compliance caused by a heavy chest wall and stiffer lungs with expanded pulmonary blood volume. In addition, respiratory muscles become inefficient. Fatty infiltration of the diaphragm may provide a partial explanation for this, but abnormal neuromuscular coupling and an unfavorable contour of the chest wall with upward displacement of the diaphragm by abdominal fat may be contributing factors.

These abnormalities are responsible for abnormal pulmonary function tests. Expiratory reserve volume (ERV) and functional residual capacity (FRC) are reduced. Consequently, breathing is more shallow with a reduced vital capacity (VC). Respiratory rate must increase to maintain minute ventilation. This breathing pattern is sufficient at rest but with effort causes a disproportionate increase in oxygen consumption worsened by an increase in relative dead space. The result is a decrease in maximum voluntary ventilation (MVV).

Shallow breathing also produces relative overventilation of the upper and underventilation of the lower lungs where perfusion is greater. The resulting ventilation-perfusion inequality is worsened if the ERV is reduced below the closing volume of the alveoli which remain collapsed but continue to be perfused. Hypoxemia is caused by these ventilation-perfusion inequalities and is worsened when the patient is in the supine position because of further reductions in ERV.

Sudden death has been recently reported in markedly obese patients.[47,51] The cause of the deaths is uncertain, but prolonged Q-T intervals on electrocardiogram[51] and an increased frequency of cardiac arrhythmias[52,53] have been reported in such patients.

Diabetes Mellitus

The association between obesity and diabetes mellitus rests on sound epidemiologic data.[31,54,56] The prevalence of diabetes increases in all age groups as relative weight increases, but the effect appears at lower relative weights in older age groups.[27] When 3751 men were followed for 10 years, a rapidly accelerating increase in the risk of diabetes was documented as initial weight increased from normal to more than 45% overweight.[19] The Framingham study found that, for each 10% change in relative weight, there was a change in blood glucose of 2.5 mg/dl in men and 1.3 mg/dl in women.[32]

The association between obesity and diabetes is also supported by a growing understanding of the mechanism through which obesity exerts its effects.[57,58] Independent of other factors known to influence insulin resistance and insulin secretion, obesity interferes with the ability of muscle and fatty tissues to take up glucose and promotes higher circulating insulin levels in response to oral glucose intake. This causes greater insulin resistance requiring increased secretion of insulin to maintain normal glucose homeostasis.[59] Insulin resistance is partly explained by a decrease in the number of insulin receptors on cell surfaces, but there are also postreceptor abnormalities in glucose transport, glucose phosphorylation, and other cellular systems.[60,61]

Gallstones

Several studies have shown an association between increasing weight and increasing prevalence of gallstones, independent of age, sex, or parity.[62-67] The abnormal cholesterol metabolism found in obese people may be responsible for this association, acting through elevated biliary cholesterol secretion and gallbladder bile that is supersaturated with cholesterol.[68,69]

Abnormalities in Sex Hormones and Reproductive Function

In both women and men, there are changes in the levels of sex hormones with obesity, but clinically important disorders have been documented only in women. In one study, women who reported irregular menstrual cycles lasting more than 36 days were more than 30 pounds heavier than those with no menstrual abnormalities, adjusting for height and age.[70] The polycystic ovary or Stein-Leventhal syndrome is associated with obesity. Multiple small cysts are found in the ovary and irregular menstrual cycles

progress to amenorrhea. Women who have had surgery for polycystic ovaries report more teenage obesity than women who have ovarian surgery for other reasons.[71]

Hyperuricemia and Gout

Increasing weight is the single most important variable associated with elevated serum uric acid levels. One study suggests that weight loss causes a decrease in uric acid levels.[8,72-74] In the Framingham study, the prevalence of gout was correlated with relative weight.[8]

Cancer

Prevalence studies suggest an association between obesity and a variety of cancers. The evidence from case-control studies is most convincing for endometrial cancer.[75-79] Obesity also has been suggested as a risk factor for breast cancer[80-88] and colon cancer.[89-91]

Osteoarthritis

Most physicians accept that excess weight is associated with osteoarthritis because of the additional stress on weight-bearing joints. Others believe that obesity is related to metabolic changes underlying development of the disease. Prospective data from the Framingham study and elsewhere confirm that excess weight leads to arthritis of the knees.[92-95]

Psychiatric and Emotional Disorders

As a group, people with mild or moderate obesity do not score differently on psychologic tests or have consistently different indices of anxiety and depression than control groups. Those with morbid obesity have no more psychopathology than others when specific criteria for psychiatric disease are used.[96-103] Nevertheless, there are emotional disturbances related to obesity found in certain subgroups of obese persons.[103,104] Almost half of juvenile-onset obese persons have a distorted body image. They perceive themselves as grotesque and loathsome and think that others view them with hostility and contempt. Dieting in young upper-class women may increase the risk of bulimia. Purging is often absent in overweight patients with bulimia.

SURGICAL COMPLICATIONS IN THE OVERWEIGHT PATIENT

Although surgeons and anesthesiologists generally agree that overweight patients have an increased risk of perioperative complications and death, few studies adequately document these beliefs.[105,106]

Surgical Mortality

There have been only three well-controlled studies of surgical mortality. In the first, 300 consecutive women weighing over 200 pounds and undergoing abdominal hysterectomy were matched with nonobese control patients undergoing the same procedure.[107] Obese patients weighed an average of 60 pounds more. There were three deaths among the obese patients and none among the controls, a difference that was not statistically significant. The second report was a cooperative study of surgical therapy for duodenal ulcer.[108] Patients were classified as obese if they weighed more than 35 pounds over their ideal weight. Of 116 obese patients, eight or seven percent died postoperatively, but only 72 or 2.7 percent of 2649 nonobese patients did so. The third report described a study of patients undergoing coronary artery bypass graft surgery in the United Kingdom, where 250 obese patients were compared to 250 age- and sex-matched control patients with a normal body-mass index.[109] The operative mortality was 0.8 percent in both groups. Others reach conflicting conclusions about relative death rates in obese and nonobese patients after inadequately controlled studies of open and laparoscopic cholecystectomy, vaginal hysterectomy, surgery for endometrial carcinoma, cesarean section, and other procedures.[110–117]

Large numbers of morbidly obese patients have undergone major surgical procedures designed to promote weight loss. The surgical mortality rate of jejunoileal bypass procedures is approximately 1.8 to 3 percent in most published studies from experienced centers, but one study described no deaths among 130 patients.[118–121] The surgical mortality rate of gastric bypass procedures is probably lower than that of jejunoileal procedures.[122–129] A recent report from a national registry of all types of surgery for obesity described a 40-day operative mortality rate of only 0.1 percent in 5178 patients.[130]

There are no studies describing the effect of preoperative weight loss on surgical mortality or complications in obese patients.

Pulmonary Complications

During surgery, morbidly obese patients experience a decrease in functional residual capacity (FRC) and thus a reduced oxygen supply during apnea.[131,132] In addition, arterial oxygen concentration (Po_2) may fall to unacceptably low levels despite inspiration of 40% oxygen.[133] Intraoperative hypoxemia is worsened when the patient is in the head-down position or when subdiaphragmatic packs are used and is not corrected by the use of positive end-expiratory pressure (PEEP).[133,134] They also experience postoperative hypoxemia that can persist for as long as five days after surgery.[135] Early postoperative hypoxemia is greater in patients with transverse abdominal incisions than with vertical incisions. It can be improved by placing the patient in a semirecumbent position.[136,137]

There is conflicting data about the incidence of postoperative atelectasis in the obese patient. In one study of patients undergoing surgery for duodenal ulcer, although criteria for diagnosing atelectasis were not described, 8.9 percent of 124 obese patients and 4.7 percent of 2695 nonobese patients developed atelectasis.[108] In contrast, a second study, also omitting criteria for diagnosis of atelectasis, reported it to be less frequent in obese (4.2 percent of 48) than in nonobese (5.9 percent of 236) female patients undergoing cholecystectomy.[110] A more recent study of consecutive cholecystectomy patients found no difference in the incidence of atelectasis and other pulmonary complications in 52 obese and 157 nonobese patients.[138] However, an increased frequency of macroatelectasis has been reported in 46 obese patients undergoing elective upper abdominal surgery and in 40 patients having elective cholecystectomy.[139,140]

Postoperative pneumonia is not more frequent in obese patients. In one controlled study, there were actually fewer postoperative pneumonias in obese patients (3.3 percent of 120) than in nonobese subjects (6.5 percent of 2532).[141] A second study with carefully defined criteria found no significant relationship between weight and the incidence of postoperative chest infections.[142] Obese patients have a larger volume of gastric contents with a lower pH than normals, and special preoperative care is recommended to prevent aspiration pneumonitis.[143–145]

Wound Complications

All seven studies examining the relationship between obesity and postoperative wound infection report a statistically significant association between the two. Though infection rates vary, the association is strengthened by the diverse nature of the studies. In a case-control study of women undergoing abdominal hysterectomy, 5.7 percent of 300 obese women and 0.8 percent of 300 nonobese women developed wound infections.[107] In a study of patients undergoing surgery for duodenal ulcer, 15 percent of 125 obese patients and 8 percent of 2695 nonobese patients experienced this complication.[108] In a study of topical antiseptic to prevent wound infection, 21 percent of 29 obese patients and 5 percent of 115 nonobese patients developed infections. Intraoperative application of povidone-iodine to the wound reduced the incidence of infection in the obese patients.[146] In a study of the value of wound drains in 250 patients with abdominal incisions, 48 percent of 23 obese and 12 percent of 26 nonobese patients developed infections. Wound drains were thought to be helpful in obese but not in nonobese patients.[147] In a study of women undergoing cesarean section, 54 percent of 61 obese and 31 percent of 68 nonobese patients developed postoperative fever thought to be due to bacterial infection.[148] In another study of consecutive patients undergoing a variety of abdominal operations, 43 percent of 73 obese and 25 percent of 396 nonobese patients developed wound sepsis.[149] A case-control study of 17 sternotomy infections in cardiac surgery patients resulted in elevated odds ratios for overweight patients, but the authors considered the results statistically inconclusive.[150]

Although few studies are adequately controlled, there are data clearly implicating obesity as a risk factor in developing wound dehiscence. This is probably due to mechanical factors and wound infection as a precursor of dehiscence.[151–155]

Postoperative Thromboembolism

The generally accepted view that obesity is associated with venous thrombosis is supported by considerable evidence.[156,157] In a study of patients undergoing surgery for duodenal ulcer, 4 percent of 124 obese and 0.7 percent of 2676 nonobese patients developed clinical thrombophlebitis.[108] Three studies have used noninvasive methods to show a higher incidence of clinically inapparent postoperative thrombosis in obese than in nonobese patients.[158–160] Prophylaxis with warfarin, but not with low-dose heparin, has been shown to be equally effective in obese and nonobese patients in preventing postoperative venous thrombosis.[161,162]

The evidence that obesity increases the risk of pulmonary embolus comes from autopsy studies of hospitalized patients and from prospective clinical studies. One such study published in 1926 reported that 25.6 percent of 156 obese and 7.9 percent of 1942 nonobese patients died of postoperative pulmonary embolism. The rate of fatal embolism increased with increasing weight.[163] Another widely quoted autopsy study found pulmonary emboli in 21.9 percent of 544 obese and 14.4 percent of 4056 nonobese patients, but the figures for those affected were not correlated with body weight.[164] Two more recent autopsy studies reported no correlation between occurrence of emboli and weight.[165,166]

Prospective clinical trials are no more conclusive. In one uncontrolled study of 167 patients with submassive or massive pulmonary emboli documented by pulmonary angiography, 30 percent were obese.[167] In a prospective study of admissions to medical and surgical services of three Philadelphia hospitals, 4.9 percent of 6527 patients had pulmonary emboli confirmed by pulmonary angiograms, autopsies, and lung scans. Relative weight was not associated with occurrence of pulmonary embolism.[168] Thromboembolism is a recognized complication of gastric and jejunoileal bypass and other procedures for obesity, but the rates vary dramatically from study to study.[118–130]

Problems with Anesthesia

Anesthesia in overweight patients is complicated by a variety of technical and, to a lesser extent, metabolic and physiologic problems.[81,114] It is difficult to establish and maintain intravenous routes for drugs and fluids. Laryngoscopy and endotracheal intubation are complicated by distorted anatomy. High pressures required for ventilation with a face mask may promote gastric aspiration by rendering the gastroesophageal sphincter incompetent. A reduced FRC may allow unexpectedly rapid decreases in arterial oxygen saturation and more rapid than normal increases in the alveolar tension of insoluble anesthetic gases.[131,132] Obese patients probably metabolize inhalational anesthetics differently, and, unless anesthesia time is limited, toxic metabolites can accumulate and cause renal and hepatic damage.[169] It is difficult to identify anatomic landmarks needed for regional and spinal anesthesia. Spinal anesthesia is further complicated by the possibility of reductions in ventilation and by uncertain requirements for anesthetic that may result from unpredictable spinal canal volumes.[170] Maintaining fluid balance is difficult because of difficulty in evaluating dehydration and hypovolemia.

SUMMARY

1. The more overweight the patient, the more likely and severe are the problems that have been described in this chapter and the more often practice should deviate from the usual pattern.

2. Extra care should be taken during the history and physical examination of the overweight patient to elicit information about the medical consequences of being overweight. These consequences include hypertension; lipid disorders; atherosclerotic vascular disease; the obesity-hypoventilation syndrome; diabetes mellitus; gallstones; gout; abnormalities of reproductive function in women; osteoarthritis; and cancer of the endometrium, breast, and colon.

3. Few of the recommendations for preoperative testing given in other chapters need be altered for the overweight patient.

4. Surgical complications are more common in the overweight than in the normal-weight patient. These complications include hypoxemia, wound infection, venous thrombosis, and perhaps, wound dehiscence and pulmonary embolism.

5. Medical and surgical problems should be managed in the overweight patient as they are in the normal-weight patient.

6. A calorie-restricted diet should not be started for the obese patient admitted for surgery. It probably will not lead to weight loss after discharge, and it may interfere with postoperative recovery. There is no evidence about the value of preoperative weight loss.

REFERENCES

1. Florey C dV: The use and interpretation of ponderal index and other weight-height ratios in epidemiological studies. *J Chronic Dis* 23:93, 1970.
2. Keys A, Fidanzia F, Karvonen MJ et al: Indices of relative weight and obesity. *J Chronic Dis* 25:329, 1972.
3. Goldburt U, Medalie JH: Weight-height indices. *Br J Prevent Soc Med* 28:116, 1974.
4. Benn RT: Some mathematical properties of weight-for-height indices used as measures of adiposity. *Br J Prevent Soc Med* 25:42, 1971.
5. Stewart AL, Brook RH, Kane RL: *Conceptualization and Measurement of Health Habits for Adults in the Health Insurance Study*, vol 2: *Overweight*. Santa Monica, The Rand Corporation, 1980, p 14.
6. *Health Implications of Obesity*. National Institutes of Health Consensus Development Conference Statement, vol 5, no 9.
7. Bray GA: Overweight is risking fate: Definition, classification, prevalence, and risks. *Ann NY Acad Sci* 499:14–28, 1987.
8. Kannel WB, Gordon T: Physiological and medical concomitants of obesity: The Framingham study, in Bray GA (ed): *Obesity in America*. Washington DC, National Institutes of Health, publ no. 79-359, 1979.
9. Westlund K, Nicolaysen R: Ten-year mortality and morbidity related to serum cholesterol. *Scand J Clin Lab Invest* 30:1, 1972.
10. Sorensen TIA, Sonne-Holm S: Mortality in extremely overweight young men. *J Chronic Dis* 30:359, 1977.
11. Lew EA, Garfinkel L: Variations in mortality by weight among 750,000 men and women. *J Chronic Dis* 32:563, 1979.
12. Drenick EJ, Bale GS, Seltzer F et al: Excessive mortality and causes of death in morbidly obese men. *JAMA* 243:443, 1980.
13. Sorlie P, Gordon T, Kannel WB: Body build and mortality in the Framingham study. *JAMA* 243:1828, 1980.
14. Comstock GW, Kendrick MA, Livesay V: Subcutaneous fatness and mortality. *Am J Epidemiol* 83:548, 1966.
15. Andres R: Effect of obesity on total mortality. *Int J Obes* 4:381, 1980.
16. Grundy SM, Greenland P, Herd A et al: Cardiovascular and risk factor evaluation of healthy American adults: A statement by an ad hoc committee appointed by the steering committee, American Heart Association. *Circulation* 75:1340A-1362A, 1987.
17. Bjorntorp P: The association between obesity, adipose tissue distribution and disease. *Acta Med Scand* 723(Suppl):121–134, 1988.
18. Bray GA: Classification and evaluation of obesities. *Med Clin N Am* 73:161–184, 1989.
19. Dublin LI: Relation of obesity to longevity. *N Engl J Med* 248:971, 1953.
20. Chiang BN, Perlman LV, Epstein FH: Overweight and hypertension. *Circulation* 39:403, 1969.
21. Kannel WB, Brand N, Skinner JJ Jr et al: Relation of adiposity to blood pressure and development of hypertension: Framingham study. *Ann Intern Med* 67:48, 1967.

22. Rimm AA, Werner LH, Yserloo BV et al: Relationship of obesity and disease in 73,532 weight-conscious women. *Public Health Rep* 90:44, 1975.

23. Beilin LJ: State of the art lecture. Diet and hypertension: Critical concepts and controversies. *J Hypertension* 5(Suppl 5):S447–S457, 1987.

24. MacMahon S, Cutler J, Brittain E et al: Obesity and hypertension: Epidemiological and clinical issues. *European Heart J* 8(Suppl B):57–70, 1987.

25. Prineas RJ: Clinical interaction of salt and weight change on blood pressure level. *Hypertension* 17(Suppl 1):143–149, 1991.

26. Selby JV, Friedman GD, Queensberry CP Jr: Precursors of essential hypertension: The role of body fat distribution pattern. *Am J Epidemiol* 129:43–53, 1989.

27. Nielson PE, Janniche H: The accuracy of auscultatory measurement of arm blood pressure in very obese subjects. *Acta Med Scand* 195:403, 1974.

28. Bray GA: The risks and disadvantages of obesity, in Bray GA: *Major Problems in Internal Medicine: The Obese Patient*. Philadelphia, Saunders, 1976, vol 9, p 215–251.

29. van Montfrans GA, van der Hoeven GMA, Karemaker JM et al: Accuracy of auscultatory blood pressure measurement with a long cuff. *Brit Med J* 295:354–355, 1987.

30. Haynes RB: Is weight loss an effective treatment of essential hypertension? The evidence against. *Can J Physiol Pharmacol* 64:825–830, 1986.

31. Kannel WB, Gordon T, Castelli WP: Obesity, lipid and glucose intolerance in the Framingham study. *Am J Clin Nutr* 32:1238, 1979.

32. Ashley FW, Kannel WB: Relation of weight change to changes in atherogenic traits in the Framingham study. *J Chronic Dis* 27:103, 1974.

33. Glueck CJ, Taylor HL, Jacobs D et al: Plasma high-density lipoprotein cholesterol: Association with measurements of body mass. *Circulation* 62(Suppl):IV62–69, 1980.

34. Heiss G, Johnson NJ, Reiland S et al: The epidemiology of plasma high-density lipoprotein cholesterol levels. *Circulation* 62(Suppl):IV116–136, 1980.

35. Osterman J, Lin T, Nankin HR et al: Serum cholesterol profiles during treatment of obese outpatients with a very low calorie diet. Effect of initial cholesterol levels. *Int J Obes* 16(1):49–58, 1992.

36. Cole TG, Bowen PE, Shcmeisser D et al: Differential reduction of plasma cholesterol by the American Heart Association Phase 3 Diet in moderately hypercholesterolemic, premenopausal women with different body mass indexes. *Am J Clin Nutr* 55(2):385–394, 1992.

37. Gordon T, Castelli WP, Hjortland C et al: Diabetes, blood lipids, and the role of obesity in coronary heart disease for women: The Framingham study. *Ann Intern Med* 87:393, 1977.

38. Keys A, Aravanis C, Blackburn H et al: *Seven Countries: A Multivariate Analysis of Death and Coronary Heart Disease*. Cambridge MA, Harvard University Press, 1980, pp 161–195.

39. The Pooling Research Group: The relationship of blood pressure, serum cholesterol, smoking habit, relative weight and ECG abnormalities to incidence of major coronary events: Final report of the pooling project. *J Chronic Dis* 31:201, 1978.

40. Hubert HB, Feinlab M, McNamara PM et al: Obesity as an independent risk factor for cardiovascular disease: A 26-year follow-up of participants in the Framingham heart study. *Circulation* 67:968–977, 1983.

41. Manson JE, Colditz GA, Stampfer MJ et al: A prospective study of obesity and risk of coronary heart disease in women. *N Engl J Med* 322(13):882–889, 1990.

42. Kannel WB, Cupples LA, Ramaswami R et al: Regional obesity and risk of cardiovascular disease; the Framingham Study. *J Clin Epidemiol* 44(2):183–190, 1991.

43. Gordon T, Kannel WB: The effects of overweight on cardiovascular diseases. *Geriatrics* 28(8):80, 1973.

44. Ostfeld AM: A review of stroke epidemiology. *Epidemiol Rev* 2:136, 1980.

45. Shinton R, Shipley M. Rose G: Overweight and stroke in the Whitehall study. *J Epidemiol Comm Health* 45(2):138–142, 1991.

46. Sharp JT, Barrocas M, Choksoverty S: The cardiorespiratory effects of obesity. *Clin Chest Med* 1:103, 1980.

47. Terry BE: Morbid obesity: Cardiac evaluation and function. *Gastroenterol Clin N Am* 16:215–222, 1987.

48. Lauer MS, Anderson KM, Kannel WB et al: The impact of obesity on left ventricular mass and geometry. The Framingham Heart Study. *JAMA* 266(2):231–236, 1991.

49. Kasper EK, Hruban RH, Baughman KL: Cardiomyopathy of obesity: A clinicopathologic evaluation of 43 obese patients with heart failure. *Am J Cardiol* 70(9):921–924, 1992.

50. Luce M: Respiratory complications of obesity. *Chest* 78:626, 1980.

51. Drenick EJ, Fisler JS: Sudden cardiac arrest in morbidly obese surgical patients unexplained after autopsy. *Am J Surg* 155:720–726, 1988.

52. Peiser J, Ovnat A, Uwyyed K et al: Cardiac arrhythmias during sleep in morbidly obese sleep-apneic patients before and after bypass surgery. *Clin Cardiol* 8:519–521, 1985.

53. Messerli FH, Nunez BD, Ventura HO et al: Overweight and sudden death: Increased ventricular ectopy in cardiopathy of obesity. *Arch Intern Med* 147:1725–1728, 1987.

54. Berger M, Muller WA, Renold AE: Relationship of obesity to diabetes: Some facts, many questions, in Katzen HM, Mahler RJ (eds): *Diabetes, Obesity and Vascular Disease*, Part I. Washington DC, Hemisphere Publishing, 1978.

55. West KM, Kalbfleisch JM: Influence of nutritional factors on prevalence of diabetes. *Diabetes* 20:99, 1971.

56. Hundley JM: Diabetes-overweight: U.S. problems. *J Am Diet Assoc* 2:417, 1956.

57. Kissebah AH, Freedman DS, Peiris AN: Health risks of obesity. *Med Clin N Am* 73:38, 1989.

58. Flack JM, Sowers JR: Epidemiologic and clinical aspects of insulin resistance and hyperinsulinemia. *Am J Med* 91(1A):11S–21S, 1991.

59. Reaven GM: Insulin-dependent diabetes mellitus: Metabolic characteristics. *Metabolism* 29:445, 1980.

60. Kolterman OG, Insel J, Saekow M et al: Mechanism of insulin resistance in human obesity: Evidence for receptor and postreceptor defects. *J Clin Invest* 65:1272, 1980.

61. Crettaz M, Jeanrenaud B: Postreceptor alterations in the states of insulin resistance. *Metabolism* 29:467, 1980.

62. Friedman GD, Kannel WB, Dawber TR: The epidemiology of gallbladder disease: Observations in the Framingham study. *J Chronic Dis* 19:273, 1966.

63. Wheeler M, Hills LL, Laby B: Cholelithiasis. A clinical and dietary survey. *Gut* 11:430, 1970.

64. Sturdevant RAL, Pearce ML, Payton S: Increased prevalence of cholelithiasis in men ingesting a serum-cholesterol-lowering diet. *N Engl J Med* 288:24, 1973.

65. Bernstein RA, Werner LH, Rimm AA: Relationship of gallbladder disease to parity, obesity, and age. *Health Serv Rep* 88:925, 1973.

66. Stampfer MJ, Maclure KM, Colditz GA et al: Risk of symptomatic gallstones in women with severe obesity. *Am J Clin Nutr* 55(3):652–658, 1992.

67. Thijs C, Knipschild P, Leffers P: Is gallstone disease caused by obesity or by dieting? *Am J Epidemiol* 135(3):274–280, 1992.

68. Bennion LJ, Grundy SM: Effects of obesity and caloric intake on biliary lipid metabolism in man. *J Clin Invest* 56:996, 1975.

69. Shaffer EA, Small DM: Biliary lipid secretion in cholesterol gallstone disease. The effect of cholecystectomy and obesity. *J Clin Invest* 59:828, 1977.

70. Fisher ER, Gregorio R, Stephan T et al: Ovarian changes in women with morbid obesity. *Obstet Gynecol* 44:839, 1974.

71. Hartz AJ, Barboriak PN, Wong A et al: The association of obesity

with infertility and related menstrual abnormalities in women. *Int J Obes* 3:57, 1979.

72. Goldbourt U, Medalie JH, Herman JB et al: Serum uric acid: Correlation with biochemical, anthropomorphic, clinical and behavioral parameters in 10,000 Israeli men. *J Chronic Dis* 33:435, 1980.

73. Nichols A, Scott JT: Effect of weight loss on plasma and urinary levels of uric acid. *Lancet* 2:1223, 1972.

74. Roubenoff R, Klag MJ, Mead LA et al: Incidence and risk factors for gout in white man. *JAMA* 266(21):3004–3007, 1991.

75. David JL, Rosenshein NB, Antunes CMF et al: A review of the risk factors for endometrial carcinoma. *Obstet Gynecol Surg* 36:107–116, 1981.

76. MacMahon B: Risk factors for endometrial cancer. *Gynecol Oncol* 2:122, 1974.

77. Elwood JM, Cole P, Rothman KJ et al: Epidemiology of endometrial cancer. *J Nat Canc Inst* 59:1055, 1977.

78. Blitzer PH, Blitzer EC, Rimm AA: Association between teenage obesity and cancer in 56,111 women: All cancers and endometrial carcinoma. *Prev Med* 5:20, 1976.

79. Elliot EA, Matanoski GM, Rosenshein NB et al: Body fat patterning in women with endometrial cancer. *Gynecol Oncol* 39(3):253–258, 1990.

80. Kelsey JL: A review of the epidemiology of breast cancer. *Epidemiol Rev* 1:74, 1979.

81. Thomas DB: Epidemiologic and related studies of breast cancer etiology. *Rev Cancer Epidemiol* 1:154, 1974.

82. Osler M: Obesity and cancer. *Dan Med Bull* 34:267–274, 1987.

83. Kinlen LJ: Fat and breast cancer. *Cancer Surveys* 6:585–599, 1987.

84. Rose DP: Dietary factors and breast cancer. *Cancer Surveys* 5:671–697, 1986.

85. Albanes D: Caloric intake, body weight, and cancer: A review. *Nutr Cancer* 9:199–217, 1987.

86. den Tonkelaar I, Seidell JC, Collette HJ et al: Obesity and subcutaneous fat patterning in relation to breast cancer in postmenopausal women participating in the Diagnostic Investigation of Mammary Cancer Project. *Cancer* 69(11):2663–2667, 1992.

87. Ballard-Barbash R, Schatzkain A, Carter CL et al: Body fat distribution and breast cancer in the Framingham study. *J Natl Canc Inst* 82(4):286–290, 1990.

88. Schapira DV, Kumar NB, Lyman GH et al: Abdominal obesity and breast cancer risk. *Ann Intern Med* 112(10):798, 1990.

89. Lee IM, Paffenbarger RS Jr: Quetelet's index and risk of colon cancer in college alumni. *J Natl Canc Inst* 84(17):1326–1331, 1992.

90. Le Marchand L, Wilkens LP, Mi MP: Obesity in youth and middle age and risk of colorectal cancer in men. *Can Causes Control* 3(4):349–354, 1992.

91. Neugut AI, Lee WC, Garbowski GC: Obesity and colorectal adenomatous polyps. *J Natl Canc Inst* 83(5):359–361, 1991.

92. Felson DT, Anderson JJ, Naimark A et al: Obesity and knee osteoarthritis: The Framingham study. *Ann Intern Med* 109:18–24, 1988.

93. Felson DT, Zhang Y, Anthony JM et al: Weight loss reduces the risk for symptomatic knee osteoarthritis in women. The Framingham study. *Ann Intern Med* 116(7):535–539, 1992.

94. Felson DT: The epidemiology of knee osteoarthritis: Results from the Framingham osteoarthritis study. *Sem Arth Rheum* 20(3)(Suppl 1):42–50, 1990.

95. Davis MA, Ettinger WH, Neuhaus JM: Obesity and osteoarthritis of the knee: Evidence from the National Health and Nutrition Examination Survey (NHANES I). *Sem Arth Rheum* 20(3)(Suppl 1):34–41, 1990.

96. Friedman J: Weight problems and psychological factors. *J Consult Clin Psychol* 23:524, 1959.

97. Weinberg N, Mendelson M, Stunkard AJ: A failure to find distinctive personality features in a group of obese men. *Am J Psychiatry* 117:1035, 1961.

98. Silverstone JT: Psychosocial aspects of obesity. *Proc R Soc Med* 61:371, 1968.

99. Crisp AH, McGuiness B: Jolly fat: Relation between obesity and psychoneurosis in a general population. *Br Med J* 4:7, 1976.

100. Moore ME, Stunkard AJ, Strole L: Obesity, social class, and mental illness. *JAMA* 118:962, 1962.

101. Holland J, Masling L, Copley D: Mental illness in lower class normal, obese, and hyperobese women. *Psychosom Med* 32:351, 1970.

102. Halmi KA, Long M, Stunkard AJ et al: Psychiatric diagnosis of morbidly obese gastric bypass patients. *Am J Psychiatry* 137:470, 1980.

103. Wadden TA, Stunkard AJ: Psychopathology and obesity. *Ann NY Acad Sci* 499:55–65, 1987.

104. Stunkard AJ: Obesity, in Kaplan HI, Freedman AM, Sadock BJ (eds): *Comprehensive Textbook of Psychiatry*, 3d ed. Baltimore, Williams & Wilkins, 1980, p 00.

105. Strauss RJ, Wise L: Operative risks of obesity. *Surg Gynecol Obstet* 146:286, 1978.

106. Fisher A, Waterhouse TD, Adams AP: Obesity: Its relation to anesthesia. *Anesthesia* 30:633, 1975.

107. Pitkin RM: Abdominal hysterectomy in obese women. *Surg Gynecol Obstet* 142:532, 1976.

108. Postlethwait RW, Johnson WD: Complications following surgery for duodenal ulcer in obese patients. *Arch Surg* 105:438, 1972.

109. Prasad US, Walker WS, Sang CT et al: Influence of obesity on the early and long-term results of surgery for coronary artery disease. *Eur J Cardiothorac Surg* 5(2):67–73, 1991.

110. Pemberton LB, Manax WG: Relationship of obesity to postoperative complications after cholecystectomy. *Am J Surg* 121:87, 1971.

111. Prem KA, Mensheha MM, McKelvey JL: Operative treatment of adenocarcinoma of the endometrium in obese women. *Am J Obstet Gynecol* 92:16, 1965.

112. Stevenson CS, Behney CA, Miller NF: Maternal death from puerperal sepsis following cesarean section. *Obstet Gynecol* 29:181, 1967.

113. Sicuranza BJ, Tisdall LH: Cesarean section in the massively obese. *J Reprod Med* 14:10–11, 1975.

114. Putnam L, Jenicek JA, Allen CR et al: Anesthesia in the morbidly obese patient. *South Med J* 67:1411, 1974.

115. Schirmer BD, Dix J, Edge SB, et al: Laparoscopic cholecystectomy in the obese patient. *Ann Surg* 216(2):146–152, 1992.

116. Unger SW, Scott JS, Unger HM et al: Laparoscopic approach to gallstones in the morbidly obese patient. *Surg Endosc* (Germany) 5(3):116–117, 1991.

117. Pratt JH, Daikoku NH: Obesity and vaginal hysterectomy. *J Reprod Med* 35(10):945–949, 1990.

118. Iber FL, Cooper M: Jejunoileal bypass for the treatment of massive obesity. Prevalence, morbidity, and short-term and long-term consequences. *Am J Clin Nutr* 30:4, 1977.

119. Bray GA, Greenway FL, Barry RE et al: Surgical treatment of obesity: A review of our experience and an analysis of published reports. *Int J Obes* 1:331, 1977.

120. Nachlas MM, Crawford DT, Pearl JM: Current status of jejunoileal bypass in the treatment of morbid obesity. *Surg Gynecol Obstet* 50:256, 1980.

121. The Danish Obesity Project: Randomized trial of jejunoileal bypass versus medical treatment in morbid obesity. *Lancet* 2(8155):1255–1258, 1979.

122. Hermreck AS, Jewell WR, Hardin CA: Gastric bypass for morbid obesity: Results and complications. *Surgery* 80:498, 1976.

123. Mason EE, Printen KJ, Blommers TJ et al: Gastric bypass for obesity after ten years experience. *Int J Obes* 2:197, 1978.

124. Griffen WO: Gastric bypass for morbid obesity. *Surg Clin N Am* 59(6):1103, 1979.

125. Pace WF, Martin EW Jr, Tetirick T et al: Gastric partitioning for morbid obesity. *Ann Surg* 190:392, 1979.

126. Benotti PN, Hollingshead J, Mascioli EA et al: Gastric restrictive operations for morbid obesity. *Am J Surg* 157:150–155, 1989.

127. Pasulka PS, Bistrian BR, Benotti PN et al: The risks of surgery in obese patients. *Ann Intern Med* 104:540–546, 1986.

128. Pories WJ, MacDonald KG Jr, Morgan EJ et al: Surgical treatment of obesity and its effect on diabetes; 10-year follow-up. *Am J Clin Nutr* 55(Suppl 2);582S–585S, 1992.

129. Benotti PN, Hollingshead J, Mascioli EA et al: Gastric restrictive operations for morbid obesity. *Am J Surg* 157(1):150–155, 1989.

130. Mason EE, Renquist KE, Jiang D: Perioperative risks and safety of surgery for severe obesity. *Am J Clin Nutr* 55(Suppl 2):573S–576S, 1992.

131. Damia G, Mascheroni D, Croci M et al: Perioperative changes in functional residual capacity in morbidly obese patients. *Br J Anesth* 60:574–578, 1988.

132. Jense HG, Dubin SA, Silverstein PI: Effect of obesity on safe duration of apnea in anesthetized humans. *Anesth Analg* 72(1):89–93, 1991.

133. Vaughan RW, Wise L: Intraoperative arterial oxygenation in obese patients. *Ann Surg* 184:35, 1976.

134. Salem MR, Balal FY, Zygmunt MP et al: Does PEEP improve intraoperative arterial oxygenation in grossly obese patients? *Anesthesiology* 48:280, 1978.

135. Vaughan RW, Engelhardt RC, Wise L: Postoperative hypoxemia in obese patients. *Ann Surg* 180:877, 1974.

136. Vaughan RW, Wise L: Postoperative arterial blood gas measurement in obese patients: Effect of position on gas exchange. *Ann Surg* 182:705, 1975.

137. Vaughan RW, Wise L: Choice of abdominal operative incision in the obese patient: A study using blood gas measurements. *Ann Surg* 181:829, 1975.

138. Poe RH, Kallay MC, Dass T, Celebic A: Can postoperative pulmonary complications after elective cholecystectomy be predicted? *Am J Med Sci* 295:29–34, 1988.

139. Latimer RG, Dickman M, Day WC et al: Ventilatory patterns and pulmonary complications after upper abdominal surgery determined by preoperative and postoperative computerized spirometry and blood gas analysis. *Am J Surg* 122:622, 1971.

140. Hansen G, Prablos PA, Steinert R: Pulmonary complications, ventilation and blood gases after upper abdominal surgery. *Acta Anaesth Scand* 21:211, 1977.

141. Postlethwait RW, Johnson WD: Complications following surgery for duodenal ulcer in obese patients. *Arch Surg* 105:438–440, 1972.

142. Presley AP, Alexander-Williams J: Postoperative chest infection. *Br J Surg* 61:448, 1974.

143. Vaughan RW, Bauer S, Wise L: Volume and pH of gastric juice in obese patients. *Anesthesiology* 43:686, 1975.

144. Illing L, Cuncan PG, Yip R: Gastroesophageal reflux during anaesthesia. *Can J Anaesth* 39(5)(part 1):466–470, 1992.

145. Vila P, Valles J, Canet J et al: Acid aspiration prophylaxis in morbidly obese patients: Famotidine versus ranitidine. *Anesthesia* 46(11):967–969, 1991.

146. Gilmore OJA, Sanderson PJ: Prophylactic interparietal povidoneiodine in abdominal surgery. *Br J Surg* 62:792, 1975.

147. Higson RH, Kettlewell MGW: Parietal wound drainage in abdominal surgery. *Br J Surg* 65:326, 1978.

148. Green SL, Sarubbi FA Jr: Risk factors associated with postcesarean section febrile morbidity. *Obstet Gynecol* 49:686, 1977.

149. Garrow JS, Hastings EJ, Cox AG et al: Obesity and postoperative complications of abdominal operations. *Br Med J* 297:181, 1988.

150. Lilienfeld DE, Vlahov D, Tenney JH et al: Obesity and diabetes as risk factors for postoperative wound infections after cardiac surgery. *Am J Infect Control* 16:3–6, 1988.

151. Schmitz HE, Beaton JH: Wound disruption and its management. *Am J Obstet Gynecol* 43:806, 1942.

152. Efron G: Abdominal wound disruption. *Lancet* 1(7399):1287–1291, 1965.

153. Reitamo J, Moller C: Abnorminal wound dehiscence. *Acta Chir Scand* 138:170, 1972.

154. Keill RH, Keitzer WF, Nichols WK et al: Abdominal wound dehiscence. *Arch Surg* 106:573, 1973.

155. Helmkamp BF: Abdominal wound dehiscence. *Am J Obstet Gynecol* 128:803, 1977.

156. Tibutt DA, Chesterman CN: Pulmonary embolism: Current therapeutic concepts. *Drugs* 11:151, 1976.

157. Moser KM: Pulmonary embolism. *Am Rev Resp Dis* 115:829, 1977.

158. Kakkar W, Howe CT, Nicholaides AN et al: Deep vein thrombosis of the leg. Is there a "high risk" group? *Am J Surg* 120:527, 1970.

159. Clayton JK, Anderson JA, McNicol GP: Preoperative prediction of postoperative deep vein thrombosis. *Br Med J* 4:910, 1976.

160. Sue-Ling HM, Johnston D, McMahon MJ et al: Preoperative identification of patients at high risk of deep venous thrombosis after elective major abdominal surgery. *Lancet* 1(8491):1173–1176, 1986.

161. Wille-Jorgensen P, Ott P: Predicting failure of low-dose prophylactic heparin in general surgical procedures. *Surg Gynecol Obstet* 171(2):126–130, 1990.

162. Lemos MJ, Sutton D, Hozack WJ, et al: Pulmonary embolism in total hip and knee arthroplasty. Risk factors in patients on warfarin prophylaxis and analysis of the prothrombin time as an indicator of warfarin's prophylactic effect. *Clin Orthop* 282:158–163, 1992.

163. Snell AM: The relation of obesity to fatal post-operative pulmonary embolism. *Arch Surg* 15:237, 1927.

164. Coon WW: Risk factors in pulmonary embolism. *Surg Gynecol Obstet* 143:385, 1976.

165. Havig O: Pulmonary thromboembolism: Clinicopathological correlations and multiple regression analysis of possible risk factors. *Acta Chir Scand Suppl* 478:48, 1977.

166. Cullen DJ, Nemeskal AR: The autopsy incidence of acute pulmonary embolism in critically ill surgical patients. *Intens Care Med* 12(6):399–403, 1986.

167. Bell WR, Simon TL, DeMets DL: The clinical features of submassive and massive pulmonary emboli. *Am J Med* 2:355, 1977.

168. Sigel B, Justin JR, Gibson RF et al: Risk assessment of pulmonary embolism by multivariate analysis. *Arch Surg* 114:188, 1979.

169. Young SR, Stoelting RK, Peterson C et al: Anesthetic biotransformation and renal function in obese patients during and after methoxyflurane or halothane anesthesia. *Anesthesiology* 42:451, 1979.

170. Vaughan RW: Anesthetic considerations in jejunoileal small bowel bypass for morbid obesity. *Anesth Analg* 53:421, 1974.

34 ANESTHESIA AND SURGERY IN THE PATIENT WITH LIVER DISEASE

Ronnie C. Parker

Frank H. Brown

Patients with liver disease frequently require surgery for complications of their disease and for a variety of related reasons. Liver disease is associated with an increased incidence of conditions that require surgical intervention, including hernias, gallstones, and peptic ulcer disease.[1-4] Furthermore, morbidity and mortality rates following general anesthesia and surgical procedures are higher in these patients,[5] and many abuse ethanol or drugs with their attendant risks of trauma and infection. Some investigators estimate that 5 to 10 percent of all patients with liver disease undergo surgery in the last two years of their lives, and two large reviews state that 4 to 16 percent of all cirrhotics die from postoperative complications.[6,7] Evaluation of the surgical patient with hepatic disease is complex because of the multiple synthetic and metabolic functions of the liver essential in maintaining homeostatic balance during the stress of surgery.

This chapter reviews the pathophysiologic effects of anesthesia and surgery on hepatic function and the evidence that patients with acute and chronic liver disease have increased operative morbidity and mortality. Preoperative risk assessment and stratification is discussed in detail as the basis for recommendations important in preparing patients with liver disease for surgery and hopefully ensuring optimal surgical outcome. Discussions of specialized procedures such as portasystemic shunting, hepatic resection, and liver transplantation are beyond the scope of this chapter.

EFFECTS OF ANESTHESIA AND SURGERY ON THE LIVER

Numerous investigators have found that many patients demonstrate detectable abnormalities in the liver function tests after surgery and anesthesia.[8-22] These changes are usually minor and transient, and their clinical significance is uncertain.

Postoperative liver function test abnormalities are often difficult to interpret and may be multifactorial in etiology. Several studies have shown that fever, sepsis, burns, multiple trauma, hemor-

rhage, and shock can each cause liver dysfunction.[23-30] Hepatic function in the surgical patient may be compromised even before surgery begins.

The contribution of anesthesia to frequently noted postoperative disturbances in liver tests remains unclear and is difficult to separate from the effects of the operative procedure itself.[31-34] Brouhoult and Gillquist found that anesthesia itself had no effect on postanesthetic serum transaminase levels in patients who had received halothane for angiography.[35] However, Stevens et al. administered various anesthetics to healthy volunteers and documented minor abnormalities in liver function tests with several agents.[36]

Most data on the effect of specific anesthetics on serum liver function tests are derived from studies of anesthetics used during various surgical procedures. In a study of 43 patients undergoing vaginal hysterectomy, the bromsulphthalein (BSP) clearance and other liver function tests were measured before and during the procedure.[37] General but not spinal anesthesia caused significant deterioration in BSP clearance and minor elevations in serum gamma-glutamyltranspeptidase levels without detectable changes in the other liver enzyme concentrations measured.

Nitrous oxide has little effect on hepatic function. In a study of eight patients anesthetized with nitrous oxide and oxygen, indocyanine green (ICG) clearance did not significantly change until other anesthetics were added.[38] In another study of 100 patients undergoing total hip replacement[39] there were no abnormalities in biochemical tests in patients receiving nitrous oxide.

There is little evidence that any anesthetic agent, with the possible exception of chloroform which is no longer used, is a direct hepatotoxin.[40] This is supported by some studies that fail to show a correlation between duration of anesthesia and postoperative liver function test abnormalities and by others showing no significant differences among various inhalational anesthetics in their effect on hepatic function.[11,13,15,16,19,21,30,41-43] In a study of 41 patients requiring repeated anesthesia with halothane for genitourinary surgery, there was no obvious relationship between the number of anesthetics or the total duration of anesthesia and disturbances in serum liver tests.[44] Despite case reports of hepatotoxicity associated with enflurane,[45,46] repeated use of it may cause fewer abnormalities than halothane.[47-49] Isoflurane, the least metabolized of the volatile anesthetic agents, may therefore be preferred in patients with liver disease.[50-52] In a study of 11 infants and children given daily isoflurane for radiotherapy, there were no alterations in serum liver function tests.[53]

The effects of various anesthetic techniques, whether local, regional, spinal, or general, have been studied in patients undergoing similar operations. Some investigators have suggested that local and spinal anesthesia interfere less with liver function than general anesthesia, but others have been unable to demonstrate statistically significant differences among techniques and conclude that factors other than anesthesia are probably more important.[8,13,19,21,41,54]

Solely intravenous techniques have been reported to cause more severe derangements in hepatic function than more balanced techniques did.[55] However, with alteration in the timing of administration of the intravenous agents, no detectable hepatic function impairment can be documented.[56]

Anesthetic agents may affect liver function by decreasing liver perfusion. Cyclopropane, which is no longer in use, reduces hepatic blood flow by approximately one-third by increasing splanchnic vascular resistance through its effect on the sympathetic nervous system. Halothane causes a similar reduction in hepatic blood flow by causing systemic vasodilation and a decrease in cardiac output. Methoxyflurane, also not in current use, lowers systemic and splanchnic perfusion pressure and may cause portal venoconstriction, thereby reducing hepatic blood flow by approximately 50%.[57] Spinal and lumbar epidural agents reduce hepatic blood flow by reducing arterial pressure, but have little or no effect on splanchnic vascular resistance.[57-59]

The effects of anesthesia are difficult to separate from other intraoperative factors that influence blood flow in patients undergoing surgery.[57-59] Positive-pressure ventilation, hypocapnia, and hypercapnia all increase splanchnic vascular resistance and decrease hepatic blood flow.[60] Hypotension, hemorrhage, systemic hypoxemia, and vasoactive drugs also reduce blood flow. In addition, traction on abdominal viscera during surgery produces reflex-mediated dilation of splanchnic capacitance vessels, systemic hypotension, and reduced blood flow.[61]

The significance of these reductions in hepatic blood flow is unclear. Although all anesthetics decrease splanchnic oxygen consumption, they cause a relatively greater reduction in hepatic blood flow, resulting in lower hepatic vein oxygen content and possible liver hypoxia.[57-59] Price and associates evaluated this hypothesis by measuring hepatic venous lactate-to-pyruvate ratios in anesthetized healthy volunteers but were unable to demonstrate evidence of hypoxia.[62]

In summary, although anesthetics themselves may exert minor hepatotoxic and hemodynamic effects, marginal changes in hepatic blood flow and oxygenation may become clinically significant when other intraoperative factors compromise hepatic perfusion. Patients with cirrhosis and hepatitis already have decreased hepatic blood flow. Therefore, they may be more sensitive to changes in hepatic blood flow and hypoxia associated with anesthesia and surgery and liver disease.[11]

In a number of studies, the frequency and magnitude of abnormalities in postoperative serum liver function tests correlate more closely with the nature and extent of surgery than with the type of anesthesia used.[10,11,63,64] For example, Killen found postoperative elevations in serum transaminase levels in 35 percent of patients after herniorrhaphy, 65 percent after laparotomy, 75 percent after biliary surgery, and 90 percent after thoracotomy.[18] Similarly, Hobson et al. documented more than twofold elevations in postoperative levels of AST in 75 percent of patients undergoing biliary and upper abdominal surgery, 17 percent undergoing lower abdominal procedures, and 4 percent undergoing minor procedures such as breast biopsy.[17] Similar data have been presented by other investigators,[9-11,65] and the high incidence of abnormalities after biliary tract or upper abdominal surgery has been repeatedly emphasized.[12,21,23,66-69]

Histologic and functional studies provide additional evidence that anesthesia and surgery may result in liver damage.[70] In one study, liver biopsies performed at the end of major abdominal procedures revealed evidence of acute inflammation in all of the patients, but control biopsies performed at the beginning of the operation were normal. Others have found that anesthesia of long duration and severe operative trauma may give rise to lesions suggestive of hepatitis.[71]

It is therefore clear that underlying illness, injury, anesthesia, and surgery may all contribute in varying degrees to functional impairment and morphologic changes in the liver. The type and extent of surgery appear to be more important than the technique and duration of anesthesia or the choice of agent in the pathogenesis of these changes. Hepatic dysfunction seen is generally mild, transient, and clinically insignificant. However, in patients with underlying acute or chronic liver disease, these changes may contribute to clinically apparent hepatic decompensation and potentially to greater operative risk.

POSTOPERATIVE MORTALITY IN PATIENTS WITH LIVER DISEASE

Compromise of the many synthetic and metabolic functions of the liver results in an increased incidence of infection, abnormal hemostasis, abnormal drug metabolism, and impaired protein and glucose synthesis, even without the added metabolic burdens of anesthesia and surgery. Frequently, associated anemia, fluid and electrolyte disturbances, malnutrition, or portal hypertension further complicate the situation. However, there are relatively few data documenting increased operative risk in patients with liver disease, or correlating the type and severity of liver disease with postoperative morbidity and mortality. Most data are derived from studies of patients undergoing portasystemic shunting procedures, and these patients represent a highly select group undergoing a specific operation directly affecting the liver and hepatic blood flow. Although there is a growing body of literature on the risk factors of patients with cirrhosis, many of the studies suffer from small sample size, lack of controls, little or no statistical analysis, and lack of prospective evaluation.

Acute Hepatitis

Stone clearly states that "active hepatitis (whether alcoholic or viral) is uniformly associated with a poor prognosis and has therefore become an almost absolute contraindication to surgery,"[72] and others have more recently repeated the admonishment against performing elective surgery in patients with acute hepatitis.[73,74] However, the evidence for this is equivocal.

In a study of three patients with viral hepatitis undergoing laparotomy, Shaldon and Sherlock documented slow postoperative recovery in all and serious deterioration of hepatic function in one.[75] Byrne cited an operative mortality rate of 33 percent in patients with hepatitis at Boston City Hospital.[76] Of 12 patients with viral hepatitis undergoing surgery in the study of Turner and Sherlock, five died after surgery, and four others suffered hepatic decompensation, developed ascites, and recovered only after protracted illness.[77]

Harville and Summerskill reviewed 42 patients with viral hepatitis and 16 patients with drug-induced hepatitis who were taken to laparotomy.[78] Among those with viral hepatitis, four or 9.5 percent died, and another five or 11.9 percent suffered major complications. The combined morbidity and mortality rate was 21.4 percent. Hargrove presented two cases of patients with chronic active hepatitis who died after laparotomy and suggested that surgery and anesthesia may have adverse effects on the course of the disease.[79] Greenwood et al. studied 12 patients with alcoholic hepatitis who underwent open liver biopsy, in some cases during abdominal surgery, and documented a postoperative mortality rate of 58 percent.[80] Orloff et al. found that patients with an elevated serum SGOT level had a higher mortality rate after portasystemic shunt surgery than those with normal levels.[81] Mikkelsen and Kein found that the degree of acute hyaline necrosis found on liver biopsy closely correlated with operative death in patients undergoing shunt procedures.[82,83]

However, other investigators have questioned the significance of hepatitis as a risk factor. Strauss et al. performed elective surgery to drain the common duct in 73 patients with hepatitis and reported no deaths in the immediate postoperative period.[84] Bourke et al. reported that three patients with hepatitis subjected to laparotomy suffered no adverse consequences.[85] Among 14 patients with acute viral hepatitis and 16 patients with chronic active hepatitis in the series of Hardy and Hughes, there were zero and two deaths, respectively.[86] The authors concluded that their "observations do not confirm the view that laparotomy is necessarily dangerous in viral hepatitis, but neither do they suggest that caution is unjustified." Based on available data, this assessment seems reasonable.

Alcoholic Hepatitis

Patients with severe alcoholic hepatitis do not tolerate surgery well, but those with mild disease usually undergo nonabdominal surgery without mishap. One study of 30 patients with mild alcoholic hepatitis[87] defined by a history of heavy alcohol ingestion and two or more specific clinical or biochemical criteria documented that all tolerated a variety of procedures well.

Chronic Hepatitis

Chronic active hepatitis has been reported to affect outcome adversely.[79] However, in a retrospective study of 20 patients with chronic active hepatitis undergoing 34 different operative procedures, no patient developed new postoperative ascites, jaundice, or encephalopathy, and there was no operative mortality.[88] The authors concluded that surgery is tolerated well in the asymptomatic patient with chronic active hepatitis. Chronic persistent hepatitis is not associated with increased risk.

Cirrhosis

Cirrhosis has long been associated with a high operative mortality rate. Hughson documented a death rate of 60 percent in patients with cirrhosis undergoing omentopexy in 1927, and Henrikson reported a postoperative mortality rate of 55 percent in similar patients undergoing various operations in 1936.[89,90] More recently, Jackson et al. cited an overall operative mortality rate of 5 to 7 percent for major procedures.[2] In 104 patients with cirrhosis, Lindenmuth and Eisenberg documented a mortality rate of 6.7 percent and an overall complication rate of 25 percent, with most complications occurring in patients with more severe disease.[91] Cayer and Sohmer compared a group of cirrhotics dying after nonshunt surgery with survivors and found evidence of greater hepatic dysfunction in those who died, suggesting that severity of cirrhosis correlates with operative death.[92] Similarly, Wirthlin et al. reported an overall surgical mortality rate of 57 percent in cirrhotics with nonvariceal gastroduodenal bleeding and demonstrated a higher death rate in those with more severe disease.[93]

Obstructive Jaundice

The observation that excessive hyperbilirubinemia increases operative risk in patients undergoing procedures for benign and malignant obstructive jaundice has been repeatedly confirmed. Other risk factors include malnourishment and malignancy. In one study of 929 patients with obstructive jaundice, the operative mortality rate was 13 percent.[94] Risk factors derived from a multivariate analysis included a hematocrit level under 30%, a serum bilirubin level above 200 μg/liter, and malignancy. If all three factors were present, the mortality rate was 60 percent. If all were absent, the rate was less than 5 percent. Denning et al. studied 57 patients undergoing surgery with serum bilirubin levels above 5 mg/dl on admission.[95] Those who underwent preoperative transhepatic drainage had fewer complications than those who did not, but there was no difference in operative mortality between the two groups. In 129 patients with hyperbilirubinemia undergoing biliary tract or pancreatic surgery and receiving vitamin K, prophylactic antibiotics, mannitol, and oral deoxycholate, the overall mortality rate was 4.7 percent.[96] The rate was 10.5 percent in those with serum bilirubin levels above 200 μg/liter. Those who died all had hematocrit levels above 30%. Six developed renal dysfunction.

In another study of patients undergoing biliary or pancreatic surgery, preoperative percutaneous transhepatic biliary drainage was performed with and without nutritional hyperalimentation. In those undergoing drainage alone, the mortality rate was 12.5 percent. However, the rate was 3.5 percent in those receiving hyperalimentation before the procedure.[97] It should be noted that operations to relieve biliary obstruction are themselves associated with a high rate of complications and a mortality rate of 5 to 10 percent.

RISK ASSESSMENT AND STRATIFICATION

In evaluating patients with liver disease before surgery, it is important to know which elements of the history, physical examination, and laboratory data best predict the magnitude of operative risk. For those with cirrhosis, there are two studies of patients undergoing nonshunt surgery that prove useful. Cayer and Sohmer found

TABLE 34–1. Child's Classification

	Class A	Class B	Class C
Bilirubin (mg/dl)	< 2.0	2.0–3.0	> 3.0
Albumin (g/dl)	> 3.5	3.0–3.5	< 3.0
Ascites	None	Easily controlled	Poorly controlled
Encephalopathy	None	Mild	Advanced
Nutritional status	Excellent	Good	Poor

that the presence of ascites, hypoalbuminemia, a prolonged prothrombin time, and anemia were correlated with increased operative mortality.[92] Jaundice and abnormal liver function tests were not significant predictors. Hepatomegaly predicted a better prognosis for cirrhotic patients, a finding that has been confirmed by others as well.[81,98] In the study by Wirthlin et al., cirrhotic patients undergoing emergency surgery for gastroduodenal bleeding were more likely to die if they had a history of cirrhosis, varices, or ascites, but the presence of ascites on physical examination was not a predictor.[93] The death rate was directly correlated with the serum bilirubin concentration, blood ammonia level, and prothrombin time, and was inversely related to the serum albumin level. The serum bilirubin concentration was felt to be the most reliable indicator.

A larger number of studies attempting to predict operative mortality from the findings of preoperative evaluation have been performed in patients undergoing portasystemic shunting, and several authors have proposed multifactorial indices to estimate surgical risk.[81,99–101] The most widely used index is that proposed by Child.[102] (See Table 36–1.) It is empirically derived and uses clinical assessment of the state of nutrition, the presence or absence of ascites, and serum levels of bilirubin and albumin to place patients in one of three groups. Several early studies showed that this classification correlates well with operative mortality in shunt surgery.[102,103]

More recent studies of patients with cirrhosis undergoing portasystemic shunt procedures confirm that the severity of underlying liver disease is the major determinant of operative death but suggest that there are other factors. In one study of 286 patients with a postoperative complication rate of 52.1 percent and a mortality rate of 14.6 percent, emergency surgery was associated with

higher mortality.[104] In another study, operative mortality in 121 shunted cirrhotic patients was associated with preoperative serum bilirubin and BUN levels, but these were no better than Child's criteria in predicting mortality. In another group of patients undergoing peritoneovenous shunting, Fulenwider et al.[105] documented similarly high rates of morbidity and mortality. Only the preoperative serum level of bilirubin proved to be a good predictor of mortality.

Although Child's criteria were originally designed to predict the operative risk of patients undergoing portasystemic shunting, Nolan and Stone have found them useful in predicting outcome in other major surgical procedures, including hepatic resection.[72] Moreover, Pugh et al. have proposed a modification in the criteria, adding prolongation of the prothrombin time and omitting assessment of nutritional status.[106] (See Table 36–2.) Patients who score five to six points are considered to be good operative risks (grade A), those with seven to nine points moderate risks (grade B), and those with 10 to 15 points poor operative risks (grade C). This classification predicted operative mortality in Pugh's series of patients undergoing transection of the esophagus for bleeding varices. In another study of patients undergoing cholecystectomy, there were no deaths in those in Child's class A and 23.5 percent of those in Child's class C died.[107] Other studies have confirmed the utility of the classification in predicting mortality in patients undergoing biliary tract surgery and cholecystectomy.[108,109] In a study of 100 cirrhotic patients, Garrison et al. used stepwise multivariate analysis to identify variables predicting survival in those undergoing cholecystectomy and procedures on the gastroduodenal complex.[110] Predictors included the serum albumin level, the presence of infection, the protime and intraoperative transfusion requirements. However, none of these proved better than Child's classification.

On the other hand, other investigators have not found Child's classification useful in predicting outcome in procedures other than those for variceal bleeding and have devised other systems to assess risk.[111,112] In a recent study of 54 patients with cirrhosis undergoing colectomy, yet another scoring system was used, identifying clinically evident encephalopathy, hemoglobin level, and serum albumin level to be the best predictors of mortality.[113] Moreover, others have found the correlation between expected predictors and outcome to be inconsistent. In a study of 33 cirrhotic patients undergoing biliary tract surgery, some with normal liver

TABLE 34–2. Grading of Severity of Liver Disease—Pugh's Criteria

Clinical and Biochemical Measurements	Points Scored for Increasing Abnormality		
	1	2	3
Encephalopathy (grade)*	None	1 and 2	3 and 4
Ascites	Absent	Slight	Moderate
Bilirubin (mg/dl)	1–2	2–3	> 3
Albumin (g/dl)	3.5	2.8–3.5	< 2.8
Prothrombin time (seconds prolonged)	1–4	4–6	> 6
For primary biliary cirrhosis:			
Bilirubin (mg/dl)	1–4	4–10	> 10

*According to grading of Trey C, Burns DG, Saunders SJ in *N Engl J Med* 274:473, 1966.

function tests and normal platelet counts and coagulation parameters experienced significant bleeding.[114] In others with hyperbilirubinemia and prolonged coagulation times, surgery was uncomplicated.

Investigators are continuing to study variables to predict mortality more accurately in patients with liver disease in a variety of settings. These efforts may be useful in selecting the optimal time for liver transplantation.[115–126] Parameters studied include formation of the lidocaine metabolite monoethylglycinexylidide (MEGX),[115] ICG clearance,[115,121] caffeine clearance,[115] aminopyrine breath analysis,[116,119] galactose elimination,[118] and amino acid clearance.[126] Other prognostic indicators may include the hepatic vein pressure gradient,[120] the presence of large esophageal varices at endoscopy,[120] hepatic venous hemoglobin oxygen saturation,[122] measurement of liver volume,[123] the APACHE II score,[124] and excretion of a water load.[125]

Despite these efforts, a consistent relationship between clinical or laboratory assessment and operative mortality has not as yet been established. In 1964, Welch et al. stated that no single test or combination of tests could be relied upon to predict survival.[98] Four years later, Jackson et al. concluded that "the prognosis for survival in cirrhotics cannot at present be predicted in clinical, laboratory or physiologic studies alone and that the ultimate outcome in an individual patient is not easily determined prior to an operation."[2] These conclusions are still applicable today.

PREOPERATIVE EVALUATION AND PREPARATION

Preoperative evaluation of the patient with liver disease has several objectives. The type and severity of liver disease must be determined and the risk of surgery estimated. Potentially reversible disturbances such as encephalopathy or coagulopathy should be defined and treated to minimize operative risk and postoperative complications. As always, preoperative evaluation begins with a careful medical history and physical examination. Particular attention should be paid to the presence of jaundice, hepatosplenomegaly, ascites, and encephalopathy and to assessment of nutritional state. Laboratory evaluation should include an electrocardiogram; chest x-ray; urinalysis; complete blood count; platelet count; prothrombin time; and determination of serum electrolyte, blood urea nitrogen, creatinine, glucose, and standard liver enzyme levels. Serologic testing for hepatitis may be useful in identifying the risk of infection to others. Bleeding times and blood ammonia levels are not generally indicated. Some have suggested that arterial blood gas measurements, pulmonary function tests, and cardiac output determinations precede portasystemic shunting.[127]

Determining the specific type of liver disease is important in decisions regarding the timing of surgery. It is generally recommended that patients with acute viral hepatitis defer elective surgery until one month after liver function tests have normalized.[128,129] While some have recommended that elective procedures be postponed in patients with alcoholic hepatitis until serial liver function tests are normal,[129] those with mild disease can probably undergo surgery without mishap. In those with chronic active hepatitis, documentation of disease quiescence for at least three months prior to operative intervention has been suggested.[129] However, surgery seems to be tolerated well in asymptomatic patients. At the present time, there is no data to support routine screening of all patients for occult liver disease with serum liver function tests.

Even though the Child-Pugh classification is not ideal, it is the best studied and most valid of the predictors. All patients with cirrhosis should therefore be classified according to these criteria. Only those in group A should be considered fit for anesthesia and surgery.[72,130] For those in group B or C, elective surgery should be deferred to allow for preoperative preparation and optimization of their medical condition.

Hepatic Encephalopathy

Evaluation and treatment of hepatic encephalopathy is indicated before surgery. Although it has not been studied as an independent risk factor, overt encephalopathy should be brought under control in all but emergency surgery. In one group of patients undergoing elective portacaval shunting procedures, encephalopathy occurred spontaneously in 23 percent.[131]

Evidence of hepatic encephalopathy requires careful examination and assessment of mental status. Examination for the presence of asterixis alone is not adequate. Frequently, several precipitating causes can be found, including hypokalemia, metabolic alkalosis, infection, gastrointestinal bleeding, and the use of potent analgesics. Treatment of encephalopathy includes lactulose or neomycin administered orally or in retention enemas.

Preoperative management of patients with severe liver disease but no encephalopathy is less straightforward. Some have recommended prophylactic treatment to prevent postoperative encephalopathy.[132,133] Routine bowel preparation for abdominal surgery with antibiotics and protein restriction imposed by inability to eat may in themselves reduce the incidence of encephalopathy.

Ascites

Ascites is common in patients with chronic liver disease and complicates anesthesia and surgery. Massive accumulation of ascites impairs diaphragmatic movement, decreases functional residual capacity, and promotes atelectasis. Since ascitic fluid is in equilibrium with fluid in the interstitial and intravascular spaces, sudden decompression of ascites can lead to fluid shifts, pooling in the splanchnic venous system, and hypotension.[134] Ascites should be treated with bed rest, sodium restriction, appropriate use of diuretics, and paracentesis as needed.

In one study, 39 percent of patients with cirrhosis and no previously recognized ascites developed ascites after upper-abdominal surgery.[135] The development of ascites correlated with the severity of liver disease and estimated blood loss. Intractable ascites development was thought to be due to additional mechanisms, such as lymphatic vessel leakage from the surgical site. In some cases, the development of massive ascites was the initial sign of otherwise unsuspected liver cirrhosis.[136]

Coagulopathy

The prothrombin time is frequently prolonged in patients with liver disease. Vitamin K-dependent coagulation factors synthesized by the liver (II, VII, IX, and X) and protein C are deficient in those with advanced liver disease[137] or jaundice and in those who receive long courses of oral antibiotics for bowel sterilization or treatment of infection or encephalopathy.[129] All patients with a prolonged prothrombin time should receive parenteral vitamin K before surgery. Those with severe liver dysfunction may not respond to vitamin K and require adequate amounts of fresh frozen plasma. Patients with alcohol-induced bone marrow depression or hypersplenism generally do not require platelet transfusions, but platelets may be needed for emergency surgery in patients with platelet counts low enough to predispose them to excessive bleeding.

Nutritional Concerns

Many patients with chronic liver disease are malnourished, and there may be nutritional problems unique to those with severe disease. Although gastrointestinal protein absorption is normal in patients with cirrhosis, oral protein intake must be limited because it may precipitate or worsen encephalopathy. Intravenous amino acids have the theoretical advantage of bypassing intestinal bacterial degradation by which most ammonia is produced. However, when conventional intravenous amino acid solutions were first given to cirrhotic patients, encephalopathy worsened.[138]

Chronic hepatocellular failure is associated with low blood levels of branched-chain amino acids and high tyrosine concentrations in the brain. Tyrosine may be metabolized by the brain to false neurotransmitters and cause some of the neuropsychiatric complications observed in patients with liver disease. Experimental solutions containing high concentrations of branched-chain amino acids and low concentrations of aromatic amino acids have been proven useful in animals and humans in some but not all studies.[139,140] In one prospective randomized trial, Kanematsu et al. studied the postoperative use of branched-chain amino acid solutions in patients with cirrhosis.[141] They failed to show that these solutions were any more effective in preventing hepatic encephalopathy than standard nutritional solutions. Experiments in animals suggested that ketoanalogs of amino acids are incorporated into protein and promote positive nitrogen balance without the hazard of encephalopathy.[142]

The use of high-fat diets as a method of caloric supplementation is also limited in patients with cirrhosis in whom impaired bile-salt synthesis limits fat digestion and absorption. Substitution of medium-chain triglycerides is not recommended because of studies documenting elevated serum octanoate concentrations in encephalopathic patients.[143] This may be due to the inability of the body to utilize medium-chain fatty acids or to incomplete oxidation of long-chain fatty acids.

In a study of 35 severely malnourished cirrhotic patients, total enteral nutrition proved better than an isocaloric isonitrogenous low-sodium standard oral diet when the Child-Pugh classifications, serum albumin levels, and in-hospital mortality were examined.[144] In a separate study of patients with alcoholic liver disease, biochemical test abnormalities resolved more quickly when casein-based tube-fed solution was given for four weeks.[145] Another study also noted improvement in liver function when special attention was paid to diet.[146]

Although there are encouraging experimental studies that may find clinical application in the future, current nutritional support of patients with severe liver disease is limited to the provision of adequate carbohydrate, maximal tolerable protein, and perhaps branched-chain amino acid solutions. Since patients with liver disease have little or no hepatic glycogen stores, glucose infusions should therefore be started before surgery to prevent intraoperative hypoglycemia and continued in the postoperative period.[147] Se-

verely malnourished patients may benefit from specific preoperative nutritional assessment by consultants in the field. Some investigators have suggested that postoperative total parenteral nutrition with special formulations may be useful in patients with liver dysfunction,[148] but their effect on clinical outcome has not yet been rigorously studied.

Electrolyte Abnormalities

Patients with chronic liver disease frequently have electrolyte disturbances including hyponatremia, hypokalemia, and metabolic alkalosis due to secondary hyperaldosteronism, diuretic therapy for ascites, prolonged vomiting, or nasogastric suction. Since these disturbances may be associated with increased operative risk and may precipitate encephalopathy, they should be treated before surgery and monitored thereafter.[81]

Metabolism of Anesthetic and Paralytic Agents

The metabolism of anesthetic agents may be abnormal in patients with liver disease due to decreased hepatic enzymatic function, changes in the volume of distribution, or alterations in protein binding. These alterations may or may not be clinically significant. For example, disposition of midazolam, despite its mainly hepatic elimination, is only slightly impaired in patients with cirrhosis, and the incidence of side effects is not increased when a single dose is given.[149] The clearance rate of etomidate is normal, but the distribution volume and elimination half-life are increased twofold. An infusion rate of 0.2 mg/kg/min for one hour or less is clinically safe in patients with severe cirrhosis, but considerable variations in the time to return to consciousness can be expected.[150] Cirrhotic patients showed no change in the elimination half-life of fentanyl[151] and thiopentone.[152]

Vecuronium does not appear to be metabolized differently in patients with alcoholic and other types of liver disease,[153] but the duration of neuromuscular blockade is prolonged. Thiopentone pharmacokinetics are normal in chronic alcoholics even though higher initial doses are sometimes required, and cross-tolerance to ethanol has been postulated to explain this phenomenon. Finally, the pharmacokinetics and action of atracurium do not appear to be altered. However, due to the possibility of enzyme induction in some hepatic processes, it is often difficult to predict how an individual patient will respond to a given dose of anesthetic, and careful monitoring is therefore mandatory.[154]

Obstructive Jaundice

Because of the relationship between the serum bilirubin level and the risk of operation in patients with obstructive jaundice, some have recommended routine preoperative biliary decompression with percutaneous catheters.[95,155,156] However, the utility of these procedures has not been definitively shown to reduce operative risk. In a retrospective study of 109 patients, Norlander found no difference between those who underwent the procedure and those who did not.[157] Moreover, some randomized prospective trials also show that preoperative percutaneous drainage does not reduce operative risk and may even increase it.[158,159] Another prospective study suggests that preoperative drainage improves renal function and decreases operative morbidity, but the complications associated with the technique may outweigh its benefits.[160] Various other investigators confirm that the morbidity and mortality of the procedure are not inconsequential.[161–164]

Some investigators have attempted to identify subgroups of patients who may benefit from drainage procedures. In one study, the antipyrine elimination half-life was used to predict outcome of percutaneous transhepatic biliary drainage and was shown to be potentially useful,[165] and other investigators have confirmed this. However, at this time, data are insufficient to recommend routine percutaneous drainage before surgery in patients with obstructive jaundice.

POSTOPERATIVE COMPLICATIONS: PREVENTION AND MANAGEMENT

A higher-than-normal postoperative morbidity rate in patients with liver disease can be expected in five areas: wound healing; bleeding; infection; deterioration of hepatic function, including encephalopathy; and the potential for developing renal failure.

Wound Healing

Abnormal wound healing can be anticipated because of associated abnormalities in protein synthesis, anemia, and poor nutritional status. Excessive bleeding or infection of surgical wounds may also impair healing. In addition, ascites also imposes a mechanical stress on abdominal wounds.

In experimental studies in rats, the presence of jaundice predicts histologic evidence of delayed wound healing and decreased wound-burst strength.[166] Ellis and Heddle found three cases of abdominal wound dehiscence and four incisional hernias among 21 jaundiced patients. In these patients, the wound failure rate was 33 percent compared to 5.2 percent among 305 nonjaundiced controls.[167] Similarly, Irvin et al. noted wound dehiscence or incisional hernias in 27.1 percent of patients undergoing laparotomy for jaundice, while only 4.3 percent of anicteric controls experienced difficulty in wound healing.[168]

Factors other than jaundice have been implicated in poor wound healing. In the review by Keill et al., anemia and hypoproteinemia rather than jaundice were found to be the significant factors.[169] Reitamo and Moller also found that anemia, hypoproteinemia, and factors increasing abdominal pressure like ascites correlated best with dehiscence.[170] However, there were too few patients with jaundice or abnormal liver function in the study to support definitive conclusions.

Wound healing has also been studied in patients with acute viral hepatitis and cirrhosis. Marx reported five cases of patients with acute viral hepatitis undergoing laparotomy, among which were two episodes of dehiscence.[171] Yonemoto and Davidson examined wound healing in 16 cirrhotic patients undergoing herniorrhaphy and found only one wound complication.[1] In another series of 104 operative procedures in cirrhotics, there were 13 wound complications with five cases of impaired healing of intestinal anastomoses and one case of wound dehiscence.[91] Serum protein levels did not correlate with wound complications, and the presence of ascites did not affect wound healing.

In patients with obstructive jaundice, wound healing may be impaired.[167,172] Wound dehiscence occurs in 2 to 4 percent of patients with obstructive jaundice, and incisional hernias occur in 10 to 12.5 percent. However, one study[173] found decreased wound healing to be related to nutritional status, malignancy, and postoperative sepsis but not to serum bilirubin levels. Askew[174] noted improved wound-bursting strength in rats with ligated bile ducts treated with taurocholate, but there are no such studies in humans.

Prophylactic antibiotics reduce the incidence of wound infection and other septic complications after biliary surgery. Antibiotic prophylaxis in patients undergoing biliary surgery should be effective against both the coliforms commonly found in bile and staphylococcus species.

Excessive Bleeding

Abnormal hemostasis is frequently found in patients with liver disease. The liver produces all clotting factors except factor VIII. Low plasma levels of one or more of factors II, V, VII, IX, and X are found in 70 to 85 percent of patients with liver disease entering the hospital.[175] Protein C concentrations are also depressed in patients with advanced liver disease.[137] Thrombocytopenia frequently occurs because of suppression of platelet production by alcohol or hypersplenism. Circulating platelets may be functionally impaired, and abnormal aggregation has been demonstrated.[176] Abnormal fibrin polymerization and increased catabolism of fibrinogen, prothrombin, and plasminogen have also been reported and may contribute to defective coagulation.[177,178] In patients with advanced cirrhosis, hyperfibrinolysis may increase the risk of gastrointestinal hemorrhage.[179] Portal hypertension may also cause increased vascularity and bleeding during abdominal surgery.

Despite these theoretical considerations, there is little evidence of a significant increase in operative or postoperative bleeding in patients with liver disease. This may reflect selection of patients and/or careful preoperative preparation. In Lindenmuth's series of 28 procedures in patients with prothrombin levels of 70% or less, not a single case of abnormal bleeding could be attributed to an abnormal prothrombin time alone, and in no instances could an increase in complications or death be attributed to hemorrhage.[91] However, there may be an increased frequency of DIC in patients with obstructive jaundice.[180]

Gastrointestinal hemorrhage occurs in 6 to 14 percent of patients undergoing surgery for obstructive jaundice, and antacids may not be effective in preventing peptic gastroduodenal ulceration. Intravenous ranitidine or oral sucralfate may offer better prophylaxis.[181] It has been suggested that antacids may be more effective once bleeding has been documented.[182]

Infection

Although liver disease is thought to lower resistance to infection, there is little evidence documenting an increased incidence of wound or other postoperative infections in these patients.[183]

Deterioration of Hepatic Function

The risk of deterioration of hepatic function after surgery in patients with liver disease is unclear. Kiéri-Szántó and Lafleur reviewed the cases of 45,000 anesthetized patients and found that 60 percent of the postoperative hepatic complications occurred in 94 patients with preexisting liver disease.[184] They concluded that existing liver disease increased the risk of postoperative hepatic complications by a factor of 500. Similar data have been presented by others.[185,186]

Hepatic encephalopathy is an especially common complication in patients with cirrhosis.[112,187] The diagnosis and management of hepatic encephalopathy in the postoperative setting is the same as in the nonsurgical patient.[188] Potent analgesics should be given with caution because hypoalbuminemia and impaired drug metabolism can result in more prolonged or pronounced effects and precipitate overt encephalopathy.

Renal Failure

Acute renal failure is not an uncommon postoperative complication in patients with liver disease. Although the differential diagnosis is much the same in these patients as in other surgical patients, several specific clinical conditions deserve mention. Aminoglycoside nephrotoxicity should be considered in patients receiving neomycin for hepatic encephalopathy. Although the drug is thought to remain in the bowel lumen, as much as 3 percent of the dose may be absorbed.

Hepatorenal syndrome refers to progressive oliguria and azotemia in patients with severe decompensated liver disease in whom other causes of renal failure have been excluded. It is characterized by a concentrated urine, a low urinary sodium concentration of less than 10 meq/liter, and a benign urine sediment. The pathogenesis is uncertain but appears to be related to an abnormal distribution of renal blood flow with a marked decrease in perfusion of the cortex despite normal total renal blood flow. This may be due to vasoconstriction of cortical vessels and intrarenal shunting of blood. Renal histology is normal, and affected kidneys function normally when transplanted into patients without liver disease, suggesting a functional basis for the disorder.[189] This theory is further supported by case reports of improved renal function after liver transplantation.[190]

Various treatment regimens for hepatorenal syndrome have been tried with little success, including volume expansion with colloid, prostaglandin inhibitors, dopamine, portasystemic shunting, and hemodialysis.[191–194] Peritoneojugular shunting has been reported to be effective, but its value remains unproved.[195] The hepatorenal syndrome is associated with a high mortality.

Many investigators report a high incidence of postoperative renal failure in patients with obstructive jaundice.[196] This is regarded by some as a distinct entity and by others as representative of hepatorenal syndrome. Direct nephrotoxic effects of bilirubin, bile salts, or endotoxin absorbed from the bowel because of decreased bile-salt excretion have been implicated. Dawson has studied this particular variant of renal failure and has found a significant correlation between preoperative serum bilirubin levels and postoperative decline in creatinine clearance.[197] Deterioration in renal function may be prevented by forced diuresis with mannitol. Another type of acute renal failure following hepatic artery ligation for hepatic tumors has also been described.[198]

Postoperative renal failure in nonjaundiced individuals with liver disease is rare. However, 60 to 75 percent of patients with obstructive jaundice experience a fall in glomerular filtration rate after surgery. Renal failure occurs in 6 to 18 percent of jaundiced patients and carries a mortality rate of 32 to 100 percent. Various factors have been implicated in the development of renal failure in patients with obstructive jaundice, including hypovolemia, hypotension, bile salt damage, poor preoperative renal function, inadequate nutrition, intravascular coagulopathy, and increased serum levels of bilirubin.[199] Bowel preparation with antibiotics was found to confer no protective benefit.[200] However, preoperative oral administration of bile salts has proven beneficial in two small studies.[201,202]

Mannitol has been used to prevent renal failure in patients with obstructive jaundice. However, its benefit has not been clearly demonstrated. In a recent randomized trial,[203] 31 patients with obstructive jaundice were studied, of whom 65 percent had a creatinine clearance of less than 70 ml/min. No relationship was found between serum bilirubin levels and preoperative renal function or between serum bilirubin concentrations and decreases in creatinine clearance. Postoperative creatinine clearance declined significantly in those treated with mannitol but remained essentially unchanged in those who had not received mannitol. Three or 9.7 percent of patients died of acute renal failure. If mannitol is used, it is necessary to ensure adequate preoperative hydration.[199]

SUMMARY

1. Abnormalities in one or more liver function tests are frequently found following anesthesia and surgery in patients without liver disease. Such abnormalities occur with greater frequency and are of greater magnitude in patients with preexisting liver disease. Anesthetic technique, choice of agent, and duration of anesthesia may play a role in the development of postoperative liver function abnormalities, but the type and extent of surgery may be more important determinants. These abnormalities are generally mild, transient, and clinically insignificant.

2. None of the anesthetic agents in current use is a direct hepatotoxin. All reduce hepatic blood flow which may be further compromised by several other intraoperative factors. Reduction in hepatic blood flow may be related to postoperative liver function abnormalities and histologic changes.

3. Although the data are not conclusive, patients with both acute and chronic liver disease appear to have a higher-than-normal risk of postoperative complications and death. The magnitude of operative risk for patients with acute hepatitis may not be so great as previously feared. Some patients with asymptomatic chronic active hepatitis, those with mild alcoholic hepatitis, and those with chronic persistent hepatitis usually tolerate surgery well. The magnitude of operative risk for patients with cirrhosis is directly related to the severity of their disease.

4. Preoperative evaluation of the patient with liver disease should include a careful history and physical examination. Laboratory evaluation should include a platelet count, prothrombin time, and liver function tests. In patients with acute hepatitis or unexplained chronic liver disease, appropriate hepatitis serologies should be performed.

5. Elective surgery should be delayed in patients with acute viral hepatitis, severe alcoholic hepatitis, and advanced forms of chronic hepatitis.

6. Patients with chronic liver disease should be classified according to the Child-Pugh's criteria. Only those in group A should be considered fit for elective surgery. Those in group B or C should be carefully prepared for surgery to minimize risk.

7. Preoperative preparation should focus on diagnosis and treatment of clotting abnormalities, electrolyte disturbances, and hepatic encephalopathy. Attempts should also be made to reduce ascites and improve nutritional status. Preoperative decompression of obstructive jaundice is controversial.

8. Postoperative complications occurring more frequently in patients with liver disease than in others include atelectasis and pneumonia, upper gastrointestinal bleeding, deterioration of hepatic function, wound complications, and acute renal failure. Most patients should receive prophylactic antacids in the perioperative period. The prophylactic use of mannitol should be considered for patients with obstructive jaundice who have an especially high risk of acute renal failure.

9. Although patients with liver disease have an increased risk of postoperative complications and death, careful preoperative assessment and preparation and aggressive treatment of postoperative complications reduce the risk.

REFERENCES

1. Yonemoto RH, Davidson CS: Herniorrhaphy in cirrhosis of the liver with ascites. *N Engl J Med* 255:733, 1956.
2. Jackson FJ, Christopher EB, Peternel WW et al: Preoperative management of patients with liver disease. *Surg Clin N Am* 48:907, 1968.
3. Finucci G, Tirelli M, Bellon S et al: Clinical significance of cholelithiasis in patients with decompensated cirrhosis. *J Clin Gastroenterol* 12(5):538–541, 1990.
4. Mosnier H, Farges O, Vons C et al: Gastroduodenal ulcer perforation in the patient with cirrhosis. *Surg Gynecol Obstet* 174(4):297–301, 1992.
5. Blundell CR, Earnest DL: Medical evaluation of the patient with liver disease prior to surgery. *Contemp Anesth Pract* 4:123–169, 1981.
6. Wallach JB, Hyman W, Angrist AA: The cause of death in patients with Laënnec's cirrhosis. *Am J Med Sci* 234:56, 1957.
7. Ratnoff OD, Patek AJ: Natural history of Laënnec's cirrhosis. *Medicine* 21:259, 1942.
8. Geller W, Tagnon H: Liver dysfunction following abdominal operation. *Arch Intern Med* 86:908, 1950.
9. Tagnon HJ, Robbins GJ, Nichole MP: The effect of surgical operations on the bromosulfalein retention test. *N Engl J Med* 238:356, 1948.
10. Engstrand L, Friberg O: On function of liver as affected by various operations and anesthetics. *Acta Chir Scand Suppl* 97:104, 1945.
11. French AB, Bares TP, Fairlie CS et al: Metabolic effects of anesthesia in man. *Ann Surg* 135:145, 1952.
12. Ayres PR, Williard RB: Serum glutamic oxaloacetic transaminase level in 266 surgical patients. *Ann Intern Med* 52:1279, 1960.
13. Fairlie CW, Bares TP, French AB et al: Metabolic effects of anesthesia in man. IV: A comparison of the effects of certain anesthetic agents on the normal liver. *N Engl J Med* 244:615, 1957.
14. Evans C, Evans M, Pollack AJ: The incidence and causes of postoperative jaundice. *Br J Anaesth* 46:520, 1974.
15. Dawson B, Adson MA, Dockerty MB et al: Hepatic function tests: Postoperative changes with halothane or diethyl ether anesthesia. *Mayo Clin Proc* 41:599, 1966.
16. Little DM, Barbour CM, Given JB: The effects of fluothane, cyclopropane, and ether anesthesia on liver function. *Surg Gynecol Obstet* 107:712, 1958.
17. Hobson RW, Conant C, Fleming A et al: Postoperative serum enzyme patterns. *Milit Med* 136:624, 1971.
18. Killen DA: Serum enzyme elevations: A diagnostic test for acute myocardial infarction during the early postoperative period. *Arch Surg* 96:200, 1968.
19. Pohle FJ: Anesthesia and liver function. *Wis Med J* 47:476, 1948.
20. Thompson DS, Geifenstein FF: Enzyme patterns reflecting hepatic response to anesthesia and operations. *South Med J* 67:69, 1974.
21. Kalow B, Rogoman E, Sims FH: A comparison of the effects of halothane and other anaesthetic agents on hepato-cellular function in patients submitted to elective operations. *Can Anaesth Soc J* 23(1):71–79, 1976.
22. Person DA, Judge RD: Effect of operation on serum transaminase levels. *Arch Surg* 77:892, 1958.
23. Hicks MH, Holt HP, Guerrant JL et al: The effect of spontaneous and artificially induced fever on liver function. *J Clin Invest* 27:580, 1948.
24. Eley A, Hargrove T, Lambert HD: Jaundice in severe infections. *Br Med J* 2:75, 1965.
25. Hartman FW, Romence HL: Liver necrosis in burns. *Ann Surg* 118:402, 1943.
26. Walker J, Saltonstall H, Rhoads JE et al: Toxemia syndrome after burns. *Arch Surg* 52:177, 1946.
27. Gilmore JP, Roggard HA: Liver function following thermal injury. *Am J Physiol* 98:491, 1960.
28. Shoemaker WC, Szanto PB, Fitch LB et al: Hepatic physiologic and morphologic alteration in hemorrhagic shock. *Surg Gynecol Obstet* 118:828, 1964.
29. Ellenberg M, Osserman KE: The role of shock in the production of central liver necrosis. *Am J Med* 11:170, 1951.
30. Nunes G, Blaisdell W, Margurettin W: Mechanism of hepatic dysfunction following shock and trauma. *Arch Surg* 100:546, 1970.
31. Defalque RJ: The first delayed chloroform poisoning. *Anesth Analg* 47:374, 1968.
32. Little DM, Welstone HJ: Anesthesia and the liver. *Anesthesiology* 25:815, 1964.
33. Carney FMT, Van Dyke RA: Halothane hepatitis: A critical review. *Anesth Analg* 51:135, 1972.
34. Dykes MH (ed): Anesthesia and the liver. *Int Anesth Clin* 8:175, 1970.
35. Brouhoult J, Gillquist J: Serum ornithine carbanyl transferase activity in man after halothane and spinal anesthesia with and without systolic blood pressure fall. *Acta Chir Scand* 135:113, 1969.
36. Stevens WC, Egar EI, Joas TA et al: Comparative toxicity of isoflurane, halothane, fluoroxene, and diethyl ether in human volunteers. *Can Anaesth Soc J* 20:357, 1973.
37. Massarrat S, Massarrat S: Transient liver deterioration induced by general anesthesia. *Acta Hepato-Gastroenterologica* 26(2):106–111, 1979.
38. Abdel Salam AR, Drummond GB, Bauld HW et al: Clearance of indocyanine green as an index of liver function during cyclopropane anaesthesia and induced hypotension. *Brit J Anaesth* 48(3):231–238, 1976.
39. Lampe GH, Wauk LZ, Whitendale P et al: Nitrous oxide does not impair hepatic function in young or old surgical patients. *Anesth Analg* 71(6):606–609, 1990.
40. Klatskin G: Symposium on toxic hepatitis. *Gastroenterology* 38:789, 1960.
41. Collins WL, Fabian LW: Transaminase studies following anesthesia. *South Med J* 57:55, 1964.
42. Akdikman SA, Flanagan TV, Landmesser CM: A comparative study of SGPT changes following anesthesia with halothane, methoxyflurane and other inhalational agents. *Anesth Analg* 45:819, 1966.
43. Dodson ME, Richards TG: A prospective study of changes in liver function after operation under two forms of general anesthesia. *Br J Anaesth* 44:47, 1942.
44. McEwan J: Liver function tests following anaesthesia. *Brit J Anaesth* 48(11):1065–1070, 1976.

45. Ona FV, Patanella H, Ayub A: Hepatitis associated with enflurane anesthesia. *Anesth Analg* 59(2):146–149, 1980.

46. Paull JD, Fortune DW: Hepatotoxicity and death following two enflurane anaesthetics. *Anaesthesia* 42(11):1191–1196, 1987.

47. Allen PJ, Downing JW: A prospective study of hepatocellular function after repeated exposures to halothane or enflurane in women undergoing radium therapy for cervical cancer. *Brit J Anaesth* 49(10):1035–1039, 1977.

48. Johnston SB, Fee JP, Black GW et al: Liver function following repeated anaesthesia—method of study and interim results. *Acta Anaesth Scand Suppl* 71:12–14, 1979.

49. Eger EI 2d, Calverley RK, Smith NT: Changes in blood chemistries following prolonged enflurane anesthesia. *Anesth Analg* 55(4):547–549, 1976.

50. Giler S, Eshel Y, Pinkhas J et al: Elevation of serum xanthine oxidase activity following halothane anesthesia in man. *Experientia* 33(10):1356–1358, 1977.

51. Brown BR Jr, Gandolfi AJ: Adverse effects of volatile anaesthetics. *Br J Anaesth* 59(1):14–23, 1987.

52. Stoelting RK, Blitt CD, Cohen PJ et al: Hepatic dysfunction after isoflurane anesthesia. *Anesth Analg* 66(2):147–153, 1987.

53. Jones RM, Diamond JG, Power SJ et al: A prospective study of liver function in infants and children exposed to daily isoflurane for several weeks. *Anaesthesia* 46(8):686–688, 1991.

54. Schmidt CR, Unrich RJ, Chesky JE: Clinical studies of liver function. I: The effect of anesthesia and certain surgical procedures. *Am J Surg* 57:43, 1942.

55. Blunnie WP, Zacharias M, Dundee JW et al: Liver enzyme studies with continuous intravenous anaesthesia. *Anaesthesia* 36(2):152–156, 1981.

56. Lees N: Experience with etomidate as part of a total intravenous anaesthetic technique. *Anaesthesia* 38(Suppl):70–73, 1983.

57. Batchelder BM, Cooperman LH: Effects of anesthetics on splanchnic circulation and metabolism. *Surg Clin N Am* 55:787, 1975.

58. Ngai SH: Current concepts in anesthesiology: Effect of anesthetics on various organs. *N Engl J Med* 302:564, 1980.

59. Cooperman LH: Effects of anaesthetics on the splanchnic circulation. *Br J Anaesth* 44:967, 1972.

60. Winso O, Biber B, Gustavason B et al: Portal blood flow in man during graded positive end-expiratory pressure ventilation. *Intens Care Med* 12:80–85, 1986.

61. Torrance HB: Liver blood flow during operation on the upper abdomen. *J Coll Surg Edinb* 2:216, 1957.

62. Price HL, Davidson IA, Clement AJ et al: Can general anesthesia produce splanchnic visceral hypoxia by reducing regional blood flow? *Anesthesiology* 27:24, 1966.

63. Clarke RS, Doggart JR, Lavery T: Changes in liver function after different types of surgery. *Br J Anaesth* 48(2):119–128, 1976.

64. Griffiths HWC, Ozguc L: Effects of chloroform and halothane anesthesia on liver function in man. *Lancet* 1:246, 1964.

65. Nickell WK, Albritten FF: Serum transaminase content related to tissue injury. *Surgery* 42:240, 1957.

66. Kelley JL, Campbell DA, Brandt RL: The recognition of myocardial infarction in the early postoperative period. *Arch Surg* 94:673, 1967.

67. Fisk AA, Thomas RG, Maurukas J: Serum transaminase values after cholecystectomy, hysterectomy, and operation on the fractured hips. *Am J Med Sci* 236:33, 1958.

68. Craig HK, Butch WL, McGowan JM: Effect of biliary operation on the liver. *Arch Surg* 37:609, 1938.

69. Giler S, Sperling O, Brosh S et al: Elevated serum xanthine oxidase activity following biliary tract and gastric surgery. *Int Surg* 61(3):153–155, 1976.

70. Zanicheck N, Chalmers TC, Davidson CS: Pathologic and functional changes in the liver following upper abdominal operations (abstract). *Am J Med* 7:409, 1949.

71. Edlund YA, Zettergren LSW: Microstructure of the liver in biliary tract disease and notes on the effect on the liver of anesthesia, intubation, and operation trauma. *Acta Chir Scand* 113:201, 1957.

72. Stone HH: Preoperative and postoperative care. *Surg Clin N Am* 57:409, 1977.

73. Conn M: Preoperative evaluation of the patient with liver disease. *Mt Sinai J Med* 58(1):75–80, 1991.

74. Gholson CF, Provenza JM, Bacon BR: Hepatologic considerations in patients with parenchymal liver disease undergoing surgery. *Am J Gastroenterol* 85(5):487–496, 1990.

75. Shaldon S, Sherlock S: Virus hepatitis with features of prolonged retention. *Br Med J* 2:734, 1957.

76. Leevy CM: Intrahepatic cholestasis. *Am J Surg* 97:132, 1959.

77. Turner MD, Sherlock S: The management of jaundice, in Smith R, Sherlock S (eds): *Surgery of the Gall Bladder and Bile Ducts*. London, Butterworths, 1964, pp 67–68.

78. Harville DD, Summerskill WHJ: Surgery in acute hepatitis. *JAMA* 184:257, 1963.

79. Hargrove MD Jr: Chronic active hepatitis: Possible adverse effect of exploratory laparotomy. *Surgery* 68(5):771–773, 1970.

80. Greenwood SM, Leffler CT, Minkowitz S: The increased mortality rate of open liver biopsy in alcoholic hepatitis. *Surg Gynecol Obstet* 34:600, 1972.

81. Orloff MJ, Chandler JG, Carters AC et al: Emergency portacaval shunt treatment for bleeding esophageal varices. *Arch Surg* 108:293, 1974.

82. Mikkelsen WP, Kein WH: The influence of acute hyaline necrosis in survival after emergency and elective portacaval shunt. *Major Prob Clin Surg* 14:233, 1974.

83. Mikkelsen WP: Therapeutic portacaval shunt: Preliminary data on controlled trial and morbid effects of acute hyaline necrosis. *Arch Surg* 108:302, 1974.

84. Strauss AA, Strauss SF, Schwartz AH et al: Decompression by drainage of the common bile duct in subacute and chronic jaundice. A report of 73 cases with hepatitis or concomitant biliary duct infection as cause. *Am J Surg* 97:137, 1959.

85. Bourke JB, Cannon P, Retchie HD: Laparotomy for jaundice. *Lancet* 2:521, 1967.

86. Hardy KJ, Hughes ESR: Laparotomy in viral hepatitis. *Med J Aust* 1:710, 1968.

87. Zinn SE, Fairley HB, Glenn JD: Liver function in patients with mild alcoholic hepatitis, after enflurane, nitrous oxide-narcotic, and spinal anesthesia. *Anesth Analg* 64(5):487–490, 1985.

88. Runyon BA: Surgical procedures are well tolerated by patients with asymptomatic chronic hepatitis. *J Clin Gastroenterol* 8(5)542–544, 1986.

89. Hughson W: Portal cirrhosis with ascites and its surgical treatment. *Arch Surg* 15:418, 1927.

90. Henrikson EC: Cirrhosis of the liver. *Arch Surg* 32:413, 1936.

91. Lindenmuth WW, Eisenberg MM: The surgical risk in cirrhosis of the liver. *Arch Surg* 86:235, 1963.

92. Cayer D, Sohmer MF: Surgery in patients with cirrhosis. *Arch Surg* 71:828, 1955.

93. Wirthlin LS, Urk HV, Malt RB et al: Predictors of surgical mortality in patients with cirrhosis and nonvariceal gastroduodenal bleeding. *Surg Gynecol Obstet* 139:65, 1974.

94. Pain JA, Cahill CJ, Bailey ME: Perioperative complications in obstructive jaundice: Therapeutic considerations. *Br J Surg* 72:942–945, 1985.

95. Denning DA, Ellison EC, Carey LC: Preoperative percutaneous transhepatic biliary decompression lowers operative morbidity in patients with obstructive jaundice. *Am J Surg* 141(1):61–65, 1981.

96. Greig JD, Krukowski ZH, Matheson NA: Surgical morbidity and mortality in 129 patients with obstructive jaundice. *Br J Surg* 75:216–219, 1988.

97. Foschi D, Cavagna G, Callioni F et al: Hyperalimentation of jaundiced patients on percutaneous transhepatic biliary drainage. *Br J Surg* 73(9):716–719, 1986.

98. Welch HF, Welch CS, Carter JH: Prognosis after surgical treatment of ascites: Results of side-to-side shunt in 40 patients. *Surgery* 56:75, 1964.

99. Linton RR: The selection of patients for portacaval shunts. *Ann Surg* 134:433, 1951.

100. McDermott W: The double portacaval shunt in the treatment of chronic ascites. *Surg Gynecol Obstet* 110:457, 1960.

101. Malt RA: Portasystemic venous shunts. *N Engl J Med* 295:24, 1976.

102. Child CG: *The Liver and Portal Hypertension.* Philadelphia, Saunders, 1964.

103. Turcotte JG, Lambert MJ: Variceal hemorrhage, hepatic cirrhosis, and protacaval shunts. *Surgery* 73:810, 1973.

104. Fegiz G, Bracci F, Trenti A et al: Operative morbidity after shunt surgery for portal hypertension. *Int Surg* 70(4):301–303, 1985.

105. Fulenwider JT, Smith RB 3d, Redd SC et al: Peritoneovenous shunts. Lessons learned from an eight-year experience with 70 patients. *Arch Surg* 119(10):1133–1137, 1984.

106. Pugh RNH, Murray-Lyon IM, Dawson JL et al: Transection of the oesophagus for bleeding oesophageal varices. *Br J Surg* 60:646, 1973.

107. Bloch RS, Allaben RD, Walt AJ: Cholecystectomy in patients with cirrhosis. A surgical challenge. *Arch Surg* 120:669–672, 1985.

108. Cryer HM, Howard DA, Garrison RN: Liver cirrhosis and biliary surgery: Assessment of risk. *South Med J* 78:138–141, 1985.

109. Kogut K, Aragoni T, Ackerman NB: Cholecystectomy in patients with mild cirrhosis. A more favorable situation. *Arch Surg* 120:1310–1311, 1985.

110. Garrison RN, Cryer HM, Howard DA et al: Clarification of risk factors for abdominal operations in patients with hepatic cirrhosis. *Ann Surg* 199(6):648–655, 1984.

111. Gill RA, Goodman MW, Golfus GR et al: Aminopyrine breath test predicts surgical risk for patients with liver disease. *Ann Surg* 198(6):701–704, 1983.

112. Doberneck RC, Sterling WA Jr, Allison DC: Morbidity and mortality after operation in nonbleeding cirrhotic patients. *Am J Surg* 146(3):306–309, 1983.

113. Metcalf A, Dozois RR, Wolff BG et al: The surgical risk of colectomy in patients with cirrhosis. *Dis Col Rec* 30:529–531, 1987.

114. Schwartz, S: Biliary tract surgery and cirrhosis: A critical combination. *Surgery* 90:577, 1981.

115. Oellerich M, Burdelski M, Lautz HU et al: Lidocaine metabolite formation as a measure of liver function in patients with cirrhosis. *Therap Drug Monitoring* 12(3):219–226, 1990.

116. Merkel C, Bolognesi M, Bellon S et al: Aminopyrine breath test in the prognostic evaluation of patients with cirrhosis. *Gut* 33(6):836–842, 1992.

117. Merkel C, Bolognesi M, Finucci GF et al: Indocyanine green intrinsic hepatic clearance as a prognostic index of survival in patients with cirrhosis. *J Hepatol* 9(1):16–22, 1989.

118. Albers I, Hartmann H, Bircher J et al: Superiority of the Child-Pugh classification to quantitative liver function tests for assessing prognosis of liver cirrhosis. *Scand J Gastroenterol* 24(3):269–276, 1989.

119. Beuers U, Jager F, Wahllander A et al: Prognostic value of the intravenous ^{14}C-aminopyrine breath test compared to the Child-Pugh score and serum bile acids in 84 cirrhotic patients. *Digestion* 50(3–4):212–218, 1991.

120. Gluud C, Henriksen JH, Nielsen G: Prognostic indicators in alcoholic cirrhotic men. *Hepatology* 8(2):222–227, 1988.

121. Hemming AW, Scudamore CH, Shackleton CR, Pudek M, Erb SR: Indocyanine green clearance as a predictor of successful hepatic resection in cirrhotic patients. *Am J Surg* 163(5):515–518, 1991.

122. Kainuma M, Nakashima K, Sakuma I et al: Hepatic venous hemoglobin oxygen saturation predicts liver dysfunction after hepatectomy. *Anesthesiology* 76(3):379–386, 1992.

123. Zoli M, Cordiani MR, Marchesini G et al: Prognostic indicators in compensated cirrhosis. *Am J Gastroenterol* 86(10):1508–1513, 1991.

124. Gagner M: Value of preoperative physiologic assessment in outcome of patients undergoing major surgical procedures. *Surg Clin N Am* 71(6):1141–1150, 1991.

125. Cosby RL, Yee B, Schrier RW: New classification with prognostic value in cirrhotic patients. *Min Electr Metab* 15(5):261–266, 1989.

126. Clowes GH Jr, McDermott WV, Williams LF et al: Amino acid clearance and prognosis in surgical patients with cirrhosis. *Surgery* 96:675–685, 1984.

127. Kaplan JA, Betner RL, Bripps RD: Hypoxia hyperdynamic circulation and the hazards of general anesthesia in patients with hepatic cirrhosis. *Anesthesiology* 35:427, 1971.

128. Leibowitz S: Guidelines to clearing patients with liver disease for surgery. *Mt Sinai J Med* 4:539, 1977.

129. Iwatsuki S, Geis WP: Hepatic complications. *Surg Clin N Am* 57:1335, 1977.

130. Stunin I: Preoperative assessment of the patient with liver dysfunction. *Br J Anaesth* 50:25, 1978.

131. Pomier-Layrarques G, Huet PM, Infante-Rivard C et al: Prognostic value of indocyanine green and lidocaine kinetics for survival and chronic hepatic encephalopathy in cirrhotic patients following elective end-to-side portacaval shunt. *Hepatology* 8:1506–1510, 1988.

132. Seifkin AD, Bolt RJ: Preoperative evaluation of the patient with gastrointestinal or liver disease. *Med Clin N Am* 631:1309, 1979.

133. Editorial: Liver disease and anesthesia. *Br Med J* 1:1374, 1978.

134. Cooperman LH, Wollman H, Marsh ML: Anesthesia and the liver. *Surg Clin N Am* 57:421, 1977.

135. Brown MW, Burk RF: Development of intractable ascites following upper abdominal surgery in patients with cirrhosis. *Am J Med* 80(5):879–883, 1986.

136. Liel Y, Fraser GM: Massive postoperative ascites: A presenting symptom of liver cirrhosis. *Israel J Med Sci* 21:634–635, 1985.

137. Bell H, Odegaard OR, Andersson T et al: Protein C in patients with alcoholic cirrhosis and other liver diseases. *J Hepatol* 14(2–3):163–167, 1992.

138. Fisher JE, Yoshimina N, Aguirre A et al: Plasma amino acids in patients with hepatic encephalopathy: Effect of amino acid infusion. *Am J Surg* 27:40, 1974.

139. Fisher JE, Rosen HM, Ebeid AM et al: The effect of normalization of plasma amino acids on hepatic encephalopathy in man. *Surgery* 80:77, 1976.

140. Freund H, Yoshimina N, Fisher JE: Chronic hepatic encephalopathy: Long-term therapy with a branched-chain amino acid–enriched elemental diet. *JAMA* 242:347, 1979.

141. Kanematsu T, Koyanagi N, Matsumata T et al: Lack of preventive effect of branched-chain amino acid solution on postoperative hepatic encephalopathy in patients with cirrhosis: A randomized, prospective trial. *Surgery* 104(3):482–488, 1988.

142. Maddrey WC, Weber FL, Coulter AW et al: Effect of ketoanalogues of essential amino acids in portal-systemic encephalopathy. *Gastroenterology* 71:190, 1976.

143. Rabinowitz JL, Staeffen J, Aumonier P et al: A method for serum octanoate in hepatic cirrhosis and hepatic encephalopathy. *Clin Chem* 23:2202, 1977.

144. Cabre E, Gonzalez-Huix F, Abad-Lacruz A et al: Effect of total enteral nutrition on the short-term outcome of severely malnourished cirrhotics. A randomized controlled trial. *Gastroenterology* 98(3):715–720, 1990.

145. Kearns PJ, Young H, Garcia G et al: Accelerated improvement of alcoholic liver disease with enteral nutrition. *Gastroenterology* 102(1):200–205, 1992.

146. Mezey E, Caballeria J, Mitchell MC et al: Effect of parenteral amino

acid supplementation on short-term and long-term outcomes in severe alcoholic hepatitis: A randomized controlled trial. *Hepatology* 14(6):1090–1096, 1991.

147. Strunin L, Davies JM: The liver and anaesthesia. *Can Anaesth Soc J* 30(2):208–217, 1983.

148. Okuno M, Nagayama M, Takai T et al: Postoperative total parenteral nutrition in patients with liver disorders. *J Surg Res* 39(2):93–102, 1985.

149. Trouvin JH, Farinotti R, Haberer JP et al: Pharmacokinetics of midazolam in anaesthetized cirrhotic patients. *Br J Anaesth* 60(7):762–767, 1988.

150. van Beem H, Manger FW, van Boxtel C et al: Etomidate anaesthesia in patients with cirrhosis of the liver: Pharmacokinetic data. *Anaesthesia* 38(Suppl):61–62, 1983.

151. Haberer JP, Schoeffler P, Couderc E et al: Fentanyl pharmacokinetics in anaesthetized patients with cirrhosis. *Br J Anaesth* 54(12):1267–1270, 1982.

152. Couderc E, Ferrier C, Haberer JP et al: Thiopentone pharmacokinetics in patients with chronic alcoholism. *Br J Anaesth* 56(12):1393–1397, 1984.

153. Arden JR et al: Vecuronium in alcoholic liver disease: A pharmacokinetic and pharmacodynamic analysis. *Anesthesiology* 68:771–776, 1988.

154. McEvedy BA, Shelly MP, Park GR: Anaesthesia and liver disease. *Br J Hosp Med* 36(1):26–34, 1986.

155. Koyama K, Takagi Y, Ito K et al: Experimental and clinical studies on the effect of biliary drainage in obstructive jaundice. *Am J Surg* 142(2):293–299, 1981.

156. O'Connor MJ: Mechanical biliary obstruction. A review of the multisystemic consequences of obstructive jaundice and their impact on perioperative morbidity and mortality. *Am Surgeon* 51(5):245–251, 1985.

157. Norlander A, Kalin B, Sundblad R: Effect of percutaneous transhepatic drainage upon liver function and postoperative mortality. *Surg Gynecol Obstet* 155(2):161–166, 1982.

158. Pitt HA, Gomes AS, Lois JF et al: Does preoperative percutaneous biliary drainage reduce operative risk or increase hospital cost? *Ann Surg* 201:545–553, 1985.

159. Pellegrini CA, Allegra P, Bongard FS et al: Risk of biliary surgery in patients with hyperbilirubinemia. *Am J Surg* 154:111–117, 1987.

160. Smith RC, Pooley M, George CR et al: Preoperative percutaneous transhepatic internal drainage in obstructive jaundice: A randomized, controlled trial examining renal function. *Surgery* 97(6):641–648, 1985.

161. Sirinek KR, Levine BA: Percutaneous transhepatic cholangiography and biliary decompression. Invasive, diagnostic, and therapeutic procedures with too high a price? *Arch Surg* 124(8):885–888, 1989.

162. Rosen J, Young SC, Berman J et al: Management of malignant obstructive jaundice. *J Surg Oncol* 40(4):256–260, 1989.

163. Rypins EB, Bitzer LG, Sarfeh IJ et al: The role of percutaneous transhepatic internal biliary drainage in preoperative patients. *Am Surgeon* 53(10):562–564, 1987.

164. McPherson GA, Benjamin IS, Hodgson HJ et al: Preoperative percutaneous transhepatic biliary drainage: The results of a controlled trial. *Br J Surg* 71(5):371–375, 1984.

165. Ramesh VS, Kochhar R, Garg SK et al: Antipyrine elimination test as a guideline for selecting patients for transhepatic biliary drainage. *J Gastroenterol Hepatol* 5(3):219–222, 1990.

166. Bayer I, Ellis HJ: Jaundice and wound healing: An experimental study. *Br J Surg* 63:392, 1976.

167. Ellis H, Heddle R: Does the peritoneum need to be closed at laparotomy? *Br J Surg* 64:733, 1977.

168. Irvin TT, Vassilakis JS, Challopadhylay DK et al: Abdominal wound healing in jaundiced patients. *Br J Surg* 65:521, 1978.

169. Keill RH, Keitzer WF, Nichols WK et al: Abdominal wound dehiscence. *Arch Surg* 106:573, 1973.

170. Reitamo J, Moller C: Abdominal wound dehiscence. *Acta Chir Scand* 138:170, 1972.

171. Marx GF: Unsuspected preoperative hepatic dysfunction. *Int Anesthesiol Clin* 8:369, 1970.

172. Arnaud JP, Humbert W, Eloy MR et al: Effect of obstructive jaundice on wound healing. An experimental study in rats. *Am J Surg* 141(5):593–596, 1981.

173. Armstrong CP, Dixon JM, Duffy SW et al: Wound healing in obstructive jaundice. *Br J Surg* 71(4):267–270, 1984.

174. Askew AR, Bates GJ, Balderson G: Jaundice and the effect of sodium taurocholate taken orally upon abdominal wound healing. *Surg Gynecol Obstet* 159:207–209, 1984.

175. Losowsky M, Simmons AV, Mitoszewski K: Coagulation abnormalities in liver disease. *Postgrad Med* 53:117, 1973.

176. Ballard HS, Marcus AJ: Platelet aggregation in portal cirrhosis. *Arch Intern Med* 136:316, 1976.

177. Green G, Thompson JM, Dymock IW et al: Abnormal fibrin polymerization in liver disease. *Br J Haematol* 34:427, 1976.

178. Verstroete M, Vermglen J, Collen D: Intravascular coagulation in liver disease. *Ann Rev Med* 25:447, 1974.

179. Violi F, Ferro D, Basili S et al: Hyperfibrinolysis increases the risk of gastrointestinal hemorrhage in patients with advanced cirrhosis. *Hepatology* 15(4):672–676, 1992.

180. Kunz A, Amor H, Hortnagi H et al: Disseminated intravascular coagulation and lethal macrothrombosis in a patient with carcinoma of the biliary tract. *Dtsch Med Wschr* 99:2643–2647, 1974.

181. Knight A, Bihari D, Tinker J: Stress ulceration in the critically ill patient. *Br J Hosp Med* 33(4):216–219, 1985.

182. Priebe HJ, Skillman JJ, Bushnell LS et al: Antacid versus cimetidine in preventing acute gastrointestinal bleeding. *N Engl J Med* 302:426, 1980.

183. Gaines KC, Sonell MF: Host resistance in liver disease—its evaluation and therapeutic modification. *Med Clin N Am* 63:495, 1979.

184. Kiéri-Szántó M, Lafleur F: Postanesthetic liver complications in a general hospital: A statistical study. *Can Anaesth Soc J* 10:531, 1963.

185. Dykes MHM, Walzer SG: Preoperative and postoperative hepatic dysfunction. *Surg Gynecol Obstet* 124:747, 1967.

186. Marx GF, Nagayoski M, Shoukos JA et al: Unsuspected infectious hepatitis in surgical patients. *JAMA* 205:169, 1968.

187. Kanematsu T, Takenaka K, Matsumata T et al: Limited hepatic resection effective for selected cirrhotic patients with primary liver cancer. *Ann Surg* 199(1)51–56, 1984.

188. Najarian JS, Harper HA, McCorkle HJ: The diagnosis and clinical management of hepatic coma in surgical patients. *Am J Surg* 96:172, 1958.

189. Kamel MH, Cobuin JW, Mimis MM et al: Transplantation of cadaveric kidney from patients with hepatorenal syndrome: Evidence for the functional nature of renal failure in advanced liver disease. *N Engl J Med* 280:1367, 1969.

190. Iwutsuki S, Popovitzer MM, Corman JL et al: Recovery from hepatorenal syndrome after orthotopic liver transplantation. *N Engl J Med* 289:1155, 1973.

191. Tristani FE, Cohn JN: Systemic and renal hemodynamics in oliguric hepatic failure: Effect of volume expansion. *J Clin Invest* 46:1894, 1967.

192. Bennet WM, Keefe E, Melnyk C et al: Response to dopamine hydrochloride in hepatorenal syndrome. *Arch Intern Med* 135:964, 1975.

193. Fisher JE, Foster GS: Survival from acute hepatorenal syndrome following splenorenal shunt. *Ann Surg* 184:22, 1976.

194. Aregan S, Sweeney T, Keistein MD: Hepatorenal syndrome: Recovery after portacaval shunt. *Ann Surg* 181:847, 1975.

195. Leveen HH, Wapnick S, Grosberg S et al: Further experience with peritoneo-venous shunt for ascites. *Ann Surg* 184:574, 1976.

196. Dawson JL: The incidence of postoperative renal failure in obstructive jaundice. *Br J Surg* 52:663, 1965.

197. Dawson JL: Postoperative renal function in obstructive jaundice: Effect of a mannitol diuresis. *Br Med J* 1:82, 1965.
198. Kim DK, Penneman R, Kallum B et al: Acute renal failure after ligation of the hepatic artery. *Surg Gynecol Obstet* 143:391, 1976.
199. Allison ME, Prentice CR, Kennedy AC et al: Renal function and other factors in obstructive jaundice. *Br J Surg* 66:392–397, 1979.
200. Hunt PS, Korman MG, Hansky J et al: Acute gastric ulceration—a prospective study of incidence and results of management. *Austr NZ J Med* 10(3):305–308, 1980.
201. Cahill CJ: Prevention of postoperative renal failure in patients with obstructive jaundice—the role of bile salts. *Br J Surg* 70:590–595, 1983.
202. Evans HJR, Torrealba V, Hudd C et al: The effect of preoperative bile salt administration on postoperative renal function in patients with obstructive jaundice. *Br J Surg* 69:706–708, 1982.
203. Gubern JM, Sancho JJ, Simon J et al: A randomized trial on the effect of mannitol on postoperative renal function in patients with obstructive jaundice. *Surgery* 103(1):39–44, 1988.

35 THE SURGICAL PATIENT WITH CEREBROVASCULAR DISEASE

James R. Brorson

Howard I. Hurtig

Francisco A. Gonzalez-Scarano

Cerebrovascular disease is the third most common cause of death in the United States, killing 85,000 and disabling a million or more patients annually.[1] Stroke can be a devastating complication of an otherwise successful surgical procedure. Identifying those with an increased risk of stroke before surgery is therefore important in patient management since surgical correction of carotid stenosis may benefit some patients. In this chapter we discuss the risks of cerebrovascular disease in the surgical patient and briefly cover surgical treatment of occlusive cerebrovascular disease.

CEREBROVASCULAR RISKS IN THE OPERATIVE PATIENT

Clinical findings and noninvasive carotid artery imaging have been used to assess risk of stroke in patients undergoing surgery. Several potential mechanisms have been implicated in focal perioperative ischemia:

1. Intraoperative hypoperfusion in the territory of a stenotic cerebral vessel;[2]
2. Embolism of thrombus, atherosclerotic material, or gas during vascular procedures;
3. Postoperative thrombosis of cerebral vessels due to a postoperative hypercoagulable state; and
4. Cardiogenic embolization due to transient cardiac arrhythmias, especially atrial fibrillation.

In addition to focal stroke, significant hypoperfusion can cause severe hypoxic-ischemic damage and a variety of more subtle neuropsychologic deficits, particularly in cases with prolonged periods of time on cardiopulmonary bypass.[3,4] Because coronary artery bypass grafting surgery (CABG) is a common procedure with a relatively high risk of stroke, most studies evaluating risk of stroke have been done in this population. Some information is available for other vascular procedures and for nonvascular general surgery. A summary of these findings is found in Tables 35–1 and 35–2.

Cardiac Surgery

In CABG, retrospective studies have consistently documented overall stroke rates of approximately 1 percent (see Table 35–1), whereas prospective studies show a risk of about 5 percent.[2,3,5] In some, subgroups of patients with increased stroke rates have been identified. Gardner et al.[6] and Reed et al.[7] retrospectively reviewed a combined total of over 9000 patients undergoing CABG and independently found that a history of previous stroke or transient ischemic attack (TIA) was a strong predictor of increased perioperative risk. One study demonstrated a strong association between the risk of stroke and age. Patients over 70 had a rate of 6.3 percent compared to an overall rate of 1.8 percent.[6] Operative factors such as an extended period of time over 120 minutes on cardiopulmonary bypass and hypotension also increased the risk of stroke. In addition, other cardiovascular conditions such as congestive heart failure, mitral regurgitation, and aortic sclerosis have been found to increase the chance of stroke, probably by serving as sources of emboli to the brain.[6,7] Since atherosclerosis is a generalized process, a history of stroke or TIA has repeatedly been identified as a strong predictor of increased cardiac mortality both in nonsurgical patients and among those undergoing CABG.[8,9]

In addition to the risk of stroke, diffuse cerebral ischemia with subtle neurological and neuropsychological injury can occur as a direct hemodynamic complication of cardiopulmonary bypass. Shaw et al. found frequent intellectual impairment in patients after CABG. Eighty-nine or 29 percent of 312 were symptomatic, and 23 or 7 percent were overtly disabled, significantly more than

TABLE 35–1.   Neurologic Complications of Coronary Artery Bypass Grafting (CABG)

Study	Number of Patients	Stroke Rate	Findings and Risk Factors
Breuer, 1980 (Prospective)	400	—	10% developed diffuse CNS deficits, 5.7% focal CNS lesions
Gonzalez-Scarano, 1981 (Retrospective)	1427	0.8%	No risk factors
Coffey, 1983 (Retrospective)	1669	0.8%	Associated with carotid bruits and peripheral vascular disease
Gardner, 1985 (Retrospective)	3279	Overall, 1.8% Over 70 years old 6.3%	Increased risk associated with pump time, prior stroke, aortic disease and hypotension
Brener, 1987 (Prospective)	4047	No carotid disease 1.9% Unilateral stenosis 5.9% Carotid occlusion 15.6% (includes strokes and TIA's)	Stratified by noninvasive carotid evaluation
Shaw, 1987 (Prospective)	312	4.8%	79% had early neuropsychologic complications, 17% discharged with neurological disability
Reed, 1988 (Retrospective)	5915	Overall 1.03% With bruit 2.9%	Increased risk with previous stroke, CHF, MR, bruit, long pump time

Source: Adapted from chapter references 2, 3, 5, 7, 78, and 79.

among a control group of vascular surgery patients.[3] Another prospective study of CABG patients documented diffuse neurologic deficits in 10 percent, most of which were not functionally significant.[5] Cardiac valvular surgery also imposes a well-recognized risk of cerebral ischemia and anoxia.

Most studies support the impression that neurologic complications in coronary or valvular heart surgery are due to either intraoperative hypotension or particulate emboli associated with the use of cardiopulmonary bypass, in which neuropsychologic deficits correlate with long pump times.[4,10-12] Percutaneous transluminal coronary angioplasty (PTCA) does not require bypass and carries a significantly lower risk of stroke and other neurological complications. Galbreath et al. reported that only 0.2 percent of 1968 patients undergoing PTCA experienced stroke or TIA.[13] This procedure provides an attractive alternative to CABG in patients with cerebrovascular risk factors.

TABLE 35–2.   Neurologic Complications of Noncardiac Surgery

Study	Number of Patients	Type of Surgery	Stroke Rate	Comments
Carney, 1977	248	Aorto-iliac reconstruction	1.6%	No strokes in 35 patients with bruits 2 strokes in patients with TIA's
Evans, 1978	588	Major vascular procedures	0.8%	No strokes in 92 patients with bruits
Treiman, 1973	246	Abdominal-aortic	1.2%	No strokes in 40 patients with bruits
Barnes, 1981 (Prospective)	116	Aortic and peripheral vascular	0.9%	Single stroke contralateral to stenotic carotid
Vogt, 1982 (Retrospective)	66	Brachiocephalic reconstruction	3%	Most patients had cerebrovascular indications for surgery
Ropper, 1982 (Prospective)	735	General elective surgery	0.7%	All 5 strokes in CABG patients; no correlation with bruits
Hertzer, 1984	714	Peripheral vascular	0.4%	Prophylactic CEA performed in 54 patients
Galbreath, 1986	1968	Percutaneous transluminal coronary angioplasty	0.2% including TIAS's	

Source: Adapted from chapter references 13–15 and 17–20.

Vascular Surgery

Patients undergoing vascular procedures have the same risk factors as those with coronary artery disease and have a risk of stroke ranging from 0.4 to 3 percent in published studies (see Table 35–2). The presence of a cervical bruit does not indicate an increased rate of stroke in these patients.[14–17] The highest rates of perioperative stroke are not surprisingly found in brachiocephalic and vertebral artery reconstruction performed for cerebrovascular disease[18] or in procedures involving aortic clamping with its accompanying risks of hypotension and embolism.[14,17]

Nonvascular Surgery

Little information is available regarding the risk of stroke in nonvascular surgical procedures. In one study of a mixed population undergoing vascular and nonvascular procedures, the rate of stroke was low, and there were no strokes among the 568 patients having nonvascular procedures.[16]

Carotid Bruits

The physical examination has proved less valuable than the clinical history in predicting the risk of perioperative stroke. The presence of a carotid bruit is an obvious concern, but carotid bruits are neither sensitive nor specific indicators of hemodynamically significant carotid stenosis. Barnes and Marszalek found that of 314 preoperative patients, 54 had significant carotid stenosis of greater than 50% on screening carotid ultrasound examination, but only one-third of the 54 had carotid bruits.[19] Conversely, fewer than 25 percent of 48 bruits correlated with significant stenosis.

It is therefore not surprising that patients with asymptomatic carotid bruits undergoing vascular surgery have not exhibited a higher stroke rate than those without bruits.[14–17] Although the prevalence of asymptomatic cervical bruits in patients undergoing vascular surgery is high at 14 to 20 percent, the rate of perioperative stroke in these patients is not significantly different from the overall rate of 0.7 to 1.6 percent.[14–17] Even among patients undergoing emergency surgery for abdominal aortic aneurysm who experience prolonged hypotension, the presence of carotid bruits has no predictive value in assessing the risk of stroke.[17] In an uncontrolled study, Hertzer et al. reported a rate of perioperative stroke of only 0.4 percent in patients undergoing peripheral vascular reconstruction after prophylactic carotid endarterectomy (CEA) and CABG.[20] However, most authors do not recommend preoperative angiography or carotid endarterectomy in asymptomatic patients with carotid bruits who are evaluated for peripheral vascular surgery.[14,15,17] One large retrospective study of patients undergoing CABG did document a fourfold increase in the risk of perioperative stroke or TIA in patients with carotid bruits. However, previous histories of stroke or TIA, congestive heart failure, or mitral regurgitation were still stronger risk factors.[7]

A history of cerebrovascular disease or an incidental cervical bruit is a better predictor of perioperative cardiac mortality than of stroke in patients undergoing CABG. In one study, the perioperative and primarily cardiac mortality of cardiovascular surgery was 18.2 percent in those with and 2.1 percent in those without bruits.[19]

Noninvasive Studies

Evaluations of the predictive value of preoperative noninvasive carotid imaging have not been uniform. Barnes and Marszalek documented carotid stenosis of > 50% using carotid ultrasound in 41 of 314 patients undergoing coronary or peripheral arterial surgery, but the two postoperative carotid ischemic events in the series were not in the distribution of stenotic vessels.[19] Similarly, Breslau et al. found that no strokes occurred in 102 patients undergoing CABG with stenotic carotid lesions detected by ultrasound.[21] In contrast, Brener et al. demonstrated a significant increase in the incidence of stroke or TIA in asymptomatic patients undergoing cardiac surgery who had significant carotid disease on noninvasive evaluation. The risk was 20.5 percent in those with occluded carotid arteries, 5.9 percent in those with unilateral carotid stenosis, and 1.9 percent in those without carotid disease.[2] Thus, for procedures carrying a high risk of perioperative stroke, noninvasive carotid screening may be warranted.

Timing of Surgery Following Stroke

Little is known about the risk of stroke in patients with a recent history of a stroke or TIA and how soon such patients may undergo surgery following their cerebrovascular event. In patients undergoing carotid endarterectomy (CEA) following stroke, the perioperative mortality rate is 44 percent in patients having surgery less than 24 hours after a stroke, 14 percent in those operated on within two weeks of stroke, and 6 percent in those in whom surgery was postponed for two weeks.[22] CEA performed during progressive stroke carries a mortality rate of 47 percent.[22] Hemorrhage into recently infarcted brain tissue or further ischemia due to disordered cerebrovascular autoregulation are the main hazards associated with CEA done immediately after stroke.

Most authors now recommend waiting at least two weeks[23] and preferably three to four weeks[24] after a mild stroke with good recovery before evaluating patients for CEA. It is unclear if these guidelines derived from experience with CEA apply to stroke victims who require another type of surgery. However, unless the operation is urgently needed, it seems prudent to postpone all invasive procedures for at least a month after a stroke or TIA, during which time appropriate diagnostic and therapeutic decisions can be made.

PREVENTION OF STROKE IN THE SURGICAL PATIENT

The prevention of perioperative cerebrovascular complications depends on careful patient selection and skillful surgical techniques. The increased perioperative risk of stroke during vascular procedures in elderly patients and in those with a previous history of stroke or TIA requires careful and comprehensive preoperative cardiovascular assessment before coronary or major peripheral vascular surgery.[6] Appropriate medical therapy to prevent stroke should be instituted when indicated. Increasing evidence supports anticoagulation with low-dose warfarin in most patients with nonvalvular atrial fibrillation[25] and in those with diseased or prosthetic heart valves. Antiplatelet agents, usually aspirin in a dose of 325 mg or less daily, are often indicated for secondary prevention of stroke following previous stroke or TIA and for primary prevention of myocardial infarction.[26] Other agents such as warfarin or ticlopidine[27] may be required for the treatment of patients who fail aspirin therapy. The perioperative management of anticoagulant and antiplatelet therapy is discussed below. Surgical therapy for cerebrovascular disease, most often CEA, should also be considered and is also discussed below.

PERIOPERATIVE MANAGEMENT OF ANTITHROMBOTIC THERAPY

Minimizing overall operative risk in patients already taking antithrombotic agents requires balancing the increased risk of surgical hemorrhagic complications against those of perioperative thromboembolism.

Anticoagulants

Recommendations for patients on warfarin are tailored to the specific indications for anticoagulation. The risk of thromboembolism is highest in patients with prosthetic mitral valves. In the three- to five-day period when warfarin is discontinued, heparin[28] and perhaps also antiplatelet agents like aspirin in a dose of 75 mg daily or dipyridamole in a dose of 300 mg daily[29] are recommended. Heparin can be discontinued six hours before surgery, and coagulation times can be checked one hour before the procedure. Heparin can be resumed 6 to 12 hours after surgery until a therapeutic protime is reestablished on warfarin. In those with prosthetic aortic valves, warfarin should be stopped three days before surgery, and heparin should be given until six hours before the operation.[29] Postoperative heparin is required only if the patient cannot resume taking warfarin within 48 hours. Some suggest that preoperative coverage with heparin is not necessary for patients with aortic prosthetic valves.[28,30] When warfarin is prescribed for nonvalvular indications like nonrheumatic atrial fibrillation, it can probably be safely discontinued for the immediate perioperative period beginning three days before surgery without heparin replacement.[29] For dental[31] or cataract[32] surgery, warfarin can be continued during the perioperative period with minor risks of reversible hemorrhagic complications.

Antiplatelet Agents

Antiplatelet agents are frequently prescribed for patients with atherosclerotic heart or cerebrovascular disease and are found in many over-the-counter remedies. A number of investigators have reported an increased rate of complications during CABG in patients taking low-dose aspirin preoperatively.[31,33] These range from increased blood loss and transfusion requirements[31,33,34] to an increased frequency of pericardial tamponade[35] or bleeding requiring reoperation.[36] An increased incidence of bleeding has also been observed in patients on aspirin undergoing transurethral resection of the prostate[37] but not in those undergoing a range of general surgical[35] and dental[38] procedures. In contrast to aspirin, preoperative dipyridamole reduced[39] and sulfinpyrazone did not increase[34] the risk of bleeding in patients undergoing CABG. The effects of ticlopidine in the surgical setting are as yet unknown.

Recommendations regarding perioperative management of anti-

platelet therapy depend on the surgical procedure. Several days are required for normalization of thromboxane B2 levels and bleeding times after even a single dose of aspirin.[35] In CABG patients, all aspirin products should be discontinued one week or more before surgery. Resuming it six hours after surgery may actually increase the rate of graft patency.[34] In other procedures, guidelines are less well defined. However, it is prudent to discontinue aspirin before any elective procedure in which blood loss is a concern.

CAROTID ENDARTERECTOMY

Although over 140,000 carotid endarterectomies are performed annually in North America,[40] the procedure has often been criticized as excessively risky[41] or inappropriately performed.[42] However, in the proper setting, CEA can be the most effective means available for preventing stroke.

Natural History of Carotid Artery Disease

The alleged benefits of CEA must be viewed in the context of the natural history of arteriosclerotic carotid artery disease. The incidence of stroke associated with carotid stenosis is three times greater in patients experiencing TIA's than in those who are asymptomatic. The risk of stroke is highest in the month following an initial TIA.[43] Therefore, the rate of stroke in those with symptomatic lesions depends on whether patients are entered into a study soon after their initial TIA or after a stable pattern of recurrent TIA's has been established. The definition of what constitutes a significant degree of carotid stenosis varies from 50% to 90% in different series. Some studies look at rates of stroke ipsilateral to carotid lesions while others look at total stroke rates. The heterogeneity of these studies must be considered when surveying results.

Most studies of asymptomatic carotid disease record an annual stroke rate ranging between one and two percent, whether the carotid lesion was identified by auscultated bruit or by stenosis > 50% seen on carotid ultrasound or doppler studies (see Table 35–3).[43,44] When the location of the stroke is considered in relation to that of the carotid lesion, most strokes occur in the distribution of the contralateral carotid and vertebrobasilar arteries.[44,45] If the carotid disease is stratified by degree of stenosis, those with severe stenosis of > 80% have a higher stroke rate of 3 to 6 percent per year.[46,47] Progressive carotid stenosis documented with sequential studies also predicts a higher incidence of stroke, particularly in the first year. Attempts by one group to use positron emission tomography (PET scanning) to identify a subgroup at higher risk were unsuccessful.[48]

Annual rates of stroke following TIA range from three percent to eight percent (see Table 35–3), and they occur more often in the distribution of the identified carotid lesion. Patients are most vulnerable in the several weeks following the initial TIA theoretically because of the presence of fresh thrombus at the site of the carotid lesion.[49] The greater risk of stroke in patients with symptomatic carotid disease supports the contention that CEA is appropriate soon after the occurrence of a TIA. Alternatively, antiplatelet therapy with aspirin or ticlopidine has also been shown to reduce the incidence of stroke following TIA's.[27]

TABLE 35–3. Carotid Endarterectomy: Medical versus Surgical Management of Carotid Disease

Study	Risk Group	Length of Follow-up (yrs)	Number of Patients		Average Stroke Incidence in Follow-up* (%/yr)	
			Medical	Surgical	Medical	Surgical
Fields, 1970 (Randomized)	TIA	3.5	147	169	3.6	1.0
Hertzer, 1986 (Nonrandomized prospective)	Asymptomatic stenosis > 50%	3	195	95	2.6	1.7
Hertzer, 1986 (Nonrandomized prospective)	Symptomatic stenosis > 50%	3	126	85	2.6	1.6
Bernstein, 1987	Amaurosis fugax	3.8	—	128	—	0.4
Moneta, 1987	Asymptomatic high-grade stenosis (> 80%)	2	73	56	9.5	2.0
ECST, 1991 (Multicenter randomized trial)	Symptomatic stenosis < 30%	3	155	219	1.7	2.1
	Symptomatic stenosis > 70%	3	323	455	7.3	1.6
NASCET, 1991 (Multicenter randomized trial)	Symptomatic stenosis > 70%	2	331	328	6.1	0.8

*Excludes perioperative strokes.

Source: Adapted from chapter references 57–59 and 63–65.

Risks of Carotid Endarterectomy

Carotid endarterectomy carries serious risks including stroke and death. The reported rate of these complications varies widely from 2 percent to 21 percent,[50,51] as summarized in Table 35–4. The most favorable outcomes are reported by surgeons tabulating their personal experiences in which perioperative stroke rates of 1.5 to 3 percent and mortality rates of less than one percent are seen in large series.[43,50,52] Surveys that include all surgeons in a community tend to show higher rates of stroke and death. One recent study found combined stroke-mortality rates of 9.4 percent, 9.6 percent, and 12.4 percent at three geographic sites. The surgical indications were considered inappropriate in 32 percent of the cases.[53] A community-based review of hospitals in Cincinnati reported an operative risk of stroke of 8.6 percent and a mortality rate of 2.8 percent.[42] Easton and Sherman found those rates to be 14.5 percent and 6.6 percent, respectively, in two other community hospitals, but a follow-up study five years later revealed that the rates had dropped substantially.[54] In contrast, rates were 2.1 percent and 1.6 percent, respectively, in patients undergoing CEA by trained vascular surgeons in a community-wide survey of over 8000 cases in Cleveland.[41] Clearly, surgical technique and experience can reduce the complication rate of CEA.

Age and underlying vascular stability are important determinants of risk in CEA. DeWeese et al. reported a dangerously high mortality of 47 percent when surgery was performed in patients with progressive stroke. In those with progressive stroke, the rate was 44 percent when CEA was performed less than 24 hours after the stroke and 14 percent when done within two weeks. The authors urged that CEA not be performed in these settings.[22] Elderly or medically unstable patients carry higher operative risks, and the mortality of CEA is known to be higher in patients with coronary artery disease.[55]

Effectiveness of Carotid Endarterectomy

Given the significant and highly variable risks of CEA, it is clear that, to be of benefit, CEA must be performed with relatively few operative complications in carefully selected patients with a high risk of stroke.[56] A number of nonrandomized studies over two decades have attempted to define appropriate patients for CEA. CEA's performed after TIA's,[43,50,57] amaurosis fugax,[58] or mild strokes[59,60] appear to reduce rates of stroke when compared with historical control patients. Ischemia recurs more frequently in patients undergoing CEA for vertebrobasilar TIA's, suggesting that CEA has little therapeutic value in patients with TIA's originating in the posterior circulation.[61] CEA provides no significant benefit for patients with asymptomatic carotid stenosis,[20] although trends toward efficacy are reported in patients with bilateral carotid disease or higher-grade stenosis.[20,62] Unfortunately, all of these nonrandomized studies suffer from potential selection bias in allocating patients to surgical or medical therapy. In addition, the statistics are often obscured by failure to include perioperative strokes and death when comparing patients treated surgically with those managed medically.

An early effort at a randomized controlled study was made in 1970 by the Joint Study of Extracranial Vascular Disease Group. More than 1000 patients were divided into medical and surgical

TABLE 35–4.   Carotid Endarterectomy: Operative Risks of CEA

Study	Number of Patients	Risk Group	Stroke Rate (%)	Mortality Rate (%)
Fields, 1970 (Prospective)	169	TIA's	7.7	3.6
Easton, 1977 (Community-based)	228	Mixed	14.5	6.6
Carmichael, 1980 (Personal series)	467	Mixed	3	0.2
Fode, 1986 (Multicenter review)	3328	Mixed	4.2	2.0
Rubin, 1988 (Community-based vascular surgeons)	8535	Mostly TIA's	2.1	1.6
Winslow, 1988 (Geographic-based review)	1302	Mixed	6.4	3.4
ECST, 1991 (Multicenter randomized trial)	219	Symptomatic stenosis < 30%	4.6% stroke or death	
	455	Symptomatic stenosis > 70%	7.5% stroke or death	
NASCET, 1991 (Multicenter randomized trial)	328	Symptomatic stenosis > 70%	5.2	0.6

Source: Adapted from chapter references 41, 52–54, 63–65, and 80.

groups.[63] Among the patients with TIA's, there was a significant increase in asymptomatic survival in those who survived surgery. However, the perioperative mortality and stroke rates of 3.6 percent and 7.7 percent, respectively, nullified the advantage of surgical treatment. When perioperative events were included, the total stroke and mortality rates in an average follow-up period of 42 months were similar in the operated and nonoperated groups with combined stroke-mortality rates of 26.6 percent and 25 percent, respectively. However, by modern standards, the methodology of the Joint Study was inadequate to measure the efficacy of CEA in preventing stroke.

The European Carotid Surgery Trial (ECST)[64] and the North American Symptomatic Carotid Endarterectomy Trial (NASCET)[65] were published in 1991. Both of these multicenter trials examined patients with recent nondisabling strokes or TIA's and ipsilateral carotid stenosis in well-designed prospective randomized controlled studies. Patients were stratified by the degree of carotid stenosis as measured by angiography. Carotid surgery was performed with low rates of perioperative stroke and mortality. In patients with 70% to 99% stenosis, both studies showed large reductions of annual stroke rates after surgery to less than 2 percent compared to over 6 percent in medically treated patients (see Table 35–4). Even when operative risks were considered, both studies showed significant improvement in the rates of ipsilateral stroke, all stroke, and stroke and death at two years in NASCET and three years in ECST in patients undergoing CEA. Thus, two studies independently support the beneficial role of CEA in symptomatic patients with high-grade ipsilateral carotid stenosis of at least 70% when the surgery can be performed with a low complication rate.

The ECST also examined patients with mild stenosis of 0 to 29% and showed that the complications of surgery outweighed any benefits accrued from the procedure. Studies are still ongoing in those with moderate stenosis of 30% to 69%, and practitioners are cautioned not to extrapolate the results in patients with severe stenosis to those with lesser degrees of stenosis[40] or to submit patients to surgery if the procedure cannot be performed with low complication rates. The effectiveness of CEA in asymptomatic patients remains unanswered. Although a case can be made for CEA in those with high-grade or progressive stenosis, most asymptomatic patients should be treated medically until further information is available.[66]

Prophylactic Carotid Endarterectomy

Much of the work on cerebrovascular disease in surgical patients has focused on the role of prophylactic CEA in patients with carotid disease undergoing CABG. The studies reviewed above and listed in Table 35–1 suggest that patients with a history of TIA or stroke and those with significant carotid obstruction documented by noninvasive studies may have a significantly higher risk of stroke during CABG and may benefit from prophylactic CEA. However, Brener et al. found that CEA offered no significant protection against stroke in patients with asymptomatic carotid disease when performed simultaneously with CABG.[2] They recommended that combined cardiac and carotid surgery be reserved for patients with symptomatic carotid disease and severe cardiac disease. There are no randomized controlled studies to document the efficacy of prophylactic CEA before CABG in such patients with symptomatic disease. However, given the efficacy of CEA in symptomatic carotid stenosis in general, both operations may be considered in this setting.

Although some have reported a greater incidence of stroke when CEA and CABG are done together rather than in two stages with CEA preceding CABG,[5] authors of most recent series advocate the combined over the staged procedure because of decreased risk of perioperative myocardial infarction (MI) and death. A meta-analysis combining the results of 20 different series published between 1972 and 1985 found that, among 1483 patients, 1161 had a combined procedure with a stroke rate of 2.8 percent, a perioperative MI rate of 3.8 percent, and a mortality rate of 4.7 percent. The 322 patients who had a CEA followed by CABG had a similar stroke rate of 3.1 percent, but a higher rate of perioperative MI at 11.8 percent and a higher mortality rate at 11.1 percent.[67] Similarly, a review of 1546 patients undergoing CEA found that operative mortality increased from 1.5 percent in those without to 18.2 percent in those with symptomatic coronary artery disease. Those with angina who underwent a prior or simultaneous CABG had a mortality rate of 3 percent.[55]

A rational approach to the patient with both coronary and carotid artery disease is to assess the merit of each procedure individually. Carotid endarterectomy is warranted only in those patients with neurological symptoms ipsilateral to a stenotic carotid artery or, according to some authors, in those with bilateral carotid disease.[68] In such patients, a combined procedure is advocated when unstable angina, left main coronary artery obstruction, or diffuse multivessel coronary disease mandates urgent CABG. When CABG is not urgent, these authors recommend performing CEA first.[68,69] However, given the high perioperative mortality in patients with angina, CEA should be considered with caution in this situation. An option that may eventually prove to be superior is to perform percutaneous transluminal coronary angioplasty (PTCA), which carries a demonstrably lower risk of stroke, followed by CEA when it is clearly indicated.

Some investigators support prophylactic CEA in patients scheduled for peripheral vascular surgery who have severely stenotic carotid vessels,[20] and this can be recommended for those who are symptomatic.[64,65] In patients undergoing nonvascular surgical procedures, the risk of perioperative stroke is low, and carotid disease should be managed as in the general population, with proper medical therapy or prophylactic CEA if indicated.

Conclusions Regarding Carotid Endarterectomy

A summary of guidelines for the application of CEA can be formulated as follows:

1. CEA should be performed only in centers at which complication and mortality rates have been demonstrated to be low.

2. CEA is possibly indicated for patients with carotid stenosis of at least 70% who have had TIA's or minor strokes in the appropriate carotid distribution.

3. In patients with mild symptomatic stenosis of less than 30%, CEA is not beneficial, and the benefits of CEA in those with moderate symptomatic stenosis of 30% to 69% are as yet unproven.

4. Endarterectomy for asymptomatic carotid stenosis has not been rigorously demonstrated to be of value, but may be beneficial in a subgroup of patients with severe or progressive stenosis of $> 80\%$.

Contraindications to CEA include acute cerebral infarction, stroke in evolution, carotid occlusion, severe ipsilateral carotid siphon disease, limited life expectancy, and high operative risk from concurrent medical problems.[24]

OTHER SURGICAL TREATMENTS OF CEREBROVASCULAR DISEASE

A variety of other surgical techniques to treat atherosclerotic obstruction of the arteries supplying the brain have become popular despite lack of definite validation of their efficacy in preventing stroke. Some helpful guidelines for their appropriate application can be offered.

Extracranial–Intracranial Bypass Surgery

Superficial temporal artery–middle cerebral artery bypass for cerebrovascular disease of the internal carotid artery (ICA) or proximal middle cerebral artery (MCA) has been performed with technical success since 1967. Its use has been recommended in various situations, including ICA or MCA occlusions in which CEA is contraindicated.[70] In a recent landmark multicenter randomized study, 1377 patients were followed after bypass for an average of 55.8 months.[71,72] Postoperative mortality and major stroke rates were only 0.6 percent and 2.5 percent, respectively, and the early graft patency rate was 96 percent. However, there was no overall improvement in any of the specific outcome measures—stroke, death, or improvement in functional status.[71] The results have been criticized because large numbers of additional eligible patients undergoing bypass at these centers were not included in the study.[73] Nevertheless, data clearly suggest that there are no indications for the procedure at the present time.[71]

Surgical Treatment of Vertebrobasilar Disease

Because of difficulties with anatomic inaccessibility of the vertebral and basilar arteries, attempts at surgical correction of lesions in these arteries have been less frequent. However, arteriosclerotic occlusive lesions at the origin of the vertebral artery have been treated safely and effectively with endarterectomy and anastomosis or implantation of the vertebral to the subclavian artery.[74] In one study, 12 symptomatic patients underwent vertebral endarterectomy for lesions lying within the second portion of the vertebral artery from C6 to T1.[75] Although 2 of the 12 required reoperation, the others experienced symptomatic improvement.

Other procedures for vertebrobasilar stenosis include unroofing in cases where the arteries are compressed by cervical spondylosis or fibrous bands, occipital-anterior inferior cerebellar artery anastomosis, and venous or synthetic grafting.[18,75] In a study of 100 patients undergoing various reconstructive procedures on branches of the brachiocephalic arteries, most patients had symptomatic improvement. However, there was significant operative morbidity in those requiring a transthoracic approach but no mortality and a stroke rate of only 3 percent in those undergoing extrathoracic procedures.[18] Although controlled evaluation of these highly individualized procedures is difficult, selective application in appropriate symptomatic patients by experienced surgeons may be of benefit.

Other Approaches to Cerebrovascular Disease

Percutaneous transluminal balloon angioplasty of the carotid and vertebral arteries has been attempted on a limited scale. Several case reports have described successful carotid angioplasty for narrowing due to fibromuscular dysplasia[76] or arteritis. Successful vertebral basilar artery angioplasty has been reported in patients with progressive vertebral basilar ischemia unresponsive to anticoagulant therapy,[77] but its use has not been widely accepted.

SUMMARY

1. The risk of stroke is low in surgical procedures that do not involve the heart or other major vascular structures.

2. The risk of stroke or diffuse cerebral ischemia is higher in patients undergoing coronary artery bypass grafting (CABG) and other vascular procedures, especially those requiring cardiopulmonary bypass. Prolonged bypass and intraoperative hypotension confer additional risk.

3. All surgery should be postponed, if possible, in the setting of recent stroke or TIA.

4. Although carotid stenosis may increase the risk of stroke during cardiac or vascular procedures, the most important risks are a previous history of cerebrovascular disease, advanced age, and the presence of cardiac lesions that can serve as sources of emboli.

5. Medical management of patients with an increased risk of stroke requires treatment of medical conditions such as hypertension and diabetes mellitus and selected application of anticoagulant and antiplatelet agents. However, preoperative use of these agents increases the rate of perioperative hemorrhagic complications.

6. CEA is more likely to be beneficial when performed at centers with low rates of perioperative stroke and mortality. Other vascular procedures intended to restore the cerebral circulation have not been shown to be efficacious in rigorous trials.

7. If there are strong indications for both carotid endarterectomy (CEA) and CABG, a combined procedure may carry the lowest risk.

REFERENCES

1. Adams R, Victor M: *Principles of Neurology*, 3rd ed. New York, McGraw-Hill, 1985.
2. Brener B, Brief D, Alpert J et al: The risk of stroke in patients with asymptomatic carotid stenosis undergoing cardiac surgery: A follow-up study. *J Vasc Surg* 5:269–279, 1987.
3. Shaw P, Bates D, Cartlidge N et al: Neurologic and neuropsychological morbidity following major surgery: Comparison of coronary artery bypass and peripheral vascular surgery. *Stroke* 18:700–707, 1987.
4. Sotaniemi KA, Mononen H, Hokkanen TE: Long-term cerebral outcome after open-heart surgery. A five-year neuropsychological follow-up study. *Stroke* 17:410, 1986.
5. Breuer AC, Hanson MR, Furlan AJ et al: Central nervous system complications of myocardial revascularization. A prospective analysis of 400 patients (abstract). *Stroke* 11:136, 1980.
6. Gardner TJ, Horneffer PJ, Manolio TA: Stroke following coronary artery bypass grafting: A ten-year study. *Ann Thorac Surg* 40:574–581, 1985.
7. Reed GL, Singer DE, Picard EH et al: Stroke following coronary artery bypass surgery. A case-control estimate of the risk from carotid bruits. *N Engl J Med* 319:1246–1250, 1988.
8. Hoffmann RG, Blumlein SL, Anderson AJ et al: The probability of surviving coronary bypass surgery. Five-year results from 1718 patients. *JAMA* 243:1341–1344, 1980.
9. Lawrie GM, Morris GC, Baron A et al: Determinants of survival 10 to 14 years after coronary bypass: Analysis of preoperative variables in 1448 patients. *Ann Thorac Surg* 44:180–185, 1987.
10. Carella F, Travaini G, Contri P et al: Cerebral complications of coronary bypass surgery: A prospective study. *Acta Neurol Scand* 77:158–163, 1988.
11. Bass RM, Longmore DB: Cerebral damage during open heart surgery. *Nature* 222:30, 1969.
12. Branthwaite MA: Prevention of neurological damage during open heart surgery. *Thorax* 30:258, 1975.
13. Galbreath C, Salgado ED, Furlan AJ et al: Central nervous system complications of percutaneous transluminal coronary angioplasty. *Stroke* 17:616–619, 1986.
14. Carney WI, Stewart WB, DePinto DJ et al: Carotid bruit as a factor in aortoiliac reconstruction. *Surgery* 81:567–570, 1977.
15. Evans WE, Cooperman MT: The significance of asymptomatic unilateral carotid bruit in preoperative patients. *Surgery* 83:521–522, 1978.
16. Ropper AH, Wechsler LR, Wilson LS: Carotid bruit and the risk of stroke in elective surgery. *N Engl J Med* 307:1388–1399, 1982.
17. Treiman RL, Foran RF, Shore EH et al: Carotid bruit: Significance in patients undergoing an abdominal operation. *Arch Surg* 106:803–805, 1973.
18. Vogt DP, Hertzer NR, O'Hara PJ et al: Brachiocephalic arterial reconstruction. *Ann Surg* 196:541–552, 1982.
19. Barnes RW, Marszalek PB: Asymptomatic carotid disease in the cardiovascular surgical patient: Is prophylactic endarterectomy necessary? *Stroke* 12:497–500, 1981.
20. Hertzer NR, Beven EG, Young JR et al: Incidental asymptomatic carotid bruits in patients scheduled for peripheral vascular reconstruction: Results of cerebral and coronary angiography. *Surgery* 96:535, 1984.
21. Breslau PJ, Fell G, Ivey TD et al: Carotid arterial disease in patients undergoing coronary bypass operations. *J Thorac Cardiovasc Surg* 82:765–767, 1981.
22. DeWeese JA, Rob CG, Satran R et al: Endarterectomy for atherosclerotic lesions of the carotid artery. *J Cardiovasc Surg* 12:299–308, 1971.
23. DeWeese JA: Management of acute strokes. *Surg Clin N Am* 62:467–472, 1982.
24. Ferguson GG: Extracranial carotid artery surgery. *Clin Neurosurg* 29:543–574, 1982.
25. Ezekowitz MD, Bridgers SL, James KE et al: Warfarin in the prevention of stroke associated with nonrheumatic atrial fibrillation. *N Engl J Med* 327:1406–1412, 1992.
26. Steering Committee of the Physicians' Health Study Research Group: Final report on the aspirin component of the ongoing Physicians' Health Study. *N Engl J Med* 321:129–135, 1989.
27. Hass WK, Easton JD, Adams HP Jr et al: A randomized study comparing ticlopidine hydrochloride with aspirin for the prevention of stroke in high-risk patients. *N Engl J Med* 321:501–507, 1989.

28. Katholi RE, Nolan SP, McGuire LB: The management of anticoagulation during noncardiac operations in patients with prosthetic heart valves. A prospective study. *Am Heart J* 96:163, 1978.

29. Travis S, Wray R, Harrison K: Perioperative anticoagulant control. *Br J Surg* 76:1107–1108, 1989.

30. Tinker JH, Tarhan S: Discontinuing anticoagulant therapy in surgical patients with cardiac valve prosthesis; observations in 180 patients. *JAMA* 239:738–739, 1978.

31. Taggart DP, Siddiqui A, Wheatley DJ: Low-dose preoperative aspirin therapy, postoperative blood loss and transfusion requirements. *Ann Thorac Surg* 50:424–428, 1990.

32. Bodnar AG, Hutter AM: Anticoagulation in valvular heart disease preoperatively and postoperatively. *Cardiovasc Clin* 14:247–264, 1984.

33. Toronsian M, Michelson EL, Morganroth J et al: Aspirin- and coumadin-related bleeding after coronary-artery bypass graft surgery. *Ann Intern Med* 89:325–328, 1978.

34. Sethi GK, Copeland JG, Goldman S et al: Implications of preoperative administration of aspirin in patients undergoing coronary artery bypass grafting. *J Am Coll Card* 15:15–20, 1990.

35. Ferraris VA, Swanson E: Aspirin usage and perioperative blood loss in patients undergoing unexpected operations. *Surg Gyn Obst* 156:439–442, 1983.

36. Ferraris VA, Ferraris SP, Lough FC et al: Preoperative aspirin ingestion increases operative blood loss after coronary artery bypass grafting. *Ann Thorac Surg* 45:71–74, 1988.

37. Watson CJ, Deane AM, Doyle PT et al: Identifiable factors in post-prostatectomy hemorrhage: The role of aspirin. *Br J Urol* 66:85–87, 1990.

38. Pawlak DF, Itkin AB, Lapeyrolerie FM et al: Clinical effects of aspirin and acetaminophen on hemostasis after exodontics. *J Oral Surg* 36:944–947, 1978.

39. Teoh KH, Christakis GT, Weisel RD et al: Dipyridamole preserved platelets and reduced blood loss after cardiopulmonary bypass. *J Thorac Cardiovasc Surg* 96:332–341, 1988.

40. Barnett HJM, Barnes RW, Clagett GP et al: Symptomatic carotid artery stenosis; a solvable problem. North American symptomatic carotid endarterectomy trial. *Stroke* 23:1048–1053, 1992.

41. Rubin JR, Pitluk HC, King TA et al: Carotid endarterectomy in a metropolitan community: The early results after 8535 operations. *J Vasc Surg* 7:256–260, 1988.

42. Brott T, Thalinger K: The practice of carotid endarterectomy in a large metropolitan area. *Stroke* 15:950, 1984.

43. Whisnant JP, Sandok BA, Sundt TM: Carotid endarterectomy for unilateral carotid system transient cerebral ischemia. *Mayo Clin Proc* 58:171–175, 1983.

44. Wolf PA, Kannel WB, Sorlie P et al: Asymptomatic carotid bruit and the risk of stroke. The Framingham study. *JAMA* 245:1442–1445, 1981.

45. Durward QJ, Ferguson G, Barr H: The natural history of asymptomatic carotid bifurcation plaques. *Stroke* 4:459–464, 1982.

46. Hennerici M, Hulsbomer H, Hefter H et al: Natural history of asymptomatic extracranial arterial disease. Results of a long-term, prospective study. *Brain* 110:777–791, 1987.

47. Chambers BR, Norris JW: Outcome in patients with asymptomatic neck bruits. *N Engl J Med* 315:860–865, 1986.

48. Powers WJ, Tempel LW, Grubb RL: Influence of cerebral hemodynamics on stroke risk: One-year follow-up of 30 medically treated patients. *Ann Neurol* 25:325–330, 1989.

49. Harrison MJG, Marshall J: The finding of thrombus at carotid endarterectomy and its relationship to the timing of surgery. *Br J Surg* 64:511–512, 1977.

50. Nunn DB: Carotid endarterectomy in patients with territorial transient ischemic attacks. *J Vasc Surg* 8:447–452, 1988.

51. Toole JF, Yuson CP, Janeway R et al: Transient ischemic attacks: A prospective study of 225 patients. *Neurology* 28:746–753, 1978.

52. Carmichael JD: Carotid surgery in a community hospital: 467 consecutive operations. *Arch Surg* 115:937–939, 1980.

53. Winslow CM, Solomon DH, Chassin MR et al: The appropriateness of carotid endarterectomy. *N Engl J Med* 318:721–727, 1988.

54. Easton JD, Sherman DG: Stroke and mortality rate in carotid endarterectomy: 228 consecutive operations. *Stroke* 8:565–568, 1977.

55. Ennix CL, Lawrie GM, Morris GC et al: Improved results of carotid endarterectomy in patients with symptomatic coronary disease: An analysis of 1546 consecutive carotid operations. *Stroke* 10:122–124, 1979.

56. Chambers BR, Norris JW: The case against surgery for asymptomatic carotid stenosis. *Stroke* 15:964–969, 1984.

57. Hertzer NR, Flanagan RA, O'Hara PJ et al: Surgical versus nonoperative treatment of symptomatic carotid stenosis. *Ann Surg* 204:163–171, 1986.

58. Bernstein EF, Dilley RB: Late results after carotid endarterectomy for amaurosis fugax. *J Vasc Surg* 6:333–340, 1987.

59. Rubin JR, Goldstone J, McIntyre KE Jr et al: The value of carotid endarterectomy in reducing the morbidity and mortality of recurrent stroke. *J Vasc Surg* 4:443–449, 1986.

60. Rosenthal D, Borrero E, Clark MD et al: Carotid endarterectomy after reversible ischemic neurologic deficit or stroke: Is it of value? *J Vasc Surg* 8:527–534, 1988.

61. McNamara J, Heyman A, Silver D et al: The value of carotid endarterectomy in treating transient cerebral ischemia of the posterior circulation. *Neurology* 27:682–684, 1977.

62. Moneta GL, Taylor DC, Nichols SC et al: Operative versus nonoperative management of asymptomatic high-grade internal carotid artery stenosis: Improved results with endarterectomy. *Stroke* 18:1005–1010, 1987.

63. Fields WS, Maslenikov V, Meyer JS et al: Joint study of extracranial arterial occlusion: V. Progress report of prognosis following surgery or nonsurgical treatment for transient cerebral ischemic attacks and cervical carotid artery lesions. *JAMA* 211:1993–2003, 1970.

64. European Carotid Surgery Trialists' Collaborative Group: MRC European surgery trial: Interim results for symptomatic patients with severe (70–90%) or with mild (0–29%) carotid stenosis. *Lancet* 337:1235–1243, 1991.

65. NASCET Collaborators: Beneficial effect of carotid endarterectomy in symptomatic patients with high-grade carotid stenosis. *N Engl J Med* 325:445–453, 1991.

66. Veterans Administration Cooperative Study Group: Role of carotid endarterectomy in asymptomatic carotid stenosis. *Stroke* 17:534–539, 1986.

67. Barnes RW: Asymptomatic carotid disease in patients undergoing major cardiovascular operations: Can prophylactic endarterectomy be justified? *Ann Thorac Surg* 42(Suppl):S36–S40, 1986.

68. Jones EL, Craver JM, Michalik RA et al: Combined carotid and coronary operations: When are they necessary? *J Thorac Cardiovasc Surg* 87:7–16, 1984.

69. Graor RA, Hertzer NR: Management of coexistent carotid artery and coronary artery disease. *Stroke* 19:1441–1444, 1988.

70. Whisnant JP, Sundt TM, Fode NC: Long-term mortality and stroke morbidity after superficial temporal artery–middle cerebral artery bypass operation. *Mayo Clin Proc* 60:241–246, 1985.

71. EC/IC Bypass Study Group: Failure of extracranial–intracranial arterial bypass to reduce the risk of ischemic stroke. Results of an international randomized trial. *N Engl J Med* 313:1191–1200, 1985.

72. Haynes RB, Mukherje J, Sackett DL et al: Functional status changes following medical or surgical treatment for cerebral ischemia. Results of the extracranial–intracranial bypass study. *JAMA* 257:2043–2046, 1987.

73. Sundt TM: Was the international randomized trial of extracranial–intracranial arterial bypass representative of the population at risk? *N Engl J Med* 316:814–816, 1987.

74. Thevenet A, Ruotolo C: Surgical repair of vertebral artery stenoses. *J Cardiovasc Surg* 25:101–110, 1984.

75. Diaz FG, Ausman JI, Shrontz C et al: Surgical correction of lesions affecting the second portion of the vertebral artery. *Neurosurgery* 19:93–100, 1986.

76. Dublin AB, Baltaxe HA, Cobb CA: Percutaneous transluminal carotid angioplasty in fibromuscular dysplasia. *Neurosurg* 59:162–165, 1983.

77. Smith HC, Sundt TM, Pipgras DG et al: Transluminal angioplasty for vertebral basilar artery stenosis, in Kaltenbach M et al (eds): *Transluminal Coronary Angioplasty and Intracoronary Thrombolysis.* Berlin, Springer-Verlag, 1982, pp 209–219.

78. Gonzalez-Scarano F, Hurtig HI: Neurologic complications of coronary artery bypass grafting: Case-control study. *Neurology* 31:1032–1035, 1981.

79. Coffey CE, Massey EW, Roberts KB et al: Natural history of cerebral complications of coronary artery bypass graft surgery. *Neurology* 33:1416–1421, 1983.

80. Fode NC, Sundt TM, Robertson JT et al: Multicenter retrospective review of results and complications of carotid endarterectomy in 1981. *Stroke* 17:370–375, 1986.

36 SURGERY IN THE PATIENT WITH NEUROLOGIC DISEASE

Steven L. Galetta

Eric C. Raps

Michael E. Selzer

A variety of neurologic disorders may affect the management of surgical patients and require special treatment in the perioperative period. This chapter discusses surgery in those with known neurologic disease. Neurologic dysfunction may also arise as a complication of surgery or anesthesia, and this situation is considered in Chap. 71.

NEUROLOGIC DISEASES

Epilepsy

The prevalence of recurrent seizures is 0.5 to 1 percent of the general population.[1] Seizures may be *generalized* or *partial*. The most common generalized seizures are major motor or *grand mal* and absence or *petit mal*. The latter occur almost exclusively in children. Partial seizures may be simple motor or sensory, consisting of involuntary movements of or abnormal sensations referable to one part of the body, or complex. Complex partial seizures have many manifestations, including automatic patterned movements such as lip smacking or facial grimacing. The common feature of complex partial seizures, however, is alteration in awareness causing patients to lose effective contact with the environment, to answer questions inappropriately or not at all, and to experience complete or partial amnesia for the episode. Because the outward manifestations of complex partial seizures may be nothing more than staring, they are often confused with petit mal. However, the two can be readily distinguished by clinical presentation and electroencephalography.[2]

The occurrence of a major motor seizure can complicate a surgical procedure and increase the risk of morbidity and mortality. It is therefore important that patients with preexisting seizure disorders be identified and that their anticonvulsant medications be continued. If the patient has no oral intake on the day of surgery, anticonvulsants must be given parenterally. In the case of phenytoin and phenobarbital, the usual daily dose can be administered intravenously in normal saline at a rate no greater than 50 mg/min. However, carbamazepine and valproic acid are not available in parenteral form at present, but a parenteral form of carbamazepine is currently under development. Patients taking one of these drugs should be loaded with phenytoin in a dose of 18 mg/kg and maintained on 4 to 8 mg/kg in three divided doses until they resume eating. Those who are allergic or intolerant to phenytoin may be loaded with phenobarbital in a dose of 6 mg/kg. If the patient is allergic to both phenytoin and phenobarbital and the risk of major motor seizures is high, premedication with prednisone in a dose of 60 mg/day for two days usually prevents allergic reactions. It is safest to load the patient orally one or two days before surgery and to give maintenance doses intravenously during the perioperative period. However, in emergency cases the loading may be performed intravenously with the same doses.

It is vital that intravenous loading proceed at a slow rate because of the danger of hypotension or asystole. In the case of phenytoin, this appears to be due primarily to the effects of the propylene glycol diluent,[3] but phenytoin itself may contribute to asystole.[4] Overly rapid administration of phenobarbital may lead to respiratory arrest or hypotension. Serum levels should be maintained in the upper half of the therapeutic range (15 to 20 μg/ml for phenytoin and 30 to 40 μg/ml for phenobarbital) in order to minimize the risk of intraoperative seizures. Phenytoin and phenobarbital are usually effective for all common types of seizures except true absences which require ethosuximide or valproic acid, not available in parenteral form. However, pure absence seizures pose little threat, and their treatment can be safely interrupted until after surgery. Rectal valproate provides another therapeutic option if needed.

Seizures in patients without a history of seizures may occur during surgery and are usually related to a particular anesthetic agent or drug.[5,6] Some anesthetics like enflurane and ketamine may cause seizures during induction and following anesthesia. Isoflurane and halothane have potent anticonvulsant activity with little proconvulsive effect.[5,6] Seizures after surgery are generally not related to the effects of anesthesia and should prompt diagnostic study including electrolyte levels and neurologic consultation. Control of seizures in the postoperative period primarily involves correcting the underlying etiology. Persistent seizures may require a short course of anticonvulsant therapy. When an isolated seizure occurs in the perioperative period without cause, it is not necessary to initiate anticonvulsants.

Multiple Sclerosis

Multiple sclerosis (MS) is a chronic progressive disease of unknown etiology characterized by exacerbations at irregular intervals.[7] Each exacerbation usually lasts one to two weeks and is followed by remission of variable degree. Ultimate long-term disability results from accumulation of residual deficits at the end of each exacerbation. The first attack usually occurs in the third or fourth decade. When onset is later, the course tends to be more rapid with fewer remissions. The pathology consists of plaques of demyelination and lymphocytic infiltration in a perivenular distribution.

Neurological deficits are the result of axonal conduction block due to the destruction of myelin. The axons and neuronal cell bodies are unaffected. Patients may have a wide variety of deficits, including spasticity and weakness in any distribution. The spasticity may make surgery difficult and require the administration of neuromuscular blocking agents in circumstances where they might not otherwise be indicated.

Patients already on baclofen for spasticity should not be withdrawn from medication abruptly because of the risk of withdrawal seizures and hallucinations. If the patient is not expected to be able to take oral medications after surgery, it is advisable to switch to diazepam before the procedure. Patients with MS who are wheelchair-bound or bedridden pose special problems for postoperative management and require physical and respiratory therapy to avoid decubitus ulcers, atelectasis, and aspiration pneumonia.

There is no substantial evidence for a causal relationship between the onset or worsening of MS and surgery or injury. However, rises in body temperature in the perioperative period may cause temporary worsening of symptoms. This is not due to formation of additional plaques of demyelination. At higher temperatures, electrical impulses in nerve fibers become shorter in duration, and a partially demyelinated marginally conducting nerve fiber may become totally blocked.[8] When body temperature returns to normal, nerve function reverts to baseline. Hyperthermic reactions to anesthesia and postoperative infections can therefore lead to temporary worsening of the patient's condition.

One of the common manifestations of spinal cord involvement with MS is urinary retention. Patients are usually able to void either spontaneously or by applying external pressure to their bladders during remissions. After surgery, some may experience temporary total retention due to fever or other factors. They can be treated with intermittent catheterization with the expectation that their condition will improve. Cholinergic agents such as urecholine can be tried but are usually not effective.

Parkinsonism

Parkinsonism is a syndrome of muscle rigidity, resting tremor, slowness of movements termed bradykinesia, blunting of facial expression, and postural instability.[9] The basic pathophysiology of parkinsonism is degeneration of the dopamine-containing neurons in the substantia nigra and consequent loss of dopaminergic input to the caudate and putamen. It is believed that, in the basal ganglia, there is a normal balance between the actions of dopamine and acetylcholine. When dopaminergic input is reduced, cholinergic activity is unopposed and may account for some of the symptoms. Administration of anticholinergic agents such as benztropine mesylate (Cogentin) and trihexyphenidyl hydrochloride (Artane) may be helpful. More effective treatment with levodopa and the dopamine agonist bromocriptine help by increasing dopaminergic input and restoring balance between the two neurotransmitters.

There are several underlying causes of parkinsonism. Idiopathic parkinsonism or Parkinson's disease is the most common. However, even idiopathic Parkinson's disease may have more than one etiology. In recent years, patients with Parkinson's disease have been found to have an unexpectedly high incidence of dementia not noted in original clinical descriptions.[10,11] It occurs in about 15 percent of patients and is both clinically and pathologically indistinguishable from Alzheimer's disease.[12] These cases may therefore represent a different disease. Other etiologies of parkinsonism include viral encephalitis, cerebral infarction, and toxins like phenothiazines and other antidopaminergic neuroleptics. In addition, a Parkinson's-like syndrome can be caused by chronic manganese intoxication.

Dopamine, the active metabolite of L-dopa, can complicate anesthesia by causing hypotension, hypertension, or cardiac arrhythmias and should be discontinued the night before surgery.[13,14] In severe cases, the resulting rigidity and bradykinesia increase the risk of pneumonia, atelectasis, and decubitus ulcers. Respiratory complications can be aggravated by sialorrhea and respiratory dyskinesias. It is advisable to anticipate the degree of respiratory compromise by obtaining an arterial blood gas determination and pulmonary function tests before surgery. Because suspension of therapy may threaten recovery, it is important to resume treatment as soon as the patient can eat. Anticholinergics like benztropine mesylate in a dose of 0.5 to 1 mg twice daily may be given intramuscularly during the perioperative period without serious cardiovascular risk.

If a satisfactory treatment regimen has not been established previously, patients should be started on a combination of L-dopa and carbidopa (Sinemet). This is available in various dose combinations of 10 or 25 mg of carbidopa and 100 or 250 mg of L-dopa. Carbidopa is an inhibitor of the enzyme dopa decarboxylase that converts L-dopa into the active metabolite dopamine. While dopamine and carbidopa do not cross the blood-brain barrier, L-dopa does so readily. Concomitant treatment with carbidopa reduces peripheral conversion of L-dopa to dopamine and thereby reduces its most serious side effects.

Dopamine has been shown to cause hypertension by binding to alpha-adrenergic receptors in vascular smooth muscle.[13] In some patients, this is outweighed by its effect on dopamine receptors in the renal and mesenteric vasculature, causing vasodilatation and hypotension. Dopamine can also bind to myocardial beta-adrenergic receptors and cause arrhythmias. Therefore, only combinations containing 25 mg of carbidopa should be used. A good starting dose is 25 mg of carbidopa with 100 mg of L-dopa orally three times daily taken with meals to reduce nausea. The daily dose can be increased by one tablet per day and the formula switched to 25/250 tablets until a good therapeutic effect is achieved or the patient develops toxicity. The total daily carbidopa dose should be at least 75 mg. Total daily L-dopa doses may range from 400 to 600 mg in early symptomatic cases, but doses as high as one gram daily may be necessary in more advanced cases.

The rate of dose increase suggested above is more rapid than that employed in the outpatient setting, and patients may develop toxic side effects like nausea at much lower doses than they will eventually tolerate. If desired, dosing can begin with as little as one-half tablet of 25/100 mg twice daily and increased gradually. Other signs of L-dopa toxicity include chorea, restlessness, hallucinations, vivid dreaming, and increased libido.

In the outpatient setting, many neurologists begin therapy with anticholinergic agents because of their efficacy in reducing resting tremor. However, the main concerns in surgical patients are bradykinesia and rigidity seen in more advanced cases which are less responsive to anticholinergic drugs. If therapy must be initiated urgently, L-dopa should be used alone. Amantadine, another commonly used antiparkinsonian agent, should be used with caution in surgical patients because it may precipitate congestive heart failure. It may also cause nausea, insomnia, hallucinations, peripheral edema, and orthostatic hypotension.

Recent studies suggest that in previously untreated patients, the dopamine D_2 receptor agonist bromocriptine provides the same therapeutic effect as carbidopa/L-dopa with fewer side effects.[15] Unfortunately, the effectiveness of bromocriptine therapy alone is not sustained after the first few months. Many experts now advocate that both agents be administered when initiating treatment, using the lower recommended doses to achieve therapeutic results.[16] Bromocriptine therapy can be started at 1.25 mg/day, and the daily dose increased by 1.25 mg as rapidly as tolerated. With this combination, most patients are adequately controlled at total daily doses of no more than 400 mg of L-dopa and 20 mg of bromocriptine. The main toxic side effects of bromocriptine are nausea and hypotension.

The most recent innovation in the treatment of Parkinson's disease is the use of the monoamine oxidase B (MAO-B) inhibitor selegiline (Eldepryl). By reducing the rate of degradation of dopamine in the brain, it increases and prolongs the effectiveness of a given dose of L-dopa and allows a 20% to 30% reduction in total daily dose. Preliminary findings suggest that the drug may slow the progression of the disease, at least in its early stages.[17] MAO-B is thought to generate neurotoxic free-oxygen radicals. The inhibition of MAO-B by selegiline may prevent the accumulation of free radicals in dopaminergic neurons and slow the rate of their destruction. Some neurologists are using selegiline in a dose of 5 mg orally twice daily as part of their initial therapy. With doses under 10 mg/day, ingestion of tyramine-containing foods does not evoke hypertensive crises. The concomitant use of meperidine and selegiline can cause stupor, fever, and rigidity and is therefore strictly contraindicated.

NEUROMUSCULAR DISEASES

Myasthenia Gravis

Myasthenia gravis is an autoimmune disorder of the neuromuscular junction characterized by fluctuating weakness of the extraocular, facial, bulbar, and extremity muscles. The disorder has an incidence of 1 in 100,000 with a bimodal distribution.[18] Females are commonly affected in the second and third decades, but men have a tendency to develop the disorder later in life.[19] The underlying pathogenic mechanism lies in the generation of antibodies against nicotinic acetylcholine receptors. The diagnosis of myasthenia can be established clinically and can be confirmed by an intravenous edrophonium (Tensilon) test. Other useful laboratory tests include the serum antiacetylcholine receptor antibody test and electromyography using repetitive stimulation.

Management of this disorder begins with the administration of an anticholinesterase. Pyridostigmine (Mestinon) is most commonly used in a starting dose of 30 mg orally every four hours. Maximum benefit is usually reached with doses of 120 mg every three to four hours. Higher doses may precipitate cholinergic crisis manifested by increased weakness. Major side effects of anticholinesterases include abdominal cramping and diarrhea. The antimuscarinic drug atropine (or an equivalent drug) may be given in a dose of 0.4 to 0.6 mg orally or intravenously with each dose of pyridostigmine to treat these symptoms without affecting the nicotinic benefits of the anticholinesterase at the neuromuscular junction. Pyridostigmine may be discontinued before surgery and restarted when the patient resumes oral intake. In those patients unable to take oral medications, anticholinesterase agents can be given intravenously or intramuscularly at appropriate doses outlined in Table 36–1.

The two major immunosuppressive drugs, corticosteroids and azathioprine, are most often used in patients who have had a poor response to anticholinesterases. Response to corticosteroids may take several weeks, and initiation of treatment may be marked by a transient worsening of weakness. Therefore, routine administration of "stress" dose steroids to patients with myasthenia not already on them is not recommended. When prednisone is used, the usual starting dose is 1 mg/kg, but some authorities suggest lower doses with gradual increases to avoid initial deterioration.[20] Azathioprine is also an effective immunosuppressive agent that may avoid the use of steroids. However, improvement usually takes 6 to 12 weeks of therapy and is not maximal until 6 to 15 months.[19] Since azathioprine may cause bone marrow suppression and hepatitis, periodic complete blood counts and liver function studies are necessary. The starting dose is 50 mg/day orally with increases to 2.5 mg/kg/day.

TABLE 36–1. Parenteral and Oral Conversion Formulas for Myasthenia Gravis

Drug	Dose		Route	Frequency
Pyridostigmine	60	mg	PO	q 3–4 h
(Mestinon)	2	mg	IV, IM	q 3–4 h
Neostigmine	15	mg	PO	q 3–4 h
(Prostigmin)	0.5	mg	IV, IM	q 3–4 h

Plasmapheresis can transiently improve function in myasthenics by removing antiacetylcholine receptor antibodies. Improvement may occur during the initial exchange but is usually delayed for several days. Benefits may last weeks to months. Plasmapheresis is reserved for the severely ill patient who is undergoing thymectomy, awaiting the response of immunosuppressive agents, or experiencing respiratory insufficiency. Complications of plasma exchange include vein thrombosis, hypovolemia, paresthesias, electrolyte imbalance, and the removal of plasma-bound drugs.[21] Intravenous gamma globulin is a new therapy also available for the severely ill myasthenic patient.

Thymic hyperplasia is seen in the vast majority of myasthenics, but 10 percent of patients harbor a thymoma.[22] Thymectomy produces a partial or complete remission in up to 80 percent of patients.[23,24] Many centers advocate thymectomy in patients with generalized myasthenia under the age of 60. Thymectomy is not recommended for ocular myasthenia alone. Immediately following thymectomy, some patients may require less pyridostigmine, but most of the benefits of the procedure are delayed for months or perhaps years.

Several exogenous factors may cause deterioration of function, including thyrotoxicosis and pregnancy. In addition, there are many drugs that impair neuromuscular transmission that should not be used unless absolutely necessary (see Table 36–2).[25]

The most feared complication of myasthenia is respiratory failure which may be abrupt in onset. Serial measurement of the vital capacity is essential to determine when mechanical ventilation is required. When the vital capacity falls below 15 ml/kg, almost all patients should be electively intubated. Local or regional anesthesia should be used whenever possible. When general anesthesia is required, small doses of nondepolarizing agents like atracurium or vecuronium can be used for paralysis with appropriate monitoring.[26] Succinylcholine may cause prolonged neuromuscular blockade and is metabolized poorly in the presence of anticholinesterase agents.[27]

Eaton-Lambert Syndrome

Eaton-Lambert syndrome is a presynaptic neuromuscular disorder, frequently but not exclusively seen in patients with oat-cell carcinoma.[28] Individuals with this disorder present with muscle weakness, but the ocular, respiratory, and bulbar musculature is usually spared. Patients may be sensitive to depolarizing and nondepolarizing anesthetic agents.[27,29] Eaton-Lambert syndrome is occasionally first noted in the postoperative period in patients who require pro-

TABLE 36–2. Drugs That May Worsen Myasthenia Gravis

Aminoglycoside and other antibiotics
  gentamcin, tobramycin, neomycin, polymyxin, kanamycin,
  clindamycin, streptomycin, netilmicin, amikacin

Antiarrhythmics   quinine, quinidine, procainamide, propranolol, verapamil
Anesthetics   lidocaine, procaine, cocaine, methoxyflurane
Analgesics   morphine, meperidine
Psychoactive   lithium, phenothiazines, amitriptyline
Others   phenytoin, magnesium salts, chloroquine, penicillamine

Source: Adapted from Adams SL, Mathews J, and Grammer LC.[25]

longed ventilation after neuromuscular blocking agents have been used.[30] It is important to be aware of all of the drugs that can impair neuromuscular transmission and produce increased muscle weakness in these patients. Treatment with 3,4-diaminopyridine and plasmapheresis yields variable results.

Myotonic Dystrophy

Myotonic dystrophy is an autosomal dominant disorder characterized by myotonia (impaired muscle relaxation) and weakness, primarily affecting the distal musculature. Associated findings include frontal balding, gonadal atrophy, cardiac conduction abnormalities, respiratory insufficiency, and cataracts. Weakness of the bulbar musculature can lead to dysphagia, dysarthria, and aspiration. Myotonia can be elicited by percussion in almost any muscle and is manifested by a delay in relaxation. Electromyography reveals prolonged bursts of muscle action potentials in response to brief stimuli.

Cardiac conduction abnormalities are common in myotonic dystrophy. In one series, 17 of 26 patients had first degree atrial-ventricular block. Other conduction abnormalities include right bundle branch block, left anterior hemiblock, and left bundle branch block.[31] Conduction irregularities in the myotonic patient undergoing surgery merit continuous cardiac monitoring in the perioperative period. Patients may require a temporary pacemaker before surgery. Anesthetic agents that depress the myocardium should be avoided if possible to avoid precipitating congestive failure.[32]

Respiratory compromise may result from weakness or myotonia of the respiratory musculature. Patients may also experience increased respiratory depression following general anesthesia. If possible, opiates, benzodiazapines, and barbiturates should be avoided.[32] Aggressive pulmonary toilet is essential in these patients. Treatment of the myotonia may be accomplished with procainamide, quinine, or phenytoin. Phenytoin may be the best agent in these patients since it shortens the P-R interval on the electrocardiogram.[33]

Guillain-Barré Syndrome

The Guillain-Barré syndrome (GBS) is an inflammatory demyelinating polyradiculoneuropathy characterized by acute areflexic quadraparesis.[34] Many patients describe an antecedent viral illness, and the disorder may rarely follow surgery.[35] Diagnosis of GBS can be made from the history and confirmed by nerve conduction studies and cerebrospinal fluid examination. A rise in the cerebrospinal fluid protein concentration without an associated pleocytosis is characteristic of GBS but may take several days to develop. Autonomic disturbances are frequent and include tachycardia, hypertension, hypotension, ileus, urinary retention, and arrhythmias.[36]

Patients often require admission to an intensive care unit for serial measurements of blood pressure and cardiac monitoring. Management requires close attention to nutritional needs, electrolyte abnormalities (particularly the syndrome of inappropriate secretion of antidiuretic hormone), skin changes, and bowel and bladder function. Insufficient eyelid closure due to facial paralysis may result in corneal injury, particularly during sleep. Artificial tears and ointments may help prevent these complications, and the lids may also be taped closed with thin paper tape at bedtime. Subcutaneous heparin therapy and the use of pneumatic boots may help prevent deep-vein thrombosis. Monitoring of respiratory status with serial measurements of vital capacity is essential. A drop in the vital capacity to the 15 ml/kg range heralds impending respiratory failure and is an indication for elective intubation.[37] Hypoxia and hypercarbia occur late and do not reliably predict respiratory failure.

Plasmapheresis is the mainstay of therapy in GBS and is most clearly indicated in those with difficulty walking or more pronounced neurologic dysfunction. In one study, patients treated with plasmapheresis required shorter periods of respiratory support and improved more rapidly.[38] Corticosteroids have not proved effective.[39] Simple surgical procedures such as placement of a tracheostomy or gastrostomy do not appear to worsen the disorder.[40]

Autonomic Dysfunction

Autonomic dysfunction may be seen in a variety of peripheral nerve disorders, particularly those associated with diabetes. Signs of autonomic disturbance include orthostatic hypotension, arrhythmias, anhydrosis, unreactive pupils, gastroparesis, impotence, and hypotonic bladder. A diagnosis of autonomic failure may be established by documenting orthostatic blood pressure in the absence of volume depletion, supersensitivity of the pupils to 0.125% pilocarpine, decreased sweating, and marked changes in rate on electrocardiogram during deep breathing.

Therapy of orthostatic hypotension includes the use of pressure stockings and discontinuing agents that may precipitate autonomic dysfunction. Fludrocortisone (Florinef) may also be helpful by increasing fluid retention and potentiating norepinephrine release.[41] Other useful agents include indomethacin, cimetidine,[42] and pindolol.[43] Gastroparesis may be treated with metoclopramide before meals and at bedtime. Patients with bladder dysfunction are urged to void on a fixed schedule using suprapubic pressure. Chronic intermittent catheterization may be necessary in severe cases.

Management of patients with autonomic dysfunction may be especially difficult in the perioperative period because of disturbed cardiovascular reflexes.[44–46] Patients may have fixed heart rates that are poorly responsive to anticholinergic agents and disordered respiratory control.[44,45] It is important to distinguish those with central autonomic dysfunction (Shy-Drager syndrome) from those with peripheral nerve abnormalities.[44] Those with the latter may be overly sensitive to direct-acting adrenergic agents like phenylephrine, while those with the former have a normal response.[44] Some have advocated the use of fentanyl for general anesthesia to decrease the risk of hypotension associated with inhalational agents.[44] Continuous monitoring of blood pressure, arterial blood gas measurements, and pulmonary artery pressures greatly assists management of these patients.

Amyotrophic Lateral Sclerosis

Amyotrophic lateral sclerosis (ALS) is a neurologic disorder characterized by weakness due to upper and lower motor neuron degeneration which is variable in extent and distribution. Sensation remains unimpaired. The diagnosis is made clinically, and there are no confirmatory laboratory tests. Electromyography may be helpful, and typically shows widespread denervation with fasciculations in both upper and lower extremities. Involvement of the lower brainstem motor nuclei may result in bulbar symptoms of dysphagia, dysarthria, and respiratory failure. The disorder tends to affect men slightly more than women and carries a median

survival rate of about four years.[47] The most common causes of death are cardiopulmonary arrest and bronchopneumonia.

Management of surgical patients with ALS is multidisciplinary. Respiratory status can be maximized by using incentive spirometry and chest physical therapy. Pulmonary function studies are helpful to exclude a superimposed treatable disorder like bronchospasm.[48] Abnormalities may mimic those of emphysema, with increased residual volume, reduced expiratory reserve volume, and maximal voluntary ventilation.[49] When possible, local or regional anesthesia is preferable to general anesthesia to avoid problems with respiratory weaning.

Since dysphagia may result in repeated aspiration, a feeding gastrostomy or jejunostomy may be required. Patients with ALS usually tolerate these minor procedures without difficulty. Mild hypoxia may be seen in stable patients with ALS. However, severe hypoxia and CO_2 retention are late signs of respiratory failure.[48]

INTRACRANIAL HYPERTENSION

Increased intracranial pressure (ICP) may be seen in surgical patients either as a preexisting condition or as a complication of anesthesia. Commonly encountered causes of elevated intracranial pressure include mass lesions of the brain, like tumor or abscess; and diffuse cerebral edema, as seen in fulminant hepatic failure, ischemia and anoxia, communicating and noncommunicating hydrocephalus, and trauma. The Monro-Kellie doctrine, formulated 150 years ago, views the cranium as a rigid container consisting of largely incompressible substances—brain, blood, and cerebrospinal fluid.[50] Intracranial hypertension, with its concurrent risk of diminished cerebral perfusion, results when an excess in one of these compartments is generated and the capacity of the intracranial vault to accommodate these perturbations, formally known as intracranial compliance, is exceeded. Injury to brain substance results when ICP causes alterations in intracranial perfusion, direct compression of nervous tissue, or herniation of intracranial contents.

Trauma

Accidents constitute the fourth leading cause of death in the United States, with an annual incidence of 48 per 100,000.[51] In the absence of rapidly deepening coma or evolving neurologic dysfunction, respiratory and hemodynamic stabilization are first priorities in injured patients. While only 20 percent of patients with head injuries require operative intervention, prompt neurosurgical and/or neurologic consultation to assess and follow the examination is essential. Most trauma units follow strict algorithms in dealing with such patients, and these include computerized tomography (CT) of the head as an early part of the evaluation.[52,53]

Intracranial hypertension and compartmental herniation can occur on the basis of epidural, subdural, subarachnoid, or intracerebral hemorrhage or contusion. Shearing injuries causing diffuse axonal injury may result in coma with or without associated deep midline hemorrhage.[54,55] Seriously injured patients with head trauma resulting in intracranial hypertension are managed according to the same principles outlined below. Adequate airway protection achieved by endotracheal intubation, hyperventilation, and appropriate use of hyperosmotic agents remain the mainstays of therapy. An intubation sequence utilizing sodium thiopental and intravenous lidocaine attenuates the increment in intracranial pressure commonly seen in this procedure. Palmer et al. advocate the early use of subarachnoid screws to assess intracranial pressure in such patients,[56] but this approach remains controversial. A small group of trauma patients may require simultaneous neurosurgical and general surgical intervention.

Diagnostic Considerations

Wakefulness is defined by both level of consciousness or arousal and the content and integrity of cognitive function or awareness. Normal cerebral function is dependent upon adequate cerebral blood flow and more specifically a cerebral perfusion pressure at or above 40 torr.[57,58] Autoregulatory mechanisms used to maintain cerebral perfusion pressure (equal to the mean arterial pressure minus the ICP) often fail in the setting of trauma, labile systemic blood pressure, hemorrhage, or infarction, and focal or generalized cerebral edema may supervene. Although the use of intracranial pressure monitoring devices has facilitated the measurement of cerebral perfusion pressure, serial neurologic examinations remain a sensitive noninvasive method to assess changes in intracranial pressure.

Rising ICP initially produces a change in level of consciousness, although early deterioration may be subtle. This decline in wakefulness occurs as a result of bilateral hemispheric dysfunction and/or compression of diencephalic or midbrain structures with consequent impairment of the reticular activating system. The level of neurologic function may be correlated with clinical signs (see Table 36–3). A few simple questions repeated at regular intervals and changed slightly to prevent memorization of the answers is often a sensitive test for early changes in level of consciousness in the awake patient.

As ICP rises, shifts in intracranial contents may develop, and if uninterrupted may lead to one of several herniation syndromes (see Table 36–4). Recognition of these dramatic changes must be prompt if intervention is to be effective. Herniation occurs when pressure differentials form either within the intracranial vault or between the intracranial vault and the spinal cord. Unilateral hemispheric tumor, hemorrhage, edema, or infection, alone or in combination, may result in a shift of one hemisphere beneath the falx cerebri. This syndrome of subfalcian herniation produces a change in level of consciousness and often progressive psychomotor retardation as limbic structures are disrupted. In the acute setting, lateral shifts of the brain, as measured by displacement of the pineal gland on CT scan, correlate with levels of consciousness.[59]

Intracranial hypertension due to mass lesions often leads to the syndrome of uncal herniation, in which the medial edge of the temporal lobe is forced through the opening of the tentorium separating the cerebral hemispheres from the posterior fossa. As herniation progresses, patients usually develop ipsilateral third nerve dysfunction, with the affected eye pointing down and out, and early pupillary dilation as well as progressive decline in wakefulness. This may be followed by contralateral or ipsilateral hemiparesis, depending on which cerebral peduncle is more compressed.

Diffuse elevation in ICP, particularly in the setting of widespread cerebral edema, results in central herniation. This is characterized by early decline in the level of consciousness due to disruption of the reticular activating system as it ascends from the upper pons to the thalamus. As the caudal brainstem and cerebellar tonsils are compressed through the rigid foramen magnum, profound bradycardia and associated systemic hypertension may occur and is known as Cushing's reflex. This is often a late manifestation of high ICP and may occur concurrently with Cheyne-Stokes respirations, an apneustic or hyperventilatory respiratory pattern, or, in the preterminal stage, ataxic breathing.

The approach to patients with elevated ICP depends on periodic reassessment of the state of consciousness, pattern of breathing, pupillary function, reflex eye movements, and motor response to a variety of stimuli.

Fulminant Hepatic Failure

With the advent of successful orthotopic liver transplantation, surgeons increasingly see patients with fulminant hepatic failure (FHF) and associated intracranial hypertension. FHF is defined by the onset of hepatic encephalopathy within two to eight weeks of the appearance of jaundice.[60] Pathologic studies have shown diffuse cerebral edema in over 80 percent of patients with FHF.[61,62] Less fulminant forms of liver failure have a lower incidence of cerebral edema, and this complication rarely occurs in patients with encephalopathy due to chronic liver disease. Diffuse cerebral edema is the major cause of mortality in patients with FHF await-

TABLE 36–3. Level of Neurologic Function Related to Clinical Signs

Level	Clinical Signs
Cerebral hemisphere	Higher intellectual function Purposeful movements
Diencephalon (thalamus)	Eye opening Decorticate posturing (arms flexed, legs extended)
Mesencephalon (midbrain)	Pupillary reflex (CN II → CN III) Decerebrate posturing (arms and legs extended)
Pontomesencephalic	Oculocephalics Calorics (CN VIII, VI, III, and medial longitudinal fasciculus)
Pontine	Corneal reflex (CN V → CN VII) Apneustic breathing
Medulla	Gag reflex (CN IX, X) Ataxic breathing

Source: Adapted from Plum F, and Posner JB.[73]

TABLE 36–4. Herniation Syndromes

	Respirations	Pupils	Eye Movements	Motor Response
Uncal Herniation				
Early	Normal	Dilated ipsilateral but reactive	Full	Purposeful
Late	Cheyne-Stokes or central neurogenic hyperventilation	Fixed and dilated	CN III palsy	Decorticate evolving to decerebrate
Central Herniation				
Early diencephalic	Normal or Cheyne-Stokes	Normal or small	Full	Purposeful
Late diencephalic	Cheyne-Stokes	Small, reactive	Full	Decorticate
Mesencephalic	Central neurogenic or Cheyne-Stokes	Fixed, mid-position	Dysconjugate internuclear ophthalmoplegia	Decerebrate
Low pontine	Agonal or ataxic	Fixed	None	None or reflexive

Source: Adapted from Plum F, and Posner JB.[73]

ing liver transplantation.[62,63] Patients may evolve from an encephalopathic state to decerebrate posturing as central herniation progresses. The associated rise in ICP results primarily from breakdown of the blood-brain barrier by accumulated toxins normally degraded by the liver.

This form of intracranial hypertension is notoriously difficult to treat and generally proves refractory to hyperventilation therapy and steroids. Treatment with hyperosmolar solutions like mannitol has demonstrated some efficacy, albeit in small series.[64] Some investigators have used charcoal hemoperfusion to remove toxic substances from the circulation with equivocal results.[65] More recently, intracranial pressure monitoring using an LADD epidural system has been utilized to assist in the care of patients with fulminant hepatic failure and deep coma.[66] Controlled studies demonstrating the benefit of this technique await completion.

Effects of Anesthetic Agents on ICP

The effects of various anesthetic agents on intracranial pressure (ICP) and subsequent neurologic function are complex. Intravenous barbiturates and narcotics combined with nitrous oxide remain popular for neurosurgical anesthesia. While nitrous oxide has little effect on cerebral blood flow, it can further increase ICP when the pressure is high initially.[67] Halothane, enflurane, and isoflurane all increase ICP. When enflurane was administered to dogs in which ICP had already been increased by an epidural balloon, there was further significant rise in ICP and associated fall in cerebral perfusion pressure.[68] A review of inhalational anesthetic use in neurosurgery has concluded that isoflurane is the best choice for most neurosurgical patients.[69] This agent seems to produce the smallest incremental increase in ICP and the smallest decrement in cerebral perfusion pressure. Gordon et al. also showed isoflurane to be safe in intracranial surgery, provided that hyperventilation maintains adequate hypocapnea.[70]

Treatment of Intracranial Hypertension

Prompt therapy for elevated ICP can often reverse what might initially seem to be a hopeless situation. Basic tenets of treatment area as follows:

1. Insure adequate airway and oxygenation.
2. Maintain adequate mean arterial pressure, avoiding the use of hypoosmolar fluids.
3. Hyperventilate the patient to a PCO_2 of 25 to 30 torr and maintain it at that level to produce an immediate although transient reduction in ICP.
4. Achieve isovolemic hyperosmolarity using osmotic agents like mannitol. Hypovolemia and an associated fall in mean arterial pressure should be avoided because they may compromise cerebral perfusion pressure. Normal saline together with an initial dose of 1 g/kg of 20% mannitol intravenously is the best combination. Subsequent doses of 0.25 to 0.5 g/kg every three to six hours should follow, titrated to either ICP or serum osmolarity of 310 to 315 milliosmoles.
5. Hypoxia is a potent stimulus to increased cerebral blood flow and should be avoided. PaO_2 should be maintained at a level of > 90 torr.
6. Adequate sedation, with or without the use of neuromuscular blockade, should be used in an intensive care unit as needed. This is particularly useful before uncomfortable procedures that might result in elevated ICP. Pretreatment with 0.5 to 0.75 mg/kg of sodium pentobarbital intravenously or lidocaine administered through the endotracheal tube may be particularly helpful prior to tracheal suctioning.
7. Slight elevation of the head to 20 to 30 degrees is probably of some use in reducing ICP.

8. Intracranial hypertension refractory to these measures may sometimes respond to high-dose barbiturate therapy with either thiopental or sodium pentobarbital.

9. Serious elevations in mean arterial pressure have been associated with exacerbation of cerebral edema, particularly in areas of the brain previously damaged by hemorrhage. Sustained systemic hypertension is best treated using small intravenous doses of propranolol intermittently or continuous infusion of intravenous labetalol. Beta-blockers have the dual advantage catecholamine blockade and little or no effect on cerebral blood flow, unlike peripheral vasodilators such as nitroprusside.

10. Careful supportive care with attention to serum electrolyte levels and nutritional therapy is critical in facilitating survival.

11. Use of corticosteroids has demonstrated efficacy only in the treatment of intracranial pressure due to vasogenic edema associated with a mass lesion. Dexamethasone is recommended in this situation with an initial dose of 20 mg intravenously followed by 6 to 10 mg every six hours. The use of corticosteroids in the treatment of elevated ICP associated with head trauma or hemorrhage has failed to improve morbidity and mortality in controlled studies.[71,72]

SUMMARY

1. Patients with epilepsy taking anticonvulsants not available in parenteral form (e.g., carbamazepine) should be covered with intravenous phenytoin or phenobarbital in the perioperative period.

2. Although there is no evidence that surgery accelerates the progression of multiple sclerosis, symptoms like urinary retention may worsen transiently due to fever and require special treatment.

3. Patients with immobilizing diseases like parkinsonism have an increased risk of pneumonia and decubitus ulcers. It is important to restart antiparkinsonian agents as soon as possible after surgery, monitoring the patient carefully for hypotension.

4. Autonomic dysfunction and/or respiratory insufficiency are common features of several neuromuscular diseases and may be exacerbated by general anesthesia. Vital signs and vital capacity measurements should be monitored carefully.

5. The increase in intracranial pressure seen with general anesthesia is due to Valsalva maneuvers during intubation, carbon dioxide accumulation, or the direct effect of the anesthetic on the cerebral vasculature. Patients with reduced intracranial compliance are especially vulnerable to increases in pressure and require periodic assessment of the state of consciousness, pattern of breathing, pupillary function, reflex eye movements, and motor responses. Direct monitoring of intracranial pressure through subarachnoid screws may be helpful.

REFERENCES

1. Hauser WE, Annegers JF, Andersen EV: Epidemiology and genetics of epilepsy. *Res Publ Assoc Res Nerv Ment Dis* 61:267–294, 1983.
2. Goldenson ES (ed): The nonconvulsive epilepsies; clinical manifestations, diagnostic considerations, and treatment. *Epilepsia* 24(Suppl 1):S1–S82, 1983.
3. Al-Khudhairi D, Whitwam JG: Autonomic reflexes and the cardiovascular effects of propylene glycol. *Br J Anaesth* 58:897–902, 1986.
4. Louis S, Kutt H, McDowell F: The cardiocirculatory effects of Dilantin and its solvent. *Am Heart J* 74:523–529, 1967.
5. Modica PA, Tempelhoff R, White PF: Pro- and anticonvulsant effects of anesthetics (Part I). *Anesth Analg* 70:303–315, 1990.
6. Modica PA, Tempelhoff R, White PF: Pro- and anticonvulsant effects of anesthetics (Part II). *Anesth Analg* 70:433–444, 1990.
7. McDonald WI, Silberberg DH (eds): *Multiple Sclerosis*. London, Butterworths; 1986.
8. Schauf CL, Davis FA: Impulse conduction in multiple sclerosis: A theoretical basis for modification by temperature and pharmacological agents. *J Neurol Neurosurg Psych* 37:152–161, 1974.
9. Stern MB, Hurtig HI (eds): *The Comprehensive Management of Parkinson's Disease*. New York, PMA Publishing, 1988.
10. Lieberman A, Dziatolowski M, Coopersmith M et al: Dementia in Parkinson's disease. *Ann Neurol* 6:335–359, 1979.
11. Mayeux R, Rosenstein R, Stern Y et al: The prevalence and risk of dementia in idiopathic Parkinson's disease. *Arch Neurol* 45:260–262, 1988.
12. Boller F, Mizutani T, Roessman U et al: Parkinson's disease, dementia and Alzheimer's disease: clinicopathological correlations. *Ann Neurol* 1:329–335, 1980.
13. Goldberg L: Levodopa and anesthesia. *Anesthesiology* 34:1–2, 1971.
14. Ngai S: Parkinsonism, levodopa, and anesthesia: *Anesthesiology* 7:344–351, 1972.
15. Olanow CW, Alberts M, Staijch J et al: A randomized blinded study of low-dose bromocriptine versus low-dose carbidopa-levodopa in untreated Parkinson patients, in Fahn S, Marsden CD, Calne D et al (eds): *Recent Developments in Parkinson's Disease*. Florham Park, NJ, Macmillan Health Care, 1987, vol 2, pp 201–208.
16. Rinne UK: Early combination of bromocriptine and levodopa in the treatment of Parkinson's disease: A five-year follow-up. *Neurology* 37:826–828, 1987.
17. The Parkinson Study Group: Effect of deprenyl on the progression of disability in early Parkinson's disease. *N Engl J Med* 321:1364–1371, 1989.
18. Lisak RP: Myasthenia gravis: Mechanisms and management. *Hosp Prac* 101–109, March 1983.
19. Scadding GK, Havard CWH: Pathogenesis and treatment of myasthenia gravis. *Br Med J* 283:1008–1012, 1981.
20. Seybold ME, Drachman DB: Gradually increasing doses of prednisone in myasthenia gravis: Reducing the hazard of treatment. *N Engl J Med* 290:81–84, 1974.
21. Lisak RP, Barchi RL: *Myasthenia Gravis*. Philadelphia, Saunders, 1982.
22. Seybold ME: Myasthenia gravis: A clinical and basic science review. *JAMA* 250:2516–2520, 1983.
23. Buckingham MB, Howard FM, Bernatz PE et al: The value of thymectomy in myasthenia gravis: A computer-assisted matched study. *Ann Surg* 184:453–458, 1976.
24. Mulder DG, Graves M, Herrmann C: Thymectomy for myasthenia gravis: Recent observations and comparisons with past experience. *Ann Thorac Surg* 48:551–555, 1989.
25. Adams SL, Mathews J, Grammer LC: Drugs that may exacerbate myasthenia gravis. *Ann Emerg Med* 13:532–538, 1984.
26. Nilsson E, Meretoja OA: Vecuronium dose-response and maintenance requirements in patients with myasthenia gravis. *Anesthesiology* 73(1):28–32, 1990.
27. Mehta MP, Gengis SD, Sokoll MD: Anesthesia and neuromuscular diseases. *MEJ Anesth* 8(1):49–63, 1985.
28. O'Neill JH, Murray MF, Newsom-Davies J: The Lambert-Eaton myasthenia syndrome: A review of 50 cases. *Brain* 111:577–596, 1988.
29. Telford RJ, Hollway TE: The myasthenic syndrome: Anaesthesia in a

patient treated with 3,4-diaminopyridine. *Br J Anaesth* 64(3):363–366, 1990.

30. Macdonell RA, Rich JM, Cros D et al: The Lambert-Eaton myasthenic syndrome: A cause of delayed recovery from general anesthesia. *Arch Phys Med Rehabil* 73(1):98–100, 1992.

31. Griggs RC, Davis RJ, Anderson DC: Cardiac conduction in myotonic dystrophy. *Am J Med* 59:37–42, 1975.

32. Tanaka M, Tanaka Y: Cardiac anaesthesia in a patient with myotonic dystrophy. *Anaesthesia* 46:462–465, 1991.

33. Jozefowicz RF, Griggs RC: Myotonic dystrophy. *Neur Clin* 6(3):455–472, 1988.

34. Asbury AK: Diagnostic considerations in Guillain-Barré syndrome. *Ann Neurol* 9(Suppl 1):1–5, 1981.

35. Arnason B, Asbury AK: Idiopathic polyneuritis following surgery. *Arch Neurol* 18:500–507, 1968.

36. Lichtenfield P: Autonomic dysfunction in the Guillain-Barré syndrome. *Am J Med* 50:772–780, 1971.

37. Lisak RP, Brown MJ: Acquired demyelinating polyneuropathies. *Sem Neurol* 7(1):40–48, 1987.

38. The Guillain-Barré Study Group. Plasmapheresis and acute Guillain-Barré syndrome. *Neurology* 35:1096–1104, 1985.

39. Hughes R, Newsom-Davies J, Perkins G et al: Controlled trial of prednisolone in acute polyneuropathy. *Lancet* 2:750–753, 1978.

40. Ropper AH, Shahani BW: Diagnosis of acute areflexic paralysis in Guillain-Barré syndrome, in *Peripheral Nerve Disorders*. London, Butterworths, 1984, pp 21–45.

41. Davies B, Bannister R, Sever P et al: The pressor actions of noradrenaline, angiotensin II and saralasin in chronic autonomic failure treated with fludrocortisone. *Br J Clin Pharm* 8:253–260, 1979.

42. Stacpoole PW, Robertson D: Combination H_1 and H_2 receptor antagonist therapy in diabetic autonomic neuropathy. *South Med J* 75:634–635, 1982.

43. Frewin DB, Leonello PP, Pentale RK et al: Pindolol in orthostatic hypotension. *Med J Aust* 1:128, 1980.

44. Stirt JA, Frantz RA, Gunz EF et al: Anesthesia, catecholamines and hemodynamics in autonomic dysfunction. *Anesth Analg* 61(8):701–704, 1982.

45. Sweeney BP, Jones S, Langford RM: Anaesthesia in dysautonomia: Further complications. *Anaesthesia* 40:783–786, 1985.

46. Osborne PJ, Lee LW: Idiopathic orthostatic hypotension, midodrine, and anaesthesia. *Can J Anaesth* 38(4):499–501, 1991.

47. Curoscio JT, Mulvehall MN, Sterling R et al: Amyotrophic lateral sclerosis: Its natural history. *Neurol Clin* 5(1):1–8, 1987.

48. Braun SR: Respiratory system in amyotrophic lateral sclerosis. *Neurol Clin* 5(1):9–31, 1987.

49. Fallat RJ, Jewitt B, Bass M et al: Spirometry in amyotrophic lateral sclerosis. *Arch Neurol* 36:74–80, 1979.

50. Monro A: *Observations of the structure and function of the nervous system*. Edinborough, Creech & Johnson, 1783.

51. Frost EAM: Central nervous system trauma. *Anesth Clin N Amer* 5(3):565–585, 1987.

52. French BN, Dublin AB: The value of computerized tomography in the management of 1000 consecutive head injuries. *Surg Neurol* 7:171–183, 1977.

53. McMicken DB: Emergency CT head scans in traumatic and atraumatic conditions. *Ann Emerg Med* 1513:274–279, 1986.

54. Ropper AH, Miller DC: Acute traumatic midbrain hemorrhage. *Ann Neurol* 18:80–86, 1985.

55. Gennarelli TA, Thibault LE, Adams JH: Diffuse axonal injury and traumatic coma in primates. *Ann Neurol* 12:564–574, 1982.

56. Palmer MA, Perry JF, Fischer RF: Intracranial pressure monitoring in the acute neurologic assessment of multi-injured patients. *J Trauma* 19:497–501, 1979.

57. Jennet WB, Harper AM, Miller JE: Relation between cerebral blood flow and cerebral perfusion pressure. *Br J Surg* 57:390–396, 1970.

58. Haggental E, Lofgren J, Nilsson J: Effects of varied cerebrospinal fluid pressures on cerebral blood flow in dogs. *Acta Phys Scand* 79:262–271, 1970.

59. Ropper AH: Lateral displacement of the brain and level of consciousness in patients with an acute hemispheral mass. *N Engl J Med* 314:953–958, 1986.

60. Bernau J, Rueff B, Benhamov JP: Fulminant and subfulminant liver failure: Definitions and causes. *Sem Liver Dis* 6:97–106, 1986.

61. Silk DBA, Hanid MA, Trewby PN: Treatment of fulminant hepatic failure by polyacrylonitrate membrane haemodialysis. *Lancet* 2:1–3, 1977.

62. Williams R, Ede RJ: Hepatic encephalopathy and cerebral edema: *Sem Liver Dis* 6:107–118, 1986.

63. Hanid MA, Davies M, Mellon PJ: Clinical monitoring of intracranial pressure in fulminant hepatic failure. *Gut* 21:866–869, 1980.

64. Canalese J, Gimson AES, Davis C: Controlled trial of dexamethasone and mannitol for the cerebral edema of fulminant hepatic failure. *Gut* 23:625–629, 1982.

65. Gimson AES, Braude S, Mellon PJ: Earlier charcoal hemoperfusion in fulminant hepatic failure. *Lancet* 2:681–682, 1982.

66. Potter D, Peachey T, Eason J: Intracranial pressure monitoring during orthotropic liver transplantation for acute liver failure. *Anesth Agents Transpl Proc* 21:3528, 1989.

67. Phirman JR, Shapiro HM: Modification of nitrous oxide induced intracranial hypertension by prior induction of anesthesia. *Anesthesiology* 46:150, 1977.

68. Boop WC, Knight R: Enflusive anesthesia and changes of intracranial pressure. *J Neurosurg* 48:228–231, 1978.

69. Frost EAM: Inhalation anesthetic agents in neurosurgery. *Br J Anesth* 56:47S–56S, 1984.

70. Gordon E, Lagerkranser M, Rudehill A: The effect of isoflurane on cerebrospinal fluid pressure in patients undergoing neurosurgery. *Acta Anaesth Scand* 32:108–112, 1988.

71. Poungvarin N, Bhoopat W, Viriyovejakul A: Effects of dexamethasone in primary supratentorial intracerebral hemorrhage. *N Engl J Med* 316:1229–1233, 1987.

72. Faupel G, Revlen HJ, Muller D: Double-blind study on the effects of steroids on severe closed-head injury, in Pappius HM, Feindel W (eds): *Dynamics of Brain Edema*. Berlin, Springer-Verlag, 1976, pp 337–343.

73. Plum F, Posner JB: *The Diagnosis of Stupor and Coma*, 3d ed. Philadelphia, Davis, 1980, pp 87–175.

37 SURGERY IN THE PATIENT WITH PSYCHIATRIC ILLNESS

Joel E. Streim

Gary L. Gottlieb

Just as coexisting medical problems can complicate the care of surgical patients, psychiatric illness may also influence the perioperative course. Unfortunately, there are few studies that identify and measure the relative risk of perioperative complications or adverse outcomes in patients with specific psychiatric disorders undergoing surgery. Therefore, many of the proposed guidelines for preoperative assessment and management are based on descriptive reports and clinical experience.

Much of the literature in this area gives little attention to current psychiatric diagnostic methods. The current standard reference for clinical psychiatric diagnostic criteria is the Diagnostic and Statistical Manual of Psychiatric Disorders of the American Psychiatric Association, Third Edition–Revised (DSM III-R).[1] The DSM III-R uses an algorithmic approach to describe constellations of signs and symptoms specific to individual diagnoses. The reliability and construct validity of DSM III-R criteria have been established for many diagnoses.[2] The medical and surgical literature often describes patients with isolated psychological symptoms, personality traits, or behaviors. However, these subjects may not meet the diagnostic criteria of DSM III-R for a diagnosis of psychiatric disorder.

It is important to recognize that isolated emotional symptoms, personality traits, adaptive and maladaptive defenses, coping strategies, and other behavior patterns may affect the perioperative course. These psychological factors allow description of a profile for every patient, whether or not that person has a diagnosable psychiatric illness. Care must be taken to distinguish between the effects of psychological factors in nonpsychiatrically ill patients and the effects of psychiatric illness. Because psychological studies of surgical patients often do not apply strict diagnostic criteria for psychiatric disorders, much of what we know about the perioperative care of psychiatrically ill patients is inferred. This chapter focuses primarily on what is and what is not known about the preoperative assessment and management of surgical patients with common psychiatric disorders.

RISKS ASSOCIATED WITH PSYCHIATRIC DISORDERS IN SURGICAL PATIENTS

Anxiety Disorders

The lack of attention to diagnostic criteria for psychiatric disorders in surgical patients is exemplified in the literature on anxiety. Many have recognized that the term *anxiety* is often ambiguously defined.[3,4] Most investigators have studied anxiety as a character style (trait) or as an isolated symptom (state) in surgical patients.[5,6] Extrapolation of these findings to predict risk in patients who meet the criteria for a diagnosis of anxiety disorder is at best difficult.

The study of the relationship of preoperative anxiety level to postoperative outcome over the past 30 years has yielded contradictory and noncomparable data.[7] Janis observed that patients with moderate levels of preoperative anxiety were least likely to have emotional adjustment problems postoperatively.[8] However, those with high preoperative anxiety levels were found to display intense fear postoperatively and were often unable to derive comfort from reassurance. Patients with low preoperative anxiety levels tended to be angry and resentful after surgery and were postulated to have unrealistic expectations leaving them poorly prepared for the process of surgical recovery. Titchener and Levine also found that patients with low preoperative anxiety levels used denial excessively, resulting in maladaptive emotional responses.[9] In contrast, subsequent investigators found that patients with little preoperative anxiety were actually less likely to have postoperative emotional problems and did have realistic expectations about surgical outcome.[10] The association between preoperative anxiety and postoperative mood disturbance is supported by the finding that women undergoing hysterectomy with high preoperative anxiety scores on Spielberger's State-Trait Anxiety Inventory (STAI) were more likely to be depressed both before and after surgery.[11,12] In any case, the effects of poor postoperative emotional adjustment on physical function and on surgical outcome were not addressed in these studies.

Wolfer and Davis found no significant connections between preoperative anxiety and postoperative outcome variables.[7] Christensen found some correlation between preoperative anxiety measures and emotional states and fatigue, but preoperative anxiety failed to predict postoperative fatigue definitively.[6] More recently, Johnston and Carpenter measured preoperative anxiety using the STAI and attempted to correlate scores with postoperative outcomes, including levels of anxiety and depression, subjective pain ratings, length of hospital stay, and return to independence in self-care and activities of daily living.[5] They found that patients with low preoperative anxiety recover more slowly than those with moderate anxiety. They also found that preoperative "negative affect" predicts postoperative "negative affect," although the term "negative affect" was not clearly defined in terms of STAI scores.

In a review of studies measuring neuroticism or trait anxiety, Mathews found that about half showed a significant relationship between anxiety and parameters of surgical outcome.[4] Although some studies suggested that "high neuroticism" is correlated with postoperative pain ratings, respiratory complications, and longer hospital stays, others failed to demonstrate any clear associations. Responses to both psychological and physical stress have been shown to correlate with immune function and surgical outcomes. Linn et al. found that high-level response to stressful life events and cold-pressor stress was associated with lower lymphocyte response to mitogen stimulation and more postoperative complications and narcotic use.[13] However, the association of the stress response patterns to a profile of anxiety symptoms and specific disorders was not investigated. Several investigators have also looked for a relationship between anxiety and postcardiotomy delirium, but findings are contradictory.[14,15] Conclusions are therefore difficult to draw because of major differences among the studies in the measures used and in the populations studied.

In summary, the literature confirms that symptoms of anxiety are prevalent in surgical patients and may be related to postoperative mood states. However, effects of anxiety on parameters of surgical outcome like extent of analgesic use, length of hospital stay, or return to independent function have not been conclusively demonstrated. Furthermore, there are no evaluations of the risks associated with surgery and anesthesia in patients who meet DSM III-R criteria for generalized anxiety disorder, panic disorder, or phobias.

Clinical experience suggests that signs and symptoms of these psychiatric disorders may complicate the perioperative course or interfere with management and rehabilitation. For example, anxiety may cause tachycardia that may be deleterious in some surgical patients. Patients who are anxious about ambulating and do not engage productively in rehabilitative efforts may have an increased risk of pulmonary, thromboembolic, cardiovascular, and musculoskeletal complications. However, there are no studies assessing the risk of specific complications like pneumonia, cardiac ischemia, deep-vein thrombosis, cardiovascular deconditioning, or contractures in patients with anxiety.

Depression

As in anxiety, the literature on depression in surgical patients is inadequate. Depression is often poorly defined, and diagnostic criteria, study populations, and selection of outcome measures vary widely from study to study. Early studies demonstrated that patients with depression before surgery have a higher incidence of morbidity and mortality.[17–19] This is consistent with the known decline in immune competence associated with depression[20,21] and with findings of increased medical morbidity in depressed persons in the general population. Preoperative depression significantly increases the risk of immediate postoperative cognitive dysfunction.[22,23] By contrast, a small prospective study of heart transplant patients indicated that depressive symptoms did not predict postoperative psychiatric complications.[24]

Depressive symptoms can complicate the perioperative course and interfere with medical management and rehabilitation. Apathy and ambivalence may reduce motivation, and impaired concentration may limit participation in perioperative teaching efforts and essential activities like pulmonary toilet and physical therapy.[25] Hospital staff caring for patients who feel hopeless and appear unmotivated may themselves give up. Diminished appetite may compromise nutrition and limit wound healing.[26] However, there are no controlled studies which identify or measure the risks of these complications attributable to depressive symptoms. Ironically, Dubovsky has reported that morbidly obese patients with preoperative depression undergoing gastroplasty are more successful in losing weight after surgery than those who are not so depressed.[27]

Psychotic Disorders

Patients with psychosis may have disorganized thought processes, delusional ideas, hallucinations, and bizarre or otherwise inappropriate behavior. Such psychotic features may be present in patients with major depression, bipolar affective disorder, delusional disorder, dementia, delirium, drug intoxication, and schizophrenia.[1] Evidence of preoperative psychosis is associated with postoperative psychiatric morbidity. Morse and Litin documented postoperative delirium in 87 percent of patients with preoperative somatic delusions.[28] However, the relationship of psychosis to nonpsychiatric outcome was not studied.

Clinical experience has demonstrated ways in which psychosis may interfere with perioperative management. Patients may be uncooperative when delusional thinking incorporates unrealistic beliefs about the nature of illness or treatment.[29] For example, a patient with paranoid delusions may refuse to consent to surgery for fear that the doctors want to kill him. After surgery, he may not cooperate with incentive spirometry because he believes that hospital staff is forcing radioactivity into the room through the heating ducts. Patients with schizophrenia may have somatic delusions or misperceptions that can result in unreliable reporting of symptoms. Some schizophrenic patients have decreased pain perception or expression leading to difficulties in assessing symptoms and making diagnoses.[30]

A recent retrospective study showed that a history of serious psychiatric illness was not associated with an increased risk of poor surgical outcome.[31] Patients with chronic schizophrenia and chronic depression tolerated surgery well. Postoperative behavioral management difficulties occurred in patients who had experienced acute "severe upset" before surgery unrelated to preoperative psychiatric diagnosis. In their study of 200 institutionalized patients undergoing surgery, Cutler and Fink found that patients with chronic psychosis had no significant difference in postoperative complication rate compared to control patients.[32] Hackett and Cassem emphasize the increased risk of suicide in patients with psychotic depression,[29] but this issue has not been examined in the perioperative period. However, they believe that psychosis by itself is not a contraindication to surgery.

In contrast, Mai regards "florid psychosis" as an absolute contraindication to heart transplant surgery.[33] However, because it is difficult to find heart transplant recipients with a history of a psychotic disorder, it is not known what risk psychosis confers on surgical outcome. In a series of 25 cardiac transplant patients, 17 had a psychiatric diagnosis preoperatively, but none had a history of psychosis.[34] Two patients died in the perioperative period, but without mortality data on matched controls it is impossible to establish a relationship between psychosis or other psychiatric disorders and perioperative mortality in transplant patients.

Cognitive Impairment

Patients with cognitive impairment have higher rates of morbidity and mortality than those of the general population. This relationship has also been demonstrated in surgical populations. In a prospective study of elderly patients with hip fractures, senile dementia was associated with increased long-term mortality.[35] The presence of brain damage and cognitive impairment preoperatively has been shown to correlate with delirium in postcardiotomy patients.[36–38] In one study, preoperative impairment of concentration and abstract thinking were found to be highly predictive of fatal outcome in patients undergoing cardiac surgery.[39]

Because impaired cognition is often associated with signs and symptoms of psychosis, the whole range of perioperative problems discussed above may be encountered in these patients. However, similar data are not found in studies of surgical outcome in patients with psychosis without concomitant cognitive impairment. Furthermore, there are no published studies of cognitively impaired surgical patients in which perioperative morbidity and mortality are shown to be a function of psychotic symptoms. Nevertheless, Mai cites both "irreversible brain damage" and "florid psychosis" as absolute contraindications to heart transplant.[33] One might infer that this recommendation is based on the clinical expectation that both of these conditions predict a poor understanding of and compliance with treatment.

Cognitive impairment may also be a postoperative complication. Common examples are postanoxic encephalopathy and delirium. Many investigators have tried to identify etiologic factors underlying postoperative delirium. While specific etiology remains unclear, preoperative psychiatric illness appears to be an important risk factor in the development of postoperative delirium.[40] A meta-analysis of 18 empiric studies revealed that the magnitude of cognitive decompensation and delirium after surgery increases with the age of the patient.[41]

Patients with mental retardation also exhibit cognitive impairment, but an association between retardation and surgical complications has not been demonstrated. Cutler and Fink showed that institutionalized patients with severe retardation or a combination of retardation, chronic psychosis, and seizure disorder had a complication rate 3.5 times that of noninstitutionalized control patients.[32] Institutionalized patients were more likely to receive general anesthesia which was associated with most of the complications, length of hospital stay, and mortality. Half of the complications were atelectasis or pneumonia. Voitk also noted a high rate of pulmonary complications in severely mentally retarded patients undergoing laparotomy and attributed it to cognitive inability to

cooperate with respiratory measures.[42] He speculated that a high incidence of gastroesophageal reflux in these patients increased the likelihood of aspiration and suggested that general anesthesia be avoided when possible. Selected retarded patients may benefit from use of an indwelling epidural catheter for postoperative analgesia instead of systemic narcotics. Finally, potential problems arise from lack of cooperation due to patient misunderstanding or mistrust of the physician[43] and behavioral changes ascribed to medications.[44] A review of the perioperative risks of cardiovascular, metabolic, and other anomalies sometimes associated with mental retardation is beyond the scope of this chapter.

Somatoform Disorders

Patients who present with somatic symptoms in the absence of demonstrable disease pose a serious challenge to the physician. Although some meet diagnostic criteria for psychiatric disorders such as hypochondriasis, conversion disorder, somotoform pain disorder, body dysmorphic disorder, and somatization disorder,[1] others exhibit an amplified or exaggerated focus on somatic concerns without being psychiatrically ill.[45] Some of these patients undergo surgical treatment and are often disappointed with the result.[1,46] In a study comparing women with somatization disorders to women with major depression, the somatizers had three times as many operations and hospitalizations as the depressed patients. The authors concluded that somatizers receive excess medical and surgical care.[47] A review of patients treated for chronic back pain in a pain treatment center revealed that 68 percent had undergone disc surgery for persistent pain associated with a psychiatric problem although they did not meet accepted criteria for surgical intervention.[48] Those who had a second procedure met these criteria, but in 73 percent reoperation was needed to treat the effects of the earlier surgery.

Although few other studies attempt to quantify the morbidity of "unnecessary" surgery, there are many descriptions of patients with unexplained symptoms who have an increased risk of morbidity from invasive diagnostic tests and surgical procedures.[49–51] These patients often go "doctor shopping" and can be demanding and persistent in their pursuit of an elusive diagnosis or relief of symptoms refractory to multiple empiric trials of treatment.[52] Typically, surgery fails to relieve their symptoms, and they become angry or dissatisfied with the result.

Personality Disorders

Studies of the relationship of personality characteristics to surgical outcome have focused mainly on anxiety as a personality trait.[5] However, other personality traits complicate perioperative management. Most studies of personality factors in surgical patients have used instruments that detect traits but do not diagnose psychiatric disorders. Therefore, conclusions about surgical risks in patients with maladaptive personality traits are not entirely referable to patients who meet strict diagnostic criteria for personality disorder.

Some personality traits have been associated with dissatisfaction, strained doctor-patient relationships, and litigation,[26] or with difficulty adjusting to the result of surgery. Patients undergoing rhinoplasty with preoperative personality problems frequently have increased nervous symptoms related to unmet expectations a year after the procedure.[53] Preoperative personality characteristics in those undergoing mastectomy are related to postoperative depression, anxiety, and sexual dysfunction.[54] Long reported that nearly half of the patients who failed to obtain relief from back surgery were diagnosed as having a personality disorder.[48]

Patients with personality disorders are often uncooperative and poorly compliant with treatment protocols and rehabilitation efforts.[26] Personality disorders characterized by antisocial or aggressive behavior have been associated with poor compliance in organ transplant programs.[32] Antisocial traits are also strongly associated with alcohol abuse and with somatization disorders that can complicate surgical management.[1,55] Patients with dependent personailty traits may lack motivation to resume self-care, ambulation, and independent function. Those with narcissistic traits may presume that the job of restoring health and function is the sole responsibility of the health care team. These patients may become resentful when they are expected to participate actively in the recovery process. Obsessive-compulsive personality traits are characterized by inflexible behavior patterns and procrastination that may limit cooperation with procedures requiring departure from rigid personal routines. Patients with histrionic traits tend to have exaggerated reactions to stressful situations and may be overwhelmed by perioperative events. Their emotional and behavioral lability may interfere with their ability to cooperate optimally with perioperative care.

Although these personality characteristics or traits may be present to varying degrees in surgical patients who otherwise do not warrant a diagnosis of personality disorder, there are no systematic studies relating them to perioperative morbidity. Clinical experience suggests that psychiatric consultation is often requested for patients who do not have a history of psychiatric illness or a previous diagnosis of a personality disorder but who adapt poorly to the context of surgical treatment. Collaborative research among all members of the health care team is needed to define the risk of poor surgical outcome in this diverse group of patients.

PERIOPERATIVE RISKS AND MANAGEMENT OF PSYCHOTROPIC DRUGS

Psychotropic drugs have an important role in the effective treatment of psychiatric disorders. Their complex effects on cardiovascular and autonomic nervous system function warrant careful consideration in the perioperative period. Patients treated with psychotropic drugs may have altered responses to other medications. With proper precautions, psychotropic drugs can be managed safely in surgical patients.

Tricyclic Antidepressants

Tricyclic antidepressants (TCA's) block synaptic reuptake of norepinephrine and block vasoconstrictor postsynaptic alpha$_1$ adrenergic receptors and presynaptic alpha$_2$ receptors. They have anticholinergic effects blocking both central cholinergic and peripheral muscarinic receptors, and they slow cardiac atrioventricular conduction and cause sedation.[16,56]

Alpha$_1$ blockade may result in orthostatic hypotension and augment the hypotensive effects of peripheral vasodilators.[57] Surgical patients who develop hypertension while taking TCA's may be safely treated with vasodilators like nitroprusside or alpha-adrenergic blockers such as phentolamine, but lower doses may be required. Exaggerated blood pressure responses have been reported after administration of indirect-acting vasopressors like ephedrine to patients taking TCA's. When patients on TCA's require vasopressors during the perioperative period, direct-acting drugs like methoxamine or phenylephrine may be better choices.[16,58]

The effects of TCA's on cardiac atrioventricular conduction include P-R interval prolongation, QRS complex widening, or an increased QT/QTc on the electrocardiogram (ECG). Patients with preexisting bundle branch block have an increased risk of developing significant conduction problems when they are treated with TCA's.[57] In the absence of preexisting cardiac conduction disturbances or toxic plasma concentrations of TCA's, reports of cardiac conduction problems are rare.[59,60] However, continuous ECG monitoring in the perioperative period has been recommended for patients taking TCA's.[58]

Other cardiac effects are less clinically significant. Left ventricular function is not depressed by TCA's even in patients with preexisting congestive heart failure.[57,61,62] However, in some studies, 50 percent of patients with preexisting congestive failure treated with imipramine developed orthostatic hypotension.[63,64] Although cardiac arrhythmias may occur at toxic plasma levels, there is little convincing evidence that TCA's alone at therapeutic levels increase the risk of arrhythmia. In fact, TCA's at therapeutic plasma concentrations have significant antiarrhythmic activity similar to that of type IA compounds like quinidine and procainamide.[54,65] Chronic imipramine use in patients anesthetized with halothane and then given pancuronium has been associated with tachyarrhythmias.[66] The newer agents vecuronium and atracurium have not been associated with arrhythmias in patients taking TCA's, but continuous ECG monitoring has been recommended when these drugs are used in combination in the perioperative period.[16] Acute treatment with imipramine has also been shown to lower the dose of epinephrine required to induce ventricular arrhythmias during anesthesia with volatile agents in dogs.[67] While chronic treatment with imipramine does not do so,[68] low risk in humans can only be inferred.

Although TCA's have been thought to increase the risk of seizures in patients treated with enflurane,[69] this effect has not been substantiated. The combination of TCA's and other anticholinergic drugs may result in a wide range of adverse effects, including tachycardia, xerostomia and xerophthalmia, constipation or ileus, urinary retention, and delirium. Doses of anticholinergic drugs, including those used for premedication, may need to be reduced to avert these problems. Similarly, the antihistaminic effects of TCA's commonly cause sedation, and the combined sedative and ventilatory depressant effects of TCA's, opioids, and barbiturates may warrant dose reduction.[16] Ventilatory depressant effects of TCA's at therapeutic plasma levels do not complicate anesthesia or analgesia in humans, but lower doses of opioids and barbiturates may be effective in patients on TCA's.

When TCA's cause hemodynamic compromise or heart block, they can be discontinued abruptly. Drug withdrawal may cause insomnia, REM sleep rebound, and sometimes nightmares. Patients can be treated symptomatically with chloral hydrate or short-acting benzodiazepines. Cholinergic rebound is rare but can be treated with low doses of atropinic agents. TCA's should otherwise be tapered over one to two weeks to minimize sleep disturbances.

Chronic treatment with TCA's need not be discontinued before most elective surgery.[16,40,58] TCA's can be administered until just before surgery and resumed as soon as the patient can take oral fluids.[26] Amitriptyline and imipramine are available in parenteral form as needed. It has not been established that patients who have taken therapeutic doses of TCA's for less than one month before surgery have an increased risk of arrhythmias. Until further studies of arrhythmogenicity have been conducted, epinephrine and pancuronium should be avoided when volatile anesthetic agents are used.

Monoamine Oxidase Inhibitors

Monoamine oxidase inhibitors (MAOI's) are used primarily in the treatment of depression. They inhibit oxidative deamination of monoamine neurotransmitters, resulting in increased intraneuronal levels of epinephrine, norepinephrine, serotonin, and dopamine. Inhibition of hepatic microsomal enzymes, anticholinergic effects, orthostatic hypotension, and sedation are additional effects of MAOI's.

A major concern is the risk of severe hypertension in patients on MAOI's who take sympathomimetic drugs or ingest foods with high tyramine content. Sympathomimetic drugs or tyramine can stimulate the release of excess norepinephrine accumulated in postganglionic sympathetic nerve endings and precipitate a hypertensive crisis. This effect has been reported with tyramine,[70] ephedrine,[71] and metaraminol.[72]

The risk of severe hypertension led to earlier recommendations that MAOI's be discontinued 14 to 21 days before elective surgery to allow synthesis of new enzyme.[73–75] However, several investigators have noted that only hydrazine compounds like phenelzine, isocarboxazid, and iproniazid cause irreversible blockade of monoamine oxidase and produce effects that persist for 14 to 21 days following cessation of therapy. Nonhydrazine compounds like tranylcypromine, pargyline, and deprenyl cause reversible inhibition of monoamine oxidase, and their effects dissipate within 24 hours of their discontinuation.[58,76] Therefore, these latter drugs do not need to be discontinued more than two days before surgery.

More recent evidence indicates that even patients receiving hydrazine compounds may undergo anesthesia safely without waiting 14 to 21 days.[76–78] In a prospective study of 27 patients on chronic MAOI therapy for three months to three years and exposed to various anesthetic and surgical procedures, El-Ganzouri et al. found no adverse effects of MAOI's on blood pressure, heart rate, temperature, electrocardiogram, or degree of neuromuscular blockade.[79] They concluded that it is not necessary to discontinue MAOI's before surgery. However, patients on MAOI's for less than three months were excluded from the study because of evidence from animal experiments that short-term treatment with MAOI's, volatile anesthetics, and epinephrine used concomitantly may increase the risk of arrhythmias.[67] In addition, because of the numerous reports of adverse reactions with meperidine and indirect-acting sympathomimetic amines, they were not administered to patients in El-Ganzouri's study.

The possibility of adverse interactions between MAOI's and opioids is also of concern. Hypertension, hypotension, tachycardia, hyperthermia, respiratory depression, muscle rigidity, hyperreflexia, seizures, and coma have all been reported with the combination.[80,81] Although the mechanism of these reactions is unclear, it may be related to reduction in serotonin metabolism induced by MAOI's or inhibition of hepatic metabolism of opioids. Although most of these reports involve the use of the opioid meperidine for analgesia, some advise that narcotic-based anesthetic techniques should be avoided in patients on MAOI's.[82] Others have reported

use of narcotic anesthesia in patients taking MAOI's chronically without any adverse effect.[77,79]

Studies of large numbers of patients are required to demonstrate more conclusively that the risk of continuing MAOI's perioperatively and using narcotic-based anesthesia in these patients is sufficiently low to support these practices. However, recent studies strongly suggest that, when it is difficult or impossible to discontinue MAOI's before surgery, the risk of complications is lower than originally believed.

The risk of complications in patients on MAOI's can be further reduced by attention to a few additional principles and precautions. Since MAOI's inhibit hepatic microsomal enzyme activity required to metabolize barbiturates and opiates, it may be necessary to reduce the doses of these drugs. Although fentanyl and morphine have been used uneventfully during surgery,[79] it is recommended that opioids be avoided when hydrazine MAOI's have been given in the preceding two weeks. Barbiturates and benzodiazepines are acceptable alternatives for induction.[58] Similarly, the effects of succinylcholine may be prolonged because of decreased plasma cholinesterase activity. In this case, anesthesia can be maintained with nitrous oxide and volatile anesthetics. Although it has been postulated that inhibition of hydroxylation and oxidation may alter metabolism of volatile anesthetics in patients on MAOI's,[16] there are no reports of an increased incidence of hepatotoxicity in these patients. Sympathetic nervous system stimulation induced by hypotension, hypoxia, or indirect-acting sympathomimetic agents should be avoided to minimize the risk of hypertension or arrhythmias.[58,67] When vasopressors are required, small doses of direct-acting agents like phenylephrine or methoxamine are preferable.[82] Finally, meperidine should be avoided for postoperative analgesia in patients taking MAOI's. While morphine appears safe, alternatives including regional nerve blocks should be considered.

Neuroleptics

Neuroleptics are used primarily to treat psychotic symptoms. Psychosis may be a manifestation of schizophrenia, delusional disorders, major depression, bipolar affective disorder, dementia, delirium, and many medical illnesses. Neuroleptics can also be helpful in the management of severe agitation whether or not it is associated with psychosis.

The neuroleptics constitute a chemically heterogeneous group of major tranquilizers, including the phenothiazines, butyrophenones, thioxanthenes, indolones, and dibenzoxazepines.[83] These drugs are all antagonists of dopamine at postsynaptic receptor sites. They also block peripheral alpha-adrenergic receptors, and many cause beta-adrenergic receptor stimulation. Some have significant antihistaminic, anticholinergic, and serotonergic effects and can interfere with hypothalamic thermoregulation, especially in anesthetized patients.

The alpha-adrenergic blocking effects can cause peripheral vasodilation and hypotension. This is more common with aliphatic substituted phenothiazines like thioridazine, mesoridazine, and chlorpromazine than with other antipsychotic agents. Because reflex sympathetic vasoconstrictor responses are blunted, intraoperative volume depletion or positive pressure ventilation can cause marked hypotension in patients on neuroleptics. The hypotensive effects of neuroleptics may also be potentiated by the concomitant use of epinephrine or isoproterenol. When hypotension occurs in this situation, alpha-adrenergic agonists are the treatment of choice.[40] When beta-adrenergic stimulation results in persistent tachycardia, beta-blockers like propranolol may be used.

Concern has also been raised about the risk of neuroleptic malignant syndrome (NMS) when general anesthesia is administered to patients treated with these drugs. NMS is an adverse effect of neuroleptics characterized by hyperthermia, skeletal muscle rigidity, changing level of consciousness, and autonomic nervous system lability with fluctuating blood pressure, tachycardia, and diaphoresis. This constellation of signs is commonly associated with leukocytosis and marked elevations in serum creatine phosphokinase (CPK) levels.[84] Despite clinical similarities to malignant hyperthermia associated with general anesthesia, muscle biopsy has failed to establish that NMS and malignant hyperthermia are related.[85] Some recommend that patients with a history of NMS who require anesthesia should be managed with the same precautions as those susceptible to malignant hyperthermia,[16,86] but others have noted that such patients can tolerate general anesthesia and succinylcholine without developing malignant hyperthermia.[87] Conversely, patients susceptible to malignant hyperthermia have been given neuroleptic agents without developing NMS.[88] There are no reports of NMS caused by neuroleptics alone in patients with a history of malignant hyperthermia.

Neuroleptics may also cause sedation and extrapyramidal symptoms including tremor, skeletal muscle rigidity, dystonia, bradykinesia, and gait disturbances that impair mobility and hinder rehabilitation. These symptoms may be controlled by reducing the dose of the neuroleptic or by administering anticholinergic agents like diphenhydramine, trihexyphenidyl, or benztropine, or by giving amantadine. However, these agents do not relieve tardive dyskinesias, which are involuntary movements occurring in patients on long-term neuroleptic treatment. These movements are often irreversible and in severe cases can interfere with postoperative rehabilitation.

Akathisia is a common adverse effect of neuroleptic treatment that often goes unrecognized. It is an intense subjective sensation of restlessness and is usually manifested by motor restlessness, frequent shifting of position, and pacing. Patients who experience akathisia while they are confined to bed or otherwise immobilized have difficulty tolerating the incessant urge to move about and become severely agitated. Unfortunately, a common "therapeutic" response to agitation is to increase the amount of neuroleptic, which only serves to aggravate the akathisia. However, they often respond to discontinuation of the neuroleptic and treatment with diphenhydramine, benztropine, or lorazepam.[83] Akathisia may persist for days or weeks after the neuroleptic is stopped, and treatment with anticholinergic agents or benzodiazepines should continue for as long as necessary.

Sedation caused by neuroleptics may lower the dose requirements for induction agents. However, doses of muscle relaxants need not be altered. Opiates used for postoperative analgesia have been reported to cause excessive central nervous system and respiratory depression in patients on butyrophenones. Sedgwick suggests using small incremental doses of morphine to minimize these effects.[16]

Neuroleptics can be discontinued abruptly after an acute adverse reaction. Reemergence of psychotic symptoms or agitation is the greatest risk. Some patients on chronic therapy experience withdrawal dyskinesias after abrupt discontinuation. They can be suppressed by administering a lower dose of the neuroleptic that can then be tapered and discontinued.

Despite these problems, most side effects of neuroleptics are easily remedied. Given the complications that can be associated with untreated psychosis in the perioperative period, it is recommended that treatment with antipsychotic drugs be continued throughout the perioperative period.[16,26]

Lithium

Lithium is used principally in the treatment and prophylaxis of bipolar affective disorder. It may also be used in adjunctive or maintenance treatment of other depressive disorders. Lithium decreases the excitability of cells by reducing sodium transport during depolarization. It also indirectly reduces adenyl cyclase activity associated with a diminished response to norepinephrine at postsynaptic receptors.

Lithium has been associated with prolongation of neuromuscular blockade in dogs treated with depolarizing agents such as succinylcholine and decamethonium[89] and competitive blockers like pancuronium.[90] The action of D-tubocurarine is potentiated by lithium in cats,[91] but not in dogs.[89] There are case reports of prolonged effects of succinylcholine[92] and pancuronium[90] in humans. Although the combination of lithium and neuromuscular blocking agents is well tolerated by many, caution has been advised in their concomitant use.[16,93] Most recommended that two doses of lithium be omitted before surgery and that the initial dose of muscle relaxant be reduced.[94] However, more recently, Sedgwick has suggested that it is not necessary to discontinue lithium in this setting.[16] There is no evidence of adverse interactions between lithium and other anesthetic agents.

Dehydration and lithium toxicity are the principal risks associated with lithium use in the perioperative period. Some patients may develop nephrogenic diabetes insipidus and become dehydrated if they are subjected to fluid restriction or experience fluid loss in the perioperative period. Dehydration can lead to reduced renal clearance of lithium and toxicity. Any factors causing diminished glomerular filtration rate, negative fluid balance, or negative sodium balance can reduce renal clearance of lithium and predispose the patient to toxicity. Hypotension, congestive heart failure, restricted oral fluid intake, vomiting, diarrhea, and administration of diuretics are all such factors. Thiazide diuretics are particularly suspect. Signs of lithium toxicity include nausea, vomiting, diarrhea, lethargy, confusion, muscle weakness, dysarthria, ataxia, cardiac conduction delays and heart block, hypotension, seizures, and coma.

These risks have prompted the recommendation to discontinue lithium two or three days before major surgery and to resume lithium when renal function, fluid balance, and electrolyte status are stable.[95] However, lithium should be resumed as soon as safely possible to avoid relapses of mania or depression. In minor surgery or elective procedures, lithium need not be discontinued[58,95] so long as serum levels are in the nontoxic range, diuretics are used with caution, and the patient is well hydrated before and after the procedure. Safe perioperative management of patients on lithium includes monitoring serum sodium and lithium levels, hydration status, blood pressure, cardiac conduction, urinary output, and renal function.

Benzodiazepines

Benzodiazepines (BZ's) are the most commonly prescribed anxiolytic drugs and play a major role in anesthesia. They act by enhancing binding of gamma-aminobutyric acid (GABA) to receptors on neuronal membranes. The GABA-BZ-receptor complex opens chloride ion channels, causing membrane hyperpolarization and decreasing excitability.

BZ's may be used throughout the perioperative period to treat anxiety and agitation. They can be used with opiates for premedication or analgesia.[16] Patients who use BZ's chronically can develop tolerance and have an increased risk of serious withdrawal symptoms. They should be maintained on BZ's in adequate doses at appropriate intervals in order to avert withdrawal in the perioperative period. Equivalent doses of parenteral BZ's can be used when the patient is not eating. After surgery, BZ's can be restarted if needed, using one with a short half-life to permit precise titration or one with a longer half-life to minimize fluctuation in drug levels and avoid withdrawal.

Flumazenil is sometimes used to reverse the effects of BZ's given in the perioperative setting. In patients who have taken BZ's chronically, flumazenil can precipitate withdrawal symptoms including anxiety, agitation, tachycardia, hypertension, and seizures. It is therefore recommended that flumazenil be avoided in chronic BZ users.

EFFICACY OF NONPHARMACOLOGIC INTERVENTIONS

A number of nonpharmacologic interventions are helpful in managing psychiatric disorders in the perioperative period.[96,97] Devine and Cook reviewed 102 studies of "psychoeducational" interventions dealing with a wide range of strategies administered by different providers in a variety of patient populations with and without psychiatric symptoms.[98] Effectiveness was judged in four classes of outcome measures—recovery, relief of postoperative pain, psychological well-being, and satisfaction with care. Measures of recovery included the incidence of medical complications, postoperative respiratory function, number of days in intensive care units, incidence of postoperative behavioral problems, length of hospital stay, degree of recovery, and number of days after discharge before venturing from home. A meta-analysis confirmed positive effects in all four classes of outcome measures. Schindler et al. also found that psychotherapeutic intervention during recovery from coronary artery bypass surgery diminished postoperative medical and psychiatric morbidity, facilitated appropriate use of analgesics, and reduced the length of hospitalization.[99]

Recommended approaches for patients with anxiety include preoperative teaching, formation of therapeutic alliances in which specific concrete concerns of the patient are elicited and addressed, and supportive contact with other patients who have successfully experienced similar surgical treatment.[26] Patients who are unresponsive to these measures or who have chronic anxiety disorders often benefit from psychotherapy. Those with simple phobias who have trouble facing elective surgery may respond to behavioral therapy that may be combined with brief psychotherapy, hypnosis, and desensitization techniques.[100] Several studies have documented the positive effects of preoperative instruction on surgical outcome in terms of decreasing postoperative anxiety, need for analgesics, and medical complications, and increasing the level of function and performance of rehabilitative tasks.[101-103] However, the use of these measures in patients with specific anxiety disorders has not been evaluated in controlled trials. To reduce anxiety and improve compliance in mentally retarded patients, Voitk recommends admission 24 to 36 hours before surgery to acclimate them to the hospital environment, staff, and routines. After surgery, anxiety can be reduced by minimizing social isolation and avoiding excessive sedation.[42]

For patients with depressive disorders in which antidepressant medication or electroconvulsive therapy is not indicated or successful as a sole treatment modality, behavioral techniques and psychotherapy may be useful, particularly for those who have adjustment disorders with depressed mood. Titchener and Levine emphasize the importance of forming supportive relationships with elderly patients suffering from preoperative depression.[9] Actively suicidal patients require close nursing surveillance and safety precautions to minimize the risk of self-destructive behavior.

Management of patients with psychotic symptoms often includes interventions other than antipsychotic medication. Communication should be kept relatively simple and concrete. Efforts to build and maintain trust in professional-patient relationships are especially important when paranoid ideation is present. Involvement of trusted family members or friends may be helpful in supporting the patient and acting as liaisons between patients and hospital staff. Factors that may aggravate psychotic symptoms should be avoided whenever possible. These include dopamine agonists, anticholinergics, antiarrhythmics, and other medications associated with psychotic phenomena; interpersonal stress, including visits from people who upset the patient; and intrusive exploration of distressing psychodynamic issues that need not be addressed in the perioperative period.

There is evidence that detection of preexisting psychiatric illness in geriatric surgical patients may prevent further psychiatric complications.[104] Several studies have demonstrated that preoperative psychiatric intervention decreases the prevalence of postoperative delirium.[12,105,106] Psychiatric interventions include interviews dealing with patients' fears, education about possible procedures and complications such as confusion, and counseling on strategies for dealing with postoperative confusion. In a meta-analysis of several studies, preoperative psychiatric intervention emerged as the best way to reduce postcardiotomy delirium.[37]

Nonpharmacologic treatment of preoperative cognitive impairment in patients with delirium or dementia usually entails repeated efforts to keep the patient oriented with frequent staff contacts; simple reminders and explanations about routines and procedures; clocks and calendars; visits from and pictures of close family and friends; and familiar personal belongings. Agitation can often be managed by the constant presence of a nurse or close family member at the bedside. Adjustment of the level of environmental stimulation may also reduce agitation. For patients who are overwhelmed by external stimuli, reducing bright lights or distracting noise may improve agitation. When sensory deprivation contributes to disorientation, measures to increase stimulation like opening a curtain to allow sunlight may be helpful. Keeping the door open may reduce feelings of isolation and fearfulness. In those with cognitive impairment attributable to mental retardation, individualized nursing care to address specific needs may help the patient through the perioperative period.[44] Patients with somatization and personality disorders pose the most complex challenges to perioperative care. Close collaboration between surgical staff and the psychiatric consultant is especially useful in recognizing and managing difficulties that commonly arise in the professional-patient relationship.

PSYCHIATRIC ASSESSMENT

Since psychiatric and educational interventions can favorably affect perioperative outcome, it is important to identify patients who may benefit from mental health care. Routine psychiatric screening or assessment of all surgical patients has not proven cost-effective. However, assessment has been recommended for patients with psychiatric disorders and candidates for certain types of surgery. Many organ transplant programs have incorporated preoperative psychiatric evaluation for all patients. For some this includes extensive psychological and neuropsychological testing[24,26,107] designed to uncover and measure severity of psychiatric disorders and provide information on personality traits, self-image, coping styles, and social supports. Liaison psychiatrists may function as consultants or even as members of the transplant team.[33]

It has been recommended that all patients undergoing surgery for head and neck cancer begin the rehabilitation process in the preoperative period. This should include psychiatric evaluation to recognize preexisting personality problems, especially those related to alcohol and tobacco abuse.[108] These factors are associated with noncompliance that may likely complicate treatment. Unfortunately, morbidity attributable to noncompliance has not been formally measured in these patients.

Meyer and Jacobsson have suggested that preoperative assessment of psychosocial and psychiatric characteristics can predict psychological adaptation after rhinoplasty.[53] They identified two psychologically important groups of patients. Those with a history of trauma to the nose tended to consume large quantities of alcohol, were usually self-reliant with poorly established social relationships, and were more likely to be dissatisfied with surgical results. Those without a history of trauma tended to have signs and symptoms of anxiety and social inhibition. Those who expected surgery to improve their psychosocial situation often suffered an increase in anxiety and other psychiatric symptoms within a year of the procedure.[109] The authors suggested that preoperative psychosocial evaluation may reliably predict postoperative psychological adaptation and provide a means to avoid surgery in patients "not suited" to rhinoplasty.

Although patients with somatoform disorders have a high risk of undergoing unnecessary or repeated surgery, it has not been demonstrated that psychiatric assessment results in effective interruption of their surgery-shopping patterns.[1,51,110] Most of these patients do not perceive themselves to be psychiatrically ill and are not receptive to referral for psychiatric evaluation and treatment.[46] Innovative consultation models need to be developed to help surgeons recognize and assess these patients. In primary care settings and pain clinics, interdisciplinary team treatment has been successful in managing many of them. Referral to such programs may be more acceptable to patients requesting surgery who are reluctant to see a psychiatrist.

Psychiatric evaluation is considered a useful routine component of the assessment of morbidly obese patients who are candidates for gastroplasty or related surgical procedures.[111] It has been used to identify patients with an increased risk of postoperative psychiatric problems associated with preexisting psychiatric illness, severe situational stress, insufficient motivation, or lack of sufficient support. Some patients may be excluded from surgery or offered preoperative psychiatric treatment.[112]

Surgical patients who are mentally retarded do not routinely require evaluation by a psychiatrist, but a comprehensive psychosocial assessment is recommended.[113] Assessment by nursing and social work staff may be supplemented by a formal neuropsychological evaluation if the patient's cognitive abilities are not known. Testing may help staff individualize communication with the patient for preoperative teaching, postoperative care, and rehabilitation. If problematic behavior is identified, consultation with a psychiatrist should be sought to plan appropriate behavioral and pharmacologic management.

Consultation by a psychiatrist is often sought when patients display cognitive impairment that may interfere with their ability to make reasoned informed decisions about treatment.[114] However, psychiatric evaluation is not always necessary before obtaining informed consent from mentally retarded, demented, or delirious patients. If a member of the treatment team ascertains that the patient is able to express a preference regarding treatment and has at least a basic understanding of the nature of the medical problems, the risks and benefits of available treatment options, and the possible consequences of his decision, he or she can document this in the medical record as evidence that the patient is capable of giving informed consent to surgery and anesthesia.[115,116] The same guidelines can be applied to patients with psychosis, depression, or personality disorders, but attention must be given to psychodynamic and situational factors that can alter the judgment of these patients.[117] A severely depressed patient may clearly demonstrate comprehension and offer a reasoned argument for refusing surgery. However, his action may reflect an alteration in his usual nondepressed outlook and represent a deviation from his expected judgment. Such a patient may be legally competent to decide but medically requires psychiatric intervention and counselling for decison-making. On the other hand, patients with severe psychiatric illness may be clinically competent to decide about surgery and anesthesia but incompetent in other areas of function and decision-making.[115] Whenever there are doubts about the ability of the patient to consent to or to refuse treatment, a psychiatric consultation should be obtained.[114,118]

Beyond these special circumstances, the literature furnishes general guidelines for identifying those patients who should be evaluated by a psychiatrist before surgery. A major anesthesia textbook proposes that "preoperative psychiatric consultation may be indicated when emotional preparation for surgery is grossly unrealistic."[119] Surman indicates that preoperative psychiatric care is valuable when the patient has "unrealistic fantasies" about surgery and when a grief reaction, major affective disorder, or psychosis is suspected.[26] Those with persistent debilitating anxiety or those who deny anxiety despite evidence to the contrary should be evaluated by a psychiatrist.

We cannot predict which asymptomatic patients with a history of psychiatric illness have an increased risk of complications from surgery and anesthesia. However, it has commonly been observed that psychiatric symptoms may reemerge in the context of the stress of illness or surgery. Preoperative psychiatric assessment is appropriate for patients with a history or pattern of psychiatric symptoms that recur with stress.[26] It is reasonable to obtain preoperative psychiatric assessment in all patients with current symptoms of psychiatric disorders or in those taking psychotropic medication.

Selected patients without psychiatric problems may also benefit from preoperative psychiatric assessment, especially geriatric patients. Controlled studies in patients with hip fractures demonstrate that perioperative interventions by liaison psychiatrists are associated with significant reductions in length of hospital stay, requirements for discharge to institutional settings, and net cost reduction.[120,121]

SUMMARY

1. Comorbid symptoms of anxiety, depression, psychosis, and cognitive impairment can complicate the perioperative course. Adverse outcomes include poor cooperation with care, nutritional compromise, respiratory complications, and morbidity due to prolonged bed rest, suboptimal participation in rehabilitation, altered pain tolerance and analgesic requirements, extended length of hospital stay, and delayed return to independent function. Depression and cognitive impairment are associated with higher mortality. Somatoform and personality disorders often lead to poor cooperation with care and disruption of the doctor-patient relationship.

2. Most classes of psychotropic drugs can be safely managed in the perioperative period if their complex effects on cardiovascular and autonomic nervous system function are carefully considered. Attention to intravascular volume and hemodynamic parameters is especially important. In most situations, the benefits of continuing the drug until surgery outweigh the risks.

3. Tricyclic antidepressants block alpha$_1$ adrenergic receptors and predispose patients to hypotension. They have central and peripheral anticholinergic effects that can lead to delirium, ileus, and urinary retention. Although they slow atrioventricular conduction, they do not impair left ventricular function and rarely cause arrhythmias at therapeutic levels except in special circumstances. TCA's need not be discontinued before most elective procedures.

4. Monoamine oxidase inhibitors hinder oxidative deamination of monoamine neurotransmitters. To minimize the risk of severe hypertension, patients should not receive indirect-acting sympathomimetic agents. MAOI's cause alpha$_1$ adrenergic blockade and have anticholinergic effects similar to TCA's. They inhibit hepatic microsomal enzymes, often necessitating a reduction in the doses of barbiturates and opioids. There is controversy regarding the need to discontinue MAOI's before surgery and about the safety of using narcotic-based anesthesia in patients taking them. Use of meperidine is, however, contraindicated.

5. All neuroleptics cause alpha$_1$ adrenergic blockade, and many cause beta-adrenergic stimulation. They can cause tachycardia and hypotension in association with volume depletion, positive pressure ventilation, and concomitant use of epinephrine or isoproteronol. Volume repletion and/or alpha-adrenergic agonists can be used for hypotension and beta-blockers for tachycardia. Because neuroleptics cause dopamine-receptor blockade, they can cause extrapyramidal symptoms. Reduction in dose and treatment with anticholinergic agents and amantadine may be helpful. To avoid recurrent psychosis, neuroleptics can be continued throughout the perioperative period.

6. Lithium, used to treat bipolar affective disorders, may potentiate the effect of depolarizing and competitive neuromuscular blocking agents. The clearance of lithium can be reduced and its toxicity increased by factors that cause negative fluid balance, negative sodium balance, and decreased glomerular filtration rate. Lithium should be discontinued before major surgery and resumed when renal function, fluid balance, and electrolyte levels are stable. It need not be discontinued before minor surgery if serum levels are not in the toxic range, renal function is normal, and fluid and electrolyte status are stable.

7. A history of chronic benzodiazepine use is helpful in avoiding withdrawal symptoms of anxiety, agitation, and sympathetic hyperactivity in the perioperative period. Flumenazil, sometimes used to reverse short-acting benzodiazepines in the recovery room, should be avoided in chronic benzodiazepine users.

8. Nonpharmacologic modalities including education interventions are helpful adjuncts in treating patients with psychiatric manifestations and cognitive impairment and favorably affect many aspects of convalescence.

9. Routine psychiatric screening for all surgical patients has not been proven helpful or cost-effective. However, it is recommended for patients with evidence of psychiatric disorders and for those undergoing specific procedures such as head and neck cancer surgery, surgical treatment of morbid obesity, organ transplantation, and reconstructive or disfiguring surgery. It is also indicated in selected geriatric patients and when there is doubt about the capacity of a patient to consent to or refuse treatment.

REFERENCES

1. *Diagnostic and Statistical Manual of Mental Disorders*, 3d rev. ed. (DSM-III-R). Washington DC, American Psychiatric Association, 1987.
2. Spitzer RL, Endicott J, Robins E: Research diagnostic criteria rationale and reliability. *Arch Gen Psychiatry* 35:73–82, 1978.
3. Lipowski ZJ: Physical illness and psychopathology. *Int J Psychiatry Med* 5:483, 1974.
4. Mathews A, Ridgeway V: Personality and surgical recovery: A review. *Br J Clin Psychol* 20:243–260, 1981.
5. Johnston M, Carpenter L: Relationships between preoperative anxiety and postoperative state. *Psychological Med* 10:361–367, 1980.
6. Christensen T, Hjortsø E, Mortensen E et al: Fatigue and anxiety in surgical patients. *Acta Psychiatry Scand* 73:76–79, 1986.
7. Wolfer JA, Davis CE: Assessment of surgical patients. Preoperative emotional condition and postoperative welfare. *Nurs Res* 19:403, 1970.
8. Janis IL: *Psychological Stress*. New York, Wiley, 1958.
9. Titchener JL, Levine ML: *Surgery as a Human Experience*. New York, Oxford University Press, 1960.
10. Abram HS, Gill BF: Predictions of postoperative psychiatric complications. *N Engl J Med* 265:1123, 1961.
11. Spielberger CD, Gorsuch RL, Lushene RE: *Manual for the State-Trait Anxiety Inventory*. Palo Alto, Consulting Psychologists Press, 1970.
12. Lalinec-Michaud M, Engelsmann F: Anxiety fears and depression related to hysterectomy. *Can J Psychiatry* 30:44–47, 1985.
13. Linn BS, Linn MW, Klimas NH: Effects of psychophysical stress on surgical outcome. *Psychosom Med* 50:230–244, 1988.
14. Layne OL, Yudofsky SC: Postoperative psychosis in cardiotomy patients. *N Engl J Med* 284:518–520, 1971.
15. Kornfeld DS, Heller SS, Frank KA et al: Delirium after coronary artery bypass surgery. *J Thorac Cardiovasc Surg* 58:891, 1969.
16. Sedgwick JV, Lewis IH, Linter SPK: Anesthesia and mental illness. *Int J Psych Med* 20:209–225, 1990.
17. Kimball CP: A predictive study of adjustment to cardiac surgery. *J Thorac Cardiovasc Surg* 58:891, 1969.
18. Tufo HM, Ostfeld AM, Sheterille R: Central nervous system dysfunction following open heart surgery. *JAMA* 212:1333, 1970.

19. Kimball CP: *The Biopsychosocial Approach to the Patient.* Baltimore, Williams & Wilkins, 1981.

20. Schleifer SJ, Keller SE, Siris SG et al: Depression and immunity. Lymphocyte function in ambulatory depressed patients, hospitalized schizophrenic patients, and patients hospitalized for herniorrhaphy. *Arch Gen Psychiatry* 42:129–133, 1985.

21. Linn BS, Jensen J: Age and immune response to surgical stress. *Arch Surg* 118:405–409, 1983.

22. Morse FM, Litin EM: Postoperative delirium: A study of etiologic factors. *Am J Psychiatry* 126:388, 1969.

23. Folks OG, Freeman AM 3d, Sokol RS et al: Cognitive dysfunction after coronary artery bypass surgery: A case-controlled study. *South Med J* 81:202–206, 1988.

24. Kuhn WF, Myers B, Brennan AF et al: Psychopathology in heart transplant candidates. *J Heart Transplant* 7:223–226, 1988.

25. Kemp B: Psychosocial and mental health issues in rehabilitation of older persons, in Brody SJ, Ruff CE (eds): *Aging and Rehabilitation: Advances in the State of the Art.* New York, Springer, 1986, pp 122–158.

26. Surman OS: The surgical patient, in Hackett TP, Chassem NH (eds): *Massachusetts General Hospital Handbook of General Hospital Psychiatry*, 2d ed. Littleton, MA, PSG Publishing, 1987.

27. Dubovsky SL, Haddenhorst A, Murphy J et al: A preliminary study of the relationship between preoperative depression and weight loss following surgery for morbid obesity. *Int J Psychiatry Med* 15:185–196, 1985.

28. Morse FM, Litin EM: Postoperative delirium: A study of etiologic factors. *Am J Psychiatry* 126:388, 1969.

29. Hackett TP, Cassem NH (eds): *Massachusetts General Hospital Handbook of General Hospital Psychiatry.* St. Louis, Mosby, 1978, pp 71–72.

30. Bickerstaff LK, Harris SC, Leggett RS et al: Pain insensitivity in schizophrenic patients. A surgical dilemma. *Arch Surg* 123:49–51, 1988.

31. Solomon S, McCartney JR, Saravay SM et al: Postoperative hospital course of patients with history of severe psychiatric illness. *Gen Hosp Psychiatry* 9:376–382, 1987.

32. Cutler BS, Fink MP: Postoperative complications in patients with disabling psychiatric illness or intellectual handicaps. A case-controlled retrospective analysis. *Arch Surg* 125:1436–1440, 1990.

33. Mai FM: Liaison psychiatry in the heart transplant unit. *Psychosomatics* 28:44–46, 1987.

34. Frierson RL, Lippman SB: Heart transplant candidate rejected on psychiatric indications. *Psychosomatics* 28:347–355, 1987.

35. Davis FM, Woolner DF, Frampton C et al: Prospective, multi-centre trial of mortality following general or spinal anesthesia for hip fracture surgery in the elderly. *Br J Anaesth* 59:1080–1088, 1987.

36. Layne OL, Yudofsky SC: Postoperative psychosis in cardiotomy patients. *N Engl J Med* 284:518–520, 1971.

37. Smith LW, Dimsdale JE: Postcardiotomy delirium: Conclusions after 25 years. *Am J Psychiatry* 146:452–458, 1989.

38. Lipowski ZJ: Delirium, clouding of consciousness, and confusion. *J Nerv Ment Dis* 145:227, 1967.

39. Kilpatrick DG, Miller WC, Allain AN et al: The use of psychological test data to predict open heart surgery outcome: A prospective study. *Psychosomatic Med* 37:62, 1975.

40. Orkin FK, Cooperman LH: *Complications in Anesthesiology.* Philadelphia, Lippincott, 1982, pp 362–364.

41. Cryns AG, Grey KM, Goldstein MZ: Effects of surgery on the mental status of older persons: A meta-analytic review. *J Geriatr Psych Neurol* 3:184–191, 1990.

42. Voitk AJ: Acute abdomen in severely mentally retarded patients. *Can J Surg* 30:195–196, 1987.

43. Stiles CM: Anesthesia for the mentally retarded patients. *Orthop Clin N Am* 12:45–56, 1981.

44. Benchot RJ: Mentally retarded patients. Special needs before and after surgery. *AORN J* 44:768–780, 1986.

45. Barsky AJ: Patients who amplify bodily sensations. *Ann Intern Med* 91:63–70, 1979.

46. Ford CV: The somatizing disorders. *Psychosomatics* 27:327–337, 1986.

47. Zoccolillo MS, Cloninger CR: Excess medical care of women with somatization disorder. *South Med J* 79:532–535, 1986.

48. Long DM, Filtzer DL, DenDebba M et al: Clinical features of the failed-back syndrome. *J Neurosurg* 69:61–71, 1988.

49. Meninger KA: Polysurgery and polysurgical addiction. *Psychoanal Q* 3:173, 1934.

50. Abram HS: Psychological aspects of surgery. *Int Psychiatry Clin* 4:2, 1967.

51. Smith RG, Monson RA, Ray DC: Psychiatric consultation in somatization disorder. A randomized controlled study. *N Engl J Med* 314:1407–1413, 1986.

52. Barsky AJ: Hidden reasons some patients visit doctors. *Ann Intern Med* 94:492–498, 1981.

53. Meyer L, Jacobsson S: The predictive validity of psychosocial factors for patients' acceptance of rhinoplasty. *Ann Plast Surg* 17:513–520, 1986.

54. Meyer L, Ringberg A: A prospective study of psychiatric and psychosocial sequelae of bilateral subcutaneous mastectomy. *Scand J Plastic Reconstr Surg* 20:101–107, 1986.

55. Lilienfeld SO, Valkenburg CV, Larntz K et al: The relationship of histrionic personality disorder to antisocial personality and somatization disorders. *Am J Psychiatry* 143:718–722, 1986.

56. Schechter GL, Brase DA, Powell J: Adverse effects of tricyclic antidepressants during nasal surgery. *Otolaryngol Head Neck Surg* 90:233–236, 1982.

57. Roose SP, Glassman AH: Cardiovascular effects of tricyclic antidepressants in depressed patients with and without heart disease. *J Clin Psychiatry Monograph* 7:1–18, 1989.

58. Stoelting RK, Dierdorf SF, McCammon RL: *Anesthesia and Coexisting Disease*, 2d ed. New York, Churchill Livingstone, 1988.

59. Kantor SJ, Glassman AH, Bigger JT Jr et al: The cardiac effects of therapeutic plasma concentrations of imipramine. *Am J Psychiatry* 135:534–538, 1978.

60. Roose SP, Glassman AH, Giardina EGV et al: Tricyclic antidepressants in depressed patients with cardiac conduction disease. *Arch Gen Psychiatry* 44:273–275, 1987.

61. Veith RC, Raskind MA, Caldwell JH et al: Cardiovascular effects of tricyclic antidepressants in depressed patients with chronic heart disease. *N Engl J Med* 306:954–959, 1982.

62. Roose SP, Glassman AH, Giardina EGV et al: Nortriptyline in depressed patients with left ventricular impairment. *JAMA* 256:521–526, 1986.

63. Glassman AH, Johnson LL, Giardina EGV et al: The use of imipramine in depressed patients with congestive heart failure. *JAMA* 250:1990–2001, 1983.

64. Roose SP, Glassman AH, Giardina EGV et al: Cardiovascular effects of imipramine and bupropion in depressed patients with congestive heart failure. *J Clin Psychopharmacol* 7:247–251, 1987.

65. Giardina EGV, Biggler JT Jr: Antiarrhythmic effect of imipramine hydrochloride in patients with ventricular premature complexes without psychological depression. *Am J Cardiol* 50:172–179, 1982.

66. Edwards RP, Miller RD, Roizen MF et al: Cardiac responses to imipramine and pancuronium during anesthesia with halothane or enflurane. *Anesthesiology* 50:421–425, 1979.

67. Wong KC, Puerto AY, Puerto BA et al: Influence of imipramine and pargyline on the arrhythmogenicity of epinephrine during halothane, enflurane, or methoxyflurane anesthesia in dogs. *Life Sci* 27:2675–2678, 1980.

68. Spiss CK, Smith CM, Maze M: Halothane-epinephrine arrhythmias

and adrenergic responsiveness after chronic imipramine administration in dogs. *Anesth Analg* 63:825–828, 1984.

69. Sprague DH, Wolf S: Enflurane seizures in patients taking amitriptyline. *Anesth Analg* 61:67–68, 1982.

70. Boaks AJ, Lawrence DR, Teoh PC et al: Interactions between sympathetic amines and antidepressant agents in man. *Br J Med* 1:311–315, 1973.

71. Hirsh MS, Walter RM, Hasterlick RJ: Subarachnoid hemorrhage following ephedrine and monoamine oxidase inhibitors. *JAMA* 194:1259, 1965.

72. Horler AR, Wynne NA: Hypertensive crisis due to pargyline and metaraminol. *Br J Med* 2:460–461, 1965.

73. Perks ER: Monoamine oxidase inhibitors. *Anesthesia* 19:376–386, 1964.

74. Schwartz AJ, Wollman H: Anesthetic considerations for patients on chronic drug therapy: L-Dopa, monoamine oxidase inhibitors, tricyclic antidepressants, and propranolol. *Anesthesiology* 4:98–111, 1976.

75. Viegas OJ: Psychiatric illness, in Stoelting RK, Dierdorf SF, McCammon RL (eds): *Anesthesia and Coexisting Disease*. New York, Churchill Livingstone, 1983.

76. El-Ganzouri AR, Ivankovich AD, Braverman B et al: Should MAOI be discontinued preoperatively? *Anesthesiology* 59:A384, 1983.

77. Michaels I, Jerrins M, Shier NQ et al: Anesthesia for cardiac surgery in patients receiving monoamine oxidase inhibitors. *Anesth Analg* 63:1041–1044, 1984.

78. Wong KC: Preoperative discontinuation of monoamine oxidase inhibitor therapy: An old wives' tale. *Sem Anesthesiology* 5:145–148, 1986.

79. El-Ganzouri AR, Ivankovich AD, Braverman B et al: Monoamine oxidase inhibitors: Should they be discontinued preoperatively? *Anesth Analg* 64:592–596, 1985.

80. Cock DP, Passmore-Rowe A: Dangers of monoamine oxidase inhibitors. *Br Med J* 2:1545–1556, 1962.

81. Jenkins LC, Graves HB: Potential hazards of psychoactive drugs in association with anesthesia. *Can Anesth Soc J* 12:121–128, 1965.

82. Smith NT, Miller RD, Corbascio AW (eds): *Drug Reactions in Anesthesia*. Philadelphia, Lea & Febiger, 1981, pp 186–190.

83. Bernstein JG: *Handbook of Drug Therapy in Psychiatry*. Boston, PSG, 1983, pp 41–71.

84. Guze SH, Baxter LR: Neuroleptic malignant syndrome. *N Engl J Med* 313:163–166, 1985.

85. Tollefson G: A case of malignant neuroleptic syndrome: In intro muscle comparison with malignant hyperthermia. *J Clin Psychopharmacol* 2:266–270, 1982.

86. Denborough MA, Collins SP, Hopkinson PKC: Rhabdomyolysis and malignant hyperpyrexia. *Br Med J* 24:1878, 1984.

87. Lotstra F, Linkowski P, Mendlewicz J: General anesthesia after neuroleptic malignant syndrome. *Biol Psychiatry* 18:243–247, 1983.

88. Addonizio G, Susman V: Neuroleptic malignant syndrome and use of anesthetic agents. *Am J Psychiatry* 143:127–128, 1986.

89. Hill GE, Wong KC, Hodges MR: Lithium carbonate and neuromuscular blocking agents. *Anesthesiology* 46:122–126, 1977.

90. Borden H, Clarke MT, Katz M: The use of pancuronium bromide in patients receiving lithium carbonate. *Can Anesth Soc J* 21:79–82, 1974.

91. Basuray BN, Harris CA: Potentiation of D-tubocurarine (D-TC) neuromuscular blockade in cats by lithium chloride. *Eur J Pharmacol* 45:79–82, 1977.

92. Hill GE, Wong KC, Hodges MR: Potentiation of succinylcholine neuromuscular blockade by lithium carbonate. *Anesthesiology* 44:439–442, 1976.

93. Jefferson JW, Greist JH, Ackerman DL: *Lithium Encyclopedia for Clinical Practice*. American Psychiatric Association Press, 1983.

94. Havdala HS, Borison RL, Diamond BI: Potential hazards and applications of lithium in anesthesiology. *Anesthesiology* 50:534–537, 1979.

95. Schou M, Hippus H: Guidelines for patients receiving lithium treatment who require major surgery. *Psych J Anesth* 59:809–810, 1987.

96. Mumford E, Schlesinger HJ, Glass GV: The effect of psychological intervention on recovery from surgery and heart attacks: An analysis of the literature. *Ann J Pub Health* 72:144–151, 1982.

97. Rogers M, Reich P: Psychological intervention with surgical patients: Evaluation outcome. *Adv Psychosom Med* 15:23–50, 1986.

98. Devine EC, Cook TD: Clinical and cost-saving effects of psychoeducational interventions with surgical patients: A meta-analysis. *Res Nurs Health* 9:89–105, 1986.

99. Schindler BA, Shook J, Schwartz GM: Beneficial effects of psychiatry intervention in recovery after coronary artery bypass surgery. *Gen Hosp Psychiatry* 11:358–364, 1989.

100. Surman OS: Postnoxious desensitization: Some clinical notes on the combined use of hypnosis and systemic desensitization. *Am J Clin Hypn* 22:54–60, 1979.

101. Fortin F, Kirouac SA: A randomized controlled trial of preoperative patient education. *Lut J Nurs Studies* 13:11–24, 1976.

102. Christopherson B, Pfeiffer C: Varying the timing of information to alter preoperative anxiety and postoperative recovery in cardiac surgery patients. *Heart and Lung* 14:854–861, 1980.

103. Moss RC: Overcoming fear. A review of research on patient, family instruction. *AORN J* 43:1107–1114, 1986.

104. Gamino LA, Hunter RB, Brandon RA: Psychiatric complications associated with geriatric surgery. *Clin Geriatr Med* 1:417–422, 1985.

105. Lazarus HR, Hagens JH: Prevention of psychosis following open-heart surgery. *Am J Psychiatry* 124:1190–1195, 1968.

106. Surman OS, Hackett TP, Silverberg EL et al: Usefulness of psychiatric intervention in patients undergoing cardiac surgery. *Arch Gen Psychiatry* 30:830–835, 1974.

107. Surman OS, Dienstag JL, Cosimi AB et al: Psychosomatic aspects of liver transplantation. *Psychother Psychosom* 48:26–31, 1987.

108. Breitbart W, Holland J: Psychosocial aspects of head and neck cancer. *Sem Oncol* 15(1):61–69, 1988.

109. Meyer L, Jacobsson S: Psychiatric and psychosocial characteristics of patients accepted for rhinoplasty. *Ann Plast Surg* 19:117–130, 1987.

110. Monson RA, Smith GR: Somatization disorder in primary care. *N Engl J Med* 308:1464–1465, 1983.

111. Charles SC: Psychiatric evaluation of morbidly obese patients. *Gastroenterol Clin N Am* 16:415–432, 1987.

112. Gertler R, Ramsey-Stewart G: Preoperative psychiatric assessment of patients presenting for gastric bariatric surgery (surgical control of morbid obesity). *Aust NZ J Surg* 56:157–161, 1986.

113. Benchot RJ: Mentally retarded patients. Special needs before and after surgery. *AORN J* 44:768–780, 1986.

114. Starkman MN, Youngs DD: Psychiatric consultation with patients who refuse medical care. *Int J Psychiatry Med* 5:115–123, 1974.

115. Roth LH, Meisel A, Lidz CW: Tests of competency to consent to treatment. *Am J Psychiatry* 134:279–284, 1977.

116. Rozovsky FA: *Consent to Treatment—A Practical Guide*. Boston, Little, Brown, 1984.

117. Applebaum PS, Roth LH: Clinical issues in the assessment of competency. *Am J Psychiatry* 138:1462–1467, 1981.

118. Irwin M, Lovitz A, Marder SR et al: Psychotic patients' understanding of informed consent. *Am J Psychiatry* 142:1351–1354, 1985.

119. Rosenberg H: Postoperative emotional responses, in Orkin FK, Cooperman LH (eds): *Complications in Anesthesiology*. Philadelphia, Lippincott, 1982, pp 362–364.

120. Levitan SJ, Kornfield DS: Clinical and cost benefits of liaison psychiatry. *Am J Psychiatry* 138:790–793, 1981.

121. Strain J, Hammer JS, Lyons JS et al: Cost offset from the psychiatric liaison intervention for elderly hip fracture patients. *Psychosomatic Med* 51:261, 1989.

38 ALCOHOL AND DRUG ABUSE IN THE SURGICAL PATIENT

Gene B. Bishop

The abuse of psychoactive substances, both legal and illegal, prescribed and nonprescribed, is a significant medical and social problem. People with alcoholism and drug abuse may come to surgery either as a direct result of their substance abuse or for unrelated matters. Substance abuse can be underdiagnosed or missed entirely. It is often approached only from the point of view of end-organ damage, ignoring the disease concept and pharmacologic and behavioral effects that may influence perioperative care. Despite discomfort or distaste on the part of many physicians for treating patients with substance abuse,[1,2] substance abusers are most likely to ask for and receive help when they develop medical complications of their problem. The perioperative period thus presents a unique opportunity to diagnose substance abuse, to initiate treatment, and to aid in the management of its consequences.[2-4]

This chapter reviews general principles applicable to all substance abuse, beginning with definitions, diagnosis, and epidemiology, and then discusses the surgical risks of substance abuse. It concludes with separate discussions of alcoholism, narcotic addiction, cocaine abuse, and use of other drugs. For each substance, perioperative risks relating to intoxication, toxic effects, and withdrawal will be considered. Many people abuse more than one substance.

DEFINITIONS AND DIAGNOSIS OF SUBSTANCE ABUSE

Substance dependence has both behavioral and physiologic components.[5] Although the behavioral aspects make some physicians afraid to diagnose alcoholism, they may more readily diagnose abuse of illegal substances because societal disapproval is clearer and evidence of illegal drugs in the urine is irrefutable. However, clear criteria have been developed to separate occasional users from abusers of alcohol and other drugs and can be found in the Diagnostic and Statistical Manual of the American Psychiatric Association (DSM-III-R) shown in Table 38-1.[6]

TABLE 38-1. DSM-III-R Diagnostic Criteria for Psychoactive Substance Dependence

At least three of the following:

1. Substance often taken in larger amounts or over a longer period than the person intended
2. Persistent desire or one or more unsuccessful efforts to cut down or control substance use
3. A great deal of time spent in activities necessary to get the substance (e.g., theft), taking the substance (e.g., chain smoking), or recovering from its effects
4. Frequent intoxication or withdrawal symptoms when expected to fulfill major role obligations at work, school, or home (e.g., does not go to work because hung over, goes to school or work "high," intoxicated while taking care of his or her children), or when substance use is physically hazardous (e.g., drives while intoxicated)
5. Important social, occupational, or recreational activities given up or reduced because of substance use
6. Continued substance use despite knowledge of having a persistent or recurrent social, psychological, or physical problem that is caused or exacerbated by the use of the substance (e.g., keeps using heroin despite family arguments about it, cocaine-induced depression, or having an ulcer made worse by drinking)
7. Marked tolerance: need for markedly increased amounts of the substance (i.e., at least a 50% increase) in order to achieve intoxication or desired effect, or markedly diminished effect with continued use of the same amount

Note: The following items may not apply to cannabis, hallucinogens, or phencyclidine (PCP)

8. Characteristic withdrawal symptoms (see specific withdrawal syndrome under Psychoactive Substance-induced Organic Mental Disorders)
9. Substance often taken to relieve or avoid withdrawal symptoms

Source: Adapted from Diagnostic and Statistical Manual of Disorders, 3d rev. ed. 1987.

Simpler definitions of alcoholism emphasize development of medical, legal, occupational, or social problems from drinking.[7] A recently published definition emphasizes its progressive and fatal nature, the characteristics of impaired control and preoccupation with alcohol, and the distortion in thinking known as denial.[8] Inclusion of the behavioral effects of alcohol abuse in this definition and the DSM-III-R criteria allows early diagnosis and identification of perioperative risk before end-organ damage becomes apparent.

EPIDEMIOLOGY OF DRUG AND ALCOHOL USE

Despite recent public and media attention to other drugs, alcohol is still the most prevalent drug abused in the United States. A survey in the early 1980s showed that 13 percent of the adult population displayed symptoms of alcohol abuse at some time in their lives.[9] Current estimates show that 10 million adult Americans have alcoholism.[2] Alcohol is involved in 50 percent of nonvehicular accidents. A 1982 Georgia study showed that alcohol was a factor in 85 percent of fatal motor vehicle accidents.[2]

Studies in general hospitals show that between 10 and 50 percent of patients on medical and surgical services have alcoholism, depending on the instrument used for diagnosis.[9-13] Rates of detection vary widely with the primary service. A recent study comparing detection by trained interviewers with that of house staff and faculty in all major departments of a teaching hospital found that detection rates in obstetrics and gynecology and surgery were less than 25 percent.[19] Similar findings were confirmed in both a community hospital and a Veterans Administration hospital.[12,13] Patients on orthopedic and trauma services were less likely to have medical end-organ damage.[19] Specific consultation in regard to substance abuse was usually requested only in the most hopeless end-stage patients, and then only if the patient presented a compliance problem in the hospital.[14] Yet in the United States the death rate from trauma in alcoholics is twice that from medical complications of alcoholism such as pancreatitis and liver disease.[15] Thus, patients with early alcoholism are more likely to be seen on surgical or trauma services. They are more often young with a better prognosis for treatment.[15,16] The medical consultant, often called for other reasons, may be the first to diagnose an alcohol or drug problem.

There are no studies on the prevalence of prescription drug dependence or illegal drug use among hospitalized patients. The use of illegal psychoactive agents varies with the population served and with societal trends in drug use. In 1992, the number of cocaine addicts numbered 2.8 million, and the number of intermittent users approached 30 million. Approximately 8 to 10 million Americans have tried opiates, and about 1.2 million are addicted to them.[17]

SUBSTANCE ABUSE AND SURGICAL RISK

Clinical experience suggests that substance abusers are high-risk patients needing careful preoperative evaluation and postoperative care even when they have no obvious end-organ damage. However, data from the literature are sparse. There have been few series of patients undergoing surgery that consider the overall morbidity of alcoholism. One study examined blood alcohol levels in trauma patients. Although retrospectively there was no significant difference in mortality between patients with and without a history of heavy ingestion of alcohol before surgery, prospectively mortality was increased in patients with blood alcohol levels > 250 mg/dl.[3] A more recent series of trauma patients reported no difference in severity of injuries or morbidity and mortality when intoxicated and nonintoxicated patients were compared.[4,18]

Another study divided 614 trauma patients into four groups— those without detectable levels of blood alcohol, those with detectable levels of blood alcohol, those with serum evidence of other drugs, and those with evidence of both alcohol and drugs—and analyzed them for severity of injury, length of hospitalization, complications, and mortality. Only the group with detectable drugs had a significantly higher incidence of shock, severity of injury, and death.[19] However, serum rather than urine was used to identify drugs, decreasing the likelihood of identifying cocaine and thereby probably underestimating the prevalence of drug use in the study population.

A comparison of morbidity after colon surgery in otherwise comparable alcoholics and nonalcoholics found that alcoholics had an increased incidence of major complications, including wound rupture, bleeding, sepsis, congestive heart failure, and delirium. They also experienced a significant delay in normalization of intestinal function and stayed in the hospital 50 percent longer than the nonalcoholics.[20] In a small series of heroin addicts requiring cardiothoracic surgery for acute trauma, morbidity was higher in the addict population than in a control population with similar trauma.[21] Pulmonary edema developed in 30 percent of the addicts and in none of the controls. The incidence of wound infection was also higher in the addicts. None of the studies considered withdrawal syndromes or behavioral and management difficulties as complications of treatment.

ALCOHOLISM

Alcohol histories should reflect the effects of uncontrolled drinking rather than the quantity consumed. This should apply to patients with obvious alcoholism or to those being screened. The CAGE questionnaire shown in Fig. 38–1 is a useful screening instrument that has been shown to be accurate in detecting alcoholism in hospitalized patients.[10,22,23] Those with two or more positive responses have a high risk of alcoholism. Additional questions should search for medical effects of alcoholism and behavioral problems drawn from the DSM-III-R criteria.

Certain common problems in the preoperative period may provide clues to the diagnosis of alcoholism. Trauma,[15,24] new onset or labile hypertension, and nonspecific history of seizure with episodic use of antiseizure medications are frequently associated with alcoholism. Insomnia with requests for sedatives should

FIGURE 38–1. CAGE Questionnaire for Drinking History

C	Have you tried to *Cut* down on drinking?
A	Are you *Angry* or *Annoyed* when people criticize your drinking?
G	Do you ever feel *Guilty* about your drinking?
E	Do you ever take an *Eye* opener (drink in the morning)?

Source: Adapted from Ewing, JA: Detecting alcoholism: The CAGE questionnaire. *JAMA* 252:1907, 1984.

prompt the physician to explore the alcohol and drug history. Laboratory clues such as elevated liver function tests, increased red cell mean corpuscular volume, or thrombocytopenia, even in apparently healthy persons who do not fit alcoholic stereotypes, should raise suspicion.[25] All patients taking daily benzodiazepines should be questioned about alcohol.[26] Two-thirds of recovering women in an alcohol treatment program had received prescriptions for hypnotic and antianxiety drugs, although only half that number met criteria for abusing them.[27]

Occasionally, alcoholism will be missed in the preoperative evaluation and will present in the postoperative period. Clues to the diagnosis include increased anxiety, changes in mental status, and desire to leave the hospital against medical advice. More commonly, physiologic withdrawal symptoms lead one to consider the diagnosis. Once the diagnosis has been made, it is useful to assess perioperative risk by considering the three areas of intoxication, toxic effects, and withdrawal.

Alcohol Intoxication

Patients are frequently taken to surgery with high blood alcohol levels. In one series of 472 patients with alcohol levels > 100 mg/dl, 48 percent were taken to the operating room shortly after arrival in the emergency room.[18] Although the literature does not discuss the usefulness of blood alcohol levels, these confirm the level of intoxication for the anesthesiologist and the degree of tolerance for other physicians involved in ongoing care of the patient. For these and other medical-legal reasons, a blood alcohol level is usually obtained.

Acute intoxication is associated with several risks in the perioperative period. The acutely intoxicated patient can be a behavioral problem. Histories are suspect and inadequate, and cooperation with the physical examination may be difficult to elicit. Careful reevaluation of the history and physical examination within several hours and after surgery is important.

There are many physiologic effects of alcohol important in the perioperative period. Alcohol stimulates secretion of gastric acid and delays gastric emptying, increasing the risk of aspiration. Alcohol increases the possibility of shock, even in minor trauma without tachycardia or blood loss.[28] Animal studies have shown poor tolerance of intravascular volume loss.[29] Decreased cerebral tolerance of hypoxia has been demonstrated in nonalcoholic men given large amounts of alcohol.[30] Acute intoxication in chronic alcoholics has also been shown to increase left ventricular end-diastolic pressure in response to increases in afterload but to cause smaller increases in stroke output and work.[31] Even in the absence of cardiomyopathy, acute intoxication may compromise cardiac function in alcoholics. In animal studies, alcohol produces a dose-dependent depression of cardiac muscle contractility, the effect of which is additive to that of halothane.[32] Intoxicated patients require less anesthesia because of the concomitant effects of depressant drugs. Animal studies have shown that rats with blood alcohol levels of 240 mg/ml were anesthetized at brain halothane concentrations one-half of those required in controls.[33]

Acutely intoxicated patients who undergo emergency surgery cannot be electively detoxified. Surgery therefore subjects them to withdrawal in the postoperative period with greater potential for morbidity. Because the only treatment for acute alcohol intoxication is time, none but emergency surgery should be done in acutely intoxicated patients. In the past, these have mostly been trauma cases. However, in recent years an increasing proportion of surgery is performed on an outpatient or "same day" basis. Patients with fractures, a group with an increased risk of alcoholism, often undergo surgery in these settings.[34] The proportion of them appearing for surgery intoxicated and the consequences of early discharge are not known. Recent studies examining reasons for admission after ambulatory surgery did not consider information about substance abuse.[35]

Toxic Effects of Alcohol

Common end-organ effects of alcoholism are listed in Table 38–2. In many cases, damage is so serious that organ system dysfunction becomes the major perioperative risk factor rather than the underlying alcoholism itself. However, organ system dysfunction can be more subtle. Once the physician has identified occult alcoholism, he should use the history, physical examination, and laboratory evaluation to look for medical end-organ effects of the disease. Although some of these effects may not have implications for the surgical procedure, they support the diagnosis of alcoholism and may facilitate further treatment. The most significant impact of identifying occult alcoholism lies in alerting the anesthesiologist and other members of the treatment team to the possibility of tolerance and the potential for withdrawal.

Several medical complications of alcoholism are particularly important in the perioperative period. Actively drinking patients frequently have electrolyte abnormalities, including decreased serum levels of sodium, phosphate, and magnesium. Gastrointestinal complications include increased risk of gastritis and peptic ulcer, recurrent diarrhea, and occult or apparent liver disease. Preoperative liver function studies may be particularly useful in interpreting postoperative abnormalities. Long-term alcoholics frequently require nutritional evaluation. In addition to anemia, thrombocytopenia and coagulopathy due to decreased production of clotting factors may predispose them to bleeding. A decrease in the pulmo-

TABLE 38–2. Medical Complications of Alcoholism

Cardiac	Arrhythmias, cardiomyopathy, hypertension
Gastrointestinal	Peptic disease, esophageal varices, erosive gastritis, diarrhea, pancreatitis, alcoholic liver disease
Nutritional	Malnutrition from poor intake, vitamin and trace element deficiency
Malignancies	Oropharyngeal, laryngeal, esophageal, liver
Infectious	Aspiration pneumonia, tuberculosis
Obstetrical	Fetal alcohol syndrome
Metabolic	Ketoacidosis, hypophosphatemia, hypomagnesemia
Muscle and Bone	Rhabdomyolysis, osteoporosis, myopathy, aseptic necrosis of hip
Neurological	Acute Wernicke's syndrome, structural brain changes (dilated ventricles, widened sulci), cognitive deficits/organic brain syndromes (reversible and irreversible), peripheral neuropathy
Endocrine	Decreased testosterone, hypoglycemia, hyperglycemia
Hematologic	Anemia (iron deficiency, sideroblastic, megaloblastic, normochromic/normocytic), macrocytosis without anemia, thrombocytopenia

nary function parameters FVC and FEV_1, independent of smoking history, has been noted in chronic alcoholics.[36] In addition, alcohol decreases protective reflexes and depresses ciliary function, leukocyte mobilization rate, and functioning of alveolar macrophages.[37] Alcoholics are more susceptible to infection because of neutropenia, decreased chemotaxis, and decreased delayed hypersensitivity reactions[38] as well as nutritional neglect and impairment of lung clearance mechanisms. Early cardiomyopathy predisposes them to congestive heart failure, and more advanced cardiomyopathy increases the risk of embolic events. Asymptomatic chronic alcoholics with normal nutritional and electrolyte balance have been shown to have abnormal myocardial contractility with lower mean ejection fractions and greater mean end-diastolic diameters than controls.[39–41] Atrial and ventricular arrhythmias occur as part of the withdrawal syndrome or several days after episodes of binge drinking. Although earlier studies have failed to demonstrate decreased adrenocortical response to stress,[42] a more recent study contradicts this.[43]

The anesthesiologist must be aware not only of the medical end-organ effects of alcohol on the heart, brain, and liver, but also of the physiology and the pharmacology of alcohol as a drug in its acute and chronic use. Studies suggest that the phenomenon of tolerance may persist beyond the usual withdrawal period.[44] Alcoholics may need increased doses of anesthesia.[31,37,44,45] Hypoglycemia and hyperkalemia from rhabdomyolysis must be anticipated. Early alcoholic cardiomyopathy may present as unexplained tachycardia, atrial or ventricular ectopy, or conduction system abnormalities.[39–41] Alcohol potentiates or exerts an additive effect with many drugs used in anesthesia. Lower doses of these drugs may be necessary in intoxicated patients, but higher doses may be required in chronic alcoholics because of tolerance. Some anesthesiologists have advocated using regional anesthesia in alcoholics whenever possible,[45] but more recent reviews simply advocate careful evaluation and individualizing choice of anesthesia.[31]

Tolerance is an important consideration for all treating physicians. Drugs exhibiting cross-tolerance with alcohol include barbiturates, all of the benzodiazepines, and most central nervous system depressants. These drugs should be avoided except in specific treatment of withdrawal. To facilitate detoxification and treatment, sleep medications should be avoided when possible and antihistamines like hydroxyzine or diphenhydramine substituted for benzodiazepines.

Risk of Withdrawal

Although not all persons with alcoholism display withdrawal reactions when abstaining, alcohol withdrawal is probably the most frequent complication of alcoholism seen in hospitalized patients. Alcohol withdrawal increases anesthesia risk, obscures diagnosis, and threatens the success of recent surgical procedures. The agitated patient with undertreated delirium tremens may pull out surgical drains, incisional sutures, central lines, and catheters, and incur the hostility of hospital personnel. For these reasons, elective surgery should be delayed until detoxification is completed.[31] In more urgent situations, detoxification should begin as soon as possible before or after the procedure.

The manifestations of alcohol withdrawal can be divided into four categories: early uncomplicated withdrawal, alcoholic hallucinosis, alcohol withdrawal seizures, and delirium tremens. Early

withdrawal, occurring within six to eight hours after the last drink, is characterized by hypertension, tachycardia, tremors, irritability, insomnia, and mild gastrointestinal symptoms. Alcoholic hallucinosis is relatively rare, occurs approximately 24 hours after the last alcohol ingestion, and is characterized by hallucinations with a clear sensorium. Withdrawal seizures occur within 24 to 48 hours, are generalized, and rarely result in status epilepticus. The risk of withdrawal seizures is increased in those with a prior history of them or an underlying seizure disorder. Recently, it has been suggested that, although alcoholism predisposes patients to seizures even if they do not have an underlying central nervous system disease, such seizures may not be a manifestation of withdrawal.[46]

Delirium tremens represents the most serious manifestation of alcohol withdrawal and is characterized by increased autonomic activity manifested by fever, tachycardia, and hypertension, as well as global disorientation and hallucinations. Cardiac arrhythmias, including ventricular tachycardia, are frequent.[47] Delirium tremens usually occurs 48 to 72 hours after ingestion of alcohol but may occur later, especially if surgery intervenes. Current figures suggest a mortality rate of 1 to 5 percent[48] or higher, depending on concomitant medical or surgical problems. Risk factors for delirium tremens include a prior history of delirium tremens, age over 30, and a long history of alcohol ingestion. However, absence of these risk factors does not preclude delirium tremens. In an older study, the leading cause of death from delirium tremens was marked hyperthermia associated with vascular collapse.[49] Since that time, the mortality of delirium tremens has decreased, but the subject has not been extensively restudied.[48]

The manifestations of alcohol withdrawal may be masked after surgery, and the diagnosis can be missed, especially if alcoholism has not been previously suspected. Common signs of early withdrawal such as hypertension, tachycardia, and anxiety may be attributed to other postoperative problems. Administration of cross-tolerant drugs for anesthesia or analgesia may treat withdrawal and diminish its symptoms.

Alcohol withdrawal treatment must be individualized and titrated to the vital signs and symptoms as outlined in Table 38–3.[48,50–53] Standing orders written without frequent reevaluation of the patient risk undertreatment or oversedation. Although intravenous alcohol has been used to treat withdrawal,[54] intravenous or oral alcohol is not recommended. It has a low therapeutic ratio, cannot easily be titrated for detoxification, and is rapidly metabolized. Its use continues to promote toxic end-organ dysfunction and increases the difficulty of addressing the underlying problem of alcoholism.

Patients may experience changes in mental status or unexplained hypertension and tachycardia that may be due to inadequate treatment of withdrawal. Although not definitively demonstrated, undertreatment of withdrawal may increase the risk of delirium tremens. Risks of overtreatment and oversedation include atelectasis and aspiration, the need for additional medical interventions, and inability of the patient to comply with therapeutic regimens. Unless the patient is in delirium tremens, the goal of withdrawal treatment should be a calm cooperative patient, not one who is obtunded. Alcoholics are susceptible to other frequent causes of an altered sensorium including sepsis, infection, intracerebral bleeding, hypoxia, hypoglycemia, hepatic encephalopathy, uremia, thiamine deficiency, or withdrawal from other drugs.[48] It is common to attribute too many problems to alcoholism in the "known" alcoholic and too few to alcoholism in the undiagnosed or "less typical" patient.

TABLE 38–3. Alcohol Withdrawal Treatment

Manifestation	Goal	Treatment	Alternative Treatment
Uncomplicated withdrawal Hypertension, tachycardia, tremors, anxiety, nausea, insomnia Time: 6–8 hours after last drink	Detoxification Normal vital signs Calm cooperative patient	Oxazepam 60 mg stat then 30–60 mg PO q 4 h titrated to vital signs × 48 hours Taper doses by 25–50% each day thereafter Thiamine 100 mg IM × 1 day 100 mg IM or PO × 3 days	Lorazepam 1–2 mg IV or IM q 8 h
Delirium tremens Global disorientation, hypertension, tachycardia, fever, agitation Time: 48–72 hours after last drink	Lightly sedated patient Facilitate medical therapy Prevent self-harm	Lorazepam 1–5 mg IV until calm Repeat doses q 2–4 h as needed to maintain light sedation Discontinue in 48–72 hours when DT's resolve Thiamine as above	Diazepam 2–10 mg/5 min until calm Repeat doses as with lorazepam OR Haloperidol 5 mg IM q 2–4 h as needed to control agitation
Alcoholic hallucinosis Hallucinations with clear sensorium Time: 24 hours after last drink	Decrease hallucinations	Haloperidol 2–5 mg PO q 4 h as needed Thiamine as above	Haloperidol 0.5–2 mg IM
Seizures A. History of withdrawal seizures	Maintain seizure free Evaluate if seizure is due to withdrawal or other cause	A. Give phenytoin 100 tid × 5 days	A. Observe with no specific antiseizure treatment
B. Single self-limited withdrawal seizure 24–48 hours after last drink		B. Load with oral phenytoin; maintain pending evaluation	B. Begin evaluation, hold medication
C. Repeated seizures Time: < 48 hours after last drink		C. Load with IV phenytoin, maintain oral therapy pending evaluation	C. Administer usual alternative regimens for control of repeated seizures (barbiturates, diazepam)

Patients in delirium tremens may require intensive care monitoring. Fever, hypertension, arrhythmias, and electrolyte imbalance superimposed on end-organ alcohol damage and recent surgery combine to produce a seriously ill patient. Heavy sedation may be needed to facilitate necessary medical treatment but increases the risk of respiratory depression. Acute delirium tremens usually resolves within 72 hours. After resolution, a clouded sensorium may persist for two weeks or longer.[48]

Alcohol withdrawal also presents complications for the anesthesiologist.[31,33,44,45] Withdrawal can cause difficult and prolonged induction. If alcoholism has not been previously diagnosed, a difficult induction may be the first indication of withdrawal. One case of delirium tremens under anesthesia has been reported in a trauma patient who went to surgery 48 hours after admission and developed hypertension and fever to 104°F intraoperatively.[55] Some of the features of delirium tremens can resemble those of malignant hyperthermia, thyrotoxicosis, or neuroleptic malignant syndrome.

Recovering Persons

Patients recovering from alcohol also require special assessment in the perioperative period. They may or may not identify themselves as recovering alcoholics or as members of Alcoholics Anonymous. Many AA members have firmly held beliefs on the use of medications. Recovering alcoholics should not be given medications such as cough syrups or theophylline elixirs that contain alcohol. If possible, cross-tolerant drugs like benzodiazepines should be avoided. Although AA members remain drug-free from all sedatives and narcotics when well, they will take analgesics as necessary when ill. However, they may prefer to abstain from routinely prescribed sleep medications. Careful histories should be taken from all persons denying even occasional alcohol use to identify recovering persons, and all members of the treating team must be aware of patient preferences and the need to explain psychoactive medications.

Disulfiram, occasionally used in the long-term treatment of recovering alcoholics, has been reported to cause acute hypotension during anesthesia. Episodes may occur during stimulatory events and may be due to norepinephrine depletion.[56] The literature suggests that it is not necessary to stop the medication if it is needed, but careful intraoperative monitoring is recommended.[56]

Treatment of Alcoholism

Alcoholism is a treatable disease with an improved prognosis for relapse-free intervals if the patient has physician support and motivation.[16] The frustrations of seeing many denying or relapsing patients, anger toward uncooperative patients, and lack of knowledge of treatment approaches and options may result in too few alcoholic patients being identified and referred for treatment.[14] For many young patients on surgical services, alcoholism is their primary medical disorder and lifelong health risk. However, in one emergency room study of 346 patients involved in motor vehicle accidents, blood alcohol levels were tested in only 25 percent. Despite a median blood alcohol level of 299 mg/dl, none was referred for alcoholism counseling or treatment.[24] In hospitalized patients with alcoholism, physician-instituted treatment rates were less than 50 percent on surgery and obstetrics and gynecology services and 50 to 75 percent in medicine and neurology.[9]

Use of the CAGE questionnaire and routine screening will result in higher detection rates of alcoholism. Once the acute complications of alcoholism or surgery have been adequately managed, the patient must be informed of the diagnosis and its implications. Counseling and treatment should be offered through whatever resources are available in the hospital or the community.

DRUG ABUSE

Commonly used illegal and abused prescription drugs include narcotics, central nervous system stimulants such as amphetamines and cocaine, hallucinogens, and central nervous system depressants. Other prescription drugs with potential for abuse include steroids and diuretics. Identifying users of illegal drugs may be difficult because of their talents at deception. Identifying addiction to prescription drugs may be complicated by the patient's lack of understanding of his addiction to a legally prescribed medication. Diagnosis is greatly aided by a high level of suspicion and the ability to test the urine for drugs.

When screening for drug use, patients should be asked in a direct, nonjudgmental manner whether they are using drugs. Explaining the medical importance of correct information in preventing withdrawal or avoiding anesthesia complications facilitates gathering accurate data. Information on the drug, quantities used, method of administration, frequency and duration of use, and time of last dose should be elicited.

Correct identification of drugs with street names should be checked with knowledgeable persons or a local drug treatment facility. Because street drugs vary in purity and concentration, information on quantity of use based on number of bags cannot be used in determining doses of in-hospital medications. The cost of the patient's habit is useful if accurate information about the current street market is available from local substance abuse programs. Previous treatment efforts and withdrawal complications should be noted. Intravenous drug users should be questioned about history of hepatitis, patterns of needle use, access to clean needles, and frequency of injections, factors which have been shown to correlate with the risk of acquiring HIV infection.[57] Previous serological testing for HIV and hepatitis should be noted. Intravenous drug abusers should also be asked about recent use of "street" nonaddictive prescription drugs. Clonidine, cephalexin, and most other antibiotics are frequently bought and sold by the addict to self-treat withdrawal or prevent infection. Most of these can be demonstrated on urine testing. Knowledge of prior antibiotic use may influence early antibiotic choices in the hospital.

Clinical clues that may suggest substance abuse include unexplained weight loss, common in amphetamine and cocaine users; medication regimens containing several sedatives, anxiolytics, or analgesics; requests for specific medications by brand name; and "allergies" to all but the most potent analgesics or most euphoria-producing anxiolytics. Patients with an increased risk of iatrogenic drug dependence include those with chronic pain, anxiety or stress disorders, depression, and insomnia. Diuretic and laxative abuse is common in patients with eating disorders, and steroid abuse is encountered in young athletes.

Physical examination should document stigmata of intravenous drug abuse and signs and symptoms of withdrawal. Laboratory data should include a urine drug screen, hepatitis serology testing as appropriate, and liver function tests. Indications for HIV testing should follow accepted guidelines.[58] The pharmacology of any unusual or unfamiliar substance should be reviewed early in the hospital course to anticipate problems. Any patient in whom substance abuse is suspected should have a urine drug screen done early in the course of the hospitalization without regard to age or socio-economic status. Even if drug screen results are not available before a scheduled or emergency procedure, they are useful for verification. Morphine will be present in toxic screens 12 to 24 hours after the last dose. Quinine, used to "cut" street heroin and cocaine, will be present 5 to 10 days after last use.[59]

Narcotic Intoxication

Commonly used narcotics include heroin, synthetic opioids (propoxyphene, oxycodone, and meperidine), codeine, and methadone. Acute heroin intoxication rarely presents a problem before surgery because of its short duration and the ability of naloxone to reverse it. Decreased consciousness, miotic pupils, and respiratory depression are the hallmarks of opiate toxicity. Hypotension and tachycardia may be present, and pulmonary edema has been reported.[60,61] Treatment of opiate overdose includes airway maintenance, ventilatory support, and correction of hypoxia. Opiates depress brainstem sensitivity to carbon dioxide, leading to increased dependence on hypoxic respiratory drive. Oxygen use must be closely monitored.[61] Naloxone should be given intravenously in doses of 0.01 mg/kg of body weight every three to five minutes until the patient is arousable with a respiratory rate of 10 to 20 per minute. Acute precipitation of withdrawal should be avoided.

Heroin-induced pulmonary edema is thought to be similar in mechanism to high-altitude pulmonary edema with central nervous system–mediated systemic vasoconstriction, massive shifts of intravascular volume to the pulmonary circulation, pulmonary capillary hypertension, and fluid exudation into the alveoli and interstitium. Treatment consists of restoring consciousness, oxygenation, artificial ventilation, and positive end-expiratory pressure if needed. If treated properly, heroin-induced pulmonary edema carries a low mortality. Pulmonary edema has also been reported with methadone use but is less common.[60] Because street heroin is usually heavily mixed with quinine, patients with heroin overdoses should have appropriate electrocardiographic monitoring.

Chronic Effects of Narcotic Use

Most long-term effects of narcotic use are seen with intravenous use (see Table 38–4). As in alcoholism, once end-organ damage has occurred, medical management of these problems is similar to that of the same problems due to other causes. The evaluation should include examination of the skin for abscesses and cellulitis and a careful search for manifestations of hepatitis, tuberculosis, sexually transmitted diseases, and HIV infection. Many intravenous drug abusers have false-positive serologic tests for syphilis

TABLE 38–4. Medical Complications of Narcotic Addiction

Infections (due to intravenous drug use)	Endocarditis, abscesses/cellulitis, septic phlebitis, hepatitis (all types), tetanus, AIDS, sexually transmitted diseases, osteomyelitis, septic arthritis, necrotizing fasciitis, anaerobic infections
Cardiac	Endocarditis, arrhythmias due to quinine
Gastrointestinal	Ileus, constipation, hepatitis
Central nervous system	CNS sequelae of infectious consequences, seizures, transverse myelitis
Pulmonary	Pulmonary edema, septic emboli, "talc" lung
Renal	Glomerulonephritis, rhabdomyolysis due to immobilization or crush injuries

that should be followed up with direct treponemal antibody testing. Those with a history of bacterial endocarditis should receive preoperative antibiotic prophylaxis even in the absence of significant murmurs or residual vegetations on echocardiogram (see Chap. 43).

Whether the substance abuser is using intravenous heroin or oral propoxyphene, he or she will have developed a tolerance that will affect management of anesthesia and pain medications. Tolerance to the euphoric effects of narcotics develops more rapidly than tolerance to respiratory depressant effects. Most surgical patients require postoperative narcotic analgesia, and these agents should not be withdrawn from an addict at that time even if elective surgery is contemplated. Methadone in a dose of 10 mg intramuscularly can be used for premedication. Patients not going to surgery immediately can be switched to methadone preoperatively and detoxified later. Narcotic addicts usually have no problems with anesthesia if their "physiologic" drug requirement is met with methadone or its equivalent.[62]

The possibility of HIV infection raises questions of perioperative risk for both patient and hospital personnel. Universal precautions as recommended by the Centers for Disease Control should be used routinely to minimize potential exposures. For a discussion of specific problems in HIV infections, see Chap. 31.

Narcotic addicts are particularly susceptible to postoperative atelectasis.[43] Intestinal "pseudo-obstruction" from increased resting tone in the bowel may also develop. Treatment is conservative.

Patients maintained on chronic methadone maintenance in approved programs present special management problems when hospitalized. The patient's participation in the program and his dose of drug must be verified immediately. Hospital personnel should not attempt to alter this dose during the hospitalization.[59] Patients who are not eating may be given two-thirds of their usual dose in two divided doses intramuscularly or subcutaneously every 12 hours. A dose should be given on the morning of the surgical procedure. Patients should be reassured that they are receiving their methadone at the usual dose, and extensive discussion of dosing requirements should be avoided. These patients do not require increased analgesic dosage. However, tolerance leads to a shortened duration of action of narcotic analgesics and the need for more frequent dosing. Usual doses of postsurgical analgesics

should therefore be given in addition to methadone. PCA pumps have been successfully used in providing postoperative analgesia to methadone-dependent patients.[63] This method of delivery avoids the peaks and troughs of dosing but requires frequent assessment of hourly demand, dose, and respiratory rate.

Narcotic Withdrawal

Narcotic addicts often engage in drug-seeking behavior in the hospital because they fear withdrawal. Early reassurance by physicians regarding knowledge of withdrawal and willingness to treat to avoid discomfort will help to deter behavioral problems. Self-reporting of the amount of "habit" should be treated with healthy skepticism, especially in patients with negative urine drug testing for opiates. Treatment for withdrawal can await the development of signs and symptoms listed in Table 38–5. Patients with positive urine screens or with physical signs of withdrawal require detoxification. Addicts admitted for problems that do not require narcotics for anesthesia or analgesia can be detoxified using clonidine in the protocol outlined in Table 38–6.[64] Management of acute medical problems always takes precedence over detoxification.

Patients exhibiting withdrawal may be placed on methadone 10 to 40 mg/day in two or three divided oral doses, titrated to prevent withdrawal symptoms and avoid sedation. Additional short-acting narcotics can be given to control pain as needed, remembering that tolerance requires a higher dose and increased frequency of dosing. Patients may also need short-acting narcotics until oral methadone takes effect. The onset of action of methadone is two to four hours after oral administration and 30 to 60 minutes after parenteral administration. Vital signs should be monitored for adequacy of dosing. Doses should not be discussed with the patient. Requests to do so should be reframed to focus on symptoms or questions concerning overall care. Pentazocine (Talwin) and

TABLE 38–5. Narcotic Withdrawal Signs and Symptoms

Grade	Signs/Symptoms
0	Anxiety Drug craving
1	Yawning Diaphoresis Rhinorrhea Lacrimation Restlessness, insomnia
2	Dilated pupils Piloerection Muscle twitching, tremors Myalgias, arthralgias Abdominal pain Anorexia
3	Nausea Extreme restlessness Hypertension, tachycardia Tachypnea Fever
4	Vomiting, dehydration Diarrhea Hyperglycemia Hypotension Curled-up position

TABLE 38–6. Clonidine Detoxification for Narcotics

0.2 mg PO stat, then
0.1 mg PO q 4 h × 48 hours
0.1 mg PO q 6 h × 24 hours
0.1 mg PO q 8 h × 24 hours
0.1 mg PO q 12 h × 24 hours
Hold dose for systolic blood pressure < 90 mmHg

nalbuphine (Nubain) should never be used in patients suspected of narcotic addiction because they have both agonist and antagonist properties and can precipitate withdrawal.[59]

A protocol using buprenorphine has recently been described for narcotic withdrawal for elderly or hypotensive patients who cannot tolerate clonidine and in those requiring coexisting treatment of pain.[69] Buprenorphine is a partial agonist that blocks withdrawal from opiates. It has few adverse hemodynamic effects and provides pain relief as it blocks withdrawal. It has a long half-life and produces a mild clinically insignificant withdrawal syndrome when discontinued. Use of buprenorphine for detoxification remains controversial because of its mixed agonist and antagonist properties. If its benefit in narcotic detoxification is confirmed in further studies, it will serve as an excellent alternative to methadone in the perioperative period.

When the acute medical or surgical problem is resolved and narcotic analgesics are no longer needed, the patient receiving methadone outside a methadone maintenance program must be detoxified. Doses can be reduced by 20% every one to two days with close monitoring of withdrawal symptoms. Although this may be tedious and time-consuming and require extended hospitalization, it is illegal to continue patients on methadone outside of maintenance programs. Early involvement of an addiction specialist may facilitate postoperative detoxification in a substance abuse treatment program if acute hospital care is not needed. All patients with addiction should be offered substance abuse treatment services through social service workers, addiction specialists, or psychiatrists even if the prognosis is poor. Although kindness, knowledge, and optimal treatment of withdrawal may prevent many behavioral problems, conflicts with physicians and nursing staff may still occur, especially when the patient and treatment team have different expectations.[66] Early psychiatric or addiction specialist consultation is encouraged to offer optimal treatment to the patient and peace of mind to staff before these problems overwhelm patient care considerations.

Recovering Persons

Naltrexone, a pure narcotic antagonist similar to naloxone, is occasionally used in outpatient treatment of narcotic addicts. It is an oral agent with a narcotic blocking half-life of 20 to 30 hours. Most patients in programs wear appropriate "medical alert" jewelry. Information on its use is important to the anesthesiologist because its narcotic blocking effects can be overcome if analgesia or anesthesia is required. Physicians caring for recovering narcotic addicts undergoing surgery should discuss analgesia with them before the procedure, provide adequate pain medication, and substitute nonnarcotic analgesics when possible.

COCAINE

In the last five years, cocaine use has risen dramatically with a concomitant increase in the number of reported medical complications.[67-70] Previously taken intranasally, it is now more commonly used intravenously or smoked as pure cocaine base or "crack." There are no studies of the overall risk of cocaine use in surgical patients. However, the general risks of poor nutrition, increased susceptibility to infection, and the previously discussed risks associated with intravenous heroin apply here as well.

Medical histories in patients who acknowledge cocaine use should detail method of administration, previous complications, symptoms of sexually transmitted diseases, and HIV status. Intravenous cocaine and crack use has been associated with increased rates of prostitution and trading of sex for drugs. The number of injections of intravenous cocaine per month, unlike in heroin use, is a serious risk factor for HIV infection.[57] All users should be encouraged to undergo HIV testing and serologic testing for syphilis. Cocaine metabolites can be detected in the urine up to five days after use by inhalation, but intravenous cocaine is rapidly cleared.

Physical examination should document the usual stigmata of intravenous drug abuse. Women should have gynecologic examinations with cultures for asymptomatic gonorrhea and chlamydia, although studies to prove the benefits of this recommendation have not yet been done.

Cocaine Intoxication

Surgery should be delayed in patients with acute cocaine intoxication until the drug is metabolized. Intravenous or inhaled cocaine has a short half-life of 90 minutes. Cocaine intoxication is accompanied by increases in pulse, systolic blood pressure, and temperature. Other effects of acute cocaine intoxication are listed in Table 38–7. Arrhythmias are common, and myocardial infarction has been reported.[69] Cocaine has been used for years as a topical anesthetic in rhinolaryngologic procedures. Even in these doses it

TABLE 38–7. Medical Complications of Cocaine Use

Cardiac	Angina, arrhythmias, myocardial infarction, sudden death, rupture of ascending aorta
Gastrointestinal	Intestinal ischemia
Infectious	All complications of intravenous drug use (see Table 38–4)
	Sexually transmitted diseases (all)
Metabolic	Hyperpyrexia
Central nervous system	Seizures, cerebrovascular accident (subarachnoid hemorrhage, infarction)
Renal	Rhabdomyolysis
Pulmonary	Pulmonary edema, spontaneous pneumomediastinum and pneumopericardium, ulceration and perforation of nasal septum from intranasal use, rhinorrhea, rhinitis
Genitourinary	Increase in time to orgasm, decreased erection and ejaculation
Endocrine	Hyperprolactinemia

causes vasoconstriction of the coronary arteries, decrease in coronary blood flow, and increase in myocardial oxygen demand.[71]

Most medical effects of cocaine are the result of acute intoxication rather than chronic use. Patients requiring emergency surgery should be evaluated for evidence of acute toxicity. Electrocardiograms should be obtained regardless of age, serum creatine phosphokinase (CPK) levels should be measured when appropriate, and temperature should be closely monitored. There is no indication for administration of prophylactic antiseizure medications.

Acutely intoxicated cocaine users requiring surgery may present behavioral problems including transient panic with terror of impending death, paranoid psychosis, and hyperactivity. Obtaining informed consent may be difficult. Acute cocaine intoxication with anxiety and paranoia can be treated with oral diazepam. More severe problems, including hallucinations, extreme paranoia, or destructive behavior, require intravenous sedation and seizure prophylaxis with either intravenous diazepam in a dose of 5 mg every five minutes to a maximum of four doses or intravenous amobarbital in a dose of 20 to 85 mg to a maximum of four doses. Persistent cocaine-induced adrenergic crisis can be treated with intravenous propranolol. Protocols and recommendations are published elsewhere and should be used with the help of an addiction specialist if possible.[72]

Chronic Effects

The chronic effects of cocaine are primarily psychiatric and behavioral and include increasing agitation, dysphoria, depression, paranoia, debilitation, and loss of ability to maintain orderly activities of daily life. However, some medical complications have been described. Nasal administration has caused hyperemia of the mucosa and septal perforation, bronchitis, and obstructive and restrictive lung disease. Delayed healing and poor surgical results have been described in patients undergoing rhinoplasty.[73] In men, chronic use interferes with ability to develop an erection and ejaculation. In women, use throughout pregnancy has caused obstetrical complications.

Withdrawal

Although cocaine withdrawal is presumed not to produce a clinically significant physiologic withdrawal syndrome, it does affect several neurotransmitters including dopamine, norepinephrine, and serotonin.[67] As neurotransmitter systems become better elucidated, treatment of withdrawal dysphoria and agitation may be possible with amino acid precursors. However, such approaches remain experimental.

Withdrawal patterns are well defined. A period of extreme dysphoria which may be accompanied by paranoia and violent behavior occurs one to six hours after euphoria dissipates. Hospitalized patients undergoing surgery in this phase should be given mild sedatives. Dysphoria is followed by a "crash" characterized by hypersomnolence, hyperphagia, severe anhedonia, and depression. This phase may be difficult to recognize in the postoperative period. Psychiatric consultation should be sought if the diagnosis is unclear or management is difficult.

Cocaine-induced alteration of cardiovascular reactivity may extend beyond the period of drug use. Ambulatory electrocardiographic monitoring of male cocaine users in a drug rehabilitation unit revealed that 40 percent had transient ST-segment elevations during the first week of withdrawal.[74]

OTHER DRUGS

Changes in the popularity of various drugs make it impossible to review each of them comprehensively. Hallucinogens were used much less commonly in the 1980s than in the 1970s. Approaches to hallucinogen intoxication and information relevant to anesthesia are available elsewhere.[45,75]

Barbiturate overdose and addiction are also seen less frequently. Barbiturate withdrawal, characterized by fever, delirium, and seizures, can be fatal. Treatment of withdrawal from barbiturates or any cross-tolerant sedative hypnotic consists of administering test doses of medium-acting barbiturates, titrating to sedation, and detoxifying over a period of several weeks. Regimens are described in many substance abuse handbooks and texts.[75,76] Butalbital, a short- to intermediate-acting barbiturate, is an ingredient in the commonly prescribed combination analgesic Fiorinal. Chronic headache and migraine sufferers may be iatrogenically addicted to butalbital, and careful histories must be obtained in such patients to avoid inadvertently stopping the drug and precipitating withdrawal.

Benzodiazepines are widely prescribed and frequently abused. A national survey in 1979 indicated that close to 11 percent of adults between the ages of 18 and 79 had used benzodiazepines at least once, and 1.6 percent reported daily use for a year or more. However, the true prevalence of benzodiazepine dependence has not been determined.[77] Patients should be carefully questioned about use of sedative hypnotics, including the type of drug and frequency and duration of use. Patients addicted to benzodiazepines usually take them as prescribed, do not increase the dose to improve effect, and may have little understanding of their physiologic addiction until the drug is abruptly stopped. Urine drug screens may be helpful to verify drug use. Serum levels may be obtained if more frequent use in greater amounts is suspected.

Benzodiazepine use is so frequent in hospitalized patients that withdrawal reactions may be unintentionally treated or prevented.[78] Withdrawal symptoms of benzodiazepines are similar to those of alcohol. However, the varying half-lives and lipid solubilities of the different benzodiazepines influence the duration of the withdrawal period. Withdrawal from alprazolam can last several weeks and include seizures unresponsive to routine treatment.[79,80] Unexpected seizures occurring more than 48 hours after admission or prolonged unexplained postoperative delirium should prompt a search for evidence of nonalcohol substance abuse.[81]

For recovering benzodiazepine abusers, every effort should be made to avoid reinstituting the drug. Alternative sleep medications like diphenhydramine, hydroxyzine, or amitriptyline may be used. Setting clear goals with patients and allowing them to participate in medication decisions can be helpful.

SUMMARY

1. Chemical dependency on alcohol, prescription drugs, and illegal drugs is common but frequently overlooked in medical and surgical patients. The medical and behavioral complications of substance abuse contribute to morbidity in the perioperative period.

2. A history of alcohol use should be elicited from all patients and should be directed at the effects of drinking rather than the quantity consumed.

3. Evaluation of alcoholic patients should include a comprehensive history, physical examination, and laboratory evaluation, including complete blood count, platelet count, prothrombin time, liver function studies, and determinations of serum concentrations of electrolytes, magnesium, and phosphorus.

4. Elective surgery should be delayed until alcohol detoxification is completed. In emergency situations, detoxification should begin as early in the hospital course as possible.

5. Anesthesia requirements vary significantly in alcoholic patients and depend on the degree of intoxication, tolerance, and the presence or absence of withdrawal symptoms.

6. In eliciting a history of drug use, it is important to determine the pattern of use and method of administration to anticipate potential perioperative complications and screen for concurrent drug-induced disease.

7. Narcotic-dependent patients usually tolerate anesthesia well but usually have increased analgesic requirements. They should not be detoxified before the procedure.

8. Cocaine is rapidly metabolized and should not interfere with surgery. However, acute cocaine intoxication may require treatment with sedatives, and long-term abusers may present significant behavioral problems.

9. Patients who are illegally or iatrogenically addicted to benzodiazepines have increased anesthetic requirements and may experience postoperative withdrawal symptoms.

10. Surgical patients suffering from substance abuse need not only diagnosis and treatment of medication complications but also postoperative referral to appropriate treatment programs.

REFERENCES

1. Chappel JN, Schnoll SH: Physician attitudes: Effect on the treatment of chemically dependent patients. *JAMA* 237:2318–2319, 1977.
2. Niven RG: Alcoholism—a problem in perspective. *JAMA* 252:1912–1914, 1984.
3. Lee JF, Giesecke AH, Jenkins MT: Anesthetic management of trauma: Influence of alcohol ingestion. *South Med J* 60:1240, 1967.
4. Ward RE, Flynn TC, Miller PW, Blaisdell WF: Effects of ethanol ingestion on the severity and outcome of trauma. *Am J Surg* 144:153–157, 1982.
5. Rinaldi RC, Steindler EM, Wilford BB, Goodwin D: Clarification and standardization of substance terminology. *JAMA* 259:555–558, 1988.
6. *Diagnostic and Statistical Manual of Mental Disorders*, 3d rev. ed. (DSM-III-R). Washington DC, American Psychiatric Association, 1987.
7. Gitlow SE, Peyser HS (eds): *Alcoholism: A practical treatment guide*. New York, Grune & Stratton, 1980.
8. Morse RM, Flavin DR et al: Definition of alcoholism. *JAMA* 268:1012–1014, 1992.
9. Moore RD, Bone LR, Geller JA et al: Prevalence, detection and treatment of alcoholism in hospitalized patients. *JAMA* 261:403–407, 1989.
10. Bush B, Shaw S, Cleary P et al: Screening for alcohol abuse using the CAGE questionnaire. *Am J Med* 82:231–235, 1987.
11. West LJ, Maxwell DS, Nobel EP et al: Alcoholism. *Ann Intern Med* 100:445–456, 1984.
12. Sherin K, Piotrowski Z, Panek S et al: Screening for alcoholism in a community hospital. *J Fam Prac* 15:1091–1095, 1982.
13. Beresford T, Low D, Adduci R et al: Alcoholism assessment on an orthopedic surgery service. *Am J Bone Joint Surg* 64:730–733, 1982.
14. Dulit RA, Strain JJ: The problem of alcohol in the medical-surgical patient. *Gen Hosp Psych* 8:81–85, 1986.
15. Reyna TN, Hollis HW, Hulsebus RC: Alcohol related trauma: The surgeon's responsibility. *Ann Surg* 201:194–197, 1985.
16. Barnes HN: The etiology and natural history of alcoholism, in Barnes HN, Aronson MD, Delbanco TL (eds): *Alcoholism: A Guide for the Primary Care Physician*. New York, Springer-Verlag, 1987, pp 16–25.
17. Parran Jr. TV, Applebaum GE: Medical problems in detoxification: The experience of a general medical consult service. *Substance Abuse* 13:207–211, 1992.
18. Huth JF, Maier RV, Simonowitz DA et al: Effect of acute ethanolism on the hospital course and outcome of injured automobile drivers. *J Trauma* 23:494–498, 1983.
19. Thal ER, Bost RO, Anderson RJ: Effects of alcohol and other drugs on traumatized patients. *Arch Surg* 120:708–712, 1985.
20. Tonnesen H, Schutten BT, Jorgensen BB: Influence of alcohol on morbidity after colonic surgery. *Dis Colon Rectum* 30:549–551, 1987.
21. Camer SJ, King N, Gianelli S et al: Inappropriate response of drug addicts to cardiothoracic surgery. *NY State J Med* 72:1718, 1973.
22. Ewing JA: Detecting alcoholism: The CAGE questionnaire. *JAMA* 252:1905–1907, 1984.
23. Bernardt MW, Mumford V, Taylor C et al: Comparison of questionnaire and laboratory tests in the detection of excessive drinking and alcoholism. *Lancet* 1:325–328, 1982.
24. Chang G, Astrachan B: The emergency department surveillance of alcohol intoxication after motor vehicle accidents. *JAMA* 260:2533–2536, 1988.
25. Skinner HA, Holt S, Schuller R et al: Identification of alcohol abuse using laboratory tests and a history of trauma. *Ann Int Med* 101:847–851, 1984.
26. Busto V, Sellers EM, Sisson B et al: Benzodiazepine use and abuse in alcoholics. *Clin Pharmacol Ther* 31:207–208, 1982.
27. Schuckit MA, Morrisey ER: Drug abuse among alcoholic women. *Psychiatry* 136:607–611, 1979.
28. Swan KG, Vidaver RM, LaVigne JE et al: Acute alcoholism, minor trauma, and "shock." *J Trauma* 17:215–218, 1977.
29. Knott DH, Beard JD: The effect of chronic ethanol administration on the response of the dog to repeated acute hemorrhage. *Am J Med Sc* 254:178–188, 1967.
30. Nettles JI, Olson RN: Effects of alcohol on hypoxia. *JAMA* 194:1193–1194, 1965.
31. Bruce DL: Alcoholism and anesthesia. *Anesth Analg* 62:89–96, 1983.
32. Lee SC, Sohn YZ, Son KS: The effects of ethyl alcohol alone and with halothane in an isolated rat left ventricular papillary muscle (abstract). *Anesthesiology* 71(Suppl):A559, 1989.
33. Wolfson B, Freed B: Influence of alcohol on anesthetic requirement and acute toxicity. *Anesth Analg* 59:826–830, 1980.
34. Elvy GA, Gillesie WJ: Problem drinking in orthopedic patients. *Br Bone Joint Surg* 67B:478–481, 1985.
35. Gold BS, Kitz DS, Lecky JH et al: Unanticipated admission to the hospital following ambulatory surgery. *JAMA* 262:3008–3010, 1989.
36. Lange P, Groth S, Mortensen J et al: Pulmonary function is influenced by heavy alcohol consumption. *Ann Rev Respir Dis* 137:1119–1122, 1988.
37. Edwards R, Mosher VB: Alcohol abuse, anesthesia, and intensive care. *Anaesthesia* 35:474–489, 1980.
38. MacGregor RR: Alcohol and immune defense. *JAMA* 256:1474–1479, 1986.

39. Urbano-Marquez A, Estioch R, Navarro-Lopez F et al: The effects of alcoholism on skeletal and cardiac muscle. *N Engl J Med* 320:409–415, 1989.

40. Regan TJ: The heart, alcoholism and nutritional disease, in Hurst JW, Logue RB et al (eds): *The Heart*, 6th ed. New York, McGraw-Hill, 1986, pp 1446–1451.

41. Askanas A, Udoshi M, Sadjadi SA: The heart in chronic alcoholism: A noninvasive study. *Am Heart J* 99:9–16, 1980.

42. Margraf HW, Moyer CA, Ashford LE, Lavalle LW: Adrenocortical function in alcoholics. *J Surg Res* 7:55–62, 1967.

43. St. Haxholdt O, Johansson G: The alcoholic patient and surgical stress. *Anesthesia* 37:797–801, 1982.

44. Wolfson G: Alcohol and anesthesia, in *Refresher Courses in Anesthesiology*. American Society of Anesthesiologists, 1982, vol 10, pp 213–224.

45. Caldwell T III: Anesthesia for patients with behavioral and environmental disorders, in Katz J, Benumof J, Kadis LB (eds): *Anesthesia and Uncommon Diseases*. Philadelphia, Saunders, 1981, pp 672–677.

46. Ng SKC, Hauser A, Brust JCM et al: Alcohol consumption and withdrawal in new onset seizures. *N Engl J Med* 319:666–673, 1988.

47. Abraham E, Shoemaker WC, McCartney SF: Cardiorespiratory patterns in severe delirium tremens. *Arch Intern Med* 145:1957–1959, 1985.

48. Turner RC, Lichstein PR, Peden J Jr et al: Alcohol withdrawal syndromes: A review of pathophysiology, clinical presentation, and treatment. *J Gen Int Med* 4:432–444, 1989.

49. Tavel ME, Davidson W, Balteron TD: A critical analysis of mortality associated with delirium tremens. *Am J Med Sci* 242:18–29, 1961.

50. Holloway HC, Hales PE, Watanabe HK: Recognition and treatment of acute alcohol withdrawal syndromes. *Psych Clin N Am* 7:729–743, 1984.

51. Sellers EM, Kalant H: Alcohol intoxication and withdrawal. *N Engl J Med* 2924:757–762, 1976.

52. Liskow BI, Goodwin DW: Pharmacologic treatment of alcohol intoxication, withdrawal and dependence: A critical review. *J Stud Alcohol* 48:356–370, 1987.

53. Thompson WL, Johnson AD, Maddrey WL: Diazepam and paraldehyde for treatment of severe delirium tremens. *Ann Intern Med* 82:175–180, 1980.

54. Levesque PR: Anesthesiology, in Molitch ME (ed): *Management of Medical Problems in Surgical Patients*. Philadelphia, Davis, 1982, pp 747–772.

55. Upham W: Delirium tremens in a patient under anesthesia. *AANA J* 46:408–410, 1978.

56. Diaz J, Hill G: Hypotension with anesthesia in disulfiram-treated patients. *Anesthesiology* 5:366–368, 1979.

57. Schoenbaum EE, Hartel D et al: Risk factor for human immunodeficiency virus infection in intravenous drug users. *N Engl J Med* 321:874–880, 1989.

58. Hagen MD, Myer KB, Pauker SG: Routine preoperative screening for HIV: Does the risk to surgeon outweigh the risk to the patient? *JAMA* 259:1357–1359, 1988.

59. Fultz JM Jr, Senay EC: Guidelines for the management of hospitalized narcotic addicts. *Ann Int Med* 82:815–818, 1975.

60. Khantzian EJ, McKenna GJ: Acute toxic and withdrawal reactions associated with drug use and abuse. *Ann Int Med* 90:361–372, 1979.

61. Jaffe JH, Martin WR: Opioid analgesics and antagonists, in Gilman AG, Goodman LS, Rall TW, Murad F (eds): *The Pharmacological Basis of Therapeutics*, 7th ed. New York, Macmillan, 1985, pp 491–501.

62. Wood PR, Soni N: Anesthesia and substance abuse. *Anesthesia* 44:672–680, 1989.

63. Boyle RK: Intra- and postoperative anaesthetic management of an opioid addict undergoing Caesarean section. *Anesth Intens Care* 19(2):276–279, 1991.

64. Gold MS, Pottash AC, Sweeny DR, Kebler HD: Opiate withdrawal using clonidine. *JAMA* 243:343–346, 1980.

65. Parran TV, Adelman CL, Jasinski DR: Buprenorphine detoxification of medically unstable narcotic dependent patients: A case series. Abstract presented to AMERSA annual meeting, Nov 1989.

66. Nicolini R, Rubenstein R: Psychiatric aspects in the management of the hospitalized intravenous drug abuser, in Levine DP, Sobel JD (eds): *Infections in Intravenous Drugs Abusers*. New York, Oxford University Press, 1991, pp 68–79.

67. Gawin FH, Ellinwood EH Jr: Cocaine and other stimulants. *N Engl J Med* 318:1173–1182, 1988.

68. Cregler LL, Mark H: Medical complications of cocaine abuse. *N Engl J Med* 315:1495–1500, 1986.

69. Isner JM, Estes NAM III, Thompson PD et al: Acute cardiac events temporally related to cocaine abuse. *N Engl J Med* 315:1438–1443, 1986.

70. Roth D, Alarcon JF, Fernandez JA et al: Acute rhabdomyolysis associated with cocaine intoxication. *N Engl J Med* 319:673–677, 1988.

71. Lange RA, Cigarroa RG, Yancey CW Jr et al: Cocaine individual coronary-artery vasoconstriction. *N Engl J Med* 321:1557–1562, 1989.

72. Landry M: Update on cocaine dependence: Crack and advances in diagnostic treatment, in Smith DE, Wesson DR (eds): *Treating Cocaine Dependency*. Center City, MO, Hazleden Foundation, 1988, pp 91–116.

73. Slavin SA: Cocaine user; potential problem patient for rhinoplasty. *Plas Reconstr Surg* 86(3):436, 1990.

74. Nademanee K, Gorelick DA, Josephson MA et al: Transient ischemic episodes among cocaine users: Evidence of coronary vasospasm. *Ann Intern Med* (in press).

75. Hyman SE: Overdoses with specific psychotropic drugs, in Hyman SE (ed): *Manual of Psychiatric Emergencies*. Boston, Little Brown, 1984, pp 243–254.

76. Schuckit MA: *Drug and alcohol abuse: A clinical guide to diagnosis and treatment*, 3d ed. New York, Plenum Press, 1989.

77. Mellinger GD, Balter MB, Uhlenhut EH: Prevalence and correlates of long-term regular use of anxiolytics. *JAMA* 251:375–379, 1984.

78. Perry SW, Wu A: Rationale for the use of hypnotic agents in a general hospital. *Ann Int Med* 100:441–446, 1984.

79. Browne JL, Hauge KJ: A review of alprazolam withdrawal. *Drug Intell Clin Pharm* 20:837–884, 1986.

80. Albeck JH: Withdrawal and detoxification from benzodiazepine dependency: A potential role for clonazepam. *J Clin Psychiatry* 48(Suppl):43–47, 1987.

81. Freiberger JJ, Marsciano TH: Alprazolam withdrawal presenting as delirium after cardiac surgery. *J Cardiothorac Vasc Anesth* 5:150–152, 1991.

39 SURGERY IN THE ELDERLY

Joseph Francis, Jr.

Cast me not off in my old age;
forsake me not when my strength fails me.
—*Psalm 71*

The elderly were once considered poor candidates for surgery. Those who had surgery usually did so as a last resort or under emergency conditions, and mortality rates were consequently as high as 30 percent.[1] Improvements in surgical technique and the "demographic imperative" of an aging society[2] have demanded a new look at old beliefs. Total numbers of surgical procedures in the elderly and age-specific rates have increased dramatically. Between 1979 and 1984, age-specific rates for lens extraction and hip arthroplasty increased by 38 percent and 33 percent, respectively, among women aged 75 or older.[3] Over the same period, age-specific rates for surgery in younger age groups decreased.

Many older patients have chronic illness that may influence operative outcome. Moreover, the physiologic changes of aging can alter the presentation and affect the management of these patients. Older patients frequently have unrecognized physical and mental disability that threaten functional recovery. The complexity of these acute and chronic health needs makes perioperative medicine in the older patient uniquely challenging. This chapter reviews the existing literature on surgery in the elderly and formulates recommendations for the consultant.

SURGICAL RISK AND BENEFIT IN THE AGED

Overall Trends

Linn and Linn reviewed perioperative mortality in data from over 100 studies published between 1940 and 1980 and showed that emergency surgery carried a markedly higher mortality than elective surgery.[4] Since the elderly were more likely to undergo emergency procedures, their risk of dying was proportionately greater.[5,6] Overall mortality for elective surgery for all ages had

remained about 10 percent.[4,7] These findings reflected several factors pertinent to older patients—bias of referral,[8] sicker baseline status,[9] and need for more difficult and complex procedures.[5]

In contrast, national hospital discharge data indicate unequivocally that both overall and procedure-specific mortality rates for the elderly have fallen considerably (see Table 39–1), in some instances approaching that of younger patients.[9] In addition, difficult procedures like major abdominal and open-heart surgery are becoming commonplace even in the "old-old," those 85 and older,[10–12] and long-term survival of these patients does not differ from that of the general population.[10] No longer can it be said that advanced age makes surgery impractical.

Is Normal Aging a Surgical Risk Factor?

Physiologic changes of normal aging can affect surgical outcome and are summarized in Table 39–2.[13–17] Such changes may increase the likelihood or severity of a postoperative complication. Examples include drug toxicity from impaired renal or hepatic function and impaired cardiac compensatory mechanisms. The physiology of aging may also alter the presentation of disease. A normal serum creatinine may belie significant renal insufficiency, and diabetes mellitus may be present despite the absence of glycosuria. Some age-related changes may have an even more direct clinical impact such as slower wound healing or prostatic hyperplasia predisposing to voiding dysfunction.

Erosion of organ reserve and homeostatic function may only become evident during the stress of major surgery.[18] Resting cardiac output does not decline with age in the absence of heart disease. Cardiac output is comparable to that in younger individuals even during exercise. Despite a lower peak heart rate in older patients, stroke volume increases.[19] However, perioperative situations that decrease preload, such as venodilation, third-spacing, or blood loss, are more likely to lead to circulatory collapse in the elderly.[14]

Several points of caution must be raised before attributing surgical risk to aging physiology:

TABLE 39–1. Mortality for Selected Procedures in 1981 and Percent Change from 1972 (National Hospital Discharge Survey)

	Age 65–74		Age 75+	
Surgical procedure	Mortality (%)	Percent Change	Mortality (%)	Percent Change
Coronary bypass	4.3	−73.6	9.4	N/A
Hip arthroplasty	0.3	−72.7	4.8	−36.0
Prostatectomy	1.5	36.4	1.8	−10.0
Endarterectomy	4.3	−78.4	8.0	−63.2
Cholecystectomy	2.0	−50.0	5.2	−32.5
All surgery	3.5	−6.1	5.5	−12.5

Source: Valvona, 1985.[9]

TABLE 39–2. Selected Physiological Changes of Aging and Their Potential Clinical Significance

System	Change	Significance
General	Decreased total body water and lean mass	Increased drug toxicity
	Decreased thermoregulatory response	Increased risk of hypothermia
Skin	Slower reepithelialization and fewer dermal blood vessels	Slower wound healing ? Increased risk of pressure sores
Cardiac	Fibrosis and degeneration of pacemaking and conducting tissue	Increased risk for conduction disturbances
	Impaired early diastolic filling due to: • mitral valve thickening • decreased ventricular compliance • prolonged isovolumic relaxation	Increased risk of hypotension with dehydration, tachyarrhythmias, vasodilators
	Decreased arterial compliance	Leads to systolic hypertension and ventricular hypertrophy ? Increased susceptibility to loss of plasma volume
	Impaired compensatory mechanisms • decreased baroreceptor sensitivity • decreased target-organ response to beta-adrenergic stimulation • decreased renin, angiotensin, and aldosterone	Decreased heart rate response to stress Increased risk of hypotension
	Resting cardiac output maintained	Cardiac risk determined more by disease than age
	Exercise cardiac output maintained by increased stroke volume since maximum attainable heart rate is less	Circulatory status dependent on adequate preload/volume
Pulmonary	Altered mechanics of ventilation • loss of elastic recoil • stiffening of chest wall • increased ventilation-perfusion mismatch	Airway closure ($FEV_{1.0}$ falls by 0.2 liter per decade after age 20); decreased vital capacity and pulmonary reserve; increased reliance on diaphragmatic breathing; arterial hypoxemia (Po_2 falls 4 mm per decade after age 20)
	Decreased ventilatory response to hypercapnia	Greater potential for ventilatory failure (e.g., with sedative drugs)
	Decreased airway protection: • cough, laryngeal reflexes impaired • slower mucociliary clearance	Risk of aspiration and infection
Renal	Nephron "drop out" with loss of GFR	Prolonged half-life of drugs cleared by kidney
	Creatinine production declines due to fall in muscle mass	GFR diminished despite "normal" serum creatinine
	Delayed response to sodium deficiency	Increased risk of volume depletion
	Delayed capacity to excrete salt and water	Risk of fluid overload and hyponatremia
	Increased renal threshold for glycosuria	Urine glucoses unreliable
Immune	Thymus gland involution Impaired T-cell function	Increased risk for infection
Hepatic	Decreased blood flow and microsomal oxidation	Prolonged half-life of some drugs metabolized by liver
Endocrine	Decreased secretion and action of insulin	Hyperglycemia in response to glucose loads in nondiabetics
Other	Prostatic hypertrophy	Risk of urine retention

1. It has not been established that age-related decline in organ function significantly affects the risk of surgical complications. An example can be drawn from pulmonary physiology. $FEV_{1.0}$ decreases 200 ml each decade after age 20, leaving an average nonsmoking 80-year-old man with an $FEV_{1.0}$ of more than two liters, a threshold below which the risk of pulmonary complications is increased.[20,21] Chronic disease and lifestyle habits exert a much greater effect on organ function than aging alone. Smoking, for instance, doubles or triples the rate of decline in $FEV_{1.0}$.[20] That age is only a minor factor in the development of pulmonary complications is highlighted by a recent study showing that the risks of thoracotomy for patients over age 70 are not significantly different from those of younger patients.[22]

2. Studies of surgical risk that control for underlying chronic disease fail to demonstrate an independent effect of age on surgical risk,[21–23] and mortality among older patients free of recognizable chronic disease is very low.[24]

3. Dysfunction attributed to normal aging because it is seen in a majority of the older population may actually be a manifestation of chronic disease, especially since most studies of the physiology of aging have been cross-sectional and have not screened for occult medical conditions.[25] These early studies maintained that cardiac output decreases with age but did not screen patients for occult coronary artery disease.[26]

4. Advancing age results in increased biologic heterogeneity, making it more difficult to predict organ reserve in the individual older patient.[18] As many as a third of all individuals show no decrease in glomerular filtration rate with age;[27] therefore, the normal range of creatinine clearance in healthy older patients is wider.[28]

Can Age Improve Surgical Benefit?

In some situations, surgery may carry higher risk for older patients but may also offer significantly greater benefits, thereby "balancing" the risk/benefit ratio. Data to support this are unavailable for most procedures but are striking in the case of coronary artery revascularization. The CASS Registry documented survival rates and functional outcomes in more than 1000 patients over age 65. Although perioperative mortality was higher in the older (5.2 percent) than in the younger (1.9 percent) patients, age was not found to be an independent predictor of long-term survival when other variables were considered.[29,30] Furthermore, the older patients had better functional outcomes and longer survival free of recurrent angina, congestive heart failure, or myocardial infarction.[31] When medical therapy was compared to surgical therapy in a retrospective analysis of elderly CASS registrants, functional class and survival rates were better in the surgical group.[32] Comparable results have been obtained by other investigators in even older cohorts.[33–35]

ASSESSING RISK IN THE INDIVIDUAL PATIENT

Though data show that overall operative risk is acceptable in the elderly, it is necessary as in all patients to identify the underlying chronic disease that determines that risk.

General Measures of Risk

The earliest attempt to quantify operative risk in a global clinical assessment was the American Society of Anesthesiologists' Classification (see Table 39–3). It distinguishes high-risk from low-risk patients based on the clinician's rating of the severity of underlying chronic conditions.[36] Unfortunately, this classification is subjective and prone to considerable interobserver disagreement.[37] Many elderly fall broadly into classes II or III where overall mortality is low, and it is impossible to define risk more accurately using this scale.

Predicting Cardiac Complications

A substantial improvement in predicting operative complications and mortality can be found in Goldman's cardiac risk index (see Chap. 18). One-third of surgical patients studied were 70 or older. Although advanced age was considered an independent risk factor in the index, it is likely that age itself was acting as a surrogate for other unmeasured chronic conditions.[38,39] Several investigators have attempted to validate the cardiac risk index in elderly surgical populations.[40–42] Although the index has predictive value, it demonstrates low sensitivity and fails to identify as many as 70 percent of patients subject to serious cardiac complications.[41]

The disappointing sensitivity of the index may reflect a high prevalence of unrecognized coronary artery disease unmasked by the stress of surgery.[43] Autopsy studies show significant stenosis in at least one coronary artery in nearly 75 percent of subjects over 60, but only about half of these cases had clinically recognized disease.[44] In the Framingham study, nearly 25 percent of myocardial infarctions were initially unrecognized with an even higher proportion in older males.[45] Although the precise clinical significance of silent coronary disease is unknown,[46] Framingham participants with "silent" infarctions had as poor a prognosis as those whose events had been clinically recognized.[45]

A variety of preoperative diagnostic studies have been recommended to identify older patients with cardiac disease underestimated by clinical evaluation. These include nuclear-gated blood-pool scans to assess ejection fraction,[41,47] dipyridamole-thallium imaging for patients unable to undergo standard exercise testing,[48] and prolonged ambulatory electrocardiographic monitoring.[49] Although these techniques may be useful in stratifying elderly pa-

TABLE 39–3. Mortality in Patients Aged 80 and Older Based on ASA Classification

Class	Definition	Perioperative Mortality (%)
I	Healty patient	N/A
II	Mild systemic disease, no functional limitations	1
III	Severe systemic disease with functional limitations	4
IV	Incapacitating disease, constant threat to life	25
V	Moribund, unlikely to survive with or without operation	N/A

Source: Djokovic, 1979.[36]

tients by cardiac risk,[50] the value of interventions made on the basis of abnormalities on such tests has not been established.

Hemodynamic Risk Factors

Invasive monitoring, including pulmonary artery catheterization, has been recommended to identify abnormal hemodynamics in elderly patients. Several studies report high rates of hemodynamic abnormalities in older surgical patients undergoing high-risk procedures.[51,52] Most of these patients fall into high-risk categories based on clinical assessment. It remains unclear whether the benefits of the information obtained from routine invasive monitoring justify its attendant risks in most older patients. However, one report suggests that routine hemodynamic evaluation, adjustment of fluid status, inotropic support and intensive care unit monitoring prevent relatively few postoperative complications when used nonselectively in very elderly patients.[53]

Predicting Pulmonary Complications

The frequency of pulmonary complications, including postoperative pneumonia, atelectasis, hypoxemia, and the need for prolonged mechanical ventilation depend on several factors. These include smoking history, serum albumin level, prior respiratory disease, degree of airflow obstruction, and the type and duration of surgery, but they exclude age alone.[22,54-56] Pulmonary function test guidelines that correlate with pulmonary complications and mortality include a maximal breathing capacity less than 50% of the predicted value, $FEV_{1.0}$ less than 2 liters, and an arterial PCO_2 greater than 45 mmHg.[57] However, precise quantitation of risk by degree of abnormality is impossible.[58]

Functional Impairment as a Risk Factor

Functional impairment is a useful indicator of the presence and severity of chronic disease[59,60] and may provide a useful global assessment of risk. Gerson found that a performance-based functional test, the ability to exercise for two minutes or longer on a bicycle, had better sensitivity and specificity in predicting cardiac complications than Goldman's cardiac risk index.[41] The reasons why inability to exercise predicted cardiac complications were unclear since patients were primarily limited by joint problems, dementia, or weakness rather than by angina, claudication, or ischemic electrocardiographic changes.[61]

Functional assessment need not require specialized testing. Simple performance-based tests such as stair climbing may identify patients with a higher risk of complications after lung resection.[62] Information obtained from interviews can also be valuable. Seymour found that "active" elderly, defined as those who reported leaving their homes at least twice weekly, had fewer postoperative respiratory, cardiac, and wound complications than the homebound.[63] Poor premorbid functional status defined as inability to perform one or more activities of daily living (eating, dressing, grooming, walking, transferring, bathing, and toileting) or to engage in instrumental activities (taking medication, using the telephone, shopping, preparing meals, doing housework, and handling money) also identifies hip-fracture patients with a higher risk of postoperative complications, loss of independence, and death.[64]

SPECIAL CONSIDERATIONS FOR OLDER PATIENTS

Atypical Presentation of Disease

Clinical evaluation of the older patient is complicated by the ways in which age and other chronic conditions mask or alter the presentation of medical illness. Appendicitis carries a higher mortality rate in the elderly because of a higher incidence of perforation caused by delay in diagnosis. Fewer than half of such patients present with classic symptoms, fever, or peritoneal signs.[65,66] Similarly, nearly one-third of patients with biliary sepsis have no fever or leukocytosis, and half have a benign abdominal examination.[67] Acute confusion or delirium, discussed in Chap. 70, can also be a nonspecific presentation of surgical conditions and of serious postoperative medical complications.[68,69]

Drug Use

The elderly are more sensitive to both the intended and unintended effects of medications. Useful principles include avoiding or eliminating unnecessary drugs and "starting low, going slow" with any medication.[70] There are several age-related changes in drug disposition: lower volume of distribution for water-soluble drugs leading to increased serum concentrations; a greater proportion of body fat prolonging half-life of lipophilic drugs; decreased hepatic metabolism and renal excretion; and increased target-organ sensitivity.[71] Disease-related changes should always be considered. Decreased serum albumin levels lead to higher free serum levels of drugs that are normally protein-bound such as phenytoin, warfarin, and tolbutamide.[72] Chronic disease frequently leads to polypharmacy, multiplying possibilities of adverse drug interactions.[70]

Medications used routinely in the perioperative period such as narcotics, anticholinergic drugs, and sedative-hypnotics frequently contribute to the risk of postoperative delirium in the elderly.[68] Older patients require much lower doses of narcotics for pain relief.[73] While younger patients more often experience sedation with excessive doses, the elderly are more likely to become acutely confused or agitated.[74] Certain classes of narcotics have unique undesirable side effects. Meperidine, for instance, produces central nervous system toxicity more frequently than other opiates due to the accumulation of the metabolite normeperidine. This is particularly important in patients with renal insufficiency.[75]

Many medications have anticholinergic properties, including antipsychotics, antiparkinsonian agents, antihistamines, certain sedative-hypnotics, and some antiarrhythmics. In addition, atropine, frequently used prior to induction of anesthesia, can produce prolonged sedation in the elderly patient.[76]

Sedative-hypnotic drugs may not only cause delirium but may also increase the risk of falling and sustaining a hip fracture.[77] Benzodiazepines with long elimination half-lives like flurazepam and diazepam, as well as those with excitatory effects like triazolam, should be avoided. Lorazepam and oxazepam do not require hepatic oxidation for elimination and in low doses are probably safer for elderly patients requiring a sedative-hypnotic.[78] Antihistamines like diphenhydramine are not necessarily safer than benzodiazepines for insomnia because of their anticholinergic activity.

Seemingly innocuous medications may cause postoperative confusion in the elderly. These include nonsteroidal anti-inflammatory agents,[79] quinolone antibiotics,[80] and H_2-blockers like cimetidine and ranitidine.[81,82]

Anesthesia in Older Patients

Early reports of the superiority of local and regional anesthesia over general probably reflected the lack of adequate monitoring during surgery and suboptimal postoperative care.[83] Several randomized trials comparing general with neurolept or spinal anesthesia in elderly patients with hip fractures show no difference in mortality among the various techniques.[84–86]

Few studies have compared complications with different forms of anesthesia in the elderly. In one randomized trial of spinal and general anesthesia in hip replacement, fewer venous thromboses were detected by ^{125}I-fibrinogen scan in patients receiving spinal anesthesia.[87] Although mental performance in the immediate postoperative period is more often affected by general anesthesia,[88] choice of anesthetic has little effect on the risk of postoperative delirium or long-term cognitive performance.[89–91]

Altered pharmacokinetics and pharmacodynamics in aging increase the likelihood of adverse effects with all forms of anesthesia. Short-acting drugs such as thiopental or midazolam may produce prolonged sedation,[92] and local anesthetics such as bupivacaine may attain free serum levels high enough to produce myocardial depression.[93]

Hypothermia

Hypothermia frequently occurs during anesthesia and in the immediate postoperative period. Anesthetized patients become vasodilated and may be more sensitive to the ambient temperature of a cool operating room.[94] Elderly patients experience more pronounced and more prolonged perioperative hypothermia than younger patients.[95] This is due to intrinsic factors such as lower basal metabolic heat production as seen in hypothyroidism, diabetes, and malnutrition; peripheral vascular disease; a high ratio of surface area to body mass; and use of medications such as phenothiazines that impair thermoregulation.[96] Hypothermia depresses cardiac output and increases central venous pressure and peripheral vascular resistance, enhancing ventricular irritability, impairing tissue delivery of oxygen, and depressing ventilatory drive.[94,97]

During recovery from hypothermia, oxygen consumption increases four- to seven-fold as a result of shivering, and this can result in hypoxia, acidosis, and cardiac ischemia. Rewarming may also precipitate sudden hypotension as a result of sudden vasodilation and hypovolemia due to transcapillary leakage at low body temperature.[94] Hypothermia can be prevented by raising ambient temperature during surgery and recovery, using heated blankets, warming parenteral fluids, and humidifying and warming inspired air. For long procedures, it is advisable to carefully monitor core body temperature, most accurately performed with an esophageal or bladder probe or pulmonary artery catheter thermistor. Even rectal temperatures can be unreliable.[98]

Nutrition

Nutritional status is a major factor in wound healing and susceptibility to infections and pressure sores. Protein-calorie malnutrition is seen in approximately 20 percent of elderly inpatients.[99] In this group, serum albumin levels inversely correlate with postoperative complication and mortality rates[100,101] and may predict long-term outcome after hospitalization.[102]

The relationship between albumin levels and operative outcome is complex and does not simply reflect nutritional status. Levels show little or no decline among healthy older patients[103] but provide a sensitive indicator of disease.[104,105] Studies demonstrating increased surgical risk in elderly patients with low serum albumin levels fail to adjust for the confounding effects of underlying disease. Unfortunately, other routine measures of nutritional status such as triceps skinfold thickness, midarm muscle circumference, creatinine-height index, serum transferrin concentration, and lymphocyte count correlate poorly with serum albumin level, may not discriminate accurately between well- and malnourished elderly, or lack appropriate normal standards for this age group.[106,107]

In addition to the difficulty of diagnosing protein-calorie malnutrition in the elderly, few data support the effectiveness of nutritional intervention.[108] A recent meta-analysis of studies on perioperative parenteral nutrition demonstrated little effectiveness in unselected patients undergoing major surgery[109] but suggested a possible beneficial role in high-risk patients like malnourished elderly. Enteral feeding through small-bore soft catheters has been suggested as an alternative to parenteral hyperalimentation in patients without gastrointestinal contraindications,[110] but this can also lead to agitation, diarrhea with resultant dehydration, and aspiration in older patients.[111] A recent randomized controlled trial of jejunostomy feeding in older patients undergoing abdominal surgery showed no reduction in postoperative complications or mortality, no improvement in nutritional parameters, and a substantial rate of catheter-related complications.[112] Another trial of overnight nasogastric feedings in malnourished elderly with hip fractures demonstrated modest improvements in albumin levels, shorter hospital stays, and a trend toward lower hospital mortality in the supplemented group. However, 22 percent of patients allocated to receive overnight supplements were unable to tolerate the tube feedings.[113] Simple oral nutritional supplements in patients able to swallow may have similar benefits without the complications of nasogastric intubation.[114]

Even less is known about the effect of micronutrients upon surgical outcome in the elderly. Zinc deficiency is prevalent in the elderly and results from marginal dietary intake; impaired absorption; and conditions that lead to increased urinary zinc losses such as diabetes mellitus, alcoholism, and diuretic use.[115] Zinc deficiency can cause poor wound healing and impaired T-cell function, and supplementation has been shown to accelerate the healing of leg ulcers.[116] However, serum zinc levels are unreliable in diagnosing zinc deficiency,[115] and the role of supplementation in elderly surgical patients remains uncertain.

Firm recommendations for nutritional support in elderly surgical patients are therefore difficult to make. Preoperative nutritional support should be considered as long as delay in surgery does not worsen outcome. Chronic diseases contributing to hypoalbuminemia should be addressed. Patients should receive sufficient levels of protein, calories, and micronutrients in the perioperative period to avoid potential deficiencies and maintain balance under conditions of stress. However, use of enteral or parenteral hyperalimentation must be tempered by consideration of potential complications.

TABLE 39–4. Expected Years of Life Remaining

Age	Male	Female	Both Sexes
65	14.6	18.7	16.9
75	9.0	11.8	10.7
85	5.1	6.5	6.0

Source: Health statistics on older persons, United States, 1986.[3]

ETHICAL CONCERNS

"Ageism" in Surgery

A bias against performing surgery in the aged probably still exists due to misconceptions about the role of age in surgical risk, but the extent of this bias is difficult to quantify. A recent study of therapy for breast cancer revealed that nearly 20 percent of older patients with stage I or II breast cancer were denied appropriate surgical intervention compared with 4 percent of younger patients. This difference could not be explained by greater comorbidity in the older group[117] and is particularly distressing in view of evidence that mastectomy or local excision has a low mortality in older patients with long-term survival rates comparable to younger patients at similar stages of disease.[118]

Although some authorities have argued for limiting therapy to patients above a certain age, perhaps that of the average biological life span of 85 years,[119] Table 39–4 demonstrates that there is significant life expectancy even among the "oldest-old."[3] If surgery can improve the quality of those remaining years, there is little ethical or moral basis for denying appropriate therapy based on age alone.[120]

Role of Patient Preferences

Recent data suggest that a great deal of surgery in the elderly is done to improve quality of life rather than to increase survival. Using complex decision analysis, one study of elective prostatectomy for chronic voiding symptoms revealed that surgery led to a net loss of one month of life but a net gain of three "quality-adjusted" months of life.[121] One may reasonably conclude that patient preferences and their perception of symptoms rather than survival rates alone should assume dominant roles in decision making.

PERIOPERATIVE MANAGEMENT OF THE GERIATRIC PATIENT

The perioperative management of the older surgical patient with underlying chronic illness is similar to that for others. However, it often involves attention to a greater number of medical problems and an appreciation of the complexities of care. Specific guidelines emphasizing unique aspects of perioperative care required by the elderly are offered below.

Preoperative Assessment

The crux of the preoperative evaluation remains the comprehensive history and physical examination. Cognitive and sensory impairment may make eliciting a history more difficult, but even de-

mented patients living in the community can give reliable reports of symptoms.[122] "Listen to the patient" remains a useful tenet for the physician. Sensory function can be optimized by ensuring a well-lit and quiet environment for assessment, speaking slowly, enunciating well, sitting close to the patient to allow lipreading, and avoiding shouting at those who are hearing-impaired.[60]

Functional impairment is common in older patients and can potentially influence the immediate postoperative course and performance after hospital discharge. Performance of activities of daily living and instrumental activities should be specifically assessed either by a validated standardized questionnaire[59] or by incorporating the functional assessment into the history and physical examination.[123] This assessment should ideally be done before hospitalization when the patient is functioning at baseline so that deterioration can be readily recognized.

It is important to determine the availability of supports in the community for patients after discharge. Those with few family or friends able to provide assistance may experience functional decline.[124] Elderly patients who are functioning poorly and have few social supports may benefit from an evaluation by a social worker with experience in geriatrics.[125]

Physical findings are modified by age and concomitant disease. Systolic ejection murmurs at the base of the heart may represent aortic valve cusp sclerosis rather than hemodynamically significant valvular obstruction. However, late-peaking or long murmurs may be indicators of severe aortic stenosis even if the carotid upstroke is normal. Echocardiography and doppler studies may be necessary to establish the diagnosis.[26] Some older patients with critical aortic stenosis who are poor candidates for valve replacement may undergo noncardiac surgery safely with careful intraoperative hemodynamic monitoring[126] or after balloon valvuloplasty to temporarily increase aortic valve area.[127]

Endocarditis is increasingly a problem in the elderly due to the high prevalence of degenerative valvular disease and the possibility of bacteremia associated with oral, bowel, urinary, biliary, and pulmonary procedures.[128] If a significant murmur is present, antibiotic prophylaxis, as described in Chap. 43, should be given.

Intravascular volume status is critical in older patients because of greater dependence of cardiac output on adequate preload. Patients with congestive heart failure, for example, must not be overtreated with diuretics to the point of volume depletion. Intraoperative pulmonary artery catheterization should be considered in those patients with functionally significant cardiopulmonary problems or uncertain volume status.

Preoperative mental status should be carefully assessed to facilitate evaluation of postoperative confusional states. Because of the frequency with which mild to moderate degrees of cognitive impairment are missed,[129] performance of a brief screening mental status examination like the "mini–mental state" exam can be useful.[130] Patients with chronically impaired cognition have higher rates of postoperative delirium, increased length of stay, and death. In such patients, special care must be taken with drugs known to cause delirium. The preoperative visit provides an ideal opportunity to review medications and eliminate those that have no clear indication or might contribute to cognitive impairment.

Although routine preoperative laboratory testing has been challenged for unselected patients,[131–133] the yield of abnormalities on blood chemistries, electrocardiograms, and chest x-rays is higher for older patients.[134–136] The most appropriate testing focuses on those conditions prevalent in the older population. A fasting serum glucose level may be necessary for the diagnosis of Type II diabetes mellitus, a condition frequently undiagnosed and prevalent with age.[137] Similarly, a serum albumin level is useful in identifying patients with a greater risk of postoperative complications due to malnutrition or chronic disease. Appropriate dosing of medications can be facilitated by approximating creatinine clearance with the formula:[138]

$$\text{CrCl (ml/min)} = \frac{(140 - \text{age}) \times (\text{weight in kg})}{\text{serum creatinine} \times 72}$$

Pulmonary function testing should be considered in older patients with a history of chronic lung disease, more than a 20-pack-year history of smoking, cough, or obesity, and in those undergoing lung resection.[58] Older patients likely to develop pulmonary complications can benefit from preoperative chest physical therapy.[139]

Postoperative Management

Fatal and nonfatal complications of surgery can occur at any time after surgery and are not limited to the first few postoperative days. In one series, one-third of deaths in elderly surgical patients occurred after the first week.[24] Consultants should follow these patients throughout the hospitalization and be prepared to assist after discharge, particularly since complex surgery is now often performed in the ambulatory setting[140] or involves nursing home patients.[12]

Prompt mobilization from bed is vital. The risk of venous thromboembolism in hospitalized patients increases exponentially with age, justifying attention to prophylactic measures described in Chap. 48. Another threat of prolonged immobility is loss of ability to walk. Bed rest leads to cardiovascular deconditioning, increased risk of orthostatic hypotension, decreased coordination and balance, loss of as much as 5 percent of muscle mass per day, and joint contractures, all of which threaten independent ambulation.[141] Recumbency also contributes to urinary retention, fecal impaction, and pneumonia. When full activity is impossible, range of motion exercises and maintenance of an upright position can reduce the frequency and severity of these complications.

Voiding problems frequently accompany surgery in the elderly and are often managed with indwelling catheters that predispose the patient to urinary tract infection and gram-negative sepsis. Very short-term use of indwelling catheters in the elderly, removing them the morning after surgery, may reduce the incidence of urinary retention and bladder overdistention without increasing the rate of urinary tract infection.[142] Use of catheters for more than 48 hours must be avoided except when urinary retention cannot be practically managed by conservative measures of early mobilization and intermittent catheterization or when wounds or pressure ulcers are being contaminated by incontinent urine.[143] Patients who require short-term postoperative catheterization for more than two days but less than two weeks may benefit from antibiotic prophylaxis.[144] However, this is not recommended in patients in whom long-term catheterization is anticipated.

Serial mental status testing with brief screening instruments can help to identify delirium which may be the only clue to drug toxicity or a new medical complication. Certain subgroups of patients, including those with dementia[68] or Parkinson's disease,[145] are particularly likely to develop delirium and should be more closely monitored. The agitation and disruptiveness that may accompany delirium may compromise postoperative care. It is impor-

tant to determine the cause of the disturbance in order to treat it specifically. Behavior can often be controlled with environmental measures. These include enlisting the help of a bedside sitter or family member to reorient the patient, providing orienting stimuli like calendars and items from home, minimizing abrupt relocations, and leaving lights on at night to decrease frightening hallucinations.[68]

Occasionally, agitation can be so severe that prompt symptomatic control is vital to prevent harm to the patient or others. There is no ideal drug for older persons, although low-dose (0.5 mg) haloperidol is generally accepted as a safe and reliable regimen for short-term use with little risk of hypotension or arrhythmias even when administered intravenously.[68] In the severely disruptive, benzodiazepines (e.g., lorazepam 0.5 to 1 mg intravenously) may work synergistically with haloperidol, blunting extrapyramidal side effects and promoting sedation.[68] Physical restraints should be considered only if conservative measures have failed.[146]

SUMMARY

1. Aging alone does not significantly influence operative risk. However, chronic diseases associated with advanced age do increase that risk.

2. Perioperative management should focus on diagnosis and optimization of these conditions. Functional impairment is a useful indicator of the presence and severity of underlying disease. Standardized instruments for assessing physical function and cognition are helpful in identifying problems that may not be immediately evident.

3. In some situations, the risk of surgery may be increased in the elderly, but potential for improvement in the quality of life may be greater than the risk of the procedure. In such cases, patient preference must take precedence.

4. Acute conditions often present in an atypical or nonspecific way in the elderly. This may delay operative intervention and hinder recognition of postoperative complications.

5. "Start low, go slow" with any drug in the elderly. Narcotics, sedatives, and anticholinergic medications have a high potential for precipitating delirium. The preoperative assessment is an ideal time to review the medication history and to discontinue any drugs that have become unnecessary.

6. The type of anesthesia does not influence perioperative mortality or morbidity in older patients.

7. Malnutrition increases surgical risk in the elderly. Preoperative nutritional support should be considered if delay in surgery will not adversely affect outcome. The effectiveness of enteral and parenteral nutritional support is not established, and both modes of feeding carry significant risks.

8. Postoperative management should be continued throughout and often beyond the hospital stay since risk of complications is not limited to the immediate postoperative period.

9. Prompt mobilization from bed is vital to preserve function and avoid complications of immobility.

10. Remove indwelling urinary catheters within 48 hours except when urinary retention cannot be managed by conservative means or incontinence threatens wound healing.

11. Postoperative agitation is best managed by diagnosing and treating the underlying disturbance and using environmental measures to control behavior. Low-dose haloperidol or lorazepam can provide symptomatic control but does not substitute for a careful medical evaluation.

REFERENCES

1. Lewin I, Lerner AG, Green SH et al: Physical class and physiologic status in the prediction of operative mortality in the aged sick. *Ann Surg* 174:217–231, 1971.
2. Siegel JS, Taeuber CM: Demographic perspectives on the long-lived society. *Daedalus* 111:77–117, 1986.
3. National Center for Health Statistics: *Health statistics on older persons, United States, 1986.* DHHS publication 87-1409, Public Health Services, 1987.
4. Linn BS, Linn MW, Wallen N: Evaluation of results of surgical procedures in the elderly. *Ann Surg* 195:90–96, 1982.
5. Greenburg AG, Saik RP, Farris JM et al: Operative mortality in general surgery. *Am J Surg* 144:22–26, 1982.
6. Sandler RS, Maule WF, Baltus ME et al: Biliary tract surgery in the elderly. *J Gen Intern Med* 2:149–154, 1987.
7. Ziffren SE: Comparison of mortality rates for various surgical operations according to age groups, 1951–1977. *J Am Geriatr Soc* 27:433–438, 1979.
8. Warner MA, Hosking MP, Lobdell CM et al: Effects of referral bias on surgical outcomes: A population-based study of surgical patients 90 years of age or older. *Mayo Clin Proc* 65:1185–1191, 1990.
9. Valvona J, Sloan F: Rising rates of surgery among the elderly. *Health Aff* 4:108–119, 1985.
10. Hosking MP, Warner MA, Lobdell CM et al: Outcomes of surgery in patients 90 years of age and older. *JAMA* 261:1909–1915, 1989.
11. Edmunds LH, Stephenson LW, Edie RN et al: Open-heart surgery in octogenarians. *N Engl J Med* 319:131–136, 1988.
12. Keating HJ: Major surgery in nursing home patients: Procedures, morbidity, and mortality in the frailest of the frail elderly. *J Am Geriatr Soc* 40:8–11, 1992.
13. Rowe JW, Minaker KL: Geriatric medicine, in Finch CE, Schneider EL (eds): *Handbook of the Biology of Aging.* New York, Van Nostrand, 1985, pp 932–959.
14. Keating HJ: Preoperative considerations in the geriatric patient. *Med Clin N Am* 71:569–583, 1987.
15. Eaglstein WH: Wound healing and aging. *Clin Geriatr Med* 5:183–188, 1989.
16. Hausman PB, Weksler ME: Changes in the immune response with age, in Finch CE, Schneider EL (eds): *Handbook of the Biology of Aging.* New York, Van Nostrand, 1985, pp 414–432.
17. Williams ME: Aging of tissues and organs, in Beck JC (ed): *Geriatrics Review Syllabus: A Core Curriculum in Geriatric Medicine.* New York, American Geriatrics Society, 1991, pp 15–29.
18. Williams ME: Clinical implications of aging physiology. *Am J Med* 76:1049–1054, 1984.
19. Rodeheffer RJ, Gerstenblith G, Becker LC et al: Exercise cardiac output is maintained with advancing age in healthy human subjects: Cardiac dilatation and increased stroke volume compensate for a diminished heart rate. *Circulation* 69:203–213, 1984.
20. Sparrow D, Weiss ST: Respiratory physiology. *Ann Rev Gerontol Geriatr* 6:197–214, 1986.
21. Johnson JC: The medical evaluation and management of the elderly surgical patient. *J Am Geriatr Soc* 31:621–625, 1983.
22. Sherman S, Guidot CE: The feasibility of thoracotomy for lung cancer in the elderly. *JAMA* 258:927–930, 1987.
23. Greenburg AG, Saik RP, Pridham D: Influence of age on mortality of colon surgery. *Am J Surg* 150:65–69, 1985.
24. Palmberg S, Hirsjarvi E: Mortality in geriatric surgery. *Gerontology* 25:103–112, 1979.
25. Rowe JW, Kahn RL: Human aging: Usual and successful. *Science* 237:143–149, 1987.
26. Wei JY, Gersh BJ: Heart disease in the elderly. *Curr Probl Cardiol* 12:1–65, 1987.
27. Lindeman RD, Tobin J, Shock NW: Longitudinal studies on the rate of decline in renal function with age. *J Am Geriatr Soc* 33:278–285, 1985.
28. Rowe JW, Andres R, Tobin JD et al: Age-adjusted standards for creatinine clearance. *Ann Intern Med* 84:567–569, 1976.
29. Eaker ED, Kronmal R, Kennedy W et al: Comparison of the long-term postsurgical survival of women and men in the coronary artery surgery study (CASS). *Am Heart J* 117:71–81, 1989.
30. Gersh BJ, Kronmal RA, Frye RL et al: Coronary arteriography and coronary artery bypass surgery: Morbidity and mortality in patients aged 65 years or older. *Circulation* 67:483–491, 1983.
31. Gersh BJ, Kronmal RA, Schaff HV et al: Long-term (5 years) results of coronary bypass surgery in patients 65 years old or older: A report from the coronary artery surgery study. *Circulation* 68(Suppl II):190–199, 1983.
32. Gersh BJ, Kronmal RA, Schaff HV et al: Comparison of coronary artery bypass surgery and medical therapy in patients 65 years of age or older. *N Engl J Med* 313:217–224, 1985.
33. Acinapura AJ, Rose DM, Cunningham JN et al: Coronary artery bypass in septuagenarians: Analysis of mortality and morbidity. *Circulation* 78(Suppl I):179–184, 1988.
34. Naunheim KS, Kern MJ, McBridge LR et al: Coronary artery bypass surgery in patients aged 80 years or older. *Am J Cardiol* 59:804–807, 1987.
35. Freeman WK, Schaff HV, O'Brien PC et al: Cardiac surgery in the octogenarian: Perioperative outcome and clinical follow-up. *J Am Coll Cardiol* 18:29–35, 1991.
36. Djokovic JL, Hedley-Whyte J: Prediction of outcome of surgery and anesthesia in patients over 80. *JAMA* 242:2301–2306, 1979.
37. Owens WD, Felts JA, Spitznagel EL: ASA physical status classifications: A study of consistency of ratings. *Anesthesiology* 49:239–243 1978.
38. Goldman L: Cardiac risks and complications of noncardiac surgery. *Ann Intern Med* 98:504–513, 1983.
39. Goldman L, Caldera KL, Nussbaum SR et al: Multifactorial index of cardiac risk in noncardiac surgical procedures. *N Engl J Med* 297:845–850, 1977.
40. Cogbill TH, Landercasper J, Strutt PJ et al: Late results of peripheral vascular surgery in patients 80 years of age and older. *Arch Surg* 122:581–586, 1987.
41. Gerson MC, Hurst JM, Hertzberg VS et al: Cardiac prognosis in noncardiac geriatric surgery. *Ann Intern Med* 103:832–837, 1985.
42. Jeffrey CC, Kunsman J, Cullen DJ et al: A prospective evaluation of cardiac risk index. *Anesthesiology* 58:462–464, 1983.
43. Eagle KA, Boucher CA: Cardiac risk of noncardiac surgery. *N Engl J Med* 321:1330–1332, 1989.
44. Lakatta EG: Heart and circulation, in Finch CE, Schneider EL (eds): *Handbook of the Biology of Aging.* New York, Van Nostrand, 1985, pp 377–413.
45. Kannel WB, Abbott RD: Incidence and prognosis of unrecognized myocardial infarction: An update on the Framingham study. *N Engl J Med* 311:1144–1147, 1984.
46. Epstein SE, Quyyumi AA, Bonow RO: Myocardial ischemia—silent or symptomatic. *N Engl J Med* 318:1038–1043, 1988.
47. Lazor L, Russell JC, DaSilva J et al: Use of the multiple uptak

gated acquisition scan for the preoperative assessment of cardiac risk. *Surg Gyn Obstet* 167:234–238, 1988.

48. Boucher CA, Brewster DC, Darling RC et al: Determination of cardiac risk by dipyridamole-thallium imaging before peripheral vascular surgery. *N Engl J Med* 312:389–394, 1985.

49. Raby KE, Goldman L, Creager MA et al: Correlation between preoperative ischemia and major cardiac events after peripheral vascular surgery. *N Engl J Med* 321:1296–1300, 1989.

50. Eagle KA, Coley CM, Newell JB et al: Combining clinical and thallium data optimizes preoperative assessment of cardiac risk before major vascular surgery. *Ann Intern Med* 110:859–866, 1989.

51. Del Guercio LRM, Cohn JD: Monitoring operative risk in the elderly. *JAMA* 243:1350–1355, 1980.

52. Older P, Smith R: Experience with the preoperative invasive measurement of haemodynamic, respiratory, and renal function in 100 elderly patients scheduled for major abdominal surgery. *Anaesth Intens Care* 16:389–395, 1988.

53. Schrader LL, McMillen MA, Watson CD et al: Is routine preoperative hemodynamic evaluation of nonagenarians necessary? *J Am Geriatr Soc* 39:1–5, 1991.

54. Mitchell C, Carrahy P, Peake P: Postoperative respiratory morbidity: Identification and risk factors. *Aust NZ J Surg* 52:203–209, 1982.

55. Garibaldi RA, Britt MR, Coleman ML et al: Risk factors for postoperative pneumonia. *Am J Med* 70:677–680, 1981.

56. Tarhan S, Moffitt EA, Sessler AD et al: Risk of anesthesia and surgery in patients with chronic bronchitis and chronic obstructive pulmonary disease. *Surgery* 74:720–726, 1973.

57. Jackson CV: Preoperative pulmonary evaluation. *Arch Intern Med* 148:2120–2127, 1988.

58. Zibrak JD, O'Donnell CR, Marton K: Indications for pulmonary function testing. *Ann Intern Med* 112:763–771, 1990.

59. Rubenstein LV, Calkins DR, Greenfield S et al: Health status assessment for elderly patients. *J Am Geriatr Soc* 37:562–569, 1989.

60. Besdine RW: Functional assessment in the elderly, in Rowe JW, Besdine RW (eds): *Geriatric Medicine.* Boston, Little Brown, 1988, pp 37–51.

61. Gerson MC, Hurst JM, Hertzberg VS et al: Prediction of cardiac and pulmonary complications related to elective abdominal and noncardiac thoracic surgery in geriatric patients. *Am J Med* 88:101–107, 1990.

62. Olsen GN, Bolton JWR, Weiman DS et al: Stair climbing as an exercise test to predict the postoperative complications of lung resection: Two years' experience. *Chest* 99:587–590, 1991.

63. Seymour DG, Pringle R: Postoperative complications in the elderly surgical patients. *Gerontology* 29:262–270, 1983.

64. Magaziner J, Simonsick EM, Kashner TM et al: Predictors of functional recovery one year following hospital discharge for hip fracture: A prospective study. *J Gerontol* 45:M101–M107, 1990.

65. Burns RP, Cochran JL, Russell WL et al: Appendicitis in mature patients. *Ann Surg* 201:695–704, 1985.

66. Owens BJ, Hamit HF: Appendicitis in the elderly. *Ann Surg* 187:392–396, 1978.

67. Morrow DJ, Thompson J, Wilson SE: Acute cholecystitis in the elderly: A surgical emergency. *Arch Surg* 113:1149–1152, 1978.

68. Francis J: Delirium in older patients. *J Am Geriatr Soc* 40, 1992 (in press).

69. Black DA: Mental state and presentation of myocardial infarction in the elderly. *Ageing* 16:125–127, 1987.

70. Montamat SC, Cusack BJ, Vestal RE: Management of drug therapy in the elderly. *NEJM* 321:303–309, 1989.

71. Greenblatt DJ, Sellers EM, Shader RI: Drug disposition in the old age. *N Engl J Med* 306:1081–1088, 1982.

72. Vestal RE, Dawson GW: Pharmacology and aging, in Finch CE, Schneider EL (eds): *Handbook of the Biology of Aging.* New York, Van Nostrand 1985, pp 744–819.

73. Belleville J, Forrest W, Miller E et al: Influence of age on pain relief from analgesics. *JAMA* 217:1835–1841, 1971.

74. Leipzig RM, Goodman H, Gray G et al: Reversible, narcotic-associated mental status impairment in patients with metastatic cancer. *Pharmacology* 35:47–54, 1987.

75. Kaiko RF, Foley KM, Grabinski PY et al: Central nervous system excitatory effects of meperidine in cancer patients. *Ann Neurol* 13:180–185, 1983.

76. Smith DS, Orkin FK, Gardner SM et al: Prolonged sedation in the elderly after intraoperative atropine administration. *Anesthesiology* 51:348–349, 1979.

77. Ray WA, Griffin MR, Schaffner W et al: Psychotropic drug use and the risk of hip fracture. *N Engl J Med* 316:363–369, 1987.

78. Thompson TL, Moran MG, Nies AS: Psychotropic drug use in the elderly. *N Engl J Med* 308:132–138, 1983.

79. Goodwin JS, Regan M: Cognitive dysfunction with naproxen and ibuprofen in the elderly. *Arthr Rheum* 25:1013–1015, 1982.

80. McDermott JL, Gideonse N, Campbell JW: Acute delirium associated with ciprofloxacin administration in a hospitalized elderly patient. *J Am Geriatr Soc* 39:909–910, 1991.

81. McCarthy DM: Ranitidine or cimetidine. *Ann Intern Med* 99:551–553, 1983.

82. Cantu TG, Korek JS: Central nervous system reactions to histamine-2 receptor blockers. *Ann Intern Med* 114:1027–1034, 1991.

83. Cote J, Lapointe P: Anaesthetic management for the elderly patient. *Can Anaesth Soc J* 32:188–191, 1985.

84. Davis FM, Woolner DF, Frampton C et al: Prospective, multi-centre trial of mortality following general or spinal anaesthesia for hip fracture surgery in the elderly. *Br J Anaesth* 59:1080–1088, 1987.

85. Wickstrom I, Holmberg I, Stefansson T: Survival of female geriatric patients after hip fracture surgery. A comparison of 5 anesthetic methods. *Acta Anaesth Scand* 26:607–614, 1982.

86. David FM, Laurenson VG: Spinal anaesthesia or general anaesthesia for emergency hip surgery in elderly patients. *Anaesth Intens Care* 9:352–358, 1981.

87. Davis FM, Laurenson VG, Gillespie WJ et al: Deep vein thrombosis after total hip replacement: A comparison between spinal and general anesthesia. *J Bone Joint Surg* 71B:181–185, 1989.

88. Chung F, Meier R, Lautenschlager E et al: General or spinal anesthesia: Which is better in the elderly. *Anesthesiology* 67:422–427, 1987.

89. Ghoneim MM, Hinrichs JV, O'Hara MW et al: Comparison of psychologic and cognitive functions after general or regional anesthesia. *Anesthesiology* 69:507–515, 1988.

90. Berggren D, Gustafson Y, Eriksson B et al: Postoperative confusion after anesthesia in elderly patients with femoral neck fractures. *Anesth Analg* 66:497–504, 1987.

91. Nielson WR, Gelb AW, Casey JE et al: Long-term cognitive and social sequelae of general versus regional anesthesia during arthroplasty in the elderly. *Anesthesiology* 73:1103–1109, 1990.

92. White PF: Anesthetic techniques for the elderly outpatient. *Int Anesth Clin* 26:105–111, 1988.

93. Krechel SW: Anesthesia for surgical care of the elderly, in Meakins JL, McClaran JC (eds): *Surgical Care of the Elderly.* Chicago, Yearbook Medical 1988, pp 276–286.

94. Morrison RC: Hypothermia in the elderly. *Int Anesth Clin* 26:124–133, 1988.

95. Vaughan MS, Vaughan RW, Cork RC: Postoperative hypothermia in adults: Relationship of age, anesthesia, and shivering to rewarming. *Anesth Analg* 60:746–751, 1981.

96. Davis BB, Zenser TV: Biological changes in thermoregulation in the elderly, in Davis BB, Wood WG (eds): *Homeostatic Function and Aging.* New York, Raven Press, 157–166, 1985.

97. Heymann AD: The effect of incidental hypothermia on elderly surgical patients. *J Gerontol* 32:46–48, 1977.

98. Cork RC, Vaughan RW, Humphrey LS: Precision and accuracy of intraoperative temperature monitoring. *Anesth Analg* 62:211–214, 1983.

99. Baron RB: Malnutrition in hospitalized patients—diagnosis and treatment. *West J Med* 144:63–67, 1986.

100. Rich MW, Keller AJ, Schechtman KB et al: Increased complications and prolonged hospital stay in elderly cardiac surgical patients with low serum albumin. *Am J Cardiol* 63:714–718, 1989.

101. Agarwal N, Acevedo F, Leighton LS et al: Predictive ability of various nutritional variables for mortality in elderly people. *Am J Clin Nutr* 48:1173–1178, 1988.

102. Linn BS: Outcomes of older and younger malnourished and well-nourished patients one year after hospitalization. *Am J Clin Nutr* 39:66–73, 1984.

103. Campion EW, deLabry LO, Glynn RJ: The effect of age on serum albumin in healthy males: Report from the normative aging study. *J Gerontol* 43:M18–M20, 1988.

104. O'Keefe SJD, Dicker J: Is plasma albumin concentration useful in the assessment of nutritional status of hospital patients? *Eur J Clin Nutr* 42:41–45, 1988.

105. Friedman PJ, Campbell AJ, Caradoc-Davies TH: Hypoalbuminemia in the elderly is due to disease not malnutrition. *J Clin Exp Gerontol* 7:191–203, 1985.

106. Finucane P, Rudra T, Hsu R et al: Markers of the nutritional status in acutely ill elderly patients. *Gerontology* 34:304–310, 1988.

107. Mitchell CO, Lipschitz DA: The effect of age and sex on the routinely used measurements to assess the nutritional status of hospitalized patients. *Am J Clin Nutr* 36:340–349, 1982.

108. Cooper JK: Does nutrition affect surgical outcome? *J Am Geriatr Soc* 35:229–232, 1987.

109. Veterans Affairs Total Parenteral Nutrition Cooperative Study Group: Perioperative total parenteral nutrition in surgical patients. *NEJM* 325:525–532, 1991.

110. Heymsfield SB, Bethel RA, Ansley JD et al: Enteral hyperalimentation: An alternative to central venous hyperalimentation. *Ann Intern Med* 90:63–71, 1979.

111. Ciocon JO, Silverstone FA, Graver LM et al: Tube feedings in elderly patients. *Arch Intern Med* 148:429–433, 1988.

112. Smith RC, Hartemink RJ, Hollinshead JW et al: Fine bore jejunostomy feeding following major abdominal surgery: A controlled randomized clinical trial. *Br J Surg* 72:458–461, 1985.

113. Bastow MD, Rawlings J, Allison SP: Benefits of supplementary tube feeding after fractured neck of femur: A randomized controlled trial. *Br Med J* 287:1589–1592, 1983.

114. Delmi M, Rapin CH, Bengoa JM et al: Dietary supplementation in elderly patients with fractured neck of the femur. *Lancet* 335:1013–1016, 1990.

115. Morley JE: Nutritional status of the elderly. *Am J Med* 81:679–695, 1986.

116. Hallbook T, Lanner E: Serum zinc and healing of venous leg ulcers. *Lancet* 2:780–782, 1972.

117. Greenfield S, Blanco DM, Elashoff RM et al: Patterns of care related to age of breast cancer patients. *JAMA* 257:2766–2770, 1987.

118. Hunt KE, Fry DE, Bland KI: Breast carcinoma in the elderly patient: An assessment of operative risk, morbidity and mortality. *Am J Surg* 140:339–342, 1980.

119. Callahan D: *Setting Limits: Medical Goals in an Aging Society.* New York, Simon and Schuster, 1987.

120. Reiss R: Moral and ethical issues in geriatric surgery. *J Med Ethics* 6:71–77, 1980.

121. Barry MJ, Mulley AG, Fowler F et al: Watchful waiting versus immediate transurethral resection for symptomatic prostatism. *JAMA* 259:3010–3017, 1988.

122. David PB, Robins LN: History-taking in the elderly with and without cognitive impairment. *J Am Geriatr Soc* 37:249–255, 1989.

123. Lachs MS, Feinstein AR, Cooney LM et al: A simple procedure for general screening for functional disability in elderly patients. *Ann Intern Med* 112:699–706, 1990.

124. Cummings SR, Phillips SL, Wheat ME et al: Recovery of function after hip fracture: The role of social supports. *J Am Geriatric Soc* 36:801–806, 1988.

125. Reardon GT, Blumenfield S, Weissman AL et al: Findings and implications from preadmission screening of elderly patients waiting for elective surgery. *Soc Work Health Care* 13:51–63, 1988.

126. O'Keefe JH, Shub C, Rettke SR: Risk of noncardiac surgical procedures in patients with aortic stenosis. *Mayo Clin Proc* 64:400–405, 1989.

127. Hayes SN, Holmes DR, Nishimura RA et al: Palliative percutaneous aortic balloon valvuloplasty before noncardiac operations and invasive diagnostic procedures. *Mayo Clin Proc* 64:753–757, 1989.

128. Terpenning MS, Buggy BP, Kauffman CA: Infective endocarditis: Clinical features in young and elderly patients. *Am J Med* 83:626–634, 1987.

129. Pinholt EM, Kroenke K, Hanley JF et al: Functional assessment of the elderly: A comparison of standard instruments with clinical judgment. *Arch Intern Med* 147:484–488, 1987.

130. Folstein MF, Folstein SE, McHugh PR: "Mini-mental state": A practical method for grading the cognitive state of patients for the clinician. *J Psychiatr Res* 12:189–198, 1975.

131. Tape TG, Mushlin AI: The utility of routine chest radiographs. *Ann Intern Med* 104:663–670, 1986.

132. Goldberger AL, Okonski M: Utility of the routine electrocardiogram before surgery and on general hospital admission. *Ann Intern Med* 105:552–557, 1986.

133. Kaplan EB, Sheiner LB, Boeckmann AJ et al: The usefulness of preoperative laboratory screening. *JAMA* 253:3576–3581, 1985.

134. Boghosian SG, Mooradian AD: Usefulness of routine preoperative chest roentgenograms in elderly patients. *J Am Geriatr Soc* 35:142–146, 1987.

135. Seymour DG, Pringle R, Maclennan WJ: The role of the routine preoperative electrocardiogram in the elderly surgical patient. *Ageing* 12:97–104, 1983.

136. Hodkinson HM: Value of admission profile tests for prognosis in elderly patients. *J Am Geriatr Soc* 29:206–210, 1981.

137. Courtney DL: Diagnosis of diabetes mellitus in the elderly: A practical guide. *Clin Report Aging* 3:5–8, 1989.

138. Friedman JR, Norman DC, Yoshikawa TT: Correlation of estimated renal function parameters versus 24-hour creatinine clearance in ambulatory elderly. *J Am Geriatr Soc* 37:145–149, 1989.

139. Castillo R, Haas A: Chest physical therapy: Comparative efficacy of preoperative and postoperative in the elderly. *Arch Phys Med Rehabil* 66:376–379, 1985.

140. Gold BS, Kitz DS, Lecky JH et al: Unanticipated admission to the hospital following ambulatory surgery. *JAMA* 262:3008–3010, 1989.

141. Harper CM, Lyles YM: Physiology and complications of bed rest. *J Am Geriatr Soc* 36:1047–1054, 1988.

142. Michelson JD, Lotke PA, Steinberg ME: Urinary-bladder management after total joint-replacement surgery. *N Engl J Med* 319:321–326, 1988.

143. Kane RL, Ouslander JG, Abrass IB: *Essentials of Clinical Geriatrics,* 2d ed. New York, McGraw-Hill, 1989, pp 164–181.

144. Van der Wall E, Verkooyen RP, Mintjes-DeGroot J et al: Prophylactic ciprofloxacin for catheter-associated urinary-tract infection. *Lancet* 339:946–951, 1992.

145. Golden WE, Lavender RC, Metzer WS: Acute postoperative confusion and hallucinations in Parkinson disease. *Ann Intern Med* 111:218–222, 1989.

146. Evans LK, Strumpf NE: Tying down the elderly: A review of the literature on physical restraint. *J Am Geriatr Soc* 37:65–74, 1989.

40 SURGERY IN THE PREGNANT PATIENT

Arnold W. Cohen

Ernest M. Graham

Wadia R. Mulla

The incidence of abdominal surgery during pregnancy is 2 to 4 percent.[1] The most common reasons for surgery include appendicitis, cholecystitis, intestinal obstruction, and exploratory laparotomy. These procedures have important implications for both the mother and fetus and are often accompanied by a significant maternal morbidity and fetal morbidity and mortality. The obstetrician, surgeon, and internist must consider many factors before recommending surgery during pregnancy, and this chapter reviews many of these concerns.

PHYSIOLOGIC CHANGES OF PREGNANCY

Understanding the physiologic changes of pregnancy listed in Table 40–1 is essential to successful perioperative management. Although these changes help to maintain the pregnancy, they pose some significant problems for the surgeon and anesthesiologist. The increase in cardiac output and intravascular volume of 40 to 50 percent protects maternal hemodynamics,[2] but the resulting physiologic dilutional anemia renders the patient more prone to anemia after significant blood loss.[3] Increases in cardiac output in those with underlying heart disease predisposes them to congestive heart failure with fluid shifts or febrile illness. Rapid hydration, blood loss, and postoperative fevers therefore significantly increase surgical risk in pregnant women. As pregnancy progresses, compression of the inferior vena cava decreases preload and produces a fall in cardiac output.[4] When possible, patients should preferably be placed in the left lateral position with at least a 15% tilt. In addition, glomerular filtration rate begins to rise by the twelfth week of pregnancy and complicates medication dosing in the perioperative period.[5]

TABLE 40–1. Cardiovascular Changes in Pregnancy

Cardiac output	Increased 40–50%
Heart rate	Increased 10%
Intravascular volume	Increased 50%
Red blood cell volume	Increased 30%
Central venous pressure	No change
Pulmonary capillary wedge pressure	No change
Mean arterial pressure	No change

GENERAL PRINCIPLES OF MANAGEMENT

Surgery during pregnancy is often delayed and can result in an untoward outcome. This is due in part to hesitation to perform surgery on pregnant patients for fear of pregnancy loss or wastage, premature labor and delivery, and undiagnosed fetal distress during the procedure. However, surgery during the first trimester is often undertaken without knowledge of the pregnancy. Women of childbearing age undergoing surgery should always be considered pregnant until proven otherwise. A careful menstrual, contraceptive, and sexual history must therefore be obtained from any woman between the ages of 12 and 50 before performing any surgery, and pelvic examination should always be performed. If abdominal pain is present or there is any question of early pregnancy, a serum level or rapid urine determination of HCG should be obtained prior to the procedure. If patients are found to be pregnant with an acute abdomen, ectopic pregnancy should always be considered.

During the first trimester, medications should be selected carefully in consultation with the obstetrician. Clinically important human teratogens are listed in Table 40–2. However, commonly used medications rarely cause congenital anomalies, and a wide

TABLE 40–2. Clinically Important Human Teratogens

Alcohol	Retinoic
Aminopterin	acids
Androgenic steroids	Tetracycline
Busulfan	Thalidomide
Carbamazepine	Trimethadione
Diethylstilbestrol	Valproic acid
Phenytoin	Warfarin

TABLE 40–3. Respiratory Changes in Pregnancy

Respiratory rate	No change
Vital capacity	No change
Tidal volume	Increased 30–40%
Functional residual capacity	Decreased 20%
Expiratory reserve volume	Decreased 20%
Residual volume	Decreased 20%
Total lung capacity	Decreased 5%

range of anesthetic agents are safe during pregnancy.[1] The baseline risk of spontaneous abortion and nonobstetric surgery is 15 to 20 percent; non-obstetric surgery that is not associated with hypoxia, hypovolemia, acidosis, and severe febrile illness does not increase the risk. However, every effort should be made to maintain hemodynamic stability and administer agents with proven efficacy and safety during pregnancy.

During the second and third trimester, nonobstetric surgery carries risk of premature labor, premature delivery, and fetal distress.[6] Tocolytic agents can be used prophylactically but do not prevent premature labor or delivery in all cases. Adequate hydration and prevention of hypotension are important in preventing intraoperative fetal distress. In addition, left lateral displacement of the uterus to prevent compression of the inferior vena cava in the supine position can be accomplished by either placing a roll under the patient's right flank or adjusting the operating table appropriately.[4] Minimizing uterine manipulation is extremely important in preventing premature labor and requires planning incisions and appropriately positioning the patient. Transcutaneous monitoring of oxygen saturation is necessary to prevent hypoxia. When fetal viability becomes likely after 24 weeks of gestation, fetal heart rate monitoring should ideally be carried out during and immediately after the procedure. If evidence of uteroplacental insufficiency develops, the patient should be treated with oxygen, placed in the left lateral position, and given crystalloid fluid to increase preload and cardiac output. If these measures fail to increase the fetal heart rate, then delivering the fetus should be considered.

It is imperative that all patients undergoing surgery in the second half of pregnancy undergo continuous uterine contraction monitoring postoperatively, and intraoperative monitoring may be indicated in some situations. If premature labor is documented by uterine contractions and change in the cervix, aggressive treatment with tocolytic agents such as intravenous ritodrine, subcutaneous terbutaline, indomethacin (prior to 34 weeks gestation), or magnesium sulfate should be initiated to prevent premature delivery. After surgery, the patient should go to a unit where fetal heart rate and uterine contractions can be monitored under the supervision of trained obstetrical nursing and medical staff. Depending on the severity of the patient's condition, this can be accomplished in a surgical intensive care unit with a nurse from the labor and delivery unit or on a labor and delivery floor. Difficult decisions required to ensure the health of both mother and fetus should be made jointly by the obstetrician, internist, and surgeon.

ANESTHESIA CONSIDERATIONS

The changes in respiratory physiology occurring during pregnancy (see Table 40–3) increase the risk of general anesthesia in the mother. Increases in tidal volume and minute ventilation and de-

creases in residual volume lead to lower levels of PCO_2 and may make ventilation more difficult during induction. High levels of progesterone in pregnancy cause delayed emptying and increased acidity of gastric contents. Pulmonary aspiration of gastric contents (Mendelson's syndrome) is an acknowledged risk and is even more likely during pregnancy.[7] A nonparticulate antacid like sodium citrate given 10 to 45 minutes before anesthesia decreases the severity of pulmonary damage after aspiration without contributing the added hazard of particulate agents. The most important safeguard against aspiration is skillful intubation while cricoid pressure is applied.[8] Pregnant patients can be difficult to intubate, and there have been a significant number of maternal deaths in patients undergoing general anesthesia for cesarean section during which intubation could not be performed successfully.[9]

General anesthesia has been associated with decreased uteroplacental perfusion during induction.[10] The halogenated agents halothane, enflurane, and isoflurane, frequently used to supplement nitrous oxide, readily cross the placenta and can produce narcosis in the fetus.[11] Because halothane is infrequently associated with cardiodepressant and hypotensive effects in the mother and has been associated with hepatitis and massive hepatic necrosis probably attributable to non–dose-dependent hypersensitivity, enflurane and isoflurane are often substituted. Although an increased incidence of congenital abnormalities and fetal loss is associated with chronic exposure to halothane in rats and the chick embryo, no such risk has been demonstrated following acute exposure during surgery in humans.[12] Nonetheless, whenever possible, one should minimize exposure to any anesthetic during fetal organogenesis during days 15 to 56 and central nervous system myelinization in the seventh to ninth month.

Low-spinal anesthesia, often referred to as "saddle block," is usually administered by using 4 mg of tetracaine in a hyperbaric solution injected into the L4–L5 interspace when the patient is sitting. Although this method is intended to anesthetize only the "saddle region," it frequently produces a sensory level as high as T10. Profound hypotension and a decrease in uteroplacental perfusion may occur with significant sympathetic block. Therefore, the patient should be monitored closely during and after the induction of spinal anesthesia.

Anesthetics can be injected through a lumbar intervertebral space for lumbar epidural analgesia or the sacral hiatus and sacral canal for caudal epidural analgesia. Lumbar epidural block is more often used because less drug is required to produce adequate analgesia. The incidence of uteroplacental insufficiency with epidural anesthesia can be reduced by hydrating the mother beforehand and avoiding supine hypotension. Puncture of the dura with inadvertent subarachnoid injection may occur and may require management of high-spinal block. Headache after spinal injection is a less serious but frequently troublesome complication of inadvertent entry into the subarachnoid space. Convulsions are rare after epidural anesthesia.

DIAGNOSTIC DIFFICULTIES

One of the most significant problems associated with nonobstetric surgery during pregnancy is failure to make the correct diagnosis in a timely fashion. Delay in diagnosis rather than the underlying condition is most often the cause of maternal and fetal morbidity and mortality. Many physicians are reluctant to obtain radiographic and other diagnostic tests during pregnancy because of the possible risks to the fetus. However, radiation exposure of less than 10 rads to the pelvis does not result in an increased incidence of congenital abnormalities even when it occurs in the first trimester. Most diagnostic radiologic procedures such as intravenous pyelograms, barium enema, upper GI series, flat plate of the abdomen, and chest x-ray expose the fetus to no more than one to two rads. Pregnant women who sustain significant trauma to the pelvis and undergo multiple x-rays and fluoroscopy may be exposed to as much as five to ten rads. In this situation, careful determination of which x-rays are necessary should be made before they are obtained.

Newer diagnostic tests such as ultrasound, computerized tomography, and magnetic resonance imaging have facilitated the diagnosis of many conditions and have thereby reduced the amount of radiation otherwise required. Ultrasound and MRI are safe for both mother and fetus, and computerized tomography results in less than 0.5 rads, even if the fetus is in the direct field of exposure. This degree of exposure imposes no increased risk of congenital abnormalities or growth retardation. Radioactive isotope scanning during pregnancy may be problematic. Lung scans using technitium are safe, even during the first trimester. However, since the fetal thyroid binds iodine 200 times more avidly than the adult gland after 10 weeks of gestation, use of radioactive iodine scanning should be avoided during pregnancy. Although the risk of cretinism in newborns of mothers who have been exposed to diagnostic levels of radioactive iodine during pregnancy is not increased, larger quantities of radioactive iodine used for ablation of the thyroid after the tenth week of pregnancy can result in neonatal hypothyroidism.

Physiologic changes in laboratory parameters must be considered in diagnostic evaluations of pregnant women. The white blood cell count increases slightly during pregnancy and can rise to 25,000 cells/mm^3 with the onset of labor. However, despite this increase, the differential count should not exhibit a leftward shift. Electrolytes remain normal during pregnancy, but the blood urea nitrogen levels and creatinine are usually below 10 and 0.8 mg/dl, respectively. Creatinine clearance increases 50% and should be considered in evaluating renal disease. Liver function tests, including bilirubin and liver enzyme concentrations, remain normal except for an increase in the level of alkaline phosphatase originating from the placenta. A gamma-glutamyltranspeptidase level is helpful in differentiating liver disease from other causes of elevations in alkaline phosphatase levels. Thyroid function studies reveal an increase in T_4 and a decrease in T_3 resin binding, resulting in a normal free thyroxine index (FTI) during pregnancy. The TSH remains unchanged. Most other blood chemistries remain within normal limits.

SPECIFIC CONDITIONS

Appendicitis

Appendicitis is the most common reason for nonobstetrical abdominal surgery during pregnancy with an incidence of 1 in 1500 to 2000 pregnancies.[13] The diagnosis of appendicitis is more difficult because of the physiologic changes of pregnancy. Anorexia, nausea, vomiting, and abdominal pain are common to both appendicitis and pregnancy. In addition, the position of the appendix varies during pregnancy and becomes displaced upward by the expanding uterus.[14] Therefore, the pain associated with acute appendicitis may be different from that described in classical appendicitis. Leukocytosis as high as 12,000 cells/mm^3 during pregnancy and 25,000 cells/mm^3 during labor may further obscure the diagnosis unless there is a leftward shift.[15] The differential diagnosis of acute appendicitis includes ruptured or hemorrhagic corpus luteum, adnexal torsion, ectopic pregnancy (ruptured or unruptured), preterm labor, placental abruption, chorioamnionitis, urinary tract disease, bowel obstruction, ovarian torsion, mesenteric adenitis, pancreatitis, inflammatory bowel disease, carcinoma of the appendix, and biliary tract disease.

Treatment of appendicitis during pregnancy requires surgical intervention, and early diagnosis is imperative to prevent complications. Before surgery, pregnant patients need adequate hydration with a dextrose-containing solution to prevent ketosis. Complete blood counts with differential counts and electrolyte levels should be followed. Nasogastric suction should be initiated as necessary. During the late second or the third trimester, the patient should be positioned to achieve left lateral displacement of the uterus during surgery to prevent positional hypotension. The incision should be made over the point of maximal tenderness rather than at McBurney's point because of the upward displacement of the appendix. If the diagnosis is unclear, a midline or paramedian incision should be considered for maximal exposure and exploration. Uterine manipulation should be minimized to avoid irritation and contractions. Appropriate broad-spectrum antibiotic therapy should be instituted before surgery and continued thereafter as indicated. Tetracyclines should be avoided during pregnancy, especially during the second half. The false-positive rate of diagnosis is approximately 30 percent and should be considered acceptable in view of the high rate of complications when diagnosis is delayed.[16] Overall fetal loss due to spontaneous abortion or premature delivery is 8.7 percent in uncomplicated appendicitis, but considerably higher at 33 to 50 percent in cases complicated by rupture or peritonitis.[17] Maternal mortality is as high as 4 percent in complicated cases.[18] The morbidity and mortality associated with appendicitis during pregnancy is directly related to delay in diagnosis and reluctance to proceed with surgical intervention.

Cholecystitis

The incidence of cholecystitis in pregnancy is approximately 1 in 1000, and the rate of cholecystectomy is 1 in 1250 to 12,500.[15] The incidence of cholecystitis increases with age, gravidity, and weight. Hormonal changes associated with pregnancy affect gallbladder contractility and volume. Progesterone inhibits gallbladder contractility both directly and by inhibiting cholecystokinin.[18] The volume of the gallbladder is increased, and emptying is decreased.[18–20] Some believe that these factors may predispose women to cholelithiasis and cholecystitis during pregnancy.

The diagnosis of cholecystitis is primarily based on clinical findings. Pain is usually described as colicky, localized in the right-upper quadrant, and often accompanied by nausea and vomiting. Murphy's sign is not consistently present in pregnancy. Ultrasound of the biliary system may indicate cholelithiasis or common duct dilatation. Since leukocytosis and an elevated alkaline phosphatase level are normal in pregnancy, these laboratory parameters are less useful.

Acute cholecystitis can usually be treated medically with intravenous hydration, nasogastric suctioning, and bowel rest. If the patient remains symptomatic, exploratory laparotomy with cholecystectomy or percutaneous gallbladder drainage should be considered. Recently, laparoscopic cholecystectomy has been performed during pregnancy, but it should only be undertaken by skilled surgeons after consultation with the obstetrician. A significant risk of premature labor and fetal loss accompanies cholecystitis, and delay in diagnosis and treatment should be avoided to minimize risk to the pregnancy.

Asymptomatic cholelithiasis is common. Up to 3.5 percent of all women undergoing abdominal ultrasound have gallstones.[21] When discovered during pregnancy, asymptomatic cholelithiasis should be managed expectantly.

Intestinal Obstruction

Intestinal obstruction most often is mechanical and due to intraabdominal adhesions from previous surgery or, less commonly, intestinal volvulus of the sigmoid and cecum. Although infrequent during pregnancy, maternal morbidity and mortality can be as high as 10 to 20 percent depending on the cause of the obstruction. Delay in diagnosis and treatment increases these rates.

Obstruction usually presents with vomiting of bilious material and colicky abdominal pain, and the pain becomes more intense and more diffuse as the obstruction worsens. Dehydration and electrolyte imbalances are frequent complications. Essential radiographic examinations, including plain abdominal x-rays and contrast studies, should be performed to prevent delay or misdiagnosis.

Cardiac Surgery

If possible, cardiac surgery should be avoided during pregnancy. However, if it is necessary, medical therapy should be optimized beforehand. Mitral valvulotomy, mitral or aortic valve replacement, and other repairs of congenital cardiac malformations are generally diagnosed prior to pregnancy and repaired at that time. Coronary artery bypass grafting procedures have also been reported during pregnancy.

A detailed cardiac evaluation should be performed in all pregnant patients with evidence of cardiac dysfunction. If medical management fails, surgery should be considered. Fetal well-being and lung maturity should be assessed if the patient is near term. If the fetal lungs have adequately matured, the patient should be delivered before cardiac surgery. If the patient is still far from term, surgery can be undertaken.

The effects of cardiopulmonary bypass on the fetus have been studied. The primary fetal response is bradycardia due to decreased flow. Therefore, it is currently recommended that continuous electronic fetal monitoring be carried out during bypass. High flow with normothermic settings should be used to avoid fetal hypoxia.[22] In two studies, good maternal outcomes were reported in 21 cases. There was one stillbirth and one preterm delivery following preterm labor, and the remainder delivered without complications.[23,24]

Mitral valvulotomy has been performed during pregnancy with good results and is currently recommended for patients with de-

compensated mitral valve disease refractory to medical therapy. Other forms of thoracic surgery have been performed during pregnancy and require the same perioperative precautions against maternal hypotension and hypoxia and their subsequent effects on the fetus.

Breast Surgery

Although the prognosis of breast cancer is not altered by pregnancy, it is often diagnosed at a later stage in pregnant patients. Diagnosis is difficult in the engorged breast, and physicians are often hesitant to perform diagnostic procedures during pregnancy. The approach to a breast mass is the same as in nonpregnant patients. Fine-needle biopsy can be done in an outpatient setting, and needle localization and open-breast biopsy can be performed safely with local or general anesthesia if proper operative precautions are taken.

Either lumpectomy or modified radical mastectomy with axillary node dissection can be performed for definitive treatment during pregnancy. Breast tissue is more vascular during pregnancy, and more blood loss should be anticipated. The risks to the pregnancy and fetus are related primarily to anesthesia as previously described and to maternal hypotension from hemorrhage.

POSTOPERATIVE THROMBOPHLEBITIS

Hormonal changes of pregnancy increase the risk of deep-vein thrombophlebitis both during gestation and in the immediate postpartum period.[25] Therefore, any patients undergoing surgery during pregnancy should probably receive prophylactic heparin during and after surgery to decrease the risk of pulmonary embolism unless contraindicated. If there are other risk factors like obesity, prolonged bedrest, immobilization of a limb, previous thrombophlebitis, or a history of pulmonary embolism, prophylactic heparin should definitely be administered.[26] The dose is 5000 units subcutaneously twice daily during the first trimester, 7500 units twice daily during the second, and 10,000 units twice daily during the third.[27] If the patient develops thrombophlebitis or pulmonary embolism, full therapeutic doses should be continued throughout pregnancy and the postpartum period.[28]

SUMMARY

1. Abdominal surgery is performed in 2 to 4 percent of pregnant women, most often for appendicitis, cholecystitis, and intestinal obstruction.

2. Normal physiologic changes in pregnancy including increased intravascular volume, dilutional anemia, compression of the inferior vena cava, and increased glomerular filtration rate may complicate management.

3. Pregnancy should be documented or excluded in any woman of childbearing age with abdominal pain.

4. If indicated, abdominal surgery should not be delayed because of pregnancy.

5. In the first trimester, the baseline incidence of spontaneous abortion is 15 to 20 percent but is not increased by uncomplicated nonobstetric surgery. Drugs should be chosen carefully.

6. In the second and third trimester, nonobstetric surgery carries the risk of premature labor and delivery and fetal distress, and tocolytic agents may be useful. After 24 weeks of gestation, fetal heart rate should be monitored during the procedure. In the second half of pregnancy, uterine contractions should be monitored during and after surgery.

7. Pregnant patients undergoing general anesthesia may be more difficult to intubate and are more prone to aspiration. Halogenated anesthetics can be used but should be avoided during fetal organogenesis (days 15 to 56) and central nervous system myelinization (seventh to ninth months).

8. Accurate diagnosis of abdominal pain can be difficult to make during pregnancy. Necessary radiologic procedures should not be withheld. Ultrasound and MRI are safe for both mother and fetus. Radionuclide technitium scans are safe during pregnancy, but radioactive iodine should be avoided due to the risk of neonatal hypothyroidism.

9. Laboratory parameters like the white blood cell count and thyroid function tests must be interpreted in view of their normal changes during pregnancy.

10. Surgery for appendicitis, cholecystitis, and intestinal obstruction during pregnancy should not be delayed. Although valvular heart surgery has been successfully performed, valvular disease should be managed medically until term if possible.

11. Pregnant patients are predisposed to the development of deep-venous thrombosis and should receive prophylactic subcutaneous heparin during hospitalization.

REFERENCES

1. Brodsky JB, Cohen EN, Brown BW Jr et al: Surgery during pregnancy and fetal outcome. *Am J Obstet Gynecol* 138:1165, 1980.
2. Elkayam U, Gleicher N: Cardiovascular physiology of pregnancy, in Elkayam U, Gleicher N (eds): *Cardiac Problems in Pregnancy: Diagnosis and Management of Maternal and Fetal Disease.* New York, Liss, 1982, p 5.
3. Hyatten FE, Lind T: Volume and composition of the blood, in Hyatten FE, Lind T (eds): *Diagnostic Indices in Pregnancy.* Basel, Documenta Geigy, 1973, p 36.
4. Metcalfe J, McAnulty JH, Ueland K: Cardiovascular physiology. *Clin Obstet Gynecol* 24:693, 1981.
5. Barron WM, Lindheimer MD: Renal function during pregnancy. *Contemp Ob Gyn* May 1983: 179, 1983.
6. Shnider SM, Webster GM: Maternal and fetal hazards of surgery during pregnancy. *Am J Obstet Gynecol* 92:891, 1965.
7. Cohen S: The aspiration syndrome. *Clin Obstet Gynecol* 9:235, 1982.
8. Bowes WA: Clinical aspects of normal and abnormal labor, in Creasy RK, Resnik R (eds): *Maternal-Fetal Medicine: Principles and Practice*, 2d ed. Philadelphia, Saunders, 1989, p 534.
9. Marx GF, Finster M: Difficulty in endotracheal intubation associated with obstetric anesthesia. *Anesthesiology* 51:364, 1979.
10. Jouppila P, Kuikka J, Jouppila R et al: Effect of induction of general anesthesia for cesarean section on intervillous blood flow. *Acta Obstet Gynecol Scand* 58:249, 1979.
11. Cunningham FG, MacDonald PC, Gant NF (eds): Analgesia and anesthesia, in *Williams Obstetrics*, 18th ed. Norwalk, CT, Appleton & Lange, 1989, p 329.
12. Anonymous: Pregnancy and anesthesia (editorial). *Lancet* 2:169, 1975.
13. Hill LM, Johnson CE, Lee RA: Prophylactic use of hydroxyprogesterone caproate in abdominal surgury during pregnancy: A retrospective evaluation. *Obstet Gynecol* 46:287, 1975.
14. Hibbard L: Cesarean section and other surgical procedures, in Gabbe SG, Niebyl JR, Simpson JL (eds): *Obstetrics: Normal and Problem Pregnancies.* New York, Churchill Livingstone, 1986, p 517.
15. Bauer JL, Reis RA, Arens RA: Appendicitis in pregnancy: With changes in position and axis of the normal appendix in pregnancy. *JAMA* 98:1363, 1932.
16. Mercer B: Appendicitis, in Gleicher N, Gall S, Sibia B et al (eds): *Principles & Practice of Medical Therapy in Pregnancy*, 2d ed. New York, Appleton & Lange, 1992, p 1270.
17. Key T: Gastrointestinal disease, in Creasy RK, Resnick R (eds): *Maternal Fetal Medicine*, 2d Ed. Philadelphia, Saunders, 1989, p 1032.
18. Horowitz MD, Gomez GA, San Nesteban R et al: Acute appendicitis during pregnancy. *Arch Surg* 120:1362, 1985.
19. DeVore G: Acute abdominal pain with pregnant patient due to pancreatitis, acute appendicitis, cholecystitis or peptic ulcer disease. *Clin of Perinatology* 7:349, 1980.
20. Everson GT, Braverman DZ, Johnson ML et al: A critical evaluation of realtime ultrasound for the study of gallbladder volume and function. *Gastroenterology* 79(1):40, 1980.
21. Stalffer RA, Adams A, Uygal J et al: Gallbladder disease in pregnancy. *J Obstet Gynecol* 144:661, 1982.
22. Beck WN: Intestinal obstruction in pregnancy. *Obstet Gynecol* 43:374, 1974.
23. Levy DL, Warriner RA, Burgess GE: Fetal response to cardiopulmonary bypass. *Obstet Gynecol* 56:112, 1980.
24. Bernae JM, Miralles PJ: Cardiac surgery with cardiopulmonary bypass during pregnancy. *Obstet Gynecol Surv* 41:1, 1986.
25. Laros RK, Alger LS: Thromboembolism and pregnancy. *Clin Obstet Gynecol* 22:871, 1979.
26. Aaro LA, Juergens JL: Thrombophlebitis associated with pregnancy. *Am J Obstet Gynecol* 109:1128, 1971.
27. Whitfield LR, Lele AS, Levy G: Effect of pregnancy on the relationship between concentration and anticoagulant action of heparin. *Clin Pharmacol Therap* 34:23, 1983.
28. Sasahara AA, Sharma GVRK, Barsamian EM et al: Pulmonary thromboembolism. *JAMA* 249:2945, 1983.

41 NUTRITIONAL ASSESSMENT OF THE SURGICAL PATIENT

Steven J. Fishman

James D. Luketich

James L. Mullen

Over a decade ago, nutrition surveys reported a 10 to 50 percent prevalence of "malnutrition" among hospitalized patients.[1–2] Moreover, nutritional status often declined during hospitalization,[3] and the degree of depletion was repeatedly found to correlate with subsequent morbidity and mortality. The variability in the prevalence of malnutrition and subsequent outcomes is due to a number of factors, including the specific tests used to assess nutrition, the cutoff points chosen to define malnutrition, the definition of clinical outcome endpoints, the presence of comorbid disease states, and the types of patient populations surveyed.

As early as 1936, Studley showed that surgical outcome was related to preoperative nutritional status in 50 consecutive patients undergoing gastric resection for peptic ulcer disease.[4] In patients who had suffered weight loss of more than 20%, the mortality rate was 33 percent. In those with less severe weight loss, the rate was only 5 percent. Other early reports by Rhoads, Cannon, Neumann, and Drucker documented a relationship between malnutrition and an increased number of postoperative infections, decreased cell-mediated immunity, impaired response to shock, and poor wound healing.[5–8]

More recently, these observations have been confirmed and expanded. Seltzer documented a fourfold increase in complication rate and a sixfold increase in death rate among patients with serum albumin levels below 3.5 g/dl.[9] In addition, a weight loss of more than 10 lbs proved to be a strong predictor of surgical mortality.[10] Rombeau confirmed that weight loss and decreased serum albumin levels correlate with increased morbidity and death in patients with colorectal cancer.[11] Among patients with gastric and esophageal cancer, Saito reported an increased incidence of sepsis and death in those with decreased lower arm muscle circumference, body weight, and serum retinol-binding protein levels.[12] Kaminski found

that low serum transferrin concentrations were associated with a 2.5-fold increase in hospital mortality,[13] and Blackburn confirmed that levels below 170 mg/dl predicted increased risk of sepsis and death.[14] Mullen found that a combination of several nutritional parameters, including serum levels of albumin and transferrin and anthropometric measurements, predicted adverse postoperative outcome with greater sensitivity and specificity.[15,16] A recent review by Meguid summarizes the extensive evidence that nutritional status strongly influences clinical outcome.[17]

The clinical impact of "malnutrition" was confirmed in early studies, but specific recommendations for diagnosis and treatment remained uncertain. As the number of assessment parameters increased, the clinical value of nutritional tests became even more questionable. If many tests are used, almost all patients will manifest some abnormalities.[18] Because of this, clinicians have attempted to evaluate assessment techniques more carefully and to identify patients with clinically relevant malnutrition more precisely. Malnutrition in this context is defined as an abnormality in an objective nutritional parameter or parameters associated with increased risk of adverse clinical events, i.e., morbidity and mortality, and with decreased risk of such events when corrected. Once patients are identified in this way, assessment data may help decide which subset of patients require active therapeutic intervention. These data also serve as a reference baseline for serial monitoring over time to determine when active nutritional intervention is no longer needed.

The subset of patients with malnutrition within a patient population varies not only with demographics but also with severity of illness. In one study, a serum albumin level of < 2.5 g/dl was associated with a mortality rate of 100 percent of patients in an intensive care unit.[19] When the same cutoff value was applied to a hospitalized pediatric population, the mortality rate was only 3.5 percent.[20] These examples emphasize that any definition of clinically relevant malnutrition must be developed and evaluated in populations similar to those in which it will be applied. Misapplication abounds in the literature and in clinical practice.

Normal individuals undergoing surgery experience a period of catabolism of variable duration characterized by weight loss and negative nitrogen balance. The duration of the catabolic phase is related to the severity of the surgical trauma and associated complications and coincides with a period of at least five to seven days during which the patient usually is unable to take oral nutrition. Patients with preexisting illness (e.g., underlying malignancy) or complications of the problems requiring surgery (e.g., bowel obstruction, abscesses, or fistulas) may already be malnourished. In addition, many of them, especially those with certain malignancies, sepsis, pancreatitis, burns, and long-bone fractures, have significantly increased caloric requirements.[21–22] Moreover, surgery causes depletion of glutamine, alanine, and branched-chain amino acids in muscle, leading to depression of muscle protein synthesis and postoperative fatigue.[23–25]

A perfect test should identify all individuals who subsequently develop a nutritionally related complication and not falsely identify anyone who does not have such an event. Unfortunately, there is no such test in clinical practice. From a practical standpoint, the best test must have a high enough sensitivity not to miss any malnourished patients even at the expense of losing specificity. Overtreating carries minimal risk, and treatment-related morbidity is usually easily managed.

This chapter examines individual nutritional assessment tests and their ability to identify patients with clinically relevant malnutrition. It then presents a practical synthesis of a step-wise approach to nutritional assessment and intervention. Finally, it surveys the measures that are most useful in serial assessment during active nutritional intervention.

CLINICALLY AVAILABLE MEASURES OF NUTRITIONAL STATUS

Body Size

Body weight is often the first variable considered in the assessment of nutritional status. Current body weight (CBW) is compared to ideal body weight (IBW) and to usual body weight (UBW). As seen in Table 41–1, IBW is drawn from mortality tables controlled for age, height, and gender.[26] UBW is the patient's estimate of his own body weight when he was last well and is generally reliable and accurate.[27] Historical data in the medical record may also be helpful. These measures define changes in body weight and deviation from control values and may reflect the severity of body compartment depletion.

Extreme weight loss clearly correlates with outcome. A recent study reported that a 10-pound weight loss was associated with a 19-fold increase in mortality.[10] However, weight loss alone is not sensitive enough to serve as the sole measure of nutritional status because the specific composition of lost weight cannot be determined by simple weighing. Weight loss may indicate a loss of fat mass or lean body mass from malnutrition or may simply be due to loss of fluids. Significant depletion of lean body mass may be present with little or no change in weight. Body weight may even increase in patients with significant malnutrition, as in those with hepatic cirrhosis and ascites. Similarly, significant loss of fat

TABLE 41–1. 1983 Metropolitan Height and Weight Tables for Men and Women aged 25–29 according to frame

MEN					WOMEN				
Height (in shoes)**		Weight in Pounds (in indoor clothing)*			Height (in shoes)**		Weight in Pounds (in indoor clothing)*		
		Small Frame	Medium Frame	Large Frame			Small Frame	Medium Frame	Large Frame
Feet	Inches				Feet	Inches			
5	2	128–134	131–141	138–150	4	10	102–111	109–121	118–131
5	3	130–136	133–143	140–153	4	11	103–113	111–123	120–134
5	4	132–138	135–145	142–156	5	0	104–115	113–126	122–137
5	5	134–140	137–148	144–160	5	1	106–118	115–129	125–140
5	6	136–142	139–151	146–164	5	2	108–121	118–132	128–143
5	7	138–145	142–154	149–168	5	3	111–124	121–135	131–147
5	8	140–148	145–157	152–172	5	4	114–127	124–138	134–151
5	9	142–151	148–160	155–176	5	5	117–130	127–141	137–155
5	10	144–154	151–163	158–180	5	6	120–133	130–144	140–159
5	11	146–157	154–166	161–184	5	7	123–136	133–147	143–163
6	0	149–160	157–170	164–188	5	8	126–139	136–150	146–167
6	1	152–164	160–174	168–192	5	9	129–142	139–153	149–170
6	2	155–168	164–178	172–197	5	10	132–145	142–156	152–173
6	3	158–172	167–182	176–202	5	11	135–148	145–159	155–176
6	4	162–176	171–187	181–207	6	0	138–151	148–162	158–179

*Indoor clothing weighing 5 pounds for men and 2 pounds for women.
**Shoes with 1-inch heels.
Source: Build Study, 1979; Society of Actuaries and Association of Life Insurance Medical Directors of America, 1980. Courtesy of *Statistical Bulletin,* Metropolitan Life Insurance Company.

weight may occur with little or no loss of lean body mass, as in obese individuals who undertake a sensible weight reduction program. The rate of weight loss should also be considered. Chronic loss is usually less detrimental than a loss of equal or less magnitude occurring more acutely. Changes in body weight are only useful when the composition rate and cause of the change are considered.

Analysis of body composition allows quantitation of the size of specific body compartments. Lean body mass can be subdivided into extracellular mass (ECM) and body cell mass (BCM). The body cell mass represents the sum of all cellular components, including those that exchange oxygen, oxidize glucose, and perform work. It constitutes 40 percent of body weight in normal adults, of which 60 percent is skeletal muscle mass and 20 percent is visceral cell mass like the liver, pancreas, and kidney. The remaining 20 percent includes red blood cells and the cellular elements in cartilage, bone, tendons, and adipose tissue. Nutritional depletion always adversely affects the body cell mass. Unfortunately, there is no direct measure of body cell mass, and indirect measurements are expensive and time-consuming. However, the BCM is a valuable research tool used to evaluate and validate other more clinically practical tests.[28]

During unstressed starvation, weight loss primarily represents loss of fat and body cell mass in a ratio of 4:1. Extracellular fluid, blood volume, and bone solids remain nearly constant.[29-30] In stressed starving trauma patients, the ratio may be reversed with major loss in the body cell mass.[31]

Total Body Fat

Total body fat is composed of subcutaneous and central fractions. Subcutaneous fat represents 50 percent of total body fat, and losses from these deposits correlate with loss of total body fat. Anthropometric measurement of fat stores is an inexpensive noninvasive method to assess subcutaneous fat, and involves measuring triceps skinfold (TSF) thickness using calipers and comparing measurements to percentile standards (Table 41–2). Values in the 35th to 40th percentile represent mild fat depletion, those in the 25th to 35th percentile describe moderate depletion, and those falling below the 25th percentile define severe depletion. Preoperative depletion of fat stores as determined by triceps skinfold thickness correlates independently with poor outcome.[32] In addition, large excesses of fat stores in morbid obesity are associated with an increased rate of surgical complications. A high coefficient of variation has limited the usefulness of anthropometric measurements in static nutritional assessment of the individual patient,[33] but they have greater value when used serially over several months. Visual assessment of fat stores may well be sufficient to define this body compartment.

Skeletal Muscle Stores

Skeletal muscle contains 60 percent of total body protein and is the major site of protein catabolism and amino acid supply in malnourished patients. This compartment represents a fraction of

TABLE 41–2. Triceps Skinfold Percentiles (mm)

Age (yr)	Female Percentiles					Male Percentiles				
	5th	25th	50th	75th	95th	5th	25th	50th	75th	95th
1	6	8	10	12	16	6	8	10	12	16
2	6	9	10	12	16	6	8	10	12	15
3	7	9	11	12	15	6	8	10	11	15
4	7	8	10	12	16	6	8	9	11	14
5	6	8	10	12	18	6	8	9	11	15
6	6	8	10	12	16	5	7	8	10	16
7	6	9	11	13	18	5	7	9	12	17
8	6	9	12	15	24	5	7	8	10	16
9	8	10	13	16	22	6	7	10	13	18
10	7	10	12	17	27	6	8	10	14	21
11	7	10	13	18	28	6	8	11	16	24
12	8	11	14	18	27	6	8	11	14	28
13	8	12	15	21	30	5	7	10	14	26
14	9	13	16	21	28	4	7	9	14	24
15	8	12	17	21	32	4	6	8	11	24
16	10	15	18	22	31	4	6	8	12	22
17	10	13	19	24	37	5	6	8	12	19
18	10	15	18	22	30	4	6	9	13	24
19–25	10	14	18	24	34	4	7	10	15	22
25–35	10	16	21	27	37	5	8	12	16	24
45–55	12	20	25	30	40	6	8	12	15	25
55–65	12	20	25	31	38	5	8	11	14	22
65–75	12	18	24	29	36	4	8	11	15	22

Source: Data derived from Health and Nutrition Examination Survey data of 1971–1974, using the same population samples as those of the National Center for Health Statistics (NCHS) growth percentiles for children. Adapted from Frisancho AR: New forms of upper limb fat and muscle areas for assessment of nutritional status. *Am J Clin Nutr* 34:2540, 1981.

total body protein reserves and can be measured by biochemical and anthropometric techniques. Anthropometric estimation of muscle mass uses measurement of mid-arm circumference (MAC) and skinfold thickness to calculate mid-arm muscle circumference (MAMC) and mid-arm muscle area (MAMA):

$$MAMC \ (cm) \ = \ \frac{MAC \ (cm) \ - \ TSF \ (mm)}{10}$$

$$MAMA \ (cm^2) \ = \ \frac{(MAMC)^2}{4}$$

These derivations rely on assumptions about the geometric distribution of various tissues within the arm which may be invalid to some degree. The usefulness of these measurements may be no better than visual assessment.[34]

The calculated creatinine-height index (CHI) is a biochemical parameter that estimates skeletal muscle size. The ratio of the patient's 24-hour urinary excretion of creatinine to gender and height-matched control values, expressed as a percentage, defines the CHI. Creatinine is the breakdown product of creatine, a high-energy compound found in skeletal muscles. The quantity of creatinine excreted in the urine in a 24-hour period correlates well with skeletal muscle stores in a steady state where there is no imbalance between muscle protein synthesis and breakdown.

Some of the difficulties in measuring urinary creatinine include significant daily variation in the same individual and between individuals, the effects of dietary creatinine intake, variable extrarenal losses, difficulty in obtaining accurate 24-hour urine collections, and variability in renal clearance. To achieve a precise measurement of urinary creatinine, patients must be on a meat-free diet and have normal renal function. They must not be in a catabolic state. A CHI of 100 indicates normal excretion of creatinine and normal skeletal muscle mass. A CHI of < 80% of the predicted normal value defines skeletal muscle depletion. A decline in the CHI correlates with subjective global assessment, but a CHI of < 90% of the predicted normal value was only moderately successful in predicting adverse clinical outcome.[34]

Circulating Serum Proteins

Circulating serum proteins are synthesized and secreted by the liver. Plasma levels are primarily dependent upon adequate nutrient precursors, liver synthesis, and their circulating half-lives. Half-life is in turn determined by catabolic rate and distribution between intravascular and extravascular spaces. Nutritional factors are therefore not the sole determinants of serum levels of circulating proteins. A decline in precursor intake results in a fairly rapid decrease in the synthetic rates of all the serum proteins. However, levels of some serum proteins may be affected by levels of other vitamins and minerals. For example, transferrin levels are affected by iron and retinol-binding protein levels by vitamin A. In addition, most serum proteins are acute phase reactants, and their concentrations change in a variety of illnesses.

Despite these limitations, a number of serum proteins have been found to decline in acute and chronic starvation, although their response to nutritional repletion is more variable. The serum protein levels most commonly used in nutritional assessment are albumin, transferrin, and prealbumin. They should be viewed as complementary rather than competitive since their unique characteristics reflect different situations.

Albumin is a 65,000-dalton serum protein with a 20-day half-life. It is the major protein synthesized by the liver. Degradation occurs primarily in the liver with a minor contribution by the kidney. Forty percent of total body albumin circulates at any given time. Normal serum concentration is 3.5 to 4.5 g/dl. The primary functions of albumin are to maintain intravascular plasma oncotic pressure and serve as a carrier for enzymes, drugs, hormones, and trace elements. Because albumin has a long half-life, its serum levels are not useful in detecting acute changes in the rate of synthesis. The level declines only if nutritional deprivation is prolonged. Administration of exogenous albumin increases the serum concentration but does not indicate improvement in nutritional status.[35]

The serum albumin level is the best single predictor of outcome. Reinhardt demonstrated a linear correlation between the degree of hypoalbuminemia and the 30-day mortality rate in hospitalized patients.[36] In most studies, the chosen cutoff point of serum albumin concentration results in a high degree of specificity at the expense of sensitivity. As the cutoff level defining abnormal is lowered, the sensitivity of the test to identify clinically relevant malnutrition correctly declines from 82 percent to 20 percent, while the specificity increases from 80 percent to 99 percent.[32]

Transferrin is a 76,000-dalton serum beta-globulin with a circulating half-life of eight days. It is synthesized in the liver and has a normal serum concentration of 200 to 260 mg/dl. Transferrin transports iron in the plasma, and its iron-binding properties may also contribute to defending against bacterial infection. The serum level of transferrin is affected by both nutritional factors and iron metabolism. The transferrin level is often reported as a function of total iron-binding capacity. These two measurements are linearly related and interchangeable except in the setting of iron overload or deficiency.[37] The shorter half-life of transferrin should theoretically make it a better early marker for nutritional deprivation and repletion than albumin. However, transferrin has not been studied as extensively as albumin, and it has not shown a decided advantage over albumin as the best single test to identify clinically relevant malnutrition.[14,18,38–40]

Prealbumin is a 54,000-dalton serum protein with a half-life of two to three days. It is synthesized by the liver and normally has a serum level of 15 to 25 mg/dl. Prealbumin transports thyroxine and acts as a carrier protein for retinol-binding protein.[41] Changes in serum prealbumin levels are an early indicator of nutrient deprivation and repletion, and changes in its concentration precede those in serum albumin.[42] Measurable alterations in prealbumin levels occur within seven days of a change in nutrient intake.[43] Few studies have validated prealbumin as a prospective marker of clinical outcome. One study of 319 general surgical patients compared the ability of several serum proteins to predict outcome. All proved to be effective predictors, but prealbumin was no better than albumin or transferrin.[44]

Immunologic Function

The association between malnutrition and an increased incidence of sepsis may be partially the result of specific defects in immune function due to malnutrition. Immunocompetence depends on complex interaction between cellular and humoral components and can be measured by a variety of tests. While both cellular and humoral mechanisms are affected by malnutrition, cell-mediated immunity (CMI) is affected earlier and to a greater extent than humoral function. Impaired CMI induced by malnutrition has been demonstrated in recall to primary and secondary antigens, total peripheral lymphocyte counts, total thymus-derived cell counts, and in vitro lymphocyte response to mitogens.

Early clinical reports suggested that abnormal delayed cutaneous hypersensitivity (DCH) reactions occurred in malnourished patients and correlated with poor outcome. Some reactivity could be recovered with nutrient repletion, and patients with improvement in skin testing reactivity had better outcomes than those who remained anergic. Subsequent studies criticized these earlier reports because they did not control for age, antigen variability, or prior antigen exposure.[45] Alterations in reactivity could be found in patients with concurrent diseases or sepsis who had no other evidence of malnutrition as measured by other parameters. The use of DCH is therefore not recommended in routine clinical nutritional assessment. It remains a clear marker of clinical outcome but has limited value as a measure of nutritional status.

Protein Balance

Commonly employed measures of protein turnover include nitrogen balance studies, 3-methylhistidine excretion, and isotopic tracer studies. Nitrogen balance techniques were first described over 100 years ago and continue to be used frequently. Nitrogen balance can be calculated by subtracting nitrogen output from nitrogen intake. A positive result indicates an anabolic state with net retention of nitrogen for the day, and a negative result indicates net protein loss. Although nitrogen balance studies are theoretically simple, the test is fraught with inaccuracies. The calculations require careful measurement of nitrogen intake and meticulous 24-hour urine collections. Intake tends to be overestimated, and output is often underestimated, resulting in a falsely positive balance.[46] Extrarenal losses of nitrogen occur through the skin and gastrointestinal tract and are not routinely measured. They can be estimated at 2 to 4 g/day and added as a correction factor to measured renal losses. This practice introduces significant error in disease states like intestinal malabsorption. Accuracy can be further affected if extrarenal losses from fistulous output and wound drainage are not measured.

In measuring nitrogen output, one must also consider accumulation of nitrogen as total body urea.[46] In worsening renal insufficiency with progressive impairment of urea excretion, measurement of urinary nitrogen alone would underestimate protein catabolism. The following equation allows correction for incomplete urinary excretion of nitrogen:

$$\text{Nitrogen balance} = \text{N intake} - \text{urinary N}$$
$$\pm \text{ change in body urea N}$$

$$\text{Change in body urea N (g)} = [0.6 \times BW_i \times (SUN_f - SUN_i)]$$
$$+ [(BW_f - BW_i) \times SUN_f]$$

SUN is serum urea nitrogen (g/liter), BW is body weight (kg), and i and f are initial and final values in the measurement period. The values in the first set of brackets account for changes in serum urea concentration. Those in the second set correct for volume changes in extracellular fluid during the period of measurement.

The urinary nitrogen excretion alone is a useful but gross measure of protein catabolism. Nitrogen excretion normally amounts to

5 to 8 g/day and drops to 2 to 4 g/day after several days of unstressed starvation. In severe sepsis or trauma, urinary nitrogen excretion may be as high as 30 to 50 g/day, reflecting the loss of 1.0 to 1.5 kg of lean tissue per day.

Energy Balance

Energy balance can be viewed as energy intake minus energy expenditure. Positive energy balance means an accumulation of energy usually in the form of increased fat stores. Negative energy balance, in which expenditure exceeds intake, reflects a decrease in energy or fat stores. Metabolic rate or energy expenditure can be estimated by the Harris-Benedict equation with comparison to controls matched for age, sex, height, and weight, or it can be measured using a portable indirect calorimeter.[47] Harris-Benedict predictions of resting energy expenditure are adequate only for normal patients in which 95% of the measured rates are within 10% of the predicted values. Several modified formulae have been developed for predicting energy expenditure in certain clinical settings but are too inaccurate for clinical use.[48,49] Bedside indirect calorimetry more reliably allows measurement of resting energy expenditure (REE).

REE is measured two hours after a meal with the patient at rest for 30 minutes in the supine position. The REE is approximately 10% higher than the basal metabolic rate, which is measured in the morning after a 12-hour fast before activity commences. REE makes up approximately 75% to 80% of the total daily energy expenditure in sedentary normals but represents 80% to 90% of this expenditure in most patients.[50] Total energy expenditure in hospitalized patients is 130% of the measured resting energy expenditure. It is significantly influenced by nutrient infusions, ambient room temperature, fever, and certain disease states.

Multi-Parameter Indices

A number of multi-parameter indices have been developed to improve the clinician's ability to predict outcome.[32] These involve correlating outcomes with a large number of nutritional test results and statistically choosing combinations of tests to form the best predictive model. The Prognostic Nutritional Index (PNI) was first developed at the University of Pennsylvania to predict postoperative complications from preoperative nutritional data, and was based on retrospective analysis. Four parameters were selected by discriminant analysis and computer-based step-wise regression and incorporated into a linear predictive model:

$$PNI(\% \text{ risk}) = 158 - [16.6 \times (\text{albumin in g\%})]$$
$$- [0.78 \times (\text{triceps skinfold in mm})]$$
$$- [0.2 \times (\text{transferrin in mg\%})]$$
$$- [5.8 \times (\text{skin test reactivity scale of } 0\text{–}2)]$$

This index was validated prospectively in several surgical populations. Another index, the Nutritional Risk Index (NRI), was developed using a similar approach: NRI = (15.9 × albumin) + (0.417 × %UBW).[51] A number of investigators have developed alternative predictive indices using a combination of objective and subjective criteria.[10,34,52,53] Most rely heavily on the serum albumin concentration as the major component.

The multi-parameter indices maintain excellent sensitivity and improve specificity compared to single tests of nutritional status. When the prevalence of nutritionally-related complications is above

25 percent, 80 to 90 percent sensitivity and > 60 percent specificity in predicting clinical outcome in surgical populations can be achieved.[15,16,53,54] At lower prevalence rates in better-nourished populations, the performance of these indices declines.[32,55]

PRACTICAL NUTRITIONAL ASSESSMENT

1. Understand the patient's primary diseases and therapy. Different thresholds for initiating nutritional intervention are based on these considerations. Specific factors to consider include the likelihood of additional treatments such as chemotherapy or radiation therapy that may further affect nutritional reserves. One cannot make nutritional recommendations outside the context of the patient's current and future clinical course.

2. Determine current nutrient intake. A patient may be severely nutritionally depleted after a prolonged course of chemotherapy, but appetite and nutrient intake may return to an acceptable level long before repletion of body cell mass can be expected. Alternatively, a lesion in the upper gastrointestinal tract may abruptly interfere with nutrient intake in a patient with normal nutritional status, requiring only maintenance nutritional support until he resumes eating.

Nonprotein caloric intake can be expressed in absolute quantities and as a percent of resting energy expenditure. Protein intake is measured and expressed as grams of protein per kg of IBW or CBW, whichever is lower. This allows one to compare current with optimal intake.

3. Assess current nutritional status. The authors use current body weight, mid-arm muscle circumference, triceps skinfold, and serum protein concentrations in conjunction with the history and physical examination.

Body weight. Current body weight (CBW) is compared to the patient's usual body weight (UBW), ideal body weight (IBW), and a clinical estimate of dry body weight. Losses of > 10% of usual body weight or a CBW of < 90% of IBW are considered mild risk factors in the development of nutritionally related complications. Classical "malnutrition" is seen in the patient who has lost fat and muscle stores and is "all skin and bones."

Skeletal muscle stores. Mid-arm muscle circumference measurement and subjective visual observation are used to assess skeletal muscle stores. Patients who have an MAMC below the 25th percentile have a clinically significant decrease in skeletal muscle stores.

Fat stores. Fat stores are evaluated by measuring triceps skinfold (TSF) thickness using skinfold calipers in conjunction with the physical examination. A TSF measurement below the 25th percentile represents significant depletion of fat stores and correlates with substantial loss of subcutaneous fat.

Serum proteins. Biochemical assessment includes the measurement of serum albumin, transferrin, and prealbumin concentrations. A serum albumin level < 3.5 g/dl, transferrin level < 200 mg/dl, or prealbumin level < 15 mg/dl indicates protein depletion.

4. Determine nutritional goals. Based on the predicted clinical course, current nutrient intake, and current nutritional status, nutritional goals are set for body weight (fat stores) and protein stores. In the case of body weight, three possible goals are (1) repletion if current body weight is < 90% of IBW, (2) maintenance if current

weight is between 90% and 120% of IBW, or (3) depletion if current body weight is > 120% of IBW. For protein, the goal is maintenance or repletion depending upon the serum protein levels, skeletal muscle stores, and protein catabolic rate.

5. Define nutrient requirements of calories and protein. *Caloric requirements* are based on the metabolic rate obtained by measuring resting energy expenditure by indirect calorimetry and the nutritional goal for fat stores. Musculoskeletal activity in most hospitalized patients increases REE < 20% above baseline. This is offset by a 10% to 20% decline in energy expenditure during eight hours of sleep. Total energy expenditure (TEE) in hospitalized patients is assumed to be 130% of REE. If the nutritional goal is positive energy balance and weight gain, caloric requirements are greater than TEE. If the goal is maintenance, calories are given at the TEE level.

Protein requirement is estimated from a direct measurement of urinary nitrogen excretion or from the lesser of CBW and IBW and a factor based on clinical status. In unstressed normal patients, this usually amounts to 1.0 gm protein/kg. If assessment reveals depletion of muscle or decreased levels of serum proteins, 1.5 gm protein/kg are given. In stressed and depleted patients, 2.0 gm protein/kg of IBW or CBW, whichever is lower, are administered.

6. Make the forced feeding decision. The need for forced feeding depends on current nutritional status and comparison between current and future nutrient intake and derived nutrient requirements. The ultimate decision is influenced by the prognosis and anticipated course of the patient's illness, additional planned therapies, and the estimated impact of nutritional status on outcome. The feeding plan must fit in well with the overall treatment plan. An important factor is how soon the patient will resume adequate voluntary oral intake. If either current or future nutritional status is compromised, forced feeding should be undertaken if outcome may be otherwise jeopardized. An access route must be established and a nutrient prescription determined, as discussed in Chap. 42.

7. Monitor forced feeding. Once feeding is initiated, it is necessary to determine if the patient is receiving what was planned. Problems may arise with intravenous or gastrointestinal access and nutrient solution preparation and administration. If delivery is successful, serial nutritional assessments are necessary to determine whether to continue, alter, or discontinue feeding.

SERIAL NUTRITIONAL ASSESSMENT

Serial assessment becomes important in the context of long-term nutritional goals. Most parameters do not show consistent improvement with nutritional intervention of less than two to three weeks. However, positive nitrogen balance can be achieved within two to three days in most cases. Anthropometric assessment is performed monthly. Serum protein levels should be monitored with expected improvements based on their individual half-lives. Prealbumin levels improve after three days of repletion, and transferrin will do so within seven days. Significant improvement in albumin levels before two to three weeks is unlikely.

Changes in anthropometrics and circulating protein levels are not always sensitive or specific in measuring response to nutritional repletion, especially when attempting to assess acute response. In fact, nitrogen and caloric intake may be adequate for several weeks before a significant increase in total body nitrogen can be measured. Recent interest has centered on evaluating skeletal muscle function as a potential early indicator of response to nutritional depletion and repletion.[56]

SUMMARY

1. Malnutrition is common among surgical patients, particularly among those with underlying illness. Nutritional status often declines further in the hospital and is related to clinical course.

2. Defining and quantitating malnutrition is difficult. Changes in body weight alone or alterations in single parameters (e.g., anthropometric measures of fat and skeletal muscle, circulating serum protein levels, determination of immunologic function, or measures of protein or energy balance) may not be sufficient. Multi-parameter indices have been developed and have a higher sensitivity and specificity.

3. Practical nutritional assessment includes understanding the patient's underlying disease and course, evaluating current nutrient intake, assessing nutritional status, determining goals, and quantitating requirements. Once the decision to undertake forced feeding is made, careful monitoring and serial assessment of nutritional status is mandatory.

REFERENCES

1. Bistrian BR, Blackburn GL, Vitale J et al: Prevalence of malnutrition in general medical patients. *JAMA* 235:1567–1570, 1976.
2. Bistrian BR, Blackburn GL, Hallowell E et al: Protein status of general surgical patients. *JAMA* 230:858–860, 1974.
3. Butterworth CE Jr, Weinsier RL: Malnutrition in hospitalized patients: Assessment and treatment, in Goodhart RS, Shils ME (eds): *Modern Nutrition in Health and Disease*, 6th ed. Philadelphia, Lea & Febiger, 1980.
4. Studley HO: Percentage of weight loss: A basic indicator of surgical risk in patients with chronic peptic ulcer. *JAMA* 106:458–460, 1936.
5. Rhoads JE, Alexander CE: Nutritional problems of surgical patients. *Ann NY Acad Sci* 63:268–275, 1955.
6. Cannon PR, Wissler RW, Woolridge et al: The relationship of protein deficiency to surgical infection. *Ann Surg* 120:514–525, 1944.
7. Neumann CG, Lawlor GL, Stiehm ER et al: Immunological responses in malnourished children. *Am J Clin Nutr* 28:89–104, 1975.
8. Drucker WR, Howard PL, McCoy S: The influence of diet on response to hemorrhagic shock. *Ann Surg* 181:698–704, 1975.
9. Seltzer MH, Bastidas JA, Cooper DM et al: Instant nutritional assessment. *JPEN* 3:157–159, 1979.
10. Seltzer MH, Slocum BA, Cataldi-Belcher EL: Instant nutritional assessment: Absolute weight loss and surgical mortality. *JPEN* 6:218–221, 1982.
11. Hickman DM, Miller RA, Rombeau JL et al: Serum albumin and body weight as predictors of postoperative course in colorectal cancer. *JPEN* 4:314, 1980.
12. Saito T, Zeze K, Kuwahara A, Miyahara M, Kobayashi M: Correlations between preoperative malnutrition and septic complications of esophageal cancer surgery. *Nutrition* 6(4):303–308, 1990.
13. Kaminski MV, Fitzgerald MJ, Murphy RJ et al: Correlation of mortality with serum transferrin and anergy. *JPEN* 1:27, 1977.
14. Blackburn GL, Bistrian BR, Harvey K: Indices of protein-calorie malnutrition as predictors of survival, in Levenson SM (ed): *Nutritional*

Assessment: Present Status, Future Directions, and Prospects. Columbus, Ohio, Ross Laboratories, 1981, pp 131–137.

15. Mullen JL, Buzby GP, Waldman TG et al: Prediction of operative morbidity and mortality by preoperative nutritional assessment. *Surg Forum* 30:80–82, 1979.
16. Buzby GP, Mullen JL, Matthews DC et al: Prognostic nutritional index in gastrointestinal surgery. *Am J Surg* 139:160–167, 1980.
17. Meguid MM, Campos AC, Hammond WG: Nutritional support in surgical practice: Part I. *Am J Surg* 159:345–358, 1990.
18. Mullen JL, Gertner MH, Buzby GP et al: Implications of malnutrition in surgical patients. *Arch Surg* 114:121–125, 1979.
19. Apelgren KN, Rombeau JL, Twomey PL et al: Comparison of nutritional indices and outcome in critically ill patients. *Crit Care Med* 10:305–307, 1982.
20. Hay RW, Whitehead RG: Serum-albumin as a prognostic indicator in edematous malnutrition. *Lancet* 2:427–429, 1975.
21. Luketich JD, Mullen JL, Feurer ID et al: Ablation of abnormal energy expenditure by curative tumor resection. *Arch Surg* 125:337–341, 1990.
22. Hyltander A, Drott C, Korner U et al: Elevated energy expenditure in cancer patients with solid tumours. *Eur J Cancer* 27(1):9–15, 1991.
23. Carli F, Webster J, Ramachandra V et al: Aspects of protein metabolism after elective surgery in patients receiving constant nutritional support. *Clin Sci* 78:621–628, 1990.
24. Petersson B, Wernerman J, Waller SO et al: Elective abdominal surgery depresses muscle protein synthesis and increases subjective fatigue: Effects lasting more than 30 days. *Br J Surg* 77:796–800, 1990.
25. Carli F, Ramachandra V, Gandy J et al: Effect of general anesthesia on whole body protein turnover in patients undergoing elective surgery. *Br J Anaesth* 65:373–379, 1990.
26. *Metropolitan Life Foundation Statistical Bulletin.* New York, Metropolitan Life Foundation, 1983, vol 64, pp 2–9.
27. Stewart AL: The reliability and validity of self reported weight and height. *J Chron Dis* 35:295–309, 1982.
28. Lukaski HC: Methods for the assessment of human body composition: Traditional and new. *Am J Clin Nutr* 46:537–556, 1987.
29. Keys A, Brozek J, Henschel A et al: *The Biology of Human Starvation.* Minneapolis, University of Minnesota Press, 1950.
30. Shizgal HM: Nutritional assessment with body composition measurements. *JPEN* 11:428–478, 1987.
31. Kinney JM, Duke JH Jr, Long CL et al: Tissue fuel and weight loss after injury. *J Clin Pathol* 23(Suppl 4):65–72, 1970.
32. Dempsey DT, Mullen ML: Prognostic value of nutritional indices. *JPEN* 11:109S–114S, 1987.
33. Buzby GP, Mullen JL: Nutritional assessment, in Caldwell M, Rombeau J (eds): *Clinical Nutrition*, vol I: *Enteral and Tube Feeding.* Philadelphia, Saunders, 1984.
34. Baker JP, Detsky AS, Wesson DE et al: Nutritional assessment: A comparison of clinical judgment and objective measurements. *N Engl J Med* 306:969–972, 1982.
35. Grundman R, Meyer H: Der einfluss von operation und hamodilution auf den kolloidosmotischen druck. *Chirurg* 51:594–600, 1980.
36. Reinhardt GF, Myscofski JW, Walkens DB et al: Incidence and mortality of hypoalbuminemic patients in hospitalized veterans. *JPEN* 4:357–359, 1980.
37. Crosby LO, Giandomenico A, Mullen JL: Relationships between serum total iron-binding capacity and transferrin. *JPEN* 8:274–278, 1984.
38. Braga M, Baccari P, Scaccabarozzi S et al: Prognostic role of preoperative nutritional and immunological assessment in the surgical patient. *JPEN* 12:138–142, 1988.
39. Detsky AS, McLaughlin JR, Baker JP et al: What is subjective global assessment of nutritional status? *JPEN* 11:8–13, 1987.
40. Bozetti F, Migliavacca S, Gallus G et al: Nutritional markers as prognostic indicators of postoperative sepsis in cancer patients. *JPEN* 9:464–470, 1985.

41. Tuten MB, Wogt S, Dasse F et al: Utilization of prealbumin as a nutritional parameter. *JPEN* 9:709–711, 1985.
42. Helms RA, Dickerson RN, Ebbert ML: Retinol-binding protein and prealbumin: Useful measures of protein repletion in critically ill malnourished infants. *J Ped Gastroenterol Nutr* 5:586–592, 1986.
43. Buonpane EA, Brown RO, Boucher BA et al: Use of fibronectin and somatomedin-C as nutritional markers in the enteral nutrition support of traumatized patients. *Crit Care Med* 17:126–132, 1989.
44. Boraas M, Peterson O, Knox L et al: Serum proteins and outcome in surgical patients (abstract). *JPEN* 6:585, 1982.
45. Twomey P, Ziegler D, Rombeau R: Utility of skin testing in nutritional assessment: A critical review. *JPEN* 6:50–57, 1982.
46. Kopple JD: Uses and limitations of the balance technique. *JPEN* 11:79S–85S, 1987.
47. Jequier E: Measurement of energy expenditure in clinical nutritional assessment. *JPEN* 11:86S–89S, 1987.
48. Ireton-Jones CS, Turner WW, Baxter CR: The effect of burn wound excision on measured energy expenditure and urinary nitrogen excretion. *J Trauma* 27:217–220, 1987.
49. Lukaski HC, Mendez J: Relationship between fat-free weight and urinary 3-methylhistidine excretion in man. *Metabolism* 29:758–761, 1980.
50. Foster GD, Knox LS, Dempsey DT et al: Caloric requirements in total parenteral nutrition. *J Am Coll Nutr* 6:231–253, 1987.
51. Buzby GP, Williford UO, Peterson OL et al: A randomized clinical trial of total parenteral nutrition in malnourished surgical patients: The rationale and impact of previous clinical trials and pilot study on protocol design. *Am J Clin Nutr* 47:357–365, 1988.
52. Seltzer MH, Fletcher HS, Slocum BA et al: Instant nutritional assessment in the intensive care unit. *JPEN* 5:70–72, 1981.
53. Meguid MM, Debonis D, Meguid V et al: Complications of abdominal operations for malignant disease. *Am J Surg* 156:341–345, 1988.
54. Simms JM, Smith J, Weeds HF: A modified prognostic index based upon nutritional measurements. *Clin Nutr* 1:71–79, 1982.
55. Brenner U, Muller FM, Keller HW et al: Nutritional assessment in surgical planning. *Clin Nutr* 7:225–229, 1988.
56. Jeejeebhoy KN: Bulk or bounce—the object of nutritional support. *JPEN* 12:539–549, 1988.

PROPHYLACTIC THERAPY AND THE PREVENTION OF POSTOPERATIVE PROBLEMS

IV

42 NUTRITIONAL SUPPORT OF THE SURGICAL PATIENT

John M. Daly

Kurt P. Hofmann

Most patients can withstand the brief period of inanition associated with preoperative preparation, surgery itself, and postoperative recovery, without harmful sequelae. However, if the stresses of surgery and anesthesia are superimposed on malnutrition or the underlying disease process or procedure causes prolonged starvation, significant morbidity and mortality can result.

The incidence of malnutrition among hospitalized patients is variable. Studies using biochemical and anthropometric markers have shown that up to 50 percent of patients on surgical services are malnourished.[1,2] Increased morbidity in patients with significant weight loss prior to surgery has been documented repeatedly.[3] In 1955 Rhoads and Alexander noted that severe malnutrition was common in surgical patients, and discovered an increased incidence of postoperative infection in hypoproteinemic patients.[4] More recently, Kaminski and Mullen reported increased rates of postoperative complications and mortality in malnourished patients.[5,6] Thus, it is important to identify malnutrition in hospitalized patients and to treat it promptly.

CONSEQUENCES OF MALNUTRITION

Energy is stored as carbohydrate in the form of glycogen, protein (performing nonfuel structural or enzymatic functions), and lipid. Fat is the primary storage depot of energy in humans. During simple starvation, glycogen stores are utilized within 24 hours. Thereafter, glucose, the primary fuel for nervous tissue, is derived from gluconeogenesis. Amino acid precursors, primarily from muscle and lactate, are utilized to resynthesize glucose in the liver. Protein breakdown is avoided through the use of endogenous ketones and fatty acids by most tissues as an energy source.

In prolonged starvation, the brain is able to utilize the ketones betahydroxybutyrate and acetoacetate, and the remaining glucose and protein are spared.[7] Protein metabolism is a dynamic process of continuous synthesis and degradation involving exogenous and endogenous amino acids. Levels of those proteins essential for survival such as enzymes and immunoglobulins are maintained at the expense of muscle protein during periods of prolonged starvation. When demand for additional high-priority protein is increased by major surgery, severe trauma, or sepsis, essential proteins may become depleted enough to cause clinical deterioration and death. The goal of nutritional support is to provide exogenous calories, protein, vitamins, and minerals to preserve body cell mass and organ function.[8]

BENEFITS OF NUTRITIONAL SUPPORT

Numerous clinical studies have documented the benefit of nutritional support in surgical patients. Shizgal, using a multiple isotope dilution technique, demonstrated that total parenteral nutrition (TPN) preserved body cell mass and prevented expansion of the extracellular component that occurs in critically ill malnourished patients.[9] Williams et al. studied 70 patients after surgery for gastric cancer and showed that those who received TPN for 7 to 10 days developed significantly fewer wound complications than those who did not. However, the incidence of other infectious complications and mortality were the same in both groups.[10] Holter and Fischer demonstrated significant increase in serum albumin concentrations and decreased weight loss after surgery in patients receiving 72 hours of TPN but no difference in postoperative morbidity and mortality rates.[11]

Buzby et al. documented changes in serum transferrin concentrations after 15 days of TPN. Patients without substantial increases in these levels had a fivefold increase in morbidity.[12] Similarly, Church and Hill demonstrated that those patients achieving positive nitrogen balance on TPN had a postoperative complication rate of seven percent, and those patients with negative nitrogen balance had a rate of 73 percent.[13] Jeevanandum et al. showed that patients on TPN utilize the exogenous amino acids for protein synthesis. However, utilization efficiency was only 39% in cachectic patients, and 51% in normals.[14] It is therefore important to monitor nutritional support to determine if it is beneficial or if more aggressive medical or surgical intervention is needed before benefit can be realized.

Several retrospective clinical reviews have confirmed the benefits of TPN. In a retrospective review of 145 surgical patients, Mullen et al. found that severely malnourished patients who received seven days of preoperative TPN had a twofold decrease in postoperative complications and a sevenfold decrease in postoperative mortality compared to those who did not receive TPN.[15] Daly et al. reported that TPN administered to malnourished patients with esophageal cancer for at least five days before surgery resulted in a significant decrease in major infectious, wound, and anastomotic complications.[16] Riboli et al. found that patients with esophageal anastomotic leaks undergoing immediate reoperation had a significantly higher mortality rate than those patients treated with conservative drainage and TPN.[17]

There have also been several prospective randomized studies evaluating the effect of TPN in surgical patients (see Table 42–1). Heatley et al. found that patients with esophageal or gastric cancer who received supplemental preoperative TPN for 7 to 10 days had fewer postoperative wound infections than those who received oral diets but found no decrease in overall morbidity or mortality.[18] Thompson et al. randomized patients who had lost more than 10 pounds before surgery to receive either preoperative TPN for five days or standard hospital diets and found that postoperative morbidity and mortality were the same in both groups.[19] In a 10-day trial, Muller et al. similarly randomized 125 patients with gastrointestinal carcinoma, and found fewer postoperative complications and a lower mortality rate in those receiving TPN.[20] Foschi et al. randomized 64 jaundiced patients undergoing percutaneous transhepatic biliary drainage and reported a significant decrease in morbidity and mortality in those patients who received nutritional support.[21] Bellantone et al. demonstrated a statistically significant reduction in septic complications in nutritionally depleted patients with serum albumin levels < 3.5 g/dl and/or total lymphocyte counts of < 1500 cells/mm[3] who received seven days of preoperative parenteral nutritional supplementation.[22]

The present consensus is to delay surgery when possible to provide nutritional support to severely malnourished patients.

TABLE 42–1. Compilation of Studies Showing Decreased Surgical Complication Rates in Patients Receiving Total Parenteral Nutrition (TPN)

Author	Number of Patients	Complication Rate (%) TPN	Control
Holter (1977)	56	13	19
Moghissi (1977)	15	30	50
Heatley (1979)	74	28	25
Simms (1980)	40	—	—
Lim (1981)	19	30	50
Schildt (1981)	15	39	57
Thompson (1981)	41	17	10
Sako (1981)	69	50	56
Mueller (1982)	125	11	19
Jenson (1982)	20	—	—
Stecker (1986)	59	12.5	45
Foschi (1986)	64	18	47
Bellantone (1988)	100	5	22

Source: Modified from Redmond and Daly.[72]

Those with mild-to-moderate malnutrition should probably underg elective procedures and receive postoperative TPN if necessary The choice of nutritional support—enteral, parenteral, or both— depends on the clinical condition of the individual patient.

NUTRITIONAL REQUIREMENTS

The most precise method of determining caloric requirements i measurement of resting energy expenditure (REE) using indirec calorimetry. Because it is expensive and technically difficult, cald rimetry is not practical outside a research setting. Caloric require ments can also be calculated as the basal energy expenditur (BEE) from the Harris-Benedict formula:

Males: BEE (kcal) = 66 + [13.7 × weight (kg)] + [5 × height (cm)] − [6.8 × age (yrs)]

Females: BEE (kcal) = 655 + [9.6 × weight (kg)] + [1.7 × height (cm)] − [4.7 × age (yrs)]

Daily caloric requirements can be met by providing 1000 kca above the patient's BEE or 150% of the measured or calculate REE. In obese patients, the caloric goal is 90% to 100% of th REE. Alternatively, a nonprotein caloric intake of approximatel 30 to 40 kcal/kg/day can be given to maintain body cell mas with additional calories for those who are depleted or malnour ished.

Dietary nitrogen requirements should be provided in a ratio c approximately 1 g of nitrogen to 135 kcal of nonprotein calories. Another method of calculating nitrogen requirements is to provid 0.30 g of nitrogen or 3.1 g of amino acids[24] per kilogram of bod weight per day. Nitrogen balances should be calculated weekl with the formula:

$$N(bal) = N(in) - N(out)$$

where N(in) = dietary protein in grams/6.25 and N(out) = 24 hour urinary urea nitrogen (UUN) measurement in grams plus factor of 2 g/day for daily nonurea nitrogen losses (e.g., creatinin and ammonia) and an additional 2 g/day for fecal and skin losses The formula then becomes:[25]

$$N(bal) = N(in) \times UUN + 4$$

In patients receiving TPN, carbohydrate in the form of glucos is given to match the maximal rate of glucose oxidation an amounts to 7 mg/kg/min or 40 kcal carbohydrate/kg/day.[23] Patient who require more calories or who have severe glucose intoleranc should receive excess calories as lipid. Insulin can be added di rectly to the TPN solution or given subcutaneously to maintain th serum glucose level between 130 and 200 mg/dl. Carbohydrate provided in excess of the above amounts are not oxidized and ar stored as glycogen and fat. This leads to fatty infiltration of the liver and excess CO_2 production.[26]

Lipid emulsions in either a 10% solution providing 1 kcal/ml o a 20% solution providing 2 kcal/ml can be infused through centra or peripheral veins. Lipid solutions allow for administration o more calories in a smaller volume of water. They also provide a source of free fatty acids that can serve as a primary source o energy for most peripheral tissues. However, a minimum of 50 to 150 g of glucose should be given daily as fuel for the central nervous system.[25] Currently, 10% fat emulsions are administered in a volume of 500 ml over a six- to eight-hour period each day. Serum triglyceride levels should be monitored to ensure adequate metabolism. An ideal balance of energy requirements can be achieved by providing 30 to 50 percent of nonprotein calories as lipid. In any case, a minimum of 1500 ml of 10% lipid emulsion should be given each week to prevent essential fatty acid deficiency. All-in-one solutions allow admixtures of glucose, fat, and amino acids to be administered over a 24-hour period. It is also important to provide adequate vitamins and trace elements, as shown in Table 42–2.

Additional information on nutritional assessment and requirements is provided in Chap. 41.

Enteral Nutrition

Enteral nutritional support is preferable in patients with functioning gastrointestinal tracts. Although caloric and protein goals are attained more quickly and positive nitrogen balance is achieved earlier with TPN, several prospective randomized clinical studies have shown that enteral nutrition is equally efficacious and less expensive when used for periods of a week or more.[27,28,29] Recent animal studies have demonstrated the physiologic benefit of maintaining gastroesophageal function with enteral nutrition.[30,31,32] Absolute contraindications to enteral nutrition include gastric outlet or intestinal obstruction, enterocutaneous fistula, and toxic megacolon. Relative contraindications include severe radiation enterocolitis and short-bowel syndrome.

If a patient is unable to meet caloric needs, the initial step in nutritional support is dietary counseling and provision of palatable oral nutritional supplements. However, many patients cannot ingest enough calories even with counseling. Any patient who is moderately to severely malnourished has by definition failed oral nutrition and needs enteral nutritional support through tube feedings.[33]

Small-bore nasoenteral tubes made of silicone, rubber, or polyurethane are flexible and minimize patient discomfort. They vary in length and in bore size. Those measuring 91 cm are for nasogastric feeding, while the mercury-weighted 109 cm tubes allow the tip to pass spontaneously through the pylorus into the distal duodenum or upper jejunum. Choice of bore size is determined by the viscosity and osmolarity of the formula. Isotonic formulas flow easily through no. 8F tubes, but hypertonic formulas require 10F tubes. One should select the smallest bore tube appropriate for the given formula (see Table 42–3).

If long-term enteral nutritional support is anticipated, the solution should be infused through a gastrostomy or jejunostomy. In patients with esophageal or upper gastrointestinal anastomoses, in those predisposed to aspiration, or in those who have not tolerated

TABLE 42–2. Daily Trace Element and Vitamin Recommendations for Adults Receiving TPN

Trace	RDA	Intestinal Absorption	Recommendations
Zinc	15 mg	10–40%	2.6 mg*
Copper	2–3 mg	30%	0.1–2.8 mg**
Chromium	0.05–0.2 mg	10–25%	5–20 µg***
Manganese	2.5–5 mg	50%	0.2–3.3 mg
Selenium	0.05–0.2 mg	80%	40–120 µg
Iron	10–15 mg		0.5–7 mg
Iodine	150 µg		70–140 µg
Fluoride	1.5–4 mg		0.9–4 mg
Molybdenum	0.15–4 mg		0.02–0.03 mg
Cobalt	as part of B_{12} requirement		0.09 mg

Vitamin	RDA	Parenteral Dose
Vitamin A	2640–3300 IU	3300 IU
Vitamin D	200 IU (5 µg)	200 IU
Vitamin E	8–10 IU	10 IU
Vitamin K	0.5–1.0 µg/kg	5–10 mg weekly
Vitamin B_1	0.5 mg/1000 kcal	3.0 mg
Vitamin B_2	1.2–1.6 mg	3.6 mg
Pantothenic acid	4.0–7.0 mg	15.0 mg
Vitamin B_6	2.0–2.2 mg	4.0 mg
Vitamin B_{12}	3.0 µg	5.0 µg
Vitamin C	60 mg	100 mg
Biotin	100–200 mg	60 mg

RDA = Recommended daily allowance
  *2 mg in acute catabolic states; 6–12 mg for diarrhea or intestinal losses
 **12–24 mg for diarrhea or intestinal losses
***0.4–0.5 mg for intestinal losses
Source: Adapted from Reilly JJ, Gerhardt AL: Modern surgical nutrition. *Curr Prob Surg* 22(10):1–81, 1985.

TABLE 42–3. Nasoenteric Tubes

French Size	Composition	Lengths (cm)	Weighted Tip — None	Weighted Tip — Small Bolus	Weighted Tip — Large Bolus	Stylet Available	Radio-opaque	Brand
Large Bore								
18.0	rubber	40	X					Rob-Nell catheter (Argyle)
18.0	silicone rubber	90, 109		X		X	X	Keofeed (Hedeco)
14.6	silicone rubber	90, 109		X		X	X	Keofeed (Hedeco)
14.0	silicone rubber	105		X			X	Health Care Group (American Pharmaseal)
12.0	polyurethane	109		X		X	X	Entriflex (Biosearch)
Medium Bore								
10.0	silicone rubber	105		X	X	X	X	Health Care Group (American Pharmaseal)
	polyvinyl chloride	105	X				.	(Argyle)
9.6	silicone rubber	90, 109		X	X	X	X	Keofeed (Hedeco)
8.0	polyurethane	51, 76, 90, 109		X	X	X	X	Nutriflex, Entriflex, Dobbhoff (Biosearch)
	silicone rubber	38, 105	X	X	X	X	X	Health Care Group (American Pharmaseal)
	polyvinyl chloride	105	X					(Argyle)
	silicone rubber, polyvinyl chloride*	105		X		X	X	Duo-Tube (Argyle)
7.3	silicone rubber	75, 90, 105		X	X	X	X	Keofeed (Hedeco)
Small Bore								
6.0	silicone rubber	105		X	X	X	X	Health Care Group (American Pharmaseal)
5.0	silicone rubber	38	X			X	X	Health Care Group (American Pharmaseal)
	silicone rubber,	50		X		X		Keofeed (Hedeco)
	polyvinyl chloride	40, 90	X					(Argyle)

*polyvinyl chloride tube functions as stylet for Duo-Tube.

Source: Adapted from Hearne B, Daly JM: Enteral nutrition, in Kirkpatrick J (ed): *Nutrition and Metabolism in the Surgical Patient.* Kisco NY, Futura, 1983, with permission from the authors.

nasogastric feedings, jejunostomy tubes are preferred. Gastrostomy tubes may be inserted by the percutaneous endoscopic technique (PEG tubes) or by means of a surgical procedure under local, regional, or general anesthesia. Jejunostomy tubes are usually placed at the time of laparotomy, and the need for such a tube should be considered prior to any major abdominal operation. The recommended indications for placing a feeding jejunostomy are summarized in Table 42–4.[34]

There are four types of commercially available enteral formulas: blenderized tube-feeding formulas, nutritionally complete commercial formulas, chemically defined diets, and modular formulas. Blenderized formulas are composed of any food that can be proc-

TABLE 42–4. Recommended Indications for Placement of Feeding Jejunostomy

1. Patients who are malnourished at the time of laparotomy.
2. Patients who undergo major emergency or elective upper-abdominal procedures.
3. Patients who may receive adjuvant aggressive chemotherapy or radiation therapy after abdominal operation for cancer.
4. Patients who are multiply injured at the time of laparotomy.

Source: Adapted from Ryan JA, Page CP: Intrajejunal feeding: Development and current states. *JPEN* 8:187, 1984.

essed and often include meats, milk, vegetables, fruit, and cereal. Soy, safflower, or corn oil may be added to increase caloric density and supply essential fatty acids. Caloric concentrations vary from 0.6 to 1.3 kcal/ml, and caloric distribution is similar to that of a normal diet with 15% protein, 50% carbohydrate, and 35% fat. Nutritionally complete commercial formulas vary in their protein, carbohydrate, and fat content and provide approximately 1 kcal/ml. They are low in residue and lactose-free.

Chemically defined or elemental diets provide complete nutritional requirements in a predigested, easily absorbed form. They contain hydrolyzed protein or amino acids with enough carbohydrate and fat to provide a ratio of 150 nonprotein calories per gram of nitrogen. Fat provides a source of essential fatty acids, but medium-chain triglycerides that can be directly absorbed in the small bowel may be a source of additional calories. Modular formulas are used in patients who need special formulas or modifications of conventional enteral formulas. They consist of core modules of protein, carbohydrate, fat, vitamins, and minerals which can be combined to provide a specific nutritionally complete diet.[33]

Chemically defined or elemental diets are often used in the early postoperative period and in patients with small-bowel impairment. They are hyperosmolar and must be diluted to half strength and given at a slow rate of 40 ml/hr when feeding is initiated. The rate and concentration should be advanced slowly to allow the intestinal tract to adapt and to avoid bloating, cramping, and diarrhea (see Table 42–5). Fairfield-Smith et al. have shown that nonelemental isotonic diets are better tolerated than elemental diets in the postoperative period for most conditions except severe small-bowel impairment due to short-bowel syndrome and radiation enteritis. Most patients can be started on an isotonic nonelemental balanced liquid diet by continuous gravity drip or pump infusion. If intolerance develops, an elemental diet can be substituted.[35]

Parenteral Nutrition

Total parenteral nutrition is indicated in patients who are unable to tolerate gastrointestinal feeding or require rapid nutritional repletion because of severe malnutrition. Patients in the latter category have lost more than 12% of their body weight and have serum albumin levels of < 2.5 g/dl and serum transferrin levels of < 150 mg/dl.

A liter of TPN usually contains about 20% to 25% dextrose, 4% to 5% crystalline amino acids providing about 1000 nonprotein kcal, 6.5 to 8 g of nitrogen, electrolytes, vitamins, and minerals. Daily requirements of electrolytes include 60 to 120 meq of sodium, 60 to 100 meq of potassium, 60 to 120 meq of chloride, 8 to 10 meq of magnesium, 200 to 400 mg of calcium, and 300 to 400 mg of phosphorus. Preexisting fluid and electrolyte deficits must be corrected; ongoing urine and gastrointestinal losses must be replaced; and cardiac, hepatic, and renal dysfunction must be considered in the calculations. Vitamin and mineral requirements are listed in Table 42–2. In some hospitals, 1000 units of heparin are added to each liter of TPN to decrease the risk of catheter occlusion and subclavian vein thrombosis.

The best method to provide adults with long-term infusion of hypertonic TPN solutions is by means of an infraclavicular percutaneously inserted subclavian catheter. A chest x-ray must be obtained after insertion of the catheter and prior to infusion of the solution to verify the position of the catheter tip in the mid-portion of the superior vena cava. Silicone catheters cause the least intimal and thrombogenic reactivity. Double-lumen and triple-lumen catheters can be used when additional fluids or medications are needed.

It is vitally important to ensure careful aseptic catheter care. The dressing over the catheter insertion site should be changed every two to three days and the skin cleansed with acetone and treated with povidone-iodine ointment. Blood cultures should be drawn through the catheter and the catheter changed over a guide wire at the first sign of sepsis. The tip of the old catheter should also be cultured. A new catheter should be inserted at another site if the catheter tip and blood cultures are positive.

TPN solutions are initially infused at a slow rate of 40 ml/hr for the first day. Monitoring the urine for sugar and acetone ensures adequate metabolism of infused glucose. If the patient toler-

TABLE 42–5. Potential Complications of Enteral Nutritional Support

Complication	Prevention
Mechanical	
1. Regurgitation and aspiration	1. Elevate patient to 30° angle.
2. Tube or ostomy leak or malfunction	2. Use careful surgical technique and local care.
3. Erosion of external nares	3. Tape tube to prevent contact with nares.
4. Erosion of pharynx or esophagus	4. Use small diameter silicone rubber or polyurethane tubes.
5. Clogging of tube lumen	5. Irrigate before and after feeding with 50 ml tepid water; use appropriate bore tube with formula and mode of administration.
6. Otitis media	6. Use small-bore soft feeding tube.
Gastrointestinal	
1. Nausea, vomiting, or bloating	1. Reduce flow rate; increase time interval between intermittent feedings.
2. Diarrhea or cramping	2. Reduce flow rate; reduce formula concentration; select appropriate formula.
Metabolic	
1. Hyperglycemia and glycosuria, osmotic diuresis and hyperosmotic dehydration	1. Monitor urine for glucose and acetone; obtain blood glucose and serum electrolytes.
2. Edema	2. Monitor body weight, fluid, and salt requirements, and intake and output.
3. Prerenalazotemia	3. Monitor blood urea nitrogen and creatinine.

Source: Adapted from Hearne B, Daly JM: Enteral nutrition, in Kirkpatrick J (ed): *Nutrition and Metabolism in the Surgical Patient.* Kisco NY, Futura, 1983, with permission from the authors.

TABLE 42–6. Mechanical and Metabolic Complications of TPN

Mechanical
Pleural Space
Pneumothorax
Tension pneumothorax
Hemothorax
Hydrothorax (intrapleural infusion)
Mediastinum
Hemomediastinum
Hydromediastinum
Superior vena cava syndrome
Subcutaneous emphysema
Arterial injury (subclavian, carotid, cervical, and thoracic)
Hematoma
AV malformation
False aneurysm
Stenosis
Nerve injury (phrenic, vagus, recurrent laryngeal, brachial plexus)
Venous injury
Laceration with hemorrhage
Air embolism
Catheter embolism
Venobronchial fistula
Hepatic vein thrombosis
Superior vena cava thrombosis (pulmonary embolism)
Cardiac
Arrhythmia
Myocardial perforation (hydropericardium, tamponade)
Coronary sinus block (tamponade)
Catheter Sepsis

(Continued)

TABLE 42–6. Mechanical and Metabolic Complications of TPN (*Continued*)

Metabolic	
Complication	*Possible Etiology*
I. Carbohydrate metabolism	
A. Hyperglycemia	1. Excessive rate of glucose infusion 2. Insufficient endogenous insulin secretion 3. Sepsis 4. Glucocorticoids
B. Hyperosmolar nonketotic dehydration	1. Persistent hyperglycemia 2. Osmotic diuresis 3. Dehydration
C. Hypoglycemia	1. Abrupt interruption of TPN infusion 2. Excessive insulin
II. Amino acid metabolism	
A. Elevated BUN	1. Intrinsic renal disease 2. Dehydration 3. Excessive rate of infusion of amino acids 4. Low caloric nitrogen ratio of solution
B. Hyperammonemia	Intrinsic liver disease
III. Electrolyte and mineral metabolism	
A. Hypokalemia	Insufficient potassium intake relative to losses and anabolic requirements
B. Hypophosphatemia	Insufficient phosphate intake relative to losses and anabolic requirements
C. Hypomagnesemia	Insufficient magnesium intake relative to losses and anabolic requirements

Source: Adapted from Ryan JA: Complications of total parenteral nutrition, in Fisher JE: *Total Parenteral Nutrition.* Boston, Little Brown, 1976; and Reinhardt GF: *Surg Clin NA* 56:1283, 1977.

ates the infusion, the rate can be safely advanced to provide the calculated nutritional requirements in the second 24 hours. Patients who have elevated serum glucose levels above 200 mg/dl or significant glucosuria should receive crystalline insulin. It can be added to the solution in doses of 5 to 60 units to maintain the serum glucose level between 130 and 250 mg/dl. The infusion rate is usually tapered over 8 to 12 hours to 40 ml/hr before and during surgery. The rate can be advanced after the first postoperative day. Mechanical and metabolic complications of TPN are summarized in Table 42–6.

Peripheral Parenteral Nutrition

Parenteral solutions can be infused through peripheral veins if the osmolarity of the solution is 900 mOsm/liter or less.[36] To minimize the risk of phlebitis, butterfly needles should be used and changed every 48 hours.[37,38] Added heparin and hydrocortisone and use of inline filters also reduce the incidence of peripheral vein phlebitis.[39] Peripheral parenteral nutrition is generally used when central venous access is unavailable or as a supplement to oral or enteral feedings.

Nutritional Monitoring

Patients receiving enteral or parenteral nutritional support require careful monitoring of their vitals signs, urine fractional sugar and acetone levels, and fluid balances. Overall guidelines for nutritional monitoring are provided in detail in Table 42–7.

Home Parenteral Nutrition

Ambulatory patients unable to ingest and absorb enough calories to maintain lean body mass are candidates for home parenteral nutrition.[40] In the adult surgical population, these are patients with short-bowel syndromes due to extensive Crohn's disease, mesenteric infarction, or severe abdominal trauma. Home TPN is also indicated in patients with pseudoobstruction, radiation enteritis, carcinomatosis, necrotizing enterocolitis, and intestinal fistulae. In many, TPN will facilitate mucosal adaptation and growth, allowing eventual return to oral or enteral diets. Many patients, and particularly those with inflammatory bowel disease, experience weight gain, improvement in nutritional parameters, closing of enterocutaneous fistulae, resolution of gastrointestinal symptoms, and healing of inflammatory intestinal lesions.[41,42]

Those eligible for home TPN require extensive evaluation, teaching, and training during their hospitalization by a nutrition support team composed of a physician, psychiatrist, nurse, and pharmacist. The patient must have adequate intelligence, motivation, and family support. Instruction should cover basic nutritional principles, aseptic catheter care, and use of infusion pumps. Private home-care companies can coordinate management of home TPN and greatly simplify long-term care.

Candidates for home TPN require insertion of a long-term silastic catheter.[43] They are placed in the operating room under fluoroscopic guidance to ensure proper positioning of the tip at the junction of the superior vena cava and the right atrium. These catheters have a Dacron velour cuff just proximal to the skin exit site to allow for tissue growth and sealing of the subcutaneous catheter tract. TPN fluid can be infused over a period of 12 to 14 hours overnight to allow a more normal lifestyle. Daily electrolyte, minerals, and vitamin requirements are provided in the fluid, and fat infusions are used to reduce the carbohydrate load and provide essential fatty acids.

The complications of home parenteral nutrition are similar to those of hospitalized patients and include mechanical, infectious, metabolic, and psychosocial problems. Infectious complications proximal to the Dacron cuff usually respond well to antibiotics and local wound care. Infections of the intravascular portion of the catheter may require removal of the catheter if a trial of intravenous antibiotics effective against the cultured organism is unsuccessful. Metabolic complications due to nutritional deficiencies can be reduced by careful monitoring (see Table 42–6). Provision of vitamins and trace elements prevents unusual deficiency syndromes.[44,45] Although home TPN is costly because of the necessary patient training, equipment, supplies, and follow-up, it is approximately 50% to 70% less expensive than in-hospital care.[45]

TABLE 42–7. Guidelines for Nutritional Monitoring

Test	Initial	Stable Hospitalized Patient	Home Patient
Body weight	daily	daily	twice weekly
Output: urine	every 8 hours	daily	twice weekly
stool		daily	twice weekly
Urine glucose	every 6 hours	every 6 hours	twice weekly
Blood:			
Glucose	daily	every other day	weekly
Electrolytes	daily	every other day	monthly
BUN, creatinine	daily	weekly	monthly
Total protein, albumin, transferrin	weekly	weekly	monthly
Calcium, phoshorus	weekly	weekly	monthly
LDH, AST, Bilirubin Alkaline phosphatase	weekly	weekly	monthly
TIBC, iron	weekly	weekly	monthly
CBC, differential, prothrombin time	weekly	weekly	monthly
Triglycerides	weekly	monthly	monthly
Anthropometrics		monthly	monthly
Nitrogen balance	twice weekly	weekly	monthly

NUTRITION IN CARDIAC FAILURE

Patients with congestive heart failure who require nutritional support pose special problems. The term cardiac cachexia is used to describe patients with heart failure who suffer from protein-calorie malnutrition.[1] In the classic form, malnutrition develops as a consequence of longstanding failure. In the nosocomial type, patients with cardiac dysfunction are unable to ingest sufficient quantities of calories and protein after a surgical procedure. Contributing factors include anorexia, increased metabolic rate, and excessive loss of nutrients in the urine and stool.[46]

The goals of nutritional therapy are to stop weight loss other than necessary fluid loss, restore lean body mass, and provide adequate vitamins and minerals. As in all patients, the enteral route is preferred, but parenteral infusion can be used if necessary. Restriction of volume to 0.5 ml of water per kcal and sodium to 0.5 to 1.5 g/day is recommended.

Energy requirements are calculated from the Harris-Benedict equation. To the basal value, 15 to 25 percent is added for minimal physical activity, and 10 to 20 percent more is added for the hypermetabolism associated with severe congestive failure. Daily vitamins and minerals must be provided, and additional potassium, magnesium, and calcium are needed to replace diuretic-induced losses.[47] Nutritional repletion should be gradual to avoid volume overload.[48]

NUTRITION IN RENAL FAILURE

Renal failure in surgical patients is characterized by increased protein catabolism and inability to excrete protein breakdown products. This results in increased blood urea nitrogen levels with concurrent loss of body cell mass. Such patients are often unable to tolerate the nitrogen and volume loads of standard TPN unless they are undergoing hemodialysis or continuous arteriovenous hemofiltration.[49]

The exogenous protein provided by TPN contributes to underlying azotemia caused by underlying protein catabolism. Amino acids enter the metabolic pool from which new proteins are synthesized or are deaminated to produce urea. Protein catabolism can be reduced by providing adequate nonprotein calories. However, exogenous protein is needed to achieve positive nitrogen balance.

High-calorie, low-protein diets in patients with renal failure have been shown to result in improved nitrogen balance, weight gain, and reduction of blood urea nitrogen levels.[50,51] However, enteral nutrition is often not well tolerated in these patients due to their hypermetabolic state, underlying disease processes, and renal failure itself. Theoretically, providing high-quality protein or essential amino acids alone allows for utilization of available urea for production of nonessential amino acids. Dudrick et al. demonstrated the efficacy of parenteral administration of essential amino acids and hypertonic dextrose in patients with postoperative renal failure, and documented improvement in nitrogen balance, weight gain, and reduction in blood urea nitrogen levels.[52] Prospective randomized trials comparing essential amino acids with a balanced amino acid formula have yielded conflicting results.[53–56] Solutions containing both essential and nonessential amino acids are currently recommended with close monitoring of nitrogen balance and blood urea nitrogen levels. The formulation should provide approximately 1 g/kg/day of protein.

Daily caloric intake of 35 to 40 kcal/kg/day should be provided with 20% to 40% of the total energy content as fat. Sodium, potassium, phosphorus, magnesium, and calcium concentrations in the solution should be reduced initially, particularly if dialysis is unavailable. Recommended parameters for those on dialysis are 40 to 80 mmol/day of sodium, 20 to 40 mmol/day of potassium, 5 to

10 mmol/day of phosphorus, 2 to 4 mmol/day of magnesium, and 5 mmol/day of calcium. Frequent monitoring of serum electrolyte levels is essential.[57]

Nutritional therapy should be individualized in patients with renal failure because those with different levels of catabolism have different caloric requirements. The mortality rate in acute renal failure is increased in patients with negative caloric balance.[58] Therefore, the goal of therapy is to optimize the individual's nutritional condition to provide an opportunity for the kidneys to recover.

NUTRITION IN HEPATIC FAILURE

Hepatic failure causes numerous metabolic alterations. Changes in concentrations of neurotransmitter precursors and toxic metabolites lead to hepatic encephalopathy. Patients with encephalopathy have abnormally low levels of the branched-chain amino acids leucine, isoleucine, and valine, and high levels of the aromatic amino acids tyrosine, phenylalanine, free tryptophan, and methionine.[59] Morgan et al. compared levels of plasma leucine, isoleucine, and valine with those of phenylalanine and tyrosine and demonstrated a correlation between the ratio of the two groups of amino acids and the degree of liver disease.[60] Branched-chain amino acids are primarily metabolized in skeletal muscle, while aromatic amino acids are handled largely in the liver.

The transport of amino acids across the blood-brain barrier is regulated by amino acid concentrations in plasma. Several amino acids competitively share the same transport mechanisms. Increased concentrations of aromatic amino acids with corresponding lower levels of branched-chain amino acids allow for increased entry of aromatic amino acids into the brain.[61] Fischer and Baldessarini proposed that abnormal plasma amino acid concentrations may alter brain amino acid levels and change brain neurotransmitter levels to cause encephalopathy.[62] In addition, increased plasma levels of phenylalanine contribute to elevated levels of brain tyrosine. Accumulation of phenylalanine and tyrosine in the brain leads to elevated levels of betahydroxylated phenylethylamines including octopamine. Elevated urinary and plasma octopamine levels have been demonstrated in patients with hepatic encephalopathy.[63]

Critically ill patients with acute hepatic encephalopathy are often malnourished and require nutritional support. In patients with alcoholic cirrhosis, parenteral nutritional support has been shown to hasten clinical improvement, decrease serum bilirubin levels, and improve nutritional parameters. However, it does not change long-term morbidity and mortality.[64,65] Animal studies have demonstrated that solutions with high concentrations of branched-chain amino acids reduce the proportion of methionine and aromatic amino acids in experimentally produced encephalopathy. This results in amelioration of the encephalopathy and normalization of relative plasma amino acid levels.[66] Controlled clinical studies in patients comparing solutions enriched in branched-chain amino acids with standard therapy demonstrate improvement in encephalopathy and nutritional status in those receiving the former.[67-69] Other studies show that similar results can be obtained using such formulas either enterally or parenterally.[69-71]

Therefore, nutritional support is indicated in patients with hepatic failure and should be given enterally if possible. If given parenterally, meticulous catheter care is crucial in view of the increased risk of sepsis. Exogenous calories and nitrogen should be provided with a formula high in branched-chain and low in aromatic amino acids.

SUMMARY

1. Nutritional support decreases perioperative morbidity and mortality. Its goal is to provide exogenous calories, protein, vitamins, and minerals to preserve body cell mass and organ function.

2. Elective procedures should be postponed until nutritional status has been improved.

3. Enteral nutritional support is preferable in patients with functional gastrointestinal tract. If patients cannot take supplement orally, enteral support can be provided through a small-bore nasogastric tube for short periods of time or by way of a gastrostomy or jejunostomy for longer periods. Blenderized tube-feeding, nutritionally complete, chemically defined, or modular formulas can be used.

4. Total parenteral nutrition is indicated in patients unable to tolerate gastrointestinal feeding or in those who require rapid nutritional repletion because of severe malnutrition. TPN is best administered through a central venous catheter.

5. Patients receiving enteral or parenteral nutritional support in the hospital or at home require careful monitoring of nutritional parameters, as outlined in Table 42–7.

6. In patients with congestive heart failure, nutritional repletion should be gradual to avoid volume overload. Solutions often contain additional potassium, magnesium, and calcium to replace diuretic-induced losses. In those with renal failure, solutions containing both essential and nonessential amino acids are needed to achieve positive nitrogen balance with enough nonprotein calories to reduce protein catabolism. Solutions containing branched-chain amino acids improve encephalopathy as well as nutritional status in patients with hepatic failure.

REFERENCES

1. Hill GL, Blacket RL, Pickford I et al: Malnutrition in surgical patients. An unrecognized problem. *Lancet* 1:689–692, 1977.
2. Bistrian BR, Blackburn GL, Hallowell E et al: Protein status of general surgical patients. *JAMA* 230(6):858–860, 1974.
3. Studley HO: Percentage of weight loss: Basic indicator of surgical risk in patients with chronic peptic ulcer. *JAMA* 106:458–460, 1936.
4. Rhoads JE, Alexander CE: Nutritional problems of surgical patients. *Ann NY Acad Sci* 63:268–275, 1955.
5. Kaminski MV, Fitzgerald MJ, Murphy RJ et al: Correlation of mortality with serum transferrin and anergy. *JPEN* 1:27, 1977.
6. Mullen JL, Gertner MH et al: Implications of malnutrition in the surgical patient. *Arch Surg* 114:121–125, 1979.
7. Cahill GF: Starvation in man. *NEJM* 282:668–675, 1970.
8. Stein TP, Buzby GP: Protein metabolism in surgical patients. *Surg Cli N Am* 61(3):519–527, 1981.
9. Shizgal HM: Nutritional assessment with body composition measurements. *JPEN* 11(5):425–475, 1987.

10. Williams RH, Heatley RV, Lewis MH: A randomized, controlled trial of preoperative intravenous nutrition in patients with stomach cancer. *Br J Surg* 63:667, 1976.

11. Holter AR, Fischer JE: The effects of perioperative hyperalimentation on complications in patients with carcinoma and weight loss. *J Surg Res* 23:31–34, 1977.

12. Buzby GP, Foster J, Rosato EF: Transferrin dynamics in total parenteral nutrition. *JPEN* 3:34, 1979.

13. Church JM, Hill GL: Assessing the efficacy of intravenous nutrition in general surgical patients: Dynamic nutritional assessment with plasma proteins. *JPEN* 11(2):135–139, 1987.

14. Jeevanandum M, Legaspi A, Lowry SF et al: Effect of total parenteral nutrition on whole body protein kinetics in cachectic patients with benign or malignant disease. *JPEN* 12(3):229–236, 1988.

15. Mullen JL, Buzby GP, Matthews DC et al: Reduction of operative morbidity and mortality by combined preoperative and postoperative nutritional support. *Ann Surg* 192(5):604–613, 1980.

16. Daly JM, Massas E, Giacco G et al: Parenteral nutrition in esophageal cancer patients. *Ann Surg* 196(2):203–208, 1982.

17. Riboli EB, Bertoglio S, Arnulfo G et al: Treatment of esophageal anastomotic leakages after cancer resection. The role of total parenteral nutrition. *JPEN* 10(1):82–84, 1986.

18. Heatley RV, Williams RHP, Lewis MH: Preoperative intravenous feeding—a controlled trial. *Postgrad Med J* 55:541–545, 1979.

19. Thompson BR, Julian TB, Stremple JF: Perioperative total parenteral nutrition in patients with gastrointestinal cancer. *J Surg Res* 30:487–500, 1981.

20. Muller JM, Dienst C, Brenner U et al: Preoperative parenteral feeding in patients with gastrointestinal carcinoma. *Lancet* 1:68–71, 1982.

21. Foschi D, Cavagna G, Callion F et al: Hyperalimentation of jaundiced patients on percutaneous transhepatic biliary drainage. *Br J Surg* 73(9):716–719, 1986.

22. Bellantone R, Giovan Baltista D et al: Preoperative parenteral nutrition of malnourished surgical patients. *Acta Chir Scand* 22:249–251, 1988.

23. Smith RC, Burkinshaw L, Hill GL: Optimal energy and nitrogen intake for gastroenterological patients requiring intravenous nutrition. *Gastroenterology* 82:445–452, 1982.

24. Talikoura J: Maintenance of visceral protein levels in serum during postoperative parenteral nutrition. *JPEN* 2(6):597–601, 1988.

25. Benotti P, Blackburn GL: Protein and caloric or macronutrient metabolic management of the critically ill patients. *Crit Care Med* 7(12):520–525, 1979.

26. Wolfe KS, O'Donnell JI, Stone MD et al: Investigation of factors determining the optimal glucose infusion rate in total parenteral nutrition. *Metabolism* 29:892, 1980.

27. Muggia-Sullam M, Bower RH, Murphy RF et al: Postoperative enteral versus parenteral nutritional support in gastrointestinal surgery. A matched, prospective study. *Am J Surg* 149:106–112, 1985.

28. Fletcher JP, Little JM: A comparison of parenteral nutrition and early postoperative enteral feeding on the nitrogen balance after major surgery. *Surgery* 100(1):21–24, 1986.

29. Bower RH, Talamini MA, Sax HC et al: Postoperative enteral versus parenteral nutrition. A randomized, controlled trial. *Arch Surg* 121(9):1040–1045, 1986.

30. Paterson VM, Moore EE, Jones TN et al: Total enteral nutrition versus total parenteral nutrition after major torso injury: Attenuation of hepatic protein reprioritization. *Surgery* 104(2):199–207, 1988.

31. Alverdy JC, Aoys E, Moss GS: Total parenteral nutrition promotes bacterial translocation from the gut. *Surgery* 104(2):185–190, 1988.

32. Mochizuki H, Trocki O, Dominion L et al: Mechanism of prevention of postburn hypermetabolism and catabolism by early enteral feeding. *Ann Surg* 200(3):297–310, 1984.

33. Hearne B, Daly JM: Enteral nutrition, in Kirkpatrick J (ed): *Nutrition and Metabolism in the Surgical Patient*. Mt. Kisco NY, Futura Publishing, 1983.

34. Ryan Jr JA, Page CP: Intrajejunal feeding: Development and current states. *JPEN* 8:187, 1984.

35. Fairfield-Smith R, Abenassar R, Freeman JB et al: Rational use of elemental and non-elemental diets in hospitalized patients. *Ann Surg* 192(5):600–603, 1980.

36. Isaacs JW, Millilcon WJ, Stackhouse J et al: Parenteral nutrition of adults with a 900 milliosmolar solution via peripheral veins. *Am J Clin Nutr* 30:552–559, 1977.

37. Daly JM, Masser E, Hansen L et al: Peripheral vein infusion of dextrose l-amino acid solution + 2.0% fat emulsion. *JPEN* 9(3):296–299, 1985.

38. Masser E, Daly JM, Copeland EM et al: Peripheral vein complications in patients receiving amino acid/dextrose solutions. *JPEN* 7:159–162, 1983.

39. Bivens BA, Rapp RP, DeLuca PP et al: Final inline filtration: A means of decreasing the incidence of infusion phlebitis. *Surgery* 85:388–394, 1979.

40. Grundfest S, Steiger E: Home parenteral nutrition. *JAMA* 244:1701–1703, 1980.

41. Stokes MA, Irving MH: How do patients with Crohn's disease fare on home parenteral nutrition? *Dis Colon Rectum* 31(6):454–458, 1988.

42. Kushner RF, Shapir J, Sitrin MD: Endoscopic radiographic and clinical response to prolonged bowel rest and home parenteral nutrition in Crohn's disease. *JPEN* 10(6):568–573, 1988.

43. Broviac JW, Scribner BH: Prolonged parenteral nutrition in the home. *Surg Gyn Ob* 139:24–28, 1974.

44. Davis AT, Franz FP, Courtney DA et al: Plasma vitamins and mineral status in home parenteral nutrition patients. *JPEN* 11(5):480–485, 1987.

45. Gouttebel MC, Saint-Aubert B, Jonquet D et al: Ambulatory home parenteral nutrition. *JPEN* 11(5):475–479, 1987.

46. Quinn T, Askanaz J: Nutrition and cardiac disease. *Crit Care Clin* 3(1):167–184, 1987.

47. Heymsfield SB, Smith I, Redd S et al: Nutritional support in cardiac failure. *Surg Clin N Am* 61:635–652, 1981.

48. Weinsier RL, Krumdieck CL: Death resulting from overzealous total parenteral nutrition: The refeeding syndrome revisited. *Am J Clin Nutr* 34:393–399, 1981.

49. Feinstein EI: Nutrition in renal failure. *Adv Exp Biol* 212:297–301, 1987.

50. Giordano C: Use of exogenous and endogenous urea for protein synthesis in normal and uremic subjects. *J Lab Clin Med* 62:231–246, 1963.

51. Giovannetti S, Maggiore Q: A low nitrogen diet with proteins of high biologic value for severe chronic uremia. *Lancet* 1:1000–1003, 1964.

52. Dudrick SJ, Steiger E, Long JM: Renal failure in surgical patients. Treatment with intravenous essential amino acids and hypertonic glucose. *Surgery* 68:180–186, 1970.

53. Abel RM, Beck CH, Abbott WM et al: Improved survival from acute renal failure after treatment with intravenous essential l-amino acids and glucose. *NEJM* 288:695–699, 1973.

54. Freund H, Atamian S, Fischer JE: Comparative study of parenteral nutrition in renal failure using essential and nonessential amino acid–containing solutions. *Surg Gyn Ob* 151:652–656, 1980.

55. Leonard CD, Luke RG, Sieger RR: Parenteral essential amino acids in acute renal failure. *Urology* 6:154–157, 1975.

56. Feinstein EI, Blumenkrantz MJ, Healy M et al: Clinical and metabolic responses to parenteral nutrition in acute renal failure. *Medicine* 60:124–127, 1981.

57. Takula J: Nutrition in acute renal failure. *Crit Care Clin* 3(1):155–166, 1987.

58. Feinstein EI: Parenteral nutrition in acute renal failure. *Am J Nephrol* 5(3):145–149, 1985.

59. Fischer JE, Fanovics JM, Aguirre A et al: The role of plasma amino acids in hepatic encephalopathy. *Surgery* 78:276–290, 1975.

60. Morgan MY, Milson JP, Sherlock S: Plasma ratio of valine, leucine and isoleucine to phenylalanine and tyrosine in liver disease. *Gut* 19:1068–1073, 1978.

61. Oldendorf WH, Szabo J: Amino acid assignment to one of three blood-brain barrier amino acid carriers. *Am J Physiol* 230:94–98, 1976.

62. Fischer JE, Baldessarini RS: False neurotransmitters and hepatic failure. *Lancet* 2:75–79, 1971.

63. Monghani KK, Lanzer MR, Billing BH et al: Urinary and serum octopamine in patients with portal systemic encephalopathy. *Lancet* 2:943–946, 1975.

64. Naveau S, Pelletier G, Poynard T et al: A randomized clinical trial of supplementary parenteral nutrition in jaundiced alcoholic cirrhotic patients. *Hepatology* 6(2):270–274, 1986.

65. Diehl AM, Boitnott JM: Effect of parenteral amino acid supplementation in alcoholic hepatitis. *Hepatology* 5:57–63, 1985.

66. Rosen HM, Soeters PB, James JH et al: Influences of exogenous intake and nitrogen balance on plasma and brain amino acid concentrations. *Metabolism* 27:393–404, 1978.

67. Rossi-Fanelli F, Riggio O, Cangiano C et al: Branched-chain amino acids versus lactulose in the treatment of hepatic coma. *Dig Dis a Sci* 27:929–935, 1982.

68. Cerra FB, McMillan M, Angelico R et al: Cirrhosis, encephalopat and improved results with metabolic support. *Surgery* 94:612–61 1983.

69. Horst D, Grace ND, Conn HO et al: Comparison of dietary prote with an oral, branched-chain–enriched amino acid supplement chronic portal-systemic encephalopathy: A randomized, controlled tri *Hepatology* 4:279–287, 1984.

70. Millikan WJ, Henderson JM, Warren WD et al: Total parenteral nut tion with FO80 in cirrhotics with subclinical encephalopathy. *Ann Su 197:294–303, 1983.

71. O'Keefe SJD, Ogden J, Dicker J: Enteral and parenteral branche chain amino acid–supplemented nutritional support in patients wi encephalopathy due to alcoholic liver disease. *JPEN* 11(5):447–45 1987.

72. Redmond HP, Daly JM: Preoperative nutritional therapy in cancer p tients is beneficial, in Simmons, R (ed): *Debates in Clinical Surger vol 2. St. Louis, Mosby Year Book, 1990, pp 45–56.

43 PREVENTION OF BACTERIAL ENDOCARDITIS

Frank H. Brown

Whether or not to use prophylactic antibiotics to prevent bacterial endocarditis is one of the most common reasons for preoperative consultation. The consulting internist is frequently asked to evaluate a patient with a heart murmur, to decide if endocarditis prophylaxis is warranted, and to recommend an appropriate drug regimen. However, several surveys indicate that considerable confusion exists among clinicians concerning the proper use of antibiotics for this purpose. This chapter critically examines the scientific basis for endocarditis prophylaxis and reviews details of the latest recommendations.

RATIONALE FOR ENDOCARDITIS PROPHYLAXIS

Endocarditis remains a serious illness with a mortality rate of 14 to 46 percent even when treated.[1] The complications of the disease can be catastrophic, and, even after successful treatment, long-term sequelae can cause significant morbidity and shorten survival. Although recommendations for chemoprophylaxis have been developed in an attempt to prevent as many cases of endocarditis as possible, theoretical and clinical data suggest that only about 10 percent of cases are potentially preventable.[2,3]

The rationale for chemoprophylaxis rests on an understanding of the pathogenesis of endocarditis. Bacteremia is necessary for the development of endocarditis. Transient bacteremia with organisms capable of producing endocarditis in susceptible patients predictably occurs during the course of several diagnostic and therapeutic procedures. Appropriate antibiotics administered before the procedure may confer protection through a number of mechanisms. Experimental studies have shown that prophylactic antibiotics decrease the frequency and magnitude of bacteremia, impair bacterial adherence to damaged valvular epithelium, and inhibit the growth of bacteria lodged on heart valves.[4]

Although the rationale for chemoprophylaxis is clear, there is no definitive clinical documentation of its efficacy in preventing endocarditis in humans. The only direct comparison between susceptible patients who received prophylaxis and those who did not was reported by Taran in 1944.[5] He noted that 4 of 350 children with rheumatic heart disease who did not receive antibiotics died of endocarditis following dental extractions, while none of 220 children receiving sulfa prophylaxis developed the disease. The study was not randomized, used historical controls, lacked statistical analysis, and provides no information about the effectiveness of prophylaxis as currently practiced.

Indirect evidence that prophylaxis is effective is based on three observations. First, the administration of antibiotics before a dental procedure significantly decreases the incidence of positive blood cultures thereafter.[6-9] Second, there are relatively few reports of prophylaxis failures, and, when such reports are examined, it is clear that few used adequate prophylaxis as defined by current standards.[10] Finally, antibiotic prophylaxis has been shown to be effective in the animal model of endocarditis initially developed by Garrison and Freedman.[11] In this model, a polyethylene catheter is passed across the tricuspid or aortic valve, traumatizing the endocardium and allowing thrombus to form at the site of contact. Injected viable bacteria localize in the thrombus and multiply, leading to the formation of the typical vegetations of infective endocarditis. Various prophylactic regimens have been shown to prevent endocarditis in this experimental model.

Despite the indirect evidence that endocarditis prophylaxis may be effective, there are still questions regarding its value for the individual patient and as health care policy. Transient bacteremia is ubiquitous, occurring frequently after activities like brushing teeth or chewing candy (see Table 43–1).[12] Given the frequency of bacteremia and the relatively low incidence of endocarditis, development of endocardial infection after transient bacteremia must be exceedingly uncommon.

The only direct estimates of the risk of developing endocarditis after a procedure likely to induce bacteremia come from two studies performed before antibiotics were developed, and both suggest a relatively low risk. As noted above, Taran documented endocarditis in only 1.1 percent of unprotected children with rheumatic heart disease after dental extractions.[5] In 1942, Schwartz and

TABLE 43–1. Incidence of Bacteremia with Common Procedures.

Procedure	Incidence (%)
Dental and Upper Respiratory Tract	
Dental extraction	18–92
Tooth cleaning	0–40
Tooth brushing	0–40
Oral irrigation	7–50
Chewing of hard candy or gum	0–22
Tonsillectomy	20–38
Nasotracheal intubation	0–30
Orotracheal intubation	0–3
Rigid bronchoscopy	16
Fiberoptic bronchoscopy	0
Nasotracheal suctioning	16
Gastrointestinal	
Percutaneous liver biopsy	3–14
Peritoneoscopy	0
Rectal exam	0–4
Urologic	
Urethral catheterization	8
Catheter removal	2–30
Urethral dilation	10–33
Transurethral prostatic resection	32–46
sterile urine	11
infected urine	58
Retropubic prostatectomy	68
sterile urine	13
infected urine	82
Cystoscopy	0–22
Transrectal prostate biopsy	76
Percutaneous shock wave lithotripsy	0–14
Obstetric-Gynecologic	
Vaginal delivery	0–5
Punch biopsy of cervix	0
Intrauterine device	0–6
Suction abortion	85
Surgical	
Burn surgery	21–46
Abscess drainage	25–54
Appendectomy	21
Cholecystectomy	17
Hemorrhoidectomy	8
Miscellaneous	
Peritoneal dialysis	2–4
Hemodialysis	2–8
Cardiac catheterization	0
Angiography	0
Transesophageal echocardiography	0–17

Salman studied 98 patients with rheumatic heart disease undergoing a total of 403 extractions and found no cases of endocarditis.[13] Other estimates of risk in susceptible patients range from 1 in 10 to fewer than 1 in 100,000.[14,15] These numbers approximate the risk of a serious adverse reaction to prophylactic antibiotics. Therefore, large numbers of potentially susceptible patients must be subjected to the risk, expense, and inconvenience of prophylactic therapy to prevent a single case of endocarditis. Since the risk-benefit and cost-benefit ratios may not be favorable, the practice of administering antibiotics to prevent endocarditis remains controversial, with recommendations ranging from no antibiotics for any patient to universal prophylaxis.[16]

A randomized controlled trial would be helpful in resolving the controversy. However, Durack calculated that 10,000 patients with valvular heart disease would be required to demonstrate statistical significance if the risk of developing endocarditis were 1 in 500 and prophylaxis were 90% effective.[17] Furthermore, current ethical standards would probably preclude withholding prophylaxis from a control group. More recently, two groups of investigators have attempted to resolve the issue using case-control methods but presented disparate results. One group found the protective efficacy of antibiotics to be 91%, while the other found prophylaxis to be only 49% effective.[18,19] The American Heart Association (AHA) and the British Society for Antimicrobial Chemotherapy (BSAC) have attempted to approach the problem from another perspective by establishing formal registries of prophylaxis failures. It is hoped that these data will provide further information about the effectiveness of current regimens.

Although the issues surrounding the use of antibiotics to prevent endocarditis are not resolved, the weight of the evidence continues to support prophylaxis. The clinician is therefore faced with three basic questions in patient management: (1) For which types of heart disease should prophylactic antibiotics be administered? (2) For which procedures should they be given? (3) What drug regimens should be employed?

HEART DISEASE REQUIRING PROPHYLAXIS

There is no uniformity of opinion about which cardiac lesions make a patient sufficiently susceptible to endocarditis to require antibiotic prophylaxis. Evidence of relative susceptibility is derived from the incidence of endocarditis in patients with given lesions, the prevalence of different lesions in series of patients with endocarditis, and experimental studies of the hemodynamic characteristics of lesions susceptible to endocarditis. Most of the information comes from Rodbard's demonstration that susceptible valvular lesions are generally characterized by a high-pressure source forcing blood through a narrow orifice into a low-pressure sink, producing jet and Venturi effects that determine the distribution of vegetations.[20] These studies help explain the greater susceptibility of left-sided rather than right-sided valves, small rather than large ventricular septal defects, regurgitant lesions, and arteriovenous fistulas, and the rarity of endocarditis in uncomplicated atrial septal defects. The most common cardiovascular lesions can be divided into three categories of relative risk (see Table 43–2).[2] Several of these lesions are of sufficient interest or have provoked sufficient controversy to warrant specific mention.

Mitral Valve Prolapse

Shortly after Barlow predicted that patients with mitral valve prolapse (MVP) might be at increased risk of endocarditis,[22] case reports and small case series linking the two began to appear.[23–2] Subsequently, longitudinal evaluations of patients with mitral valve prolapse report an incidence of endocarditis ranging from 0 to 8 percent,[26–30] and surveys of patients with endocarditis found a prevalence of MVP of 12 to 29 percent.[31] Case-control studies allow a more precise estimate of the relative risk and consistently show that patients with MVP have approximately a fivefold greater risk of developing endocarditis than those in the general popula-

TABLE 43–2. Relative Risks of Cardiac Lesions

High-Risk Cardiac Lesions
 Prosthetic heart valve including bioprosthetic and homograft valves
 Valves previously affected by infective endocarditis even in the
    absence of valvular dysfunction
 Surgically created systemic–pulmonary artery shunts

Moderate-Risk Cardiac Lesions
 Congenital heart disease
    Ventricular septal defect
    Patent ductus arteriosus
    Tetralogy of Fallot
    Pulmonic stenosis
    Coarctation of the aorta
    Bicuspid aortic valve
 Rheumatic valvular disease
 Other acquired valvular heart including degenerative valve disease
 Mitral valve prolapse with risk factor(s)
 Hypertrophic cardiomyopathy
 Nonvalvular intracardiac prosthetic implants
 Indwelling intraatrial or transvalvular catheters
 Hemodialysis shunts

Low- or Negligible-Risk Cardiac Lesions
 Uncomplicated ostium secundum ASD
 Previous coronary bypass grafting
 Patent ductus arteriosus six months after closure
 ASD or VSD six months after surgical repair without residua
 Physiologic, functional, or innocent heart murmurs
 Syphilitic aortitis without aortic insufficiency
 Mitral valve prolapse without risk factors
 History of rheumatic fever without valvular dysfunction
 Permanent cardiac pacemaker
 Automatic implantable cardioverter-defibrillator

Source: Modified from the American Heart Association.[21]

tion.[32–37] However, given the low incidence of endocarditis, the absolute risk of a patient with mitral valve prolapse developing endocarditis remains quite small at approximately 1 in 7000 per year.[33]

Because the absolute risk is low and the prevalence of MVP is relatively high, questions remain about the cost-benefit and risk-benefit ratios if all patients with MVP receive prophylactic antibiotics. Two quantitative studies examining this strategy find that prophylaxis with parenteral penicillin results in a net loss of life and that prophylaxis with oral regimens is very costly.[38,39] More recent studies have attempted to identify subsets of patients with MVP with the greatest risk of endocarditis to allow more selective administration of antibiotics and decrease the costs and risks of prophylaxis. Of the risk factors summarized in Table 43–3, a preexisting systolic murmur appears to be most important. Several case-control studies have shown that patients with MVP and a systolic murmur have a relative risk of endocarditis 4 to 15 times

TABLE 43–3. Mitral Valve Prolapse

Risk Factors for Endocarditis

Clinical
 Systolic murmur
 Male gender
 Age > 45 years

Echocardiographic
 Leaflet thickening
 Leaflet redundancy
 Moderate or severe mitral regurgitation

higher than such patients without a murmur.[32–37] In fact, patients with mitral valve prolapse but no systolic murmur appear to have no greater risk of endocarditis than the general population. Patients with holosystolic murmurs may have the highest risk.

Approximately two-thirds of patients with MVP and endocarditis are men, even though mitral valve prolapse is more prevalent among women. The risk of endocarditis in men with MVP is therefore two to three times greater.[32,34,36] Likewise, two-thirds of cases of endocarditis occur in patients with MVP over the age of 45 who have a fourfold risk when compared to younger patients.[36] Significant mitral regurgitation occurs more often in men and older patients with MVP and may account for the increased risk of endocarditis in these groups. Two studies have also demonstrated the association of thickening or redundancy of the mitral leaflets on echocardiography with the risk of endocarditis.[40,41] The finding of moderate-to-severe mitral regurgitation on doppler echocardiography has also been suggested as grounds for prophylactic antibiotics.[42]

In summary, some patients with MVP have an increased risk of developing endocarditis. The absolute risk of endocarditis remains quite small, and most of the risk is confined to those with certain risk factors. Prophylactic antibiotics should be given only to patients with one or more of these clinical features and oral regimens should be used when possible. Prophylaxis is not required in patients with an isolated systolic click or "silent" prolapse.

Degenerative Valvular Disease

Degenerative valvular disease has become increasingly important as the elderly population increases in size and older patients undergo more invasive procedures. It accounts for as much as 25 percent of cardiac lesions predisposing to endocarditis in some series and as much as 50 percent in patients over 60.[43] Mortality rates of elderly patients with endocarditis can be as high as 70 percent.[44]

An aggressive approach to prophylaxis was proposed by Lichtman and Master, who noted anatomic evidence of valvular disease in more than half of autopsies on patients over 50.[45] Because clinical evidence of valvular disease was frequently absent, the investigators suggested consideration of routine prophylaxis for all patients over 50. Although this is obviously impractical and unwarranted, clinical evidence of degenerative valve disease should be carefully sought in elderly patients, and, when it is found, prophylaxis should be administered.

Other Clinical Situations

Underlying hypertrophic cardiomyopathy has been found in 5 percent of cases of endocarditis,[31] and endocarditis has occurred as a complication in 5 to 9 percent in some series of patients with hypertrophic cardiomyopathy.[46] The risk approximates that of valvular aortic stenosis, and prophylaxis is therefore warranted.

Patients successfully treated for an initial episode of endocarditis have an 8 to 17 percent chance of suffering a second episode, and 25 percent of those will experience a third.[47,48] Therefore, all patients who have recovered from endocarditis should receive prophylactic antibiotics even if there is no evidence of residual valvular disease on physical examination.

Rheumatic heart disease clearly warrants prophylaxis. However, a history of rheumatic fever without clinical evidence of valvular heart disease is not an indication for prophylaxis. Studies in patients with lupus erythematosus have shown an increased prevalence of clinically significant valvular disease[49] and an increased incidence of endocarditis.[50] These observations have led some to recommend antibiotic prophylaxis in these patients.[50,51]

A higher-than-normal incidence of bacterial endocarditis has been reported in patients with arteriovenous (AV) fistulas for hemodialysis.[52,53] Dogs with experimental AV fistulas have a high incidence of spontaneous infective endocarditis, and only a small inoculum of bacteria is required to produce endocarditis.[54,55] Because of this, Kaye has recommended that prophylactic antibiotic be given to patients with AV fistulas even if they do not have valvular heart disease.[56]

Indwelling transvalvular devices such as Swan-Ganz catheters or pacing wires have the potential to induce nonbacterial thrombotic endocarditis that can become infected in the course of bacteremia. However, the risk in patients with permanent pacemakers and implantable defibrillators is so low that prophylaxis is not recommended.[21]

Other indwelling intravascular devices such as central venous pressure lines, Hickman or catheters, LeVeen shunts, or ventriculoatrial shunts can induce right-heart lesions or become infected during the course of bacteremia. However, no quantitative estimates of risk exist, and no firm recommendations about prophylaxis can be made.

The risk of late infection in a properly functioning prosthetic valve is approximately 0.4 to 1.1 percent per year.[57] This is comparable to the risk in patients with chronic rheumatic heart disease.[58] However, the complication and mortality rates of prosthetic valve endocarditis are much higher than those of native valve endocarditis, and result in shortened survival.[59] Patients with prosthetic valves should be therefore regarded as having a high risk of infection and should definitely receive prophylaxis.

PROCEDURES REQUIRING PROPHYLAXIS

The need to administer prophylactic antibiotics before a given procedure is proportional to the risk of developing endocarditis thereafter. It is impossible to quantitate the risk of a specific procedure directly. It can only be inferred from published reports of endocarditis following and presumably caused by the procedure, and from what is known about bacteremia and its microbiology.

The incidence of bacteremia following various procedures has been reported by numerous investigators and is summarized in Table 43–1. The wide variation in some of the numbers reflects considerable differences in the timing and number of cultures drawn and the sophistication of microbiologic techniques employed in different studies. The magnitude and duration of bacteremia are important determinants in animal models, in which the occurrence of endocarditis is proportional to the size of the inoculum. In addition, measures that decrease the clearance of organisms and prolong the duration of bacteremia increase the incidence of endocarditis. In most studies of patients undergoing diagnostic or therapeutic procedures, bacteremia is short-lived and involves a relatively small inoculum.

Although anaerobes and gram-negative bacilli most frequently cause bacteremia in humans, they seldom cause endocarditis in

TABLE 43–4. Relative Risks of Common Procedures

Procedures Requiring Endocarditis Prophylaxis for All Susceptible Patients
 Oral cavity and respiratory tract
  All dental procedures likely to induce gingival or mucosal bleeding, including professional cleaning
  Tonsillectomy or adenoidectomy
  Surgical procedures or biopsy involving oral or respiratory mucosa
  Bronchoscopy with a rigid bronchoscope
  Incision and drainage of infected tissue
 Genitourinary and gastrointestinal tracts
  Esophageal dilatation
  Sclerotherapy for esophageal varices
  Gallbladder surgery
  Surgical operations involving intestinal mucosa
  Urethral catheterization in the presence of infections
  Cystoscopy
  Prostatic surgery
  Urinary tract surgery
  Vaginal hysterectomy
  Vaginal delivery in the presence of infection
  Incision and drainage of infected tissue
 Skin
  Incision and drainage of infected tissue

Procedures Requiring Prophylaxis Only for High-Risk Patients
 Nasotracheal intubation
 Endodontic procedures
 Transesophageal echocardiography
 Upper endoscopy
 Endoscopic laser therapy
 Endoscopic retrograde cholangiopancreatography
 Percutaneous endoscopic gastrostomy
 Proctosigmoidoscopy
 Colonoscopy
 Hemorrhoidal sclerotherapy
 Barium enema
 Percutaneous liver biopsy
 Brief urethral catheterization
 Extracorporeal shock wave lithotripsy
 Uncomplicated vaginal delivery
 Uterine dilatations and curettage
 Cesarean section
 Therapeutic abortion
 Sterilization procedures
 Insertion/removal of intrauterine device

Procedures Not Requiring Prophylaxis
 Angiography
 Cardiac catheterization
 Orotracheal intubation
 Adjustment of orthodontic appliances
 Shedding of primary teeth
 Tympanoplasty tube
 Flexible bronchoscopy

Source: Modified from the American Heart Association.[21]

naturally diseased valves. Gram-positive cocci and particularly streptococci have an unusual predilection for attacking these valves and account for most cases of the disease. This clinical observation has been corroborated by both in vivo and in vitro experimental data. In the animal model, a much larger inoculum of gram-negative than gram-positive bacteria is required to produce infection.[60] Using human and canine aortic valve tissue, Gould et al. demonstrated that streptococci, enterococci, and staphylococci are more adherent than most gram-negative bacilli.[61] They also showed that the adherence ratio for each strain remained constant with different concentrations of bacteria and concluded that the number of bacteria adhering to a valve is related to the duration and magnitude of bacteremia as well as to adherence.

Although no definitive statement can be made about which procedures require prophylaxis, the relative risk of a susceptible patient developing endocarditis can be inferred from reports of cases attributed to a given procedure and knowledge of the incidence, type, duration, and magnitude of bacteremia following the procedure. Based on these considerations, common procedures can be divided into three broad categories of risk (see Table 43–4). Several procedures merit specific discussion because the use of prophylaxis remains controversial, the recommendation is unclear or has recently been changed, or the situations are not specifically addressed by the guidelines published by the American Heart Association (AHA).

Gastrointestinal Procedures

The AHA previously recommended that all high-risk patients receive parenteral prophylactic antibiotics before all endoscopic procedures and barium enemas. It also recommended prophylaxis for all patients with native valvular disease prior to upper endoscopy or proctosigmoidoscopy if biopsies were performed as well as for those undergoing colonoscopy, esophageal dilatation, and sclerotherapy of esophageal varices.[62] Although most clinicians accepted the recommendations for high-risk patients, those for prophylaxis in other patients remained controversial for several reasons.[63,64] First, the risk of bacteremia following most of these procedures is low (see Table 43–5), and many of the organisms isolated from those with positive blood cultures do not usually cause endocarditis. Second, there have been very few adequately documented cases of endocarditis attributable to endoscopic procedures. Since these procedures are so frequently performed and the majority of gastroenterologists do not routinely prescribe prophylaxis, the risk of endocarditis must be low. Third, there is little or no evidence that biopsies, often decided upon during the procedure itself, increase the risk of bacteremia or endocarditis. Finally, situations in which the oral regimens could be used were poorly defined, resulting in continued emphasis on parenteral drugs.

These considerations led many individual experts, the British Society for Antimicrobial Chemotherapy, the American Society for Gastrointestinal Endoscopy, and the American Society of Colon and Rectal Surgeons to conclude that prophylaxis should be routinely recommended only for high-risk patients undergoing gastrointestinal endoscopic procedures.[63-67] In its most recently revised recommendations, the AHA does not recommend prophylaxis for most endoscopic procedures and considers it optional even in high-risk patients.[21] The two situations in which prophylactic antibiotics are still recommended for moderate-risk patients are esophageal dilatation and endoscopic sclerotherapy of esophageal varices, because both result in mucosal disruption and have a higher reported rate of bacteremia than most other procedures.[21] Some investigators have noted that rates of bacteremia are highly variable, are based on small numbers of patients, and may be reduced by changes in technique. Therefore, overall rates of bacteremia for these procedures may not be significantly different from other gastrointestinal procedures.[68,69] However, since several studies have documented high rates of bacteremia with organisms capable of causing endocarditis, the recommendation for prophylaxis is reasonable.[70,71]

Several other gastrointestinal procedures are not specifically addressed by the AHA. Endoscopic retrograde cholangiopancreatography (ERCP), with or without sphincterotomy, is associated with a low incidence of systemic bacteremia, probably due to efficiency of the liver in clearing bacteria from the portal circulation.[72,73] Prophylaxis is therefore probably not warranted except in high-risk patients. Few data are available regarding endoscopic laser therapy of upper- and lower-tract lesions or hemorrhoidal sclerotherapy. Wolf et al. documented bacteremia in 40 percent of patients undergoing laser therapy for esophagogastric carcinoma but not in those receiving laser therapy for arteriovenous malformations.[74] They postulated that bacteremia was induced by passage of the endo-

TABLE 43–5. Summary of Studies of Frequency of Bacteremia After Gastrointestinal Procedures

	Number of Procedures	Number of Cases	Bacteremia Case Range	Overall	Reports of Endocarditis
Upper GI Procedures					
Upper Endoscopy	14	972	0–12.5	5	2
Esophageal Dilation	6	103	0–100	45	2
ERCP	9	603	0–48	11	0
Variceal Sclerotherapy	10	428	0–53	16	1
Endoscopic Laser Therapy of Neoplasm	2	35	30–40	35	0
Endoscopic Laser Therapy of AVM	5	0		0	0
Percutaneous Endoscopic Gastrostomy	1	25	24	24	0
Lower GI Procedures					
Barium Enema	3	253	0–23	10	1
Double Contrast Barium Enema	1	45	0	0	0
Rigid Sigmoidoscopy	5	455	0–9.5	5	5
Flexible Sigmoidoscopy	1	100	1	1	3
Colonoscopy	15	740	0–27	4	1
Endoscopic Laser Therapy	1	20	19	19	0

scope through the tumor rather than the laser therapy itself and concluded that prophylaxis was warranted in the former situation for patients with high-risk valvular lesions. Kohler et al. found bacteremia in 19 percent of patients receiving laser treatment of stenosing colorectal lesions and recommended prophylaxis only in high-risk situations.[75] Hemorrhoidal sclerotherapy results in bacteremia in 8 percent and therefore probably warrants prophylaxis only in high-risk patients.[76] A single study of percutaneous endoscopic gastrostomy placement documented bacteremia in 24 percent, again suggesting that prophylaxis is prudent in high-risk patients.[77] Because there are no studies of the incidence of bacteremia following peroral small-bowel biopsy, no recommendations can be made.

In summary, the risk of endocarditis following gastrointestinal endoscopic procedures other than esophageal dilatation and sclerotherapy appears to be quite low. Prophylaxis using parenteral drugs is mandatory only in those with prosthetic valves or other high-risk valvular lesions. Parenteral therapy is optional in all others, and oral amoxicillin probably conveys adequate protection.

Other Procedures

The incidence of bacteremia is 0 to 3 percent following orotracheal intubation and 0 to 30 percent after nasotracheal intubation. Studies directly comparing the two have found no significant difference.[78,79] Although some have recommended antibiotic prophylaxis prior to nasotracheal intubation,[80–82] the AHA currently does not. Nasotracheal intubation probably should be avoided in those with high-risk lesions, particularly since it can result in bacteremia with staphylococci not covered by routine prophylactic regimens. Although bacteremia develops in 16 percent of patients during rigid bronchoscopy, it almost never occurs with fiberoptic bronchoscopy even when biopsies or transbronchial needle aspiration are performed.[83–85] Prophylaxis is therefore not warranted with fiberoptic bronchoscopy.

The AHA guidelines make no mention of prophylaxis for nonsurgical endodontic procedures. Procedures such as reaming, filing, or filling of root canals generally produce no detectable bacteremia. However, instrumentation beyond the apex of an infected tooth can result in bacteremia, and several cases of endocarditis have been attributed to endodontic procedures. Antibiotic prophylaxis should be reserved for high-risk patients.[86]

There has been one case report of endocarditis following extracorporeal shock-wave lithotripsy for renal calculi,[87] and two studies have shown the incidence of bacteremia to be 0 to 14 percent.[88,89] If there is evidence of infection, prophylactic antibiotics directed at the most likely bacterial pathogen are warranted in high-risk patients. Currently, there are no data regarding the risk of bacteremia associated with gallstone lithotripsy.

Transesophageal echocardiography (TEE) is being used with increasing frequency as a diagnostic study and for intraoperative monitoring of patients with cardiac disease. There has been one case report of endocarditis following TEE.[90] One study demonstrated bacteremia in 17 percent of patients,[91] but others have shown no significant bacteremia.[92] The need for prophylaxis is therefore uncertain, but it is probably advisable in high-risk patients. The AHA currently recommends prophylaxis in all susceptible patients undergoing urethral catheterization in the presence of infection.[21] However, one study of patients with chronic indwelling catheters and positive urine cultures documented a low incidence

of bacteremia even when the catheters were changed.[93] Thus, the risk of bacteremia in this situation may be lower than in the de novo placement of urinary catheters.

The AHA recommends antibiotic prophylaxis for incision and drainage of abscesses, but makes no recommendations regarding other types of dermatologic surgery. Incision and drainage of abscesses and surgery on infected tissue results in a high incidence of bacteremia, usually due to *Staphylococcus aureus*. Dermatologic surgery on clinically noninfected skin results in a low rate of bacteremia, and prophylaxis is suggested only for those with prosthetic valves or other high-risk lesions.[94,95]

There have been no prospective studies of the risk of bacteremia during interventional radiologic procedures. The AHA addresses only angiography and recommends no prophylaxis. However, a thorough review of the risk of infectious complications following a variety of procedures has been published and includes empiric recommendations for antibiotic prophylaxis in some.[96] Angiographic and vascular procedures, including angioplasty, embolization, and transcatheter implantation of caval filters, are considered clean and do not require prophylaxis even in those with prosthetic valves. All other biliary and genitourinary tract procedures and percutaneous drainage of intraabdominal collections other than simple cysts require prophylactic antibiotics, including coverage of enterococcus.

DRUG REGIMENS

A number of organizations and individual experts have proposed drug regimens to prevent endocarditis in susceptible individuals. All of these are empiric and based on theoretic considerations and secondary sources of information. Differing interpretations of the same data have resulted in important variations in the recommendations. Each of these is an attempt to approximate the characteristics of the ideal regimen listed in Table 43–6 and is based on the following considerations.

Choice of Drugs

There are no comparative trials of various antibiotic regimens. Formulation of drug regimens is based on in vitro sensitivity data, comparative trials in animal models of endocarditis, and reports of

TABLE 43–6. Characteristics of the Ideal Prophylactic Regimen

1. Effectively prevents endocarditis
2. Is applicable to all patients and procedures
3. Can be easily administered
4. Can be administered orally or parenterally
5. Can be administered in a fixed dosage
6. Can be administered as a single dose
7. Can be used for repetitive procedures
8. Has no associated complications
9. Causes few side effects
10. Has no contraindications
11. Is acceptable to patients and nursing staff
12. Requires no monitoring
13. Is inexpensive

prophylaxis failure. The most important and the most controversial of these are the animal data, which suggest that only high and sustained levels of bacteriocidal drugs were protective. This principle served as the basis for the stringent 1977 AHA recommendations that emphasized repeated doses of parenteral antibiotics.[97] However, inocula of bacteria used in animal studies exceed the magnitude of the bacteremia induced in humans by dental extraction or other procedures.[98] In addition, the use of a catheter and thrombus formation in animal studies lowers the size of inoculum required to initiate infection and makes it harder to eradicate. Because of this, infection in the animal model may be more comparable to established prosthetic valve endocarditis in humans. Finally, drug data are not comparable because rabbits excrete most antibiotics more rapidly than humans at comparable doses.

More recent studies in rabbits and rats using lower inocula of bacteria provide new insights into the mechanism of antibiotic prophylaxis of endocarditis. These experiments show that antibiotics can provide protection in the absence of bacterial killing, presumably by interference with adherence or inhibition of bacteria lodged on the valves. Bacteriostatic antibiotics or lower concentrations of bacteriocidal antibiotics may therefore be effective in preventing endocarditis.[4]

Although these data must be applied with caution, they confirm the usefulness of in vitro sensitivity data in formulating prophylactic regimens, provide new insights into the mechanisms and requirements of successful prophylaxis, and allow direct comparison of the relative efficacies of various regimens. These newer animal models provide a rigorous way to test a given antibiotic regimen and may guarantee a wide margin of safety when the results are extrapolated to humans.

Drug Administration

There are several important principles of drug administration that must be considered in formulating prophylactic regimens. These include the initiation, dosing, and duration of therapy and the route of administration. Prophylactic antibiotics should be started shortly before the planned procedure to achieve high serum levels and minimize the selection of relatively resistant organisms. It has been shown that the population of penicillin-sensitive streptococci in the saliva decreases after 24 hours of penicillin therapy and is replaced by more resistant organisms after 48 hours.[99] Premature initiation of antibiotics is unnecessary, costly, and may select re-

sistant organisms. It is important that the antibiotics be started before the procedure. "Prophylactic" antibiotics cannot be given after the fact. Drug regimens capable of preventing experimental endocarditis are ineffective when given six hours after the inoculum of bacteria.[100,101] Dosing of antibiotics should result in inhibitory or preferably bactericidal concentrations during the entire period of risk. Experimental evidence suggests that this period extends approximately nine hours from the initiation of bacteremia.[102,103] Continuation of antibiotic therapy longer conveys no additional benefit and only increases cost, risk, and inconvenience to the patient. Full doses of antibiotics should be given and should be modified only for children or patients with severely compromised renal function. Regimens may also need to be modified due to concurrent antibiotic administration for other reasons.

The route of administration is an important consideration. Oral regimens are more convenient, achieve higher compliance rates, and are less expensive than parenteral regimens. However, oral regimens may be less effective and impractical in patients undergoing intubation and general anesthesia who cannot take oral medications immediately before the procedure. Although they may be more effective, intramuscular and intravenous injections require skilled personnel for administration and are associated with more pain, higher cost, and an increased incidence of anaphylaxis. In addition, anticoagulation in patients with prosthetic valves poses a relative contraindication to intramuscular injection. Because of these considerations, effective oral regimens are most desirable for the majority of patients, but parenteral alternatives must be available for high-risk patients or those who cannot take oral medications.

Contraindications to Use

Alternative regimens must be available for patients who are allergic to penicillin or likely to harbor resistant bacteria. Resistant strains of *Streptococcus viridans* are particularly important in two clinical situations. Because patients who are chronically taking penicillin for rheumatic fever prophylaxis are not protected against endocarditis and may harbor strains of oral streptococci that are relatively resistant to penicillin, they should receive other drugs for endocarditis prophylaxis such as amoxicillin and ampicillin. Similarly, resistant oral flora may develop in patients receiving repeated courses of the penicillins for prophylaxis during sequential dental procedures. Since resistant organisms can develop within hours of a course of a prophylactic penicillin and persist for

TABLE 43–7. Recommended Standard Prophylactic Regimen for Dental, Oral, or Upper Respiratory Tract Procedures in Patients Who Are at Risk*

Drug	Dosing Regimen[†]
Standard Regimen	
Amoxicillin	3.0 g orally 1 h before procedure; then 1.5 g 6 h after initial dose
Amoxicillin/Penicillin-Allergic Patients	
Erythromycin or	Erythromycin ethylsuccinate 800 mg or erythromycin stearate 1.0 g orally 2 h before procedure; then half the dose 6 h after initial dose
Clindamycin	300 mg orally 1 h before procedure; then 150 mg 6 h after initial dose

*Includes those with prosthetic heart valves and other high-risk patients.
†Initial pediatric doses are as follows; amoxicillin, 50 mg/kg; erythromycin ethylsuccinate or erythromycin stearate, 20 mg/kg; and clindamycin, 10 mg/kg. Follow-up doses should be one half the initial dose. Total pediatric dose should not exceed total adult dose. The following weight ranges may also be used for the initial pediatric dose of amoxicillin: < 15 kg, 750 mg; 15 to 30 kg, 1500 mg; and > 30 kg, 3000 mg (full adult dose).

TABLE 43–8. Alternate Prophylactic Regimens for Dental, Oral, or Upper Respiratory Tract Procedures in Patients Who Are at Risk

Drug	Dosing Regimen*
Patients Unable to Take Oral Medications	
Ampicillin	Intravenous or intramuscular administration of ampicillin 2.0 g 30 min before procedures; then intravenous or intramuscular administration of ampicillin 1.0 g, or oral administration of amoxicillin 1.5 g, 6 h after initial dose
Ampicillin/Amoxicillin/Penicillin-Allergic Patients Unable to Take Oral Medications	
Clindamycin	Intravenous administration of 300 mg 30 min before procedure; then an intravenous or oral administration of 150 mg 6 h after initial dose
Patients Considered High Risk and Not Candidates for Standard Regimen	
Ampicillin, gentamicin, and amoxicillin	Intravenous or intramuscular administration of ampicillin 2.0 g, plus gentamicin 1.5 mg/kg (not to exceed 80 mg), 30 min before procedure; then amoxicillin 1.5 g orally 6 h after initial dose; alternatively, the parenteral regimen may be repeated 8 h after initial dose
Ampicillin/Amoxicillin/Penicillin-Allergic Patients Considered High Risk	
Vancomycin	Intravenous administration of 1.0 g over 1 h, starting 1 h before procedure; no repeated dose necessary

*Initial pediatric doses are as follows: ampicillin, 50 mg/kg: clindamycin, 10 mg/kg; gentamicin, 2.0 mg/kg; and vancomycin, 20 mg/kg. Follow-up doses should be one-half the initial dose. Total pediatric dose should not exceed total adult dose. No initial dose is recommended in this table for amoxicillin (25 mg/kg is the follow-up dose).

approximately 10 days, an alternate regimen should be used if a repeat procedure is required within this period of time.[104] Similar considerations apply to patients who have recently taken penicillins for other reasons.

Specific Regimens

Based on these considerations, a number of regimens for prophylaxis against endocarditis have been proposed. Those of the AHA are the most widely used in this country and are summarized in Tables 43–7, 43–8, and 43–9.[21] Their application in various clinical situations and alternative regimens suggested by others are considered below. Clinical situations are defined by the type of procedure and several patient-specific variables. The type of procedure determines the bacterium most likely to cause endocarditis and the drug regimen necessary to prevent infection by that organism. Dental, respiratory, and upper gastrointestinal procedures most often induce bacteremia with *Streptococcus viridans*. Biliary, lower gastrointestinal, and genitourinary procedures can induce enterococcal bacteremia. Cardiac and dermatologic surgery are most frequently associated with staphylococcal bacteremia. Patient factors that affect prophylaxis include the degree of risk posed by the cardiac disease, the ability of the patient to take oral medications, and the presence or absence of contraindications to the use of penicillin.

TABLE 43–9. Regimens for Genitourinary/Gastrointestinal Procedures

Drug	Dosing Regimen*
Standard Regimen	
Ampicillin, gentamicin, and amoxicillin	Intravenous or intramuscular administration of ampicillin 2.0 g, plus gentamicin 1.5 mg/kg (not to exceed 80 mg), 30 min before procedure; then amoxicillin 1.5 g orally 6 h after initial dose; alternatively, the parenteral regimen may be repeated once 8 h after initial dose
Ampicillin/Amoxicillin/Penicillin-Allergic Patient Regimen	
Vancomycin and gentamicin	Intravenous administration of vancomycin 1.0 g over 1 h, plus intravenous or intramuscular administration of gentamicin 1.5 mg/kg (not to exceed 80 mg), 1 h before procedure; may be repeated once 8 h after initial dose
Alternate Low-Risk Patient Regimen	
Amoxicillin	3.0 g orally 1 h before procedure; then 1.5 g 6 h after initial dose

*Initial pediatric doses are as follows: ampicillin, 50 mg/kg; amoxicillin, 50 mg/kg; gentamicin, 2.0 mg/kg; and vancomycin, 20 mg/kg. Follow-up doses should be half the initial dose. Total pediatric dose should not exceed total adult dose.

DENTAL, UPPER RESPIRATORY, OR UPPER GASTROINTESTINAL TRACT PROCEDURES (FIGURE 43–1)

Moderate-Risk Patients

No penicillin allergy or use; able to take oral medications. The AHA currently recommends that this group of patients receive two doses of amoxicillin rather than penicillin.[21] This recommendation is supported by others[105] and experimental data from animal models.[106,107] An important alternative has been proposed by the British Society for Antimicrobial Chemotherapy, consisting of a single oral dose of three grams of amoxicillin given one hour prior to the procedure.[65] Amoxicillin has a number of potential advantages over penicillin.[108] It is better absorbed from the stomach, and absorption is independent of gastric contents. It is less highly protein-bound and achieves higher serum levels. More importantly, its longer serum half-life allows the administration of a single dose since bactericidal concentrations are maintained for 10 hours. It can be administered in the practitioner's office, guaranteeing full compliance. This regimen markedly reduces the incidence of postextraction bacteremia.[109] It is effective in most animal models[110,111] but may not be entirely effective in the face of large inocula or tolerant organisms.[111,112] In addition, at least one case report of failure of single-dose amoxicillin prophylaxis has been reported.[113] The administration of a second dose of amoxicillin as recommended by the AHA or the addition of probenicid to diminish the rate of excretion have resulted in full protection.[107] In summary, single-dose amoxicillin is a reasonable alternative to the AHA standard recommendation, but may not be adequate in situations where an intense bacteremia is anticipated unless probenicid is given concomitantly or a second dose of amoxicillin is given four to six hours later.

No penicillin allergy or use; unable to take oral medications (NPO). In this situation, the AHA suggests two doses of intramuscular or intravenous ampicillin.[21] The BSAC has proposed a simpler alternative for patients undergoing general anesthesia, consisting of three grams of amoxicillin orally with probenicid four hours prior to the procedure or three grams of oral amoxicillin four hours prior to the procedure and a second dose as soon as possible thereafter.[65] These regimens should allow adequate time for gastric emptying and adequate duration of coverage while avoiding parenteral drugs.[114,115]

Penicillin allergy or use; able to take oral medications. Although the AHA recommends erythromycin for these patients,[21] its effectiveness may be less certain than other regimens. When initially tested in the rabbit model, it was effective only when the size of the inoculum was reduced.[100] Recent studies show it to be no better than placebo in reducing the incidence of postextraction bacteremia.[116,117] Hunt et al. have reported resistance to erythromycin in many strains of streptococci isolated from the oral cavity,[118] and several cases of prophylaxis failure have been reported.[10,119,120] Although it is probably reasonable to use erythromycin for prophylaxis, its margin of safety may not be so great as that of other regimens.

Appropriate dosing of erythromycin is also less certain. The AHA and others recommend one gram of erythromycin stearate or 800 mg of erythromycin ethylsuccinate before the procedure and a second smaller dose six hours later.[21] Because of concerns about its efficacy and substantial variation in drug levels, the BSAC recommends a larger dose of 1.5 grams and specifies the stearate base because of its superior bioavailability.[121] This dose is reasonably well tolerated and significantly reduces the rate of post-extraction bacteremia in humans.[122] Both of these modifications seem prudent. In addition, enteric-coated preparations should not be used for prophylaxis unless dose timings are changed, because of significant delays in absorption and achieving peak drug levels.[123]

In patients who cannot tolerate erythromycin, the AHA suggests clindamycin.[21] Although early experiments using high inocula and relatively low doses of clindamycin suggested it was ineffective,[103] a subsequent study using lower inocula and higher doses of the drug showed it to be effective and superior to erythromycin.[124] It is well tolerated and has been used in Europe for several years without reports of prophylaxis failure. Clindamycin may therefore be preferable to erythromycin in this setting.

The AHA no longer recommends cephalosporins as an alterna-

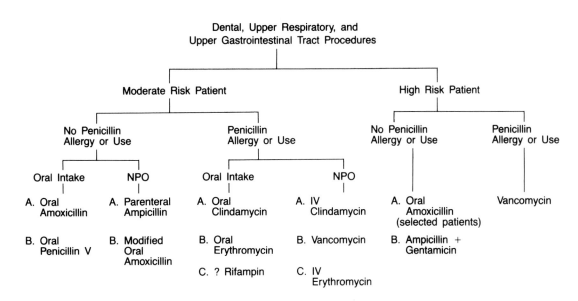

FIGURE 43–1. Dental, upper respiratory, and upper gastrointestinal tract procedures.

tive regimen.[21] Trials in animal models using high inocula showed them to be ineffective even when large doses were given.[125] A single study in animals using rifampin found it to be highly effective even when high inocula of *S. viridans* were introduced,[126] but further data are needed before it can be recommended. Newer macrolide antibiotics that theoretically might be useful for prophylaxis have not yet been adequately tested in animal models. Tetracyclines and sulfonamides are not recommended for endocarditis prophylaxis.[21]

Penicillin allergy or use; unable to take oral medications. The new AHA guidelines recommend intravenous clindamycin for such patients.[21] Vancomycin, which was previously recommended, is an acceptable alternative.[62] The BSAC recommends vancomycin and gentamicin because the combination is synergistic and more reliably bacteriocidal.[65] Intravenous erythromycin has also been suggested as an alternative.[127]

High-Risk Patients

No penicillin allergy or use; able to take oral medications. Both the AHA and BSAC now recommend the standard oral amoxicillin regimen for high-risk patients, including those with properly functioning prosthetic valves.[21,65] These regimens have been used in high-risk patients in Britain for several years without reports of prophylaxis failure. However, other investigators, noting both experimental and clinical data, have continued to recommend parenteral drugs. For this reason, the AHA has also published parenteral regimens using ampicillin and gentamicin for use in these patients and those unable to take oral medications.[21]

Penicillin allergy or use. The AHA recommends vancomycin, while the BSAC recommends vancomycin and gentamicin for the reasons discussed above.[21,65] In such high-risk patients, the addition of gentamicin is reasonable.

BILIARY, LOWER GASTROINTESTINAL, AND GENITOURINARY PROCEDURES (FIGURE 43–2)

Moderate-Risk Patients

No penicillin allergy; minor procedure. The AHA suggests two doses of oral amoxicillin in this situation but does not clearly define "minor" procedure.[62] They should probably include procedures for which prophylaxis is considered optional, such as gastro-intestinal endoscopic procedures and most gynecologic, urologic, and radiologic procedures performed in the absence of infection with low risk of bacteremia and low intensity of the bacteremia. Although single-dose amoxicillin is successful in some animal models,[112] experiments using higher inocula of enterococci have found even repeated doses of amoxicillin or ampicillin to be ineffective.[128] Therefore, the margin of safety of this regimen may not be high, and it should not be used in high-risk patients or when high rates or high intensity of bacteremia are anticipated. Interestingly, the BSAC does not offer this option.

No penicillin allergy; major procedure. The AHA recommends intramuscular or intravenous ampicillin and gentamicin as its standard regimen with a second dose of amoxicillin six hours later or a repeat parenteral dose eight hours later.[21] The BSAC recommends the combination of parenteral amoxicillin and gentamicin followed by a single dose of amoxicillin six hours later.[65] This regimen is effective in some animal models but not in those using high inocula models unless repeated doses are given over 48 hours.[128]

Penicillin allergy. There is no widely accepted oral regimen for penicillin-allergic patients undergoing low-risk procedures. Thus, all penicillin-allergic patients must receive parenteral drugs. Both the AHA and BSAC recommend vancomycin and gentamicin. This regimen is completely effective in animal models even with high inocula of enterococci.[129]

High-Risk Patients

In the high-risk patient, parenteral drugs must be used. The choice of regimen is based only on the presence or absence of an allergy to penicillin.

No penicillin allergy. As for the moderate-risk patient undergoing a major procedure, a regimen of intramuscular or intravenous ampicillin and gentamicin and a second dose following the procedure are recommended.[21]

Penicillin allergy. Vancomycin with gentamicin is the regimen of choice.[21]

CARDIAC SURGERY

The AHA offers no specific recommendations for patients undergoing open-heart surgery for the placement of prosthetic heart valves or other intracardiac or intravascular prosthetic materials.

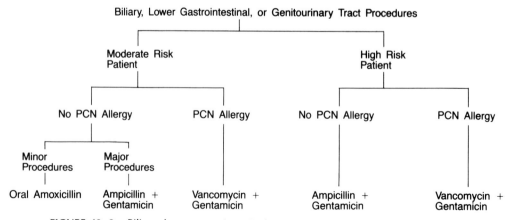

FIGURE 43–2. Biliary, lower gastrointestinal, or genitourinary tract procedures.

TABLE 43–10. Antibiotic Regimens for Cardiac Surgery

Vancomycin 15 mg/kg body weight intravenously before surgery followed by a dose of 10 mg/kg immediately after cardiopulmonary bypass

plus

Gentamicin 1.7 mg/kg body weight intravenously before surgery and repeated 8 hours later

Doses may require modification in patients with decreased renal function.

Source: Adapted from Kaye.[131]

suggests that the choice between a penicillinase-resistant penicillin or "first generation" cephalosporin plus vancomycin be based on the prevalence of staphylococcal resistance to methicillin at each institution.[21] Durack makes a similar recommendation.[130] However, Kaye points out that most cases of early prosthetic-valve endocarditis are caused by *S. epidermidis* which are resistant to all penicillins and cephalosporins and recommends vancomycin as the prophylactic agent of choice.[131] Animal studies have also demonstrated the superiority of vancomycin in preventing experimental endocarditis due to methicillin-resistant *S. epidermidis*.[132,133] Kaye also suggests the addition of gentamicin to prevent postoperative infection with enteric pathogens involving both the valve and other sites.

Doses for patients with normal renal function are summarized in Table 43–10 but may require modification in patients with compromised renal function.[131,134] Prophylaxis should be limited to minimize the risk of selecting resistant flora or superinfection.

DERMATOLOGIC SURGERY

Although the AHA suggests antibiotic prophylaxis directed against *S. aureus* for patients undergoing incision and drainage of skin abscesses, it makes no specific recommendations for high-risk patients undergoing this or for other forms of dermatologic surgery.[21] Of the empiric regimens suggested,[94,95,135–137] most call for first-generation cephalosporins despite the fact that limited animal data suggest they may be less effective than penicillinase-resistant penicillins or clindamycin.[138] Kaye's recommendations cover most clinical situations and are summarized in Table 43–11.[135] In situations with a high prevalence of methicillin-resistant coagulase-positive staphylococci, vancomycin should be employed.[135] Others suggest that vancomycin should also be used in patients undergoing dermatologic surgery with newly placed prosthetic valves in the last 60 days because of a higher risk of infection with diphtheroids.[95] In patients who are allergic to beta-lactam antibiotics, erythromycin has been suggested,[136] but clindamycin is probably a better choice.[138]

ANCILLARY MEASURES

Ancillary measures are as important as prophylactic antibiotics to minimize the risk of endocarditis in patients with valvular heart disease. Dental hygiene should be maintained, and endodontic procedures rather than extraction should be performed when possible. Application of chlorhexidine or other antiseptic agents to the gingiva before tooth extraction may reduce postextraction bacteremia. Unnecessary risks imposed by water irrigation and intrauterine devices should be avoided. All patients undergoing prosthetic heart valve replacement should have a complete dental evaluation before the procedure. Patients with a high risk of endocarditis should have orotracheal rather than nasotracheal intubation and fiberoptic rather than rigid bronchoscopy.[12,139]

It is impossible to make recommendations for all possible clinical situations. Clinicians should exercise judgment in determining the duration and choice of antibiotic(s) when special circumstances apply. Furthermore, since endocarditis may occur despite antibiotic prophylaxis, physicians and dentists should maintain a high index of suspicion in the interpretation of any unusual clinical events following the above procedures. Early diagnosis is important to reduce complications, sequelae, and mortality.[62]

SUMMARY

1. The efficacy of prophylactic antibiotics in the prevention of bacterial endocarditis has been neither proved nor disproved. However, there is sufficient indirect clinical evidence to support the continued use of antibiotics before procedures known to induce bacteremia to prevent endocarditis in susceptible patients.

2. Patients with prosthetic valves, a prior history of endocarditis, and surgically created systemic–pulmonary artery shunts have the highest risk of endocarditis. Prophylaxis is mandatory, and parenteral drugs should be used in most circumstances.

3. The risk of endocarditis in patients with mitral valve prolapse is low and confined to those with one or more clinical risk factors, including a systolic murmur, male gender, and age over 45. The presence of mitral valve leaflet thickening or redundancy and significant mitral regurgitation on echocardiography are additional risk factors. Antibiotic prophylaxis, using oral regimens when possible, should be limited to these subsets of patients.

4. The risk of bacteremia, and hence endocarditis, following most gastrointestinal endoscopic procedures is low. Prophylaxis should be given to those with high-risk lesions and considered optional in all others. Sclerotherapy of esophageal varices and esophageal dilation may carry a higher risk, and antibiotic prophylaxis is recommended for all susceptible patients undergoing these procedures.

TABLE 43–11. Antibiotic Regimens for Procedures Involving Infected Skin

Cefazolin 1 g intramuscularly 30 minutes before incision followed by Cephalexin 500 mg orally 6 hours later

Cephalexin 1 g orally 1 hour before incision followed by 500 mg doses 4 hours and 8 hours later

In patients in whom methicillin-resistant organisms are likely:

Vancomycin 1 g intravenously given over 60 minutes prior to incision

Trimethoprim 160 mg and Sulfamethoxazole 800 mg orally one hour prior to incision

Source: Adapted from Kaye.[135]

5. Amoxicillin has a number of advantages over other antibiotics and has replaced penicillin as the drug of choice for dental, upper-respiratory, and upper-gastrointestinal procedures.

6. Clindamycin is now recommended as an alternative for penicillin-allergic patients undergoing procedures likely to induce bacteremia with *Streptococcus viridans* and may be superior to erythromycin for this purpose.

7. Specific drug regimens proposed by the AHA, BSAC, and Medical Letter are rational guidelines based on currently available data.

REFERENCES

1. Bayliss R, Clarke C, Oakley CM et al: Incidence, mortality and prevention of infective endocarditis. *J Royal Coll Phys* 20:15–20, 1986.
2. Kaye D: Prophylaxis against bacterial endocarditis—a dilemma, in Kaplan EL, Taranta AV (eds): *Infective Endocarditis* American Heart Association Monograph Series, 1977, no 52, p 67.
3. Pelletier LL Jr, Petersdorf RG: Infective endocarditis. A review of 125 cases from the University of Washington Hospitals, 1963–1972. *Medicine* 56:287, 1977.
4. Bayer AS: New concepts in the pathogenesis and modalities of the chemoprophylaxis of native valve endocarditis. *Chest* 96:893–899, 1989.
5. Taran LM: Rheumatic fever in its relation to dental disease. *NYJ Dent* 14:107, 1944.
6. Schirger A, Martin WJ, Roger RQ et al: Bacterial invasion of blood after oral surgical procedures. *J Lab Clin Med* 55:326, 1960.
7. Elliott RH, Dunbar JM: Streptococcal bacteremia in children following dental extractions. *Arch Dis Child* 43:451, 1968.
8. Glazer RJ, Dankner A, Mathes SB et al: Effect of penicillin on the bacteremia following dental extraction. *Am J Med* 4:55, 1948.
9. Bender IB, Pressman RS, Tashman SG: Comparative effects of local and systemic antibiotic therapy in the prevention of postextraction bacteremia. *J Am Dent Assoc* 57:54, 1958.
10. Durack DT, Kaplan EL, Bisno AL: Apparent failures of endocarditis prophylaxis. *JAMA* 250:2318–2322, 1983.
11. Garrison PK, Freedman LR: Experimental endocarditis: I. Staphylococcal endocarditis in rabbits resulting from placement of a polyethylene catheter in the right side of the heart. *Yale J Biol Med* 42:394, 1970.
12. Everett ED, Hirschman JV: Transient bacteremia and endocarditis prophylaxis. *Ann Rev Med* 56:61, 1977.
13. Schwartz SP, Salman I: The effects of oral surgery on the course of patients with disease of the heart. *Am J Orthod* 28:331, 1942.
14. Australian Dental Association, Therapeutics Advisory Committee Report: Prevention of infective endocarditis associated with dental treatment and dental disease. *Aus Dent J* 25:51–55, 1980.
15. Pogrel MA, Welsby PD: The dentist and prevention of infective endocarditis. *Br Dent J* 139:12, 1975.
16. Oakley C: Prevention of infective endocarditis. *Thorax* 34:711–712, 1979.
17. Durack DT: Experience with prevention of experimental endocarditis, in Kaplan EL, Taranto AV (eds): *Infective Endocarditis*. American Heart Association Monograph Series, 1977, no 52.
18. Imperiale TF, Horwitz RI: Does prophylaxis prevent postdental infective endocarditis? A controlled evaluation of protective efficacy. *Am J Med* 88:131–136, 1990.
19. Van Der Meer JTM, Wijk WV, Thompson J et al: Efficacy of antibiotic prophylaxis for prevention of native-valve endocarditis. *Lancet* 339:135–139, 1992.
20. Rodbard S: Blood velocity and endocarditis. *Circulation* 28:18, 1963.
21. Dajani AS, Bisno AL, Chung KJ et al: Prevention of bacterial endocarditis. *Recommendations by the American Heart Association* 264: 2919–2922, 1990.
22. Barlow JB, Pocock WA, Marchand P et al: The significance of late systolic murmurs. *Am Heart J* 66:443–452, 1963.
23. Facquet J, Alhomme P, Raharison S: Sur la signification du souffle frequemment associe au claquement telesploligie. *Acta Cardiol* 19: 417–422, 1964.
24. Lachman AS, Bramwell-Jones DM, Lakier JB et al: Infective endocarditis in the billowing mitral leaflet syndrome. *Br Heart J* 37:326, 1975.
25. Corrigall D, Bolen J, Hancock EW et al: Mitral valve prolapse and infective endocarditis. *Am J Med* 63:215, 1977.
26. Allen A, Harris A, Leatham A: Significance and prognosis of an isolated late systolic murmur. *Br Heart J* 36:525, 1974.
27. Koch FH, Hancock EW: Ten year follow-up of forty patients with the midsystolic click/late systolic murmur syndrome. *Am J Cardiol* 37:149, 1976.
28. Appelblatt NH, Willis PW, Lenhart JA et al: Ten to forty year follow-up of 69 patients with systolic click with or without late systolic murmur. *Am J Cardiol* 35:119, 1975.
29. Mills P, Rose J, Hollingsworth J: Long-term prognosis of mitral valve prolapse. *N Engl J Med* 297:13, 1977.
30. Duren DR, Becker AE, Dunning AJ: Long-term follow-up of idiopathic mitral valve prolapse in 300 patients: A prospective study. *JACC* 11:42–47, 1988.
31. McKinsey DS, Ratts TE, Bisno AL: Underlying cardiac lesions in adults with infective endocarditis. The changing spectrum. *Am J Med* 82:681–688, 1987.
32. Clemens JD, Horwitz RI, Jaffee CC et al: A controlled evaluation of the risk of bacterial endocarditis in persons with mitral valve prolapse. *N Engl J Med* 23:776–781, 1982.
33. Hickey AJ, MacMahon SW, Wilcken DE: Mitral valve prolapse and bacterial endocarditis: When is antibiotic prophylaxis necessary? *Am Heart J* 109:431–435, 1985.
34. Devereux RB, Hawkins I, Kramer-Fox R et al: Complications of mitral valve prolapse. Disproportionate occurrence in men and older patients. *Am J Med* 81:751–758, 1986.
35. MacMahon SW, Hickey AJ, Wilcken DE et al: Risk of infective endocarditis in mitral valve prolapse with and without precordial systolic murmurs. *Am J Cardiol* 59:105–108, 1987.
36. MacMahon SW, Roberts JK, Kramer-Fox R et al: Mitral valve prolapse and infective endocarditis. *Am Heart J* 113:1291–1298, 1987.
37. Danchin N, Voiriot P, Briancon S et al: Mitral valve prolapse as a risk factor for infective endocarditis. *Lancet* 1:743–745, 1989.
38. Clemans JD, Ransohoff DF: A quantitative assessment of predental antibiotic prophylaxis for patients with mitral valve prolapse. *J Chron Dis* 37:531–544, 1984.
39. Bor DH, Himmelstein DU: Endocarditis prophylaxis for patients with mitral valve prolapse. A quantitative analysis. *Am J Med* 76:711–717 1984.
40. Nishimura RA, McGoon MD, Shub C et al: Echocardiographically documented mitral valve prolapse. Long-term follow-up of 237 patients. *N Engl J Med* 313:1305–1309, 1985.
41. Marks AR, Choong CY, Sanfilippo AJ et al: Identification of high-risk and low-risk subgroups of patients with mitral valve prolapse. *N Engl J Med* 320:1031–1036, 1989.
42. Devereux RB: Diagnosis and prognosis of mitral valve prolapse. *N Engl J Med* 320:1077–1079, 1989.
43. Uwaydah MM, Weinberg AN: Bacterial endocarditis—a changing pattern. *N Engl J Med* 273:1231, 1965.
44. Cantrell M, Yoshikawa TT: Aging and infective endocarditis. *J Amer Geri Soc* 31:216–222, 1983.
45. Lichtman P, Master AM: The incidence of valvular heart disease i

people over fifty and penicillin prophylaxis of bacterial endocarditis. *NY State J Med* 49:1693, 1949.

46. Alessandri N, Pannarale G, Del Monte F et al: Hypertrophic obstructive cardiomyopathy and infective endocarditis: A report of seven cases and a review of the literature. *Euro Heart J* 11:1041–1048, 1990.

47. Morgan WL, Bland EF: Bacterial endocarditis in the antibiotic era. *Circulation* 19:753, 1959.

48. Welton DE, Young JB, Gentry WO: Recurrent infective endocarditis. Analysis of predisposing factors and clinical features. *Am J Med* 66:932–938, 1979.

49. Galve E, Candell-Riera J, Pigrau C et al: Prevalence, morphologic types, and evaluation of cardiac valvular disease in systemic lupus erythematosus. *N Engl J Med* 319:817–823, 1988.

50. Zysset MK, Montgomery MT, Redding SW et al: Systemic lupus erythematosus: A consideration for antimicrobial prophylaxis. *Oral Surg* 64:30–34, 1987.

51. Payne G, Smith S, MacColl S, Schwartz S: Examining the need for clinical prophylactic antibiotic coverage. *Ontario Dentist* 64:21–26, 1987.

52. King LH, Bradley KP, Shires DL et al: Bacterial endocarditis in chronic hemodialysis patients: A complication more common than previously suspected. *Surgery* 69:554, 1971.

53. Ribot S, Ruthfeld D, Frankel HJ: Infectious endocarditis in maintenance hemodialysis patients: A report of four episodes among three patients. *Am J Med Sci* 264:183, 1972.

54. Lillihei LC, Robb JRR, Visscher MB: The occurrence of endocarditis with valvular deformities in dogs with arteriovenous fistulae. *Ann Surg* 132:577, 1950.

55. Lillihei LC, Shaffer JM, Spink WW et al: Role of cardiovascular stress in the pathogenesis of endocarditis and glomerulonephritis. *Arch Surg* 63:421, 1951.

56. Kaye D: Bacterial endocarditis in the presence of arteriovenous fistulae. *Am J Med Sci* 264:189, 1972.

57. Wilson WR, Danielson GK, Giuliani ER et al: Prosthetic valve endocarditis. *Mayo Clin Proc* 57:155–161, 1982.

58. Doyle EF, Spaznuolo M, Taranta A et al: The risk of bacterial endocarditis during antirheumatic prophylaxis. *JAMA* 201:129–134, 1967.

59. Ivert TSA, Dismukes WE, Cobbs CG et al: Prosthetic valve endocarditis. *Circulation* 69:223–232, 1984.

60. Freedman LR, Valone J: Experimental infective endocarditis. *Prog Cardiovasc Dis* 22:169, 1979.

61. Gould K, Ramez-Rands CH, Holmes RK et al: Adherence of bacteria to heart valve in vitro. *J Clin Invest* 56:1364, 1975.

62. Shulman ST, Amren DP, Bisno AL et al: Prevention of bacterial endocarditis. *Circulation* 70:1123A–1127A, 1984.

63. Meyer GW: Endocarditis prophylaxis and gastrointestinal procedures. *Amer J Gastroenterol* 84:1492–1493, 1989.

64. Perucca P, Meyer GW: Who should have endocarditis prophylaxis for upper gastrointestinal procedures? *Gastrointest Endosc* 31:285–287, 1985.

65. Recommendations from the Endocarditis Working Party of the British Society for Antimicrobial Chemotherapy: Antibiotic prophylaxis of infective endocarditis. *Lancet* 335:88–89, 1990.

66. Infection control during gastrointestinal endoscopy. Guidelines for clinical application. *Gastrointest Endosc* 34:37S–40S, 1988.

67. Rosen L, Abel ME, Gordon PH et al: Practice parameters for antibiotic prophylaxis—supporting documentation. *Dis Colon Rectum* 35:278–285, 1992.

68. Meyer G: Endocarditis prophylaxis for gastrointestinal procedures: A rebuttal to the newest American Heart Association recommendations. *Gastrointest Endosc* 37:201–202, 1991.

69. Meyer G: Endocarditis prophylaxis and esophageal dilation. *Gastrointest Endosc* 35:129–130, 1989.

70. Sauerbruch T, Holl J, Ruckdeschel G et al: Bacteriaemia associated with endoscopic sclerotherapy of oesophageal varices. *Endoscopy* 17:170–172, 1985.

71. Hansen CP, Westh H, Brok KE et al: Bacteraemia following orotracheal intubation and oesophageal balloon dilatation. *Thorax* 44:684–685, 1989.

72. Barr H, Youngs E, Wilkins E et al: Who should have endocarditis prophylaxis for upper gastrointestinal procedures? *Gastrointest Endosc* 32:302–303, 1986.

73. Low DE, Micflikier AB, Kennedy JK et al: Infectious complications of endoscopic retrograde cholangiopancreatography. *Arch Intern Med* 140:1076–1077, 1980.

74. Wolf D, Fleischer D, Sivak MV: Incidence of bacteremia with elective upper gastrointestinal endoscopic laser therapy. *Gastrointest Endosc* 31:247–250, 1985.

75. Kohler B, Ginsbach C, Riemann JF: Incidence of bacteremia following endoscopic laser treatment of stenosing colorectal lesions. *Gastrointest Endosc* 34:73–74, 1988.

76. Adami B, Eckardt VF, Suermann RB et al: Bacteremia after proctoscopy and hemorrhoidal injection sclerotherapy. *Dis Col Rectum* 24:373–374, 1981.

77. Sontheimer J, Salm R, Friedrich G et al: Bacteremia following operative endoscopy of the upper gastrointestinal tract. *Endoscopy* 23:67–72, 1991.

78. Gerber MA, Gastanaduy AS, Buckley JJ et al: Risk of bacteremia after endotracheal intubation for general anesthesia. *South Med J* 73:1478–1480, 1980.

79. Depoix JP, Malbezin S, Videcoq M et al: Oral intubation versus nasal intubation in adult cardiac surgery. *Br J Anaesth* 59:167–169, 1987.

80. McShane AJ, Hone R: Prevention of bacterial endocarditis: Does nasal intubation warrant prophylaxis? *Br Med J* 292:26–27, 1986.

81. Dinner M, Tjeuw M, Artusio JF: Bacteremia as a complication of nasotracheal intubation. *Anesth Analg* 66:460–462, 1987.

82. McShane AJ, Hone R: Anaesthesia and prophylaxis for infective endocarditis. *Lancet* 2:165, 1986.

83. Smith RP, Sahetya GK, Baltch A et al: Bacteremia associated with fiberoptic bronchoscopy. *NY State J Med* 83:1045–1047, 1983.

84. Haynes J, Greenstone MA: Fiberoptic bronchoscopy and the use of antibiotic prophylaxis. *Br Med J* 294:1199, 1987.

85. Witte MC, Opal ST, Gilbert JG et al: Incidence of fever and bacteremia following transbronchial needle aspiration. *Chest* 89:85–87, 1986.

86. Bender IB, Montgomery S: Nonsurgical endodontic procedures for the patient at risk for infective endocarditis and other systemic disorders. *J Endodontics* 12:400–407, 1986.

87. Kroneman OC, Brodsky MS, Mackenzie J et al: Endocarditis after lithotripsy. *Ann Intern Med* 106:777, 1987.

88. Westh H, Knudsen F, Hedengran AM et al: Extracorporeal shock wave lithotripsy of kidney stones does not induce transient bacteremia. A prospective study. *J Urol* 144:15–16, 1990.

89. Muller-Mattheis VG, Schmale D, Seewald M et al: Bacteremia during extracorporeal shock wave lithotripsy of renal calculi. *J Urol* 146:733–736, 1991.

90. Foster E, Kusumoto FM, Sobol S et al: Streptococcal endocarditis temporally related to transesophageal echocardiography. *Amer Soc Echocardiography* 3:424–427, 1990.

91. Gorge C, Erbel R, Henrichs KJ et al: Positive blood cultures during transesophageal echocardiography. *Am J Cardiol* 65:1404–1405, 1990.

92. Khandheria BK: Prophylaxis or no prophylaxis before transesophageal echocardiography? *J Amer Soc Echocardiography* 5:285–287, 1992.

93. Polastri F, Auckenthaler R, Loew F et al: Absence of significant bacteremia during urinary catheter manipulation in patients with chronic indwelling catheters. *Amer Geri Soc* 38:1203–1208, 1990.

94. Sabetta JB, Zitelli JA: The incidence of bacteremia during skin surgery. *Arch Dermatol* 123:213–215, 1987.

95. Halpern AC, Leyden JJ, Dzubow LM et al: The incidence of bactere-

mia in skin surgery of the head and neck. *J Amer Acad Dermatol* 19:112–116, 1988.

96. Spies JB, Rosen RJ, Lebowitz AS: Antibiotic prophylaxis in vascular and interventional radiology: A rational approach. *Radiology* 166:381–387, 1988.

97. American Heart Association Committee Report: Prevention of bacterial endocarditis. *Circulation* 56:139A, 1977.

98. Petersdorf RG: Antimyocardial prophylaxis of bacterial endocarditis—Prudent caution or bacterial overkill? *Amer J Med* 65:220, 1978.

99. Garrod LP, Waterworth PM: The risks of dental extraction during penicillin therapy. *Br Heart J* 24:39, 1962.

100. Petersdorf RG, Pelletier LL, Durack DT: The 1976 Paul B. Beeson Lecture: Some observations on experimental endocarditis. *Yale J Biol Med* 50:67, 1977.

101. James J, MacFarlane TW, McGowan DA et al: Failure of postbacteraemia delayed antibiotic prophylaxis of experimental rabbit endocarditis. *J Antimicrobial Chemother* 20:883–885, 1987.

102. Durack DT, Beeson PB, Petersdorf RG: Experimental bacterial endocarditis: III. Production and progress of the disease in rabbits. *Br J Exp Pathol* 54:142, 1973.

103. Pelletier LL Jr, Durack DT, Petersdorf RG: Chemotherapy of experimental streptococcal endocarditis: IV. Further observations on prophylaxis. *J Clin Invest* 56:319, 1975.

104. Leviner E, Tzukert AA, Benoliel R et al: Development of resistant oral *viridans* streptococci after administration of prophylactic antibiotics: Time management in the dental treatment of patients susceptible to infective endocarditis. *Oral Surg* 64:417–420, 1987.

105. Prevention of bacterial endocarditis. *Medical Letter* 31:112, 1989.

106. McGowan DA, Nair S, MacFarlane TW et al: Prophylaxis of experimental endocarditis in rabbits using one or two doses of amoxycillin. *Br Dental J* 155:88–90, 1983.

107. Pujadas R, Escriva E, Jane J et al: Comparative capacity of orally administered amoxicillin and parenterally administered penicillin-streptomycin to protect rabbits against experimentally induced streptococcal endocarditis. *Antimicrob Agents Chemother* 29:909–912, 1986.

108. Shanson DC: Antibiotic prophylaxis of infective endocarditis in the United Kingdom and Europe. *J Antimicrob Chemother* 20:119–131, 1987.

109. Roberts GJ, Radford P, Holt R: Prophylaxis of dental bacteraemia with oral amoxicillin in children. *Br Dent J* 162:179–182, 1987.

110. Malinverni R, Overholser CD, Bille J et al: Antibiotic prophylaxis of experimental endocarditis after dental extractions. *Circulation* 77:182–187, 1988.

111. Glauser MP, Bernard JP, Moreillon P et al: Successful single-dose amoxicillin prophylaxis against experimental streptococcal endocarditis: Evidence for two mechanisms of protection. *J Infec Dis* 147:568–575, 1983.

112. Francioli P, Moreillon P, Glauser MP: Comparison of single doses of amoxicillin or of amoxicillin-gentamicin for the prevention of endocarditis caused by *streptococcus faecalis* and by *viridans* streptococci. *J Infec Dis* 152:83–89, 1985.

113. Denning DW, Cassidy M, Dougall A et al: Failure of single-dose amoxicillin as prophylaxis against endocarditis. *Br Med J* 289:1499–1500, 1984.

114. Cannon PD, Black HJ: Antibiotic prophylaxis of infective endocarditis. *Br Dental J* 154:234, 1983.

115. Shanson DC, McNabb R, Hajipieris P: The effect of probenecid on serum amoxicillin concentrations up to 18 hours after a single 3 g oral dose of amoxicillin: Possible implications for preventing endocarditis. *J Antimicrob Chemother* 13:629–632, 1984.

116. Sefton AM, Maskell JP, Kerawala C et al: Comparative efficacy and tolerance of erythromycin and josamycin in the prevention of bacteraemia following dental extraction. *J Antimicrob Chemother* 25:975–984, 1990.

117. Cannell H, Kerawala C, Sefton AM et al: Failure of two macrolide antibiotics to prevent postextraction bacteraemia. *Br Dent J* 171:170–173, 1991.

118. Hunt DE, King TJ, Fuller GE: Antibiotic susceptibility of bacteria isolated from oral infections. *J Oral Surg* 36:527, 1978.

119. Eng RH, Wolff M, Smith SM: Failure of erythromycin in preventing bacterial endocarditis. *Arch Intern Med* 142:1958–1959, 1982.

120. Bayliss R, Clarke C, Oakley C et al: The teeth and infective endocarditis. *Br Heart J* 50:506–512, 1983.

121. Shanson DC, Tidbury P, McNabb WR et al: The pharmacokinetics and tolerance of oral erythromycin stearate compared with erythromycin ethylsuccinate: Implications for preventing endocarditis. *J Antimicrob Chemother* 14:157–163, 1984.

122. Shanson DC, Akash S, Harris M et al: Erythromycin stearate, 1.5 g, for the oral prophylaxis of streptococcal bacteraemia in patients undergoing dental extraction: Efficacy and tolerance. *J Antimicrob Chemother* 15:83–90, 1985.

123. Browning DK, Martin ME: Erythromycin preparations: Which one should be prescribed for SBE chemoprophylaxis? *Gen Dentistry* 38:216–217, 1990.

124. Glauser MP, Francioli P: Successful prophylaxis against experimental streptococcal endocarditis with bacteriostatic antibiotics. *J Infec Dis* 146:806–810, 1982.

125. Longman LP, Martin MV, Smalley JW: One and two doses of cephradine in the prophylaxis of experimental streptococcal endocarditis. *J Antimicrob Chemother* 20:557–562, 1987.

126. Malinverni R, Bille J, Glauser MP: Single-dose rifampin prophylaxis for experimental endocarditis induced by high bacterial inocula of *viridans* streptococci. *J Infec Dis* 156:151–157, 1987.

127. Shanson DC: Prophylaxis and treatment of infective endocarditis. *Drugs* 25:433–439, 1983.

128. Malinverni R, Francioli PB, Glauser MP: Comparison of single and multiple doses of prophylactic antibiotics in experimental streptococcal endocarditis. *Circulation* 76:376–381, 1987.

129. Guze PA, Kalmanson GM, Freedman LR et al: Antibiotic prophylaxis against streptomycin-resistant and susceptible *streptococcus faecalis* endocarditis in rabbits. *Antimicrob Agents and Chemother* 24:514–517, 1983.

130. Durack DT: Current issues in prevention of infective endocarditis. *Amer J Med* 78:149–156, 1985.

131. Kaye D: Prophylaxis for infective endocarditis: An update. *Ann Int Med* 104:419–423, 1986.

132. Archer GL, Vazquez GJ, Johnston JL: Antibiotic prophylaxis of experimental endocarditis due to methicillin-resistant *staphylococcus epidermidis*. *J Infec Dis* 142:725–731, 1980.

133. Wheat LJ, Smith JW, Reynolds J et al: Comparison of cefazolin, cefamandole, vancomycin, and LY146032 for prophylaxis of experimental *staphylococcus epidermidis* endocarditis. *Antimicrob Agents and Chemother* 32:63–67, 1988.

134. Farber BF, Karchmer AW, Buckley MJ et al: Vancomycin prophylaxis in cardiac operations: Determination of an optimal dosage regimen. *J Thorac Cardiovasc Surg* 85:933–940, 1983.

135. Kaye D: Prophylaxis for infective endocarditis. *Ann Int Med* 105:299–300, 1986.

136. Wagner RF, Grande DJ, Feingold DS: Antibiotic prophylaxis against bacterial endocarditis in patients undergoing dermatologic surgery. *Arch Dermatol* 122:799–801, 1986.

137. Anderson GS, Katz JH, Zier BG: Bacterial endocarditis. *J Amer Pod Med Assoc* 76:332–336, 1986.

138. Dhawan VK, Thadepalli H, Rao B et al: Chemoprophylaxis of experimental endocarditis caused by staphylococcus aureus. *J Antimicrob Chemother* 9:319–324, 1982.

139. Sipes JN, Thompson RL, Hook EW: Prophylaxis of infective endocarditis. A reevaluation. *Ann Rev Med* 28:371, 1977.

44 PROPHYLACTIC ANTIBIOTICS IN SURGERY

Margaret Trexler Hessen

Jaime Carrizosa

Elias Abrutyn

Prophylactic antibiotics have been used for years to prevent surgical infections which contribute significantly to the morbidity and mortality of surgery. Despite extensive clinical experience and the existence of a large body of literature, their use is still controversial. However, in recent years, several excellent studies have helped to define guiding principles and have identified situations in which prophylaxis appears to be effective.[1-7] This chapter reviews the principles of prophylaxis and their applications.

EVALUATING THE LITERATURE: STANDARDS FOR STUDIES OF ANTIMICROBIAL PROPHYLAXIS

The literature on the efficacy of antimicrobial prophylaxis is difficult to interpret because of marked variation in research design from study to study. Reviewing the features that characterize excellent studies enables the reader to identify those which are most informative and provides a background for understanding why studies without these features have been interpreted differently. This review is a compilation of the features detailed by several investigators.[3,8-11] Official guidelines for evaluation of perioperative antibiotic regimens have been recently developed by the Food and Drug Administration and the Infectious Disease Society of America.[12]

Studies of antimicrobial prophylaxis in surgery should be prospective, randomized, and double-blind. Major and minor hypotheses should be clearly stated at the outset. Sample size should be sufficiently large to determine whether or not significant differences exist among regimens under study. The study population should be representative of the patients undergoing a given procedure, and risk factors for infection should be equally distributed among patients in each group. Different procedures are evaluated best in separate studies. In studies combining the efficacy of an

antibiotic in several procedures, each procedure should be defined and equally distributed among the study groups. Major and minor endpoints should be explicitly defined before undertaking the study, and precise definitions of the various endpoints should be provided, particularly criteria used to define wound infection. Antibiotics used should be effective against likely offending pathogens, and the dose, route, and duration of therapy should be sufficient to provide adequate levels at least for the duration of the operation. Use of antibiotics other than those under study must be eliminated or strictly controlled. A specific period of follow-up for infection should be defined and all randomized cases that cannot be evaluated should be described. Statistical methods require careful description with clear-cut confidence intervals, particularly when comparing efficacy among treatment groups.

GENERAL PRINCIPLES OF SURGICAL PROPHYLAXIS

The use of antibiotics for prophylaxis must be clearly distinguished from therapy for proved or suspected infection and empiric therapy. Administration of antibiotics in documented infections such as pneumonia or urinary tract infection is considered therapeutic, as it is in the surgical context involving traumatic wounds, a gangrenous gallbladder, a ruptured appendix, or an ischemic bowel. In these situations, antibiotics are given to treat bacterial contamination or infection presumed to have already occurred. Antibiotics may also be given expectantly when infection is suspected but not yet proved by confirmatory studies. Therapeutic or expectant use of antibiotics must be distinguished from prophylaxis because of major differences in dosage schedule and duration of treatment.

Several principles guide the use of prophylactic antibiotics in surgery. The first rests on establishing the need for prophylaxis based on risk of infection. Prophylaxis should be considered in high-risk situations but not in those of low risk unless the consequences of infection would be disastrous. Factors that alter the risk of wound infection after contamination include age, nutritional status, the nature of the underlying disease, the presence of necrotic tissue, and changes in blood supply.[13-17] Although these parameters are difficult to measure, the standard classification of surgical procedures permits crude estimation of the risk of infection and need for prophylaxis.[18]

Clean operations are those in which aseptic technique is maintained; inflammation is not present; and the gastrointestinal, respiratory, or genitourinary tract is not entered. Such operations are usually elective, and wounds are nearly always closed by primary intention. The risk of infection in these procedures is less than five percent. Clean-contaminated operations involve entering the gastrointestinal, respiratory, or genitourinary tract, but contamination by their contents is not significant. In these operations, the risk of infection is less than 10 percent. Contaminated operations are those in which acute inflammation without exudate is found. These include procedures in which there has been a major break in aseptic technique or spillage of contents from a hollow viscus. Fresh open traumatic wounds fall into this category. The infection rate for contaminated operations is approximately 20 percent. Dirty operations include those involving old traumatic wounds and those in which an abscess, purulent material, or a perforated viscus is found. In these cases, the infection rate exceeds 30 percent.

Prophylaxis is generally not indicated in clean surgical procedures unless the consequences of infection would be catastrophic, as with infection complicating cardiac valve replacement. However, a recent study has shown prophylaxis to be beneficial in two clean procedures, breast surgery and herniorrhaphy.[19] Prophylaxis is often considered in clean-contaminated operations and is almost always used in contaminated and dirty procedures. In the latter two cases, the use of antibiotics is considered treatment of early or established infection rather than prophylaxis.

The second principle of prophylaxis requires that choice of prophylactic antibiotics be guided by consideration of those organisms most likely to cause contamination and infection in a given setting. For example, the possible role of *Staphylococcus aureus* in hip replacement and that of gram-negative organisms and anaerobes in colon surgery need to be taken into account.

The third principle states that antibiotics should be chosen on the basis of both clinical and laboratory evidence of efficacy against important potentially infecting microorganisms.[20] All antibiotic regimens are selective, and no single agent or combination is effective against all potential pathogens. Because of this, only common pathogens are covered by prophylactic antibiotics. Broad-spectrum coverage suppresses indigenous flora and selects for resistant organisms that may produce more serious infections.[21] The fourth principle requires the choice of nontoxic antibiotics with specific pharmacokinetic properties that make them especially effective in prophylaxis. Such properties are discussed in more detail below.

The fifth principle requires that the chosen antibiotic regimen be administered appropriately. Prophylaxis should be started before the procedure and, depending on the route of administration and the pharmacokinetic characteristics of the drug, administered in a dose and at a frequency expected to produce therapeutic serum levels when the incision is made.[22] Prophylaxis started earlier is probably no more effective, and long courses of antibiotics before surgery lead to selection of resistant organisms. Serum and tissue drug levels must be maintained at therapeutic levels throughout the procedure. Since some antibiotics have short half-lives, additional doses may be required during long procedures. After surgery, antibiotics should be continued only for a short time. This period is often no more than one or two days, and there is considerable evidence that a single dose is equally effective. Short-course therapy is effective in part because the bacterial load when contamination occurs is small. In addition, fibrin, necrotic tissue, compromise in blood supply, and other factors that render established infection difficult to treat are usually not present. Prolonged prophylactic courses may mask smoldering infection requiring different therapy.

The sixth principle dictates that prophylaxis be used only when its benefits outweigh its risks. Appropriately used prophylactic antibiotics designed to prevent specific infections do not prevent all postoperative infections. Pneumonia and urinary tract infection may occur even when wound infection has been successfully prevented. Prophylaxis is no substitute for meticulous surgical technique. The importance of strict aseptic technique, care in handling tissues, closure of dead spaces, and elimination of necrotic debris cannot be overemphasized.

ANTIBIOTIC SELECTION

The selection of prophylactic antibiotics is based on the type of procedure, the species of commonly involved organisms, and the pharmacokinetic and pharmacologic characteristics of the drugs. Antimicrobial agents should ideally be nontoxic, inexpensive, and bactericidal. They should be available in parenteral form, preferably for intravenous use, and achieve therapeutic levels shortly after administration. The drugs should be widely distributed in tissues, and serum half-life should allow for maintenance of therapeutic levels throughout the procedure to obviate the need for additional doses intraoperatively.[23] The therapeutic-to-toxic ratio or therapeutic index should be high. Although the clinical significance of protein-binding remains controversial, it is thought that the level of free drug and its activity are inversely related to its affinity for serum proteins.

Despite adequate serum drug levels, several other factors influence the effectiveness of prophylactic antibiotics. Drug concentrations are higher in well-perfused tissues like the heart, lung, liver, and kidney, and lower in relatively poorly perfused tissues like muscle, skin, adipose, bone, and ligaments.[23] Tissue hypoxia and acidosis may decrease the activity of some antibiotics. When bacteria like *S. aureus* are sequestered intracellularly, the effectiveness of many antibiotics is decreased because they fail to penetrate phagocytes.

Among the various drugs used in prophylaxis, cephalosporins have clear advantages. They are bactericidal with a broad spectrum of activity against organisms that include *S. aureus*, all streptococci including *S. pneumoniae*, and some enterobacteriaceae like *Escherichia coli*, *Klebsiella*, and *Proteus mirabilis*. However, they are not active against enterococci. First-generation cephalosporins are generally preferred and include cefazolin, cephalothin, cephapirin, and cephradine. Cefazolin has the longest half-life (100 minutes) and allows for less-frequent dosing every eight hours rather than every four or six hours. It can be conveniently given intramuscularly or intravenously. The second-generation cephalosporin cefoxitin is effective when activity against *Bacteroides fragilis* is needed. The third-generation cephalosporins cefotaxime ceftizoxime, ceftriaxone, ceftazidime, and cefoperazone are highly active against aerobic gram-negative rods, variably active against *Pseudomonas aeruginosa* and anaerobes, and less active than first-generation cephalosporins against gram-positive cocci involved in most wound infections. Their diminished activity against gram-positive organisms and expense dictate against their general use in prophylaxis.

The penicillinase-resistant penicillins (methicillin, nafcillin, and oxacillin) have also been used successfully in prophylaxis. They are relatively inexpensive nontoxic bactericidal agents with excellent activity against gram-positive cocci, especially *S. aureus*. Vancomycin is most reliable against methicillin-resistant staphylococci and may be indicated for prophylaxis in clean procedures in institutions where such organisms are prevalent.

CLEAN SURGERY

Orthopedic Surgery

The risk of infection in orthopedic surgery is variable, depending in part on the nature of the procedure. Most orthopedic operations can be classified as clean and carry a risk of infection under five percent. However, prophylaxis is given before clean procedures involving prosthetic devices because the consequences of infection would be especially serious. Surgical treatment of open fractures often involves a clean-contaminated procedure and usually includes the use of antibiotics. Contamination is presumed to have already occurred, and the use of antibiotics is viewed as therapeutic rather than prophylactic.

Additional measures to prevent infection in orthopedic surgery include the use of ultraviolet light, incorporation of antibiotics into bone cement, perfusion of wounds with antimicrobials through ingress and egress tubes, and measures to purify the air in the operating room, such as laminar flow. Each of these methods has been reported to be successful, but the data are not entirely convincing.

Hip Fractures

Repair of hip fractures may carry a higher incidence of infection than other clean orthopedic procedures because it involves manipulation of previously traumatized tissues and insertion of a prosthetic device. However, the benefit of prophylaxis in reducing the rate of infection is unclear. Boyd and Burke reported a reduction in deep infections among patients undergoing hip repair by methods other than total hip replacement.[24] The rate of infection was 0.8 percent in the group receiving prophylactic nafcillin and 4.8 percent in the control group, with no difference in the incidence of infected hematoma. A study by Burnett et al. showed similar efficacy with a 24-hour regimen of cephalothin.[25] Gatell et al. compared a 20-hour course of cefamandole to placebo in patients with a variety of fractures repaired with prosthetic fixation devices and found the drug to reduce the incidence of wound infections significantly.[26]

Total Joint Replacement

The rate of infection after surgical replacement of a joint may be higher because of the presence of foreign materials, including cement, or the length and difficulty of the procedure. Postoperative infections can be classified as early or late. Early infections occur within two months of surgery and are commonly caused by *S. aureus* or *S. epidermidis*. Late infections occur thereafter and are frequently due to *S. aureus*, *E. coli*, and *P. aeruginosa*. Early infections are thought to result from contamination of the wound during surgery. Late infections may also be due to contamination, but may also be a result of bacteremia unrelated to the operation.

One controlled study has shown that two weeks of prophylactic therapy with cloxacillin reduces the frequency of late infections.[27] Doyon et al. found that cefazolin given for five days perioperatively significantly reduced both early and late hip infections during a follow-up period of three to five years.[28] In three other more recent studies, a shorter regimen of cefazolin was found equally effective.[29–31] These studies appear to confirm that some late infections may be the result of contamination during surgery and that prophylaxis against *S. aureus* and *S. epidermidis* may be effective in preventing them.

Acceptable short-course prophylaxis regimens include 1 g cefazolin, 500 mg nafcillin or 2 g cephalothin given intravenously one hour before surgery and every four to six hours thereafter for 24 to 48 hours. These agents are likely to be effective against most staphylococci. Vancomycin in a dose of 1 g before surgery and one or two doses every 12 hours thereafter may be indicated in hospitals where methicillin-resistant staphylococci are prevalent. Although there are no firm data, studies of prophylaxis in other clean procedures suggest that a single dose of antibiotic may also be effective.

Prophylactic antibiotics are often used in patients who have a prosthesis in place when they undergo any operative procedure or when instrumentation associated with a high incidence of bacteremia is used. However, the value of prophylactic antibiotics in this setting is unclear. One study of 1112 patients with hip prostheses documented a low incidence of hip infection following transient bacteremia.[32]

Other Orthopedic Procedures

The use of antibiotics in other clean orthopedic procedures is probably not indicated. Pavel et al. demonstrated that the use of cephaloridine resulted in a significant reduction in the rate of wound infection in all such orthopedic procedures from 5 percent to 2.8 percent.[33,34] However, when the results were classified according to the anatomic site of surgery, the number of patients in each group was small and the differences not significant. Therefore, because the risk of infection is low and the benefit of prophylaxis minimal, the use of antibiotics in most of these procedures is not justified. However, a case can be made for prophylaxis in some types of spinal surgery like correction of scoliosis. This procedure is long and difficult, and postoperative infection has disastrous consequences. In addition, prophylactic administration of cefoxitin or an antistaphylococcal penicillin has been shown to be effective in reducing the rate of wound infection following amputation of an ischemic lower limb.[35,36]

Vascular Surgery

Most vascular surgery is clean but often involves implantation of foreign materials. The catastrophic consequences of graft infection have been cited to justify prophylaxis. *S. aureus* is the most common pathogen complicating vascular procedures, and some experimental data support the use of prophylactic antibiotics. Wilson et al. showed that preoperative cephalothin prevented graft infection in dogs when *S. aureus* was injected at the time of graft implantation.[37] Lane and Abrutyn showed that oxacillin and vancomycin reduced the frequency of infection by *S. aureus* in newly created arteriovenous fistulas in rabbits.[38]

In one large study in humans, Kaiser et al. evaluated the use of 1 g of cefazolin given preoperatively and then every six hours for four doses after surgery.[39] Rates of infection varied for different surgical procedures. None was seen in 103 patients undergoing brachial or carotid artery surgery or in 56 patients undergoing femoral artery surgery. However, in patients undergoing femoral to lower-extremity bypass procedures or abdominal aortic resection, infection rates tended to be lower with prophylaxis but not significantly so. Several subsequent studies have documented a reduction in wound infections but not necessarily in graft infections when prophylactic antibiotics are used.[40–42]

Patients undergoing vascular surgery involving the abdomen or femoral region or in whom a vascular graft is placed should therefore receive prophylaxis with a first-generation cephalosporin like cefazolin in a dose of 1 g every six hours for 24 hours intravenously. Vancomycin in a dose of 1 g given once or twice intravenously is an acceptable alternative for patients allergic to cephalosporins or in hospitals with a high incidence of infections due to methicillin-resistant *S. aureus*.[9,43] Antimicrobial prophylaxis is not recommended for percutaneous transluminal angioplasty.[44]

Although prophylaxis appears to be of some benefit in vascular procedures performed on the abdominal aorta and the vessels of the lower extremity, it remains controversial in other procedures.[45] In practice, prophylactic antibiotics are used widely in all types of vascular surgery. Additional studies of single-dose regimens are needed.

Cardiothoracic Surgery

There are no conclusive studies comparing the efficacy of antibiotic prophylaxis and placebo in preventing infection after cardiac surgery. Because of the potential severity of infections such as mediastinitis, sternal osteomyelitis, and prosthetic valve infection, most authorities recommend prophylaxis despite the clean nature of the procedures. The most frequently recommended agent is a first-generation cephalosporin. Cefazolin in a dose of 1 g intravenously before surgery and for up to 48 hours thereafter is a common regimen.[9,43] Some authors report equal or better results with the second-generation cephalosporins cefamandole and cefotaxime.[46–49] For patients allergic to cephalosporins or those in hospitals where methicillin-resistant staphylococci are prevalent, vancomycin in a dose of 1 g intravenously before surgery and for up to 48 hours thereafter can be used.

The duration of antibiotic administration in cardiac surgery remains controversial. At least one study has shown that extending the period of prophylaxis beyond 48 hours does not improve results.[50] An earlier study of patients undergoing valve replacement found that a single dose of antibiotic was as effective as a 20-dose regimen.[51] However, some surgeons prefer to continue prophylaxis until thoracostomy tubes and other drains are removed. The most important factor is probably maintenance of therapeutic antibiotic levels in tissue for the duration of the operation. If the procedure lasts longer than the usual dosing interval of the antibiotic, an

additional dose should be given at the appropriate time during surgery.[48]

Antimicrobial prophylaxis is not routinely recommended for pacemaker placement, chest tube insertion,[52–54] or percutaneous transluminal angioplasty. Several studies address the issue of prophylaxis for other noncardiac thoracic procedures such as elective pulmonary resection and repair of trauma and are summarized by Mandal et al.[55] The efficacy of prophylaxis in pulmonary resection is controversial. Antibiotics may reduce the incidence of postoperative wound infection but not that of pneumonia or empyema. Some authorities therefore recommend a regimen of cefazolin in a dose of 1 g every six hours for 24 hours intravenously.[9,43] However, most studies do not support the use of prophylactic antibiotics in the surgical treatment of chest trauma.

Neurosurgery

Neurosurgical procedures are classified as clean and carry low infection rates. Tenney et al. found great variability in rates depending on the type of operation, ranging from 1 percent in some procedures to 10 percent after resection of a glioma.[56] However, most studies do not stratify patients as selectively and evaluate prophylaxis in a variety of procedures taken together. In a study that was neither blind nor controlled, Malis et al. reported no infections in 1732 patients receiving systemic vancomycin and gentamicin and wound irrigation with streptomycin.[57] These results were confirmed by Geraghty and Feely, who documented significant reduction in infection in patients receiving prophylaxis with the same regimen.[58] In a controlled trial, Young and Lawner documented fewer postoperative wound infections with a regimen of cefazolin and gentamicin given immediately before surgery and repeated every six hours intraoperatively for the duration of the operation.[59] More recently, Bullock et al. showed a similar benefit with prophylactic piperacillin in elective neurosurgical procedures.[60] Another study showed that a single dose of vancomycin successfully reduced the rate of bone flap infections in patients undergoing craniotomy.[61] Recently, Djindjian et al. documented a decrease in wound infections in patients given prophylactic oxacillin undergoing clean neurosurgical procedures lasting over two hours.[62] At present, although prophylactic antibiotics are often used, their benefits in clean neurosurgical procedures remain incompletely established. Several thorough reviews of the literature are available.[63–65] Several studies have addressed the need for prophylactic antibiotics in the setting of cerebrospinal fluid shunt placement, and most investigators find no benefit.[66–68]

Other Clean Surgery

Platt et al. showed that 1 g of cefonicid, a highly protein-bound cephalosporin with a long half-life, is effective in reducing infection rates after herniorraphy and breast procedures including excision of masses, mastectomy, reduction mammoplasty, and axillary node dissection.[19]

CLEAN-CONTAMINATED SURGERY

Surgery of the Colon and Rectum

Elective colorectal surgery is performed in areas of heavy bacterial colonization with a high probability of peritoneal contamination.

Rates of postoperative infection range between 10 percent and 50 percent. Prophylactic antibiotic regimens fall into three major categories: intestinal antisepsis, systemic prophylaxis, and irrigation with topical antibiotics.[69] Numerous regimens involving different antimicrobial agents and combinations of modalities have been proposed.

Intestinal Antisepsis

Mechanical cleansing and administration of oral antibiotics before surgery have been used to reduce the intraluminal mass of aerobic and anaerobic bacteria. Mechanical cleansing transiently reduces the bacterial load by removing large amounts of feces from the colon. Although it does not sterilize the colon, it reduces the incidence of wound infection and sepsis after colorectal surgery. The most commonly used regimen includes a low-residue diet for the first 24 to 48 hours followed by a liquid diet for 24 hours, cathartics, and enemas. Enemas are usually composed of saline solutions to reduce electrolyte losses. In recent years, the use of orally administered isotonic lavage has largely replaced traditional mechanical cleansing.[70]

Mechanical cleansing has been combined with oral antibiotics to reduce the bacterial load further. The combination is more effective than mechanical cleansing alone and is the standard of practice in colorectal surgery. Several studies have shown that mechanical cleansing or orally administered lavage and combinations of neomycin and erythromycin, neomycin and tetracycline, neomycin and metronidazole, or kanamycin and metronidazole given for one or two days before surgery reduce the infection rate from approximately 30 to 40 percent in patients given mechanical cleansing alone to 8 to 10 percent.[70–82] Other combinations are neomycin with sulfathalidone and erythromycin with kanamycin.[73,83,84] The most widely used regimen consists of 1 g of neomycin and 1 g of erythromycin base given during the afternoon and evening before surgery at 1 PM, 2 PM, and 11 PM. No enemas are given the evening before surgery, but the patient evacuates three hours before going to the operating room.

Systemic Antibiotics

Several studies have evaluated the benefit of systemic without oral antibiotics.[85–91] The use of a first-generation cephalosporin alone or in combination with an oral regimen has been evaluated in a number of trials. Although some show a significant reduction in wound infection with the cephalosporin alone, most do not. Moreover, the addition of such an agent to an oral regimen is of no benefit.[82,83,86,91,92] In the well-designed Veterans Administration Cooperative Study, the infection rate was 39 percent in patients given parenteral cephalothin and 6 percent in those given oral neomycin and erythromycin with or without cephalothin.[86]

Failures with systemic first-generation cephalosporins have been attributed to lack of activity against *Bacteroides* species. A recent study documents the necessity of activity against both anaerobes and gram-negative aerobes in achieving effective prophylaxis.[93] Consequently, parenteral cefoxitin provides effective prophylaxis when used as a single agent.[89,94] The combination of gentamicin and metronidazole given parenterally is equally effective.[95]

Topical Antibiotics

A third modality of prophylaxis in colorectal surgery is irrigation with antibiotic solutions. Because the benefit of this practice has not been evaluated in rigorous well-controlled studies, firm conclusions cannot be drawn.[96] Injection of antibiotics into the incision has been found promising in a few studies, but further investigation is needed.[97,98] Absorption of these agents can occur, and toxic compounds like neomycin should be avoided.

Gastroduodenal Surgery

The overall rate of infection after gastroduodenal surgery ranges from 3 percent to 28 percent with an average of about 10 percent. The benefit of antibiotic prophylaxis is difficult to assess, but one study showed that a three-dose course of cephaloridine, now no longer available, effectively reduces the rate.[82]

Patients undergoing gastroduodenal surgery can be stratified into low- and high-risk groups.[99] Low-risk patients have no impairments in normal host defenses and, for example, have normal bowel motility and gastric acid production. They undergo primarily elective procedures such as surgery for bleeding duodenal ulcer unresponsive to medical therapy. Risk may be low because of the relatively sterile acid environment of the stomach. Organisms found in the stomach include low numbers of streptococci, lactobacilli, and staphylococci, and occasionally anaerobic bacteria or enterobacteriaceae. Patients who have received long-term therapy with H_2 antagonists, omeprazole, or antacids may also have an increased risk because of increased bacterial colonization associated with decreased gastric acidity. In contrast, high-risk patients have clearly compromised host defenses and undergo extensive procedures for gastric carcinoma, peptic ulcer disease with obstruction, and acute hemorrhage from gastric or duodenal ulcer.

Using this classification in 109 patients undergoing gastroduodenal surgery, Lewis et al. found no organisms or only grampositive cocci in the gastric contents of low-risk patients and gram-positive cocci, gram-negative rods, anaerobic streptococci, and *Candida* species in the stomachs of high-risk patients. Identification of isolated organisms allowed prediction of both risk and etiology of infection.[100,101] Examination of infection rates in different gastroduodenal procedures supports separation of patients into low- and high-risk groups. Infection rates of 3 to 10 percent are seen in duodenal ulcer surgery and 16 to 48 percent in procedures involving perforated gastric ulcer, gastric tumor, and acute gastrointestinal hemorrhage.

In studying the benefit of prophylactic antibiotics, Nichols et al. determined the effect of antimicrobials on the incidence of postoperative sepsis in high-risk patients undergoing gastroduodenal surgery.[102] Patients who received three doses of cefamandole beginning one hour before surgery had an infection rate of five percent, and those given a placebo had a rate of 35 percent. At present, it is therefore advisable to consider prophylaxis only in patients with a high risk of infection, although some recommend it for gastric bypass surgery and percutaneous endoscopic gastrostomy as well.[43] Cefazolin in a dose of 1 g intramuscularly or intravenously as above is a reasonable choice.

Biliary Tract Surgery

The role of prophylactic antibiotics in biliary surgery is unclear. Several investigators have evaluated prophylaxis primarily in elective procedures and found it to be beneficial.[103–111] In separate studies, gentamicin, tobramycin with lincomycin, intravenous trimethoprim-sulfamethoxazole, and cefazolin, even in single doses, have been shown to be effective. However, the risk of infection in otherwise healthy patients undergoing biliary surgery with or without incidental cholelithiasis is low.

As in gastroduodenal surgery, it is useful to assign patients undergoing biliary tract surgery to low- and high-risk groups. Patients in the high-risk category include those over 70 and those with acute cholecystitis, obstructive jaundice, common duct stones with or without jaundice, or a recent history of fever or chills. These patients should receive preoperative prophylactic antibiotics.

The risk of infections is also high if bacteria are present in the bile. Infected bile contains 10^4 to 10^8 organisms including *E. coli*, enterococci, and *S. aureus*, which frequently cause infection after biliary surgery. In contrast, the rate of infection in patients with uncontaminated bile is about two percent. The need for prophylaxis in patients with none of the above risk factors can be determined by an intraoperative gram stain of the bile. The bile can be cultured during surgery to guide therapy if infection develops.[104]

Antibiotics used in the prophylaxis of biliary surgery are often chosen on the basis of their hepatic excretion. However, when obstruction is present, drug levels in bile are undetectable. A reasonable prophylactic regimen in high-risk patients is cefazolin in a dose of 1 g before surgery and every six to eight hours thereafter for a total of 24 hours. Gentamicin and other nephrotoxic antibiotics are not recommended for routine use.

Gynecologic Surgery

Abdominal Hysterectomy

The use of prophylactic antibiotics in abdominal hysterectomy remains controversial. Rates of postoperative infection vary depending on the definition of morbidity used. For example, the frequency of wound and deep-pelvic infection is about 10 to 15 percent, but the overall complication rate approaches 40 percent when "febrile or operative morbidity" and other infections like those of the urinary tract and pneumonia are included. "Febrile or operative morbidity" is often defined as temperature elevation over 38°C on two separate occasions at least six hours apart during a defined period after surgery excluding the first 24 hours. This definition varies among studies, making comparisons among them difficult. Moreover, because proven infections are relatively uncommon, most studies rely on evaluation of this variably defined parameter. An additional problem is the difficulty of defining the precise nature of an infection (e.g., wound infection or pelvic cellulitis) even when it is clearly present.

Several studies support the use of cephalosporins for prophylaxis.[112–114] In a prospective study of cephalothin, Allen et al. reported a reduction in the rate of febrile morbidity from 41 percent to 14 percent and decreased length of hospital stay in the treated group.[112] Ohm and Galask showed that cephaloridine given on the day of surgery followed by cephalexin for four days thereafter reduced operative morbidity from 39 percent to 15 percent but did not affect length of stay.[113] However, patient groups were small and the differences were not statistically significant. Resistant organisms were recovered from patients receiving antibiotics. Grossman et al. compared penicillin and cefazolin prophylaxis in abdominal and vaginal hysterectomy.[114] There were fewer infections in those treated with antibiotics undergoing abdominal hysterectomy, but there were no differences in febrile morbidity or duration of hospital stay.

Although these studies suggest that prophylaxis may be beneficial, the data are not entirely convincing. Moreover, other investigators have failed to demonstrate such benefit, and a recent review discusses these studies in detail.[115] Therefore, until the role of antibiotic prophylaxis in abdominal hysterectomy is better defined, it is reasonable to use cefoxitin in a dose of 2 g or cefazolin in a dose of 1 g intravenously before the procedure.

Vaginal Hysterectomy

The incidence of complications following vaginal hysterectomy likewise varies with the definition of the term, the type of procedure, and perhaps the age of the patient. Infection is often difficult to document after vaginal hysterectomy, and reduction in febrile or operative morbidity is therefore frequently used as an outcome measure. However, if febrile morbidity is excluded, the incidence of wound infections, including those of the vaginal cuff, pelvic cellulitis, and adnexal abscesses, is high and ranges from 12 percent to 64 percent. This rate justifies evaluation of the potential benefits of prophylaxis.

Initial studies of antibiotic prophylaxis using intramuscular chloramphenicol or a combination of penicillin and streptomycin showed a reduction in febrile morbidity. The combination was more effective than chloramphenicol alone. When cephalosporins were introduced, their use in prophylaxis yielded good results. Allen et al. showed that cephalothin given on the day of surgery and for three days thereafter reduced febrile morbidity.[112] Studying the efficacy of cefazolin given just before surgery and six and 12 hours thereafter, Polk documented decreased rates of pelvic infection from 21 percent to 2 percent.[116] Febrile morbidity and length of hospital stay were also reduced in patients given cefazolin. Grossman et al. showed that cefazolin given before surgery and every six hours thereafter for a total of 48 hours was also effective.[114]

Several studies have evaluated the efficacy of shorter courses of prophylactic antibiotics.[117–126] Ledger et al. showed that cephaloridine given only on the day of surgery was as effective as a regimen of cephaloridine before surgery with cephalexin for five days thereafter.[117] Mendelson et al. found that a single 2-g dose of cephradine was as effective as 1 g given preoperatively and every six hours after surgery for 24 hours.[118] Lett et al. obtained comparable results with a single 1-g dose of cefazolin just before surgery or a regimen of three preoperative doses of cephaloridine 10 hours apart.[119]

Many other regimens have been evaluated in vaginal hysterectomy. Jennings administered cefazolin before surgery and cephalexin thereafter until the urinary catheter was removed.[120] Biven et al. and Ohm and Galask used combined cephalothin-cephalexin regimens for five days.[121,122] Roberts and Homesley used carbenicillin in a dose of 2 g every six hours for five days.[123] Bolling and Plunkett used either ampicillin or tetracycline for seven days.[125] More complicated regimens designed to provide broader coverage to include anaerobic flora with gentamicin and clindamycin or metronidazole are not more efficacious, but further comparative trials are required. Studies involving combinations of beta-lactam antibiotics and beta-lactamase inhibitors are ongoing. The spectrum of these drugs includes gram-negative aerobes, streptococci, and anaerobes.

Two recent comprehensive reviews conclude that prophylaxis is useful in vaginal hysterectomy and can be accomplished with a single dose of a cephalosporin before surgery.[9,127] Cefazolin in a dose of 1 g intramuscularly or intravenously one hour before the procedure is therefore recommended. Antibiotic prophylaxis for elective abortion is the same.

Cesarean Section

The risk of infection following cesarean section is increased by difficult labor, rupture of membranes, and the need for emergency surgery. In these situations, postoperative infection rates range from 45 percent to 85 percent compared to 10 percent in elective cases.[115] Several studies address prophylaxis but are not discussed here in detail. In summary, recent work supports the use of a first-generation or, less preferably, a second-generation cephalosporin given in one to three doses beginning at the time the cord is clamped.[128–130]

Urologic Surgery

The effects of prophylactic antibiotics on the frequency of postoperative fever, urinary tract infection, gram-negative bacteremia, and epididymitis and on length of hospitalization have been studied in patients undergoing prostatectomy. Various studies have evaluated several antibiotics including cephalosporins, aminoglycosides, trimethoprim-sulfamethoxazole, nitrofurantoin, and combination regimens.[131–140] However, as in other procedures, the role of prophylaxis remains unclear.

The two major risk factors in the development of postoperative infection following transurethral resection of the prostate are bacteriuria at the time of surgery and the presence of an indwelling catheter. Most studies show a clear reduction in infectious complications when bacteriuria is treated for 24 to 48 hours before surgery. A single preoperative dose may also be effective.[43,141] However, short courses have resulted in high recurrence rates of infection. Some advocate continuing antibiotics until the catheter is removed if this can be accomplished within two to four days after surgery.[137] Despite conflicting studies, antimicrobial prophylaxis is probably not indicated in patients with sterile urine. Larsen et al. have reviewed these and other studies evaluating prophylaxis in a variety of urologic procedures.[142]

Clear-cut data on appropriate prophylaxis in radical prostatectomy, now a more commonly performed procedure, are not yet available. However, cefazolin may be useful since the bowel is not entered and anaerobic coverage is not needed.

Head and Neck Surgery

Most authorities agree that antimicrobial prophylaxis is indicated for major head and neck surgery when mucosal surfaces are involved. Several reviews of the literature have been published recently.[65,143] Most regimens include agents or combinations effective against usual upper-airway flora including streptococci and anaerobes. Some recommend additional coverage of gram-negative bacilli. The latter organisms are not normal upper-airway flora, but may colonize the nasopharynx in chronically ill or debilitated patients and contribute to wound infections after head and neck surgery.

Appropriate regimens include cefazolin with and without metronidazole or clindamycin[144,145] or clindamycin with or without gentamicin. Third-generation cephalosporins are also effective.[146] Several studies support limiting the duration of prophylaxis to 24 hours.[147,148]

SUMMARY

1. Clean operations are those in which (1) the gastrointestinal, respiratory, or genitourinary tract is not entered; (2) aseptic technique is maintained; and (3) inflammation is not found. Antibiotic prophylaxis is usually not necessary in clean procedures but is often considered when prosthetic devices are implanted. In one study, prophylaxis has been shown to be beneficial in herniorraphy and some procedures on the breast.

2. Clean-contaminated operations are those in which the gastrointestinal, respiratory, or genitourinary tract is entered, but contamination is not significant. Prophylaxis should be considered.

3. Infection rates for contaminated and dirty operations exceed 20 percent and 30 percent, respectively. Antibiotics are used as treatment of established infection.

4. Prophylactic antibiotics are not recommended in most clean orthopedic procedures except in placement of a prosthesis or other foreign body.

5. Prophylaxis is recommended in vascular procedures involving the abdominal aorta or vasculature of the lower extremities, particularly when prosthetic materials are used.

6. Although cardiothoracic procedures are considered clean, the catastrophic effects of postoperative wound infection justify antibiotic prophylaxis. A cephalosporin is usually used.

7. The benefits of antimicrobial prophylaxis in neurosurgical procedures remains unclear.

8. Colorectal surgery requires prophylaxis including mechanical cleansing or peroral isotonic lavage with oral or systemic antibiotics or both. Oral neomycin and erythromycin or a systemic cephalosporin can be used.

9. Patients undergoing gastroduodenal or biliary tract surgery can be clinically considered as having either a high or a low risk of infection. Prophylaxis with a cephalosporin is recommended only in high-risk patients.

10. The low frequency and mild severity of infections following abdominal hysterectomy suggest that routine prophylaxis is not justified at present. However, more data are needed.

11. Prophylaxis with a single preoperative dose of a cephalosporin is recommended in vaginal hysterectomy and cesarean section.

12. Patients undergoing prostatectomy with bacteriuria should be given antibiotics for 24 to 48 hours before surgery. Those with sterile urine do not require antibiotics. Closed drainage systems should be used when possible. Irrigation of the bladder with neomycin-polymyxin solutions is not recommended.

13. Prophylaxis in head and neck surgery is recommended when the oropharyngeal space is entered. A first-generation cephalosporin with or without additional coverage for anaerobes is effective.

REFERENCES

1. Kunin CM: Veterans Administration ad hoc interdisciplinary advisory committee on antimicrobial drug usage: I. Prophylaxis in surgery. *JAMA* 237:1003, 1977.
2. Hurley DL, Howard P, Hahn HH: Perioperative prophylactic antibiotics in abdominal surgery. *Surg Clin N Am* 59:919, 1979.
3. Hirshman JV, Inui TS: Antimicrobial prophylaxis: A critique of recent trials. *Rev Infect Dis* 2:1, 1980.
4. Chodak GW, Plaut ME: Use of systemic antibiotics for prophylaxis in surgery. *Arch Surg* 112:326, 1977.
5. DiPiro JT, Record KE, Schanzenbach KS et al: Antimicrobial prophylaxis in surgery. Part I. *Am J Hosp Pharm* 38:320, 1981.
6. Nichols RE: Use of prophylactic antibiotics in surgical practice. *Am J Med* 70:686, 1981.
7. Platt R, Kaiser AB (eds): International symposium on perioperative antibiotic prophylaxis. *Rev Infect Dis* 13(Suppl 10):S779, 1991.
8. Norden C: A critical review of antibiotic prophylaxis in orthopedic surgery. *Rev Infect Dis* 5:928, 1983.
9. Kaiser AB: Antimicrobial prophylaxis in surgery. *N Engl J Med* 315:1129, 1986.
10. Platt R: Antibiotic prophylaxis in surgery. *Rev Infect Dis* 6:S880, 1984.
11. Conte J: Antibiotic prophylaxis: Nonabdominal surgery, in Remington JS, Swartz MN (eds): *Current Clinical Topics in Infectious Diseases.* Cambridge, MA, Blackwell Scientific Publications, 1989, pp 254–305.
12. Gorbach SL, Condon RE, Conte JE Jr et al: Evaluation of new anti-infective drugs for surgical prophylaxis. *C Infect Dis* 15(Suppl):S313, 1992.
13. Miles AA, Miles EM, Burke J: The value and duration of defense reactions of the skin to the primary lodgement of bacteria. *Br J Exp Pathol* 38:79, 1957.
14. Polk HC: Prevention of surgical wound infection. *Ann Intern Med* 89:770, 1978.
15. Nahai R, Lamb JM, Havican RG et al: Factors involved in disruption of intestinal anastomoses. *Am Surg* 43:45, 1977.
16. Cruse P: Infection surveillance: Identifying the problem and the high-risk patient. *South Med J* 70:4, 1977.
17. Mishriki SF, Law DJW, Jeffrey PJ: Factors affecting the incidence of postoperative wound infection. *J Hosp Inf* 16:223, 1990.
18. National Academy of Sciences, National Research Council, Division of Medical Sciences, Ad Hoc Committee of the Committee on Trauma and Postoperative Wound Infection: The use of ultraviolet radiation of the operating room and of various other factors. *Ann Surg* 70(Suppl):8, 1977.
19. Platt R, Zaleznik DF, Hopkins CC et al: Perioperative antibiotic prophylaxis for herniorrhaphy and breast surgery. *N Engl J Med* 322:153, 1990.
20. Moellering RC Jr, Kunz LV, Poitras JW et al: Microbiologic basis for the rational use of prophylactic antibiotics. *South Med J* 70(Suppl):8, 1977.
21. Garibaldi RA, Cushing D, Lerer T: Risk factors for postoperative infection. *Am J Med* 91(Suppl 3B):158S, 1991.
22. Classen DC, Evans RS, Pestotnik SL et al: The timing of prophylactic administration of antibiotics and the risk of surgical wound infection. *N Engl J Med* 325:281, 1992.
23. Neu HC: Clinical pharmacokinetics in preventive antimicrobial therapy. *South Med J* 70(Suppl):14, 1977.
24. Boyd RF, Burke JF, Colton T: A double-blind clinical trial of prophylactic antibiotics in hip fractures. *Am J Bone Joint Surg* 55A:1252, 1973.
25. Burnett JW, Gustilo RB, Williams DN et al: Prophylactic antibiotics in hip fractures: A double-blind, prospective study. *Am J Bone Joint Surg* 62A:457, 1980.
26. Gatell JM, Riba J, Loranzo ML et al: Prophylactic cefamandole in orthopedic surgery. *Am J Bone Joint Surg* 66A:1219, 1984.
27. Carlsson AS, Lidgren L, Lindberg L: Prophylactic antibiotics against early and late deep infections after total hip replacement. *Acta Orthop Scand* 48:405, 1977.
28. Doyon F, Evrard J, Mazas F et al: Long-term results of prophylactic cefazolin versus placebo in total hip replacement. *Lancet* 1:860, 1987.
29. Hughes SPF: The use of antibiotics in orthopedic surgery: Total joint single versus multiple dose prophylaxis. *Orth Rev* 16:209, 1987.
30. Williams DN, Gustilo RB: The use of preventive antibiotics in orthopedic surgery. *Clin Orth Rehab Res* 190:83, 1984.
31. Pollard JP, Hughes SPF, Scott JE et al: Antibiotic prophylaxis in total hip replacement. *Br Med J* 1:707, 1979.
32. Ainscow DAP, Denon RA: The risk of haematogenous infection in total joint replacement. *Br J Bone Joint Surg* 66B:580, 1984.
33. Pavel A, Smith RL, Ballard A et al: Prophylactic antibiotics in clean orthopedic surgery. *Am J Bone Joint Surg* 56A:777, 1974.
34. Pavel A, Smith RL, Ballard A et al: Prophylactic antibiotics in elective orthopedic surgery: A prospective study of 1591 cases. *South Med J* 70:50, 1977.
35. Sonne-Holm S, Boeckstyns M, Menck H et al: Prophylactic antibiotics in amputation of the lower extremity for ischemia. A placebo-controlled, randomized trial of cefoxitin. *Am J Bone Joint Surg* 67:800, 1985.
36. Moller BN, Krebs B: Antibiotic prophylaxis in lower limb amputation. *Orthop Scand* 56:327, 1985.
37. Wilson SE, Wang S, Gordon HE: Perioperative antibiotic prophylaxis against vascular graft infection. *South Med J* 70:68, 1977.
38. Lane T, Abrutyn E: Induction and prevention of experimental arteriovenous fistula infections. *Antimicrob Agents Chemother* 16:638, 1979.
39. Kaiser AB, Clayson KR, Mulherin JL et al: Antibiotic prophylaxis in vascular surgery. *Ann Surg* 188:283, 1978.
40. Hasselgren PO, Ivarson L, Risberg B et al: Effects of prophylactic antibiotics in vascular surgery: A prospective, randomized, double-blind study. *Ann Surg* 200:86, 1984.
41. Worning AM, Frimodt-Moller N, Ostri P et al: Antibiotic prophylaxis in vascular reconstructive surgery: A double-blind placebo-controlled study. *J Antimicrob Chemother* 17:105, 1986.
42. Bennion RS, Hiatt JR, Williams RA et al: A randomized prospective study of perioperative antimicrobial prophylaxis for vascular access surgery. *J Cardiovasc Surg* 26:270, 1985.
43. Anonymous: Antimicrobial prophylaxis in surgery. *Med Letter* 31:105, 1989
44. Spies JB, Rosen RJ, Lebowitz AS: Antibiotic prophylaxis in vascular and interventional radiology: A rational approach. *Radiology* 166:381, 1988.
45. Pitt HA, Postier RG, MacGowan WAL et al: Prophylactic antibiotics in vascular surgery: Topical, systemic, or both. *Ann Surg* 192(3):356, 1980.
46. Slama TG, Sklar S, Misinski J et al: Randomized comparison of cefamandole, cefazolin, and cefotaxime prophylaxis in open heart surgery. *Antimicrob Agents Chemother* 29:744, 1986.
47. Abbate M, Lomeo A, Ubo E et al: Antibiotic prophylaxis in cardiac surgery: A randomized study using cephalexin and cefotaxime. *Clin Trials J* 21:348, 1984.
48. Ariano RE, Zhanel GC: Antimicrobial prophylaxis in coronary artery bypass surgery: A critical appraisal. *DICP* 25:478, 1991.
49. Kaiser AB, Petracek MR, Lea JW IV et al: Efficacy of cefazolin, cefamandole, and gentamicin as prophylactic agents in cardiac surgery. *Ann Surg* 206:791, 1987.

50. Goldmann DA, Hopkins CC, Karchmer AW et al: Cephalothin prophylaxis in cardiac valve surgery: A prospective, double-blind comparison of two-day and six-day regimens. *J Thoracic Cardiovasc Surg* 73:470, 1977.

51. Conte JE Jr, Cohen SN, Benson BR, Elashoff RM: Antibiotic prophylaxis and cardiac surgery: A prospective double-blind comparison of single-dose versus multiple-dose regimens. *Ann Intern Med* 76:943, 1972.

52. Bluhm G, Nordlander R, Ransjo V: Antibiotic prophylaxis in pacemaker surgery: A prospective double-blind trial with systemic administration of antibiotic versus placebo at implantation of cardiac pacemaker. *PACE* 9:720, 1986.

53. LeBlance KA, Tucker WY: Prophylactic antibiotic and closed-tube thoracostomy. *Surg Gyn Obstet* 160:259, 1985.

54. Neugebauer MK, Fosburg RG, Trummer MJ: Routine antibiotic therapy following pleural space intubation. *J Thorac Cardiovasc Surg* 61:882, 1971.

55. Mandal AK, Montano J, Thadepalli H: Prophylactic antibiotics and no antibiotics compared in penetrating chest trauma. *J Trauma* 25:639, 1985.

56. Tenney JH, Vlahov D, Saleman M et al: Wide variation in risk of wound infection following clean neurosurgery: Implications for perioperative antibiotic prophylaxis. *J Neurosurg* 62:243, 1985.

57. Malis LM: Prevention of neurosurgical infection by intraoperative antibiotics. *Neurosurgery* 5:339, 1979.

58. Geraghty J, Feely M: Antibiotic prophylaxis in neurosurgery: A randomized controlled trial. *J Neurosurg* 60:724, 1984.

59. Young RF, Lawner PM: Perioperative antibiotic prophylaxis for prevention of postoperative neurosurgical infection: A randomized clinical trial. *J Neurosurg* 60:701, 1987.

60. Bullock R, van Dellen JR, Ketelbey W et al: A double-blind placebo-controlled trial of perioperative prophylactic antibiotics for elective neurosurgery. *J Neurosurg* 69:687, 1988.

61. Blomstedt GC, Kytta J: Results of a randomized trial of vancomycin prophylaxis in craniotomy. *J Neurosurg* 69:216, 1988.

62. Djindjian M, Lepresle E, Homs JB: Antibiotic prophylaxis during prolonged clean neurosurgery: Results of a randomized double-blind study using oxacillin. *J Neurosurg* 73:383, 1990.

63. Dempsey R, Rapp P, Young B et al: Prophylactic parenteral antibiotics in clean neurosurgical procedures: A review. *J Neurosurg* 69:52, 1988.

64. Haines SJ: Efficacy of antibiotic prophylaxis in clean neurosurgical operations. *Neurosurgery* 24:401, 1989.

65. Shapiro M: Prophylaxis in otolaryngologic surgery and neurosurgery: A critical review. *Rev Infect Dis* 13(Suppl 10):S858, 1991.

66. Fan-Havard P, Nahata MC: Treatment and prevention of infections of cerebrofluid shunts. *Clin Pharm* 6:866, 1987.

67. Rieder MJ, Franch TC, DelMaestro RF et al: The effect of cephalothin prophylaxis on postoperative ventriculoperitoneal shunt infection. *CMAJ* 136:935, 1987.

68. Schmidt K, Gjerns F, Osgaard O et al: Antibiotic prophylaxis in cerebrospinal fluid shunting: A prospective randomized trial in 152 hydrocephalic patients. *Neurosurgery* 17:1, 1985.

69. Polk HC Jr: Antibiotic prophylaxis in surgery of the colon. *South Med J* 70(Suppl):27, 1971.

70. Gorbach SL: Antimicrobial prophylaxis for appendectomy and colorectal surgery. *Rev Infect Dis* 13(Suppl 10):815, 1991.

71. Nichols RL, Condon RE: Preoperative preparation of the colon. *Surg Gynecol Obstet* 132:323, 1971.

72. Nichols RL, Condon RE, Gorbach SL et al: Efficacy of preoperative antimicrobial preparation of the bowel. *Ann Surg* 176:227, 1972.

73. Nichols RL, Broido P, Condon RE et al: Effect of preoperative neomycin-erythromycin intestinal preparation on the incidence of infectious complication following colon surgery. *Ann Surg* 178:453, 1973.

74. Clarke JS, Condon RE, Bartlett JE et al: Preoperative oral antibiotics reduce septic complications of colorectal operations: Results of a prospective, randomized double-blind clinical study. *Ann Surg* 186:251, 1977.

75. Bartlett JG, Condon RE, Gorbach SL et al: Veterans Administration cooperative study on bowel preparation for elective colorectal operations: Impact of oral antibiotic regimen on colonic flora, wound irrigation cultures and bacteriology of septic complications. *Ann Surg* 188:249, 1978.

76. Vargish T, Crawford LC, Stallings RA et al: Randomized prospective evaluation of orally administered antibiotics in operations on the colon. *Surg Gynecol Obstet* 146:193, 1978.

77. Washington JA II, Dearing WH, Judd ES et al: Effect of preoperative antibiotic regimen on development of infection after intestinal surgery: Prospective, randomized, double-blind study. *Ann Surg* 180:562, 1974.

78. Judd ES: Preoperative neomycin-tetracycline preparation of the colon for elective operations. *Surg Clin N Am* 55:1325, 1975.

79. Matheson DM, Arabi L, Baxter-Smith D et al: Randomized multicentre trial of oral bowel preparation and antimicrobials for elective colorectal operations. *Br J Surg* 65:597, 1978.

80. Arabi Y, Dimock R, Burdon DW et al: Influence of bowel preparation and antimicrobials on colonic flora. *Br J Surg* 65:555, 1978.

81. Goldring J, McNaught W, Scott A et al: Prophylactic oral antimicrobial agents in elective colonic surgery. *Lancet* 2:997, 1975.

82. Gillespie E, McNaught W: Prophylactic oral metronidazole in intestinal surgery. *J Antimicrob Chemother* 4(Suppl):29, 1978.

83. Rosenberg IL, Graham NG, Donibal FT et al: Preparation of the intestine in patients undergoing major large bowel surgery, mainly for neoplasms of the colon and rectum. *Br J Surg* 58:266, 1971.

84. Wapnick S, Guinto R, Reizis I et al: Reduction of postoperative infection in elective colon surgery with preoperative administration of kanamycin and erythromycin. *Surgery* 85:315, 1979.

85. Polk LC, Lopez-Mayor JF: Postoperative wound infection: A prospective study of determinant factors and prevention. *Surgery* 66:97, 1969.

86. Stone HH, Hooper CA, Kolb LD et al: Antibiotic prophylaxis in gastric, biliary and colonic surgery. *Ann Surg* 184:443, 1976.

87. Stokes EJ, Waterworth PM, Franks V et al: Short-term routine antibiotic prophylaxis in surgery. *Br J Surg* 61:739, 1974.

88. Lewis RT, Allan CM, Goodall RG et al: Antibiotics in surgery of the colon. *Can J Surg* 21:339, 1978.

89. Condon RE, Bartlett JG, Nichols RL et al: Preoperative prophylactic cephalothin fails to control septic complications of colorectal operations: Results of controlled clinical trial. A Veterans Administration Cooperative Study. *Am J Surg* 137:68, 1979.

90. Crenshaw CA, Gaugles E, Webber CE et al: Cephalothin-tobramycin as a preventive antibiotic combination. *Surg Gynecol Obstet* 147:713, 1978.

91. Lewis RT, Allan CM, Goodall RG et al: Are first-generation cephalosporins effective for antibiotic prophylaxis in elective surgery of the colon? *Can J Surg* 26:504, 1983.

92. Panichi G, Pantosti P, Guinichi G et al: Cephalothin, cefoxitin, or metronidazole in elective colonic surgery? A single-blind randomized trial. *Dis Colon Rectum* 185:783, 1982.

93. The Norwegian Study for Colorectal Surgery: Should antimicrobial prophylaxis in colorectal surgery include agents effective against both anaerobic and aerobic microorganisms? A double-blind study. *Surgery* 97:402, 1985.

94. Kaiser A, Herrington J, Jacobs J et al: Cefoxitin versus erythromycin, neomycin, and cefazolin in colorectal operations: Importance of the duration of the procedure. *Ann Surg* 198:525, 1983.

95. McDonald PJ, Karran SJ: A comparison of intravenous cefoxitin and a combination of gentamicin and metronidazole as prophylaxis in colorectal surgery. *Dis Colon Rectum* 26:661, 1983.

96. Pollack AV, Fromme K, Evans M: The bacteriology of primary wound sepsis in potentially contaminated abdominal operations: The effect of irrigation, povidone-iodine and cephaloridine on the sepsis rate assessed in clinical trial. *Br J Surg* 65:76, 1978.

97. Taylor TV, Walker NS, Masson RC et al: Preoperative intraparietal (intraincisional) cefoxitin in abdominal surgery. *Br J Surg* 69:461, 1982.

98. Dixon JM, Armstrong JP, Duffy SW et al: A randomized prospective trial comparing the value of intravenous and preincisional cefamandole in reducing postoperative sepsis after operations upon the gastrointestinal tract. *Surg Gynecol Obstet* 158:303, 1984.

99. Stone HH: Gastric surgery. *South Med J* 70(Suppl):35, 1977.

100. Lewis RT: Wound infection after gastroduodenal operations: A ten-year review. *Can J Surg* 20:435, 1977.

101. Lewis RT, Allan CM, Goodall RG et al: The discriminate use of antibiotic prophylaxis in gastroduodenal surgery. *Am J Surg* 138:640, 1979.

102. Nichols RL, Smith JW, Webb WR: Efficacy of antibiotic prophylaxis in high-risk gastroduodenal operations. Abstract #627. 20th Interscience Conference in Antimicrobial Agents and Chemotherapy. New Orleans, LA, 1980.

103. Chetlin SH, Elliott DW: Biliary bacteremia. *Arch Surg* 102:303, 1977.

104. Chetlin SH, Elliott DW: Preoperative antibiotics in biliary surgery. *Arch Surg* 107:319, 1973.

105. Keighley MRB, Baddeley RM, Burdon DW et al: A controlled trial of parenteral prophylactic therapy in biliary surgery. *Br J Surg* 62:275, 1975.

106. Keighley MRB: Prevention of wound sepsis in gastrointestinal surgery. *Br J Surg* 2:462, 1978.

107. McLeish AR, Keighley MRB, Bishop HM et al: Selecting patients requiring antibiotics in biliary surgery by immediate gram stains in bile at operation. *Surgery* 81:473, 1977.

108. Elliott DW: Biliary tract surgery. *South Med J* 70:31, 1977.

109. Strachan CJL, Black J, Powis SJA et al: Prophylactic use of cefazolin against wound sepsis after cholecystectomy. *Br Med J* 1:1254, 1977.

110. Morran C, McNaught W, McArdle CS: Prophylactic co-trimoxazole in biliary surgery. *Br Med J* 2:462, 1974.

111. Griffiths DA, Shorey BA, Simpson RA et al: Single-dose preoperative antibiotic prophylaxis in gastrointestinal surgery. *Lancet* 2:325, 1976.

112. Allen JL, Rampone JF, Wheeless CR: Use of a prophylactic antibiotic in elective major gynecologic surgery. *South Med J* 71:251, 1978.

113. Ohm MJ, Galask RP: The effect of antibiotic prophylaxis on patients undergoing total abdominal hysterectomy: I. Effect on morbidity. *Am J Obstet Gynecol* 125:442, 1976.

114. Grossman JH III, Greco TP, Minkin JP et al: Prophylactic antibiotics in gynecologic surgery. *Obstet Gynecol* 53:537, 1979.

115. Crumbleholme WR: Use of prophylactic antibiotics in obstetrics and gynecology. *Clin Obstet Gyn* 31:466, 1988.

116. Polk BF, Tager IB, Shapiro M et al: Randomized clinical trial of perioperative cefazolin in preventing infection after hysterectomy. *Lancet* 1:437, 1980.

117. Ledger WJ, Sweet RL, Headington JT: Prophylactic cephaloridine in the prevention of postoperative infections in premenopausal women undergoing vaginal hysterectomy. *Am J Obstet Gynecol* 115:776, 1973.

118. Mendelson J, Portnoy J, DeSaint VJR et al: Effect of single and multidose cephaloridine prophylaxis on infectious morbidity of vaginal hysterectomy. *Obstet Gynecol* 53:31, 1979.

119. Lett WJ, Ansbacher R, Davison BL et al: Prophylactic antibiotic for women undergoing vaginal hysterectomy. *J Reprod Med* 19:51, 1977.

120. Jennings RH: Prophylactic antibiotics in vaginal and abdominal hysterectomy. *South Med J* 71:251, 1978.

121. Biven MD, Neufeld J, McCarty WD: The prophylactic use of Keflex and Keflin in vaginal hysterectomy morbidity. *Am J Obstet Gynecol* 122:169, 1975.

122. Ohm MJ, Galask RP: The effect of antibiotic prophylaxis on patients undergoing vaginal operations and the effect on morbidity. *Am J Obstet Gynecol* 123:590, 1975.

123. Roberts JM, Homesley HD: Low-dose carbenicillin prophylaxis for vaginal and abdominal hysterectomy. *Obstet Gynecol* 52:83, 1978.

124. Holman JF, McGowan JE, Thompson JD: Perioperative antibiotics in major elective gynecologic surgery. *South Med J* 71:417, 1978.

125. Bolling DR, Plunkett GD: Prophylactic antibiotics for vaginal hysterectomies. *Obstet Gynecol* 41:689, 1973.

126. Matthews DD, Agarwal V, Gordon AM et al: A double-blind trial of single-dose chemoprophylaxis with co-trimoxazole during vaginal hysterectomy and repair. *Br J Obstet Gynecol* 86:737, 1979.

127. Brown EM: Systemic antimicrobial prophylaxis in hysterectomy. *J Antimicrob Chemother* 20:143, 1987.

128. Wong R, Gee C, Ledger W: Prophylactic use of cefazolin in monitored obstetric patients undergoing cesarean section. *Obstet Gynecol* 51:407, 1978.

129. Hawrylyshyn PA, Bernstein P, Papsin FR: Short-term antibiotic prophylaxis in high-risk patients following cesarean section. *Am J Obstet Gynecol* 145:285, 1983.

130. Carlson C, Duff P: Antibiotic prophylaxis for cesarean section; is an extended-spectrum agent necessary? *Obstet Gynecol* 76:343, 1990.

131. Gonzales R, Wright R, Blackard CE: Prophylactic antibiotics in transurethral prostatectomy. *J Urol* 116:203, 1976.

132. Morris MJ, Golavski D, Guinnesa MDG et al: The value of prophylactic antibiotics in transurethral prostatic resection: A controlled trial with observations on the origin of postoperative infection. *Br J Urol* 48:479, 1976.

133. Hills HN, Bultitude MI, Eykyn S: Co-trimoxazole in prevention of bacteriuria after prostatectomy. *Br Med J* 2:498, 1976.

134. Gibbons RP, Stark RA, Correa RJ et al: The prophylactic use and misuse of antibiotics in transurethral prostatectomy. *J Urol* 119:381, 1978.

135. Herr HW: Use of prophylactic antibiotics in the high-risk patient undergoing prostatectomy: Effect on morbidity. *J Urol* 109:686, 1973.

136. Berger SA, Nagar H: Antimicrobial prophylaxis in urology. *J Urol* 120:319, 1978.

137. Chodak GW, Plaut ME: Systemic antibiotics in urologic surgery: A critical review. *J Urol* 121:695, 1979.

138. Ruebush TK II, McConville JH, Calia FH: A double-blind study of trimethoprim-sulfamethoxazole prophylaxis in patients having transrectal needle biopsy of the prostate. *J Urol* 122:492, 1976.

139. Korbel EI, Maher PO: Use of prophylactic antibiotics in urethral instrumentation. *J Urol* 116:744, 1976.

140. Slavis SA, Miller JB, Golji H et al: Comparison of single-dose antibiotic prophylaxis in uncomplicated transurethral resection of the prostate. *J Urol* 147:1303, 1992.

141. Grabe M: Antimicrobial agents in transurethral prostatic resection. *J Urol* 138:245, 1987.

142. Larsen EH, Gasser TC, Madsen PO: Antimicrobial prophylaxis in urologic surgery. *Urol Clin N Am* 13:591, 1986.

143. Weber RS, Callendar DL: Antibiotic prophylaxis in clean-contaminated head and neck oncologic surgery. *Ann Otol Rhinol* 101:16, 1992.

144. Seagle MB, Duberstein LF, Gross CW et al: Efficacy of cefazolin as a prophylactic antibiotic in head and neck surgery. *Otolaryngology* 86:568, 1978.

145. Robbins LT, Byers RM, Cole R et al: Wound prophylaxis with metronidazole in head and neck surgical oncology. *Laryngoscope* 98:803, 1988.

146. Johnson JT, Yu VL: Antibiotic use during major head and neck surgery. *Ann Surg* 207:108, 1988.

147. Johnson JT, Schuller DE, Silver F et al: Antibiotic prophylaxis in high-risk and neck surgery: One-day versus five-day therapy. *Otol Head and Neck Surg* 95:554, 1986.

148. Fee WE, Glenn M, Handen C et al: One day versus two days of prophylactic antibiotics in patients undergoing major head and neck surgery. *Laryngoscope* 94:612, 1984.

45 PREVENTION OF ADVERSE REACTIONS TO RADIOGRAPHIC CONTRAST MEDIA

William H. Matthai, Jr.

Over ten million radiologic procedures requiring iodinated contrast media are performed annually.[1] Depending on the definition used, adverse reactions occur in 5 to 36 percent of patients.[2-9] The majority of these reactions, such as nausea and vomiting, are minor and do not require treatment.[2,4] Most others, e.g., mild urticaria, are often easily managed in the radiology suite by physicians involved in the procedure.[2] Clinically significant reactions occur in less than 0.4 percent of procedures[3-5,10] and include volume overload, contrast-induced renal failure, and anaphylactoid reactions.

RISK FACTORS

Identifying patients with increased risk of contrast-mediated adverse reactions is difficult. Most agree that those with a prior allergic reaction to contrast agents are more likely to experience a subsequent adverse event.[3,5,10-15] Anxiety, nausea, vomiting, and vasomotor phenomena like flushing, tingling, warmth, or burning are common side effects of contrast administration and do not increase the risk of a repeat reaction. Cardiac disease has been identified as another important risk factor in a number of studies of patients undergoing noncardiac angiography.[3,10] In recent studies of contrast agent use in cardiac angiography, patients with advanced cardiac disease or unstable cardiac conditions have the

greatest risk.[6,7] A history of asthma or generalized allergy,[3,5,10] female gender,[6,16] and advanced age have been inconsistently associated with adverse events. These clinical variables are poorly predictive of important adverse reactions because of their high prevalence and the low incidence of reactions. Nevertheless, these clinical data are often used in balancing the overall risk and benefit of a contrast study (see Table 45-1).

VOLUME OVERLOAD

The administration of contrast agents introduces a significant osmotic load resulting in a fluid shift into the intravascular space. Increases in intravascular volume are directly proportional to the volume and osmolality of the contrast agent used.[17-19] Even newer "low osmolality" contrast agents have osmolalities two to three times that of serum. After a bolus injection of contrast material, intravascular volume increases by 3 to 20 percent, resulting in a net change of several hundred milliliters.[18]

Some degree of dyspnea occurs in one to two percent of patients after receiving contrast material,[6,7] and over 50 percent of severe contrast agent reactions are accompanied by dyspnea.[3] While some of these may represent anaphylactoid reactions with bronchospasm or laryngeal edema, most are due to pulmonary congestion from volume overload.[13] Patients who develop such problems are unable to compensate for rapid infusion of volume into the intravascular space and commonly include those with markedly abnormal left ventricular function or baseline intravascular volume overload and those with abnormal renal function. If contrast agent administration cannot be avoided in such patients, volume status should be optimal before the procedure, and a low-osmolality contrast agent should be used in as little volume as possible. If dyspnea develops, appropriate therapy for pulmonary edema should be given. However, the possibility that dyspnea may be a manifestation of an anaphylactoid reaction must always be considered.

TABLE 45-1. Relative Risk of an Adverse Event Following Contrast Agent Administration

Risk Factor	Relative Risk	References
Prior contrast reaction	3.2–6.3	3, 5
Cardiac disease	2.3–5.4	3, 14
Generalized allergies	1.7–2.3	3, 5, 14
Unstable angina	1.2–3.1	6, 7
Female gender	1.0–2.3	3, 6, 9, 14
Age > 60 years	1.0–2.2	2, 3, 6, 14

447

CONTRAST-INDUCED NEPHROPATHY

Acute renal failure following contrast agent administration is one of the major causes of hospital-acquired renal failure. Contrast-induced nephropathy has been variously defined as an increase in the baseline serum creatinine concentration by 25% to 50% or a rise in the baseline level by 1 mg/dl after other causes of acute renal failure have been excluded. The mechanism of contrast-induced nephropathy has not been clearly defined but may involve altered systemic and renal hemodynamics or direct renal injury.[20,21] Preexisting renal insufficiency is probably the most significant predictor of contrast-induced deterioration in renal function.[22-25] Other factors include diabetes mellitus, low cardiac output, intravascular volume depletion, and the volume of contrast media used.[23-26] Of these factors, the volume status of the patient and the volume of contrast material used are the two most amenable to adjustment before the procedure. In patients with baseline renal insufficiency, especially when other risk factors are present, the appropriate radiographic examination most likely to minimize exposure to contrast media should be chosen. Echocardiography can sometimes replace contrast left ventriculography, and magnetic resonance imaging can often serve instead of contrast aortography.

Patients should be adequately but carefully hydrated before a contrast agent is administered. Particular care is required in hydrating patients with elevated serum creatinine levels, and it must not be a reflex reaction. Some with congestive heart failure or renal dysfunction may be unable to tolerate hydration before the procedure as well as the volume load induced by the contrast material. Only patients who are clinically dehydrated require hydration before a contrast study. The role of mannitol or diuretics in preventing contrast-induced nephropathy is unclear, and no recommendation can be made for their use.[23,27,28] Use of low-osmolality contrast agents may reduce the incidence of renal insufficiency but has not been shown to reduce the need for dialysis.[29,30]

The incidence of contrast-induced nephropathy varies depending on the definition used. It is rare in patients with normal renal function.[24,31,32] In those with a baseline serum creatinine level above 1.5 mg/dl and diabetes mellitus, approximately 25 percent develop a 50% increase in serum creatinine concentration.[29] When renal dysfunction occurs, a rise in serum creatinine level is usually evident within 24 to 48 hours and peaks in three to five days. Oliguria is uncommon, and dialysis is required in less than 10 percent of cases.[21] Once contrast-induced nephropathy occurs, no identifiable treatment has been found to alter its course.

ANAPHYLACTOID REACTIONS

Anaphylactoid reactions occur in one to two percent of patients receiving angiographic contrast media,[33] but severe reactions are seen in less than 0.1 percent.[10,13] They are called anaphylactoid because they mimic IgE-mediated anaphylactic reactions, producing varying degrees of urticaria, angioedema, bronchospasm, or hypotension. However, the actual mechanism of these reactions is unknown. They may be due to nonimmunologic activation of the complement system, coagulation cascade or kinin system activation, or to release of histamine.[34,35]

Patients with a history of an anaphylactoid reaction to contrast

media have the highest risk of a subsequent reaction. Repeat reactions are seen in approximately six percent of patients receiving effective premedication.[36-38] This figure may be lower if patients receive both premedication and nonionic contrast agents.[35] Only those with a documented history of such reactions to contrast agents clearly merit special management. A "seafood allergy" should not be considered equivalent to a contrast-agent sensitivity and has not been shown to carry increased risk.

An optimal pretreatment regimen for preventing anaphylactoid reactions to contrast media has not been definitively identified, but corticosteroids and H_1 blockers like diphenhydramine are widely recommended.[35-37] At least two 32-mg doses of methylprednisolone or its equivalent should be administered orally at approximately 12 and 2 hours before contrast agent exposure.[39] A single dose given just prior to injection of contrast material is not protective.[39] Some recommend another dose six hours before the procedure.[36,37] Ephedrine in a dose of 25 mg orally one hour before the procedure,[37] or an H_2 blocker like cimetidine[40] may offer added protection. Because ephedrine is a sympathomimetic agent, it is contraindicated in patients with cardiac disease. A reasonable prophylactic regimen is outlined in Table 45–2. There are no data indicating that use of high-osmolality contrast media with adequate premedication is less safe than using nonionic contrast material. However, many clinicians prefer nonionic contrast media in patients who have had anaphylactoid reactions to contrast agents in the past. Informed consent should always be obtained, and intubation apparatus should be immediately available.

Because prophylactic pretreatment is not effective in all patients, alternative imaging modalities should always be considered in patients with prior contrast reactions. Use of nonionic contrast material may reduce but does not eliminate the risk of a reaction. Moreover, reactions can occur after nonvascular administration of contrast material as in hysterosalpingography[40] or retrograde pyelography,[42] and the patients with increased risk undergoing these procedures should also be pretreated. However, the risk of reactions to contrast following extravascular administration is probably lower than that following intravascular use.[36]

When contrast reactions occur, treatment should be guided by the type and severity of the reaction. Patients who develop anxiety, nausea, vomiting, or vasomotor phenomena require only reassurance and observation. Patients with mild urticaria can be treated with diphenhydramine in a dose of 50 mg intravenously and observed. It is important to follow these patients carefully for development of other anaphylactoid phenomena. Those with major reactions causing hemodynamic or ventilatory compromise with hypotension or bronchospasm should be treated as one would treat anaphylactic shock with volume resuscitation, epinephrine, bronchodilators, oxygen, and ventilatory support as dictated by the

TABLE 45–2. A Pretreatment Regimen for Patients with a History of a Reaction to Contrast Agent Exposure

Prednisone, 40 mg PO 13, 7, and 1 hour before procedure
Diphenhydramine, 50 mg IV 1 hour before procedure
Consider: Ephedrine 25 mg PO 1 hour before procedure (contraindicated in patients with cardiac disease)
Cimetidine 300 mg PO qid (or its equivalent)
Use of nonionic contrast media

severity of the reaction. Most reactions to contrast agents occur during or immediately after administration. Less commonly, reactions may occur several hours after the procedure, but reactions beginning after 24 hours are probably not related to the contrast material.

SUMMARY

1. Iodinated contrast agents may cause minor vasomotor phenomena, volume overload, renal insufficiency, or anaphylactoid reactions that vary in severity.

2. Patients with a history of contrast agent allergy and those with cardiac disease are most likely to have reactions. A history of asthma or generalized allergy, female gender, and advanced age may be associated with adverse reactions. Alternative studies to avoid contrast exposure should be considered in patients with prior contrast reactions.

3. Dyspnea occurs in one to two percent of patients undergoing contrast studies and may indicate volume overload induced by the osmotic load of the contrast material. Patients with baseline volume overload or compromised left ventricular function are most likely to develop pulmonary congestion requiring diuretic therapy. Dyspnea may also be a manifestation of an anaphylactoid reaction.

4. Renal insufficiency following contrast agent administration occurs most often in patients with baseline renal dysfunction. Other risk factors include diabetes mellitus, low cardiac output, intravascular volume depletion, and the use of large volumes of contrast media. Volume-depleted patients only should be carefully hydrated before the procedure. Low-osmolality contrast agents may be associated with a lower incidence of contrast-induced nephropathy, but mannitol and diuretics do not prevent it. There is no specific treatment.

5. Anaphylactoid reactions mimic IgE-mediated anaphylaxis and are manifested by varying degrees of urticaria, angioedema, bronchospasm, and hypotension. Patients with past anaphylactoid reactions to contrast media have the greatest risk, but allergies to seafood are not predictive. If iodinated contrast cannot be avoided, such patients should receive prophylactic pretreatment with corticosteroids and antihistamines. Consideration should be given to use of nonionic contrast media, ephedrine, and H_2 blockers.

REFERENCES

1. Jacobson PD, Rosenquist CJ: The introduction of low-osmolar contrast agents in radiology: Medical, economic, legal, and public policy issues. *JAMA* 260:1586, 1988.
2. Shehadi WH, Toniolo G: Adverse reactions to contrast media. *Radiology* 137:299, 1980.
3. Katayama H, Kozuika T, Takashima T et al: Adverse reactions to contrast media: Ionic versus nonionic: A report from the Japanese Committee on the Safety of Contrast Media. *Radiology* 175:621, 1990.
4. Palmer FJ: The RACR survey of intravenous contrast media reactions. *Australas Radiol* 32:426, 1988.
5. Wolf GL, Mishkin MM, Roux SG et al: Comparison of the rates of adverse drug reactions. *Invest Radiol* 26:404, 1991.
6. Steinberg EP, Moore RD, Powe NR et al: Safety and cost effectiveness of high-osmolality as compared with low-osmolality contrast material in patients undergoing cardiac angiography. *N Engl J Med* 326:425, 1992.
7. Barrett BJ, Parfrey PS, Vavasour HM et al: A comparison of nonionic, low-osmolality radiocontrast agents with ionic, high-osmolality agents during cardiac catheterization. *N Engl J Med* 326:431, 1992.
8. Matthai WH, Krol JM, Kussmaul WG et al: A randomized double-blind trial of iohexol versus diatrizoate in cardiac angiography. *Circulation* 84:II-333, 1991.
9. Powe NR, Steinberg EP, Erikson JE et al: Contrast medium–induced adverse reactions: Economic outcome. *Radiology* 169:163, 1988.
10. Ansell G, Tweedie MCK, West CR et al: The current status of reactions to intravenous contrast media. *Invest Radiol* 15:S32, 1980.
11. Brinker JA: Selection of a contrast agent in the cardiac catheterization laboratory. *Am J Cardiol* 66:26F, 1990.
12. Matthai WH, Hirshfeld JW: Choice of contrast agents for cardiac angiography: Review and recommendations based on clinically important distinctions. *Cathet Cardiovasc Diagn* 22:278, 1991.
13. Hirshfeld JW, Kussmaul WG, DiBattiste PD et al: The safety of cardiac angiography with conventional ionic contrast agents. *Am J Cardiol* 66:355, 1990.
14. Lawrence V, Matthai WH, Hartmaier S: Comparative safety of high-osmolality and low-osmolality radiographic contrast agents: Report of a multidisciplinary working group. *Invest Radiol* 27:2, 1992.
15. Shehadi WH: Contrast media adverse reactions: Occurrence, recurrence, and distribution patterns. *Radiology* 143:11, 1982.
16. Johnson LW, Lozner EC, Johnson S et al: Complications of cardiac catheterization: Coronary arteriography 1984–1987: A report of registry of the Society for Cardiac Angiography and Interventions. I. Results and complications. *Cathet and Cardiovasc Diagn* 17:5, 1989.
17. Hine AL, Lui D, Dawson P: Contrast media osmolality and plasma volume changes. *Acta Radiol Diagn* 26:753, 1985.
18. Iseri LT, Kaplan MA, Evans MJ et al: Effect of concentrated contrast media during angiography on plasma volume and plasma osmolality. *Am Heart J* 69:154, 1965.
19. Barbe R, Kirkorian G, Amiel M: Effects of contrast media on circulating blood volume. *Acta Radiol Diagn* 21:495, 1980.
20. Byrd L, Sherman RL: Radiocontrast-induced acute renal failure: A clinical and pathophysiologic review. *Medicine* (Baltimore) 58:270, 1979.
21. Porter GA: Experimental contrast-associated nephropathy and its clinical implications. *Am J Cardiol* 66:18F, 1990.
22. Schwab SJ, Hlatky MA, Pieper KS et al: Contrast nephrotoxicity: A randomized controlled trial of a nonionic and an ionic radiographic contrast agent. *N Engl J Med* 320:149, 1989.
23. Moore RD, Steinberg EP, Powe NR: Nephrotoxicity of high-osmolality versus low-osmolality contrast media: Randomized clinical trial. *Radiology* 182:649, 1992.
24. Gomes AS, Baker JD, Martin-Paredero V et al: Acute renal dysfunction after arteriography. *Am J Radiol* 145:1249, 1985.
25. Taliercio CP, Vlietstra RE, Fisher LD et al: Risks for renal dysfunction with cardiac angiography. *Ann Int Med* 104:501, 1986.
26. Eisenberg RL, Bank WO, Hedgock MW: Renal failure after major angiography can be avoided with hydration. *Am J Radiol* 136:859, 1981.
27. Weisberg LS, Kurnik PB, Kurnik BR: Renal vasodilator drugs and the risk of radiocontrast nephropathy (RCN). *J Am Soc Nephrol* 3:731, 1992.
28. Rudnick MR, Goldfarb S, Murphy MJ: Mannitol and other prophylactic regimens in contrast media–induced acute renal failure. *Coron Art Dis* 2:1047, 1991.
29. Hill JA, Winniford M, Van Fossen DB et al: Nephrotoxicity following cardiac angiography: A randomized double-blind multicenter trial of ionic and nonionic contrast media in 1194 patients. *Circulation* 84:II-333, 1991.

30. Harris KG, Smith TP, Cragg AH: Nephrotoxicity from contrast material in renal insufficiency: Ionic versus nonionic agents. *Radiology* 179:849, 1991.

31. Miller DL, Chang R, Wells WT et al: Intravascular contrast media: Effect of dose on renal function. *Radiology* 167:607, 1988.

32. Parfrey PS, Griffiths SM, Barrett BJ et al: Contrast material-induced renal failure in patients with diabetes mellitus, renal insufficiency, or both. *N Engl J Med* 320:143, 1989.

33. Witten DM, Hirsch FD, Hartman GW: Acute reactions to urographic contrast medium: Incidence, clinical characteristics and relationship to history of hypersensitivity states. *Am J Radiol* 119:832, 1973.

34. Greenberger PA, Patterson R: Adverse reactions to radiocontrast media. *Prog Cardiovasc Dis* 21:239, 1988.

35. Lieberman P: Anaphylactoid reactions to radiocontrast material. *Ann Allergy* 67:91, 1991.

36. Greenberger PA, Patterson R, Kelly J et al: Administration of radiographic contrast media in high-risk patients. *Invest Radiol* 15:S40, 1980.

37. Greenberger PA, Patterson R, Radin RC: Two pretreatment regimens for high-risk patients receiving radiographic contrast media. *J Allergy Clin Immunol* 74:540, 1984.

38. Siegle RL, Halvorsen RA, Dillon J et al: The use of iohexol in patients with previous reactions to ionic contrast material: A multicenter clinical trial. *Invest Radiol* 26:411, 1991.

39. Ring J, Rothenberger KH, Clauss W: Prevention of anaphylactoid reactions after radiographic contrast media infusion by combined H_1 and H_2 receptor antagonists: Results of a prospective controlled trial. *Int Arch Allergy Appl Immunol* 78:9, 1985.

40. Lasser EC, Berry CC, Talner LB et al: Pretreatment with corticosteroids to alleviate reactions to intravenous contrast material. *N Engl J Med* 317:845, 1987.

41. Elias J: Systemic reaction to radiocontrast media during hysterosalpingography. *J Allergy Clin Immunol* 66:242, 1979.

42. Johenning PW: Reactions to contrast material during retrograde pyelography. *Urology* 16:442, 1980.

43. McCullough M, Davies P, Richardson R: A large trial of intravenous Conray 325 and Niopam 300 to assess immediate and delayed reactions. *Br J Radiol* 62:260, 1989.

46 PATHOGENESIS AND PREVENTION OF STRESS-RELATED MUCOSAL DISEASE

James C. Reynolds

When erosive gastritis occurs in the setting of the stress associated with surgery or life-threatening illness, it is called stress-related mucosal disease (SRMD). The term stress-related is used to contrast it with acute gastritis due to alcohol, ingestion of corrosive materials, or bile reflux and with various forms of chronic gastritis. SRMD most commonly occurs in patients suffering from severe trauma, hemorrhage, shock, sepsis, extensive burns, or multiple system organ failure.[1-4] It is also called stress erosive gastritis and, in its more advanced stages, acute hemorrhagic gastritis and stress bleeding. This chapter reviews the pathophysiology, clinical presentation, prevention, and treatment of stress-related mucosal disease. Although most prevalent in patients in surgical intensive care units, SRMD may also occur in medical and preoperative surgical patients. Distinctions between SRMD and other forms of peptic ulcer disease (PUD) are listed in Table 46–1. Epigastric pain and perforations occur uncommonly in SRMD, and the first clinical sign of SRMD is usually bleeding. More apparent bleeding occurs in 20 percent of patients, while hemodynamically significant bleeding is seen in five to seven percent.[5] In the majority of patients, bleeding is clinically insignificant. However, when serious bleeding does occur, short-term mortality exceeds 50 percent.[6]

The importance of gastric mucosal injury in patients who are stressed by serious injuries, central nervous system trauma, or burns has been recognized for years in the surgical literature. Early autopsy studies of intensive care patients who developed massive

TABLE 46–1. Distinctions Between Stress-Related Mucosal Disease and Peptic Ulcer Disease

	SRMD	PUD
Clinical Presentation		
Symptoms of pain	Uncommon	Common
Rapidity of bleeding	Slow continuous bleeding	Bleeding is phasic and rapid
Mortality associated with major bleeding episode	> 50%	7–35%
Incidence of perforation	Very rare	1–2%
Endoscopic Appearance		
Depth	Superficial	Superficial to deep
Number	Multiple	Usually solitary
Location	Acid secretory mucosa	Nonacid-secreting mucosa (antrum and duodenum)
Bleeding appearance	Diffuse mucosal oozing	Brisk bleeding from ulcer
Pathophysiology		
Importance of previous ulcer history	Unrelated	Common
Importance of concurrent illnesses on outcome	Major determinant	Limited importance unless patient is bleeding
Importance of *H. Pylori*	Not important	Found in most patients

TABLE 46–2. The Incidence of SRMD in ICU Patients

Extensive trauma	90–100%
Severe head injury	90–100%
Septic patients	100%
Thermal burns	86%
Medical intensive care unit	75%

gastrointestinal bleeding led to descriptions of Cushing's and Curling's ulcers. Later widespread use of endoscopy showed that, unless treated prophylactically, up to 100 percent of patients undergoing central nervous system surgery or trauma,[7] and 75 percent admitted to medical intensive care units,[8] have the typical endoscopic findings of stress-related mucosal disease (see Table 46–2). The incidence of SRMD is directly related to the severity of the underlying disease,[2] and mucosal lesions dramatically improve once it resolves. Increased recognition of this problem and intensive investigation has led to effective prophylactic therapy that prevents the development of lesions and bleeding in a majority of patients.[5] Such therapy can save patients from life-threatening hemorrhagic gastritis which is often refractory to medical or surgical therapy.[6]

CLINICAL, ENDOSCOPIC, AND HISTOLOGIC FEATURES

Several features distinguish SRMD from chronic peptic ulcer disease (see Table 46–1). SRMD occurs in the setting of trauma, shock, burns, sepsis, and multi-organ failure in patients with no previous history of ulcer disease. Stress lesions tend to be multiple while duodenal or gastric ulcers are usually one or two in number. The diffuse mucosal abnormality of SRMD can involve large areas of the stomach. It can be especially marked in the acid-secreting areas of the stomach in contrast to peptic ulcers that occur in the nonacid-secreting mucosa of the gastric antrum and duodenum.[6] SRMD is a superficial mucosal lesion involving the upper half of the gastric glands unlike peptic ulcers which can penetrate through the muscularis propria. Perforations occur in one to two percent of patients with gastric and duodenal ulcers but are distinctly uncommon in SRMD except in patients with severe burns.[9] Bleeding in SRMD is from venous capillaries, while peptic ulcers involve larger vessels.

The use of endoscopy has led to a clearer understanding of the natural history of SRMD. The outcome of patients with stress-related mucosal disease depends primarily on the outcome of their underlying disease. In patients who are not given prophylactic treatment, the onset of clinically significant bleeding heralds a dismal prognosis.[10] However, in those who do well, the mucosal injury is repaired without the sequelae of peptic ulcer disease. Since the lesions are superficial, fibrosis and scarring with resultant deformity or obstruction of the lumen are rarely seen. In most patients, SRMD is an acute self-limited condition while other forms of peptic ulcers are chronic and recurrent.

Upper gastrointestinal bleeding in the postoperative patient may be the result of SRMD in the gastric fundus or peptic ulcer disease in the esophagus, stomach, or duodenum.[1] Due to the patient's tenuous clinical status, radiographic evaluation is seldom possible and may miss the superficial ulcerations that characterize SRMD. Endoscopy provides direct visualization of the mucosa and can be performed rapidly, easily, and safely at the bedside. With good preparation, the diagnosis can be made with accuracy in 95 percent of cases.[11] If focal bleeding sites are seen, therapeutic heater probes or bicap can be used to cauterize the bleeding vessels.

Histologically, the lesions of SRMD are characterized by superficial damage with hemorrhage throughout a wide distribution of the stomach but with little penetration into the deeper submucosa or muscularis propria. The typical lesion is 0.5 to 2.0 mm in depth with a diameter that varies as the lesion progresses from focal 1 to 2 mm ulcers to confluent areas of 20 to 25 mm. Operative pathologic specimens reveal edema, microvascular congestion, and hemorrhage throughout the lamina propria. There is epithelial cell necrosis and mucosal sloughing down to the muscularis mucosa. Thrombosed vessels are not seen, and there is a surprising paucity of inflammatory cell reaction.[6]

PATHOPHYSIOLOGY: AN IMBALANCE BETWEEN AGGRESSIVE AND PROTECTIVE FACTORS

The mechanisms underlying the development of stress-related mucosal disease are incompletely understood. As in all forms of peptic ulcer disease, ulceration is the result of imbalance between mucosal damage induced by intraluminal contents and decrease in homeostatic protective factors. Strategies to prevent and treat stress-related mucosal disease attempt to restore the balance between these aggressive and protective factors.

Aggressive Factors

Factors that damage the mucosa of the upper gastrointestinal tract have been termed aggressive. They may be intrinsic and secreted by the upper intestinal tract or extrinsic and ingested by the patient. Intrinsic aggressive factors include acid, pepsin, and bile salts. Extrinsic factors include alcohol, aspirin, nonsteroidal anti-inflammatory drugs (NSAID's), chemotherapeutic agents, radiation, and trauma from nasogastric tubes. Aggressive factors may interact synergistically to produce more damage than they would alone. For example, damage from pepsin is enhanced when the enzyme is activated by sufficient hydrochloric acid to lower the pH below 4. Potentiation of damage can also result from enhanced back-diffusion of hydrogen ions in the presence of bile, pepsin, alcohol, and NSAID's.

Hydrochloric Acid

Acid is required in the pathogenesis of all forms of peptic ulcer disease. When acid is sufficiently suppressed, healing results in nearly all forms of the disease.[11,12] Patients with the highest rates of acid secretion are most likely to develop severe and intractable ulcerations. Those undergoing neurosurgery, those who have sustained head trauma, and those with Zollinger-Ellison syndrome are the most likely to develop severe and intractable ulcerations. The concept of "no acid, no ulcer," developed at the turn of the century, remains true today. On the other hand, bile reflux, alcohol, and a variety of caustic medications can induce mucosal damage. In patients with known achlorhydria who developed ulceration and upper-intestinal bleeding, malignancy is usually the cause.

Acid-induced damage to the underlying mucosa progresses as

hydrogen ions diffuse across the mucosa into the submucosa.[13] Underlying cellular structures including neurons, blood vessels, and inflammatory cells are highly susceptible to injury. The response to injury initiates a cascade of events that paradoxically act to promote further acid secretion. Neural injury causes release of neurotransmitters like acetylcholine. Serum proteins and blood diffuse into the lumen where intraluminal peptidases reduce them to amino acids which stimulate further acid secretion. Activation of intestinal inflammatory cells leads to release of vasoactive substances like histamine that directly stimulate parietal cell function. Davenport's original proposal that "back-diffusion of acid" is important in the evolution of most forms of peptic ulcer disease has now been widely accepted.[14] Cushing first discovered that accidental trauma or surgery on the central nervous system increases acid secretion and the incidence of peptic ulcer disease more than in healthy controls or in patients with similar postoperative "stress" from abdominal surgery.[15,16] The mechanism of ulcer disease in these patients is an increase in acid secretion related to enhanced vagal tone.[17]

While acid is the permissive factor in all patients with stress-related mucosal disease, not all patients with SRMD secrete excessive amounts of acid.[18] In fact, many patients with peptic ulcer disease, even those with duodenal ulcer, have maximal rates of acid secretion that are similar to or less than those seen in healthy controls. In those with benign gastric ulcers, peak acid secretion is even less than that seen in the normal controls. Therefore, in most cases acid secretion alone is insufficient to cause mucosal damage. One exception to this is the acid hypersecretion resulting from a gastrin-secreting tumor in the Zollinger-Ellison syndrome.

Other Aggressive Factors

Pepsin secreted from the chief cells of the antral mucosa is a potent proteolytic enzyme. In the presence of sufficient hydrochloric acid to activate pepsinogen to form pepsin, damage to exposed tissue is considerably enhanced. In addition, the potent enzymes and amphophilic bile salts secreted into the duodenum from the sphincter of Oddi can have a caustic effect on gastric and esophageal mucosa.[19] The damaging effect of bile is most noticeable in the presence of motility disorders or a gastroenterostomy. Bile salt conjugates can disrupt mucosal barriers, and lithocholic acid is the most damaging. Proteolytic enzymes, alkali, lysolecithin, and lipases also contribute to the caustic nature of bile. Duodenogastric reflux of pancreatic secretions and bile occur commonly in patients with postoperative ileus or impaired motility and in those who have undergone a gastrojejunostomy.

Protective Factors

Davenport and others found it difficult to demonstrate back-diffusion of hydrogen ions in intact mucosa. The fact that the stomach, distal esophagus, and proximal duodenum are exposed to high concentrations of acid daily in individuals without ulcers suggests that effective defensive factors must be in place. The pathophysiology of SRMD in most patients therefore involves multifactorial impairment of the mucosal defense systems in the presence of aggressive factors like acid.

The study of burn patients in surgical intensive care units has provided important clues about the mechanisms of mucosal ulceration. Despite the clear relationship between severity of burn injury and risk of peptic ulcer disease, there is an inverse relationship between the extent of surface burn and the rate of acid secretion.[18] Thus, while acid is necessary for the development of ulcer diseases and medications that block acid secretion can prevent them, mucosal damage must not be exclusively due to increased acid secretion. Burn patients under stress must develop so-called Curling's ulcers because of abnormalities in normal mucosal defense mechanisms.

Mucosal protective factors include mucus and bicarbonate secretion, prostaglandin synthesis, mucosal blood flow, and cell turnover. Bicarbonate and mucus combine to form a protective barrier that serves as the first line of defense against caustic substances in the lumen. Surface epithelial cells in the stomach are covered by mucus, and the pH of this "mucus blanket" is maintained in the neutral range by the secretion of bicarbonate. If the mucus becomes depolymerized, pepsin and other proteolytic enzymes can then degrade the mucus molecules, decrease their ability to retard diffusion of hydrogen ions into the mucosal surface, and facilitate diffusion of bicarbonate ions out toward the lumen. Epithelium cells lining the stomach are renewed every three to four days. When the rate of damage to mucosal cells exceeds the rate of renewal, ulceration develops.[20] Prostaglandins, particularly E_2 and $F_{2\alpha}$, enhance mucus and bicarbonate secretion and the reepithelialization process.[21,22] Mucosal damage has been documented in studies showing impairment of mucin secretion by bile salts and the bacterium *Helicobacter pylori*. Depolymerization of mucus underlies the development of some forms of peptic ulcers, particularly gastric ulcers.

The defensive properties of the epithelium require high blood flow to maintain oxygenation and nutrition. In shock and other low-flow states, mesenteric blood flow is shunted to the systemic circulation to maintain adequate perfusion pressure. This in turn reduces the ability of the gastric epithelium to undergo the active metabolic processes necessary for mucus and bicarbonate secretion, cell turnover, and maintenance of the mucosal ionic pumps that maintain mucosal integrity. Shunting may be severe enough to cause cellular necrosis and subsequent SRMD and acute hemorrhagic gastritis.[23] SRMD may be the result of impairment of a variety of defensive factors, but in most patients it is initiated by the reduction of mesenteric blood flow.

In summary, in SRMD the imbalance between excessive acid and an impaired mucosal barrier lies somewhere between the two etiologic extremes represented by Cushing's and Curling's ulcers. In patients with central nervous system surgery or trauma who develop Cushing's ulcers, and in those with Zollinger-Ellison syndrome, hypersecretion of acid is the principal pathophysiological abnormality. In those with severe burns who develop Curling's ulcerations or ulcers in the upper part of the stomach, a decrease in the integrity of the mucosal barrier is the major etiologic mechanism. The mechanisms of injury to the upper intestinal tract in most other patients are the result of the increased influence of aggressive factors and the decreased role of protective factors.

MANAGEMENT

The management of SRMD involves prevention, medical therapy, and surgery. Medical treatment of established SRMD is no different from prophylactic therapy except for the need to avoid further progression of the disease.[24] In all three modalities, control of the primary underlying disease process is critical. All efforts should be made to eliminate infection, support cardiac function, and enhance oxygenation. It is this emphasis that most influences prognosis and survival.

Medical Approaches to the Prevention and Treatment of SRMD

The most effective management of SRMD is prevention. Once hemodynamically significant bleeding has begun, chances of survival are less than 50 percent.[6] Prevention begins with recognition of patients with a high risk of developing SRMD. Nasogastric suction reduces the volume of gastric contents but will have no effect on pH.[25] Gastric mucosal damage by acid can be reduced by neutralizing intraluminal acid or by inhibiting its secretion. While several approaches have been shown to be effective,[26,27] no prophylactic regimen has been formally approved by the Food and Drug Administration. Nevertheless, the standard of practice at present is to give severely and acutely ill patients preventive therapy with one of the commonly used regimens listed in Table 46–3.

Treatment should not be given haphazardly to all postoperative patients or all patients admitted to an intensive care unit. While nearly all patients with extensive trauma and serious burns develop SRMD, those in cardiac intensive care units are affected less frequently (see Table 46–2). The probability of developing SRMD is proportional to the severity of the underlying disease, and factors associated with an increased risk of mucosal injury are listed in Table 46–4.[5] A greater number of risk factors increases the likelihood of developing ulceration.[5] These patients are more often the least likely to tolerate significant gastrointestinal bleeding without developing cardiac or respiratory instability.

Neutralization of acid by antacids or reduction of acid secretion with type 2 histamine receptor antagonists (H$_2$ antagonists) significantly reduces the risk of macroscopic gastritis, gross and microscopic bleeding, and mortality associated with SRMD.[5,11] When clinically significant bleeding is used as an endpoint, intermittent administrations of intravenous H$_2$ antagonists or antacids through a nasogastric tube are equally effective.[28]

TABLE 46–4. Factors Associated with an Increased Risk of SRMD

Shock
Sepsis
Severe trauma
Extensive burns (> 25% surface area)
Coagulopathy
Congestive heart failure
Myocardial infarction
Acute renal failure (Creatinine > 3.0)
Ventilatory assistance for > 24 hours
Central nervous system injury
Steroid administration
Hepatic dysfunction (Bilirubin > 5.0)

Antacids

Nasogastric administration of antacids was the first therapy shown to be effective in reducing the risk of SRMD.[29–31] Three mechanisms of action have been proposed. The most important is the neutralization or reduction of intraluminal H$^+$ ions available to diffuse across damaged or functionally impaired gastric mucosa. Acid secretion itself is not affected by antacid administration, and there is a net increase of one HCO^{3-} ion in the mucosa and submucosa for each H$^+$ ion secreted. Antacids may therefore indirectly produce a relatively alkaline environment in the submucosa. This so-called "alkaline tide" can neutralize H$^+$ ions that may reach the mucosa or submucosa through back-diffusion. Antacids may also serve to enhance mucosal defense factors by other as yet unidentified mechanisms.

To be effective, enough antacid must be given to increase gastric pH above 4 consistently. At this pH, pepsin is inactivated. Other studies suggest that raising the intraluminal pH to as near neutral as possible may have additional benefit. Clotting factors are activated at a pH of 6, and pepsin is irreversibly inactivated at a pH of 8. To achieve consistent and effective neutralization of acid, the dose of antacid must be individualized. The pH of gastric contents should be monitored throughout the day to be certain that adequate neutralization is maintained. This may require from 30 to 120 ml of antacid every two hours around the clock. Effective antacid therapy requires a well-functioning nasogastric tube and frequent attention by nursing staff.

Antacids have no effect on the action of intravenously administered drugs but may have significant side effects, particularly when administered in large doses. Diarrhea, constipation, nausea, and electrolyte disturbances are not uncommon. Administration of antacids in large volumes should be avoided in patients with recent intestinal anastamosis or evidence of functional or mechanical obstruction and in those in whom gastroesophageal reflux or aspiration is a concern. Since antacids adhere to a variety of medications, concurrent administration of such agents as digoxin, tetracycline, erythromycin, and ketoconazole should be avoided.

The risk of nosocomial pneumonia may be increased in patients receiving increased intragastric volume, particularly in those who are mechanically ventilated.[32] Antacids allow bacteria in the oral cavity to colonize areas of the upper gastrointestinal tract normally kept sterile by intraluminal acid. Antacids do not affect the vol-

TABLE 46–3. Medical Regimens That Are Commonly Used to Reduce the Incidence of SRMD

Intraluminal Treatment Regimen	
Sucralfate	1.0 grams q 6 hours
Antacids	30–120 ml q 2 hours
Intravenous Treatment Regimen	
Bolus Therapy	
Cimetidine	300 mg q 6 hours
Ranitidine	50 mg q 6 or q 8 hours
Famotidine	20 mg q 12 hours
Omeprazole	20 mg q day
Continuous Infusion	
Cimetidine	1000–1200 mg/24 hours
Ranitidine	200–300 mg/24 hours
Famotidine	50 mg/24 hours

ume of gastric secretions but do significantly increase the total volume of gastric contents when the nasogastric tube is clamped immediately after administration. The nasogastric tube itself may impair the competence of the upper and lower esophageal sphincters, particularly when frequent manipulation of the tube is necessary. These risks must be considered when large volumes of antacid are required to achieve an adequate pH.

H₂ Antagonists

Extensive study of H_2 antagonists in the treatment of SRMD has consistently shown them to be beneficial.[26] No other therapy is currently more effective in the prevention of bleeding from SRMD.[27] H_2 antagonists reduce both the volume and free hydrogen ion concentration of gastric secretions.

H_2 antagonists may be administered intermittently or in a continuous infusion. It is essential to maintain the intraluminal pH above 4 and preferably higher. When bolus dosing of cimetidine was compared to continuous infusion, the latter method was more effective in consistently maintaining the pH above 4.[33] Moreover, in most patients continuous infusion usually maintains the pH above 6.[34] Some H_2 antagonists can be administered continuously by adding them to intravenous alimentation solutions, but most patients require a separate dedicated line. It has not been established whether continuous infusion is more effective than intermittent administration of long-acting H_2 antagonists like famotidine.

H_2 receptor antagonists are generally well tolerated, but adverse effects have been reported with all of them. Adverse effects can be dose- or clearance-dependent, idiosyncratic, pH-dependent, or due to interactions with other drugs. Dose- or clearance-dependent side effects occur with high doses of relatively weak H_2 receptor antagonists or when hepatic or renal clearance mechanisms are impaired. These side effects, including altered mental status, gynecomastia, and impotence, have been reported most often with cimetidine and less frequently with more potent H_2 antagonists like ranitidine and famotidine. Altered mental status is the most important effect in acutely ill patients, particularly in elderly patients with renal or hepatic dysfunction. Adjustment of the dose reduces the incidence of these side effects.

Idiosyncratic side effects occur very rarely, in fewer than one in 10,000 patients treated, and are unpredictable. No animal models are available to elucidate their mechanism. Idiosyncratic side effects include hepatitis and leukopenia.

Nosocomial pneumonia has also been reported in patients in intensive care units treated with H_2 antagonists because of their effect in reducing intragastric acidity. However, in one study intermittent administration of intravenous H_2 antagonists was associated with fewer episodes of nosocomial pneumonia than either antacids or sucralfate.[35] This may be due to the fact that H_2 antagonists reduce gastric volume as well as acid production. The comparative effects of continuous infusion of H_2 antagonists on the incidence of nosocomial pneumonia is unclear.

Most drug-drug interactions with H_2 antagonists cause pharmacokinetic effects with no clinical significance.[36] Drugs metabolized by the cytochrome P-450 mixed-function oxidase system in the liver may be cleared less effectively in the presence of cimetidine or, to a lesser extent, ranitidine. Attention must therefore be given to the concurrent administration of H_2 antagonists with agents that have a narrow therapeutic window, particularly coumadin, phenytoin, lidocaine, theophylline, and some benzodiazepines like diaze-

pam. Famotidine and nizatidine do not interact with this enzyme system and have the least potential to influence elimination of other medications.

Proton Pump Inhibitors

Proton pump inhibitors like omeprazole are the most potent inhibitors of acid secretion. A single daily dose completely blocks acid secretion through inhibition of the K^+H^+ ATPase enzyme involved in acid secretion. Although few comparative studies are available, omeprazole is likely to be at least as effective as other regimens in reducing the incidence of SRMD.

Cytoprotective Agents

The integrity of mucosal cellular defense mechanisms can be enhanced by both specific and nonspecific interventions. Agents that enhance these mechanisms without affecting intraluminal pH are called cytoprotective agents. Sucralfate, the prototypic cytoprotective agent, has been shown to reduce the incidence of gross mucosal damage in hospitalized patients in intensive care units.[37,38] It has a unique structure composed of an aluminum salt and sucrose octasulfate. It works intraluminally through mucosal binding and has a particular affinity for damaged mucosa.

Sucralfate is safe and has little or no potential for intravascular drug-drug interactions. Less than 5% of orally administered sucralfate is absorbed. The aluminum moiety is not essential for its function but may induce constipation and bind other orally administered medications.

Other Measures to Enhance Mucosal Defense

Nonspecific measures aimed at alleviating patient stress may be extremely important. Improving blood pressure, reversing shock, and eliminating sepsis improve mesenteric blood flow. Nutritional support provides essential nutrients to support the continuous mucosal epithelialization process. Improved oxygenation supports the intense metabolic processes that underlie mucosal defense.

In addition to reducing acid secretion, H_2 antagonists enhance several mucosal defense factors, although the significance of this contribution remains unclear. Aluminum-containing antacids may also exert a cytoprotective effect that enhances healing to a greater extent than would be expected from their ability to neutralize acid alone.

Prostaglandin E_2 analogues enhance mucosal defense in laboratory animals. However, in currently recommended doses, available prostaglandin analogues enhance ulcer healing by inhibiting acid. There is little evidence that they are effective in preventing stress-induced gastritis.

Surgical Treatment of SRMD

While prophylactic medical therapy is usually effective, diffuse bleeding from well-established SRMD may continue unabated.[39] When bleeding exceeds four to five units per day despite maximal medical treatment, surgery should be considered. The only intervention that will definitely stop massive bleeding from acute erosive gastritis is total gastrectomy.[40] In severely ill patients, the mortality rate of the procedure approaches 100 percent.[41,42] Less extensive procedures have been attempted with variable success, but all are limited by the risk of recurrent bleeding and high operative mortality.

SUMMARY

1. Stress-related gastric mucosal injury is seen in 80 to 100 percent of patients admitted to surgical and trauma intensive care units. Once massive bleeding occurs, the mortality rate approaches 50 percent, and medical and surgical treatments have limited efficacy.

2. Risk factors in the development of SRMD include severe trauma, burns, central nervous system surgery, and multiorgan failure.

3. The best treatment of SRMD is prevention, including aggressive treatment of the underlying disease and prophylactic antacids and/or H_2 antagonists in large enough doses to maintain the intraluminal pH consistently above 4.

4. The cytoprotective agent sucralfate is an alternative therapy. Surgery has a limited role in patients with severe bleeding.

Acknowledgments:

The author would like to acknowledge the expert technical assistance of Kym Hepworth and Jonathan Taylor in the production of this chapter.

REFERENCES

1. Brown T, Davidson P, Larson G: Acute gastritis occurring within 24 hours of severe head injury. *Gastrointest Endosc* 35:37–40, 1989.
2. Le Gall JR, Mignon FC, Rapin M et al: Acute gastroduodenal lesions related to severe sepsis. *Surg Gynecol Obstet* 142:377–380, 1976.
3. Czaja AJ, McAlhany JC, Pruin BA: Acute gastroduodenal disease after thermal injury. *N Engl J Med* 291:925–929, 1974.
4. Schuster DP, Rowley H, Feinstein S et al: Prospective evaluation of the risk of upper gastrointestinal bleeding after admission to a medical intensive care unit. *Am J Med* 76:623–630, 1984.
5. Zinner MJ, Zuidema GD, Smith PL et al: The prevention of upper gastrointestinal tract bleeding in patients in an intensive care unit. *Surg Gynecol Obstet* 153:214–220, 1981.
6. Lucas CE, Sugawa C, Riddle J et al: Natural history and surgical dilemma of "stress" gastric bleeding. *Arch Surg* 102:266–273, 1971.
7. Larson G, Koch S, O'Dorisio B et al: Gastric response to severe head injury. *Am J Surg* 147:97–105, 1984.
8. Peura DA, Johnson LF: Cimetidine for prevention and treatment of gastroduodenal mucosal lesions in patients in an intensive care unit. *Ann Int Med* 103:173–177, 1985.
9. Pruitt BA, Goodwin CW: Stress ulcer disease in the burned patient. *World J Surg* 5:209, 1981.
10. Klein M, Ennis F, Sherlock P et al: Stress erosions: A major cause of gastrointestinal hemorrhage in patients with malignant disease. *Dig Dis* 18:167–173, 1973.
11. Sugawa C, Werner M, Hayes D et al: Early endoscopy: A guide to therapy for acute hemorrhage in the upper gastrointestinal tract. *Arch Surg* 107:133–137, 1973.
12. McAlhany Jr JC, Czaja A, Pruitt Jr B: Antacid control of complica-

tions from acute gastroduodenal disease after burns. *J Trauma* 16:645–647, 1976.
13. Skillman J, Gould SA, Chung RS et al: The gastric mucosal barrier: Clinical and experimental studies in critically ill and normal man, and in the rabbit. *Ann Surg* 172:564–582, 1976.
14. Davenport HW: Is the apparent hyposecretion of acid by patients with gastric ulcer a consequence of a broken barrier to diffusion of hydrogen ions into the gastric mucosa? *Gut* 6:513, 1965.
15. Gordon MJ, Skillman JJ, Zervas NT et al: Divergent nature of gastric mucosal permeability and gastric acid secretion in sick patients with general surgical and neurosurgical disease. *Ann Surg* 178:285–290, 1973.
16. Cushing H: Peptic ulcers and the interbrain. *Surg Gynecol Obstet* 55:1, 1932.
17. Bowen JC, Lleming WH, Thompson JC: Increased gastrin release following penetrating central nervous system injury. *Surgery* 75:720–724, 1974.
18. Harrison AM, Gaisford JC, Wechsler RL: Gastric secretion in the burned patient. *J Trauma* 12:1041–1043, 1973.
19. Davenport HW: Effect of lysolecithin, digitonin, and phospholipase upon the dog's gastric mucosal barrier. *Gastroenterology* 59:505–509, 1970.
20. Wang JY, Johnson LR: Role of ornithine decarboxylase in repair of gastric mucosal stress ulcers. *Am J Physiol* 258:G78–G85, 1990.
21. Strauss RJ, Stein T, Mandell C et al: Prevention of stress ulceration with cimetidine and carbenoxolone. *Surg Forum* 28:361, 1977.
22. Robert A: Cytoprotection by prostaglandins. *Clin Trends and Topic* 77:761–767, 1979.
23. Menguy R, Masters YF: Gastric mucosal energy metabolism and stress ulceration. *Ann Surg* 180:538–546, 1974.
24. Bruegge WFV, Peura DA: Stress-related mucosal damage; review of drug therapy. *J Clin Gastroenterol* 12:S35–S40, 1990.
25. Herrmann V, Kaminski DL: Evaluation of intragastric pH in acutely ill patients. *Arch Surg* 114:511–514, 1979.
26. Poleski MH, Spanier AH: Cimetidine versus antacids in the prevention of stress erosions in critically ill patients. *Am J Gastroenterol* 81:107–111, 1986.
27. Kingsley AN: Prophylaxis for acute stress ulcers: Antacids or cimetidine. *Am Surgeon* 51:545–547, 1985.
28. Shuman RB, Schuster DP, Zuckerman GR: Prophylactic therapy for stress ulcer bleeding: A reappraisal. *Ann Int Med* 106:562–567, 1987.
29. Hastings PR, Skillman JJ, Bushnell LS et al: Antacid titration in the prevention of acute gastrointestinal bleeding: A controlled, randomized trial in 100 critically ill patients. *N Engl J Med* 298:1041–1045, 1978.
30. McAlhany Jr JC, Czaja AJ, Pruitt Jr BA: Antacid control of complications from acute gastroduodenal disease after burns. *J Trauma* 16:645–649, 1976.
31. Simonian SJ, Curtis LE: Treatment of hemorrhagic gastritis by antacid. *Ann Surg* 184:429–434, 1976.
32. Fiddian-Green RG, Baker S: Nosocomial pneumonia in the critically ill; product of aspiration or translocation. *Crit Care Med* 19(6):763–769, 1991.
33. Ostro MJ, Russell JA, Soldin SJ et al: Control of gastric pH with cimetidine: Boluses versus primed infusions. *Gastroenterology* 89:532–537, 1985.
34. Albin M, Friedlos J, Hillman K: Continuous intragastric pH measurement in the critically ill and treatment with parenteral ranitidine. *Intensive Care Med* 11:295–299, 1985.
35. Driks MR, Craven DE, Celli BR et al: Nosocomial pneumonia in intubated patients given sucralfate as compared with antacids or histamine type 2 blockers: The role of gastric colonization. *N Engl J Med* 317:1376, 1987.
36. Reynolds JR: The clinical importance of drug interactions with antiulcer therapy. *J Clin Gastroenterol* 12(Suppl 2):S54–S63, 1990.
37. Tryba M: The risk of acute stress bleeding and nosocomial pneumonia in ventilated ICU patients: Sucralfate versus antacids. *Am J Med* 83:117, 1987.

38. Borrero E, Margolis IB, Bank S et al: Antacid versus sucralfate in preventing acute gastrointestinal bleeding. A randomized trial in 100 critically ill patients. *Am J Surg* 148:809–812, 1984.

39. Martin LF, Larson GM, Fry DE: Bleeding from stress gastritis. Has prophylactic pH control made a difference? *Am Surgeon* 51:189–193, 1985.

40. Menguy R, Gudacz T, Zajtchuk R: The surgical management of acute gastric mucosal bleeding: Stress ulcers, acute erosive gastritis, and acute hemorrhagic gastritis. *Arch Surg* 99:198, 1969.

41. Cody HS, Wichern WA: Choice of operation for acute gastric mucosal hemorrhage: Report of 36 cases and review of literature. *Am J Surg* 126:133, 1973.

42. Hubert JP, Klesman PD, Welch JS et al: The surgical management of bleeding stress ulcers. *Ann Surg* 191:672, 1980.

47 PREVENTION OF POSTOPERATIVE PULMONARY COMPLICATIONS

Gregory Tino

Reynold A. Panettieri, Jr.

Pulmonary complications are a major source of morbidity and mortality in patients who undergo surgical procedures requiring general anesthesia. Although pneumonia and atelectasis have been reported in as many as 76 percent of all postoperative patients, the overall incidence of these occurrences is difficult to assess.[1,2] These complications may be particularly devastating in patients with underlying lung disease. One review of 464 people with chronic obstructive pulmonary disease (COPD) reported a postoperative mortality rate of 7 percent, with the majority of deaths attributed to pulmonary complications.[3]

In order to prevent postoperative pulmonary complications, several important questions need to be addressed. Which patients have the highest risk? What tests predict pulmonary complications? What therapeutic modalities are useful in preventing these complications?[1,4,5] This chapter focuses on prevention of the most common pulmonary complications—atelectasis, nosocomial pneumonia, and aspiration pneumonitis.[4,6]

RISK FACTORS FOR POSTOPERATIVE PULMONARY COMPLICATIONS

A number of pulmonary and nonpulmonary risk factors contribute to postoperative respiratory complications. Decreases in arterial Po_2,[7] tidal volume,[8,9] and vital capacity[8,10,11] normally occur after major thoracic and abdominal surgery, and pulmonary complications arise from pathophysiologic extensions of these alterations, especially in high-risk patients.[4,12] Although it is difficult to identify the single most important risk factor in the development of pulmonary complications, underlying chronic obstructive pulmonary disease (COPD) and preoperative smoking are clearly associated with increased postoperative morbidity.[12–14] However, other factors such as operative site, type and duration of anesthesia, age,

obesity, and concurrent upper respiratory infection may pose substantial additional risk.

Underlying Chronic Obstructive Lung Disease

The most specific and sensitive predictor of postoperative pulmonary complications is COPD. After abdominal procedures, the incidence of pulmonary complications in patients with COPD is three times higher than in control patients.[15] In 1970, Stein and Cassara compared postoperative pulmonary complications in surgical patients with normal pulmonary function to those in patients with COPD. They defined COPD by pulmonary function criteria of an FEV_1/FVC ratio $< 70\%$, a mid-expiratory flow rate < 200 liters/min, and an arterial $Pco_2 > 45$ torr. Complications included atelectasis, pneumonia, and pulmonary embolism. The complication rate was 11 percent in control patients and 42 percent in those with COPD.[5,16] In a more recent study, Gracey et al. evaluated 157 patients with COPD and found that maximal voluntary ventilation and FEF_{25-75} of less than 50% predicted a higher risk of prolonged mechanical ventilation and other serious postoperative pulmonary complications.[17] Although the predictive value of preoperative pulmonary function testing is controversial,[1] identification of patients with limited pulmonary reserve may be useful in preventing postoperative pulmonary complications.

Hypercapnia, an indication of significant ventilatory impairment, is a hallmark of limited pulmonary reserve.[1,18,19] Patients with an elevated arterial Pco_2 experience higher rates of postoperative morbidity and mortality, especially after lung resection.[1,5,20–22] In a study of 12 patients with COPD undergoing various surgical procedures, one-half of the patients with hypercapnia required prolonged mechanical ventilation.[21]

Patients with stable well-controlled asthma do not have a significantly higher risk of complications.[12] Even steroid-dependent patients can undergo anesthesia without increased risk.[23] Preoperative measures to prevent perioperative bronchospasm should include therapeutic regimens that maximize bronchodilation, avoid high spinal anesthesia, and use techniques that promote rapid induction of anesthesia.[3,12] A detailed discussion of perioperative management of the asthmatic patient is presented in Chap. 23.

The incidence of postoperative pulmonary complications in patients with restrictive lung diseases, such as sarcoidosis and idiopathic pulmonary fibrosis (IPF), or in those with respiratory muscle weakness has not been definitively established, partly because of the heterogeneity of these disorders. Patients with restrictive disease and respiratory muscle weakness have decreased pulmonary reserve. Those with a moderate-to-severe restrictive impairment as defined by a baseline total lung capacity of < 70% of the predicted value probably should be considered to have a higher risk of postoperative pulmonary complications.

Cigarette Smoking

Early studies demonstrated that patients who smoke have a sixfold greater risk of postoperative pulmonary complications than nonsmokers.[10,24–26] In a recent prospective study, Warner et al. documented postoperative pulmonary complications in 192 patients undergoing coronary artery bypass surgery.[6] Major pulmonary complications, including bronchospasm, atelectasis, fever with purulent sputum, pneumothorax, and pleural effusion requiring thoracentesis occurred in 33 percent of smokers. Those who had stopped smoking for the longest period before surgery experienced fewer complications.[6] The incidence of untoward events rose sharply in patients who continued to smoke within two months of surgery. In addition, smokers experienced more profound oxyhemoglobin desaturation requiring supplemental oxygen in the immediate postoperative period than nonsmokers.[27]

The mechanisms by which smoking alters respiratory function and increases the risk of postoperative complications are unknown.[28–31] Smoking impairs mucous transport by inhibition of airway ciliary function.[32,33] Small airway disease has been demonstrated in smokers who have otherwise normal spirometry and is characterized by changes in the ratio of dynamic to static lung compliance.[34,35] Fortunately, short-term abstinence reverses these pathophysiologic changes.[30,31] The relationship of other adverse effects of smoking, including decrease in pulmonary surfactant,[36] increased platelet adhesiveness,[37] and interference with metabolism of concurrent drugs,[38] to postoperative pulmonary complications has not been well established.

Interestingly, for unknown reasons, an increased incidence of deep-venous thrombosis (DVT) has been noted in nonsmokers undergoing gynecologic surgery[39] and in those suffering acute myocardial infarction.[40,41] However, there are no data to suggest that patients who stop smoking for an extended period before surgery have a higher risk of DVT than nonsmokers.

Therefore, in view of the substantial evidence that smokers have a greater risk of postoperative pulmonary complications, cessation should be strongly recommended before surgery. Smoking should be discontinued at least eight weeks prior to elective surgery.[12,25,30]

Operative Site

The operative site markedly affects the risk of postoperative pulmonary complications. Cardiac, thoracic, and upper-abdominal procedures are associated with the highest risk.[1,3,13,15] Complications may be the result of greater decrements in lung volumes from phrenic nerve and diaphragmatic dysfunction. Procedures involving the lower abdomen and extremities carry relatively lower risks of pulmonary complications.[1,4,12,13,17]

Over the past several years, new alternatives to standard surgical techniques have been developed, such as limited muscle-sparing incisions for thoracic surgery, abdominal laparoscopy, and video thoracoscopy. Recent studies suggest that patients undergoing these procedures have improved postoperative pulmonary function as assessed by spirometry when compared to those undergoing conventional surgical interventions. In one study, patients undergoing limited lateral thoracotomy had significantly smaller decrements in FEV_1 and FVC after surgery than those undergoing the standard posterolateral approach.[42] In another prospective study, laparoscopic cholecystectomy was associated with improved postoperative FEV_1, FVC, and FEF_{25-75} measurements as compared to the open method.[43]

Type and Duration of Anesthesia

Although patients receiving general or spinal anesthesia have similar rates of postoperative pulmonary complications, those who have regional anesthesia fare better.[3,4,44] In addition, patients requiring prolonged general anesthesia have a higher incidence of complications.[10,12,45,46] In one study, 40 percent of patients anesthetized for more than four hours developed pneumonia compared to 8 percent of control patients.[45] Specific anesthetics may also be related to postoperative pulmonary complications. In one study, enflurane was found to increase the risk of respiratory insufficiency after surgery compared to other inhalational agents, but this has not been confirmed by others.[25] More recently, an intraoperative dose of fentanyl and halothane has been found to correlate with the incidence of immediate postoperative hypoxemia.[47] Patients who receive higher doses of halothane or fentanyl experience more profound hypoxemia than those given lower doses.

Age

Early studies indicated that elderly patients experience higher postoperative morbidity and mortality than younger patients,[4,48,49] but more recent studies question the association between age and pulmonary complications.[50–52] In a review of 209 patients undergoing elective cholecystectomy, there was no association between the age of the patient and postoperative respiratory complications.[53] Another study of patients with COPD confirmed this finding.[3] Excluding elderly patients from surgery in anticipation of pulmonary complications is not supported by available data.

Obesity

The association between obesity and increased risk of postoperative pulmonary complications is controversial. Obesity produces predictable alterations in pulmonary function, including diminished chest-wall compliance, functional residual capacity, and expiratory reserve volume.[4,13] Following surgery, these abnormalities worsen and are associated with lower vital capacity and arterial Po_2 than in nonobese patients.[54,55] Although obese patients have a higher incidence of atelectasis,[10,12] it is unclear whether or not this contributes to increased postoperative morbidity or mortality.[12,13,45]

Upper Respiratory Tract Infection

Upper respiratory tract infections (URI) are associated with significant alterations in pulmonary function in otherwise healthy patients. These include decrements in expiratory flow rate and lung diffusion capacity and increases in bronchial hyperresponsiveness to carbachol.[56-58] However, few studies have addressed the question of whether or not patients with either normal or abnormal lung function who have upper respiratory infections before surgery are more likely to experience postoperative pulmonary complications.[59] In one study of children with upper respiratory infections undergoing myringotomies under general anesthesia, there was no increase in intraoperative or postoperative pulmonary complications.[60] Despite a lack of data supporting an increased incidence of postoperative complications in adult patients with URI, elective surgery should be reconsidered in those with underlying COPD and concurrent URI.

SPECIFIC COMPLICATIONS AND THEIR PREVENTION

Because pulmonary complications have been variably defined and studied in different groups of patients, specific recommendations to prevent them are not uniform. Prevention of three important postoperative complications—atelectasis, pneumonia, and aspiration—are discussed.

Atelectasis

The contribution of atelectasis to significant morbidity and mortality is unclear, and some believe that it need not be treated in most cases.[61] Atelectasis is the most common radiographic finding in postoperative patients and may be dramatic with segmental or lobar collapse. However, patients with normal chest films also experience enough atelectasis to cause hypoxemia due to ventilation-perfusion mismatch.[4,62,63] This condition is termed microatelectasis[64] and occurs frequently, especially in obese patients undergoing upper-abdominal surgery.[4]

The pathophysiologic mechanisms underlying postoperative atelectasis are summarized in Fig. 47–1. Decreases in sigh volume and frequency and disruption of normal cough and mucociliary clearance mechanisms commonly occur after general anesthesia.[4,12,13,65] These findings, in conjunction with transient decrements in lung volumes[8,10,11,66,67] and diminished respiratory drive,[12,68] can result in loss of alveolar volume and atelectasis.

Prevention and treatment of postoperative atelectasis have focused primarily on the use of incentive spirometry and chest physiotherapy.[69] The incentive spirometer, developed over twenty years ago,[70] measures the volume of a sustained maximal inspiration to total lung capacity with an open glottis. Spirometry can be performed several times an hour to prevent alveolar unit collapse.[71] Chest physiotherapy refers to a number of techniques including chest percussion, postural drainage, and deep-breathing exercises designed to maintain lung inflation, assist mucociliary clearance, and improve ventilatory function.[72,73] However, the efficacy of these modalities remains controversial. In a controlled trial of patients undergoing cholecystectomy,[74] deep-breathing exercises, assisted cough, and postural drainage decreased pulmonary complications from 42 percent to 27 percent. In those who also received instruction and treatment before as well as after surgery, the complication rate was only 12 percent. Preoperative instruction and treatment may therefore be useful to minimize postoperative atelectasis.[2,44,75]

Simple measures like deep-breathing exercises and incentive spirometry alone may be as effective in preventing postoperative atelectasis as more complicated and costly regimens.[2,44,74] Lyager et al.[75] studied the use of deep-breathing exercises, incentive spirometry, and chest physiotherapy before and after surgery in 103 patients undergoing laparotomy. The incidence of atelectasis was marginally lower in treated patients, but chest physiotherapy provided no incremental benefit. In another prospective trial of 172 patients, Celli et al. randomized preoperative patients into four treatment groups receiving intermittent positive pressure breathing (IPPB), incentive spirometry, deep-breathing exercises, or no treatment, respectively, and determined the incidence of atelectasis, fever, and sputum production and chest pain in each group.[44] The incidence of these complications was 48 percent in the control group and 21 to 22 percent in each of the others. There were no significant side effects from incentive spirometry or deep-breathing exercises. Hospital stay was shortened for patients who received incentive spirometry. Furthermore, Roukema et al. compared the

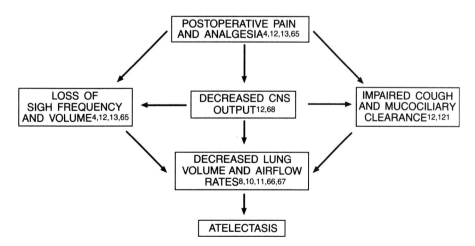

FIGURE 47–1. Pathophysiological mechanisms that may induce postoperative atelectasis.

incidence of atelectasis in patients undergoing upper-abdominal surgery who received preoperative instruction and treatment with deep-breathing exercises to control patients who received no preoperative instruction.[2] The incidence of atelectasis was 60 percent in the control group and 19 percent in the treatment group.

The utility of deep-breathing exercises and incentive spirometry in preventing postoperative atelectasis has been questioned by other investigators, especially in low-risk patients. In a prospective study of patients undergoing cholecystectomy, control patients received no specialized respiratory care, and others were treated with deep-breathing exercises and incentive spirometry after surgery.[76] No differences were found in oxygenation, spirometry results, radiographic findings, or clinical examination. In summary, although the efficacy of incentive spirometry and deep-breathing exercises in all postoperative patients remains controversial, they appear to decrease postoperative atelectasis in some patients, especially if initiated preoperatively.[2,4,12,13,18]

Another study evaluated a more aggressive approach to prevention of postoperative atelectasis, combining smoking cessation, bronchodilators, antibiotics, and chest percussion in patients with normal lung function and in those with COPD.[5] Although the independent value of each modality was not assessed, there were significant decreases in overall length of hospital stay, postoperative atelectasis, and mortality in high-risk patients receiving treatment. Whether this approach is applicable to patients with a low risk of postoperative pulmonary complications is unclear.

Pain contributes to atelectasis in postoperative patients. The use of opiate analgesia enables patients to breathe more deeply and cough more effectively.[12,77] In general, epidural or intravenous injection is more efficacious than the intramuscular route.[78] In one study, patients treated with epidural morphine after laparotomy had shorter hospital stays and fewer pulmonary complications than those receiving intramuscular morphine.[79] It is important to avoid oversedation which may compromise the airway and ventilatory drive. In elderly patients in this situation, chest percussion[80] and early mobilization[81] may be useful as adjunctive therapy. Recent studies have also determined that adequate analgesia and diminished respiratory compromise may be achieved with the use of intercostal nerve blocks in patients undergoing thoracic surgery.[82]

Intermittent positive pressure breathing (IPPB) delivered by face mask has been used to decrease atelectasis in patients after surgery,[83] but its utility remains unclear. One study reported a decrease in the incidence of postoperative atelectasis and pneumonia from 19.5 percent to 2.5 percent in individuals treated with IPPB and isoproterenol before surgery.[84] Gracey et al. prospectively documented a decrease in postoperative atelectasis in patients with COPD who received 48 hours of preparation that included IPPB, bronchodilators, theophylline, and oral hydration.[17] Alternatively, Van de Water found IPPB to be inferior to incentive spirometry in patients undergoing elective adrenalectomy.[85] Other studies have confirmed that IPPB is no better than other modalities in preventing postoperative atelectasis.[44,86–89] Since IPPB therapy is costly and may cause significant complications such as abdominal distension and barotrauma,[44] it cannot be recommended as part of a routine prophylactic regimen.

Nasal continuous positive airway pressure (CPAP) is widely used in adults with obstructive sleep apnea and may have broader application in preventing postoperative atelectasis. In neonates recovering from respiratory distress syndrome (RDS), nasal CPAP has been successful in decreasing atelectasis.[90] It also appears to reverse refractory atelectasis in nonsurgical patients.[91] Stock et al. reported more rapid increases in FRC and fewer radiographic abnormalities and signs of atelectasis in postoperative patients treated with nasal CPAP than in those receiving incentive spirometry or deep-breathing exercises.[92] However, the incidence of pneumonia in the two groups was similar. The use of nasal CPAP in preventing postoperative pulmonary complications appears promising but has not been adequately studied.

Pneumonia

Postoperative nosocomial pneumonia is the most serious pulmonary complication and contributes to prolonged mechanical ventilation and mortality.[45,93,94] Recent studies have emphasized the difficulty in diagnosing nosocomial pneumonia, especially in intubated patients.[95,96] There is discordance between clinical signs of pneumonia (changes in sputum, infiltrates on chest films, and worsening hypoxemia) and subsequent autopsy findings.[95] Nonetheless, pneumonias account for 15 percent of nosocomial infections, and one-half of these occur in postoperative patients.[94] In 12 to 53 percent of such patients, aerobic gram-negative bacilli are the causative organisms.[94,97,98] The Centers for Disease Control estimates that the rate of nosocomial pneumonia is 75 to 80 cases per 1000 patient discharges. Lower-respiratory infection ranks third after urinary tract and wound infections on hospital surgical services.[99]

Identifying patients with a high risk of postoperative pneumonia is the key to its prevention. In one large series, Garibaldi prospectively studied the incidence of pneumonia in 520 patients undergoing chest and abdominal surgery. Diagnostic criteria included fever above 38°C for two days, purulent sputum, and abnormalities on examination and chest x-ray suggestive of alveolar consolidation. Ninety-one patients or 17.5 percent were diagnosed with pneumonia.[45] A history of smoking, low serum albumin concentration, and more severe underlying disease as determined by a standard classification predicted postoperative pneumonia regardless of age, sex, or weight (see Table 47–1).[100]

Other conditions that predispose patients to pneumonia include hematogenous spread from distant sites of infection, atelectasis, dehydration, upper-airway colonization with gram-negative bacteria, and inadequate bronchial mucociliary clearance.[4,94] Previous antibiotic therapy has not been shown to play a significant role.[93,97] In the 1960s, respiratory therapy equipment, particularly reservoir nebulizers, was linked to several outbreaks of nosocomial pneumonia.[93,101–103] The availability of disposable ventilator tubing and respiratory therapy equipment has virtually eliminated this problem.[93,104]

In order to minimize the risk of postoperative pneumonia, therapy should be aimed at preserving pulmonary defense mechanisms

TABLE 47–1. Risk Factors for Development of Postoperative Pneumonia[45,100]

1. Severity of underlying disease as characterized by serum albumin of < 3.0 mg/dl and ASA (American Society of Anesthesiology) preoperative physical status classification of 3–4
2. Smoking history
3. Preoperative hospital stay greater than 2–7 days
4. Duration of surgery more than 2–4 hours
5. Thoracic or upper-abdominal surgical site

and preventing oropharyngeal colonization with bacteria and subsequent aspiration into the lower respiratory tract.[94,97] Data suggest that deep-breathing exercises and incentive spirometry are useful especially if combined with preoperative teaching.[2,44,75] The value of prophylactic antibiotics to diminish upper-airway colonization with bacteria is controversial. In one study, 298 surgical patients in intensive care units were treated with inhalational polymyxin B in an effort to prevent pneumonia from *Pseudomonas aeruginosa*. Ten patients developed pneumonia with resistant organisms, resulting in a mortality rate of 64 percent.[105] Other studies have also failed to show any benefit from prophylactic antimicrobial therapy.[106] However, it is indicated in patients with infected sputum or exacerbations of chronic bronchitis.[5,13,57] Chest percussion and IPPB therapy are not useful.[107]

Aspiration Pneumonitis

In 1946, Mendelson described a syndrome of dyspnea, tachypnea, and hemodynamic instability attributed to aspiration of gastric secretions in women after cesarean section.[108] Unfortunately, aspiration pneumonitis continues to be a major source of postoperative morbidity. Aspiration is a consequence of disruption of normal laryngeal or glottic function and occurs more often in unconscious or anesthetized patients. Pulmonary parenchymal damage results from contamination of the lower respiratory tract by oropharyngeal secretions, gastric acid, or foreign matter. The incidence of aspiration pneumonitis in patients undergoing general anesthesia is 4 to 26 percent and higher in patients who have not fasted and in those undergoing upper-abdominal or emergency procedures.[109,110] Mortality rates from aspiration pneumonitis in postoperative patients can be as high as 70 percent.[111]

Preventive modalities include identification of high-risk patients, use of regional anesthesia when possible, suppression of postoperative nausea and vomiting,[112,113] and induction and intubation of the patient in a seated position with cricoid tracheal pressure.[114] The use of nasogastric tubes also contributes to the development of aspiration pneumonitis. One study documented regurgitation in 22 percent of patients with nasogastric tubes.[110] Although avoiding the use of these tubes may decrease the incidence of aspiration, gastric distention with large residual volumes has also been associated with aspiration pneumonitis.[111]

Aspiration of gastric contents with a pH of less than 2.5 and/or volumes of 25 ml or more have been associated with pulmonary parenchymal damage.[108,111] Pharmacologic agents to increase gastric pH and lower volume have been used in an effort to decrease the incidence of aspiration. Anticholinergic drugs like atropine and glycopyrrolate do little to change gastric volume or pH.[115] In most cases, antacids increase pH but unreliably affect gastric emptying. They can result in significant pneumonitis if aspirated.[109,116] Cimetidine and other H_2 receptor antagonists successfully increase gastric pH[115,117-119] but have not been shown to reduce the incidence of aspiration. There appears to be no difference in efficacy among the commonly used H_2 receptor antagonists.[120] A combination of H_2 receptor antagonists and metaclopramide or domperidone, agents that increase gastric motility, may decrease both acidity and volume. In surgical patients randomized to groups receiving either no therapy, cimetidine alone, metaclopramide alone, or a combination of both, those treated with combination therapy exhibited a gastric pH of greater than 5 and volumes less than 25 ml.[118]

TABLE 47–2. Perioperative Therapy for the Prevention of Pulmonary Complications in the Surgical Patient

Clearly Beneficial
1. Smoking cessation at least eight weeks prior to elective surgery
2. Deep-breathing exercises and incentive spirometry pre- and postoperatively with preoperative patient instruction on proper technique
3. Maximization of preoperative lung function including treatment of apparent bronchospastic disease
4. Induction and intubation of high-risk patients in a sitting position
5. Adequate analgesia

Potentially Beneficial
1. Early ambulation postoperatively
2. Antibiotic therapy for patients with infected sputum
3. H_2 receptor antagonists
4. Weight reduction for morbidly obese patients
5. Chest percussion

Questionably Beneficial
1. IPPB
2. Nasal CPAP therapy

However, the impact of this therapy on the overall incidence of aspiration pneumonitis was not assessed.

SUMMARY

1. Chronic obstructive pulmonary disease and smoking are potent risk factors in the development of postoperative pulmonary complications.

2. Atelectasis is the most common postoperative pulmonary complication. Deep-breathing exercises, incentive spirometry, and preoperative instruction in these techniques are the most useful and cost-effective measures to prevent postoperative atelectasis and pneumonia. Chest percussion, IPPB, and prophylactic antibiotics are not useful (see Table 47–2).

3. Aspiration pneumonia is associated with significant morbidity and mortality. Unnecessary use of nasogastric tubes may predispose patients to aspiration, but gastric distention with large volumes should be avoided. A combination of H_2 antagonists and pharmacologic agents that increase gastric motility, like metaclopramide, reduce gastric pH and volume but have not been shown to decrease the incidence of aspiration pneumonitis.

REFERENCES

1. Zibrak JD, O'Donnell CR, Marton K: Indications for pulmonary function testing. *Ann Intern Med* 112:763–771, 1990.
2. Roukema JA, Carol EJ, Prins JG: The prevention of pulmonary complications after upper abdominal surgery in patients with noncompromised pulmonary status. *Arch Surg* 123:30–34, 1988.
3. Tarhan S, Moffitt EA, Sessler AD et al: Risk of anesthesia and surgery in patients with chronic bronchitis and chronic obstructive pulmonary disease. *Surgery* 74:720–726, 1973.
4. Tisi GM: Preoperative evaluation of pulmonary function: Validity, indications and benefits. *Am Rev Respir Dis* 119:293–310, 1979.

5. Stein M, Cassara EL: Preoperative pulmonary evaluation and therapy for surgery patients. *JAMA* 211:787–790, 1970.

6. Warner MA, Offord DP, Warner ME et al: Role of preoperative cessation of smoking and other factors in postoperative pulmonary complications: A blinded prospective study of coronary artery bypass patients. *Mayo Clin Proc* 64:609–616, 1989.

7. Bjork VO, Hilty HS: The arterial oxygen and carbon dioxide tension during the postoperative period in cases of pulmonary resections and thoracoplasties. *J Thorac Surg* 27:455–467, 1954.

8. Beecher HK: The measured effect of laparotomy on the respiration. *J Clin Invest* 12:639–650, 1933.

9. Ford GT, Whitelaw WA, Rosenal TW et al: Diaphragm function after upper abdominal surgery in humans. *Am Rev Respir Dis* 127:431–436, 1983.

10. Latimer RG, Dickman M, Day WC et al: Ventilatory patterns and pulmonary complications after upper abdominal surgery determined by preoperative and postoperative computerized spirometry and blood gas analysis. *Am J Surg* 122:622–632, 1971.

11. Ali J, Weisel RD, Layug AB et al: Consequences of postoperative alterations in respiratory mechanics. *Am J Surg* 128:376–382, 1974.

12. Jackson CV: Preoperative pulmonary evaluation. *Arch Intern Med* 148:2120–2127, 1988.

13. Mohr DN, Jett JR: Preoperative evaluation of pulmonary risk factors. *J Gen Intern Med* 3:277–287, 1988.

14. Pedersen T, Eliasen K, Henriksen E: A prospective study of risk factors and cardiopulmonary complications with anaesthesia and surgery: Risk indicators of cardiopulmonary morbidity. *Acta Anaesth Scand* 34:144–155, 1990.

15. Wightman JAK: A prospective survey of the incidence of postoperative pulmonary complications. *Br J Surg* 55:85–91, 1968.

16. Stein M, Koota GM, Simon M et al: Pulmonary evaluation of surgical patients. *JAMA* 181:765–770, 1962.

17. Gracey DR, Divertie MB, Didier ER: Preoperative pulmonary preparation of patients with chronic obstructive pulmonary disease: A prospective study. *Chest* 76:123–129, 1979.

18. Tisi GM: Preoperative identification and evaluation of the patients with lung disease. *Med Clin N Am* 71:399–412, 1987.

19. Burrows B, Earle RH: Prediction of survival in patients with chronic airway obstruction. *Am Rev Respir Dis* 99:865–872, 1969.

20. Van Nostrand D, Kjelsberg MO, Humphrey EW: Preresectional evaluation of risk from pneumonectomy. *Surg Gynecol Obstet* 127:306–312, 1968.

21. Milledge JS, Nunn JF: Criteria of fitness for anaesthesia in patients with chronic obstructive lung disease. *Br Med J* 3:670–673, 1975.

22. Cain HD, Stevens PM, Adaniya R: Preoperative pulmonary function and complications after cardiovascular surgery. *Chest* 76:130–135, 1979.

23. Oh SH, Patterson R: Surgery in corticosteroid-dependent asthmatics. *J Allergy Clin Immunol* 53:345–351, 1974.

24. Morton HJV: Tobacco smoking and pulmonary complications after operation. *Lancet* 1:368–370, 1944.

25. Warner MA, Divertie MB, Tinker TH: Preoperative cessation of smoking and pulmonary complications in coronary artery bypass patients. *Anesthesiology* 60:380–383, 1984.

26. Holtz B, Bake B, Sixt R: Prediction of postoperative hypoxemia in smokers and nonsmokers. *Acta Anaesth Scand* 23:411–418, 1979.

27. Tait AR, Kyff J, Crider B et al: Changes in arterial oxygen saturation in cigarette smokers following general anaesthesia. *Can J Anaesth* 37:423–428, 1990.

28. Roughton FJW, Darling RC: The effect of CO on the oxyhemoglobin dissociation curve. *Am J Physiol* 141:17–31, 1944.

29. Stedman RL: The chemical composition of tobacco and tobacco smoke. *Chemother Rev* 68:153–207, 1968.

30. Pearce AC, Jones RM: Smoking and anesthesia: Preoperative abstinence and perioperative morbidity. *Anesthesiology* 61:576–584, 1984.

31. Jones RM: Smoking before surgery: The case for stopping. *Br Med J* 29:1763–1764, 1985.

32. Dalhamm T, Rylander R: Ciliostatic action of cigarette smoke. *Acta Otolaryngol* 81:379–382, 1965.

33. Hilding AC: On cigarette smoking, bronchial carcinoma and ciliary action. II. *N Engl J Med* 254:1155–1160, 1956.

34. Tockman M, Menkes H, Colten B et al: A comparison of pulmonary function in male smokers and nonsmokers. *Am Rev Respir Dis* 114:711–722, 1976.

35. Martin RR, Lindsay D, Despas P et al: The early detection of airway obstruction. *Am Rev Respir Dis* 111:119–125, 1975.

36. Finley TN, Ladman AJ: Low yield of pulmonary surfactant in cigarette smokers. *N Engl J Med* 286:223–227, 1972.

37. Bierenbaum MD, Fleischman AI, Stier A et al: Effect of cigarette smoking upon in vivo platelet function in man. *Thromb Res* 12:1051–1057, 1978.

38. Miller RR: Effects of smoking on drug action. *Clin Pharmacol Ther* 22:749–756, 1977.

39. Clayton JK, Anderson JA, McNicol GP: Effect of cigarette smoking on subsequent postoperative thromboembolic disease in gynaecological patients. *Br Med J* 2:402, 1978.

40. Handley AJ, Teather D: Influence of smoking on deep-venous thrombosis after myocardial infarction. *Br Med J* 3:230–231, 1974.

41. Marks P, Emerson PA: Increased incidence of deep-vein thrombosis after myocardial infarction in nonsmokers. *Br Med J* 3:304–306, 1974.

42. Lemmer JH, Gomez MN, Symreng T et al: Limited lateral thoracotomy: Improved postoperative pulmonary function. *Arch Surg* 125:873–877, 1990.

43. Frazee RC, Roberts JW, Okeson GC et al: Open versus laparoscopic cholecystectomy: A comparison of postoperative pulmonary function. *Ann Surg* 213:651–654, 1991.

44. Celli BR, Rodriguez KS, Snider GL: A controlled trial of intermittent positive pressure breathing, incentive spirometry and deep breathing exercises in preventing pulmonary complications after abdominal surgery. *Am Rev Respir Dis* 130:12–15, 1984.

45. Garibaldi RA, Britt MR, Coleman ML et al: Risk factors for postoperative pneumonia. *Am J Med* 70:677–680, 1981.

46. Knudsen J, Ruben H: Pulmonary complications after 154 transthoracic operations requiring more than 8 hours of anaesthesia. *Br J Anaesth* 46:752–755, 1974.

47. Canet J, Ricos M, Vidal F: Early postoperative arterial oxygen desaturation: Determining factors and response to oxygen therapy. *Anesth Analg* 69:207–212, 1989.

48. Klug TJ, Macpherson RC: Postoperative complications in the elderly surgical patient. *Am J Surg* 97:713–717, 1959.

49. Zeffren SE, Hartford CE: Comparative mortality for various surgical operations in older versus younger age groups. *J Am Geriat Soc* 20:485–489, 1972.

50. Edmunds LH, Stephenson LW, Edie RN et al: Open heart surgery in octogenarians. *N Engl J Med* 319:131–136, 1988.

51. Mohr DN: Estimation of surgical risk in the elderly: A correlative review. *J Am Geriat Soc* 31:99–102, 1983.

52. Sherman S, Guidot CE: The feasibility of thoracotomy for lung cancer in the elderly. *JAMA* 258:927–930, 1987.

53. Poe RH, Kallay MC, Tulsi D et al: Can postoperative pulmonary complications after elective cholecystectomy be predicted? *Am J Med Sci* 295:29–34, 1988.

54. Vaughn RN, Engelhart RC, Wise L: Postoperative hypoxemia in obese patients. *Ann Surg* 180:877–882, 1974.

55. Catenacci AJ, Anderson JD, Boersma D: Anesthetic hazards of obesity. *JAMA* 175:657–665, 1961.

56. O'Connor SA, Jones DP, Collins JV et al: Changes in pulmonary function after naturally acquired respiratory infection in normal persons. *Am Rev Respir Dis* 120:1087–1093, 1979.

57. Hall WJ, Hall CB, Speers DM: Respiratory syncytial virus infection in adults: Clinical, virologic and serial pulmonary function studies. *Ann Intern Med* 88:203–205, 1978.

58. Horner GJ, Gray FD: Effect of uncomplicated presumptive influenza on the diffusing capacity of the lung. *Am Rev Respir Dis* 108:866–869, 1973.

59. Fennelly ME, Hall GM: Anaesthesia and upper respiratory tract infections—a nonexistent hazard? *Br J Anaesth* 64:535–536, 1990.

60. Tait AR, Knight PR: The effects of general anesthesia on upper respiratory tract infections in children. *Anesthesiology* 67:930–935, 1987.

61. O'Donohue WJ: Prevention and treatment of postoperative atelectasis. Can it and will it be adequately studied? *Chest* 87:1–2, 1985.

62. Benumof JL: Mechanism of decreased blood flow to atelectatic lung. *J Appl Physiol* 46:1047–1048, 1979.

63. Ravin WB: Value of deep breathing in reversing postoperative hypoxemia. *NY State J Med* 66:244–249, 1966.

64. Prys-Roberts E, Nunn JF, Dobson RH et al: Radiologically undetectable pulmonary collapse in the supine position. *Lancet* 2:399–401, 1967.

65. Egbert LD, Bendixen HH: Effect of morphine on breathing pattern. *JAMA* 188:485–488, 1964.

66. Anscombe AR, Buxton RS: Effect of abdominal operations on total lung capacity and its subdivisions. *Br Med J* 2:84–87, 1958.

67. Meyers JR, Lembeck L, O'Kane H et al: Changes in functional residual capacity of the lung after operation. *Arch Surg* 110:576–583, 1975.

68. Dureuil B, Viires N, Cantineau JP et al: Diaphragmatic contractility after upper abdominal surgery. *J Appl Physiol* 61:1775–1780, 1986.

69. O'Donohue WJ: National survey of the usage of lung expansion modalities for the prevention and treatment of postoperative atelectasis. *Chest* 87:76–80, 1985.

70. Bartlett RH, Gazzaniga AB, Geraghty TR: The yawn maneuver: Prevention and treatment of postoperative pulmonary complications. *Surg Forum* 72:196–199, 1971.

71. Murray JF: Indications for mechanical aids to assist lung inflation in medical patients. *Am Rev Respir Dis* 122(Suppl):121–126, 1980.

72. Rochester DF, Goldberg SK: Techniques of respiratory physical therapy. *Am Rev Respir Dis* 122(Suppl):133–137, 1980.

73. Menkes H, Britt J: Physical therapy: Rationale for physical therapy. *Am Rev Respir Dis* 122(Suppl):127–131, 1980.

74. Thoren L: Postoperative pulmonary complications: Observations on their prevention by means of physiotherapy. *Acta Chir Scand* 107:194–205, 1954.

75. Lyager S, Weinberg M, Rajani N et al: Can postoperative pulmonary condition be improved by treatment with the Bartlett-Edwards incentive spirometry after upper abdominal surgery? *Acta Anaesth Scand* 23:312–319, 1979.

76. Schweiger I, Gamulin Z, Forster A et al: Absence of benefit of incentive spirometry in low-risk patients undergoing cholecystectomy: A controlled randomized study. *Chest* 85:652–656, 1986.

77. Bromage PR: Spirometry in assessment of analgesia after abdominal surgery. *Br Med J* 2:589–593, 1955.

78. Cuschieri RT, Morran CG, Howie JC et al: Postoperative pain and pulmonary complications: Comparison of three analgesic regimens. *Br J Surg* 72:495–498, 1985.

79. Rawal N, Sjostrand U, Christoffersson E et al: Comparison of intramuscular and epidural analgesia in the grossly obese: Influence on postoperative ambulation and pulmonary function. *Anesth Analg* 63:583–592, 1984.

80. Kiriloff LH, Owens GR, Rogers RM et al: Does chest physical therapy work? *Chest* 88:436–444, 1985.

81. Grodsinsky C, Brush BE, Ponka JC: Postoperative pulmonary complications in the geriatric age group. *J Am Geriat Soc* 22:407–412, 1974.

82. Chan VW, Chung F, Cheng DC et al: Analgesic and pulmonary effects of continuous intercostal nerve block following thoracotomy. *Can J Anaesth* 36:733–739, 1991.

83. Noehren TH, Lasry JE, Legteri LJ: Intermittent positive pressure breathing for the prevention and management of postoperative pulmonary complications. *Surgery* 43:658–662, 1958.

84. Anderson WH, Dorsett BE, Hamilton G: Prevention of postoperative pulmonary complications: Use of isoproterenol and intermittent positive pressure breathing on inspiration. *JAMA* 186:763–766, 1963.

85. Van de Water JM, Watring WG, Linton LA et al: Prevention of postoperative pulmonary complications. *Surg Gynecol Obstet* 135:229–233, 1972.

86. Baxter WD, Levine RS: An evaluation of intermittent positive pressure breathing in the prevention of postoperative complications. *Arch Surg* 98:795–798, 1969.

87. Cottrell JE, Siker ES: Preoperative intermittent positive pressure breathing in patients with chronic obstructive lung disease: Effect on postoperative complications. *Anesth Analg* 52:258–262, 1973.

88. Ali J, Serrette C, Wood LDH et al: Effect of postoperative intermittent positive pressure breathing on lung function. *Chest* 85:192–196, 1984.

89. Pontoppidan H: Mechanical aids to lung expansion in nonintubated surgical patients. *Am Rev Respir Dis* 22(Suppl):109–119, 1980.

90. Engelke SC, Roloff DW, Kuhns LR: Postextubation nasal continuous positive airway pressure: A controlled study. *Am J Dis Child* 136:359–361, 1982.

91. Duncan SR, Negrin RS, Mihm FG et al: Nasal continuous positive airway pressure in atelectasis. *Chest* 92:621–624, 1987.

92. Stock MC, Downs JB, Gauer PK et al: Prevention of postoperative pulmonary complications with CPAP, incentive spirometry and conservative therapy. *Chest* 87:151–157, 1985.

93. Gross PA, Neu HC, Antwerpen CV et al: Deaths from nosocomial infections: Experience in a university hospital and a community hospital. *Am J Med* 68:219–223, 1980.

94. Eickhoff TC: Pulmonary infections in surgical patients. *Surg Clin N Am* 60:175–183, 1980.

95. Andrews CP, Coalson JJ, Smith JD, Johanson WG: Diagnosis of nosocomial bacterial pneumonia in acute, diffuse lung injury. *Chest* 80:254–258, 1981.

96. Fabon JY, Chastre J, Hance AJ et al: Detection of nosocomial lung infection in ventilated patients. Use of a protected specimen brush and quantitative culture techniques in 147 patients. *Am Rev Respir Dis* 138:110–116, 1988.

97. Johanson WG, Pierce AK, Sanford JP: Nosocomial respiratory infections with gram-negative bacilli. The significance of colonization of the respiratory tract. *Ann Intern Med* 77:701–706, 1972.

98. Eickhoff TC, Brachman PS, Bennett JV et al: Surveillance of nosocomial infections in community hospitals. *J Infect Dis* 120:305–317, 1969.

99. Centers for Disease Control: National nosocomial infections. Study Report. *Annual Summary 1976*, February 1978.

100. Djokovic JL, Hedley-Whyte J: Prediction of outcome of surgery and anesthesia in patients over 80. *JAMA* 242:2301–2306, 1979.

101. Reinarz JA, Pierce AK, Mays BB et al: The potential role of inhalation therapy equipment in nosocomial pulmonary infection. *J Clin Invest* 44:831–839, 1965.

102. Phillips I: *Pseudomonas aeruginosa* respiratory tract infection in patients receiving mechanical ventilation. *J Hyg* 65:229–235, 1967.

103. Sanders CV, Luby JP, Johanson WG et al: *Serratia marcescens* infections from inhalation therapy medications: Nosocomial outbreaks. *Ann Intern Med* 73:15–21, 1970.

104. Pierce AK, Sanford JP, Thomas GD et al: Long-term evaluation of decontamination of inhalational therapy equipment and the occurrence of necrotizing pneumonia. *N Engl J Med* 282:528–531, 1970.

105. Feeley TW, Dumoulin GC, Hedley-Whyte J et al: Aerosol polymyxin

and pneumonia in seriously ill patients. *N Engl J Med* 293:471–475, 1975.

106. Thulbourne T, Young MH: Prophylactic penicillin and postoperative chest infections. *Lancet* 2:907–909, 1962.
107. Graham WGR, Bradley DA: Efficacy of chest physiotherapy and intermittent positive pressure breathing in the resolution of pneumonia. *N Engl J Med* 299:624–627, 1978.
108. Mendelson CC: The aspiration of stomach contents into the lungs during obstetrical anesthesia. *Am J Obstet Gynecol* 52:191–205, 1946.
109. Carlsson C, Islander G: Silent gastropharyngeal regurgitation during anesthesia. *Anesth Analg* 60:655–657, 1981.
110. Berson W, Adriani J: Silent regurgitation and aspiration during anesthesia. *Anesthesiology* 15:644–649, 1954.
111. Maliniak K, Vakil AH: Preanesthetic cimetidine and gastric pH. *Anesth Analg* 58:309–313, 1979.
112. Rothenberg DM, Parnass SM, Litwack K et al: Efficacy of ephedrine in the prevention of postoperative nausea and vomiting. *Anesth Analg* 72:58–61, 1991.
113. Leeser J, Lip H: Prevention of postoperative nausea and vomiting using ondansetron, a new selective 5-HT$_3$ receptor antagonist. *Anesth Analg* 72:751–755, 1991.
114. Deepak M, Paust J: Antacids and cricoid pressure in prevention of fatal aspiration syndrome. *Lancet* 15:582–583, 1979.
115. Toung T, Cameron JL: Cimetidine as a preoperative medication to reduce the complications of aspiration of gastric contents. *Surgery* 87:205–208, 1980.
116. Newson AJ: The effectiveness and duration of preoperative antacid therapy. *Anaesth Intens Care* 5:214–217, 1977.
117. Coombs DW, Hooper D, Colton D: Acid-aspiration prophylaxis by use of preoperative oral administration of cimetidine. *Anesthesiology* 51:352–356, 1979.
118. Manchikanti L, Marreno TC, Roush JR: Preanesthetic cimetidine and metoclopramide for acid aspiration prophylaxis in elective surgery. *Anesthesiology* 61:48–54, 1984.
119. Husemeyer RD, Davenport HT, Rajesekaran T: Cimetidine as a single oral dose for prophylaxis against Mendelson's syndrome. *Anaesthesia* 33:775–778, 1978.
120. Vila P, Valles J, Canet J et al: Acid aspiration prophylaxis in morbidly obese patients: Famotidine versus ranitidine. *Anaesthesia* 46:967–969, 1991.
121. Newhouse M, Sanchin J, Brenenstock J: Lung defense mechanisms. *N Engl J Med* 295:990–998, 1976.

48 PREVENTION OF POSTOPERATIVE THROMBOEMBOLIC DISEASE

Thomas D. Painter

Frank H. Brown

Thromboembolic disease is a major cause of postoperative morbidity and mortality. Approximately 30 percent of patients undergoing general surgery develop thrombosis in the deep-venous system (DVT), and the number is even higher in those undergoing pelvic or orthopedic surgery. More than 30 percent of DVT occur in the postoperative setting.[1,2] Postoperative pulmonary embolism (PE) accounts for about 15 percent of all postoperative mortality,[3] and the incidence of fatal postoperative PE may exceed 25,000 cases per year.[4] Most occur in patients with a good prognosis who would otherwise have been expected to recover from surgery.

More than 25 years ago, these potentially lethal postoperative complications were shown to be preventable.[5] The Council on Thrombosis of the American Heart Association has calculated that the application of available methods of prophylaxis to patients over 40 undergoing general surgery could save 4000 to 8000 lives per year.[6] However, recent surveys show a disturbing lack and inappropriate utilization of thromboprophylatic measures.[7–9] This is often due to doubt about the efficacy and safety of available methods of prophylaxis, perhaps arising from a cumbersome number of frequently contradictory studies on the subject. The purposes of this chapter are to review the pathogenesis of postoperative venous thrombosis, evaluate data on the efficacy and safety of prophylactic methods, and make specific recommendations regarding their use in different clinical situations.

PATHOGENESIS OF POSTOPERATIVE VENOUS THROMBOSIS

In 1856, Virchow proposed a triad of factors thought to be important in thrombogenesis.[10] These factors included stasis, injury to the vessel wall, and increased coagulability.

Stasis of blood in the veins of the legs undoubtedly occurs both during and after surgery.[11,12] Anesthesia causes a decrease in arterial perfusion, venodilation, and loss of the pumping action of the calf muscles.[13–15] Venous flow decreases after surgery with pro-

longed periods of immobility. Stasis undoubtedly plays an important role in postoperative thrombogenesis but cannot cause clot formation by itself. Stagnant blood isolated between two ligatures in a normal vein will remain fluid for hours.[16] However, in the presence of vessel wall injury or hypercoagulability, stasis contributes to thrombus formation by decreasing the clearance of activated clotting factors and facilitating fibrin formation.[17]

Normal vascular endothelium is not thrombogenic. However, injury causes adherence of platelets to the vessel wall and activation of the coagulation system resulting in fibrin formation. Hip surgery is unique in its high incidence of isolated proximal venous thrombosis.[18,19] Direct trauma to the vein, thermal injury from the heat of polymerizing acrylic, and local depletion of fibrinolytic factors can cause endothelial damage that may underlie clot formation. Vessel injury probably plays a small role in most other cases of postoperative DVT. Pathological studies show that thrombi almost always lie over intact endothelium and contain few if any platelets.[20,21] However, subtle forms of endothelial damage may occur in the absence of direct surgical trauma. In any case, vessel wall injury appears to be the least important factor in the initiation of postoperative thrombosis except in the setting of hip surgery.

Surgery has long been thought to induce a hypercoagulable state contributing to the high incidence of postoperative venous thrombosis. Many changes in the coagulation and fibrinolytic systems occur in the perioperative period, but their significance is uncertain. These include increases in the platelet count and platelet adhesiveness,[22] increased concentrations of several coagulation factors,[23–25] and possible activation of clotting factors due to release of tissue thromboplastin from surgical trauma.

The coagulation system is undoubtedly activated frequently in response to minor trauma, but uncontrolled thrombus formation is normally prevented by regulatory mechanisms. These include neutralization of activated clotting factors by inhibitors, clearance of activated clotting factors by the liver, and activation of the fibrinolytic system. In the postoperative period, the concentration of antithrombin III decreases,[26–28] and perioperative venous stasis may result in decreased activation of protein C.[29] Stasis also impedes hepatic clearance of activated clotting factors. The activity of the fibrinolytic system is decreased in the postoperative period ("fibrinolytic shutdown"), and several studies have documented a decrease in some of the laboratory indices of fibrinolysis during surgery.[30-35] These parameters are more depressed in patients who develop venous thrombosis than in those who do not.[34-36]

In summary, during and after surgery there are changes in venous flow, the venous endothelial surface, and the coagulation system. Endothelial damage and platelet adhesion appear to be relatively unimportant except in hip surgery. Activation of the coagulation system and decreased neutralization and clearance of activated clotting probably result in at least locally increased concentrations of activated factors. In the presence of venous stasis, activated clotting factors are potent stimuli to thrombogenesis. These mechanisms probably account for the initiation of postoperative venous thrombosis.

Natural History of Perioperative Venous Thrombosis

Although as many as 15 percent of surgical patients develop DVT before the procedure,[37] most occur during surgery or in the early postoperative period.[38] About 50 percent of cases develop within the first 24 hours of surgery,[49] and 80 percent do so within the first 72 hours.[40] Some risk persists for at least 10 days following general surgery[41] and 18 days after hip procedures[42] and can extend beyond discharge from the hospital.[43] Therefore, to be effective, a prophylactic agent must be given preoperatively and continued through surgery for the duration of the period of risk. Early discontinuation probably accounts for late or rebound thrombosis.

^{125}I-fibrinogen scanning shows that more than 90 percent of postoperative thrombi originate in the calves,[39,44-48] usually beginning in the valve cusps or sinusoids of the soleal plexus.[20] Isolated thrombi in the proximal veins are unusual but do occur in about 10 percent of patients undergoing pelvic surgery and 15 to 20 percent of those undergoing hip surgery.[18,19] Most calf-vein thrombi undergo spontaneous lysis and estimates of the incidence of propagation to the proximal venous system vary from 4 to 22 percent.[38,49]

The risk of embolization following DVT is approximately 15 to 20 percent but varies with the location of the thrombus.[1] Calf-vein thrombi embolize in only 0 to 4 percent of cases or cause clinically insignificant emboli.[49-51] However, one autopsy study attributed one-third of significant emboli to thrombosis in the calves.[52] The risk of embolization of proximal thrombi is much higher. Approximately 50 percent of femoral-vein and 66 percent of pelvic-vein thrombi embolize. The mortality rate in those who suffer a PE is approximately 10 percent.[53]

Aside from pulmonary embolism, the major complication of deep-venous thrombosis is postphlebitic syndrome and chronic venous insufficiency. In nonsurgical patients with femoral thrombosis, as many as 80 percent suffer long-term morbidity from chronic venous insufficiency.[54] However, the risk of developing secondary changes in the leg after perioperative DVT has not been exhaustively studied. In one study, there was no clear correlation between the presence of postoperative thrombi as documented by venography and subsequent leg symptoms over several years.[55-57]

STRATEGIES FOR THE PREVENTION OF FATAL PULMONARY EMBOLISM

There are three diagnostic and therapeutic strategies to reduce the risk of fatal embolism. The traditional approach is based on clinical recognition of DVT and nonlethal PE. Patients suspected of having thromboembolic disease are studied to confirm the diagnosis and treated with full-dose anticoagulation. This strategy is suboptimal for several reasons. First, clinical recognition of both DVT and PE is notoriously unreliable. As few as 20 percent of patients with fatal pulmonary emboli (FPE) exhibit premonitory signs or symptoms suggestive of DVT or nonfatal emboli.[58] Second, treatment of documented DVT is not completely effective in preventing subsequent embolization. Most patients sustaining FPE die within the first one or two hours before the diagnosis can be made and treatment instituted.[59,60] Finally, this strategy substitutes the substantial risks of full anticoagulation for the much lower risks of prophylactic therapy. This approach has been shown to be both expensive and ineffective in preventing loss of life.[61,62]

A second strategy involves surveillance with noninvasive screening tests to allow early diagnosis and treatment of DVT to prevent FPE. This strategy is dependent on the accuracy of the surveillance technique. For example, although fibrinogen scanning is accurate in diagnosing calf-vein thrombosis, it is unreliable in detecting clot in the proximal veins and could not be used with confidence in patients undergoing pelvic and hip surgery. All patients with positive scans would require additional studies such as venography or impedance plethysmography to diagnose proximal propagation requiring full anticoagulation. This strategy has been shown to be extremely expensive.[62,63]

The third strategy involves identifying patients with a high risk of postoperative thrombosis and administering prophylactic therapy to them. This is the most cost-effective approach, but its cost-effectiveness is directly proportional to the precision with which patients with increased risk can be identified.

Assessment of the Risk of Postoperative Venous Thrombosis

Every preoperative evaluation should include an assessment of the risks of postoperative thromboembolic complications inherent in the patient and the procedure. The duration of surgery is one important factor. Risk is low after procedures lasting less than 30 minutes but increases linearly with the length of the operation[64] and is proportional to the duration of postoperative immobilization.[53] In addition, general anesthesia may carry a higher risk than subarachnoid block and epidural analgesia, which are associated with increased venous flow.[65,66] The site and extent of surgery is another important factor. For example, although the risk of venous thrombosis is increased in many orthopedic operations, arthroscopic procedures involving the knee carry a low risk of calf thrombi and are not associated with proximal DVT.[67]

Other factors that increase the risk of postoperative venous thrombosis are listed in Table 48–1. Age appears to be the single most important variable.[68] Risk begins to rise at age 40 and steadily increases thereafter. Possible reasons include decreased mobility, venous dilation, and decreased fibrinolytic capacity. Previous

TABLE 48–1. Risk Factors for Postoperative
Thromboembolic Disease

Age > 40
Previous venous thrombosis
Malignancy
Obesity
Estrogens, including oral contraceptives
Postoperative infection
Congestive heart failure
Varicose veins
Stroke or acute spinal cord injury
Pregnancy and parturition
Orthopedic and pelvic surgery
General surgery of more than 30 minutes duration
Prolonged immobilization

DVT increases the risk of recurrent thrombosis by a factor of three.[69] Those with malignancy have a risk 1.5 to 3 times that of patients with benign disease.[69,70] Obesity increases the risk by 50 percent.[68] Oral contraceptives and other estrogens do so presumably by depressing antithrombin III activity.[71,72] If possible, oral contraceptives should be discontinued at least one month prior to elective surgery and other methods substituted.[73] Varicose veins may not be an independent risk factor in the development of venous thrombosis but are associated with advanced age, obesity, and prior thrombosis. There are no preoperative laboratory tests of the coagulation system that predict the development of postoperative thrombosis.[74-76]

The incidence of thrombosis increases with the number of risk factors present.[53] A number of attempts have been made to quantitate cumulative risk more precisely using relatively complicated point systems,[77-80] but unfortunately most of these indices have not been helpful. A simpler index based on age and body weight has been developed and applied to general surgical patients, and satisfactory results were obtained with the index when low-dose heparin was administered only to those deemed high-risk.[81] Although this index is easier to use and has produced encouraging initial results, further evaluation is needed.

Thus, while precise quantification of risk and selective use of prophylaxis are desirable, the risk of thromboembolic complications in a given patient cannot be assessed with accuracy. Because of this, universal prophylaxis for all patients over age 40 has been recommended.[59]

THROMBOPROPHYLAXIS: METHODS AND APPLICATION

The decision to initiate thromboprophylaxis and the choice of method must be based not only on the risk of thromboembolic complications but also on the characteristics of available methods. The choice of prophylaxis therefore depends on analysis of data on the safety and efficacy of each method in a given clinical setting.

Unfortunately, the literature on the safety and efficacy of the various prophylactic methods is voluminous, frequently contradic-

tory, and pervaded with methodologic problems that complicate evaluation of individual studies and comparison of different studies. These problems include differences in choices of endpoints, diagnostic studies, criteria for diagnosis, patient populations, and prophylactic regimens.

Individual studies suffer from various methodological problems, including failure to use adequate sample size, specify diagnostic criteria, provide appropriate controls, perform statistical analysis, limit concurrent medications, and provide proper blinding. The last two are particularly important in evaluating bleeding complications of anticoagulants when subjective endpoints such as wound hematoma are used and the concurrent use of drugs like aspirin are not taken into account.

Despite these caveats, clinicians rely on the literature to make decisions regarding the safety and efficacy of the various thromboprophylactic methods. These regimens can be divided into physical or mechanical methods aimed at reducing venous stasis, and pharmacologic methods that reduce the coagulability of blood.

Physical Methods of Thromboprophylaxis

Physical methods of thromboprophylaxis include leg elevation, early ambulation, passive foot flexion, graduated compression stockings, electrical calf-muscle stimulation, and intermittent pneumatic compression. Although most of them are simple, inexpensive, and free of bleeding complications, they vary greatly in efficacy. Leg elevation,[82,83] early ambulation, and passive foot flexion[84] are not consistently effective in preventing postoperative thromboembolic events. Active exercise with a bed bicycle and electrical calf-muscle stimulation[85] have been found to be impractical in most circumstances.

Graduated Compression Stockings

Graduated compression of the leg with external pressures of 18 mmHg at the ankle decreasing to 8 mmHg at the upper thigh has been shown to increase mean flow in the femoral vein.[86] The thigh-length thromboembolic deterrent (TED) stocking is designed to produce such a gradient and can be used in 95 percent of patients.[87] It significantly increases femoral venous blood flow velocity[88] and clearance of radiocontrast material.[89]

There are few controlled studies on the efficacy of graduated compression stockings in preventing postoperative DVT in general surgical patients. Although they appear to be of some value in some patients, their efficacy is less certain in those with an increased risk of thromboembolic disease.[43,90] Some additional benefit has been demonstrated when they are used in conjunction with low-dose heparin (LDH)[91,92] or dextran.[93]

External Pneumatic Compression (EPC)

Intermittent pneumatic compression, the most effective of the mechanical methods of thromboprophylaxis, was first used in 1959.[94] Cuffs, boots, or stockings are cyclically inflated and deflated with compressed air. Several devices are available and differ in design, cycle length, pressure applied, and method of applying pressure. They improve pulsatile venous flow[95] and may cause activation of the fibrinolytic system.[96] Evaluating the efficacy of EPC is particularly difficult because of differences in the devices and duration of application. However, EPC has been proven effective in general surgical, gynecologic, urologic, and neurosurgical patients. Since EPC causes no increase in postoperative bleeding, it may be the method of choice in eye surgery or neurosurgery. EPC is not effective if compression is applied only during surgery or for less than 48 hours thereafter. It is therefore recommended that EPC be continued for the duration of the period of risk.[97]

The efficacy of EPC in high-risk patients has been questioned, with conflicting data in patients with malignancy[40,98] and in those undergoing orthopedic surgery[99] and neurosurgery.[100] More recent studies of patients undergoing hip surgery have demonstrated the efficacy of thigh-length devices with sequential compression,[101,102] but, until further studies are performed, EPC cannot be recommended in this setting. With these exceptions, EPC is generally effective in preventing DVT but has not yet proven so in reducing the incidence of PE or FPE by itself.

Pneumatic compression boots are considered safe, but acute compartment syndrome has been reported when a device malfunctioned and excessive pressure was applied.[103] Patient acceptance has been limited because prolonged use may cause excessive warmth and sweating,[64] but newer models have overcome some of these problems. EPC cannot be used in procedures involving the lower leg and is contraindicated in patients with severe peripheral vascular disease and in those with suspected DVT.

Pharmacologic Methods of Prophylaxis

Low-Dose Heparin (LDH)

Soon after its discovery, heparin in therapeutic doses was found to be effective in preventing postoperative venous thrombosis. However, because full anticoagulation with heparin is complicated by the risk of bleeding and requires careful monitoring, low-dose heparin regimens were developed.[104] These consist of the subcutaneous administration of doses of heparin that do not alter coagulation studies, thereby reducing the risk of bleeding and the need for monitoring.

Only trace amounts of heparin are required to accelerate the neutralization of activated factor Xa by antithrombin III.[105] This may explain why LDH is less effective when the coagulation system has already been previously activated, as in patients with hip fracture or extensive trauma. In addition to its effect on antithrombin III, heparin may also decrease platelet aggregation and blood viscosity.[106]

Most studies of LDH prophylaxis use 5000 units of subcutaneous heparin 12 hours before surgery and 5000 units subcutaneously every 8 or 12 hours thereafter. There is no difference in efficacy between the two regimens,[106] but more bleeding complications occur with more frequent administration. Therefore, 5000 units every 12 hours is recommended.

The duration of therapy has varied in clinical trials. Short courses limited to the early postoperative period have not been effective in preventing thrombosis after discontinuation of the drug. Heparin prophylaxis should therefore be continued until discharge from the hospital. Although administration of fixed low doses of heparin results in wide variation in blood heparin levels among patients[107] and occasionally prolongs the partial thromboplastin time in some individuals,[108] routine monitoring of coagulation studies is unnecessary.[6] However, the prothrombin time, partial thromboplastin time, and platelet count should be checked before initiating therapy.

Other methods of administering LDH have recently been introduced. These include perioperative intravenous heparin[109] and an ultra-low-dose regimen (1 mg/kg/hr).[110] Both regimens have proved effective in small series of patients but require further study.

The efficacy of LDH in preventing DVT after general surgery has been analyzed in a large number of studies. In patients undergoing general surgery, the preponderance of evidence confirms the effectiveness of LDH in reducing the incidence of calf-vein thrombosis.[111] More importantly, LDH has been shown to reduce the incidence of PE[112] and FPE[113] in general surgical patients.

Similar results have been demonstrated in patients undergoing gynecologic surgery.[113] However, patients undergoing surgery for gynecologic cancer may not be protected.[114] They have a higher risk of DVT because they have malignancy, are older, and usually undergo longer procedures involving extensive pelvic dissection. LDH is effective in urologic procedures other than open prostatectomy. The results in open prostatectomy have generally been unsatisfactory[115] and are attributed to the extent of pelvic surgery often performed for malignancy in older patients. LDH may not be able to counteract the large amounts of tissue thromboplastin released during the procedure.

Few trials of LDH have been conducted in neurosurgical patients because of the fear of bleeding complications. In one study, the incidence of DVT was significantly reduced with no increase in bleeding complications.[116,117] However, the data are not yet sufficient to recommend the use of LDH in this setting.

The efficacy of LDH in orthopedic surgery has been most thoroughly studied in patients undergoing surgical repair of hip fracture or elective hip replacement. Results in these high-risk patients are disappointing. Although ^{125}I fibrinogen scanning demonstrates significant reduction in DVT in patients treated with LDH, the incidence remains unacceptably high, particularly in those undergoing surgery for hip fracture. Moreover, ^{125}I scans may overestimate the benefit of LDH because they are unreliable in detecting proximal iliofemoral thrombosis that is particularly common without associated calf thrombosis in these patients. In addition, fibrin in the surgical wound can interfere with interpretation of the scan. Thus, studies that rely on fibrinogen scanning alone or use venography only in patients with positive scans may underestimate the incidence of clinically important proximal thrombi. Although one study demonstrated a significant decrease in the frequency and extent of proximal thrombosis with LDH,[118] others have shown reductions only in calf thrombi. Studies using routine venography have demonstrated no benefit of LDH.[119] There is also no convincing evidence that LDH is effective in preventing pulmonary embolism in orthopedic patients.[120]

The lack of efficacy of LDH in this setting may be due to several factors. Trauma to muscle and soft tissue may release tissue thromboplastin or platelet factor 4 in amounts too great to be neutralized by low doses of heparin. Hip surgery can also lead to endothelial injury and platelet aggregation, mechanisms not usually seen in other procedures and perhaps not amenable to inhibition by LDH. Hip surgery more often involves older patients and longer periods of immobility. In procedures for hip fractures, the coagulation system may be activated by the injury itself, and thrombi may form before LDH is administered.

Attempts have been made to improve the efficacy of LDH in orthopedic surgery using heparin in increased doses. Regimens of 5000 units given every eight rather than every 12 hours afford more protection but are associated with increased bleeding. Adjusted-dose regimens in which the amount given is based on plasma heparin levels or partial thromboplastin times result in larger total daily doses.[121,122] Although this method requires more monitoring than standard LDH prophylaxis, initial results have been encouraging.[122]

The major complication of LDH is intraoperative or postoperative bleeding. The incidence of bleeding ranges from 0 to 27 percent[123] and occurs more often when heparin is given every eight hours. Excessive bleeding has most often been described as increased formation of wound hematomas, but double-blind studies have failed to confirm this finding.[58] In fact, these studies have generally failed to demonstrate a significant overall increase in bleeding, transfusion requirements, or adverse outcomes due to bleeding in patients treated with LDH.[58] However, LDH has been associated with hematuria and occasional hematomas at injection sites.

The major reservation concerning the use of LDH in neurosurgical patients is the possibility of intracranial hemorrhage. There is little literature on this subject presumably because prophylactic anticoagulation has been attempted so infrequently. In one study of 58 neurosurgical patients treated with standard LDH, none had significant intracranial hemorrhage.[124] In another study examining patients with intracranial hemorrhage, those treated with LDH actually had a lower incidence of rebleeding than control patients but did not benefit in terms of prevention of thrombosis.[125]

There are several less-common complications of LDH therapy. Thrombocytopenia can develop approximately three days after heparin administration. It is not related to dose or route of administration, and has been reported in patients receiving LDH prophylaxis[126] and in those with a history of heparin-induced thrombocytopenia who are subsequently treated with LDH.[127] Hyperkalemia has been reported[128] and is due to suppression of plasma aldosterone levels by the drug. Patients with diabetes mellitus and chronic renal insufficiency have a higher risk of this complication. LDH rarely causes allergic reactions and skin necrosis.

Since the use of low-dose heparin has not been extensively studied in spinal surgery and other neurosurgical procedures, other forms of thromboprophylaxis should be considered. Because of even a small risk of bleeding, LDH should not be used in patients undergoing eye surgery, in those receiving spinal anesthesia, and in those who have sustained major trauma. It should not be given to patients who have taken aspirin or other antiplatelet agents before surgery or to those with a known or suspected bleeding diathesis. It should be used with caution, if at all, in patients with known or suspected endocarditis or pericarditis.

Low-Dose Heparin–Dihydroergotamine (LDH-DHE)

Dihydroergotamine (DHE) is an ergot alkaloid that causes constriction of venous capacitance vessels and alters peripheral vascular resistance and arterial flow. It has been shown to increase venous flow rates as much as 200 percent[129] and therefore presumably acts by reducing stasis. It has been speculated that DHE may prevent subtle endothelial damage by reducing venodilation.[130] No definite effects on the coagulation or fibrinolytic systems have been demonstrated. DHE is most often used in combination with LDH. The two drugs have different modes of action, and their effects are additive. The usual dosage of DHE is 0.5 mg subcutaneously, generally given in combination with 5000 units of heparin two hours before surgery and every 12 hours thereafter.

In patients undergoing general,[131,132] gynecologic,[133] and urologic surgery,[134] there is no compelling evidence that LDH-DHE is superior to other methods of prophylaxis. However, in elective hip surgery, the combination is more effective than LDH alone in reducing the incidence of DVT.[135–137] There are no data on the safety or efficacy of LDH-DHE in patients undergoing neurosurgery and insufficient data on its effectiveness in preventing proximal thrombosis, PE, and FPE.

LDH-DHE is associated with more adverse reactions than LDH alone, and the only fixed-drug combination has been withdrawn from the market.[138] There are case reports of significant arterial spasm in patients receiving DHE,[139,140] resulting in mesenteric infarction, stroke, skin and muscle necrosis, and ischemia of the extremities. The precise role of DHE in these complications is not entirely clear since some of the patients studied had associated sepsis, trauma, or hypotension. The incidence of these complications is less than 0.01 per 1000 patients treated.[141] Most studies document no cardiac complications, and animal experiments show that myocardial blood flow is unchanged. Minor side effects include numbness and tingling of the fingers or toes, myalgia, weakness, transient tachycardia or bradycardia, rashes, nausea, vomiting, pruritus, and edema. Hypertension, fever, bronchospasm, and anaphylaxis have also been reported.[138]

LDH-DHE is contraindicated in the same situations as LDH. In addition, the combination should not be given to patients with sepsis, hypotension, vasospastic disorders, significant peripheral vascular disease, severe hypertension, recent myocardial infarction, or angina. Unlike heparin, it is contraindicated in pregnancy. It should be used with caution, if at all, in patients receiving beta-blockers or dopamine, which can increase the toxicity of ergot alkaloids.[142]

The cost to the pharmacist for a seven-day supply of the fixed combination of LDH-DHE is four to five times greater than that of LDH alone.

Dextran

Dextran was originally developed during World War II as a plasma substitute. It was subsequently shown to have an antithrombotic effect[129] and has been used primarily in Europe in the prophylaxis of thrombotic disease. Its effects include expanding intravascular volume, decreasing blood viscosity, decreasing platelet adhesiveness,[143] reducing factor VIII activity, and accelerating the inhibition of factor Xa by antithrombin III.

Dextran requires intravenous administration in a dose of 500–1000 ml on the day of surgery. The higher dose may be more effective. Several studies have reported efficacy with infusions given only on the day of surgery, while others have recommended that additional infusions be given every other day for the duration of the period of risk. Two dextran preparations of different molecular weights are currently available, dextran 40 and dextran 70. Although they are metabolized differently, there is little evidence that one preparation is significantly more effective than the other.[110]

Dextran does not cause a significant reduction in postoperative venous thrombosis after general or gynecologic surgery and is therefore less effective than low-dose heparin. In patients undergoing elective hip procedures, dextran produces no significant reductions in DVT but is surprisingly more effective in surgery for hip fractures.[144] However, there is no evidence that dextran is superior to other prophylactic methods. Data on its effectiveness in reducing the incidence of PE and FPE are inconclusive.

Dextran has been associated with a number of serious adverse effects, including allergic reactions ranging from mild to fatal cases of anaphylaxis. The incidence of serious allergic reactions is less than one percent.[145] They can be prevented by hapten inhibition,[146] in which the patient is pretreated with low-molecular-weight dextran to block antibody binding sites and prevent aggregation when the higher-molecular-weight compounds are infused. There have been some reports of increased postoperative bleeding but not with newer dextran preparations in doses of less than 1.5 g/kg body weight. Dextran can also cause in vitro clumping of erythrocytes and interfere with crossmatching of blood. In expanding intravascular volume, it can exacerbate or precipitate congestive heart failure in susceptible patients. Acute renal failure has been reported in patients with dehydration, hypotension, and pre-existing renal insufficiency. It should not be given to patients with asthma or a history of a previous allergic reaction to dextran. It is contraindicated in neurosurgical patients who may have defects in the blood-brain barrier. The osmotic effect of dextran can cause increases in intracranial pressure.[147]

Dextran requires intravenous administration and is at least three times the cost of LDH prophylaxis.

Warfarin

Warfarin produces anticoagulation by inhibiting the synthesis of the vitamin K-dependent coagulation factors II, VII, IX, and X. The time of initiation of warfarin varies from study to study and ranges from 14 days before to four days after surgery. In most trials, warfarin is started shortly after surgery and is therefore not truly prophylactic except in preventing propagation of clot.

Although not rigorously studied, warfarin is more effective the earlier it is initiated and should be started before surgery if possible. The ideal duration of warfarin therapy is unknown. One study documented late pulmonary embolism after discontinuation of anticoagulation, leading to the recommendation that warfarin be routinely continued for three months after hip surgery.[148]

The dose of warfarin must be individualized with close monitoring of the prothrombin time (PT). In most studies, attempts have been made to achieve a prothrombin time of 1.5 to 2 times the control value. There have been limited trials of a low-dose warfarin regimen in which elevations in prothrombin time are maintained at 1.2 to 1.4 times the control value and of an ultra-low-dose schedule in which patients are given a fixed dose of one mg per day. These latter two methods have yielded encouraging initial results but require further study.[149,150]

Although warfarin has been studied in most surgical settings, it should only be used in high-risk patients when safer and equally effective alternatives are not feasible. Warfarin has been shown to be an effective prophylactic agent in high-risk patients undergoing major urologic surgery.[151] It also reduces the incidence of DVT and may also decrease the incidence of FPE after hip surgery.[152-154]

The major risk of oral anticoagulants is hemorrhage. The incidence of severe hemorrhage is two to seven percent, with a mortality rate of less than 0.1 percent.[52] The risk of bleeding is lower when therapy is started after surgery and is proportional to the prolongation of the PT. When the PT is within the therapeutic range, bleeding is generally confined to the operative site. With greater degrees of anticoagulation, the risk of spontaneous bleeding, including intracranial and retroperitoneal hemorrhage, increases substantially. However, despite the appreciable risk of severe and even fatal hemorrhage with oral anticoagulants, it is lower than that of FPE in patients undergoing hip surgery. Since overall mortality is decreased with warfarin, its prophylactic use in this setting can be justified.[155]

Oral anticoagulants should be used with caution and careful monitoring and only in high-risk patients in whom the risk of thromboembolism exceeds that of bleeding. They are contraindicated in patients with known bleeding, uncontrolled hypertension, active peptic ulcer disease, or a bleeding diathesis. They are also contraindicated in patients undergoing neurosurgical procedures, eye surgery, spinal anesthesia, or spinal surgery. They should not be given to patients who have sustained intracranial or visceral trauma and should be used with caution, if at all, in patients taking antiplatelet agents or other drugs that significantly interact with them.

Oral anticoagulants themselves are relatively inexpensive and are comparable in cost to LDH. However, monitoring of the prothrombin time increases the cost substantially.

Low-Molecular-Weight Heparin (LMWH)

The biologic effects of heparin depend on its molecular weight. Commercially available heparin consists of components with molecular weights ranging from 3000 to 40,000 daltons, with an average of 15,000.[156] Studies on heparin fractions of different molecular weights have shown increasingly potent inhibition of factor Xa with decreasing molecular weight.[157] However, other effects on the clotting system decrease with decreasing molecular weight. Animal studies support the hypothesis that LMWH has greater antithrombotic activity but is associated with less bleeding than standard preparations.

When compared to standard LDH regimens in general surgical[158-160] and gynecologic patients,[161] LMWH is equally effective in preventing venous thrombosis. In those with hip fractures, LMWH significantly reduces the rate of venous thrombosis[162,163] and has been shown to be as or more effective than LDH.[164,165] In one study, LMWH and warfarin were compared in patients with hip fractures, and those receiving LMWH had lower rates of venous thrombosis.[166] Standard doses of LMWH do not produce excessive bleeding.[167,168] LMWH allows a simplified dosing schedule requiring only a single injection before surgery and one daily during the remainder of the hospitalization.

The cost of LMWH is about twice that of standard heparin therapy.

Other Modalities

Several other methods have been investigated in a number of small series. DHE has been given in combination with LMWH but has not yet been found to be superior to the heparin compound alone. Aspirin and other antiplatelet agents have not proved effective in reducing DVT.[169] In addition, tocainide has been largely ineffective.[170]

Drugs that have shown promise and merit further investigation include ancrod,[171] lidocaine,[172] antithrombin III,[173] and defibrinotide.[174] Several semisynthetic heparin analogues have been developed, and initial clinical trials suggest that they are as effective as LDH and dextran in preventing postoperative thrombosis.[175] In patients undergoing hip surgery, ancrod, a defibrinating enzyme derived from snakes,[171] and lidocaine, which inhibits leukocyte adhesion,[172] have proved effective in reducing the incidence of postoperative thrombosis. Since the hypercoagulable state during and after surgery is accompanied by a decrease in antithrombin III levels, attempts have been made to administer it with low-dose heparin.[173] Defibrinotide, an agent with profibrinolytic and antithrombotic but not anticoagulant effects, has also been utilized.[174]

Caval interruption or insertion of a Greenfield filter does not prevent postoperative DVT but may prevent PE. Although its use in selected patients has been recommended,[176,177] it is justified only in high-risk patients with contraindications to anticoagulants or documented pulmonary embolism while fully anticoagulated.

SUMMARY OF COMPARATIVE TRIALS AND RECOMMENDATIONS

Review of controlled trials of the safety and efficacy of various prophylactic modalities allows formulation of recommendations for prophylaxis of postoperative thromboembolic disease in various clinical settings. These recommendations are summarized in Table 48-2 and serve as general guidelines for patients undergoing surgery. The assessment of the risk of thromboembolic complications, the decision to use prophylactic measures, and the choice of regimen must be made on an individual basis. A given patient may present a set of circumstances warranting rational deviation from these guidelines. Since none of the various methods is totally effective, clinicians must maintain a high index of suspicion of thromboembolic disease even in patients receiving prophylactic therapy.

General Surgery

Patients undergoing general surgery do not have a uniform risk of developing postoperative thromboembolism, but can be stratified into three broad categories. Low-risk patients are under age 40, undergo relatively short procedures, and have no other risk factors. Early ambulation and graded compression stockings are sufficient prophylaxis. Most surgical patients fall into the moderate risk category because they are over 40, undergo longer procedures, and have associated risk factors like obesity. Modalities with demonstrated efficacy in general surgical patients include EPC, LDH, LDH-DHE, dextran, and oral anticoagulants. The risk of bleeding with oral anticoagulants exceeds the risk of thromboembolism in this group of patients and is not warranted. EPC and LDH have comparable efficacy, and LDH-DHE may be marginally more effective. Although dextran may be equally effective as LDH in preventing FPE, it is less effective than LDH in preventing DVT. Moreover, because dextran is more difficult to administer, associated with more adverse reactions, and more expensive than LDH, it should not be considered the method of choice. Any of the three remaining modalities—EPC, LDH, or LDH-DHE—are acceptable. EPC is more cumbersome and not as well accepted by patients as LDH. LDH-DHE is more expensive than LDH and carries greater risk. Therefore, LDH remains the prophylactic method of choice.

TABLE 48-2. Recommendations for Thromboprophylaxis

Procedures	Recommended Prophylaxis	Alternative Methods
General Surgery		
1. Low risk: age < 40	Graduated compression stockings	Early ambulation
2. Moderate risk: age > 40 and surgery > 30 minutes	LDH	EPC
3. High risk: age > 40 and previous history of DVT or extensive surgery for malignancy	LDH (q 8 h) or LDH-DHE	Continuous heparin infusion or EPC plus LDH or low-dose warfarin
Gynecologic Surgery		
1. Benign disease	LDH	EPC
2. Malignant disease	EPC	See high-risk general surgery
Urologic Surgery	EPC	Warfarin
Neurosurgery	EPC	None
Orthopedic Surgery		
1. Elective hip surgery	LDH-DHE or LMWH	Dextran or warfarin
2. Hip fracture	Warfarin or LMWH	Dextran
3. Knee surgery	EPC or warfarin	Aspirin

High-risk patients having general surgery are older, undergo prolonged surgery often for extensive malignancy, or have a previous history of thromboembolic disease. There are few data to guide the choice of prophylaxis in this group. Empiric recommendations include LDH in a dose of 5000 units subcutaneously every eight hours instead of every 12; LDH-DHE; continuous intravenous heparin infusion to maintain a PTT of 1.2 to 1.5 times the control value; LDH in combination with EPC; and low-dose warfarin started at the time of surgery to maintain a PT 1.2 to 1.5 times the control value.[178]

Gynecologic Surgery

Because there have been relatively few comparative trials in gynecologic patients and they are more often included in studies of general surgical patients, the recommended approach is similar in the two groups. LDH therapy is the first choice, although LDH-DHE and EPC are effective alternatives. Dextran offers no advantage over LDH and may be less effective. LMWH may also be effective but has not been extensively studied. Standard LDH prophylaxis may not be sufficient in patients undergoing surgery for pelvic malignancy. Although EPC is effective in this situation,[179] the regimens listed above for high-risk patients undergoing general surgery should be considered. A single study has demonstrated benefit from warfarin.[152]

Urologic Surgery

There are few comparative trials in urological patients and little experience with modalities like LDH-DHE, dextran, and aspirin. LDH is effective in patients undergoing transurethral resection of the prostate but is less reliable in those undergoing open prostatectomy. External pneumatic compression and warfarin are effective in these patients and are the methods of choice.

Neurosurgery

There are relatively few options for prophylaxis in neurosurgical patients. Limited data suggest that LDH is safe and effective in these patients,[180] and one review recommends it in those undergoing elective neurosurgical procedures.[147] However, until there are further studies with larger numbers of patients, LDH cannot be recommended for routine use. EPC remains the method of choice because of its efficacy and lack of bleeding complications.

Orthopedic Surgery

Elective Hip Surgery

The recommended agents with demonstrated efficacy in elective hip surgery include LDH-DHE, warfarin, and LMWH. Patients with a high risk of thromboembolism such as those with a history of DVT or PE should receive warfarin. Adjusted-dose heparin and sequential external pneumatic compression with a thigh-length device are promising alternatives but require further study. The efficacy of dextran and aspirin has not been demonstrated.

Hip Fractures

Warfarin and LMWH are effective in reducing the rate of DVT in patients with hip fractures and are recommended as first choices.

Dextran can be used alternatively in those with contraindications to anticoagulation. Further study of LDH-DHE, adjusted-dose heparin, and EPC is needed.

SUMMARY

1. Postoperative venous thrombosis and pulmonary embolism remain major causes of excessive morbidity and mortality related to surgical procedures.

2. Patients with the greatest risk of DVT and PE are those undergoing joint replacement surgery involving the lower extremity.

3. Patients with no increased risk of perioperative thrombosis include those under 40, those undergoing brief operative procedures, those undergoing head and neck surgery, and those undergoing arthroscopy of the knee.

4. In patients undergoing general surgery and most types of gynecologic and urologic surgery, effective methods of thromboprophylaxis include low-dose heparin, low-dose heparin with dihydroergotamine, and external pneumatic compression stockings.

5. In patients undergoing open prostatectomy surgery, external pneumatic compression and warfarin have been shown to be effective.

6. In patients undergoing neurosurgery, the risk of bleeding has limited the study of LDH therapy in thromboprophylaxis. Therefore, the recommended method remains external pneumatic compression stockings.

7. Patients undergoing joint replacement surgery in the lower extremity should receive thromboprophylaxis with the combination of low-dose heparin and dihydroergotamine, low-molecular-weight heparin, warfarin, or external pneumatic compression stockings.

REFERENCES

1. Nylander G, Olivecrona H, Hedner U: Earlier and concurrent morbidity of patients with acute lower leg thrombosis. *Acta Chir Scand* 143:425, 1977.
2. Bell WR, Simon TL, DeMets DL: The clinical features of submassive and massive pulmonary emboli. *Am J Med* 62:355, 1977.
3. Bell W, Zuidema G: Low-dose heparin—concern and perspectives. *Surgery* 85:469, 1979.
4. Van De Water JM: Preoperative and postoperative techniques in the prevention of pulmonary complications. *Surg Clin N Am* 60:1339 1980.
5. Sevitt S, Gallagher NG: Prevention of venous thrombosis and pulmonary embolism in injured patients. *Lancet* II:981, 1959.
6. Council on Thrombosis of the American Heart Association: Prevention of venous thromboembolism in surgical patients by low-dose heparin. *Circulation* 55:423A, 1977.
7. Bergqvist D: Prevention of postoperative deep-vein thrombosis in Sweden: Results of a survey. *World J Surg* 4:489, 1980.
8. Conti S, Daschbach M: Venous thromboembolism prophylaxis: A survey of its use in the United States. *Arch Surg* 117:1036, 1982.
9. Piement GD, Wessinger SJ, Harris WH: Survey of prophylaxis against venous thromboembolism in adults undergoing hip surgery VTED prophylaxis. *Surg Clin Orthop* 223:188, 1987.
10. Virchow R: *Gesammelte Abhandlugen zur Wissenschaftlichen Medizin.* Von Meidinger Sohn, Frankfurt, 1856.

11. Nicolaides AN, Kakkar VV, Field ES et al: Venous stasis and deep-vein thrombosis. *Br J Surg* 59:713, 1972.

12. Lindstrom B, Ahlman H, Jonsson O et al: Blood flow in the calves during surgery. *Acta Chir Scand* 143:335, 1977.

13. Bird AD: The effect of surgery, injury, and prolonged bed rest on calf blood flow. *Aust NZ J Surg* 41:374, 1972.

14. Comerota AJ, Stewart GJ, Alburger PD et al: Operative venodilation: A previously unsuspected factor in the cause of postoperative deep-vein thrombosis. *Surg* 106:301, 1989.

15. Almen T, Nylander G: Serial phlebography of the normal lower leg during muscular contraction and relaxation. *Acta Radiol* 57:264, 1962.

16. Hewson W. *Experimental Inquiries: 1. An Inquiry into the Properties of the Blood, with Some Remarks on Some of Its Morbid Appearances, and an Appendix Relating to the Discovery of the Lymphatic System in Birds, Fish and the Animals Called Amphibians*. London, Cadell, 1771.

17. Wessler S: The role of stasis in thrombosis, in Sherry S, Brinkhouse KM, Genlon E et al: (eds): *Thrombosis*. Washington, National Academy of Science, 1969.

18. Hamilton HW, Crawford JS, Gardiner JH et al: Venous thrombosis in patients with fracture of the upper end of the femur. A phlebographic study of the effects of prophylactic anticoagulation. *J Bone Joint Surg* 52B:268, 1970.

19. Harris WH, Salzman E, Athanasoulis C et al: Comparison of 125I-fibrinogen count scanning with phlebography for detection of venous thrombi after elective hip surgery. *N Engl J Med* 292:665, 1975.

20. Sevitt S: The structure and growth of valve-pocket thrombi in femoral veins. *J Clin Path* 27:517, 1974.

21. Stewart GJ, Stern HS, Lynch PR et al: Responses of canine jugular veins and carotid arteries to hysterectomy: Increased permeability and leucocyte adhesions and invasion. *Thromb Res* 20:473, 1980.

22. Warren R, Lauridsen J, Belko J: Alterations in numbers of circulating platelets following surgical operation and administration of adrenocorticotropic hormone. *Circulation* 7:481, 1953.

23. Ygge J: Studies on blood coagulation and fibrinolysis in conditions associated with an increased incidence of thrombosis. Methodological and clinical investigations. *Scand J Haematol* 11(Suppl):1, 1970.

24. Godal HC: Quantitative and qualitative changes in fibrinogen following major surgical operations. *Acta Med Scand* 171:687, 1962.

25. Egeberg O: Changes in the coagulation system following major surgical operations. *Acta Med Scand* 171:679, 1962.

26. Aberg M, Nilsson IM, Hedner U: Antithrombin III after operation. *Lancet* II:1337, 1973.

27. Olsson P: Variations in antithrombin activity in plasma after major surgery. *Acta Chir Scand* 126:24, 1963.

28. Stathatkis N, Papayannis AG, Gardikas CD: Postoperative antithrombin III concentration. *Lancet* I:430, 1973.

29. Esmon CT, Esmon ML, Saugstad J et al: Activation of protein C by complex between thrombin and endothelial cell surface protein, in Nossel HL, Vogel HJ (eds): *Pathobiology of the Endothelial Cell*. New York, Academic, 1982.

30. Nicolaides AN, Clark CT, Thomas RD et al: Fibrinolytic activator in the endothelium of the veins of the lower limb. *Br J Surg* 63:881, 1976.

31. Sue-Ling HM, Johnston D, Verheijen JH et al: Indicators of depressed fibrinolytic activity in preoperative prediction of deep-venous thrombosis. *Br J Surg* 74:275, 1987.

32. Aranda A, Paramo JA, Rocha E: Fibrinolytic activity in plasma after gynecological and urological surgery. *Haemostasis* 18:129, 1988.

33. Gomez MJ, Carroll RC, Hansard RM et al: Perioperative fibrinolytic kinetics. *Curr Surg* Nov/Dec:476, 1987.

34. Sorensen J, Lars B, Lassen M et al: Association between plasma levels of tissue plasminogen activator and postoperative deep-vein thrombosis—influence of prophylaxis with a low molecular weight heparin. *Thromb Res* 59:131–138, 1990.

35. Jorgensen L, Lind B, Hauch O et al: Thrombin-antithrombin III-complex and fibrin degradation products in plasma: Surgery and postoperative venous thrombosis. *Thromb Res* 59:69–76, 1990.

36. Gitel SN, Stephenson RC, Wessler S: In vitro and in vivo correlation of clotting protease activity: Effect of heparin. *Proc Natl Acad Sci USA* 74:3028, 1977.

37. Rodzynek JJ, Damien J, Huberty M et al: Incidence of preoperative deep-venous thrombosis in abdominal surgery. *Br J Surg* 71:731, 1984.

38. Kakkar VV, Howe CT, Flanc C et al: Natural history of postoperative deep-vein thrombosis. *Lancet* II:230, 1969.

39. Flanc C, Kakkar VV, Clarke MB: The detection of venous thrombosis of the legs using 125I-labelled fibrinogen. *Br J Surg* 55:742, 1968.

40. Roberts VC, Cotton LT: Prevention of postoperative deep-vein thrombosis in patients with malignant disease. *Br Med J* 1:358, 1974.

41. Kakkar VV: Prevention of venous thromboembolism. *Clin Hematol* 10:543, 1981.

42. Sikorski JM, Hampson WG, Staddon GE: The natural history and aetiology of deep-vein thrombosis after total hip replacement. *J Bone Joint Surg* 63:171, 1981.

43. Clarke-Pearson DL, Jelovsek FR, Creasman WT: Thromboembolism complicating surgery for cervical and uterine malignancy: Incidence, risk factors, and prophylaxis. *Obstet Gynecol* 61:87, 1983.

44. Fossard DP, Kakkar VV, Corrigan TP et al: The origin of deep-vein thrombosis: A phlebography study. *Br J Surg* 61:332, 1974.

45. McLachlin J, Patterson JC: Some basic observations on venous thrombosis and pulmonary embolism. *Surg Gynecol Obstet* 93:1, 1951.

46. Stamatakis JD, Kakkar VV, Lawrence D et al: The origin of thrombi in the deep veins of the lower limb. A venographic study. *Br J Surg* 65:449, 1978.

47. Nicolaides AN, O'Connell JD: Origin and distribution of thrombosis in patients with clinical deep-vein thrombosis, in Nicolaides AN (ed): *Thromboembolism*. Lancaster, Medical and Technical Publishing, 1975.

48. Brouse NL, Thomas ML: Source of nonlethal pulmonary emboli. *Lancet* 1:258, 1974.

49. Clarke-Pearson DL, Synan IS, Colemen E et al: The natural history of postoperative venous thromboemboli in gynecologic oncology: A prospective study of 382 patients. *Obstet Gynecol* 148:1051, 1984.

50. Bell WR, Simon TL: Current status of pulmonary thromboembolic disease: Pathophysiology, diagnosis, prevention and treatment. *Am Heart J* 103:329, 1982.

51. Moser KM, LeMoine JR: Is embolic risk conditioned by location of deep-venous thrombosis? *Ann Intern Med* 94:439, 1981.

52. Havig O: Deep-vein thrombosis and pulmonary embolism. An autopsy study with multiple regression analysis of possible risk factors. *Acta Chir Scand* 478(Suppl):–95, 1977.

53. Moser KM: Thromboembolic disease in the patient undergoing urologic surgery. *Urol Clin N Am* 10:101, 1983.

54. O'Donnell T, Browse N, Burnaud K et al: The socioeconomic effects of an idiofemoral venous thrombosis. *J Surg Res* 22:483, 1977.

55. Francis CW, Ricotta JJ, Evarts CM et al: Long-term clinical observations and venous functional abnormalities after asymptomatic venous thrombosis following total hip or knee arthroplasty. *Clin Orthop* 232:271, 1988.

56. Lindhagen A, Bergqvist D, Hallbook T et al: Venous function five to eight years after clinically suspected deep-venous thrombosis. *Acta Med Scand* 217:289, 1985.

57. Browse NL, Clemenson G, Thomas ML: Is the postphlebitic leg always postphlebitic? Relation between phlebographic appearances of deep-vein thrombosis and late sequelae. *Br Med J* 281:1167, 1980.

58. Evans DS: The early diagnosis of thromboembolism by ultrasound. *Ann R Coll Surg Engl* 49:225, 1971.

59. Doran FSA, White M, Drurz M: A clinical trial designed to test the relative value of two simple methods of reducing the risk of venous stasis in the lower limbs during surgical operation, the danger of

thrombosis and a subsequent pulmonary embolus with a survey of the problem. *Br J Surg* 57:20, 1970.

60. Kakkar VV: The current status of low-dose heparin in the prophylaxis of thrombophlebitis and pulmonary embolism. *World J Surg* 2:3, 1978.

61. Oster G, Tuden RL, Colditz GA: A cost-effectiveness analysis of prophylaxis against deep-vein thrombosis in major orthopedic surgery. *JAMA* 257:203, 1987.

62. Hull RD, Hirsh J, Sackett DL et al: Cost-effectiveness of primary and secondary prevention of fatal pulmonary embolism in high-risk surgical patients. *CMA Journal* 127:990, 1982.

63. Salzman E, Davies G: Prophylaxis of venous thromboembolism. Analysis of cost-effectiveness. *Ann Surg* 191:207, 1980.

64. Borow M, Goldson H: Postoperative venous thrombosis: Evaluation of five methods of treatment. *Am J Surg* 141:245, 1981.

65. Modig J, Borg T, Karlstrom G et al: Thromboembolism after total hip replacement: Role of epidural and general anesthesia. *Anesth Analg* 62:174, 1983.

66. Modig J, Hjelmstedt A, Sahlstedt B et al: Comparative influences of epidural and general anaesthesia on deep-venous thrombosis and pulmonary embolism after total hip replacement. *Acta Chir Scand* 147:125, 1981.

67. Stringer MD, Steadman CA, Hedges AR et al: Deep-vein thrombosis after elective knee surgery. *J Bone Joint Surg* 71B:492, 1989.

68. Nicolaides AN, Irving D: Clinical factors and the risk of deep-venous thrombosis, in Nicolaides AN (ed): *Thromboembolism. Aetiology, Advances in Prevention and Management.* Baltimore, University Park Press, 1975.

69. Coon WW: Epidemiology of venous thromboembolism. *Ann Surg* 186:149, 1977.

70. Spires J, Byers R, Sanches E: Pulmonary thrombosis after head and neck surgery. *South Med J* 82:1111–1115, 1989.

71. Vesser MP, Doll R, Fanburn AS et al: Postoperative thromboembolism and the use of oral contraception. *Br Med J* 3:123, 1970.

72. Greene GR, Sarlwell PE: Oral contraceptive use in patients with thromboembolism following surgery, trauma or infection. *Am J Public Health* 62:680, 1972.

73. DeStefano F, Peterson HB, Ory HW et al: Oral contraceptives and postoperative venous thrombosis. *Am J Obstet Gynecol* 143:227, 1982.

74. Dhall TZ, Shah GA, Ferguson IA et al: Preoperative blood tests in prediction of postoperative deep-vein thrombosis. *Thromb Res* 27:143, 1982.

75. Sixma JJ: Techniques for diagnosing prethrombotic states. A review. *Thromb Haemost* 40:252, 1978.

76. Blanchard SA, Sirridge M: Deep-venous thrombosis in surgical patients: Possible laboratory predictors. *South Med J* 78:1161, 1985.

77. Tubiana R, Duparc J: Prevention of thromboembolic complications in orthopaedic and accident surgery. *J Bone Joint Surg* 43B:7, 1961.

78. Breneman J: A formula for predicting and a device for preventing postoperative thromboembolic disease. *Angiology* 14:437, 1963.

79. Laaksonen VA, Arola MKJ, Hannelin M et al: Effect of anaesthesia on the incidence of postoperative lower-limb thrombosis. *Ann Chir Gynecol Fenn* 62:304, 1973.

80. Tammisto T, Palmu A, Elfving G et al: Postoperative thromboembolism after different modes of artificial respiration. *Acta Chir Scand* 136:39, 1970.

81. Lowe GDO, McArdle BM, Carter DC et al: Prediction and selective prophylaxis of venous thrombosis in elective gastrointestinal surgery. *Lancet* 1:409, 1982.

82. Sigel B, Edelstein A, Felix R et al: Compression of the deep-venous system of the lower leg during inactive recumbency. *Arch Surg* 106:38, 1973.

83. Hartman T, Altner P, Freeark R: The effect of limb elevation in preventing venous thrombosis. A venographic study. *J Bone Joint Surg* 52:1618, 1970.

84. DeNardo SJ, DeNardo GL: [123]Iodine-fibrinogen scintigraphy. *Sem Nucl Med* 7:245, 1977.

85. Rosenberg IL, Evans M, Pollock AV: Prophylaxis of postoperative leg-vein thrombosis by low-dose subcutaneous heparin or preoperative calf-muscle stimulation: A controlled clinical trial. *Br Med J* 1:649, 1975.

86. Sigel B, Edelstein A, Savitch L et al: Type of compression for reducing venous stasis. A study of lower extremities during inactive recumbency. *Arch Surg* 110:171, 1975.

87. Allan A, Williams JT, Bolton JP et al: The use of graduated compression stockings in the prevention of postoperative deep-vein thrombosis. *Br J Surg* 70:172, 1983.

88. Inada K, Shirai N, Hayashi M et al: Postoperative deep-venous thrombosis in Japan. Incidence and prophylaxis. *Am J Surg* 145:775, 1983.

89. Lewis C, Antoine J, Mueller C et al: Elastic compression in the prevention of venous stasis. A critical reevaluation. *Am J Surg* 132:739, 1976.

90. Barnes R, Brand R, Clarke W et al: Efficacy of graded-compression antiembolism stockings in patients undergoing total hip arthroplasty. *Clin Orthop Rel Res* 132:61, 1978.

91. Thorngren S: Low-dose heparin and compression stockings in the prevention of postoperative deep-venous thrombosis. *Br J Surg* 67:482, 1980.

92. Jorgensen P, Hauch O, Dimo B et al: Venous thrombosis after acute abdominal operation. *Surg Gynecol Obstet* 172:44–48, 1991.

93. Bergqvist D, Lindblad B: The thromboprophylactic effect of graded elastic compression stockings in combination with Dextran 70. *Arch Surg* 119:1329, 1984.

94. Brush B, Wylie J, Block M et al: A device for the prevention of phlebothrombosis and pulmonary embolism. *Henry Ford Hosp Med J* 7:27, 1959.

95. Tarnay T, Rohr P, Davidson A et al: Pneumatic calf compression, fibrinolysis, and the prevention of deep-venous thrombosis. *Surg* 88:489, 1980.

96. Summaria L, Caprini JA, McMillan R et al: Relationship between postsurgical fibrinolytic parameters and deep-vein thrombosis in surgical patients treated with compression devices. *Am Surg* 54:156, 1988.

97. Butson R: Intermittent pneumatic calf compression for prevention of deep-venous thrombosis in general abdominal surgery. *Am J Surg* 142:525, 1981.

98. Hills NH, Pflug JJ, Jeyasignh K et al: Prevention of deep-vein thrombosis by intermittent pneumatic compression of calf. *Br Med J* 1:131, 1972.

99. Hull R, Delmore TJ, Hirsh J et al: Effectiveness of intermittent pulsative elastic stockings for the prevention of calf and thigh vein thrombosis in patients undergoing elective knee surgery. *Thromb Res* 16:37, 1979.

100. Turpie AG, Hirsh J, Gent M et al: Prevention of deep-vein thrombosis in potential neurosurgical patients: A randomized trial comparing graduated compression stockings alone or graduated compression stockings plus intermittent pneumatic compression with control. *Arch Intern Med* 149:679, 1989.

101. Hartman JT, Pugh JL, Smith RD et al: Cyclic sequential compression of the lower limb in prevention of deep-venous thrombosis. *J Bone Joint Surg* 64:1059, 1982.

102. Woollson ST, Watt JM: Intermittent pneumatic compression to prevent proximal deep-venous thrombosis during and after total hip replacement. *J Bone Joint Surg* 73A(4):507–512, 1991.

103. Werbel GB, Shybut GT: Acute compartment syndrome caused by a malfunctioning pneumatic-compression boot. A case report. *J Bone Joint Surg* 68A:1445, 1986.

104. Sharnoff JG: Results in the prophylaxis of postoperative thromboembolism. *Surg Gynecol Obstet* 123:303, 1966.

105. Wessler S, Yen ET: Theory and practice of minidose heparin in surgical patients: A status report. *Circulation* 47:671, 1973.

106. Erdi A, Thomas DP, Kakkar VV et al: Effect of low-dose subcutaneous heparin on whole-blood viscosity. *Lancet* II:342, 1976.

107. Brozovic M, Sterling Y, Abbosh J: Plasma heparin levels after low-dose subcutaneous heparin in patients undergoing hip replacement. *Br J Haematol* 31:561, 1975.

108. Clarke-Pearson DL, DeLong ER, Synan IS et al: Complications of low-dose heparin prophylaxis in gynecologic oncology surgery. *Obstet Gynecol* 64:689, 1984.

109. Sharrock N, Biren W, Salvati E et al: The effect of intravenous fixed-dose heparin during total hip arthroplasty on the incidence of deep-vein thrombosis. *J Bone Joint Surg* 72A:1456–1461, 1990.

110. Negus D, Friedgood A, Cos SJ et al: Ultra-low-dose intravenous heparin in the prevention of postoperative deep-vein thrombosis. *Lancet* I:891, 1980.

111. An International Multicentre Trial: Prevention of fatal postoperative pulmonary embolism by low doses of heparin. *Lancet* II:45, 1975.

112. Kiil J, Kiil J, Axelsen F et al: Prophylaxis against postoperative pulmonary embolism and deep-vein thrombosis by low-dose heparin. *Lancet* I:1115, 1978.

113. Clark-Pearson D, DeLong E, Synan I et al: A controlled trial of two low-dose heparin regimens for the prevention of postoperative deep-vein thrombosis. *Obstet Gynecol* 75:684–689, 1990.

114. Clarke-Pearson DL, Coleman RE, Synan IS et al: Venous thromboembolism prophylaxis in gynecologic oncology: A prospective, controlled trial of low-dose heparin. *Am J Obstet Gynecol* 145:606, 1983.

115. Halverstadt DB, Albert DD, Kroovand RL et al: Anticoagulation in urologic surgery. *Urology* 9:617, 1977.

116. Cerrato D, Ariano C, Fiacchino F: Deep-vein thrombosis and low-dose heparin prophylaxis in neurosurgical patients. *J Neurosurg* 49:378, 1978.

117. Barnett H, Clifford J, Llewellyn R: Safety of mini-dose heparin administration for neurosurgical patients. *J Neurosurg* 57:27, 1977.

118. Sagar S, Stamatakis JD, Higgins AF et al: Efficacy of low-dose heparin in prevention of extensive deep-vein thrombosis in patients undergoing total-hip replacement. *Lancet* I:151, 1976.

119. Harris WH, Salzman EW, Athanasoulis C: Comparison of warfarin, low-molecular-weight dextran, aspirin, and subcutaneous heparin in prevention of venous thromboembolism following total hip replacement. *J Bone Joint Surg* 56:1552, 1974.

120. Williams JW, Eikman EA, Greenberg SH et al: Failure of low-dose heparin to prevent pulmonary embolism after hip surgery or above the knee amputation. *Ann Surg* 188:468, 1978.

121. Pollar L, Taberner DA, Sandilands DG et al: An evaluation of APTT monitoring of LDH dosage in hip surgery. *Thromb Haemost* 47:50, 1982.

122. Leyvraz PF, Richard J, Bachmann F et al: Adjusted versus fixed-dose subcutaneous heparin in the prevention of deep-vein thrombosis after total hip replacement. *N Engl J Med* 309:954, 1983.

123. Pachter L, Riles T: Low-dose heparin: Bleeding and wound complications in the surgical patient. A prospective randomized study. *Ann Surg* 186:660, 1977.

124. Bostrom S, Holmgren E, Jonsson O et al: Postoperative thromboembolism in neurosurgery: A study on the prophylactic effect of calf muscle stimulation plus dextran compared to low-dose heparin. *Acta Neurochir* 80:83, 1986.

125. Dickmann U, Voth E, Schicha H et al: Heparin therapy, deep-vein thrombosis and pulmonary embolism after intracerebral hemorrhage. *Klin Wochenschr* 66:1182, 1988.

126. Hrushesky W: Subcutaneous heparin-induced thrombocytopenia. *Arch Intern Med* 138:1489, 1978.

127. Laster J, Elfrink R, Silver D: Reexposure to heparin of patients with heparin-associated antibodies. *J Vasc Surg* 9:677, 1989.

128. Edes TE, Sunderrajan EV: Heparin-induced hyperkalemia. *Arch Intern Med* 145:1070, 1985.

129. Rieckert H: Primare therapieziele bei der hypotonen fehlregulation. *Fortschr Med* 89:173, 1971.

130. The Multicenter Trial Committee: Prophylactic efficacy of low-dose dihydroergotamine and heparin in postoperative deep-venous thrombosis following intraabdominal operations. *J Vasc Surg* 1:608, 1984.

131. The Multicenter Trial Committee: Dihydroergotamine-heparin prophylaxis of postoperative deep-vein thrombosis. A multicenter trial. *JAMA* 251:2960, 1984.

132. Wille-Jorgensen P, Kjaergaard J, Thorup J et al: Heparin with and without dihydroergotamine in prevention of thromboembolic complications of major abdominal surgery. A randomized trial. *Arch Surg* 188:926, 1983.

133. Hohl MK, Luscher DP, Annaheim M et al: Dihydroergotamine and heparin or heparin alone for the prevention of postoperative thromboembolism in gynecology. *Arch Gynecol* 230:15, 1980.

134. Hansberry KL, Thompson IM, Bauman J et al: A prospective comparison of thromboembolic stockings, external sequential pneumatic compression stockings and heparin sodium/dihydroergotamine mesylate for the prevention of thromboembolic complications in urological surgery. *J Urol* 145:1205–1208, 1991.

135. Lowe LW: Venous thrombosis and embolism. *J Bone Joint Surg* 63:155, 1981.

136. Lahnborg G: Effect of low-dose heparin and dihydroergotamine prophylaxis on frequency of postoperative deep-vein thrombosis in patients undergoing posttraumatic hip surgery. *Acta Chir Scand* 146:319, 1980.

137. Schondorf TH, Weber U: Heparin in orthopaedic surgery. Prevention of deep-vein thrombosis in orthopaedic surgery with the combination of low-dose heparin plus either dihydroergotamine or dextran. *Scand J Haematol* 36(Suppl):126, 1986.

138. Dihydroergotamine-heparin to prevent postoperative deep-vein thrombosis. *Med Letter* 27:45, 1985.

139. Seifert KB, Blackshear WM, Cruse CW et al: Bilateral upper-extremity ischemia after administration of dihydroergotamine-heparin for prophylaxis of deep-venous thrombosis. *J Vasc Surg* 8:410, 1988.

140. Ashenburg RJ, Phillips DA: Ergotism as a consequence of thromboembolic prophylaxis. *Radiology* 170:375, 1989.

141. Krupp P, Majer M: Ergotism and heparin-dihydroergotamine prophylaxis. *Lancet* 1:1302, 1982.

142. Borgstrom S, Gelin L-E, Zederfeldt B: The information of vein thrombi following tissue injury. *Acta Chir Scand* 242(Suppl):247, 1959.

143. Jansen H: Postoperative thromboembolism and its prevention with 500 ml dextran given during operation. With a special study of the venous flow pattern in the lower extremities. *Acta Chir Scand* 427(Suppl):1, 1972.

144. Bergqvist D, Efsing HO, Hallbook T et al: Thromboembolism after elective and posttraumatic hip surgery—a controlled prophylactic trial with dextran and low-dose heparin. *Acta Chir Scand* 145:213, 1979.

145. Gruber UF, Saldeen T, Brokop T et al: Incidences of fatal postoperative pulmonary embolism with dextran 70 and low-dose heparin. An International Multicentre Study. *Br Med J* 280:69, 1980.

146. Messmer K, Ljungstrom K-G, Gruber U et al: Prevention of dextran-induced anaphylactoid reactions by hapten inhibition. *Lancet* I:975, 1980.

147. Powers SK, Edwards MSB: Prophylaxis of thromboembolism in the neurosurgical patient: A review. *Neurosurgery* 10:509, 1982.

148. Swierstra BA, Stibbe J, Schouten HJA: Prevention of thrombosis after hip arthroplasty; a prospective study of preoperative oral anticoagulants. *Acta Orthop Scand* 59(2):139, 1988.

149. Guyer RD, Booth RE, Rothman RH: The detection and prevention of pulmonary embolism in total hip replacement. *J Bone Joint Surg* 64A:1040, 1982.

150. Poller L, McKernan A, Thomson JM et al: Fixed minidose warfarin: A new approach to prophylaxis against venous thrombosis after major surgery. *Br Med J* 295:1309, 1987.

151. Chandhoke PS, Gooding GAW, Narayan P: Prospective randomized trial of warfarin and intermittent pneumatic leg compression as pro-

phylaxis for postoperative deep-venous thrombosis in major urological surgery. *J Urol* 147:1056–1059, 1992.

152. Doran FSA, Drury M, Sivyer A: A simple way to combat the venous stasis which occurs in the lower limb during surgical operations. *Br J Surg* 51:486, 1964.

153. Powers PJ, Gent M, Jay RM et al: A randomized trial of less intense postoperative warfarin or aspirin therapy in the prevention of venous thromboembolism after surgery for fractured hip. *Arch Intern Med* 149:771, 1989.

154. Francis CW, Pellegrini VD, Marder VJ et al: Comparison of warfarin and external pneumatic compression in prevention of venous thrombosis after total hip replacement. *JAMA* 267(21):2911–2915, 1992.

155. Clagett GP, Salzman E: Prevention of venous thromboembolism. *Prog Cardiovasc Dis* 17:345, 1975.

156. Johnson EA, Mallory B: The molecular weight range of mucosal heparin preparations. *Carbohydr Res* 51:119, 1976.

157. Holmes E, Kurachi K, Soderstrom G: The molecular weight dependence of the rate-enhancing effect of heparin on the inhibition of thrombin, factor Xa, factor IXa, factor XIa and kallikrein by antithrombin. *Biochem J* 193:395, 1981.

158. The European Fraxiparin Study (EFS) Group: Comparison of low molecular weight heparin and unfractionated heparin for the prevention of deep-vein thrombosis in patients undergoing abdominal surgery. *Br J Surg* 75:1058, 1988.

159. Bergqvist D, Burmark US, Frisell J et al: Low molecular weight heparin once daily compared with conventional low-dose heparin twice daily. A prospective double-blind multicentre trial on prevention of postoperative thrombosis. *Br J Surg* 73:204, 1986.

160. Liezorovicz A, Picolet H, Peyrieux JC et al: Prevention of perioperative deep-vein thrombosis in general surgery: A multicentre double-blind study comparing two doses of logiparin and standard heparin. *Br J Surg* 78:412–416, 1991.

161. Monreal M, Lafoz E, Navarro A et al: A prospective double-blind trial of a low-dose heparin once daily compared with conventional heparin three times daily to prevent pulmonary embolism and venous thrombosis in patients with hip fracture. *J Trauma* 29:873, 1989.

162. Turpie AGG, Levine MN, Hirsh J et al: A randomized controlled trial of low-molecular-weight heparin (Enoxaparin) to prevent deep-vein thrombosis in patients undergoing elective hip surgery. *N Engl J Med* 315:925, 1986.

163. Turpie AG: Efficacy of a postoperative regimen of enoxaparin in deep-vein thrombosis prophylaxis. *Am J Surg* 161:532–536, 1991.

164. Leyvraz PF, Bachmann F, Hoek J et al: Prevention of deep-vein thrombosis after hip replacement: Randomised comparison between unfractionated heparin and low molecular weight heparin. *Br Med J* 303:543–548, 1991.

165. Planes A, Vochelle N, Gaola M et al: Efficacy and safety of a perioperative enoxaparin regimen in total hip replacement under various anesthesias. *Am J Surg* 161:525–531, 1991.

166. Gerhart TN, Yett HS, Robertson LK et al: Low-molecular-weight heparinoid compared with warfarin for prophylaxis of deep-vein thrombosis in patients who are operated on for fracture of the hip. *J Bone Joint Surg* 73A(4):494–501, 1991.

167. Samama M, Bernard P, Bonnardot JP et al: Low molecular weight heparin compared with unfractionated heparin in prevention of postoperative thrombosis. *Br J Surg* 75:128, 1988.

168. Levine M, Hirsh J, Gent M et al: Prevention of deep-vein thrombosis after elective hip surgery. *Ann Intern Med* 114:545–551, 1991.

169. Handin RI, Valeri CR: Hemostatic effectiveness of platelets stored at 22°C. *N Engl J Med* 285:238, 1971.

170. Modig J, Borg T, Karlstrom G et al: Effects of tocainide, an oral analogue of lidocaine, on thromboembolism after total hip replacement. *Upsala J Med Sci* 86:269, 1981.

171. Lowe GDO, Campbell AF, Meek DR et al: Subcutaneous ancrod in prevention of DVT after operation for fractured neck of femur. *Lancet* II:698, 1978.

172. Cooke ED, Bowcock S, Lloyd MJ et al: Intravenous lidocaine in prevention of deep-venous thrombosis after elective hip surgery. *Lancet* II:797, 1977.

173. Francis CW, Pellegrini VD, Harris CM et al: Antithrombin III prophylaxis of venous thromboembolic disease after total hip or total knee replacement. *Am J Med* 87(Suppl):3B–61S, 1989.

174. Ferrari A, Dindeli M, Sellaroli C: Preventing postoperative deep-venous thrombosis in gynecological surgery with defibrinotide. *Int Surg* 75:184–188, 1990.

175. Bergqvist D, Efsing HO, Hallbook T et al: Prevention of postoperative thromboembolic complications. A prospective comparison between dextran 70, dihydroergotamine-heparin and a sulphated polysaccharide. *Acta Chir Scand* 146:559, 1980.

176. Kusminsky RE, Medine S, Abu-Rahma AF et al: Prophylactic inferior vena cava clipping in colonic surgery. *Dis Colon Rectum* 25:108, 1982.

177. Vaughn BK, Knezevich S, Lombardi AV et al: Use of the Greenfield filter to prevent fatal pulmonary embolism associated with total hip and knee arthroplasty. *J Bone Joint Surg* 71A:1542, 1989.

178. Dommering M: Low-dose heparin prophylaxis in herniorrhaphy? A prospective trial in bleeding complications. *Arch Chir Neerl* 31:57, 1979.

179. Clarke-Pearson DL, Synan IS, Hinshaw WM et al: Prevention of postoperative venous thromboembolism by external pneumatic calf compression in patients with gynecologic malignancy. *Obstet Gynecol* 63:92, 1984.

180. Bynke O, Hillman J, Lassvik C: Does perioperative external pneumatic leg muscle compression prevent postoperative venous thrombosis in neurosurgery? *Acta Neurochir* 88:46, 1987.

49 DRUG METABOLISM, REACTIONS, AND INTERACTIONS IN THE SURGICAL PATIENT: PREVENTION OF MEDICATION-INDUCED MORBIDITY

Kathleen M. Guarnieri

Bernadette Pastewski McKeon

Many patients undergoing surgery today have multiple medical problems and are taking a variety of both prescription and over-the-counter drugs. In addition, they may receive as many as 5 to 10 additional medications during anesthesia and surgery, making drug reactions and interactions almost inevitable. The incidence of adverse reactions is seven percent in patients taking 6 to 10 drugs and 40 percent in those taking 10 to 20.[1,2] The frequency of acute withdrawal from medications before surgery is 74 percent in patients undergoing emergency surgery and 44 percent in those undergoing elective procedures.[3] Before the patient goes to the operating room, it is important to decide when to stop and restart these medications. The clinical implications of these decisions on anesthetic management should not be underestimated.

This chapter begins with a brief discussion of the preoperative assessment of the medication history. The remainder discusses drug metabolism and adverse reactions most common in the perioperative period as well as interactions of drugs with commonly used anesthetics. Emphasis is placed on clinical implications and prevention of drug-induced morbidity in the perioperative setting. Descriptions of drug-drug and drug-disease reactions and interactions in nonsurgical patients are discussed elsewhere.[4–6]

PREOPERATIVE ASSESSMENT OF MEDICATION HISTORY

Preoperative assessment of the surgical patient provides an opportunity to assess anesthetic risk, identify current prescription and over-the-counter medications, and clarify any previous adverse drug reactions. Identifying anesthetic risk is difficult because operative complications are often the result of multiple factors including the anesthetic agent, the complexity of the procedure, coexisting diseases, and other factors like smoking, obesity, increased age, and alcoholism. Many of these factors affect the metabolism of current medications and newly administered drugs in the perioperative period.

A good medication history includes information about prescription and over-the-counter medications. The trade name of a drug may be useful because some generic products contain different fillers, stabilizers, and dyes. In addition to dose, frequency, and route of administration, it is important to obtain information regarding the length of time the medications have been prescribed, the reason for the medications, and how compliant the patient has been in taking them. This information is important in predicting the likelihood of withdrawal symptoms in the perioperative period.

Over-the-counter preparations are frequently overlooked and can contribute to significant morbidity. For example, drugs containing aspirin can prolong the bleeding time and increase bleeding in surgical patients.[7] Since many analgesic and cold medications contain aspirin, consultation with a pharmacist is often helpful. *The Handbook of Nonprescription Drugs* is another good resource for information about the ingredients in such preparations.[7]

Determining the nature of past adverse drug reactions is important to clarify whether they involved life-threatening immunologic reactions like anaphylaxis or expected side effects. Adverse drug reactions can be classified into those that are predictable with known side effects and toxicities and those that are unpredictable and representative of true drug allergy, pseudoallergy, or idiosyncratic reactions.[8–10] Drug toxicity and side effects represent extensions of the desired pharmacologic effects or chemical properties of a drug or its metabolite. Idiosyncratic reactions are often particularly difficult to manage since their underlying mechanisms are usually unknown. True drug allergy or hypersensitivity is usually the result of an immunologic reaction, in which a drug or its metabolite forms a complex with a host protein and stimulates an immune response.[10] Classic type I immediate hypersensitivity consists of a broad range of anaphylactic manifestations that includes urticaria, edema, bronchospasm, and hemodynamic collapse. Type II involves antibody-mediated cytotoxicity to cellular elements of the blood. Type III consists of immune-complex disease with skin rash, proteinuria, and hematologic abnormalities. In type IV or delayed hypersensitivity, the drug-protein conjugate is recognized by T-lymphocytes that subsequently mediate clinical manifestations of fever, anemia, nephritis, dermatitis, and arthritis.[8–10] Pseudoallergic reactions probably involve nonimmunologic mechanisms in which the drug causes mast cells to release histamine.[8,9]

ADVERSE DRUG REACTIONS IN THE SURGICAL PATIENT

Adverse drug reactions and interactions that occur during induction of general anesthesia may include tachycardia, hypotension, bronchospasm, or cardiovascular collapse. These reactions may be complications of over- or underdosage, well-characterized side effects, or unpredictable allergic phenomena. Drug interactions are frequently the result of polypharmacy. Some of these interactions can actually be beneficial, as in the use of the muscle relaxant properties of isoflurane to reduce the dose of pancuronium, or hazardous, as in the effect of chronic cocaine abuse in enhancing the cardiac irritability of halothane.[1] In general, anesthetic agents can be classified into four categories: (1) inhalation anesthetics; (2) intravenous anesthetics; (3) local anesthetics; and (4) anesthetic supplements such as muscle relaxants and anticholinergic drugs. Their effects in the perioperative period are discussed below.

Inhalation and Intravenous Anesthetics

The cornerstones of general anesthesia are the inhalation and intravenous anesthetics. Inhalation anesthetics include both the gaseous agent nitrous oxide and volatile liquids such as halothane, enflurane, isoflurane, desflurane, and sevoflurane. Methoxyflurane, an older volatile agent, is often mentioned but rarely used because of its fluoride-induced nephrotoxicity. Intravenous anesthetics include barbiturates, opioids, benzodiazepines, and miscellaneous drugs like ketamine, etomidate, and propofol.

Depth of anesthesia usually depends on and is proportional to the concentration of the anesthetic in the central nervous system (CNS).[11] Concentration gradients from alveoli to blood and to the CNS determine the level of anesthesia when inhalational agents are administered. In addition, general anesthetics depress myocardial and respiratory function.[11] Altering the hepatic metabolism or renal elimination of anesthetics may prolong CNS and systemic depressant effects and cause adverse reactions and toxicity.

Inhalational agents depress cardiac output and myocardial contractility in a dose-dependent fashion.[11,12] Isoflurane produces the least depression of cardiac output and at low enough concentrations may produce none. The effect of halothane and enflurane on cardiac output parallels reductions in blood pressure. Conversely, nitrous oxide causes a mild increase in cardiac output that is probably due to its weak sympathomimetic effect.[13]

Intravenous agents exert various effects on blood pressure and myocardial function. Except for meperidine, even large doses of opioids have little effect on these parameters.[14] Barbiturates like thiopental or methohexital, used for induction of anesthesia, produce modest reductions in blood pressure, venous return, and cardiac output. Propofol can significantly decrease systolic and diastolic blood pressure, cardiac index, and pulmonary capillary wedge pressure. However, ketamine, a phencyclidine derivative used for induction and maintenance of anesthesia, causes cardiovascular stimulation through direct stimulation of the sympathetic nervous system, an effect that may be absent when catecholamines are depleted.[15] Benzodiazepines (e.g., midazolam and diazepam) and etomidate produce minimal changes when used alone for induction. Because of their stability, benzodiazepines are frequently used with opioids in patients with cardiovascular disease. However, benzodiazepines should be titrated slowly to avoid direct myocardial depression and hypotension.[16]

Morphine, unlike other opioids such as fentanyl, sufentanil, and alfentanil, can release histamine when used in high doses. Except for meperidine, opioids can cause bradycardia, probably by stimulating the vagal nucleus in the medulla. Bradycardia is particularly marked with sufentanil. Opioids do not sensitize the heart to the cardiac dysrhythmic effects of catecholamines.[14]

Inhaled anesthetics and most intravenous agents produce dose-dependent and drug-specific respiratory depression. Most inhaled agents increase the rate of breathing but decrease the tidal volume as drug concentration increases, ultimately causing decreases in minute ventilation and increases in $PaCO_2$. All anesthetics produce some degree of dose-related depression in the ventilatory response curve to carbon dioxide, and large doses usually obliterate the response entirely.[17]

Anesthetics also depress the ventilatory response to hypoxia. Knill et al. demonstrated that doses of halothane, enflurane, and isoflurane that do not produce anesthesia markedly depress the hypoxic response in humans, and higher concentrations abolish the response completely. Nitrous oxide significantly depresses the hypoxic response as well. Inhaled agents also attenuate the usual synergistic effect of arterial hypoxemia and hypercapnia in stimulating ventilation.[18] It is therefore particularly important to monitor patients who are just recovering from anesthesia. They may appear to be resting comfortably, but subanesthetic levels of an inhalational agent can cause diminished ventilatory response to arterial hypoxemia.

Barbiturates and opioids also depress medullary ventilatory centers. Barbiturates usually produce transient apnea during induction of anesthesia. When breathing resumes, it is characterized by a slow rate and a reduced tidal volume. Opioids produce rapid and sustained dose-dependent ventilatory depression. Frequency of breathing is decreased while tidal volume is often increased. Fentanyl, alfentanil, and sufentanil can frequently cause muscle rigidity when rapidly injected intravenously. The rigidity often accompanies induction and can interfere with positive pressure ventilation before intubation. Opioid-induced muscle rigidity can be avoided by pretreatment with a small dose of a nondepolarizing muscle relaxant or treated with a paralyzing dose of any type of muscle relaxant. It can also be terminated by administration of an opioid antagonist like naloxone.[19]

Inhalation anesthetics cause some degree of neuromuscular blockade, in decreasing order: isoflurane > enflurane > halothane > nitrous oxide.[20] However, intravenous agents cause little if any neuromuscular blockade.

The halogenated anesthetics and intravenous agents undergo biotransformation in the liver and/or kidney. Degradation of inhalational anesthetics occurs in the liver by oxidation, dehalogenation, and conjugation. Reductive anaerobic metabolism of inhaled anesthetics is rare and occurs to a significant degree only with halothane.[21] Except for inorganic fluoride, the metabolites are not considered toxic.[21]

Toxicity of inhaled anesthetics often reflects the direct effects of the parent molecule or metabolites on the liver, kidneys, or reproductive system.[21] The toxic effects on the liver and kidney are discussed below in the section on drug-drug interactions. There is some evidence that inhaled anesthetics cause an increased incidence of spontaneous abortion in female operating-room personnel. However, there has not been any evidence that inhaled anesthetics have a significant effect on germ cells in humans or that they are mutagenic or carcinogenic.[22]

Adverse hematologic reactions due to inhalational anesthetics have been reported only after prolonged exposure to nitrous oxide. These reactions include suppression of all bone marrow elements after 48 hours of exposure. No bone marrow suppression has been noted after only 24 hours.[23]

When hypersensitivity reactions to general anesthetics occur, barbiturates are frequently implicated. The incidence of thiopental-induced hypersensitivity is about 1 in 14,000 to 29,000.[24] Thiopental may cause either pseudoallergic reactions or IgE-mediated reactions. Positive skin testing for anaphylaxis and RAST have been suggested to predict such reactions.[9,10]

Local Anesthetics

Systemic toxicity, neurotoxicity, and allergic reactions are rare but important side effects of local anesthetics. Systemic toxicity is most frequent and accounts for the majority of complications and deaths.[25]

Local anesthetics are classified as aminoesters and aminoamides (see Table 49–1). The aminoesters have an ester link between the aromatic end of the molecule and the intermediate chain, while the aminoamides have an amide linkage. The ester compounds are metabolized by plasma pseudocholinesterase, and the amide compounds undergo enzymatic degradation in the liver. Ester derivatives of paraaminobenzoic acid are more likely to cause allerguc reactions.[26]

Local anesthetics given parenterally may cause swelling at the injection site that is often due to local irritation, improper injection technique, or concomitant use of local vasoconstrictors.[25] When applied topically, some of them may also cause irritation. A nonimmunologic reaction consisting of inflammation, edema, and ulceration may result from direct irritation and appear after one or more applications. Prolonged or repeated local contact can cause immunologic sensitization, probably mediated by IgE.[25]

Local neural toxicity has been reported. In most cases, nerve damage is related to mechanical trauma following intraneural injection or contamination of the solution. Several reports of prolonged sensory and motor deficits have been reported after the

TABLE 49–1. Local Anesthetic Agents

Esters	
Agent	Clinical Use
Cocaine	Topical anesthesia
Benzocaine	Topical anesthesia
Procaine	Local infiltration, spinal
Chloroprocaine	Local infiltration, peripheral nerve block, epidural
Tetracaine	Topical anesthesia, spinal

Amides	
Agent	Clinical Use
Lidocaine	Topical anesthesia, local infiltration, intravenous nerve block, peripheral nerve block, epidural, spinal
Prilocaine	Local infiltration, intravenous nerve block, peripheral nerve block, epidural
Etidocaine	Local infiltration, peripheral nerve block, epidural
Mepivacaine	Local infiltration, peripheral nerve block, epidural
Bupivacaine	Local infiltration, peripheral nerve block, epidural, spinal

accidental intrathecal administration of chloroprocaine.[26] Animal studies suggest that the localized neural irritation may be due to the low pH and presence of sodium bisulfite preservative in solutions of the agent rather than to the drug itself.[26] Vasoconstrictors such as epinephrine, used to prolong the effect of local anesthetics, can cause necrosis and gangrene, particularly in the fingertips and toes in patients with peripheral vascular disease.[25]

Local anesthetic agents can produce central nervous system and cardiovascular toxicity. Most systemic reactions are due to high plasma concentrations of the drug that can develop after accidental intravascular injection during nerve blocks or, less often, absorption from tissue injection sites. In the case of lidocaine, peak plasma concentrations of 3 to 5 mcg/ml can cause nausea, vomiting, dizziness, and tinnitus, but levels above 5 mcg/ml can be associated with generalized tonic-clonic seizures and subsequent CNS depression.[27] CNS toxicity caused by ester-type agents is usually self-limited because they are rapidly hydrolyzed by plasma esterases, but amide-type local anesthetics require hepatic degradation and can therefore produce longer-lasting effects. The relative CNS toxicities of these agents are proportional to their anesthetic potencies.[28]

Local anesthetics can produce profound cardiovascular effects by acting directly on the heart and peripheral vasculature and indirectly on autonomic nerve fibers. Doses used for most regional procedures result in peak blood concentrations that generally do not have cardiodepressant effects. However, inadvertent rapid intravenous injection or excessive doses can cause significant depression of myocardial contractility and peripheral vasodilatation leading to profound hypotension and circulatory collapse. Potent lipid-soluble agents like bupivacaine are more cardiotoxic than the less potent and less lipid-soluble drugs like lidocaine. In addition, cardiac arrhythmias have been observed, particularly in those who are pregnant, following rapid intravenous injection of bupivacaine. Bupivacaine in a concentration of 0.75% is no longer recommended for epidural anesthesia in obstetrical patients, and its use in intravenous regional anesthesia should be avoided.[26]

Methemoglobinemia and cyanosis are unique to prilocaine and can occur when it is used in high doses. It is therefore advisable to limit the dose to 600 mg. Methemoglobinemia can be rapidly reversed by intravenous administration of methylene blue.[29,30]

Hypersensitivity reactions to local anesthetics occur in less than one percent of patients and are more frequent with ester-type than with amide-type agents. Multiple-dose vials of some amide-type agents contain the preservative methylparaben, which may cause allergic reactions.[26] Patients who have experienced anaphylactoid or other symptoms thought to be due to ester-type anesthetics can usually receive amide-type agents. If there is doubt, provocative dose testing can be performed. Detailed methods are outlined elsewhere.[9,29,31]

Anesthetic Supplements

Neuromuscular Blocking Agents

Neuromuscular blocking agents (NMBA's) supplement general anesthesia by inducing flaccid paralysis of skeletal muscle through the selective inhibition of neurochemical transmission at the neuromuscular junction.[32] Nondepolarizing agents such as D-tubocurarine, pancuronium, atracurium, doxacurium, and vecuronium competitively inhibit acetylcholine binding at postjunctional membrane receptors.[33] Depolarizing agents such as succinylcholine bind to postjunctional membranes and produce persistent depolarization and desensitization of the receptors to acetylcholine.[32]

Although the sequence of muscle relaxation to paralysis is similar with both types of NMBA's, there is considerable variability in dose response. Repeated doses of nondepolarizing agents can produce a cumulative effect, but depolarizing agents usually cause partial tachyphylaxis. Because of the lingering sensitivity of nondepolarizing agents, supplemental doses should be reduced by 30% to 50% to prevent prolonged postoperative paralysis and apnea.[32]

In view of this variability, identifying patients with unusual sensitivity to average doses of muscle relaxants is important. Factors contributing to prolonged paralysis and apnea include concomitant administration of drugs with neuromuscular blockade activity like aminoglycosides, altered electrolyte balance, hypothermia, reductions in pH, and complicating diseases like renal and hepatic insufficiency.[33]

The adverse effects of NMBA's are extensions of their pharmacologic activities. There are predictably profound effects on the cardiovascular system and the eye. Effects on the heart and peripheral circulation are mediated by stimulation or inhibition of either nicotinic receptors in autonomic ganglia or muscarinic receptors in the sinus node, or by systemic histamine release.[32] Maximal cardiovascular effects are usually seen within one to five minutes following an intravenous injection. When circulatory changes occur after more than five minutes, other causes should be considered.

D-tubocurarine and, to a lesser extent, metocurine, atracurium, and mivacurium produce hypotension by causing systemic histamine release. Pancuronium increases blood pressure and heart rate by 10 to 15 percent through vagolytic effects and sympathetic nervous system stimulation. Succinylcholine may produce either bradycardia or tachycardia. Tachycardia results from stimulation of autonomic nervous system ganglia. Severe sinus bradycardia, nodal rhythms, and asystole are more common in patients who receive repetitive doses of the drug at short intervals. Intravenous administration of atropine one to three minutes before succinylcholine reduces the likelihood of these cardiac effects. Vecuronium, doxacurium, and pipecuronium have little or no cardiovascular side effects.[33]

Succinylcholine can also cause hyperkalemia, trismus, myalgias, and increased intraocular, intragastric, and intracranial pressure. The exaggerated release of potassium in response to succinylcholine is well described. In some settings such as spinal cord injury or burns, hyperkalemia may be severe enough to cause cardiac arrest. Patients with crush injury, nerve damage, and neuromuscular disease are also susceptible to hyperkalemia. Patients with renal failure, however, do not have an increased risk of hyperkalemia from succinylcholine if the baseline potassium is normal.

Postoperative skeletal muscle myalgias occur more frequently after use of succinylcholine in minor surgery, especially in young adults who ambulate early. Prior administration of a subparalyzing dose of a nondepolarizing muscle relaxant appears to prevent or attenuate the myalgias. Succinylcholine also can cause varying degrees of trismus in the masseter muscles, especially in pediatric patients. About 50 percent of those with masseter muscle rigidity may be susceptible to malignant hyperthermia.[33]

A transient increase in intraocular pressure occurs after administration of succinylcholine, peaking two to four minutes after injection and subsiding after six minutes. In patients with open-eye injuries, the drug can theoretically cause extrusion of intraocular contents but rarely does so.[34] Increases in intragastric pressure are variable and may be related to the amount of muscle fasciculations noted. Succinylcholine can also transiently increase intracranial pressure. In both cases, a small subparalyzing dose of a nondepolarizing agent before succinylcholine is given can attenuate or prevent these responses.[33]

Anaphylactoid reactions are related to release of histamine by NMBA's. D-tubocurarine has the highest propensity to release histamine, metocurine does so to a lesser extent, and atracurium and mivacurium do so the least. Most anaphylactoid reactions occur after high-dose rapid intravenous injection. Succinylcholine causes minimal release of histamine, while pancuronium, gallamine, vecuronium, pipecuronium, and doxacurium do not release any.[33]

Anticholinergics

Anticholinergic agents are frequently used as part of routine preanesthetic care because of their antisialagogue and vagolytic actions. Although some have argued that routine administration of these drugs is unnecessary, many practicing anesthesiologists still routinely use them.[35,36]

Most adverse effects of anticholinergics are dose-related extensions of their pharmacologic activities and primarily involve the cardiovascular system, gastrointestinal tract, and the eye. Some cardiovascular effects may not be dose-related, depending on the use of concomitant anesthetic drug administration. In adults, doses of atropine of 0.4 to 0.6 mg generally cause proportional increases in heart rate. The heart rate does not increase above 130 to 150 beats per minute with doses above 3 mg. The arrhythmogenic potential of anticholinergic agents is difficult to predict at a given dose. Arrhythmogenicity appears to be dependent on the type of anesthetic. Atrioventricular dissociation, nodal rhythms, and ventricular extrasystoles are frequently reported with atropine and scopolamine. The frequency of arrhythmias with atropine at doses of 0.4 mg is 17 percent when halothane anesthesia is used.[37] Glyco pyrrolate inhibits salivation and sweating at doses of 0.2 mg, at which cardiovascular effects are minimal.[38]

The gastrointestinal effects of atropine, scopolamine, and glycopyrrolate are decreased peristalsis, delayed gastric emptying, and a reduction in lower esophageal sphincter pressure.[39,40] Intragastric pH and esophageal sphincter pressures are important considerations since surgical patients are often prone to aspiration. The effect of glycopyrrolate on increasing gastric pH is minimal. Nonparticulate antacids or H_2 antagonists in combination with metoclopramide are therefore recommended.

Since anticholinergic agents may cause mydriasis and cycloplegia, they have been avoided in patients with glaucoma. However, they are now used more commonly in this setting without significant ophthalmologic morbidity.

The CNS effects of anticholinergic agents are thought to be manifestations of toxicity rather than adverse reactions. Both atropine and scopolamine are tertiary ammonium compounds that penetrate the blood-brain barrier. Anticholinergics given in recommended preanesthetic doses usually produce little or no CNS effects. However, in elderly patients, doses as low as 0.4 mg can cause prolonged postoperative sedation. Scopolamine is eight times more potent than atropine in this regard. Therefore, the recommended preanesthetic dose of scopolamine (0.2 to 0.4 mg) may produce confusion, lethargy, and prolonged sleep, even in normal patients.[39]

Anticholinergic psychosis is characterized by excitation and hyperactivity, alternating with depression and somnolence. Other clinical manifestations include intense vasoconstriction, hot dry skin, ophthalmologic signs, hallucinations, delirium, generalized tonic-clonic seizures, and sometimes coma. Deaths have rarely been reported. CNS effects occur with cumulative doses exceeding 5 to 10 mg of atropine. No CNS effects are seen with glycopyrrolate because its highly polar quaternary ammonium structure does not allow penetration of the blood-brain barrier.[38] Physostigmine, a centrally active cholinesterase inhibitor, is recommended to treat some of the clinical manifestations of anticholinergic toxicity. It is also effective in reversing the residual postoperative sedative effects of atropine and scopolamine.[35]

DRUG-DRUG INTERACTIONS

The mechanisms of drug interactions can help provide a basis for understanding the resulting pharmacologic effects. These mechanisms can be classified into six categories.[5,41-45] The first involves the development of physical and chemical incompatibilities when two or more drug solutions are combined to form an admixture. The next four correspond to the four processes of pharmacokinetics—absorption, distribution, metabolism, and elimination.[42,45] The rate of absorption of one drug can be altered by the administration of another, and the route of drug administration can also affect the time course of interaction. Drug distribution and interaction with receptors can be affected by protein-binding displacement. The volume of distribution also affects the rate of drug movement among tissue compartments and sites of drug activity. Enzyme induction and inhibition by a drug can alter the plasma concentration of others that are metabolized by the affected enzyme system. Elimination of a drug can be affected by urinary pH, underlying renal and hepatic function, and concomitant use of other drugs that may be toxic to the kidney or liver. Finally, drug

interactions can be influenced by pharmacodynamics involving quantification of drug effect. Modification of drug activity at a receptor site can alter its pharmacologic activity.[45] Coexisting disease may also influence pharmacologic effect and predispose patients to drug-disease interactions.

Physical and Chemical Incompatibilities

Physical incompatibilities between two drugs can be identified by visible alterations such as discoloration of the admixture or formation of a precipitate that may represent inactivation of one or both of the drugs.[46,47] Chemical incompatibilities involve inactivation of one or both agents in the solution mixture without visible changes.[46] Decreased drug concentration may also be the result of adsorption onto the surface of polyvinylchloride bags or intravenous tubing.[46,47] Barbiturates are drugs that are commonly associated with physical and chemical incompatibilities because of their low pKa and high pH.[45-47] Diazepam and chlordiazepoxide are both physically and chemically incompatible with several other intravenous medications, and concomitant mixing and administration with other agents should be avoided.[47]

Drug Absorption

The rate of absorption or receptor uptake of a drug may be altered by another drug.[5,41-43] For local anesthetics, absorption is affected by blood flow and the pH at the site of injection, as well as the total volume and concentration of the drug.[48] Epinephrine-induced vasoconstriction decreases systemic absorption and prolongs local anesthetic effect. Local anesthetics with a pKa near 7.4 usually penetrate and act more rapidly.[48] For inhalational anesthetics, use of more than one inhalational agent may alter the diffusion characteristics of another, producing the so-called "second gas effect."[49] The addition of nitrous oxide can accelerate the rate of alveolar uptake of halogenated anesthetics and produce a more rapid induction.

Drug Distribution

Drug distribution can be affected by displacement of one protein-bound drug by another, allowing an increased amount of free drug to interact with receptors.[42] The pharmacologic effect of the displaced drug increases until balance is once again achieved by increased elimination.

The volume of distribution of a drug is important in characterizing drug movement from blood and blood vessel-rich tissue to peripheral tissue compartments to achieve a steady-state volume.[45] A large steady-state volume indicates that a large proportion of the drug has moved from plasma to tissue, and a small steady-state volume indicates limited tissue penetration.[45] Altered distribution of some drugs can be affected by the patient's age or the lipid-solubility of the drug. For example, morphine, with its low lipid-solubility, has a slower onset of activity than alfentanil.[45]

Drug Metabolism

Some drugs can induce or inhibit enzymes needed to metabolize other drugs, thereby affecting their plasma concentrations and pharmacologic effects.[42] It usually takes a week or more before the maximal effects of enzyme induction are noticed. When the drug is discontinued, enzyme induction gradually dissipates, depending upon the elimination half-life of the drug and the decline in enzyme activity. However, patients who are chronically taking enzyme inducers with a long elimination half-life, such as phenobarbital, exhibit sustained enzyme induction for several days to weeks after the drug is stopped. Other barbiturates, phenytoin, and rifampin also induce hepatic enzymes.[42,49] Cigarette smoking induces hepatic cytochrome P450-IA enzymes and can alter pharmacologic response.[42] Drugs that are affected by enzyme induction include warfarin, tricyclic antidepressants, cyclosporine, corticosteroids, beta-blockers, disopyramide, mexiletine, neuroleptics, quinidine, theophylline, thyroid hormone, and verapamil.[42]

Anesthetic-induced hepatotoxicity and nephrotoxicity are often attributed to increased production of toxic metabolites resulting from enzyme induction. However, a study of surgical patients in whom enzyme induction was documented failed to show an increased incidence of toxicity. Genetic factors seem to be the most important determinant of drug metabolizing enzyme activity.[49]

The effects of hepatic enzyme inhibitors can be evident within the first 24 hours after administering the drug, and dissipation of effects is also rapid. Hepatic enzyme inhibitors include amiodarone, cimetidine, erythromycin, diltiazem, ethanol, ketoconazole, monoamine oxidase inhibitors, quinidine, and verapamil.[42] For example, cimetidine decreases the clearance of diazepam and lidocaine by inhibiting hepatic cytochrome P-450 enzymes, resulting in a more pronounced and prolonged pharmacologic effect.[49]

Biotransformation is another mechanism that affects drug metabolism. For example, all halogenated anesthetics undergo biotransformation in the liver, leading to formation of immunoreactive proteins that can sensitize patients to subsequent exposure to halothane and related anesthetics. Halothane may damage the liver directly, or cytochrome P-450 enzymes may biotransform the anesthetic to a metabolite that can serve as a hapten in antibody-dependent cell-mediated cytotoxicity.[49,50] Work in animals has confirmed that structural and functional hepatic damage caused by halothane occurs only when enzyme induction and hypoxia produce large concentrations of reductive metabolites.[51]

Drug Elimination

Drugs can be eliminated through renal excretion and respiratory ventilation. Drug elimination by the kidneys is affected by systemic or urinary pH and renal function. Renal excretion of phenobarbital and fluoride ions from the metabolism of some halogenated anesthetics is enhanced by alkaline urinary pH.[5,49] Increased serum concentrations of fluoride ions can induce kidney dysfunction that subsequently affects elimination of other drugs dependent on renal excretion.

Increased blood levels of inorganic fluoride from hepatic biotransformation of halogenated anesthetics has been implicated in methoxyflurane nephrotoxicity. Methoxyflurane, rarely used now, can cause direct dose-related tubular injury and lead to nephrogenic diabetes insipidus. The severity depends on the dose of methoxyflurane, hepatic metabolism of the anesthetic, and variations in sensitivity to fluoride ion.[49]

When degraded, enflurane produces less inorganic fluoride than methoxyflurane and has not been associated with obvious renal dysfunction. Although some clinicians avoid enflurane in patients with preexisting renal disease, Mazze et al. has shown no detectable reduction in renal function in patients with chronic renal disease undergoing elective procedures under enflurane or halothane anesthesia.[52] Metabolism of halothane and isoflurane to fluoride ions is thought to be insufficient to produce nephrotoxicity.[21]

Drug Pharmacodynamics

Pharmacodynamic drug interactions involve modification of receptor activity when two or more drugs with similar binding capacities bind to the same receptor site. Pharmacologic effects can be additive or antagonistic and are usually rapid in onset.[42] For example, naloxone antagonizes the CNS depressant effects of opiate narcotics by blocking the narcotic receptor. The pharmacologic effect of NMBA's can be potentiated and prolonged by other NMBA's, potent inhalation anesthetics, calcium channel blockers, lithium, magnesium, procainamide, quinidine, and certain antibiotics.[42,49] Aminoglycosides and polymyxins are most often implicated. Aminoglycosides can be ranked in decreasing order of their effect: neomycin > streptomycin > netilmicin > kanamycin = amikacin > gentamicin = tobramycin.[53,54]

Halothane has been reported to sensitize the heart to catecholamines and increase the risk of arrhythmias.[49] Isoflurane does not sensitize the heart to catecholamines; enflurane does so but somewhat less than halothane.[49] Drugs such as theophylline that stimulate sympathetic activity may also produce arrhythmias during halothane anesthesia.[49,55]

DRUG-DISEASE INTERACTIONS

Several disease states affect the metabolism of drugs in the perioperative period. These include cardiovascular disease such as coronary artery disease, arrhythmias, and hypertension; pulmonary disease including asthma and chronic obstructive pulmonary disease; neurologic disease including seizures and stroke; and psychologic disorders. The following section discusses these disease states, their implications for anesthesia and drug therapy, and recommendations for perioperative drug management. The specific disease entities of malignant hyperthermia and pseudocholinesterase deficiency are discussed in Chap. 6.

Cardiovascular Disease

Antihypertensive and Antianginal Drugs

The large category of antihypertensives includes diuretics, catecholamine or sympathetic receptor-blocking drugs, calcium channel blockers, angiotensin-converting enzyme inhibitors, centrally acting agents, and direct vasodilators. Except in the case of diuretics, patients with hypertension remain more hemodynamically stable during anesthesia if they are maintained on antihypertensives until the procedure. Intravenous, sublingual, or transdermal agents are substituted until oral intake is sufficient enough for resumption of oral medications.[1,2]

If continued in the immediate preoperative period, diuretics can cause significant volume depletion and electrolyte imbalance. Hypokalemia increases the incidence of arrhythmias during anesthesia, increases the toxicity of digitalis, enhances the action of nondepolarizing muscle relaxants, sensitizes the heart to succinylcholine, and increases the likelihood of paralytic ileus.[2] Thiazide and loop diuretics can also produce hyponatremia, hypomagnesemia, hyperglycemia, and metabolic alkalosis. Potassium-sparing diuretics are usually associated with hyperkalemia and hyponatremia.[56] It is therefore recommended that diuretics be withheld on the morning of surgery in patients on long-term therapy. Pre operative volume and potassium replacement should be given as appropriate.

The abrupt discontinuation of beta-blockers can cause marked increases in sympathetic stimulation manifested by anxiety, nausea, vomiting, palpitations, rapidly increasing rebound hypertension, angina, and occasionally acute myocardial infarction in those with underlying coronary artery disease.[2] A similar withdrawal syndrome can be seen with clonidine, methyldopa, and reserpine.

It is now accepted that continuing beta-blockers until the time of surgery conveys no increased risk and is more likely to be beneficial if used throughout the perioperative period. Beta-blockers can prevent arrhythmias from surges in catecholamine levels due to stresses like endotracheal intubation and surgical incision. The cardiovascular response to hypoxia remains intact with beta-blockers. For patients who cannot eat for more than eight hours after surgery, propranolol can be given intravenously either intermittently or as a continuous infusion. Alternatively, intravenous metoprolol or labetalol can be substituted. When oral intake is resumed, the patient's usual dose of beta-blocker can be resumed.[2]

Hydralazine is a direct vasodilator that relaxes vascular smooth muscle and can therefore exacerbate the hypotensive effect of anesthetics. It is often combined with a beta-blocker to avoid the tachycardia associated with the use of hydralazine alone. The hypotensive effect of hydralazine may last 18 to 24 hours after it is discontinued.[2] It should be continued up until and including the morning of surgery. Since it is available in oral and parenteral forms, it can be useful in maintaining blood pressure control in the perioperative period. The parenteral dose is smaller than the oral dose and ranges from 5 to 20 mg every two to four hours.[57]

Minoxidil is a potent vasodilator that can cause reflex increases in heart rate, cardiac index, and fluid retention.[58] Like hydralazine, it may be given on the morning of surgery. If the patient is not eating and requires blood pressure control, other parenteral agents are required.

Patients already taking nitrates for coronary artery disease should receive them in some dosage formulation throughout the perioperative period. Nitroglycerin ointment can be used, but requires some drug-free interval to avoid tachyphylaxis. Intravenous nitroglycerin requires continuous invasive hemodynamic monitoring.[2,59]

Angiotensin-converting enzyme (ACE) inhibitors provide effective therapy of hypertension, and some are approved for treatment of congestive heart failure. In combination with general anesthetics, they can produce significant intraoperative hypotension that can usually be corrected with volume expansion. They can also cause elevations in serum potassium levels by decreasing aldosterone secretion. These elevations are usually mild but can be exaggerated with concurrent acidosis, hemolysis, acute tissue necrosis, or acute renal failure. Serum potassium levels should therefore be checked before surgery. Acute withdrawal of captopril has been reported to cause rebound hypertension.[2,59] ACE inhibitors should be continued until the morning of surgery. Enalaprilat, the active metabolite of enalapril maleate, is available in an intravenous dosage formulation for postoperative blood pressure control if needed.

Alpha-methyldopa, clonidine, and guanabenz are antihypertensive agents that act on central alpha$_2$ receptors. Stimulation of these receptors decreases sympathetic tone from the central nervous system to the peripheral nervous system. Alpha-methyldopa reduces total peripheral resistance without significantly affecting cardiac output and heart rate. Used alone, it can cause fluid retention and weight gain and is commonly used in combination with a diuretic.[59] An intravenous dosage formulation is available. Both alpha-methyldopa and clonidine may decrease requirements for volatile anesthetics.[60,61]

Abrupt discontinuation of clonidine can cause rebound hypertension.[62] Rebound hypertension is usually mild but can be severe and produce a hypertensive crisis in patients receiving as little as 0.2 mg daily.[63] Withdrawal symptoms usually begin 8 to 20 hours after the last dose.[59] Clonidine should be continued until the morning of surgery. Until oral medication can be resumed, transdermal clonidine can be substituted.[2] Guanabenz has properties similar to clonidine but fewer side effects. Withdrawal symptoms have also been reported.[59]

Prazosin causes selective inhibition of alpha$_1$ adrenergic receptors and is often combined with a diuretic or beta-blocker to treat hypertension. No major adverse effects have been reported with prazosin during surgery or anesthesia.[2] It can be continued until the day of surgery and resumed thereafter.

When administered in large doses, reserpine can produce significant refractory hypotension during anesthesia. However, use of this agent in small doses in combination with other antihypertensives reduces the likelihood of drug interactions.[64] It may be continued until the morning of surgery and resumed thereafter. Like alpha-methyldopa and clonidine, it reduces requirements for volatile anesthetics.[60]

Guanethidine decreases blood pressure by inhibiting peripheral sympathetic activity and was used in patients with severe hypertension before newer antihypertensives were developed.[59] It does not cross the blood-brain barrier and does not affect volatile anesthetic requirements.[65] It can be continued until surgery and resumed thereafter as needed.

Calcium channel blockers have been associated with a number of interactions with general anesthetics. The combination of inhalational anesthetics such as halothane, isoflurane, or enflurane and calcium channel blockers can produce mild hemodynamic depressant effects. Nifedipine decreases peripheral vascular resistance, while verapamil depresses myocardial contractility and interferes with atrioventricular conduction in anesthetized patients.[2]

Nifedipine and verapamil also cause a mild decrease in blood pressure and peripheral vascular resistance when narcotics are used concomitantly during anesthesia. Verapamil and nifedipine can also potentiate the effects of depolarizing and nondepolarizing NMBA's, but the clinical significance of this is unclear. There is no evidence that patients on chronic therapy with these agents have an increased anesthetic risk without other coexisting complicating factors. Calcium channel blockers should be given on the day of surgery and at regular intervals.[2] Verapamil and diltiazem are available in both oral and parenteral forms, and nifedipine can be given sublingually or orally.

Antiarrhythmic Drugs

Patients already undergoing therapy for significant arrhythmias such as ventricular tachycardia or rapid supraventricular tachyarrhythmia should be treated continuously throughout the perioperative period.[2] Those with infrequent atrial or ventricular premature contractions or controlled atrial fibrillation should continue oral antiarrhythmics until the day of surgery. If the arrhythmia becomes problematic during the perioperative period, an intravenous preparation can be used with appropriate monitoring.

Antiarrhythmics are divided into four classes. Class I consists of membrane stabilizers like quinidine, procainamide, disopyramide, lidocaine, tocainide, mexiletine, and the newer agents encainide and flecainide; class II consists of beta-blockers; class III includes antifibrillatory agents like bretylium and amiodarone; and class IV consists of the calcium channel blockers.[66] Class II and IV agents are discussed above in the section on antihypertensive agents.

The class I agent quinidine is used to treat both atrial and ventricular arrhythmias. It can be administered orally or parenterally, but acute hemodynamic effects can follow parenteral administration. It has a short half-life of six to seven hours and therefore requires dosing every six to eight hours in most patients.[66] Oral quinidine may be given until the morning of surgery. Intravenous lidocaine can be used prophylactically or if significant ventricular arrhythmias develop intraoperatively. Propranolol or verapamil can be substituted for treatment of supraventricular arrhythmias. Quinidine interacts with digoxin and may result in digoxin toxicity, which can depress myocardial contractility.[2]

Procainamide can be used to treat ventricular and supraventricular arrhythmias and, like quinidine, can cause significant myocardial depression and hypotension when administered intravenously. Its half-life varies markedly between three and six hours. It is usually safe to give the last dose of oral procainamide on the morning of surgery. Ventricular arrhythmias occurring thereafter can be treated with intravenous lidocaine or procainamide, and supraventricular arrhythmias can be treated with intravenous procainamide, propranolol, or verapamil.[2]

Disopyramide is effective in the treatment of supraventricular and ventricular tachyarrhythmias.[66] It exerts a negative inotropic effect which may be troublesome in some patients with preexisting congestive heart failure. It has marked anticholinergic effects, including constipation and urinary retention. The elimination half-life is approximately seven hours. It can be discontinued on the night before surgery, and intravenous lidocaine or procainamide can be substituted as needed.[2]

Lidocaine is the prototype of the class Ib drugs and is useful in the acute treatment of almost all types of ventricular arrhythmias except those precipitated by an abnormally prolonged Q-T interval.[66] Tocainide and mexiletine are class Ib drugs similar to lidocaine, but specifically developed for oral use with half-lives of 12 to 16 hours. Tocainide does not significantly depress myocardial contractility. A dose of either may be given on the morning of surgery in hopes of maintaining a therapeutic blood level. If oral intake is not resumed, intravenous lidocaine can be substituted.[2] The class Ic drugs—encainide and flecainide—are used for control of ventricular arrhythmias and can be used like other class I agents.

Class III antifibrillatory agents include bretylium and amiodarone. Bretylium is an intravenous drug used to treat refractory ventricular tachycardia or fibrillation. If a patient is on an intravenous infusion of the drug before surgery, he should continue it throughout the perioperative period. Little is known about interactions of bretylium with anesthetic agents. Because it blocks release of catecholamines, chronic therapy with bretylium has been associated with hypersensitivity to vasopressors.[66]

Amiodarone is an oral agent used to control life-threatening ventricular arrhythmias such as recurrent ventricular fibrillation or hemodynamically unstable ventricular tachycardia. Its use is limited by potentially fatal toxicities. It is a potent myocardial depressant that can cause atropine-resistant bradycardia, severe hypotension, and A-V nodal blockade. Because of its long half-life, discontinu-

ing amiodarone the night before surgery offers little in terms of ameliorating possible side effects.[66]

Cardiac glycosides are used primarily in patients with congestive heart failure and certain arrhythmias and are often useful to slow the ventricular response rate in atrial fibrillation or flutter. Digitalis preparations have a narrow therapeutic index. The risk of toxicity increases with hypokalemia. Digoxin can be continued orally or intravenously in the perioperative period. Although digoxin levels may be helpful in management, monitoring heart rate and rhythm are more important.[67]

Pulmonary Disease

The most commonly used pulmonary medications are bronchodilators and corticosteroids. The sympathomimetic drugs like albuterol, metaproterenol, terbutaline, and theophylline can interact with volatile anesthetics, especially halothane, and cause cardiac arrhythmias. A drug level should be obtained before surgery in all patients taking theophylline preparations. When levels exceed 20 mcg/ml, toxic side effects such as gastrointestinal symptoms, arrhythmias, or seizures may appear. All oral bronchodilators should be given on the day of surgery. Aerosol inhalers are useful before the procedure because they deliver medication directly to its site of action with minimal systemic toxicity.[68] When aminophylline is given intravenously, the rate of infusion should be decreased 30 to 50 percent during the procedure because of decreased inactivation of theophylline by the liver due to decreased hepatic blood flow under general anesthesia.[68]

Corticosteroid supplementation should be administered to any patient on suppressive doses of steroids (greater than 7.5 mg of prednisone or the equivalent) for longer than two weeks within the previous year. Details of appropriate steroid coverage is discussed in Chap. 26. Patients using inhaled steroids do not require supplemental coverage.[68]

Endocrine Disorders

Insulin or oral hypoglycemics for diabetes mellitus, supplemental steroids for a variety of diseases, and thyroid replacement are the most commonly encountered endocrine drugs in the perioperative period. Patients with diabetes mellitus face a series of potential problems. Uncontrolled diabetes can result in ketoacidosis, hyperosmolar coma, impairment of wound healing, and altered white cell function. In the surgical context, tight control of serum glucose levels should be avoided since the morbidity associated with hypoglycemia can be more severe than that of mild hyperglycemia.

Insulin-dependent diabetics can undergo most procedures with smaller-than-usual doses of insulin if an infusion of glucose is administered during the procedure. Specifically, one-third or one half of their usual daily dose of intermediate-acting insulin can be given subcutaneously on the morning of surgery, with a continuous intravenous infusion of 5% dextrose at a rate of 2 mg/kg/hr during and just after surgery.[2] Serum glucose levels should be measured before the infusion is begun, before induction of anesthesia, one hour after each bolus of insulin is given, and again in the recovery room. Subsequent doses of regular insulin can be given intravenously based on a sliding scale as detailed in Chap. 24. Insulin-dependent patients undergoing brief minor surgery under local anesthesia can hold their morning insulin until after the procedure provided that surgery is performed early in the morning and that the patient can resume oral intake following the operation.[2]

A continuous insulin drip can also be used in insulin-dependent diabetics undergoing major procedures. Plasma glucose and potassium levels are determined on the morning of surgery. An infusion of 5% dextrose is begun at 100 ml/hr, and an insulin drip of 25 units in 250 ml of normal saline can be "piggy-backed" into the infusion. The number of units per hour can be derived by dividing the plasma glucose in mg/dl by 150 and measuring the blood glucose every hour with a glucometer. For those patients who are obese or on steroids, the denominator is 100.[69]

Noninsulin-dependent diabetics on oral hypoglycemics require discontinuation of these agents the evening before surgery. Longer-acting agents like chlorpropamide can produce hypoglycemia for 24 to 36 hours and should be discontinued earlier. A fasting blood sugar level should be measured on the day of surgery and an intravenous solution of normal saline or 5% dextrose in half-normal saline chosen based on the result. Depending on the length of the procedure, glucose levels should be measured every four to six hours until oral intake is resumed. Significantly elevated sugars above 300 mg/dl should be treated with regular insulin on a sliding scale.[69]

Hypothyroidism is treated with oral desiccated thyroid extract or synthetic thyroid hormone. Patients who are clinically euthyroid with normal plasma concentrations of thyroid-stimulating hormone can continue their replacement dose of thyroid hormone until the morning of surgery. L-thyroxine has a half-life of seven days, allowing it to be restarted after the procedure. Parenteral thyroxine can be used if the patient cannot eat for an extended period of time.[2]

Elective surgery should be postponed until the patient is euthyroid, but more urgent procedures can be safely done in patients who are mildly hypothyroid. Anesthetic concerns include the following:

1. Hypothyroid patients can be sensitive to depressant drugs and require smaller doses of anesthetics and analgesics;

2. Ventilatory responses to hypoxemia and hypercarbia are blunted and hypoventilation is common;

3. Hyponatremia, hypothermia, and hypoglycemia are common;

4. The cardiovascular system is hypodynamic, and baroreceptors are unresponsive;

5. Drug metabolism is slowed, especially for opioids;

6. Intravascular volume is decreased;

7. Gastric emptying is delayed;

8. Normocytic anemia is common; and

9. The incidence of primary adrenal insufficiency is increased, necessitating exogenous administration of cortisol.[70,71]

Although some feel that parenteral triiodothyronine is more appropriate for emergency treatment of severe hypothyroidism,[70] intravenous L-thyroxine is the treatment of choice by most endocrinologists. The treatment of hypothyroidism in the surgical setting is discussed in detail in Chap. 26.

Hyperthyroidism is considered more dangerous than hypothyroidism in the perioperative period because of the possibility of thyroid storm. Elective surgery should therefore be postponed until the patient is clinically and chemically euthyroid. The combined use of beta-blockers and potassium iodine is effective in rendering most patients euthyroid in 10 days, but most endocrinologists prefer to treat patients with antithyroid drugs for six to eight weeks, sometimes giving oral iodide solution for 7 to 10 days before the procedure. When surgery cannot be delayed in patients with mild hyperthyroidism, beta-blockers should be administered to reduce sympathetic nervous system activity,[70] and antithyroid medication can be given postoperatively. The perioperative management of patients with more severe hyperthyroidism in the perioperative period is discussed in Chap. 25.

Formerly hyperthyroid patients who have been rendered euthyroid can usually interrupt therapy safely to undergo surgery. About 50 percent of patients on antithyroid therapy for a year or more and one-third of those on short-term therapy for five months or less remain in remission. The medication should be continued until the day of surgery and resumed orally or through a nasogastric tube within 24 hours of surgery.

Occult adrenal insufficiency is the major hazard in surgical patients taking supraphysiologic doses of steroids and can lead to hypotension, cardiovascular collapse, and death. The degree of adrenal suppression depends on dose, dosage schedule, route of administration, and duration of therapy. Although treatment with up to 40 mg of prednisone per day for less than a week does not usually cause significant long-term suppression, doses of 7.5 mg or more for longer can produce suppression requiring up to nine months off the drug for full recovery of the hypothalamic-pituitary-adrenal axis to occur.[2] Supplemental corticosteroids are usually given to patients suspected of decreased adrenal reserve. A variety of regimens have been proposed for different types of surgical procedures.[72] Steroid coverage is discussed in detail in Chap. 26.

Neurologic Disease

All anticonvulsants should be continued until the time of surgery and should be resumed as quickly as possible thereafter. If an intravenous form of the drug is not available, phenytoin or phenobarbital can be substituted as discussed in Chap. 36. Phenytoin should be slowly given intravenously at a rate not to exceed 50 mg/min due to its hypotensive effects. If control of seizures has been adequate in the year before surgery, it is unnecessary to repeat blood levels or an electroencephalogram before the procedure. If control has been poor, surgery should be postponed until stable therapeutic levels are achieved and seizures are controlled.[2]

Anticoagulant Therapy

Perioperative management of patients on oral anticoagulants can be difficult because of the risk of bleeding and thromboembolism in patients with prosthetic heart valves, ventricular aneurysms, atrial fibrillation, an enlarged left atrium, or recurrent deep-venous thrombosis or pulmonary embolism.[2] For elective or emergency minor procedures like dental extractions, patients with a high risk of thrombosis should continue full-dose anticoagulation. Patients with a lower risk of thrombosis may either continue the drug or discontinue it for two or three days before the procedure and resume it thereafter.[2] Those requiring emergency major surgical procedures require vitamin K the day before surgery or fresh frozen plasma on the day of the procedure until the prothrombin time is normal or within two seconds of the control value. In high-risk patients, full-dose intravenous heparin should be resumed about 12 hours after the procedure if surgically feasible. Oral agents can be restarted three to five days thereafter when the patient is eating. For lower-risk patients, there is less urgency to start full-dose heparin if the patient can resume oral anticoagulants soon.[2,73]

For major elective procedures, high-risk patients should discontinue oral anticoagulants one or two days beforehand. If necessary, vitamin K can be used to normalize the prothrombin time.[2,73] Continuous intravenous heparin is recommended to protect the patient from thromboembolic disease in the perioperative period. It can be discontinued three to four hours before surgery to ensure normal coagulation during the procedure.[73,74] In lower-risk patients, oral anticoagulation can be discontinued two to three days beforehand and restarted three to five days after the procedure if the patient is eating.[2,73]

Protamine sulfate is commonly used during cardiac catheterization and cardiopulmonary bypass to neutralize the anticoagulation effects of heparin. However, the incidence of adverse reactions to the drug ranges from 10 percent to 34 percent.[9,10] Although the exact mechanism is unknown, hypotheses include pseudoallergic reactions, activation of complement with development of anaphylatoxins, and IgE-mediated reactions.[10] Clinical manifestations resemble those of anaphylaxis.

Aspirin impairs platelet function by irreversibly acetylating the enzyme cyclooxygenase and inhibiting the synthesis of thromboxane A_2, a platelet aggregating prostaglandin. Aspirin is commonly used by patients with coronary artery and cerebrovascular disease. Although a single dose can affect platelet function for 7 to 10 days, the correlation between aspirin therapy, bleeding time, and perioperative bleeding has not been fully established.[2,75] In general, aspirin should be discontinued at least seven days before elective surgery in which normal hemostasis is critical. In emergency cases, a bleeding time should be performed.[2] If it is significantly prolonged, surgery should be postponed as long as possible until hematology consultation is obtained. If postponement is impossible, platelet transfusion should be considered. The role of DDAVP in this setting is unclear.[75] Nonsteroidal anti-inflammatory agents have similar effects on platelet function but exert a more readily reversible effect, making significant bleeding less likely. They have a short half-life and can be stopped one or two days before surgery.[2]

Psychotropic Medications

Tricyclic antidepressants prolong sleeping time, potentiate some antihypertensives like guanethidine, increase the likelihood of cardiac arrhythmias in combination with halothane and pancuronium, and exert unwanted anticholinergic activity.[76] Despite these interactions, tricyclic antidepressants need not be discontinued before surgery. They require several weeks to take effect but are eliminated relatively rapidly. Therefore, one might consider a discontinuation of the drug for 72 hours, but the risk of recurrent depression may be greater than that of any untoward drug reaction.[77]

Monoamine oxidase inhibitors (MAOI's) interact with a variety of medications during anesthesia. For example, in combination with MAOI's, meperidine can produce hypertensive crisis, convulsions, and hyperpyrexic coma. Some recommend that MAOI's be discontinued two weeks before surgery in elective cases.[78] When this is not feasible, the following guidelines may be helpful:

1. Adequate premedication with benzodiazepines to alleviate anxiety and sympathetic nervous system overactivity;
2. Use of fentanyl or morphine instead of meperidine;
3. Use of enflurane or isoflurane anesthesia instead of halothane;
4. Careful use of epidural or spinal anesthesia as needed;
5. Treatment of intraoperative hypotension with fluid and small doses of direct-acting sympathomimetic amines like phenylephrine if needed;
6. Treatment of intraoperative hypertension with small doses of direct-acting vasodilators like nitroprusside; and
7. Consideration of placement of an arterial line.[78,79]

Phenothiazines, butyrophenones, and benzodiazepines have relatively long half-lives and infrequent side effects. They can usually be discontinued the day before surgery without adverse effects and resumed in their regular doses after surgery.

SUMMARY

1. All patients, and especially those with underlying medical illness who are taking a number of medications, should undergo a careful detailed medication history as the best way to avoid drug reactions and interactions in the perioperative period. Patients should be questioned about prescription and over-the-counter medications.

2. Adverse drug reactions can be classified into those that are predictable and consist of known side effects or toxicity and those that are unpredictable and representative of true drug allergy, pseudoallergy, or idiosyncratic reactions.

3. All clinicians caring for surgical patients should have a working knowledge of the major organ side effects of and interactions among commonly used general anesthetics, local anesthetics, neuromuscular blocking agents, and premedications.

4. Interactions between drugs (drug-drug interactions) are likely to occur in patients already taking medications who receive an average of 5 to 10 more drugs in the perioperative period. A basic understanding of pharmacologic principles and frequent review of the medication list can help avoid problems.

5. The effects of medications on underlying diseases can be altered by surgery and anesthesia (drug-disease interactions), requiring appreciation of the consequences of initiating and/or discontinuing medications in the perioperative period.

REFERENCES

1. Cullen BF: Drug interactions and anesthesia: A review. *Anesth Analg* 58:413–423, 1979.
2. Cygan R, Waitzkin H: Stopping and restarting medications in the perioperative period. *J Gen Int Med* 2:270–283, 1987.
3. Duthie D: Concurrent drug therapy in patients undergoing surgery. *Anaesthesia* 42:305, 1987.
4. *Evaluations of Drug Interactions*, St. Louis, PDS Publishing, 1992, p 2/0.01–2/74.

5. *Drug Interaction Facts*, 2d ed. St. Louis, Lippincott, 1990, pp 122–125, 337, 364, 394, 557–577, 667–684.

6. Dukes M, Beeley L (eds): *Side Effects of Drugs Annual 15*. Amsterdam, Elsevier, 1991, pp 101–108.

7. VanTyle WK: Internal analgesics, in Feldman E (ed): *Handbook of Nonprescription Drugs*, 9th ed. Washington, American Pharmaceutical Association, 1990, pp 557–589.

8. Thomassen D: Effect of stress on drug hypersensitivity. *Drug Safety* 6:235, 1991.

9. Anderson J: Allergic reactions to drugs and biological agents. *JAMA* 268:2845, 1992.

10. Weiss M: Drug allergy. *Clin Allergy* 76:857, 1992.

11. Ngai SH: Current concepts in anesthesiology: Effect of anesthetics on various organs. *N Engl J Med* 302:564, 1980.

12. Merin RG: Effect of anesthetic drugs on myocardial performance in man. *Ann Rev Med* 28:75, 1977.

13. Stoelting RK, Miller RD: *Basics of Anesthesia*, 2d ed. New York, Churchill Livingstone, 1989, pp 47–56.

14. Stoelting RK, Miller RD: *Basics of Anesthesia*, 2d ed, pp 69–79.

15. Stoelting RK, Miller RD: *Basics of Anesthesia*, 2d ed, p 78.

16. Stanley TH: New developments in intravenous anesthesia. *ASA Refresher Course Lectures* 233:1–6, 1989.

17. Stoelting RK, Miller RD: *Basics of Anesthesia*, 2d ed, pp 43–47.

18. Stevens WC, Kingston HG: Inhalation anesthesia, in Barash PG, Cullen BF, Stoelting RK: *Clinical Anesthesia*, 2d ed. Philadelphia, Lippincott, 1992, p 446.

19. Stoelting RK, Miller RD: *Basics of Anesthesia*, 2d ed, pp 69–79.

20. Stoelting RK, Miller RD: *Basics of Anesthesia*, 2d ed, pp 100–101.

21. Stoelting RK, Miller RD: *Basics of Anesthesia*, 2d ed, pp 57–67.

22. Berman ML, Holaday DA: Inhalation anesthetic metabolilsm and toxicity, in Barash PG, Cullen PF, Stoelting RK (eds): *Clinical Anesthesia*, 1st ed. Philadelphia, Lilppincott, 1989, p 334.

23. Kripke BJ, Talario L., Shah NK et al: Hematologic reaction to prolonged exposure to nitrous oxide. *Anesthesiology* 47:342, 1976.

24. Whitwam JG: Adverse reactions to IV induction agents. *Br J Anaesth* 50:77, 1978.

25. DeJong R: Toxic effects of local anesthetics. *N Engl J Med* 286:975, 1972.

26. Covino BG: The pharmacologic basis for choosing a local anesthetic. *ASA Refresher Course Lectures* 131:1–5, 1990.

27. Adriani J, Naraghi M: Etiology and management of adverse reactions to local anesthetics. *J Am Med Wom Assoc* 33:367, 1978.

28. Covino BG, Vassallo HG: *Local Anesthetics: Mechanism of Action in Clinical Use*. Orlando, Grune & Stratton, 1976, pp 123–125.

29. Stoelting RK, Miller RD: *Basics of Anesthesia*, 2d ed, pp 87–88.

30. Olson M, McEvoy G: Methemoglobinemia induced by local anesthetics. *Am J Hosp Pharm* 38:89, 1981.

31. Incaudo G, Schatz M et al: Administration of local anesthetics to patients with a history of prior adverse reactions. *J Allergy Clin Immunol* 61:339, 1978.

32. Ali H, Savarese JJ: Monitoring of neuromuscular function. *Anesthesiology* 45:216–249, 1976.

33. Stoelting RK, Miller RD: *Basics of Anesthesia*, 2d ed, pp 91–106.

34. Libonati MM, Leahy JJ, Ellison N: The use of succinylcholine in open eye surgery. *Anesthesiology* 62:637–640, 1985.

35. White PF: Pharmacologic and clinical aspects of preoperative medication. *Anesth Analg* 65:967–968, 1986.

36. Mirakhur RK, Dundee JW, Connolly JDR: Studies of drugs given before anesthesia—anticholinergic premedicants. *Br J Anaesth* 51:339–345, 1979.

37. Jones R, Deutsch S, Turndorf H: Effects of atropine on cardiac rhythm in conscious and anesthetized man. *Anesthesiology* 22:67, 1961.

38. Mirakhur R, Dundee J, Jones C: Evaluations of the anticholinergic actions of glycopyrronium bromide. *Br J Clin Pharmacol* 5:77, 1978.

39. Mirakhur R: Anticholinergic drugs. *Br J Anaesth* 51:671, 1979.

40. Brocke-Ulre J, Rubin J, Welman S et al: The effect of glycopyrrolate on the lower esophageal sphincter. *Can Anaesth Soc J* 25:144, 1978.

41. *PDR–Drug Interactions and Side Effects Index*, 46th ed. Montvale NJ, Medical Economics Data, 1992, pp 214–216, 359, 383–384, 441–442, 452–453, 807, 886–887, 1002–1004, 1017–1018.

42. Hansten P, Horn J: *Drug Interactions & Updates*, Malvern PA, Lea & Febiger, 1992, pp 1–27.

43. *Handbook of Adverse Drug Interactions. The Medical Letter on Drugs and Therapeutics*. New Rochelle NY, The Medical Letter, 1992, pp 4–5, 119–120.

44. Evans W, Schentag J, Juskow W: *Applied Pharmacokinetics*, 2d ed. Spokane, Applied Therapeutics, 1986, pp 1–8, 139–206.

45. Stanski D: The contribution of pharmacokinetics and pharmacodynamics to clinical anesthesia care. *Can J Anaesth* 35:542, 1988.

46. Kramer W, Inglott A, Cluxton R: Physical and chemical incompatibilities of drugs for IV administration. *Drug Intell Clin Pharm* 5:211, 1971.

47. Trissel L (ed): *Handbook on Injectable Drugs*, 6th ed. Bethesda, American Society of Hospital Pharmacy, 1990.

48. McCaughey W: Adverse effects of local anesthetics. *Drug Safety* 7:178, 1992.

49. *AMA Drug Evaluations Annual*, 1992. Chicago, American Medical Association, 1992, pp 149–163, 165–206.

50. Neuberger J: Halothane and hepatitis, incidence, predisposing factors and exposure guidelines. *Drug Safety* 5:28, 1990.

51. Shingu K, Eger EI II, Johnson BH et al: Effect of oxygen concentration, hyperthermia, and choice of vendor on anesthetic induced hepatic injury in rats. *Anesth Analg* 62:146–150, 1983.

52. Mazze RI, Sicvenpiper TS, Stevenson J: Renal effects of enflurane and halothane in patients with abnormal renal function. *Anesthesiology* 60:161–163, 1984.

53. Pittinger C, Adamson R: Antibiotic blockade of neuromuscular function. *Ann Rev Pharmacol* 12:169, 1972.

54. Hashimato Y, Shima T, Matsukawa S et al: A possible hazard of prolonged neuromuscular blockade by amikacin. *Anesthesiology* 49:219, 1978.

55. Roizen M, Stevens W: Multiform ventricular tachycardia due to the interaction of aminophylline and halothane. *Anaesth Analg* 57:738, 1978.

56. Cheng EY, Kay J: *Manual of Anesthesia and the Medically Compromised Patient*. Philadelphia, Lippincott, 1990, p 145.

57. *Physicians Desk Reference*, 46th ed. Montvale NJ, Medical Economics, 1992, pp 855–857.

58. Pettinger WA: Minoxidil and the treatment of severe hypertension. *N Engl J Med* 303:922–926, 1980.

59. Miller ED: Antihypertensive therapy, in Kaplan JA (ed): *Cardiac Anesthesia*, 2d ed. New York, Grune & Stratton, 1987, pp 401–402.

60. Miller RD, Way WL, Eger EI II: The effects of alpha-methyldopa, reserpine, guanethidine, and iproniazid on minimum alveolar anesthetic requirement (MAC). *Anesthesiology* 29:1153–1158, 1968.

61. Bloor BC, Flacke WE: Reduction in halothane anesthetic requirements by clonidine, an alpha-adrenergic agonist. *Anesth Analg* 61:741–745, 1982.

62. Bruce DL, Croley TF, Lee JS: Preoperative clonidine withdrawal syndrome. *Anesthesiology* 51:90–92, 1979.

63. O'Connor DE: Accelerated acute clonidine withdrawal syndrome during coronary artery bypass surgery. *Br J Anaesth* 53:431–433, 1981.

64. Craig DB, Bose D: Drug interactions in anesthesia: Chronic antihypertensive therapy. *Can Anaesth Soc J* 31:580–589, 1984.

65. Stoelting RK, Miller RD: *Basics of Anesthesia*, 2d ed, p 37.

66. Davis RF: Etiology and treatment of perioperative cardiac dysrhythmias, in Kaplan JA (ed): *Cardiac Anesthesia*, 2d ed, pp 442–440.

67. Roizen MF: Anesthetic implications of concurrent diseases, in Miller RD (ed): *Anesthesia*, 3d ed. New York, Churchill Livingstone. 1990, p 874.

68. Coursin DB, Croy S, Goelzer SL: Pulmonary disorders, in Cheng EY, Kay J (ed): *Manual of Anesthesia and the Medically Compromised Patient*. Philadelphia, Lippincott, 1990, pp 157–167.

69. Kay J: Endocrine disorders, in Cheng EY, Kay J (ed): *Manual of Anesthesia and the Medically Compromised Patient*, pp 362–369.

70. Stoelting RK, Miller RD: *Basics of Anesthesia*, 2d ed, pp 329–333.

71. Kay J: Endocrine disorders, in Cheng EY, Kay J (ed): *Manual of Anesthesia and the Medically Compromised Patient*, pp 378–386.

72. Kay J: Endocrine disorders, in Cheng EY, Kay J (ed): *Manual of Anesthesia and the Medically Compromised Patient*, pp 376–378.

73. Cade JF, Hunt P, Stubbs KP et al: Guideline for the management of oral anticoagulant therapy in patients undergoing surgery. *Med J Aust* 2:292–294, 1979.

74. Pennock JL: Perioperative management of drug therapy. *Surg Clin NA* 63-5:1049–1056, 1983.

75. Rodgers RPC, Levin J: A critical reappraisal of bleeding time. *Sem Throm Hemo* 16-1:1–20, 1990.

76. Sladen RN: Anemia, bleeding disorders, and transfusion therapy, in Cheng EY, Kay J (eds): *Manual of Anesthesia and the Medicallky Compromised Patient*, pp 453–455.

77. Lawson NW: Autonomic nervous system physiology and pharmacology, in Barash PG, Cullen BF, Stoelting RK (eds): *Clinical Anesthesia*, 2d ed, pp 363–364.

78. Haddox JD: Psychiatric disorders and their treatment, in Cheng EY, Kay J (eds): *Manual of Anesthesia and the Medically Compromised Patient*, pp 598–604.

79. Wells DG, Bjorksten AR: Monoamine oxidase inhibitors revisited. *Can J Anaesth* 36-1:64–74, 1989.

50 SURGERY IN THE PATIENT WITH COMMUNICABLE DISEASE: PREVENTION OF DISEASE TRANSMISSION

Frank Kroboth

This chapter reviews issues involving transmission of infection between patient and surgeon. There are three major areas of importance:

1. Diseases commonly transmitted or discussed among health care professionals, including hepatitis B (HBV) and human immunodeficiency virus (HIV) infection. Other retroviruses like human T-cell leukemia virus type I are transmitted by dirty needles but are not as yet prevalent.[1] HIV type II and unexplained T-lymphocyte–depleting organisms may also become more prominent.[2,3]

2. Diseases of less frequent concern in the West but reported as risks to the surgeon or hospital community, including cytomegalovirus disease, malaria, Creutzfeldt-Jakob disease, trypanosomiasis, babesiosis, viral hemorrhagic fevers, and syphilis.

3. Diseases, including some of the above, which require isolation or official reporting. Two such diseases in this category, tuberculosis and meningococcal infection, are discussed in detail. General reference appendices are provided.

This chapter excludes infections transmitted to the patient through transplantation[4] and from local skin infections of the surgeon.

DISEASES OF MOST COMMON CONCERN

Viral Hepatitis

A practicing surgeon's risk of contracting hepatitis B infection over a period of 40 years is 30 to 40 percent, and that of becoming a chronic carrier is about 4 percent.[5] The two most important components of physician protection are utilizing universal precautions and taking hepatitis B vaccine before exposures. Universal precaution measures were defined precisely by the Centers for Disease Control (CDC) in 1987 and 1988.[6,7] All patients should be regarded as potential carriers of bloodborne infection. Blood, certain body fluids, and instruments exposed to them should be handled with extreme care. Feces, sputum, sweat, nasal secretions, urine, vomitus, and breast milk carry a lower risk of infection but should be handled in the same way when contaminated with blood. Universal precautions should be viewed as additional measures to standard infection control practices like isolation of patients with certain diseases. Protective barriers are commonly used in the surgical arena, but eyewear is frequently neglected. Implementing universal precautions increases hospital costs by 15 percent,[8] but in larger studies 26 to 37 percent of injuries could have been avoided by proper infection control techniques.[9,10] In addition, hepatitis B vaccine should be given to all nonimmune physicians who have potential contact with body fluids or needles.

The CDC has provided recommendations for the prevention of hepatitis B.[11–14] The 1985 guidelines in Table 50–1 define high-risk contacts,[14] and those from 1990 in Table 50–2 outline treatment options following exposure.[13] Some additional points should be made:

1. By definition, anyone who is exposed is a candidate for hepatitis B vaccine if not already immunized.

2. Both hepatitis B immune globulin (HBIG) and hepatitis B vaccine if indicated should be given as soon as possible after exposure. Testing for immune status is useful only if it does not delay treatment for more than seven days.

3. If an exposed physician or health care worker refuses vaccination, an additional dose of HBIG is recommended one month after exposure.

491

TABLE 50–1. Prevalence of Hepatitis B Serologic Markers in Various Population Groups

Population Group	Prevalence of Serologic Markers of HBV Infection	
	HBsAg (%)	All Markers (%)
High Risk		
Immigrants/refugees from areas of high HBV endemicity	13	70–85
Clients in institutions for the mentally retarded	10–20	35–80
Users of illicit parenteral drugs	7	60–80
Homosexually active men	6	35–80
Household contacts of HBV carriers	3–6	30–60
Patients of hemodialysis units	3–10	20–80
Intermediate Risk		
Health-care workers— frequent blood contact	1–2	15–30
Prisoners (male)	1–8	10–80
Staff of institutions for the mentally retarded	1	10–25
Low Risk		
Health-care workers— no or infrequent blood contact	0.3	3–10
Healthy adults (first-time volunteer blood donors)	0.3	3–5

TABLE 50–2. Recommendations for Hepatitis B Prophylaxis Following Percutaneous or Permucosal Exposure

Exposed Person	Treatment When Source Is Found to Be:		
	HBsAg-Positive	HBsAg-Negative	Source Not Tested or Unknown
Unvaccinated	HBIG × 1* and initiate HB vaccine†	Initiate HB vaccine†	Initiate HB vaccine†
Previously vaccinated Known responder	Test exposed for anti-HBs 1. If adequate,§ no treatment 2. If inadequate, HB vaccine booster dose	No treatment	No treatment
Known nonresponder	HBIG × 2 or HBIG × 1 plus 1 dose HB vaccine	No treatment	If known high-risk source, may treat as if source were HBsAg-positive
Response unknown	Test exposed for anti-HBs 1. If inadequate,§ HBIG × 1 plus HB vaccine booster dose 2. If adequate, no treatment	No treatment	Test exposed for anti-HBs 1. If inadequate,§ HB vaccine booster dose 2. If adequate, no treatment

*HBIG dose 0.06 ml/kg IM.

†HB vaccine dose—see text.

§Adequate anti-HBs is ≥ 10 SRU by RIA or positive by EIA.

4. If HBIG is unavailable, serum immune globulin in a dose of 0.06 ml/kg may be of some benefit.

5. The CDC recommendations should be applied with judgment. For example, in the case of a needlestick from an unknown patient in a setting in which nearly all patients carry hepatitis B, exposure might logically be considered "known."

6. The dose of Recombivax-HB is 10 mcg per inoculation and that of Engerix-B is 20 mcg per inoculation for nonimmunized adults. The efficacy of these is similar to that of plasma-derived vaccine.[14,15]

7. If a patient to whom the physician is exposed demonstrates both surface antigen and antibody in his serum, he should be considered possibly infectious. One longitudinal study documented that 19 percent of such patients became seronegative for antibody on later testing.[16]

Response to vaccine is a common question among health care personnel. Approximately 90 percent of recipients of plasma-derived vaccine develop adequate antibody levels, which then decline over time to immeasurable levels in 10 to 15 percent.[11] Protection persists even after levels of antibody are no longer detectable.[17]

Some believe that nonresponders or low-level responders should receive revaccination with a booster dose.[18–20] This means that determination of immune status must be performed after all vaccinations. The CDC recommends such an approach in health care workers with an increased risk of percutaneous exposure. Antibody status should be assessed one to six months after the vaccination. A single booster dose is successful in up to 20 percent of persons with inadequate initial response. Three additional doses raise the success rate to 50 percent. Therefore, one or more additional doses are recommended for nonresponders.[13] Booster doses are also recommended in most cases when antibody status of previously vaccinated persons is found to be inadequate (see Table 50–2).

The CDC does not at present recommend routine antibody assessment years after the primary series or mandatory boosters unless actual exposure occurs. However, patients on hemodialysis should have their antibody status checked yearly and be revaccinated when titers fall below 10 mIU/ml.[21] The Surgical Infection Society arbitrarily recommends revaccination every five years for all persons.[22]

Prophylaxis against hepatitis C after needlestick is even less clear. Studies of immunoglobulin prophylaxis have been inconclusive. The CDC recommends that "it may be reasonable to administer" immunoglobulin in a dose of 0.06 ml/kg after a needlestick from a patient believed to have hepatitis C.[13] Now that diagnosis is available for chronic infection, some recommend that health care workers with accidental percutaneous exposure undergo serologic evaluation.[23] If the patient cannot be identified or has elevated serum ALT levels or antihepatitis C virus antibody titers, these parameters can be measured in the health care worker and repeated in three to six months if initially negative.

Measures to prevent hepatitis B infection are advisable after exposure to a source of hepatitis D. No immunoglobulin need be given to hospital workers exposed to hepatitis A unless there is fecal contact during an outbreak of the disease.[13]

Physician-to-patient transfer of hepatitis virus has been well studied.[24] Recent recommendations for hepatitis B–infected physicians have been included in HIV policy statements. The CDC recommends that health care workers who have detectable levels of e-antigen perform invasive procedures with informed consent only if cleared by an expert panel.[25]

HIV Infection

Recommendations regarding the prevention of transmission of HIV to health care workers during invasive procedures have been published by the CDC.[12,26] Percutaneous exposure through needle and sharp-object injury occurs with disturbing frequency in all types of surgery. Several studies have documented that glove perforations occur in over 30 percent of procedures.[27–30] Moreover, in two studies, glove wearers were aware of the perforations only 39 percent and 60 percent of the time, respectively.[28,29] Double-gloving decreases the risk of perforation to skin layer by two-thirds or more.[27,31–33] A variety of modified surgical techniques and special care during wound closure may also decrease injury.[29,34–37] Although not all glove tears involve skin penetration, estimates of percutaneous injury vary between 1.7 percent and 15.4 percent.[38,39]

Data from 10 studies reveal that the risk of transmission of HIV from needlestick injury is 0.37 percent. The risk from a single mucous membrane exposure to infected blood is 0.32 percent or even lower.[8,40] In a CDC surveillance study, none of 103 workers with mucous membrane or nonintact skin contact seroconverted within 180 days.[10] However, special care should be taken if the worker has open or weeping skin lesions.[41] Transmission in the course of usual ward activities is exceedingly small.[42] Of 106 health care workers exposed to body fluids other than blood in the CDC surveillance study, none seroconverted.[10] Transmission by aerosolized bone has not been adequately studied.[43] Therefore, the surgeon's primary concern should be parenteral exposure to infected blood or body fluids. The rate of HIV transmission is orders of magnitude smaller than that of hepatitis B, but the possible outcome if infection develops is at least an order of magnitude more serious.

Compounding the fear of HIV infection is the lack of any substantive treatment available to surgeons or health care personnel. Public health issues dictate that the HIV and hepatitis B serological status of the patient and the surgeon be determined at the time of exposure.[12] Any acute febrile illness suffered by the surgeon in the 12 weeks after exposure should be reported. If the patient has serologic evidence of HIV infection or refuses testing, the surgeon should obtain follow-up testing at 6, 12, and 26 weeks after the injury. The surgeon should take strict precautions to prevent transmission of HIV, especially in the first 12 weeks. This includes refraining from donating blood, engaging in unprotected sex, or breastfeeding. The question of continuing practice during this period has not been adequately addressed.[12,44] Patients with risk factors for HIV infection should at times be considered infected even if serologic testing is negative, since recent data suggest that high-risk individuals may remain seronegative by conventional antibody testing for up to 42 months.[45,46] Given the number and complexity of the issues involved, health centers should consider providing a central information service. In some centers, needlestick hotlines and postexposure testing protocols have proven helpful and are simple to maintain once consensus is reached and on-site personnel are trained to respond.

The use of prophylactic zidovudine (AZT) after parenteral exposure to HIV rests on data from animal studies. In retrovirus infection in cats and mice, AZT administered within hours of exposure favorably altered the course of infection, suppressing viremia in mice and abrogating viral replication in cats.[47,48] However, there are no data indicating that HIV reacts similarly in humans.[40] Postexposure prophylaxis against simian immunodeficiency virus in primates has not been shown to be successful.[44] The manufacturers of AZT instituted a study to test its effectiveness in this setting, but difficulty in recruiting enough subjects limited their progress.[40,49]

Hospital employee health services and physicians of exposed workers face the decision of whether or not to use AZT empirically. Model programs at the National Institutes of Health (NIH) and the University of California at San Francisco have been undertaken.[40] They depend on the ability and willingness to educate exposed workers quickly about the rationale for using AZT, its toxicity, and the possible mutagenic and teratogenic effects. The actual risk of a given exposure should be considered. Obtaining informed consent is recommended. Two publications listed in the bibliography may serve as adjuncts in further educating workers.[40,44] The health care worker must ultimately decide whether or not to take the drug. The regimen recommended by the NIH is 200 mg every four hours orally for 42 days. Blood counts and serum chemistry determinations should be monitored frequently.

The issue of counseling surgeons and health care workers who become infected is mired in medical-legal debate. The American Medical Association's Council on Ethical and Judicial Affairs has said that "if no risk (of transmission) exists, disclosure of the physician's medical condition to his or her patients will serve no rational purpose; if a risk does exist, the physician should not engage in the activity. The Council recommends that the afflicted physician disclose his condition to colleagues who can assist in the individual assessment of whether the physician's medical condition or the proposed activity poses any risk to patients."[50]

In July 1991, the CDC issued a policy statement on preventing transmission of HBV and HIV to patients.[25] (See Fig. 50–1.) In summary, it recommends that health care workers who perform exposure-prone procedures know their HIV and hepatitis B e-antigen status. If positive for either, they should not perform such procedures unless they are counseled by an expert review panel and receive informed consent from patients. The Surgical Infection Society does not agree with restrictions based on HIV serology,[22] and the National Commission on AIDS has concluded similarly.[51] At this time, the definition of "exposure-prone procedures" is problematic[52–54] because CDC recommendations fall short of providing a specific procedural listing.

Lack of data prevents more concrete recommendations. Aside from the well-publicized cases of HIV infection contracted from a Florida dentist, conclusive evidence of transmission from health care worker to patient has been deemed impossible in 15,795 cases reviewed by the CDC as of May 1992. Most consider the physicians with HIV infection to be of little or no risk to patients if no invasive procedures are performed. In the absence of state laws defining exposure-prone procedures, each one should be carefully reviewed by the CDC as of May 1992.[55] Most consider the physicians with HIV infection to be of little or no risk to patients if no settlements concluded that infected physicians can continue to practice, but should limit the "performance of seriously invasive

- All health care workers (HCWs) should adhere to universal precautions, including the appropriate use of hand washing, protective barriers, and care in the use and disposal of needles and other sharp instruments. HCWs who have exudative lesions or weeping dermatitis should refrain from all direct patient care and from handling patient-care equipment and devices used in performing invasive procedures until the condition resolves. HCWs should also comply with current guidelines for disinfection and sterilization of reusable devices used in invasive procedures.

- Currently available data provide no basis for recommendations to restrict the practice of HCWs infected with HIV or HBV who perform invasive procedures not identified as exposure-prone, provided the infected HCWs practice recommended surgical or dental technique and comply with universal precautions and current recommendations for sterilization/disinfection.

- Exposure-prone procedures should be identified by medical/surgical/dental organizations and institutions at which the procedures are performed.

- HCWs who perform exposure-prone procedures should know their HIV antibody status. HCWs who perform exposure-prone procedures and who do not have serologic evidence of immunity to HBV from vaccination or from previous infection should know their HBsAg status and, if that is positive, should also know their HBeAg status.

- HCWs who are infected with HIV or HBV (and are HBeAg positive) should not perform exposure-prone procedures unless they have sought counsel from an expert review panel and been advised under what circumstances, if any, they may continue to perform these procedures.* Such circumstances would include notifying prospective patients of the HCW's seropositivity before they undergo exposure-prone invasive procedures.

---

*The review panel should include experts who represent a balanced perspective. Such experts might include all of the following: a) the HCW's personal physician(s), b) an infectious disease specialist with expertise in the epidemiology of HIV and HBV transmission, c) a health professional with expertise in the procedures performed by the HCW, and d) state or local public health official(s). If the HCW's practice is institutionally based, the expert review panel might also include a member of the infection-control committee, preferably a hospital epidemiologist. HCWs who perform exposure-prone procedures outside the hospital/institutional setting should seek advice from appropriate state and local public health officials regarding the review process. Panels must recognize the importance of confidentiality and the privacy rights of infected HCWs.

FIGURE 50–1. CDC Policy Statement on Preventing Transmission of HBV and HIV to Patients.

procedures," use strict infection control procedures, and allow supervision by their physicians and institutions.[56]

A similarly unanswered question for both the infected health care worker and his or her counseling physician is at what point immune status becomes compromised enough to avoid contact with the great variety of pathogens in the hospital. A counselor must also assess mental and emotional competence to practice even if the physician is still physically able to do so.

IMPORTANT DISEASES OF LESS FREQUENT CONCERN

Cytomegalovirus (CMV)

Information about transmission of cytomegalovirus (CMV), a member of the herpesvirus group, is limited.[57] Children in day care centers transmit CMV to each other and to employees after prolonged or intimate contact.[58] CMV is also transmitted by blood transfusion.[59] In one study, the seroconversion rate in newborn nursery and other nursing personnel was 3.3 percent per year and was no higher than in middle-class mothers in the same community. Risk is higher after intimate contact than in usual occupational settings.[60]

A recent epidemiologic study examined the seroconversion rate in health care workers in a large city hospital where most had been exposed to patients with AIDS.[61] The annual conversion rate was 5.4 percent and was similar to conversion rates in the community documented in other studies. A similar study failed to substantiate an increased risk of CMV infection in caregivers in pediatric hospital settings.[62] Therefore, even after exposure to a high-risk population, occupational risk is low.

Although CMV infection is clinically mild or asymptomatic in most adults, infants may develop cytomegalovirus inclusion disease. A vaccine is available that is immunogenic in women of child-bearing age.[63] However, because the risk of infection in health care workers is similar to that in mothers in the community, it is reasonable simply to wash carefully after contact with saliva, blood, stool, tears, or soiled articles from high-risk patients.[64,65]

Creutzfeldt-Jakob Disease (CJD)

Creutzfeldt-Jakob disease (CJD) is a subacute degeneration of the central nervous system caused by a transmissible virus-like agent without nucleic acid content.[66] A rare variant of CJD, the Gerstmann-Straussler syndrome, is also a transmissable disease.[67] Interest has centered around possible transmission to the surgeon in view of documented spread to patients from infected grafts, corneae, brain electrodes, and growth hormone extracts.[68] The agent is resistant to usual sterilization techniques, progresses relentlessly, and is as yet untreatable.[69–72] Disease has been reported in a neurosurgeon, a pathologist, and two histopathology technicians.[73]

Although CJD is transmissable to animals and humans, its prevalence in physicians is not increased.[74] There has been no documented passage of infection by way of respiratory, oral, venereal, or percutaneous routes.[71] In infected individuals, the agent is present in central nervous system tissue and cerebrospinal fluid. It can be found in lower titer in liver, lung, lymph node, kidney, urine, and white blood cells.[75] Guidelines for the surgical team are drawn from several sources:[72,75,76]

1. Tissues from elderly demented patients should not be used for transplantation or blood donation.

2. Specimens from suspected patients should be well-labeled.

3. Exposed skin should be washed for several minutes with 1 N sodium hydroxide.

4. The site of a needlestick should be cleansed promptly with an iodine or phenolic antiseptic.

5. Patients do not need special isolation.

6. Contaminated reusable materials should be vigorously decontaminated. Effective regimens include steam autoclaving at 121°C at 15 lb/in^2 for four to five hours or combining autoclaving and 1 N sodium hydroxide washing.[70,76]

Malaria

Although malaria is seen rarely in this country, *Plasmodium malariae* can persist in the blood in asymptomatic patients for over 50 years.[77] Malaria is a documented transfusion-related disease and has been reported after needlestick with an incubation period of 4 to 17 days.[78,79] Personnel exposed by skin puncture to blood from patients with known malarial infection should receive prophylactic therapy appropriate to the species.[78] When needlestick involves high-risk patients with no known disease (e.g., those from endemic areas, those with a past history of malaria, or those who use illegal drugs), malaria should be kept in mind as a possible etiology if future symptoms develop.

Trypanosomiasis

Trypanosomiasis has been recently reported in the United States after transfusion,[80,81] and is presumably related to immigration from endemic areas. Although needlestick or mucosal transmission has occurred in laboratory exposures,[79] at this point in time it is only important to be aware of the remote possibility of infection. Chemoprophylaxis is reasonable only in documented exposures carrying more than "slight risk." Similar recommendations have been made in the literature for laboratory personnel.[82]

It has been suggested that immigrants from endemic areas be serologically screened for asymptomatic chronic Chagas' disease. If screening becomes routine, more information about the risk of needlestick and mucosal exposure will be needed. The present chemotherapeutic agents, nifurtimox or benznidazole, are not entirely effective and have toxic side effects.[83] Although African trypanosomiasis has been reported after transfusion, needlestick carries only a potential risk of transmitting the disease.[79]

Babesiosis

Babesiosis, a malaria-like protozoan disease, has been reported after transfusion in the northeastern United States.[84,85] There are no documented incidents of needlestick transmission.[79] The illness is usually mild in patients with normal splenic function. Therefore, no particular precautions are warranted at this time.

Viral Hemorrhagic Fevers

Viral hemorrhagic fevers are a group of diseases very rarely seen in North America. In four of these—Lassa fever, Ebola disease, Marburg disease, and Crimean-Congo hemorrhagic fever—person-to-person spread in hospital settings has been documented.[86,87] These diseases should be kept in mind in patients from endemic areas of Africa, Asia, and eastern Europe, or in virology laboratory workers who develop a serious unknown viral illness. If one of them is suspected, extensive isolation precautions are necessary. Surgeons operating on these patients should wear protective eyewear and a double set of gloves and seek advice from the CDC.[86] The reader is referred to general material on the disease and specific case reports for further information.[86–91]

Syphilis

The threat of syphilis to surgeons and health care personnel has been described since the early part of the century.[92] Transmission to physicians by direct contact and needlestick has been well documented. When the site of inoculation was inapparent, the disease was called syphilis d'emblée or syphilis without recognized contact. Fingers were particularly vulnerable, especially in physicians who performed "bare-handed" vaginal examinations and operated without gloves. The eyelid could also be affected by inadvertent wiping with a contaminated examining hand.

Most of the hygienic recommendations of the past are now universal practice. Many contacts carry a low risk of infectivity. Chances of transmission are lower if the patient has been infected for a long period of time, and risk nears zero after five years. In the preantibiotic era, one or two doses of arsenical therapy was believed to reduce the risk of transmission substantially in the earlier, more infectious stages of the disease.[92] Therefore, after needlestick injury from a known high-risk patient, thorough cleansing, RPR determination, and follow-up testing and consideration of antibiotic therapy are appropriate.

Other Diseases

Transmission of leishmaniasis and toxoplasmosis by needlestick has been described in a laboratory but not a clinical setting.[79] Transfusion-related rickettsial infections have been reported,[93] but remain a remote possibility. Lyme disease can potentially be transmitted by transfusion,[94] but in one follow-up study of 14 exposed recipients no one developed clinical or serologic evidence of disease.[95] There are no reports of needlestick transmission of Lyme disease.

DISEASES REQUIRING ISOLATION OR CASE REPORT

Many illnesses require isolation of the patient or notification of local health departments. Appendix A is reproduced in modified form from the CDC Guidelines for Isolation Precautions in Hospitals.[96] Its alphabetical format allows quick reference to suspected diseases. Pediatric material has been omitted. The six major categories of isolation or precaution are strict isolation, contact isolation, respiratory isolation, tuberculosis isolation, enteric precautions, and drainage/secretion precautions (DSP).

Although nomenclature may vary slightly in different hospitals, techniques are similar and are fully described in the CDC Guidelines. In addition, protective isolation is another category applicable to some patients with agranulocytosis, severe dermatitis, extensive burns, and some hematologic and oncologic diseases. Universal precautions have been substituted for blood and body fluid precautions in the original table. These apply to all patients, and precautions required for specific diseases are additive.

Two more frequently encountered diseases requiring isolation are tuberculosis and meningococcal infection. Two important questions raised are how long isolation is needed and what measures should be taken by exposed health care personnel.

Meningococcal Infection

Recommendations for meningococcal disease are reasonably consistent. Many hospitals and the CDC recommend at least one day of effective therapy before isolation is discontinued.[96] Aside from household contacts, hospital personnel having "intimate" contact

with affected patients are advised to take prophylactic antibiotic therapy. Intimate contact includes mouth-to-mouth resuscitation or close contact with oral secretions. The presently recommended prophylactic regimen for adults is rifampin in a dose of 600 mg twice daily orally for two days.[97]

Tuberculosis

Tuberculosis exposure and isolation raise several interesting questions. Droplet nuclei produced by coughing, sneezing, or talking are most often responsible for infection. The frequency of such events, radiographic extent of disease, presence of cavitation, and involvement of the upper airway are determinants of infectivity.[98] Prolonged exposure in an infectious environment is thought to be the major risk factor in developing infection.[99] Some investigators estimate that breathing contaminated air for 800 hours is required to infect a hospital worker.[100] These data were derived by reviewing tuberculin conversion rates in hospital and sanitarium nurses, and correlate well with those of guinea pigs placed in an air outflow tract of a tuberculosis ward. It has also been estimated that 22 percent of household contacts of smear-positive index cases become infected.[101] Recent literature has pointed out the shortcomings of standard surgical masks in protecting people from droplet nuclei. Masks with adequate face seals that can be reused as needed cost about three times as much as standard masks.[102]

Patients probably become noninfectious after two weeks of appropriate therapy for sensitive organisms even if smears are still positive.[98,103] Two weeks constitute a reasonable minimal period of isolation for patients with active disease. Decreased cough, sputum production, fever, and number of acid-fast bacilli on smear should confirm clinical response. Patients who fail initial therapy and require retreatment should show signs of improvement before isolation is discontinued.[96] Smears and cultures may remain positive for many months after initiation of treatment, depending on smear status and presence or absence of cavitation at the time of presentation.[104] The CDC recommends that a patient taken out of isolation not be put in a room with other patients until 3 daily smears are negative.[105] If a health care provider has significant exposure to a patient with active tuberculosis in whom proper precautions have not been taken, a PPD skin test should be placed if not already done recently, and repeated in one week if negative and again two to three months later if still negative.

Several factors should be considered if the PPD is positive. About 3.3 percent of patients develop active disease in the first year after conversion, and 5 to 15 percent do so over the rest of their lives.[99] Since most active disease develops in the first two years after infection, it is useful to know whether a positive test represents recent conversion. This information is easy to obtain if PPD testing is done frequently. However, if testing has not been done for many years, the booster phenomenon may obscure proper interpretation; mild or no reaction may make proper interpretation of the result difficult. This phenomenon occurs when there is no reaction or a mild reaction to the first skin test after a long interval but a full response to one performed soon thereafter, and it should not be construed as recent conversion. Therefore, high-risk individuals who have a mild reaction to a first PPD test after several years should have the test repeated a week later. A positive repeat test then indicates earlier infection. It should be appreciated that isoniazid (INH) is only 60 to 80 percent effective in preventing disease in most studies.[99]

The American Thoracic Society recommendations for preventing asymptomatic infected individuals without such disease on chest x-ray from developing active disease depend on whether or not they are over or under the age of 35. The risk of INH-induced hepatotoxicity rises with age and must be balanced against the risk of active disease, which is highest in the two years after infection. Those who have converted in the last two years should receive prophylactic therapy with INH regardless of age. If a patient has a positive test that is thought to be old and has not been treated, he should receive INH if he is under 35 but not if he is older unless there are circumstances indicating a higher risk of developing active disease. Such factors include radiographic evidence of old disease, diabetes mellitus, past gastrectomy, steroid or immunosuppressive treatment, renal failure, and malnutrition. Possible additions to the list include silicosis, hematologic malignancy, and AIDS or seropositivity to HIV.[106] Some have argued for reducing the cut-off age from 35 years to 20 or 25 to achieve a proper risk-benefit ratio.[99]

The usual prophylactic dose of INH is 300 mg daily for 12 months, but a six-month course may be nearly as effective. Before beginning therapy, the patient should be questioned about previous INH therapy, reactions to the drug, chronic or acute liver disease, use of alcohol and potentially interactive drugs, peripheral neuropathy, and pregnancy. Monthly clinical monitoring for signs of INH toxicity is mandatory, and patients over 35 should have periodic serum transaminase determinations.[106] Although physician conversion rates during and after medical school are falling, compliance with recommended INH regimens among physician converters is low.[107]

Since 1985, the incidence of tuberculosis has risen, largely due to HIV-infected patients developing the disease. The incidence of disease resistant to multiple drugs has also increased. In a survey in 1991, 3.3 percent of cases were resistant to both isoniazid and rifampin, with even higher rates in some locales.[108] Patients who are immunocompromised, inadequately treated, or exposed to drug-resistant TB have a higher risk of developing resistant strains.[109] The CDC has issued detailed algorithms to stratify the risk of patients exposed to drug-resistant TB and to determine the need for multidrug therapy.[110] (See Table 50–3 and Fig. 50–2.) Knowledge of drug sensitivities of isolated organisms and expert consultation are recommended in choosing therapeutic regimens.

Diseases of Reportable Status

Reportable diseases vary among the individual states. Certain disorders are then reported to federal authorities for surveillance purposes. Appendix B serves as an example and lists diseases currently reportable in Pennsylvania. Questions specific to other jurisdictions can be addressed to hospital infection control committees or the local health departments.

SUMMARY

1. Surgeons and other exposure-prone health care workers should be immunized against hepatitis B virus. Those who are not immune should receive hepatitis B immune globulin (HBIG) promptly after exposure as well as the standard vaccine course.

2. Hepatitis C exposure should be followed with serial serologic tests. Administration of serum immunoglobulin at the time of the exposure may be beneficial.

3. The risk of HIV transmission from percutaneous exposure is small but real. Universal precautions, double-gloving, and appropriate surgical techniques decrease the risk.

4. An organized institutional program for proper serologic testing, counseling, follow-up, and provision of vaccine, HBIG, immune globulin, AZT, or other prophylactic measures is recommended.

5. Surgeons infected with hepatitis B or HIV are in a difficult position regarding performance of exposure-prone procedures and should seek counsel from hospital risk management committees, personal physicians, and perhaps an attorney.

TABLE 50–3. Likelihood of Infection with Multidrug-resistant *Mycobacterium Tuberculosis* Among Contacts Thought to Be Newly Infected*

Infectiousness of the Source MDR-TB† Case	Closeness and Intensity of MDR-TB Exposure	Contact's Risk of Exposure to Drug-susceptible TB	Estimated Likelihood of Infection with Multidrug-resistant *M. tuberculosis*§
+	+	−	High
+	−	−	High-intermediate
−	+	−	High-intermediate
−	−	−	Intermediate
+	+	+	Intermediate
+	−	+	Low-intermediate
−	+	+	Low-intermediate
−	−	+	Low

Key: + = high; − = low.

*Anergic contacts should be considered likely to be newly infected if there is evidence of contagion among contacts with comparable exposure.

†MDR-TB = multidrug-resistant tuberculosis.

§Multidrug preventive therapy should be considered for persons in high, high-intermediate, and intermediate categories.

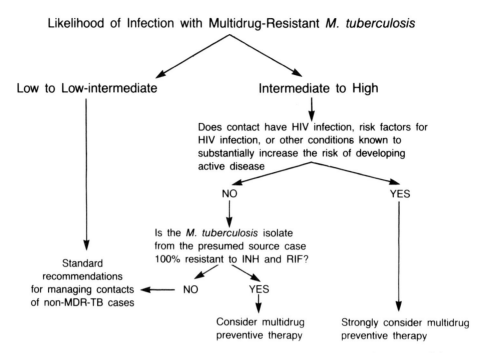

FIGURE 50–2. Approach to selecting drug regimens for preventive therapy candidates by likelihood of infection with multidrug-resistant *Mycobacterium tuberculosis* and by likelihood that persons will develop active tuberculosis.

HIV = human immunodeficiency virus; INH = isoniazid; RIF = rifampin; MDR-TB = multidrug-resistant tuberculosis.

6. CMV and Creutzfeldt-Jakob disease are best prevented by careful technique and proper cleansing.

7. Malaria, babesiosis, and trypanosomiasis are remote risks in the health care environment. Viral hemorrhagic fevers do constitute a genuine risk but are rarely seen.

8. Needlestick-acquired syphilis and Lyme disease are presently not significant concerns. If an individual is exposed to blood of a high-risk patient, serologic follow-up and antibiotic therapy are reasonable.

9. The incidence of tuberculosis has been rising since 1985. Periodic skin testing should be performed in all health care workers. Patients suspected of having active tuberculosis should be isolated immediately. Prophylactic INH is indicated for recent skin test conversion due to susceptible organisms. The incidence of multidrug-resistant tuberculosis requires specialized regimens for treatment and prophylaxis.

10. In addition to adhering to universal precautions, physicians should follow proper isolation procedures and disease-reporting guidelines at all times. Hospital infection control committees may be helpful in this regard.

APPENDIX A

Disease	Category
Abscess, etiology unknown	
Draining, major	Contact
Draining, minor	DSP
AIDS	Universal
Amebiasis, dysentery	Enteric
Anthrax	DSP
Arthropod-borne viral fevers	Universal
Babesiosis	Universal
Brucellosis, draining, minor	DSP
Campylobacter gastroenteritis	Enteric
Cellulitis, draining	DSP
Chickenpox	Strict
Chlamydia trachomatis infection	DSP
Cholera	Enteric
Closed-cavity infection	DSP
Clostridium perfringens	
(except food poisoning)	DSP
Colorado tick fever	Universal
Conjunctivitis	DSP
Coxsackievirus	Enteric
Creutzfeldt-Jakob	Universal
Croup	Contact
Decubitus ulcer, infected	
Major	Contact
Minor or limited	DSP
Dengue	Universal
Diarrhea, acute, infectious etiology	
suspected	Enteric
Diphtheria	
Cutaneous	Contact
Pharyngeal	Strict
Echovirus disease	Enteric
Eczema vaccinatum	Contact
Encephalitis or encephalomyelitis	Enteric
Endometritis	
Group A streptococcal	Contact
Other	DSP
Enterocolitis	
Clostridium difficile	Enteric
Staphylococcus	Enteric
Enteroviral infection	Enteric
Epiglottis due to H. influenzae	Resp
Erythema infectiosum	Resp
Escherichia coli gastroenteritis	Enteric
Furunculosis—staphylococcal	DSP
Gas gangrene	DSP

Disease	Isolation
Gastroenteritis, infectious	Enteric
German measles	Contact
Giardiasis	Enteric
Hand, foot, and mouth disease	Enteric
Hemorrhagic fevers	Strict
Hepatitis, viral	
Type A	Enteric
Type B	Universal
Non-A, Non-B	Universal
Unspecified type	Universal
Herpangina	Enteric
Herpes simplex	
Mucocutaneous	Contact
Recurrent mucocutaneous	DSP
Herpes zoster	
Immunocompromised patient or disseminated	Strict
Normal patient, local	DSP
Impetigo	Contact
Jakob-Creutzfeldt	Universal
Keratoconjunctivitis, infectious	DSP
Lassa fever	Strict
Leptospirosis	Universal
Malaria	Universal
Marburg virus disease	Strict
Measles (rubeola)	Resp
Meningitis	
Aseptic	Enteric
Hemophilus influenzae	Resp
Neisseria meningitidis	Resp
Meningococcal pneumonia	Resp
Meningococcemia	Resp
Multiply-resistant organisms	Contact
Mumps	Resp
Mycobacteria, atypical	
Pulmonary	None
Wound	DSP
Necrotizing enterocolitis	Enteric
Norwalk agent	Enteric
Parainfluenza	Contact
Pediculosis	Contact
Pertussis	Resp
Plague	
Bubonic	DSP
Pneumonic	Strict
Pleurodynia	Enteric
Pneumonia	
Chlamydia	DSP
Meningococcal	Resp
Multiply-resistant bacterial	Contact
Staphylococcus aureus	Contact
Streptococcus, group A	Contact
Poliomyelitis	Enteric
Rabies	Contact
Rat-bite fever	Universal
Relapsing fever	Universal
Respiratory syncytial virus	Contact
Ritter's disease	Contact
Rotavirus infection	Enteric
Rubella	Contact
Salmonellosis	Enteric
Scabies	Contact
Scalded skin syndrome	Contact
Shigellosis	Enteric
Smallpox (variola)	Strict
Spirillium minus disease	Universal
Staphylococcal disease	
Skin, wound, or burn infection	
Major	Contact
Minor or limited	DSP
Enterocolitis	Enteric
Pneumonia or lung abscess	Contact
Scalded skin syndrome	Contact
Toxic shock syndrome	DSP
Streptobacillus moniliformis	Universal
Streptococcal disease (group A)	
Skin, wound, or burn infection	
Major	Contact
Minor or limited	DSP
Endometritis	Contact
Pharyngitis	DSP
Pneumonia	Contact
Scarlet fever	DSP
Syphilis	
Skin and mucous membrane	DSP + Universal
Toxic shock syndrome	DSP
Trachoma, acute	DSP
Tuberculosis	
Extrapulmonary, draining lesion	DSP
Extrapulmonary, meningitis	None
Pulmonary, confirmed or suspected	Tuberculosis
Tularemia	
Draining lesion	DSP
Pulmonary	None
Typhoid fever	Enteric
Vaccinia	
At vaccination site	DSP
Generalized	Contact
Varicella	Strict
Variola (smallpox)	Strict
Vibrio parahaemolyticus	Enteric
Viral diseases	
Pericarditis, myocarditis, or meningitis	Enteric

APPENDIX B

The Following Diseases Must Be Reported as Soon as Diagnosis Is Made

Acquired immuno-deficiency syndrome	Mumps
	Neonatal hypothyroidism
Amebiasis	Pertussis (whooping cough)
Animal bite	Phyenylketonuria
Anthrax	Plague
Botulism	Poliomyelitis
Brucellosis	Psittacosis (Ornithosis)
Campylobacter	Rabies
Cholera	Reye's syndrome
Diphtheria	Rheumatic fever
Encephalitis	Rickettsial diseases
Food poisoning	Rocky Mountain spotted fever
Giardiasis	Rubella (German measles) and congenital rubella syndrome
Gonococcal infections	
Guillain-Barré syndrome	
Hemophilus influenzae type B (HIB)	Salmonellosis
	Shigellosis
Hepatitis, non-A non-B (C)	Smallpox
Hepatitis, viral A & B	Syphilis—all stages
Histoplasmosis	Tetanus
Influenza	Toxic shock syndrome
Kawasaki syndrome	Toxoplasmosis
Lead poisoning	Trichinosis
Legionnaires' disease	Tuberculosis—all forms
Leptospirosis	Tularemia
Lyme disease	Typhoid
Lymphogranuloma venereum	Viral infections
Malaria	Yellow fever
Measles	Yersinia
Meningitis—all types	*Also:* Any unusual disease occurrence
Meningococcal disease	

REFERENCES

1. Kaplan JE, Litchfield B, Rouault C et al: HTLV-1-associated myelopathy associated with blood transfusion in the United States. *Neurology* 41:192–197, 1991.
2. O'Brien TR, George JR, Epstein JS et al: Testing for antibodies to human immunodeficiency virus type 2 in the United States. *MMWR* 41(RR-12):1–9, 1992.
3. CDC: Unexplained CD4+ T-lymphocyte depletion in persons without evident HIV infection—United States. *MMWR* 41:541–546, 1992.
4. Gottesdiener KM: Transplanted infections: Donor-to-host transmission with the allograft. *Ann Intern Med* 110(12):1001–1016, 1989.
5. Lemmer JH: Hepatitis B as an occupational disease of surgeons. *Surg Gynecol Obstet* 159(July):91–100, 1984.
6. CDC: Recommendations for prevention of HIV transmission in health-care settings. *MMWR* 36(25 Supp):35–185, 1987.
7. CDC: Update: Universal precautions for prevention of transmission of human immunodeficiency virus, hepatitis B virus, and other bloodborne pathogens in health-care settings. *MMWR* 37(24):377–388, 1988.
8. Becker CE, Cone JE, Gerberding J: Occupational infection with human immunodeficiency virus (HIV). *Ann Intern Med* 110(8):653–656, 1989.
9. Anonymous: National surveillance program on occupational exposure to the human immunodeficiency virus among health care workers in Canada. *CMAJ* 138:31–33, 1988.
10. Marcus R: CDC Cooperative Needlestick Surveillance Group: Surveillance of health care workers exposed to blood from patients infected with the human immunodeficiency virus. *N Engl J Med* 319(17):1118–1123, 1988.
11. Immunization Practices Advisory Committee: Update on hepatitis B prevention. *Ann Intern Med* 107:353–357, 1987.
12. CDC: Guidelines for prevention of transmission of human immunodeficiency virus and hepatitis B virus to health care and public-safety workers. *MMWR* 38(S-6):1–37, 1989.
13. Immunization Practices Advisory Committee (ACIP): Protection against viral hepatitis. *MMWR* 39(RR-2):1–26, 1990.
14. Immunization Practices Advisory Committee (ACIP): Recommendations for protection against viral hepatitis. *MMWR* 34(22):313–340, 1985.
15. Andre FE: Summary of safety and efficacy data on a yeast-derived hepatitis B vaccine. *Am J Med* (3A):14S–20S, 1987.
16. Tsang T-K, Blei AT, O'Reilly DJ et al: Clinical significance of concurrent hepatitis B surface antigen and antibody positivity. *Dig Dis Sci* 31(6):620–624, 1986.
17. Hadler SC, Francis DP, Maynard JE et al: Long-term immunogenicity and efficacy of hepatitis B vaccine in homosexual men. *N Engl J Med* 315(4):209–214, 1986.
18. Hollinger FB: Factors influencing the immune response to hepatitis B vaccine, booster dose guidelines, and vaccine protocol recommendations. *Am J Med* 87(3A):36S–40S.
19. Jilg W, Schmidt M, Deinhardt F, Zachoval R: Hepatitis B vaccination: How long does protection last? *Lancet* (Aug):458, 1984.
20. Anonymous: Immunization against hepatitis B. *Lancet* (Apr):875–876, 1988.
21. Immunization Practices Advisory Committee: Hepatitis B virus: A comprehensive strategy for eliminating transmission in the United States through universal childhood vaccination. *MMWR* 40(RR-13):1–25, 1991.
22. Davis JM, Demling RH, Lewis FR et al: The Surgical Infection Society's policy on human immunodeficiency virus and hepatitis B and C infection. *Arch Surg* 127:218–221, 1992.
23. National Hepatitis Detection and Treatment Program: *Consensus on HCV Testing and Treatment.* Secaucus NJ, Advanced Therapeutics Communications, 1992.
24. Weber DJ, Joffmann KK, Rutala WA: Management of the healthcare worker infected with human immunodeficiency virus: Lessons from nosocomial transmission of hepatitis B virus. *Infect Control Hosp Epidemiol* 12:625–630, 1991.
25. CDC: Recommendation for preventing transmission of human immunodeficiency virus and hepatitis B virus to patients during exposure-prone invasive procedures. *MMWR* 40(RR-8):1–9, 1991.
26. CDC: Recommendations for preventing transmission of infection with human T-lymphotropic virus type III/lymphadenopathy-associated virus during invasive procedures. *JAMA* 256(10):1257–1262, 1986.
27. McLeod GG: Needlestick injuries at operations for trauma. *Br J Bone Joint Surg* 71-B(3):489–491, 1989.
28. Sim AJW, Dudley HAF: Surgeons and HIV. *Br Med J* 296(Jan):80, 1988.
29. Brough SJ, Hunt TM, Barrie WW: Surgical glove perforations. *Br J Surg* 75(Apr):317, 1988.
30. Godin MS, Lavernia CJ, Harris JP: Occult surgical glove perforations in otolaryngology head and neck surgery. *Arch Otolaryngol Head Neck Surg* 117:910–913, 1991.
31. McCue SF, Berg EW, Saunders EA: Efficacy of double-gloving as a barrier to microbial contamination during total joint arthroplasty. *J Bone Joint Surg* 63-A(5):811–813, 1981.
32. Gani JS, Anseline PF, Bissett RL: Efficacy of double versus single gloving in protecting the operating team. *Aust NZ J Surg* 60:171–175, 1990.
33. Dodds RDA, Barker SGE, Morgan NH et al: Self-protection in surgery: The use of double gloves. *Br J Surg* 77:219–220, 1990.
34. Hussain SA, Latif ABA, Choudhary AA: Risk to surgeons: A survey of accidental injuries during operations. *Br J Surg* 75(4):314–316, 1988.
35. Royle JP: AIDS and the vascular surgeon. *J Cardiovasc Surg* 33:139–142, 1992.
36. Raahave D, Bremmelgaard A: New operative technique to reduce surgeons' risk of HIV infection. *J Hosp Infect* 18(SA):177–183, 1991.
37. Wright JG, McGeer AJ, Chyatte D et al: Mechanisms of glove tears and sharp injuries among surgical personnel. *JAMA* 266(12):1668–1671, 1991.
38. Hagen MD, Meyer KB, Pauker SG: Routine preoperative screening for HIV. *JAMA* 259(9):1357–1359, 1988.
39. Nichols RL: Percutaneous injuries during operation. *JAMA* 267(21):2938–2939, 1992.
40. Henderson DK, Gerberding JL: Prophylactic zidovudine after occupational exposure to the human immunodeficiency virus: An interim analysis. *J Infect Dis* 160(2):321–327, 1989.
41. Krieger JN: The acquired immunodeficiency syndrome: Prudent precautions for the practicing urologist. *J Urol* 139(Apr):801–802, 1988.
42. Henderson DJ: HIV infection: Risks to health care workers and infection control. *Nurs Clin N Am* 23(4):767–777, 1988.
43. Schecter WP: HIV transmission to surgeons. *Occup Med* 4:65–69.
44. CDC: Public Health Service statement on management of occupational exposure to human immunodeficiency virus, including considerations regarding zidovudine postexposure use. *MMWR* 39(RR-1):14, 1990.
45. Imagawa DT, Lee MH, Wolinsky SM et al: Human immunodeficiency virus type I infection in homosexual men who remain seronegative for prolonged periods. *N Engl J Med* 320(22):1458–1462, 1989.
46. Wolinsky SM, Rinaldo CR, Kwok S et al: Human immunodeficiency virus type I (HIV-I) infection a median of 18 months before a diagnostic Western blot. *Ann Intern Med* 111(12):961–972, 1989.
47. Tavares L, Roneker C, Johnston K et al: 3'-Azido-3'-deoxythymidine in feline leukemia virus-infected cats: A model for therapy and prophylaxis of AIDS. *Cancer Res* 47(June):3190–3194, 1987.
48. Ruprecht RM, O'Brien LG, Rossoni LD et al: Suppression of mouse viraemia and retroviral disease by 3'-azido-3'-deoxythymidine. *Nature* 323(Oct):467–469, 1986.
49. LaFon SW, Nusinoff-Lehrman S, Barry D: Prophylactically adminis-

tered retrovir (R) in health care workers potentially exposed to the human immunodeficiency virus. *J Infect Dis* 158(2):503, 1988.

50. Council on Ethical and Judicial Affairs: Ethical issues involved in the growing AIDS crisis. *JAMA* 259(9):1360–1361, 1988.

51. Cooper C: Panel opposes physician disclosure of HIV infection. *Int Med News* 15;1,50, 1992.

52. Kalkwarf K: CDC open meeting to discuss invasive procedures under consideration for designation as exposure-prone and nonexposure-prone. *J Dent Educ* 55:810–813, 1992.

53. Lo B, Steinbrook R: Health care workers infected with human immunodeficiency virus. *JAMA* 267:1100–1105, 1992.

54. Check WA: Do HIV-infected doctors pose a threat to patients? A daunting question for medicine. *ACP Observer* Jan 1992.

55. CDC: Update: Investigations of patients who have been treated by HIV-infected health-care workers. *MMWR* 41:344–346, 1992.

56. Gostin LO: The AIDS litigation project. *JAMA* 263(15):2086–2093, 1990.

57. Interview with Sergio Stagno: Isolation precautions for patients with cytomegalovirus infection. *Pediatr Infect Dis* 1(3):145–147, 1982.

58. Adler SP: Molecular epidemiology of cytomegalovirus: Viral transmission among children attending a day care center, their parents, and caretakers. *J Pediatr* 112(3):366–372, 1988.

59. Ho M: Cytomegalovirus, in Mandell GL, Douglas RG, Bennett JE (eds): *Principles and Practice of Infectious Diseases*, 3d ed. New York, Churchill Livingstone, 1990, pp 1159–1172.

60. Dworsky ME, Welch K, Cassady G et al: Occupational risk for primary cytomegalovirus infection among pediatric health care workers. *N Engl J Med* 309(16):950–953, 1983.

61. Gerberding JL, Bryant-LeBlanc CE, Nelson K et al: Risk of transmitting the human immunodeficiency virus, cytomegalovirus, and hepatitis B virus to health care workers exposed to patients with AIDS and AIDS-related conditions. *J Infect Dis* 156(1):1–8, 1987.

62. Balcarek KB, Bagley R, Cloud GA et al: Cytomegalovirus infection among employees of a children's hospital. *JAMA* 263(6):840–844, 1990.

63. Fleisher GR, Starr SE, Friedman HM et al: Vaccination of pediatric nurses with live attenuated cytomegalovirus. *Am J Dis Child* 136(Apr):294–296, 1982.

64. Embil JA, Pereira LH, Manley K et al: Prevalence of cytomegalovirus antibodies in the personnel of a children's hospital, Halifax, Nova Scotia. *Can J Public Health* 79 (Nov/Dec):455–457, 1988.

65. Committee on Infectious Diseases and Immunization, Canadian Paediatric Society: Cytomegalovirus: An occupational hazard? *Can Med Assoc J* 131(Oct):730, 1984.

66. Prusiner SB: Prions and neurogenerative diseases. *N Engl J Med* 317(25):1571–1581, 1987.

67. Masters CL, Gajdusek C, Gibbs CJ: Creutzfeldt-Jakob disease virus isolations from the Gerstmann-Straussler syndrome. *Brain* 104:559–588, 1981.

68. Thadani V, Penar PL, Partington J et al: Creutzfeldt-Jakob disease probably acquired from a cadaveric dura mater graft. *J Neurosurg* 69:766–769, 1988.

69. Tateiski J, Tashima T, Kitamoto T: Inactivation of the Creutzfeldt-Jakob disease agent. *Ann Neurol* 24(3):466, 1988.

70. Tamai Y, Taguchi F, Miura S: Inactivation of the Creutzfeldt-Jakob disease agent. *Ann Neurol* 24(3):466–467, 1988.

71. Brown P: An epidemiologic critique of Creutzfeldt-Jakob disease. *Epidemiol Rev* 2:113–135, 1980.

72. Gajdusek DC, Gibbs CJ, Asher DM et al: Precautions in medical care of, and in handling materials from, patients with transmissable virus dementia (Creutzfeldt-Jakob disease). *N Engl J Med* 297(23):1253–1258, 1977.

73. Brown P, Preece MA, Will RG: "Friendly fire" in medicine: Hormones, homografts and Creutzfeld-Jakob disease. *Lancet* 340:24–27, 1992.

74. Schoene WC, Masters CL, Gibbs CJ et al: Transmissable spongiform encephalopathy (Creutzfeldt-Jakob disease). *Arch Neurol* 38:473–477, 1981.

75. Rosenberg RN, White CL, Brown P et al: Precautions in handling tissues, fluids, and other contaminated materials from patients with documented or suspected Creutzfeldt-Jakob disease. *Ann Neurol* 19(1):75–77, 1986.

76. Lehrich JR, Tyler KL: Slow infections of the central nervous system, in Mandell GL, Douglas RG, Bennett JE (eds): *Principles and Practice of Infectious Diseases*, 3d ed. New York, Churchill Livingstone, 1990, pp 769–777.

77. Wyler W: Plasmodium species (malaria), in Mandell GL, Douglas RG, Bennett JE (eds): *Principles and Practice of Infectious Diseases*, 3d ed. New York, Churchill Livingstone, 1990, pp 2056–2066.

78. Cannon NJ, Walker SP, Dismukes WE: Malaria acquired by accidental needle puncture. *JAMA* 222(11):1425, 1972.

79. Lettau LA: Nosocomial transmission and infection control aspects of parasitic and ectoparasitic diseases. Part II. Blood and tissue parasites. *Infect Control Hosp Epidemiol* 12:111–121, 1991.

80. Grant IH, Gold JW, Wittner M et al: Transfusion-associated acute Chagas disease acquired in the USA. *Ann Intern Med* 111:849–851, 1989.

81. Nickerson P, Orr P, Schroeder ML et al: Transfusion-associated *Trypanosoma cruzi* infection. *Ann Intern Med* 111:851–853, 1989.

82. Brener Z: Laboratory-acquired Chagas disease: An endemic disease among parasitologists? in Morel C (ed): *Genes and Antigens of Parasites*, 2d ed. Rio de Janeiro, Fundacao Oswaldo Cruz, 1984, pp 3–9.

83. Kirchhoff LV: *Trypanosoma* species (American trypanosomiasis Chagas disease): Biology of *Trypanosomas*, in Mandell GL, Douglas RG, Bennett JE (eds): *Principles and Practice of Infectious Diseases*, 3d ed. New York, Churchill Livingstone, 1990, pp 2077–2084.

84. Popovsky MA, Lindberg LE, Syrek AL, Page PL: Prevalence of babesia antibody in a selected blood donor population. *Transfusion* 28(1):59–61, 1988.

85. Mintz ED, Anderson JF, Cable RG et al: Transfusion-transmitted babesiosis: A case report from a new endemic area. *Transfusion* 31:365–368, 1991.

86. CDC: Management of patients with suspected viral hemorrhagic fever. *MMWR* 37(S-3):1–15, 1988.

87. Campbell BA, Pequegnat D, Clayton AJ: A hospital contingency plan for exotic communicable diseases. *Infect Control* 5(12):565–569, 1984.

88. Johnson KM: Markuz and ebola viruses, in Mandell GL, Douglas RG, Bennett JE (eds): *Principles and Practice of Infectious Diseases*, 3d ed. New York, Churchill Livingstone, 1990, pp 1303–1306.

89. Heymann DL, Weisfeld JS, Webb PA et al: Ebola hemorrhagic fever: Tandala, Zaire, 1977–1978. *J Infect Dis* 142(3):372–376, 1980.

90. Emond RTD, Evans B, Bowen ETW et al: A case of ebola virus infection. *Br Med J* 27(Aug):541–544, 1977.

91. Van Eeden PJ, Joubert JR, Van DeWal BW et al: A nosocomial outbreak of Crimean-Congo haemorrhagic fever at Tygerberg hospital. *S Afr Med J* 68:711–717, 1985.

92. Stokes JH, Beerman H, Ingraham NR: *Modern Clinical Syphilology: Diagnosis, Treatment. Case Study*. 3d ed. Philadelphia, Saunders, 1944, pp 468–505.

93. Shulman IA, Appleman MD: Transmission of parasitic and bacterial infections through blood transfusion within the U.S. *Cirt Rev Clin Lab Sciences* 28:447–459, 1991.

94. Aoki SK, Hollard PV: Lyme disease—another transfusion risk? *Transfusion* 29:646, 1989.

95. Weiland T, Kuhnl P, Darda C et al: Retrospective study of a borrelliosis-infected blood donor. *Beitrage zur Infusionstherapie* 28:32–34, 1991.

96. Garner JS, Simmons BP: Guideline isolation precautions in hospitals:

Table A. Category-specific isolation precautions. *Infect Control* 4(4):261–325, 1983.

97. CDC: Meningococcal disease—United States, 1981. *MMWR* 30(10): 113–115, 1981.

98. Johnston RF, Wildrick KH: "State of the art" review. The impact of chemotherapy on the care of patients with tuberculosis. *Am Rev Respir Dis* 109:636–664, 1974.

99. Des Prez RM, Heim CR: Myocobacterium tuberculosis, in Mandell GL, Douglas RG, Bennett JE (eds): *Principles and Practice of Infectious Disease*, 3d ed. New York, Churchill Livingstone, 1990, pp 1877–1906.

100. Riley RL: The J Burns Amberson lecture. Aerial dissemination of pulmonary tuberculosis. *Am Rev Tuberculol* 76(6):931–941, 1957.

101. Comstock GW: Epidemiology of tuberculosis. *Am Rev Respir Dis* 125(3):8–15, 1982.

102. Charney W, Fisher J, Ishida C: The inefficiency of surgical masks for protection against droplet nuclei tuberculosis. *J Occup Med* 33:943–944, 1991.

103. Rouillon A, Perdrizet S, Parrot R: Transmission of tubercle bacilli: The effects of chemotherapy. *Tubercle* 57:275–299, 1976.

104. Kim TC, Blackman RS, Heatwole KM et al: Acid-fast bacilli in sputum smears of patients with pulmonary tuberculosis. *Am Rev Respir Dis* 129:264–268, 1984.

105. CDC: Guidelines for preventing the transmission of tuberculosis in health care settings, with special focus on HIV-related issues. *MMWR* 39(RR-17):21 1990.

106. American Thoracic Society and The Centers for Disease Control: Treatment of tuberculosis and tuberculosis infection in adults and children. *Am Rev Respir Dis* 134:355–363, 1986.

107. Barrett-Connor E: The epidemiology of tuberculosis in physicians. *JAMA* 241(1):33–38, 1979.

108. CDC: National action plan to combat multidrug-resistant tuberculosis. *MMWR* 41(RR-11):1–48, 1992.

109. CDC: Nosocomial transmission of multidrug-resistant tuberculosis among HIV-infected persons—Florida and New York, 1988–1991. *MMWR* 40:585–592, 1991.

110. Vallarino ME, Dooley SW, Geiter LJ et al: Management of persons exposed to multidrug-resistant tuberculosis. *MMWR* 41(RR-11):59–71, 1992.

51

ALTERNATIVES TO HOMOLOGOUS TRANSFUSION AND THE PREVENTION OF TRANSFUSION-ASSOCIATED DISEASE

David F. Friedman

Leslie E. Silberstein

Modern blood collection and banking procedures, including exclusive use of volunteer donors, screening for infectious diseases, duplicate ABO blood grouping, cross-matching, and strict record-keeping protocols, make the transfusion of blood components relatively safe. However, transfusion is not entirely without risk, and some of the problems related to clerical errors, transmission of infectious diseases, hemolytic and nonhemolytic transfusion reactions, alloimmunization and graft-versus-host disease are discussed in Chap. 66.

This chapter discusses strategies available to the physician to minimize or avoid these risks. It focuses on reducing exposure to homologous transfusion donated by persons other than the recipient by critically reevaluating the indications for transfusion and substituting autologous for homologous blood products. In addition, specific pharmacologic interventions can reduce or eliminate the need for transfusion in certain clinical situations. Although synthetic blood substitutes are currently being developed, their use is limited by significant technical problems and toxicities. Public concern about the risks of blood transfusion makes it imperative to be familiar with alternative therapies and to discuss their use with patients.

THE THRESHOLD FOR TRANSFUSION

Red Cells

Most physicians agree that symptomatic anemia in patients with ongoing bleeding or in those who have undergone surgery is a reasonable indication for red cell transfusion. However, there is controversy regarding the proper threshold or "trigger" for transfusion in asymptomatic mildly anemic patients. The traditional requirement of having a hemoglobin level over 10 g/dl before surgery or maintaining that level in the immediate postoperative period has been questioned because of increased concern about the risks of transfusion. In a stable patient, it is often possible to accept a lower hemoglobin and provide supportive care.

Simple widely accepted criteria for red cell transfusion do not exist. One way to judge the physiologic impact of anemia is to determine the adequacy of oxygen delivery to meet the requirements of the tissues. In experimental hemodilution in animals, oxygen delivery is maintained at hematocrit levels as low as 20%.[1] However, delivery depends not only on the hematocrit level but also on blood volume, cardiac output, pulmonary function, and vascular supply. Unfortunately, there is no easy objective measurement that takes all of these variables into account. The best clinical index of the adequacy of oxygen delivery to meet demand is the total body oxygen extraction estimated from the difference between the arterial and central mixed venous blood oxygen contents.[2] This parameter is not determined routinely because a true measurement of mixed venous blood oxygen content requires use of a central venous catheter.

The decision to transfuse mildly anemic asymptomatic or mildly symptomatic patients is usually made on the basis of the hematocrit level and clinical judgment.[3] Many factors related to the underlying disease and its therapy influence this decision. Compensated normovolemic anemia is tolerated by many patients with chronic renal failure or chronic hemolytic anemia who may function normally with hemoglobin levels of 7 to 8 g/dl or less. However, others with reduced cardiac or pulmonary reserve may not tolerate a hemoglobin level under 12 g/dl. The physiologic stress of surgery and its complications may increase demand for oxygen beyond delivery capacity in some anemic patients who were formerly well-compensated.[4] On the other hand, there are several series describing patients undergoing surgery with hemoglobin levels under 10 g/dl who suffered no morbidity attributable to anemia.[5] There is also considerable experience with intraoperative hemodilution in selected patients in whom hematocrit levels have been safely reduced to 30% and below.

In 1988, the National Institutes of Health Consensus Development Conference on the Perioperative Use of Red Cells proposed the following guidelines:[6]

1. Healthy patients with a hemoglobin level over 10 g/dl rarely require red cell transfusion.
2. Patients with acute anemia and a hemoglobin level under 7 g/dl frequently require red cell transfusion.
3. Some patients with chronic anemia tolerate hemoglobin levels under 7 g/dl.
4. The decision to transfuse depends on clinical judgment aided by available laboratory data.

These guidelines are more a reflection of the problems in deciding on standardized indications for red cell transfusion than a solution to them. They serve to remind the physician that the benefits of red cell transfusion in an individual patient must be considered carefully before risks are incurred.

Fresh Frozen Plasma

Transfusion of fresh frozen plasma carries many of the same risks of homologous red cell transfusion including the potential of transmitting viral disease. However, the indications for plasma are usually much clearer. In general, plasma products are indicated for replacement of coagulation factors and should not be used for volume expansion when crystalloid or colloid solutions will serve. While defining coagulation disorders may be difficult, screening prothrombin and partial thromboplastin time determinations provide simple indications of the need for plasma therapy. Fresh frozen plasma or plasma products are often required in congenital and acquired disorders of coagulation such as hemophilia, von Willebrand's disease, and disseminated intravascular coagulation. It is sometimes reasonable to transfuse plasma when clotting times are prolonged and bleeding is ongoing, suspected, or anticipated, even if the underlying reason is unclear.

Platelets

Severe thrombocytopenia, with or without evidence of bleeding, is the most common indication for platelet transfusion. Disorders of platelet funtion may be indications for platelet transfusion when the platelet count is normal. Congenital disorders of platelet function are quite rare, but platelet dysfunction can be an acquired state in uremia, with aspirin ingestion, and after cardiopulmonary bypass. The risks of platelet transfusion are the same as those posed by administration of other homologous blood products. However, because most patients receive more readily available random-donor platelets harvested from 6 to 8 units of blood drawn from several donors, the number of donor exposures in each transfusion is increased severalfold when compared to transfusions of red cells or plasma. Single-donor platelets reduce the number of exposures per transfusion but require more complicated apheresis techniques that may not be readily available.

Prophylactic use of platelet transfusion also increases the risks of exposure. Although a platelet count of 20,000/mm³ is commonly used as the threshold for transfusion in many patients with cancer, this single "trigger value" has been questioned because it may unnecessarily increase the risk of exposure.[7] Higher or lower threshold levels may be more appropriate in certain other clinical settings. For example, patients with intracranial pathology or those facing surgery often receive platelet transfusions when counts are higher, while many patients receiving chemotherapy may not have so high a risk of bleeding and therefore may not require transfusions until their counts fall to 5000 or 10,000/mm³. Similarly, these lower threshold counts are often chosen in disease states lilke idiopathic thrombocytopenic purpura (ITP) or thrombotic thrombocytopenic purpura (TTP), in which transfused platelets are more likely to be rapidly destroyed. The decision to transfuse platelets thus remains highly individualized, and the goal in patients who are bleeding should be to stop the hemorrhage rather than to restore a certain platelet count.

AUTOLOGOUS TRANSFUSION

The use of autologous blood avoids the risks of transmitting infectious diseases, alloimmunization, and graft-versus-host disease associated with homologous transfusion. Autologous transfusion does not avoid the risks related to clerical errors, contamination, or alteration during storage, which are fortunately rare. The process of donating blood for autologous use carries minimal risk. The number of autologous donations made in the United States has risen substantially in the past five years. In some clinical settings, offering the patient the option of donating autologous blood is considered the standard of care, and, in a few states, informing a patient of this option is mandated by law. Blood can be collected and returned by three methods: predeposit, intraoperative hemodilution, and blood salvage.[8]

Autologous Predeposit

Autologous predeposit refers to the donation of one or more units of whole blood before a surgical procedure during which red cell transfusion may be necessary. This method is safely used in many patients undergoing orthopedic, spinal, vascular, transplant, or plastic surgery, and in selected patients undergoing coronary bypass grafting and valve replacement who would not be hemodynamically compromised by donation. In addition, autologous donation has been performed safely in the third trimester of pregnancy in anticipation of a complicated delivery in patients with placenta previa. It is safe in otherwise healthy elderly patients and in children as young as eight years old.

One unit of whole blood or about 500 ml is collected, separated into packed red cells and plasma, and stored usually in liquid form at 4°C until the procedure. Smaller volumes are withdrawn from children. Serial donations can be made to accumulate several units. Healthy donors who are not iron-deficient may be able to replace red cell mass fast enough to donate one unit of blood every three days without an appreciable fall in hematocrit. However, patients are more commonly phlebotomized about once a week and deferred if the hematocrit is below 33% just before donation. Pregnant women are more frequently deferred because of a low hematocrit level.[9] All donors are given oral iron supplementation.

Red cells collected in appropriate preservative solution (AdSol) can be stored in liquid form for up to 42 days at 4°C. Most patients can therefore donate two to four units within the time limitation imposed by the shelf-life of the first unit.[10] Although the last unit may be drawn as close as 72 hours before surgery, a period of two weeks is preferable to allow time for the hematocrit level to normalize. Freezing autologous red cells to extend shelf-life adds to the expense and is usually done only for patients with rare blood group antigens or multiple red cell alloantibodies for whom finding suitable homologous blood would be difficult or impossible.

The patient's overall health must be considered before recommending autologous predeposit. Phlebotomy of one unit of whole blood is safe in healthy volunteer blood donors who meet the standard donor screening criteria published by the American Association of Blood Banks.[11] Recognizing that these criteria may be too rigorous to apply to autologous donors, the 14th Edition of the Standards of the American Association of Blood Banks recommends that the patient's physician give consent for the procedure, donation be deferred if the hematocrit level is under 33% or if the patient is bacteremic, and donations be spaced at least three days apart and end at least three days before surgery. A major concern is that the underlying disease may increase the risk of morbidity from donating blood. For example, acute loss of 500 ml of blood might be hazardous in patients with significant cardiovascular or pulmonary disease. They may not tolerate the hemodynamic changes of vasovagal reactions to blood donation that are seen in one to two percent of first-time blood donors. Those with severe aortic stenosis are particularly vulnerable. The risks of phlebotomy in pregnant women and unborn fetuses are generally thought to be minimal, but there are no large studies to support this assumption. Individuals with chronic medical problems like renal failure or rheumatoid arthritis may have a blunted erythropoietic response that prevents rapid replacement of red cell mass and leaves them significantly more anemic at the time of surgery. Such patients often cannot make donations as frequently as healthy donors. In those with potentially unstable conditions, like angina pectoris, the risks of delaying surgery to collect autologous blood must be weighed against the benefits of avoiding homologous transfusion.

There are several small published series from autologous blood donor programs that address these safety issues. Healthy patients have successfully deposited autologous blood before orthopedic, urologic, vascular, and plastic procedures. Patients with coronary artery disease and valvular heart disease[12,13] and pregnant women requesting predeposit for routine or complicated deliveries[8] have also done well. However, although complication rates in these reports are low, the numbers of patients studied are relatively small. Physician approval was obtained in all cases, but criteria for approval were not standardized. Adverse events similar to those seen in volunteer donors, lightheadedness and vasovagal reactions, occurred in fewer than five percent.[13] Rare anecdotal reports of more serious adverse events like myocardial ischemia do not establish that the donation was the etiology of the complication.

There are clear-cut recognized contraindications to autologous donation. Patients who may be bacteremic should not donate to avoid infecting the autologous unit. In cancer patients, there is concern about the theoretic possibility of reinfusing viable metastatic tumor cells. Patients receiving such drugs as cytotoxic agents should also avoid donation for similar reasons. Severe aortic stenosis and unstable angina pectoris are also considered contraindications to autologous blood donation. In summary, it is sometimes difficult to estimate the risk of autologous donation in individual patients. While it appears to be low in prudently selected patients, it is probably higher than in healthy volunteer donors.

Coordinating the collection and delivery of autologous blood products presents several logistic problems not encountered when homologous blood is used. The surgeon must find out how many units were collected to be sure that enough blood is available for the procedure. If the date of surgery is changed, some of the units may become outdated. If blood is not collected at the hospital where surgery will take place, the bloodbank at the hospital must be informed in time to obtain the blood from the collection center. In considering autologous donation, the physician should recognize that certain procedures like spinal fusion and hip replacement are likely to require transfusion, while others like appendectomy, uncomplicated cesarean section, and vaginal delivery are not. Patient and physician together must decide if the risk, cost, and effort required for autologous donations are warranted.

Intraoperative Hemodilution

Intraoperative hemodilution is a technique used by some anesthesiologists to reduce exposure to homologous blood. In the operating room just before surgery, a predetermined volume of whole blood is collected from the patient and replaced with colloid or crystalloid to maintain normovolemia. In some reports, the hematocrit level has been reduced to as low as 20%. The blood is anticoagulated, labeled, stored in the operating room, and reinfused as needed or at the end of the procedure. Blood lost during surgery has a lower hematocrit after hemodilution, and, if stored autologous cells are subsequently reinfused, net loss of red cell mass is smaller. With a higher postoperative hematocrit, the need for transfusion of homologous red cells is reduced or avoided entirely. Reinfused blood contains clotting factors and fresh viable platelets that may provide a hemostatic advantage.

Intraoperative hemodilution may not be appropriate for patients with underlying cardiovascular, cerebrovascular, or pulmonary disease, or for those with infections or malignancies. If the volume removed is replaced with crystalloid, the patient may be hypervolemic when the autologous blood is reinfused. In addition, the quantity of autologous red cells made available by this technique is limited by the preoperative hematocrit and often can substitute for no more than two homologous units. On the other hand, intraoperative hemodilution requires less advanced planning and coordination of services than predeposit, and has been used successfully in orthopedic, general, and vascular procedures in both adults and children.[5]

Intraoperative Salvage

Intraoperative red cell salvage involves collecting blood lost in the operative field for immediate reinfusion. Some techniques employ simple suction and a blood filter for reinfusion. Others use semi-automated cell washers to remove debris, aggregated cells, and activated clotting factors, and concentrate the red cells before reinfusion. The latter techniques involve specialized equipment and disposable plastic ware and require trained personnel to remain in the operating room throughout the operation to monitor the salvage procedure. Intraoperative salvage is most useful when large losses of blood are expected because it makes autologous red cells available for reinfusion in a short period of time.[14]

Intraoperative blood salvage has been used in trauma, cardiac, vascular, obstetric, orthopedic, and liver transplant surgery and can reduce the need for homologous red cell transfusion by 40 to 70 percent.[15,16] The technique does not reliably recover platelets or clotting factors and may therefore result in dilutional thrombocytopenia and coagulopathy. Theoretically, reinfusion of activated clotting factors can cause hemorrhage and disseminated intravascular coagulation. Moreover, some systems may traumatize red cells enough to cause hemolysis and reinfusion of free hemoglobin and red cell stroma. Air embolism has also been reported.

Intraoperative blood salvage is contraindicated when the operative field is potentially infected, as in bowel surgery, drainage of an abscess, or removal of an infected prosthesis. Salvage is also contraindicated in cancer surgery because of the possibility of reinfusing potentially viable metastatic tumor cells. However, these contraindications may not apply in massive hemorrhage caused by trauma when salvage may be the best source of rapidly available red cells.

PHARMACOLOGIC ALTERNATIVES

Certain drugs and synthetic blood substitutes have been used in specific clinical situations to reduce the need for homologous blood products. Crystalloid and colloid can be used in limited quantities in place of blood products and are discussed in the previous section.

DDAVP

DDAVP, or desmopressin, is a synthetic analog of the posterior pituitary hormone vasopressin.[17,18] It has been shown to raise plasma levels of von Willebrand's factor and factor VIII procoagulant activity by as much as threefold by causing their release from preformed reserves in the vascular endothelium. The effect of DDAVP is transient, usually lasting about four hours. However, it has been used successfully in patients with certain forms of von Willebrand's disease and in those with mild and moderate hemophilia A in whom levels of endogenous factor VIII are low but detectable. DDAVP transiently corrects the bleeding tendency in these patients and can obviate the need for factor replacement with cryoprecipitate or factor VIII concentrate in minor surgical procedures.

DDAVP has also been reported to correct the bleeding time in some patients with hepatic cirrhosis,[19] platelet functional defects, and chronic renal failure[20] and to reduce bleeding after cardiac surgery in patients with no documented underlying bleeding disorder. However, these effects are controversial, and several studies of DDAVP used in coronary bypass surgery[21–24] and spinal fusion for scoliosis[25] have demonstrated no reduction in surgical blood loss attributable to it. The drug should be used only after consultation with a hematologist because it is contraindicated in some forms of

von Willebrand's disease and is of no value in other variants of the disease. It is also not helpful in most hemophiliacs with very low endogenous levels of factor VIII.

Recombinant Erythropoietin

Recombinant human erythropoietin has been used to stimulate endogenous red cell production and can reduce or eliminate the need for homologous red cell transfusion in certain clinical settings.[26] It is primarily indicated in the anemia of chronic renal failure. Many such patients, whether or not on dialysis, produce insufficient erythropoietin and are therefore transfusion-dependent. Maintenance erythropoietin replacement by subcutaneous injection reduces or eliminates the need for red cell transfusion and improves the overall quality of life in many of these patients.[27]

Erythropoietin has also been used in conjunction with autologous red cell predeposit and can increase the volume of red cells donors can bank before surgery by as much as 42 percent.[28] However, erythropoietin is not used routinely for autologous blood collection because the required volume of blood can almost always be obtained without it if the collections are scheduled far enough in advance. Preliminary studies have demonstrated that erythropoietin may be of benefit in reducing requirements for transfusion in premature infants.[29,30] It has also been used in patients with anemia related to chronic inflammatory disease and in those with cancer[31,32] and has been shown to be of value in reducing the need for transfusion and improving the quality of life in patients with HIV infection.[33]

Other Hematopoietic Growth Factors

Several other recombinant human growth factors, including G-CSF, GM-CSF, IL-1, IL-3, IL-6, and stem cell factor (c-kit ligand), have been shown to affect hematopoiesis in vitro and in vivo.[34–36] There is synergy among these factors in stimulation, proliferation, and differentiation of hematopoietic cells. The most extensive and successful clinical trials have focused on treatment of congenital and acquired neutropenia, and G-CSF and GM-CSF have become important components of the supportive care of many neutropenic patients.[37] The impact of growth factors on homologous transfusion has been modest because homologous transfusion of white cells for which these factors may substitute is relatively infrequent. These agents reduce the rate of infectious complications in neutropenic patients and may therefore indirectly contribute to further reductions in homologous transfusion. Other human recombinant growth factors, alone or in combination, are under study as alternatives to chronic red cell transfusion therapy in certain congenital anemias and may prove to have wide applicability in reducing the need for homologous red cells. Unfortunately, none of the factors characterized to date appears to have a significant clinically useful effect on platelet production.

SYNTHETIC BLOOD SUBSTITUTES

Perfluorochemicals

Perfluorochemicals (PFC's) are organic liquids that can carry 10 to 20 times as much dissolved oxygen as water at high partial pressures of oxygen. PFC-based products have been developed as possible substitutes for transfused red cells and have been tested to a limited extent in patients injured in battle and in those who refuse transfusion on religious grounds. Although they increase arterial oxygen content, maximum doses of PFC used in clinical trials increase oxygen delivery by the equivalent of only 0.5 g/dl of hemoglobin. They have had no effect on clinical outcome in patients with mild or severe acute anemia.[38] The limitations of PFC's include insolubility in water, short intravascular half-life, requirement for high FiO_2, and potential adverse effects on the reticuloendothelial system.[39] Their use remains experimental, and the currently available product (Fluosol-DA) has been licensed only for use in coronary artery balloon dilation procedures to augment myocardial oxygenation distal to the inflated balloon.

Synthetic Hemoglobin

There are ongoing efforts to create synthetic and semisynthetic preparations of chemically modified hemoglobin with oxygen-carrying properties similar to those of native red cells. Chemical modifications are required to prolong the intravascular dwell time of free soluble hemoglobin preparations and reduce their oxygen affinity to approximate the oxygen loading and unloading characteristics of hemoglobin in the red cell. Other limitations include nephrotoxicity of small concentrations of tetrameric soluble hemoglobin and potential effects on the reticuloendothelial system. As an alternative to soluble hemoglobin harvested from outdated human red cells, attempts have been made to encapsulate hemoglobin in synthetic membranes and produce human hemoglobin in bacteria by recombinant DNA technology. At present, there is no synthetic hemoglobin product being tested in clinical trials.[39]

SUMMARY

1. Exposure to homologous blood products can be reduced by considering a higher threshold for transfusion in surgical patients with mild anemia and using autologous blood products whenever possible.

2. Intraoperative hemodilution and red cell salvage are safe and effective measures to conserve autologous red cells and thereby reduce the need for homologous transfusion.

3. DDAVP has a well-defined role as a substitute for plasma products in a small subset of patients with congenital bleeding disorders, including some forms of von Willebrand's disease and hemophilia A.

4. Recombinant erythropoietin is a useful treatment for the anemia of chronic renal failure and other chronic disease and can be used as an adjunct to autologous blood collection.

REFERENCES

1. Gould SA, Sehgal LR, Rosen AL et al: Surgery with transfusions: The surgeon's viewpoint, in Carlson and Golub (eds): *Limiting Homologous Exposure: Alternative Strategies*. Arlington VA, American Association of Bloodbanks, 1989, pp 71–86.
2. Gould SA, Rice CL, Moss GS: The physiologic basis of the use of blood and blood products. *Surg Ann* 16:13–38, 1984.
3. Friedman BA, Burns BL, Schork MA: An analysis of blood transfusion of surgical patients by sex: A quest for the transfusion trigger. *Transfusion* 20(2):179–188, 1980.
4. Carson JL, Spence RK, Poses RM et al: Severity of anaemia and operative mortality and morbidity. *Lancet* 1(8588):727–729, 1988.
5. Stehling LC: Surgery without transfusion: The anesthesiologist's viewpoint, in Carlson and Golub (eds): *Limiting Homologous Exposure: Alternative Strategies*. Arlington VA, American Association of Bloodbanks, 1989, pp 87–106.
6. NIH Consensus Conference: Perioperative red blood cell transfusion. *JAMA* 260(18):2700–2703, 1988.
7. Beutler E: Platelet transfustions: The 20,000/mm³ trigger. *Blood* 81:1411–1413, 1993.
8. National Blood Resource Education Program Expert Panel: The use of autologous blood. *JAMA* 263(3):414–417, 1990.
9. Kruskall MS, Leonard S, Klapholz H: Autologous blood donation during pregnancy: Analysis of safety and blood use. *Obst Gyn* 70:938–940, 1987.
10. Toy PTCY, Strauss RG, Stehling LC et al: Predeposited autologous blood for elective surgery. *N Engl J Med* 316:517–520, 1987.
11. Widmann FK, AABB Standards Committee: *Standards for Blood Banks and Transfusion Services*, 13th ed. Arlington VA, American Association of Blood Banks, 1989, pp 3–10.
12. Love TR, Hendren WG, O'Keefe DD et al: Transfusion of predonated autologous blood in elective cardiac surgery. *Ann Thorac Surg* 43:508–512, 1987.
13. Mann M, Sacks HJ, Goldfinger D: Safety of autologous blood donation prior to elective surgery for a variety of potentially "high risk" patients. *Transfusion* 23:229–232, 1983.
14. Popovsky MA, Devine PA, Taswell HF: Intraoperative autologous transfusion. *Mayo Clin Proc* 60:125–134, 1985.
15. Giordano GF, Goldman DS, Mammana RB et al: Intraoperative autotransfusion in cardiac operations. *J Thorac Cardiovasc Surg* 96:382–386, 1988.
16. Giordano GF, Wallace BA: Intraoperative autotransfusion: A review, in Carlson and Golub (eds): *Limiting Homologous Exposure: Alternative Strategies*. Arlington VA, American Association of Bloodbanks, 1989, pp 57–70.
17. Mannucci PM: Desmopressin: A nontransfusional form of treatment for congenital and acquired bleeding disorders. *Blood* 72(5):1449–1460, 1988.
18. Manucci PM: Desmopressin: A nontransfusional hemostatic agent. *Ann Rev Med* 41:55–64, 1990.
19. Cattaneo M, Tenconi P, Alberca I et al: Subcutaneous desmopressin (DDAVP) shortens the prolonged bleeding time in patients with liver cirrhosis. *Thromb Haemost* 64:358–360, 1990.
20. Soslau G, Schwartz AB, Putatunda B et al: Desmopresin-induced improvement in bleeding times in chronic renal failure patients correlates with platelet serotonin uptake and ATP release. *Am J Med Sci* 300:372–379, 1990.
21. Andersson TLG, Solem JO, Tengborn L et al: Effects of desmopressin acetate on platelet aggregation, von Willebrand factor and blood loss after cardiac surgery with extracorporeal circulation. *Circulation* 81:872–878, 1990.
22. Hackmann T, Gascoyne RD, Naiman SC et al: A trial of desmopressin (1-desamino-8-D-arginine vasopressin) to reduce blood loss in uncomplicated cardiac surgery. *N Engl J Med* 321:1437–1443, 1989.
23. Hedderich GS, Petsikas DJ, Cooper BA et al: Desmopressin acetate in uncomplicated coronary artery bypass surgery; a prospective randomized clinical trial. *Can J Surg* 33:33–36, 1990.
24. LoCicero J, Massad M, Matano J: Effect of desmopressin acetate on hemorrhage without identifiable cause in coronary bypass patients. *Am Surg* 57:165–168, 1991.
25. Guay J, Reinberg C, Poitras B et al: A trial of desmopressin to reduce blood loss in patients undergoing spinal fusion for idiopathic scoliosis. *Anesth Analg* 75:405–410, 1992.

26. Erslev AJ: Drug therapy; erythropoietin. *N Engl J Med* 324:1339–1344, 1991.

27. Eschbach JW, Egrie JC, Downing MR et al: Correction of the anemia of end-stage renal disease with recombinant human erythropoietin. *N Engl J Med* 316:73–78, 1987.

28. Goodnough LT, Rudnick S, Price TH et al: Increased preoperative collection of autologous blood with recombinant human erythropoietin therapy. *N Engl J Med* 321(17):1163–1168, 1989.

29. Ohls RK, Christensen RD: Recombinant erythropoietin compared with erythrocyte transfusion in the treatment of anemia of prematurity. *J Ped* 119:781–788, 1991.

30. Shannon KM, Mentzer WC, Abels RI et al: Recombinant human erythropoietin in the anemia of prematurity: Results of a placebo-controlled pilot study. *J Ped* 118:949–955, 1991.

31. Ludwig H, Fritz E, Kotzmann H et al: Erythropoietin treatment of anemia associated with multiple myeloma. *N Engl J Med* 322:1693–1699, 1990.

32. Miller CB, Jones RJ, Piantadosi S et al: Decreased erythropoietin response in patients with the anemia of cancer. *N Engl J Med* 322:1689–1692, 1990.

33. Fischl M, Galpin JE, Levine JD et al: Recombinant human erythropoietin for patients with AIDS treated with zidovudine. *N Engl J Med* 322:1488–1493, 1990.

34. Erickson N, Quesenberry PJ: Regulation of erythropoiesis. *Med Clin N Am* 76:745–755, 1992.

35. Groopman JE, Molina J-M, Scadden DT: Hematopoietic growth factors; biology and clinical applications. *N Engl J Med* 321:1449–1459, 1989.

36. Robinson BE, Quesenberry PJ: Hematopoietic growth factors: Overview and clinical applications, parts I, II, and III. *Amer J Med Sci* 300:163–170, 237–244. 311–321, 1990.

37. Lieschke GJ, Burgess AW: Granulocyte colony–stimulating factor and granulocyte macrophage colony–stimulating factor, parts I and II. *N Engl J Med* 327:28–35, 99–106, 1992.

38. Gould SA, Rosen AL, Sehgal LR et al: Fluosol-DA as a red-cell substitute in acute anemia. *N Engl J Med* 314:1653–1656, 1986.

39. Zuck TF: The quest for a blood substitute: In 1990, an unfulfilled promise, in Nance SJ (ed): *Transfusion Medicine in the 90's.* Arlington VA, American Association of Bloodbanks, 1990, pp 181–199.

PART V

POSTOPERATIVE COMPLICATIONS: A PROBLEM-ORIENTED APPROACH

52 APPROACH TO THE PATIENT WITH POSTOPERATIVE FEVER

George H. Talbot

Stephen J. Gluckman

Fever may develop after any procedure, and always accompanies extensive operations such as those involving the heart.[1] Often no etiology is identified. Garibaldi et al., in a prospective study of 871 patients undergoing general surgery, documented that 81 or 9 percent developed fever above 38°C orally on two consecutive days for which no etiology was ever found.[2] The majority became febrile within the first two days after surgery. Those who developed fever later more often had postoperative wound, urinary, or respiratory infection. Galicier and Richet observed postoperative fever with a rectal temperature over 38°C for more than 48 hours in 78 or 13.7 percent of 570 patients, and in 22 or 28 percent of these no cause was found.[3] Fever with no documented infection began earlier and resolved sooner than that of infectious etiology. In both studies, patients undergoing "dirty" procedures were excluded. Finally, Klimeck et al. found that infection often could not be documented in women who developed fever after obstetric or gynecologic procedures.[4] The rate of infection in those undergoing cesarean section, vaginal delivery, abdominal hysterectomy, vaginal hysterectomy, or dilatation and suction curettage who subsequently developed fever was less than 50 percent.

The causes of postoperative fever fall into three categories. In the first are general causes not necessarily related to the specific surgical procedure. Examples include intravenous catheter phlebitis, drug fever, and deep-venous thrombosis. The second category is related to the nature of the procedure and includes sternal wound infection after open-heart surgery or bacterial meningitis following craniotomy. The third group includes those causes that occur with the same frequency in the nonsurgical population. Most postoperative fevers fall into the first two categories.

GENERAL CAUSES OF POSTOPERATIVE FEVER

General causes of postoperative fever include both infectious and noninfectious processes. Many consider fever in the context of its temporal relation to the procedure. However, although certain complications are more likely to occur at one particular time than another, overdependence on such thinking may lead to misdiagnosis. It is preferable to approach each patient individually, keeping the following processes in mind.

Wound Infection

Wound infection, whether superficial or deep, is a major cause of postoperative fever. Systemic and local abnormalities decrease host resistance and predispose the patient to wound infection. Systemic abnormalities include: (1) extremes of age; (2) nutritional abnormalities including obesity and malnutrition; (3) glucose intolerance; (4) adrenocorticosteroid excess or deficiency; (5) shock and decreased perfusion; (6) some malignancies and their treatment with irradiation and chemotherapy; and (7) aberrations in the function of the reticuloendothelial system, immunoglobulin production, and cell-mediated immunity.[5] Local factors are often more important and include the presence of necrotic tissue, decreased local perfusion, hematoma formation, tissue dead space, and foreign bodies.[5]

These factors predispose to colonization by bacteria from either exogenous or endogenous sources.[5] Environmental sources of bacteria include air, equipment, and personnel in the operating room; the patient's own skin; and postoperative surroundings. Current technology and techniques have diminished the danger of external sources, but infection from endogenous sites by direct contact or hematogenous spread remains a major concern.[5] The risk of developing wound infection is directly related to the degree of contamination at surgery.[6] Other factors contributing to a higher infection rate include prolonged surgery, longer preoperative hospitalization, and infection at a remote site.[7,8]

When wound infection is suspected, a gram stain and culture of the drainage or aspirated material are crucial.[9] Polymorphonuclear leukocytes and organisms on the stain are highly indicative of infection. Staphylococci including both *S. aureus* and coagulase-negative varieties are major offenders in clean surgery.[9] Polymicrobial infection involving aerobes and anaerobes occurs frequently when respiratory, gastrointestinal, or genitourinary flora contaminate the surgical site.[9,10] In selected cases, mycobacteria or fungi may be the offending agents.[11,12]

Hematoma Formation

Hematoma formation can complicate almost any surgical intervention, especially in vascular and orthopedic procedures. In one study, fever was attributed to hematoma in four or 0.01 percent of 570 febrile patients after general surgery.[3] Distinguishing hematoma formation from wound abscess may be difficult because both may look like localized areas of inflammation. In addition, an originally bland hematoma may evolve into an overt suppurative process after bacterial superinfection. When significant occult bleeding complicates intraabdominal or intrathoracic surgery, the diagnosis is even harder to establish but should be suspected when fever is accompanied by a falling hemoglobin, hyperbilirubinemia, and elevated lactate dehydrogenase levels without evidence of external blood loss or abnormal hepatic function. Careful aseptic needle aspiration of accessible hematomas may differentiate a hematoma from a seroma or wound abscess. However, violation of a closed space may itself introduce bacteria and should be done only after careful consideration.

Pulmonary Disorders

Pulmonary disorders, including atelectasis, aspiration pneumonia, and empyema are among the most common causes of postoperative fever. They are discussed fully in Chap. 57.

Deep-Venous Thrombosis and Pulmonary Embolism

Deep-venous thrombosis with or without pulmonary embolism should alway be considered in febrile patients after surgery. Physical examination can be misleading in diagnosing thrombophlebitis in the lower extremities and useless when prostatic or other pelvic veins are involved. Similarly, pulmonary embolism may occur without the classic signs and symptoms. A normal lung scan or pulmonary angiogram essentially excludes the diagnosis of clinically important pulmonary embolism. However, "high" or "low" probability readings can be wrong approximately 15 percent of the time. In a patient with a suspicious history, a "low" probability lung scan may require further evaluation.[13,14] Lower extremity venography, serial impedance plethysmography, duplex doppler flow studies, and pulmonary angiogram all have roles in approaching this problem.[13,15] A hectic fever curve suggestive of sepsis or the absence of overt focal signs should not lead one to dismiss the possibility of thromboembolic disease.[16]

Intravenous Catheters

Intravenous catheters can cause fever by infectious or noninfectious mechanisms. In the latter case, fever can be the result of irritation by the catheter itself or by infused fluids, including certain antibiotics and hypertonic nutritional solutions.[17] Irritation is usually apparent with peripherally placed lines. Pyogenic infection, including overt suppurative thrombophlebitis, may complicate a preexistent chemical phlebitis or may arise de novo.[17–19] The factors predisposing to pyogenic infection include the duration of catheterization, the number of catheter lumens, and the composi-

tion of the infusate.[20,21] In some cases, the diagnosis may not be evident on inspection, and local signs and symptoms may be absent.[22] Hyperalimentation lines in large central veins are frequently major offenders,[20,23] and suppurative thrombophlebitis may also complicate central venous catheterization.[21,24]

S. aureus, coagulase-negative staphylococci, and gram-negative rods may be responsible for pyogenic phlebitis.[17,20,21] In addition, various fungi, including *Candida albicans*, *Candida alabrata*, and *Malassezia furfur* may colonize central lines and cause septicemia, disseminated infection, and death.[17,24–31] Documentation of invasive fungal disease may be difficult, but persistently positive blood cultures after removal of the catheter and fungal endophthalmitis are the most specific indicators.[32] Bacterial endocarditis is an infrequent but important complication of infection in vascular lines.[33]

Contamination of plastic administration sets or solutions occurs infrequently.[17] This is difficult to establish in an individual patient but should be considered if an outbreak of septicemia due to a single organism develops in the hospital. Hydrophilic gram-negative rods and yeasts are most frequently isolated in such situations.[17] Indwelling hemodynamic pressure monitoring catheters are also a potential source of infection.[34,35] Semiquantitative cultures of venous and arterial catheter tips have been useful in determining the source of bacteremia when a catheter is in place.[36]

Urinary Tract Infection

Urinary tract infection must always be considered a potential source of fever, particularly in those requiring prolonged urethral catheterization.[37] The incidence of infection increases with the duration of catheterization, and after three weeks virtually all patients become colonized whether or not they have received "suppressive" antibiotics. It is often difficult to distinguish colonization from infection. Bacteriuria with pyuria in a febrile patient without another source of fever should be treated presumptively as infection. Significant fever usually suggests upper tract involvement. Males may also develop fever from catheter-associated prostatitis or epididymitis. The development of urinary tract infection in catheterized patients is associated with nearly a threefold increase in mortality.[38] A urinalysis and urine culture are first-line diagnostic tests in most febrile postoperative patients.

Drug-Related Causes

Drug-induced fever should always be considered,[39,40] and some agents are more likely to cause temperature elevation than others. These are listed in Table 52–1.[39,41] Concomitant rash or eosinophilia support the diagnosis but are frequently not present. Patients with drug fever may feel and look better than their temperature curves suggest. Repeated intramuscular injections of analgesics causing "sterile abscesses" have also been associated with fever.[42]

When drug fever is suspected, possibly offending medications should be discontinued. If an indispensable medication is likely to be at fault, one must decide whether the risks of continued administration outweigh those of withdrawal or substitution with another agent. In the absence of severe rash or interstitial nephritis, continuation of an offending but indispensable drug may be safer. Under special circumstances, cautious rechallenge with a previously discontinued medication may confirm the diagnosis of drug fever.

TABLE 52–1. Medications Associated with Fever

Antimicrobials

Penicillins	Isoniazid
Cephalosporins	Amphotericin B
Sulfonamides	Rifampin
Nitrofurantoin	

Antihypertensive and Cardiovascular Agents

Hydralazine	Quinidine
Thiazides	Procainamide
Alpha-methyldopa	Furosemide

Other Agents

Allopurinol
Diphenylhydantoin
Iodides
Propylthiouracil
Salicylates

Endocrinologic Causes

Endocrinologic causes of fever are rare, sometimes precipitated by the stress of surgery and anesthesia.[43] Acute adrenal insufficiency may cause fever and refractory hypotension, occasionally with concomitant eosinophilia and acid-base disturbances. Signs of Addison's disease such as hyperpigmentation may not be present. A pheochromocytoma may cause postoperative fever, labile hypertension, flushing, nausea, vomiting, and tachycardia. Finally, thyroid storm may develop postoperatively with high fever and hypermetabolism. Though uncommon, these entities are important because they are life-threatening if untreated and remediable if appropriate therapy is instituted promptly.

Malignant Hyperthermia

Malignant hyperthermia is a rare disorder of skeletal muscle that can cause postoperative fever.[44] This genetically transmitted disease of abnormal sarcoplasmic calcium release is classically induced by muscle relaxants like succinylcholine. Inhalation anesthetics and other factors including high ambient temperatures, emotional excitement, injury, infection, and exercise have also been implicated. Although hyperthermia usually begins 10 to 30 minutes after induction of anesthesia, it may be delayed until several hours after surgery.

Temperatures in malignant hyperthermia are usually between 39°C and 42°C but can reach 44°C to 46°C. The anesthesiologist may note incomplete muscle relaxation with increased muscle fasciculations. Tachypnea, tachycardia, other tachyarrhythmias, and cyanosis follow. Skeletal muscle rigidity occurs in 80 percent of patients, and acidosis, hypoxemia, hyperglycemia, hyperphosphatemia, hypocalcemia, and hyperkalemia may be seen. Myoglobinemia and subsequent myoglobinuric acute renal failure often supervene. Rapid recognition of this syndrome may save the patient if cooling procedures and dantrolene are instituted immediately, but the mortality rate remains 30 to 40 percent.[44]

Transfusion Reactions

Transfusion reactions commonly cause postoperative fever.[45] They can occur after administration of any component of blood and are attributed to antibodies directed toward the cells. Fever, often with rigors, is usually the only clinical manifestation. Such reactions rarely lead to serious consequences. However, acute intravascular hemolysis, a rare cause of transfusion-related fever due to ABO incompatibilities, is more serious and can progress to shock, renal failure, and disseminated intravascular coagulation.

Febrile reactions after blood transfusion may be due to microorganisms. If blood becomes infected during storage and handling, fever and shock may result from infusion of preformed endotoxin or viable bacteria.[46] If fever occurs during or immediately after a transfusion, the product should be returned to the blood bank for examination. Other infections transmitted by transfused blood include hepatitis B, hepatitis C, cytomegalovirus (CMV), Epstein-Barr virus (EBV), human immunodeficiency virus (HIV), human T-cell leukemia virus type I (HTLV-I), syphilis, malaria, babesiosis, Chagas' disease, brucellosis, and toxoplasmosis.[47] In these cases, fever generally develops well after the transfusion.

Liver Disease

Liver disease resulting in postoperative fever may be due to drugs, infectious agents, tissue hypoxia following hypotension, passive congestion, direct trauma, biliary obstruction, and hyperalimentation therapy for chronic malnutrition. Halothane was once a prominent cause of postoperative hepatitis[48] but is now used less commonly. Since several other drugs can cause hepatic injury,[49,50] it is wise to review the medication list. Hepatitis C and CMV are the most common infectious causes of postoperative hepatitis.[51,52]

Disseminated Candidiasis

Candidemia, a well-recognized complication of vascular catheterization, may be easy to recognize and treat. However, disseminated candidiasis without candidemia is more difficult to diagnose. It should be suspected in severely ill patients in intensive care units who remain persistently febrile with negative cultures despite empiric broad-spectrum antibacterial therapy.[29,30,53]

Toxic Shock Syndrome

Epidemic toxic shock syndrome (TSS) associated with menstruation was recognized in 1980, and the role of toxin-producing *S. aureus* was defined soon thereafter.[54] Subsequently, cases of nonmenstrual TSS were observed with toxigenic *S. aureus* infection of surgical wounds and other sites.[55–58] Although rare, nonmenstrual TSS should be suspected in febrile postoperative patients with purulent incisional drainage who develop the characteristic fever, hypotension, and diffuse erythematous rash with subsequent desquamation. TSS is often accompanied by diarrhea, myalgias, vomiting, conjunctivitis, pharyngitis, edema, and strawberry tongue. Postpartum cases have also occurred. Laboratory findings include leukocytosis, thrombocytopenia, hypocalcemia, and elevated serum levels of creatinine, creatine phosphokinase, liver enzymes, and total bilirubin. Therapy includes incision and drainage of the infected area, antistaphylococcal antibiotic therapy, and other supportive measures. Since TSS has been caused by methicillin-resistant *S. aureus* (MRSA) and coagulase-negative staphylococci that can also be methicillin-resistant, vancomycin may be appropriate first-line therapy in many institutions.

Clostridium Difficile–Associated Diarrhea

Clostridium difficile causes a spectrum of illness, ranging from mild diarrhea to fatal pseudomembranous colitis.[59,60] Fever is common and occasionally develops before gastrointestinal symptoms. Etiologic factors include antibiotic exposure, advanced age, hospitalization in intensive care units, and upper GI instrumentation.[61] An assay for *C. difficile* toxin in the stool is often an appropriate part of an evaluation of postoperative fever.

Sinusitis and Otitis

Sinusitis is an important diagnostic consideration in patients who have had nasotracheal intubation. Linden et al. diagnosed 19 cases in a six-month study of patients in a surgical intensive care unit.[62] Multiple trauma was noted in 14 of 19 affected patients. Sinusitis was diagnosed approximately one week after intubation. Isolated organisms included *S. aureus*, *H. influenzae*, hospital-acquired gram-negative bacilli like *P. aeruginosa* and anaerobes, and infection was frequently polymicrobial. Bacterial otitis media is occasionally seen in patients receiving long-term mechanical ventilation.[63] Intubated postoperative patients with fever therefore require otorhinolaryngologic evaluation and plain sinus x-rays or computerized tomographic scans. Since the organisms are difficult to predict in this setting, sinus aspiration or tympanocentesis is often necessary for microbiological diagnosis and proper drainage.

CAUSES OF FEVER IN SPECIFIC TYPES OF SURGERY

Cardiac Surgery

Fever lasting several days is common after cardiac surgery[1] and can persist for more than a week in as many as 36 to 73 percent of patients.[64] More often the fever remains unexplained and is self-limited. Pien et al. found that infected patients are more likely to exhibit fever beyond the third postoperative day.[65] Less than 10 percent of the uninfected patients had fever after the fourth postoperative day, and by the ninth day only four percent had a temperature above 38°C. They concluded that fever after the third day should prompt a search for deep infection. In addition to the usual infections seen after any procedure, major concerns after cardiac surgery include prosthetic valve endocarditis (PVE), sternal wound infection, and mediastinitis.

Prosthetic valve endocarditis can be divided into early and late forms on the basis of onset before or after 60 days following surgery.[66] Late PVE resembles natural valve endocarditis in its course and microbiology.[66] Early PVE is more often fulminant and is commonly due to staphylococci, gram-negative rods, or fungi. In addition to fever, chills, and new or changing murmurs, patients may demonstrate shock, uncontrollable septicemia, refractory congestive heart failure, and manifestations of major systemic emboli. Signs of longstanding endocarditis such as Roth's spots, splenomegaly, and clubbing are absent. Conjunctival petechiae may be observed in noninfected patients after cardiac surgery, making this finding nonspecific. Though sustained bacteremia after prosthetic valve surgery should always lead one to consider endocarditis, Sande et al. found it to be uncommon.[67] Almost all of the 22 patients in his series had an obvious extracardiac source of fever.[67]

Bacteremias occurred early in the course, 70 percent were caused by gram-negative rods, and none of the patients developed a changing murmur.[67]

The incidence of wound infection after median sternotomy ranges from 0.7 percent to 1.5 percent with an associated mortality rate of 13 percent to 33 percent.[68] The major organisms are *S. aureus* and *S. epidermidis*, although many other hospital-acquired pathogens have been reported. Demmy et al. found that only male sex and the presence of pulmonary disease were statistically independent predictors of sternal wound infection.[68] The presentation of sternal wound infection is variable, depending on the virulence of the organism and the extent of infection.[11,69,70] Less aggressive pathogens cause chronic fever, sternal instability or tenderness, or persistent drainage, and clinical illness may not be evident for weeks or months. However, infection may develop quickly with high fever, toxemia, wound dehiscence, and extrusion of overt pus when more virulent pathogens are involved. Since the incision is contiguous to the sternum, osteomyelitis and mediastinal infection may supervene. In all cases of sternal wound purulence, the possibility of deep infection should be entertained. Successful management may require surgical exploration to delineate and drain involved areas.

Mediastinitis complicating open-heart surgery appears one to three weeks after surgery[70,71] and occurs in 0.5 to 4.0 percent of patients.[70] Outbreaks have been associated with cross-contamination by critical care nurses[72] and nasal carriage of a methicillin-resistant *S. aureus* by a surgical resident.[73] The incubation period is usually 4 to 30 days.[70] Fever and bacteremia can antedate obvious local wound infection. The diagnosis may be difficult to establish if there is no purulence in the wound or drainage tubes. The pericardial sac may be involved as well. Less frequent problems involve infection of cardiac suture lines, patches, and pacemaker wires, and recurrent cellulitis of the saphenous vein donor site.[74,75] Right-sided native valve endocarditis can complicate flow-directed pulmonary artery catheterization.[76]

The postperfusion syndrome occurs in about 3 to 10 percent of patients undergoing cardiopulmonary bypass and begins in the second month after surgery.[64] Features include fever and hepatosplenomegaly, atypical lymphocytosis, and abnormalities in hepatic function. Current data implicate cytomegalovirus infection. The course of the disease is rarely serious, and spontaneous resolution occurs over a period of several weeks.

One noninfectious cause of fever that may be overdiagnosed is the postcardiotomy or postpericardiectomy syndrome. It can occur two to three weeks after surgery but can also develop as early as one week or as late as 5 to 10 months later.[64,77] It consists of fever, substernal pain, pericardial and pleural friction rubs, and a variety of nonspecific laboratory abnormalities including leukocytosis, elevated sedimentation rate, cardiomegaly on chest x-ray, and electrocardiographic manifestations of pericarditis. Currently accepted clinical criteria require that patients have persistent or recurrent fever beyond the seventh postoperative day in association with a pericardial friction rub. Defined in this way, the incidence of the syndrome has been documented to be as low as 6.2 percent.[64] Livelli et al. noted that leukocytosis, pleuritic chest pain, pericardial rubs, pleural effusion, and mediastinal widening on chest x-ray were as common in afebrile as in febrile patients.[1] The presence or absence of any of these features therefore does not predict which patients will develop recurrent pericarditis after discharge. The authors suggested that the term "postpericardiotomy syndrome" be reserved for those few patients with late illness.

Neurosurgery

Central nervous system infections are of particular concern in patients on neurosurgical services.[78] Those with major penetrating or nonpenetrating craniospinal trauma have a high risk of bacterial meningitis due to overt communication with the subarachnoid space. In some cases, communication is occult. Cerebrospinal fluid (CSF) fistulas occur in 3 to 50 percent of all cases of nonpenetrating head trauma.

In patients with closed head trauma, meningitis may occur within the first 72 hours after the injury. *Pneumococcus* is the usual pathogen, but other organisms like *H. influenzae* may be involved.[79] In penetrating injury or after surgical intervention, gram-negative rods or *S. aureus* are more common. Meningitis may occur after several days. Prophylactic antibiotics may affect the incidence and type of infectious sequelae, but data from controlled studies of this issue are lacking.

Patients undergoing neurosurgical procedures for indications other than trauma also have a risk of developing bacterial meningitis. Fever is usually present, but classic signs of meningitis such as headache, nuchal rigidity, and decreased level of consciousness may be absent or difficult to interpret because of the underlying illness. Seizures and focal signs correlate with poor prognosis. The only way to confirm the diagnosis is by examining the CSF. A high opening pressure and elevation of the protein concentration and leukocyte count in the fluid are often found in meningitis but may occur after uncomplicated neurosurgery. However, hypoglycorrhachia generally means infection. In the above study, it was documented in 85 percent of infected patients but only rarely found in others. The most frequent pathogens are *S. aureus*, coagulase-negative staphylococci, enterococci, and gram-negative rods.

The presentation of ventricular shunt infection is variable.[80,81] Symptomatic infection usually occurs within the first month or two after surgery. Patients often appear acutely ill with fever, lethargy, meningismus, and evidence of local wound infection, but none of these findings may be present. Tenderness over the valve and tubing is a frequent finding. Patients can also present with symptoms and signs of shunt malfunction rather than infection, and occasionally demonstrate no clinical findings despite persistently positive cultures drawn from the tubing or valve. Patients with infected ventriculoperitoneal shunts may develop abdominal pain with pseudocyst formation. Hypocomplementemic glomerulonephritis and a syndrome mimicking bacterial endocarditis with low-grade fever and splenomegaly may rarely occur in patients with ventriculoatrial shunts.

Predisposing factors include extremes of age, history of more than two shunting procedures, congenital malformations, normal-pressure hydrocephalus, and a suboptimal infection record in the operating surgeon. The type of shunt, whether ventriculoatrial or ventriculoperitoneal, and the use of prophylactic antibiotics do not appear to affect the incidence of infection. Fever immediately after shunt procedures is common and does not predict subsequent infection.

Examination of the CSF obtained from the shunt or the lumbar subarachnoid space is critical. The opening pressure and protein concentration are usually elevated. White blood cell counts and glucose concentration are usually abnormal in patients with shunt infection but are less dramatic than in patients with meningitis not related to a shunt. Culture reveals staphylococcal species in over 50 percent, but gram-negative rods and other species can be found. George et al. found no difference between bacteria isolated in early infection occurring less than 30 days after surgery and in late infection occurring thereafter.[80] Organisms usually considered to be contaminants like anaerobic diphtheroids may be pathogens in infections of prosthetic implants.[82] Mixed aerobic and anaerobic enteric flora cultured from a ventriculoperitoneal shunt suggest the presence of bowel perforation by the distal tip of the tubing.[83]

Meningitis can occur when external ventriculostomies are in place.[84] A snug fit between the tubing and the dura to minimize leakage of CSF and strict maintenance of a closed system are important to avoid infection. The duration of catheter placement and use of prophylactic antibiotics may play a role in the development of infection, but prospectively acquired data have not been accumulated to answer this question.

A syndrome of aseptic meningitis following posterior fossa surgery has been described.[85,86] Patients demonstrate clinical and laboratory findings indistinguishable from those of bacterial infection, but cultures of the CSF are negative. This syndrome usually occurs within 48 hours of surgery but may not appear for several weeks. Patients do not respond to antibiotics, but steroid therapy improves the clinical picture. Infections should be carefully excluded.

Vascular Grafts

Major infections occur in one to six percent of vascular grafts.[87–89] Many of these are not clinically apparent in the immediate postoperative period. Features are variable and include fever, chills, sweats, or bacteremic shock; local inflammation; alterations in flow through the graft with either overt thrombosis and distal ischemia or petechiae distal to the graft; and breakdown of the suture line with false aneurysm formation and external or internal hemorrhage. Acute gastrointestinal bleeding may result from fistula formation between the proximal end of an abdominal aortic graft and the bowel. Although *S. aureus* and gram-negative organisms are sometimes implicated, coagulase-negative staphylococci currently are the most common isolates.[88]

Graft infection develops as a consequence of direct contamination during the procedure or, more rarely, bacterial seeding from a distant site after surgery. Grafts are most susceptible to bacterial infection in the immediate postoperative period when formation of a new intimal lining has not been completed. Other important factors include the type of graft, location of the graft, the type of suture material, and the use of prophylactic antibiotics. The highest rates of infection are seen in grafts in the femoral and inguinal regions. The presence of remote infection at the time of surgery and the development of extraprosthetic infection after surgery pose additional risk.

When graft infection is suspected, blood cultures, wound cultures, arteriography, noninvasive imaging with ultrasound, CT or MRI scan, and occasionally sinography may be helpful in confirming the diagnosis. More recently, isotopic imaging has been utilized.[90] Management usually involves removal of the graft, but occasionally a combination of aggressive local therapy and long-term antibiotic treatment may suppress though rarely eradicate the infection.

Obstetrical Procedures and Gynecologic Surgery

Fever in the postpartum patient raises the possibility of infectious complications, especially endometritis.[91,92] The patient usually develops fever and lower abdominal pain and tenderness shortly after the appearance of foul-smelling purulent vaginal discharge. There is often a history of premature rupture of the membranes, difficult delivery, or amnionitis. Bacteremia, septic shock, and death may supervene.

Endometritis is usually a polymicrobial process involving aerobes, anaerobes, and chlamydia. In addition, *Mycoplasma hominis* has been implicated in some patients.[92] Because of the difficulty in obtaining endometrial cultures that have not been contaminated by cervical flora, antimicrobial therapy is usually empiric. Wound infection and urinary tract infection are also common in this setting.[92]

Compared to vaginal delivery, cesarean section is more frequently associated with postoperative fever. Conditions predisposing to fever include antepartum risk factors such as high parity, greater-than-average age, and concurrent medical problems, and intrapartum factors such as significant bleeding, prolonged rupture of membranes before delivery, and internal monitoring.[93–95] Postpartum patients can develop pelvic abscesses, but they are more common after gynecologic procedures.[96,97] Subgluteal and retropsoas abscesses after paracervical and pudendal nerve block anesthesia and epidural infections following regional anesthesia have been described.

Septic abortion is encountered less frequently since abortion laws have been liberalized. However, infection following therapeutic abortion still occurs, and the same vaginal microflora are usually implicated.[98] Though extremely uncommon, the most dramatic form of infection is clostridial myonecrosis of the uterus characterized by acute toxemia, shock, disseminated intravascular coagulation, and hemolysis. However, a gram stain suggestive of *Clostridium perfringens* must be interpreted carefully, since these organisms may normally colonize the female genital tract.[98] Only in the appropriate clinical setting does this finding require aggressive therapy.

Gynecological procedures are frequently complicated by fever and overt infection. The incidence, which increases with the extent of the procedure, is lowest after laparotomy and abdominal hysterectomy and highest after extensive procedures like radical vulvectomy and pelvic exenteration. Urinary tract and wound infections are common. Pelvic cellulitis, necrotizing fasciitis, and abscess formation are more serious complications and may lead to bacteremia and death.[92,99] Abscesses are more common after vaginal than abdominal surgery. Purulent collections may be found in the vaginal cuff, cul-de-sac, or adnexae.

Ovarian abscesses are especially common after vaginal hysterectomy but may follow other types of pelvic surgery or develop in the puerperium. Vaginal cuff abscesses usually occur early in the postoperative period, while deeper pelvic abscesses, whether ovarian, tubal, or in the cul-de-sac, present later. Abscesses characteristically cause fever and pain. However, intraperitoneal collections may produce a progressive enlarging mass or lead to catastrophic rupture, peritonitis, and sepsis.

Patients with fever, pelvic symptoms, or bacteremia in whom an abscess cannot be found by repeated internal examination and ultrasonography are considered to have pelvic cellulitis. Antibiotic therapy alone is curative in this group, while a drainage procedure is often necessary in patients with true abscess formation. In either case, a mixture of aerobic and anaerobic bacterial pathogens is most often isolated.

Because septic pelvic thrombophlebitis is so difficult to document, its true incidence and clinical presentation are not easy to define.[92,100] It must be considered in postoperative patients who have no identifiable abscess or extragenital source of infection who remain febrile despite administration of broad-spectrum antibiotics active against pelvic flora. Some persistently febrile patients, often with few pelvic or extrapelvic signs and symptoms, defervesce and improve clinically after treatment with heparin. A trial of anticoagulation may thus be considered diagnostic as well as therapeutic. Unless a patient has a documented pulmonary embolism or thrombosed pelvic veins are visualized at laparotomy, the diagnosis can only be inferred from the response to heparin. Fever should abate within 48 to 72 hours. Lack of response should lead to consideration of other diagnoses.

Urologic Surgery

Urologic patients often require indwelling urethral catheters after surgery, which predispose them to bacteriuria.[101] However, bacteriuria does not necessarily mean symptomatic infection, and not all symptomatic urinary tract infections produce fever. A positive urine culture, especially without pyuria, may not correctly identify the cause of postoperative fever. On the other hand, bacteriuria does predispose the patient to bacteremia,[102] which is more likely to occur if preoperative urinary catheterization has been performed or if prostatitis is present.

Other complications of lower urinary tract surgery or indwelling urethral catheters include acute bacterial prostatic abscess, epididymitis, and orchitis. These are readily recognizable in responsive patients, but when the patient cannot describe symptoms one must include them in the differential diagnosis of postoperative fever. Osteomyelitis of the pubic symphysis is a less-common complication that can occur more than two weeks after surgery.[103] This must be distinguished from osteitis pubis, a noninfectious process, which may also present with low-grade fever, pubic pain, leukocytosis, and radiographic evidence of bone destruction.[104] Sinus tract formation with purulent drainage or isolation of a pathogenic bacterium from a bone biopsy with histopathologic changes of osteomyelitis confirms the presence of infection. Osteomyelitis may also develop elsewhere after urologic surgery. Bacterial spread through Batson's plexus and arterial dissemination have been implicated in spread of infection to lumbar vertebrae.[105] Arterial spread is more likely when other noncontiguous osseous structures are involved. Persistent local pain and fever are the cardinal manifestations of osteomyelitis.

Upper-tract infection may also occur after surgery. Perinephric abscess is an infrequent but serious complication.[106] Bacteria associated with infections following urinary tract surgery are usually enteric organisms like *Escherichia coli*. However, hospital-acquired pathogens such as *Pseudomonas* and *Serratia* species should be considered. *S. aureus* is particularly associated with prostatic abscesses.[107]

Orthopedic Surgery

Total hip and knee replacements are being performed with increasing frequency. Fever in the first few days after surgery is nearly universal and does not predict subsequent complications. Unless accompanied by worrisome physical findings, it does not require extensive evaluation. Occasionally such "innocent" fevers last several weeks, but those persisting more than a week after surgery suggest significant complications.

Hematoma formation is particularly common and may cause fever. The patient may be uncomfortable but does not otherwise appear ill. In obvious cases, a warm tense erythematous and painful swelling develops at the incision, sometimes accompanied by local edema and purpura. It may be difficult to distinguish hematoma from wound infection, and bacterial superinfection may complicate an initially aseptic process. In selected cases, needle aspiration of the collection may be desirable. Documentation of infection may necessitate further surgery. The collection of blood may be deep and impossible to appreciate on examination. Suspicion should be raised if the postoperative hematocrit is disproportionately low for estimated operative blood loss, especially if the patient has been excessively anticoagulated.

Lower-extremity thrombophlebitis is particularly common after knee and hip surgery,[108] and must always be considered as a cause of fever.

Persistent or late fever is worrisome, especially that due to deep infection after hip replacement. Although most series report rates of 0.5 to 2.0 percent, it can occur in up to 11 percent of cases.[109] Previous hip surgery with or without infection increases risk, while the use of prophylactic antibiotics and laminar air flow in the operating room decrease it.[109] Hematoma formation and drainage may also predispose patients to infection, but spontaneous drainage may itself be the result of infection.

Deep hip infection should be suspected when the patient continues to experience pain after the immediate postoperative period. When it develops in the first three months after surgery, it often results in prolonged postoperative fever and other signs of infection. Late infection may be manifested only by persistent and worsening pain without fever or signs of inflammation. Approximately 40 to 50 percent of all infections fall into the early group. Presentation of late infection may be delayed for months or even years.[110]

The major etiologic pathogens are *S. aureus* and coagulase-negative staphylococci.[110] The latter cause a more indolent process, but the former can also underlie smoldering infection.[111] The incidence of gram-negative bacterial infection in hip prostheses has increased in recent years. The pathogenesis and presentation of infection after knee replacement parallels that of the hip.[112]

Compound fractures requiring surgery are particularly prone to infection. In one series, 15 percent of open fractures, 22 percent of open joint wounds, and 50 percent of open soft-tissue injuries became infected.[113] Many of these wounds were already infected at the time of hospital admission. Although others have not documented as high a rate of overt infection, they have confirmed the high incidence of bacterial contamination, providing a good rationale for the use of prophylactic antibiotics.[114,115]

Abdominal Surgery

Fever is common after abdominal surgery and is usually due to infection, with wound infection predominating. Intraabdominal infections after intestinal perforation involve mixed aerobic and anaerobic flora from the peritoneal cavity, the wound, and abdominal abscess in 76 percent to 82 percent of cases.[116] The predominant aerobes and facultative anaerobes are usually *E. coli* and *Strepto-*

coccus species including enterococci. The predominant anaerobes are *Bacteroides*, *Peptostreptococcus*, and *Clostridium* species,[116] suggesting that endogenous intraoperative contamination plays a major role in the pathogenesis of infection. Postoperative peritonitis is the result of preoperative contamination, as in appendiceal perforation, intraoperative contamination from either an external or internal source, an unrelated secondary disease, or a variety of postoperative complications including breakdown of an anastomotic site.[117]

When infection becomes localized, an intraperitoneal, retroperitoneal, or visceral abscess forms.[118] Like peritonitis, it may be a consequence of the primary disease process requiring surgery, the surgical procedure, or an intercurrent illness. Visceral abscesses usually form in the liver but may occur in the pancreas, spleen, or kidneys. Retroperitoneal abscesses are less commonly associated with surgery but may develop anteriorly in the retroperitoneal space when procedures are performed in the presence of established infection.

Subphrenic abscesses are well described in the literature. The use of antibiotics has transformed their once fulminant course into a more insidious, chronically debilitating, and often occult process.[119] At the turn of the century, they were most often the result of perforated gastric ulcer and appendicitis but are now more often sequelae of biliary and gastric surgical procedures. Responsible microorganisms are derived from the gastrointestinal tract. Fever, chills, and pain are frequent but not invariable findings. Symptoms and signs are commonly referable to the chest as well as the abdomen and together constitute the so-called thoracoabdominal complex. Similarly, radiographs may reveal abnormalities above the diaphragm such as atelectasis, pneumonitis, effusion, and empyema and others below it like air fluid levels, limited diaphragmatic motion, and hepatic displacement. Ultrasonography, MRI scanning, and computerized tomography are the best modalities for noninvasive diagnosis.

Postsurgical febrile complications relating to the pancreas may arise from both infectious and noninfectious processes.[120] Acute postoperative pancreatitis is usually the result of intraoperative trauma to the pancreas or to surrounding structures such as the biliary tree and stomach. Injury may be so slight as to be inapparent except in retrospect. The incidence of pancreatitis after gastric resection has been reported to be as high as 3 percent. Pancreatitis may also result from surgery at distant and even extraabdominal sites, but its pathogenesis in such cases is unclear. In either event, the patient may present with minimal findings or may exhibit the full-blown syndrome of fever, abdominal pain and tenderness, and ileus. Extraabdominal findings include adult respiratory distress syndrome, arthritis, and rash. Intraoperative trauma to the pancreas may also result in pseudocyst formation. Pseudocysts may be associated with fever, but persistent fever in a toxic patient suggests possible bacterial superinfection of a cyst or overt abscess formation.

SUMMARY: CLINICAL APPROACH TO THE FEBRILE POSTOPERATIVE PATIENT

Certain generalizations are applicable to the evaluation of most patients. It is helpful to approach postoperative fever in a rational stepwise fashion as outlined below to avoid overlooking possible sources.

1. Thorough history and chart review with particular attention to:
   a. preoperative course and preexisting medical and surgical problems;
   b. medications administered, especially anesthetics and antibiotics;
   c. nature of the surgical procedure including whether performed under elective or emergency conditions;
   d. intraoperative and postoperative complications;
   e. presence and time of placement of vascular and urinary catheters as well as other tubes and monitoring devices;
   f. timing of transfusion of blood products;
   g. history of allergies.

2. Physical examination with particular attention to:
   a. the operative site and contiguous areas;
   b. the presence of catheters and indwelling monitoring devices as well as areas around their entry points;
   c. signs suggestive of deep-vein thrombosis, pulmonary embolism, or hematoma formation;
   d. decubiti due to pressure necrosis or sterile abscesses from intramuscular injections;
   e. the lower respiratory tract.

3. Initial laboratory evaluation including:
   a. urinalysis, urine gram stain, and culture;
   b. sputum gram stain and culture if sputum is available;
   c. gram stain and culture of wound exudate or drainage from closed systems such as pleural or mediastinal tubes with anaerobic culture when the specimen can be properly obtained;
   d. blood cultures;
   e. complete blood count with differential;
   f. chest x-ray.

4. If an infectious etiology is apparent at this point or the patient is toxic, antimicrobial therapy is warranted.

5. If no diagnosis is apparent, one should consider:
   a. changing and culturing all intravascular catheters;
   b. withdrawing medications suspected of causing fever;
   c. liver function tests.

6. More extensive tests may often be helpful and are occasionally crucial. These include radiographic contrast studies, radionuclide scanning, venography, arteriography, MRI scanning, and computerized tomography.

THERAPY

It is impossible to provide specific recommendations for empiric antimicrobial therapy in all febrile postoperative patients since such a wide variety of clinical problems may cause fever. Nonetheless, the following generalizations may be considered:

1. Fever alone is not an indication for immediate antimicrobial therapy. If the patient does not appear toxic and if no source of infection is identified clinically, antibiotics may be withheld pending further data. If a source is found on initial evaluation, therapy should be instituted at once with antibiotic selection determined by gram stain results and an understanding of the pathogens likely to be involved in a specific situation.

2. Empiric antibiotic therapy is more easily justified and broad antimicrobial coverage is reasonable if the patient appears ill. If a patient is desperately ill, coverage should be extended to include all reasonably possible organisms.

3. Whenever possible, empiric therapy should be based on the results of a gram-stained specimen from the infected site.

4. Infections developing in the hospital are more likely to be caused by relatively resistant pathogens than are infections occurring outside the hospital.

5. If a gastrointestinal or gynecologic source is likely, coverage for *B. fragilis* should be included.

6. Empiric antifungal therapy should be considered in selected patients with a high risk of candidiasis.

Once an initial regimen has been initiated, further therapeutic and diagnostic decisions depend on accumulated laboratory data and the response to therapy. Persistent undefined fever should prompt repeated thorough physical examinations and judicious repetition of basic laboratory tests. Change or removal of indwelling lines or monitoring devices may be life-saving. Discussions among all involved physicians are crucial when more invasive diagnostic or therapeutic interventions are considered.

REFERENCES

1. Livelli FD Jr, Johnson RA, McEnany MT et al: Unexplained in-hospital fever following cardiac surgery. Natural history, relationship to the postpericardiotomy syndrome, and a prospective study of therapy with indomethacin versus placebo. *Circulation* 57:968, 1978.
2. Garibaldi RA, Brodine S, Matsumiya S et al: Evidence for the noninfectious etiology of early postoperative fever. *Infect Control* 6:273, 1985.
3. Galicier C, Richet H: A prospective study of postoperative fever in a general surgery department. *Infect Control* 6:487, 1985.
4. Klimeck JJ, Ajemian ER, Gracewski JG et al: A prospective analysis of hospital-acquired fever in obstetric and gynecologic patients. *JAMA* 247:3340, 1982.
5. Cruse PJE: Wound infections: Epidemiology and clinical characteristics, in Simmons RL, Howard RJ, Henriksen A (eds): *Surgical Infectious Diseases*. New York, Appleton Century Crofts, 1982, p 929.
6. Olson M, O'Connor M, Schwartz ML: Surgical wound infections. A five-year prospective study of 20,193 wounds at the Minneapolis Veterans Administration Medical Center. *Ann Surg* 199:253, 1989.
7. Haley RW, Culver DH, Morgan WM et al: Identifying patients at high risk of surgical wound infection. A simple multivariate index of patient susceptibility and wound contamination. *Am J Epidemiol* 121:206, 1985.
8. Edwards LD: The epidemiology of 2056 remote site infections and 1966 surgical wound infections in 1865 patients: A four-year study of 40,923 operations at the Rush-Presbyterian-St. Luke's Hospital, Chicago. *Ann Surg* 184:758, 1976.
9. Stone HH: Infection in postoperative patients. *Am J Med* 81(Suppl 1A):39, 1986.

10. Rotstein OD, Pruett TL, Simmons RL: Mechanisms of microbial synergy in polymicrobial surgical infections. *Rev Infect Dis* 7:151, 1985.
11. Kuritsky JW, Bullen MG, Broome CV et al: Sternal wound infections and endocarditis due to organisms of the *Mycobacterium fortuitum* complex. *Ann Intern Med* 98:938, 1983.
12. Kraug WE, Valengtein PN, Corey GR: Purulent pericarditis caused by *Candida*: Report of three cases and identification of high-risk populations as an aid to early diagnosis. *Rev Infect Dig* 10:34, 1988.
13. Kelly MA, Carson JL, Palevsky HI et al: Diagnosing pulmonary embolism: New facts and strategies. *Ann Intern Med* 114:300, 1991.
14. PIOPED Investigators: Value of the ventilation/perfusion scan in acute pulmonary embolism. *JAMA* 263:2753, 1990.
15. Moser KM: Venous thromboembolism. *Am Rev Resp Dis* 141:235, 1990.
16. Murray HW, Ellis GC, Blumenthal DS et al: Fever and pulmonary thromboembolism. *Am J Med* 67:232, 1979.
17. Maki DG, Goldman DA, Rhame FS: Infection control in intravenous therapy. *Ann Intern Med* 79:867, 1973.
18. Stein JM, Pruitt BA: Suppurative thrombophlebitis. A lethal iatrogenic disease. *N Engl J Med* 282:1453, 1970.
19. Muengter AM: Septic thrombophlebitis. A surgical disorder. *JAMA* 230:1010, 1974.
20. Hilton E, Haglett TM, Borenstein MT et al: Central catheter infections: Single- versus triple-lumen catheters. Influence of guide wires on infection rates when used for replacement of catheters. *Am J Med* 84:667, 1988.
21. Verghese A, Widrich WC, Arbeit RD: Central venous septic thrombophlebitis—the role of medical therapy. *Medicine* 64:394, 1985.
22. Freeman R, King B: Recognition of infection associated with intravenous catheters. *Br J Surg* 62:404, 1975.
23. Armstrong CW, Mayhall GC, Miller KB et al: Prospective study of catheter replacement and other risk factors for infection of hyperalimentation catheters. *J Infect Dis* 154:808, 1986.
24. Strinden WD, Helgerson RB, Maki DG: *Candida* septic thrombosis of the great central veins associated with central catheters. Clinical features and management. *Ann Surg* 202:653, 1985.
25. Harvey RL, Myers JP: Nosocomial fungemia in a large community teaching hospital. *Arch Intern Med* 147:2117, 1987.
26. Bross JE, Talbot GH, Maislin G et al: Risk factors for nosocomial candidemia: A case control study in patients without leukemia. *Am J Med* 87:614, 1989.
27. Wey SB, Mori M, Pfaller MA et al: Risk factors for hospital-acquired candidemia. A matched case-control study. *Arch Intern Med* 149:2349, 1989.
28. Dankner WM, Spector SA, Fierer J et al: *Malassezia* fungemia in neonates and adults: Complication of hyperalimentation. *Rev Infect Dis* 9:743, 1987.
29. Marsh PK, Tally FP, Kellum J et al: *Candida* infections in surgical patients. *Ann Surg* 1982:42, 1983.
30. Solomkin JS, Flohr AM, Simmons RL: Indications for therapy for fungemia in postoperative patients. *Arch Surg* 117:1272, 1982.
31. Wey S, Mori M, Pfaller MA et al: Hospital-acquired candidemia. The attributable mortality and excess length of stay. *Arch Intern Med* 148:2642, 1988.
32. Brooks RG: Prospective study of *Candida* endophthalmitis in hospitalized patients with candidemia. *Arch Intern Med* 149:2226, 1989.
33. Terpenning MS, Buggy BP, Kaufmann C: Hospital-acquired infective endocarditis. *Arch Intern Med* 148:1601, 1988.
34. Beck-Sague CM, Jarvis WR: Epidemic bloodstream infections associated with pressure transducers: A persistent problem. *Infect Control Hosp Epidemiol* 10:54, 1989.
35. Mermel LA, Maki DG: Epidemic bloodstream infections from hemodynamic pressure monitoring: Signs of the times. *Infect Control Hosp Epidemiol* 10:47, 1989.
36. Maki D, Weise CE, Sarafin HW: A semiquantitative culture method for identifying intravenous catheter-related infection. *N Engl J Med* 296:1305, 1977.
37. Platt R, Polk BF, Murdock B et al: Risk factors for nosocomial urinary tract infection. *Am J Epidemiol* 124:977, 1986.
38. Platt R, Polk BF, Murdock B et al: Mortality associated with nosocomial urinary tract infection. *N Engl J Med* 307:637, 1982.
39. Lipsky BA, Hirschmann JV: Drug fever. *JAMA* 245:851, 1981.
40. Young EJ, Fainstein V, Musher D: Drug-induced fever: Cases seen in the evaluation of unexplained fever in a general hospital population. *Rev Infect Dis* 4:69, 1982.
41. Mackowiak PA, LeMaistre CJ: Drug fever: A critical appraisal of conventional concepts. An analysis of 51 episodes in two Dallas hospitals and 97 episodes reported in the English literature. *Ann Intern Med* 106:728, 1987.
42. Semel JD: Fever associated with repeated intramuscular injections of analgesics. *Rev Infect Dis* 8:68, 1986.
43. Simon HB, Daniels GH: Hormonal hyperthermia. Endocrinologic causes of fever. *Am J Med* 66:257, 1979.
44. Nelson TE, Flewellen EH: The malignant hyperthermia syndrome. *N Engl J Med* 309:416, 1983.
45. Pineda AA, Brzica SM, Tagwell HF: Hemolytic transfusion reaction. Recent experience in a large blood bank. *Mayo Clin Proc* 53:378, 1978.
46. Davis JP, Moser M, Hutcheson RH: *Yersinia enterocolitica* bacteremia and endotoxin shock associated with red blood cell transfusion. United States, 1987–88. *MMWR* 37:577, 1988.
47. Berkman SA: Infectious complications of blood transfusion. *Blood Rev* 2:206, 1988.
48. Carney FMT, Van Dyke RA: Halothane hepatitis: A critical review. *Anesth Analg* 51:135, 1982.
49. Kaplowitz N, Aw TY, Simon FR et al: Drug-induced hepatotoxicity. *Ann Intern Med* 104:826, 1986.
50. Onorato IM, Axerod JL: Hepatitis from intravenous high-dose oxacillin therapy. Findings in an adult inpatient population. *Ann Intern Med* 89:497, 1978.
51. Alter HJ, Purcell RH, Shih JW et al: Detection of antibody to hepatitis C virus in prospectively followed transfusion recipients with acute and chronic non-A, non-B hepatitis. *N Engl J Med* 321:1494, 1989.
52. Adler SP: Transfusion-associated cytomegalovirus infections. *Rev Infect Dis* 5:977, 1983.
53. Lewis P, Salaman RA, Aubrey DA: Management of candidiasis in the surgical patient. *Br J Clin Prac* 44:711, 1990.
54. Shands XN, Schmid GP, Dan BB et al: Toxic-shock syndrome in menstruating women: Its association with tampon use and *Staphylococcus aureus* and the clinical features in 52 cases. *N Engl J Med* 303:1436, 1980.
55. Bartlett P, Reingold AL, Graham DR et al: Toxic-shock syndrome associated with surgical wound infections. *JAMA* 247:1448, 1982.
56. Reingold AL, Shands XN, Dan BB et al: Toxic-shock syndrome not associated with menstruation. A review of 54 cases. *Lancet* 1:1, 1982.
57. Hughes D, Stapleton J: Postoperative toxic shock syndrome. *Iowa Med* 81:55, 1991.
58. Allen ST, Liland JB, Nichols CG et al: Toxic shock syndrome associated with use of latex nasal packing. *Arch Intern Med* 150:2587, 1990.
59. Gerding DN: Disease associated with *Clostridium difficile* infection. *Ann Intern Med* 110:255, 1989.
60. Gerding DW, Olson MM, Peterson LR et al: *Clostridium difficile*-associated diarrhea and colitis in adults: A prospective case-controlled epidemiologic study. *Arch Intern Med* 146:95, 1986.
61. Brown EB, Talbot GH, Axelrod PA et al: *Clostridium difficile* toxin–associated diarrhea: A case-control study. *Infect Control Hosp Epidemiol* 11:283, 1990.
62. Linden BE, Aquilar EA, Allen SJ: Sinusitis in the nasotracheally

intubated patient. *Arch Otolaryngol Head Neck Surg* 114:860, 1988.

63. Lucks D, Consiglio A, Stankiewicz J et al: Incidence and microbiological etiology of middle ear effusion complicating endotracheal intubation and mechanical ventilation. *J Infect Dig* 157:368, 1988.

64. Roses DR, Rose MR, Rapaport FT: Febrile responses associated with cardiac surgery. Relationship to the postpericardiotomy syndrome and to altered host immunologic reactivity. *J Thorac Cardiovasc Surg* 67:251, 1974.

65. Pien FD, Ho PWL, Fergusson DJ: Fever and infection after cardiac operation. *Ann Thorac Surg* 33:382, 1982.

66. Karchmer AW, Dismukes WE, Buckley J et al: Late prosthetic valve endocarditis. Clinical features influencing therapy. *Am J Med* 64:199, 1978.

67. Sande MA, Johnson WD, Hook EW et al: Sustained bacteremia in patients with prosthetic cardiac valves. *N Engl J Med* 286:1067, 1972.

68. Demmy TL, Park SB, Liebler GA et al: Recent experience with major sternal wound complications. *Ann Thorac Surg* 49:458, 1990.

69. Firmin RK, Wood A: Postoperative sternal wound infections. *Infect Surg* 6:231, 1987.

70. Grossi EA, Culliford AT, Krieger KH et al: A survey of 77 major infectious complications of median sternotomy: A review of 7949 consecutive operative procedures. *Ann Thorac Surg* 40:214, 1985.

71. Sarr MG, Gott VL, Townsend TR: Mediastinal infection after cardiac surgery. *Ann Thorac Surg* 38:415, 1984.

72. Ehrenkranz NJ, Pfaff SJ: Mediastinitis complicating cardiac operations: Evidence of postoperative causation. *Rev Infect Dis* 13:803, 1991.

73. Gaynes R, Marosok R, Mowry-Hanley J et al: Mediastinitis following coronary artery bypass surgery: A three-year review. *J Infect Dis* 163:117, 1991.

74. McHenry MC, Longworth DC, Rehm SJ et al: Infections of the cardiac suture line after left ventricular surgery. *Am J Med* 85:292, 1988.

75. Baddour LM, Bisno AL: Recurrent cellulitis after saphenous venectomy for coronary bypass surgery. *Ann Intern Med* 97:493, 1982.

76. Rowley KM, Clubb KS, Smith GJW et al: Right-sided infective endocarditis as a consequence of flow-directed pulmonary artery catheterization. A clinicopathological study of 55 autopsied patients. *N Engl J Med* 311:1152, 1984.

77. Engle MA, Gay WA Jr, McCabe J et al: Postpericardiotomy syndrome in adults: Incidence, autoimmunity, and virology. *Circulation* 64(2):58, 1981.

78. Hirgchriana JV: Meningitis following neurosurgery and blunt head trauma. *Infect Surg* 9:73, 1990.

79. Bryan CS, Jernigan FE: Posttraumatic meningitis due to ampicillin-resistant *Hemophilus influenzae*. *J Neurosurg* 51:240, 1979.

80. George R, Leibrock L, Epstein M: Long-term analysis of cerebrospinal fluid shunt infections. A 25-year experience. *J Neurosurg* 51:804, 1979.

81. McLaurin RL, Frame PT: Treatment of infections of cerebrospinal fluid shunts. *Rev Infect Dis* 9:595, 1987.

82. Everett ED, Eickhoff TC, Simon RH: Cerebrospinal fluid shunt infections with anaerobic diphtheroids (*Propionibacterium* species). *J Neurosurg* 44:580, 1976.

83. Brook I, Johnson N, Overturf GD et al: Mixed bacterial meningitis: A complication of ventriculo- and lumboperitoneal shunts. *J Neurosurg* 47:961, 1977.

84. Hickman KM, Mayer BL, Muwasiocs M: Intracranial pressure monitoring: Review of risk factors associated with infection. *Heart Lung* 19:84, 1990.

85. Carmel PW, Fraser RAR, Stein BM: Aseptic meningitis following posterior fossa surgery in children. *J Neurosurg* 41:44, 1974.

86. Kaufman HH, Carmel PW: Aseptic meningitis and hydrocephalus after posterior fossa surgery. *J Neurosurg* 41:48, 1974.

87. Goldstone J, Moore WS: Infection in vascular prostheses. Clinical manifestations and surgical management. *Am J Surg* 128:225, 1974.

88. Edmiston CE, Schmitt DD, Seabrook GR: Coagulase-negative staphylococcal infections in vascular surgery: Epidemiology and pathogenesis. *Infect Control Hosp Epidemiol* 10:111, 1989.

89. Pons VG, Wurtz R: Vascular graft infections: A 25-year experience of 170 cases. *J Vasc Surg* 13:751, 1991.

90. Insall RL, Jones NAG, Lambert D et al: New isotopic technique for detecting prosthetic arterial graft infection: 99mTc-hexametazime-labelled leucocyte imaging. *Br J Surg* 77:1295, 1990.

91. Soper DE: Postpartum endometritis. Pathophysiology and prevention. *J Reprod Med* 33(1):97–100, 1988.

92. Gibbs RS: Severe infections in pregnancy. *Med Clin N Am* 73(3):713–721, 1989.

93. Anstey JT, Sheldon GW, Blythe JG: Infectious morbidity after primary cesarean section at a private institution. *Am J Obstet Gynecol* 136:205, 1980.

94. Yonekura ML: Risk factors for postcesarean endomyometritis. *Am J Med* 78(6B):177–187, 1985.

95. Yonekura ML: Treatment of postcesarean endomyometritis. *Clin Obstet Gynecol* 31(2):488–500, 1988.

96. Ledger WJ, Campbell C, Wilson JR: Postoperative adrenal infection. *Obstet Gynecol* 31:83, 1968.

97. Livergood CH III, Addison WA: Adrenal infection as a delayed complication of vaginal hysterectomy. *Am J Obstet Gynecol* 143:596, 1982.

98. Larson B, Galask RP: Vaginal microbial flora. Composition and influences of host physiology. *Ann Intern Med* 96(Suppl 6):926, 1982.

99. Golde S, Ledger WJ: Necrotizing fasciitis in postpartum patients. A report of four cases. *Obstet Gynecol* 50:670, 1977.

100. Josey WE, Staggers SR: Heparin therapy in septic pelvic thrombophlebitis: A study of 46 cases. *Am J Obstet Gynecol* 120:228, 1974.

101. Lipsky BA: Urinary tract infections in men. Epidemiology, pathophysiology, diagnosis and treatment. *Ann Intern Med* 110:138, 1989.

102. Kreiger JW, Kaiser DL, Wenzel RP: Urinary tract etiology of bloodstream infections in hospitalized patients. *J Infect Dig* 148:57, 1983.

103. Burns JR, Gregory JG: Osteomyelitis of the pubis symphysis after urologic surgery. *J Urol* 118:803, 1977.

104. Sequeira W: Diseases of the pubic symphysis. *Sem Arthr Rheum* 16(1):21, 1986.

105. Sapico FL, Montgomerie JZ: Pyogenic vertebral osteomyelitis: Report of nine cases and review of the literature. *Rev Infect Dig* 1:754, 1979.

106. Edelstein H, McCabe RE: Perinephric abscess. Modern diagnosis and treatment in 47 cases. *Medicine* 67:118, 1988.

107. Weinberger M, Cytron S, Servadio C et al: Prostatic abscess in the antibiotic era. Department of Internal Medicine, Belilinson Medical Center, Petah Tiqva, Israel. *Rev Infect Dis* 10(2):239–249, 1988.

108. Hull RD, Ragkob GE, Gent M et al: Effectiveness of intermittent pneumatic leg compression for preventing deep-vein thrombosis after total hip replacement. *JAMA* 263:2313, 1990.

109. Michelson JF, Lotke PA, Steinberg ME: Urinary bladder management after joint replacement surgery. *N Engl J Med* 319:321, 1988.

110. Inman RD, Gallegos KV, Brause BD et al: Clinical and microbial features of prosthetic joint infection. *Am J Med* 77:47, 1984.

111. Speller DCE: Microbiology of infected joint prostheses. *Sem Orthop* 1:19, 1986.

112. Petty W, Bryan RS, Coventry MB et al: Infection after total knee arthroplasty. *Orthop Clin NA* 6:1005, 1975.

113. Dellinger EP, Miller SD, Wertz MJ et al: Risk of infection after open fracture of the arm or leg. *Arch Surg* 123:1320, 1988.

114. Benson DR, Riggins RS, Lawrence RM: Treatment of open fractures. A prospective study. *J Trauma* 23:25, 1983.

115. Roth AI, Fry DE, Polk HC: Infectious morbidity in extremity fractures. *J Trauma* 26:757, 1986.

116. Brook I: A 12-year study of aerobic and anaerobic bacteria in intraabdominal and postsurgical abdominal wound infections. *Surg Gyneco Obstet* 169:387, 1989.

117. DiPiro JT, Mansberger JA, Davis JB: Current concepts in clinical therapeutics: Intraabdominal infections. *Clin Pharm* 5:34, 1986.
118. Calandra T, Bille J, Schraeder R et al: Clinical significance of *Candida* isolated from peritoneal fluid in surgical patients. *Lancet* 2:1437, 1989.
119. Nicholas RL: Infections following gastrointestinal surgery: Intraabdominal abscess. *Surg Clin N Am* 60:197, 1980.
120. Malagelada JR, Go VLW, Remine WH et al: Postsurgical complications involving the pancreas. *Clin Gastroenterol* 8:455, 1979.

53 PERIOPERATIVE HYPOTENSION

Michael J. Neary

Hypotension in the postoperative period is a common clinical problem with a number of possible etiologies. Determining its mechanism in the individual patient can be complex and frequently requires the input of the surgeon, anesthesiologist, internist, and critical care specialist before effective therapy can be initiated. This chapter briefly reviews the physiologic determinants of blood pressure, the systematic approach to the patient with postoperative hypotension, and the variety of therapeutic modalities available. The final section deals with the special problems presented by patients undergoing cardiac surgery.

DETERMINANTS OF BLOOD PRESSURE

Guyton defines blood pressure as the force exerted by the blood against any unit area of the vessel wall.[1] The factors determining that force include the cardiac preload, inotropic state, afterload, and heart rate. (see Fig. 53–1). Preload is defined as the pressure within the ventricle before contraction. Ventricular end-diastolic pressure is dependent upon venous return to the heart and the total blood volume and its distribution. Blood distribution is determined by body position and changes exerted by gravitational forces, intrathoracic pressure, and venous tone as modulated by the sympathetic nervous system. Inotropy refers to the intrinsic contractile state of the heart and is quantified by the rate at which contractile elements shorten (dP/dt).

Afterload has been defined by Braunwald et al. as the tension in the wall of the ventricle during ejection.[2] Impedance to ventricular ejection is determined by the physioanatomical characteristics of the ventricular outflow tract and the resistance of the pulmonary and systemic vasculature. The systemic vascular resistance can be calculated by the following equation:

$$SVR = [(MAP) - (RAP) / CO] \times 80 \text{ dyne/sec/cm}^2$$

where SVR is systemic vascular resistance, MAP is mean arterial pressure, RAP is right atrial pressure, CO is cardiac output, and 80 is a conversion factor. Cardiac output can be measured at the bedside by thermodilution using a pulmonary artery catheter.

Heart rate affects blood pressure through its effect on cardiac output. At a given constant stroke volume, there is a linear relationship between heart rate and cardiac output. In patients with myocardial dysfunction unable to increase stroke volume, tachyarrhythmias decrease available time for ventricular filling during diastole and thereby reduce cardiac output. They also increase oxygen demand by the myocardium, increasing the risk of ischemia. In atrial fibrillation, in which adequate atrial contraction is absent, up to 40% of the cardiac stroke volume can be lost.

APPROACH TO THE PATIENT WITH POSTOPERATIVE HYPOTENSION

Diagnostic Considerations

Once postoperative hypotension is recognized and confirmed, a brief determination of mental status should be made to judge the adequacy of cerebral perfusion. Further physical examination should assess the quality of the heart sounds, strength of the peripheral pulses, and briskness of capillary refill as indicators of peripheral perfusion. It is important to evaluate the patient's ventilatory status and ability to protect his airway. Hypotension is often heralded by nausea, vomiting, and diminished mentation, which predispose the patient to aspiration of gastric material. The decision to institute ventilatory support is determined by a number of criteria reviewed elsewhere and is also dictated by the particulars of a given clinical situation. The use of positive pressure ventilation and positive end-expiratory pressure (PEEP) further compromise blood pressure, decreasing venous return and the dimensions of the left ventricle to limit stroke volume.

The clinician should systematically consider possible etiologies of hypotension. The following guidelines may be useful:

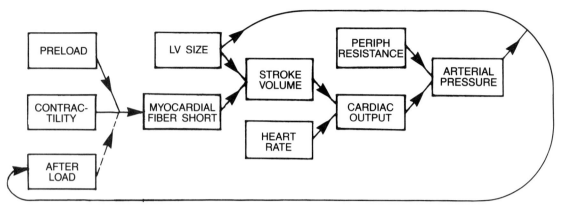

FIGURE 53–1. Factors determining systemic arterial pressure.

Source: From Braunwald E: Regulation of the circulation. *N Engl J Med* 290:1124, 1974.

1. *Is the blood pressure reading accurate?* A blood pressure cuff of improper size may distort the actual pressure. Intraarterial lines should be checked for patency and the transducers accurately zeroed.

2. *Is hypotension due to obvious or occult blood loss?* In the absence of blood-saturated dressings, unrecognized occult bleeding into a major body cavity or limb should be considered. Measurement of hemoglobin level is clearly important.

3. *Is hypotension due to myocardial dysfunction?* Patients with a history of prior myocardial infarction or multiple risk factors require special consideration. Cardiac rhythm should be evaluated and a 12-lead ECG obtained in all patients.

4. *Is hypotension due to bacteremia or sepsis?* Even in the absence of fever or leukocytosis, infection is a major consideration in many surgical settings. Appropriate cultures should be obtained and decisions regarding antibiotic therapy made promptly.

5. *Is hypotension a direct result of an anesthetic agent or technique?* Ascending subarachnoid or epidural blockade, rapid uptake of local anesthetic, or direct effects of analgesics, sedatives, or anesthetic agents should be considered.

6. *Are other pharmacologic agents responsible for hypotension?* Medication lists should be reviewed to look for antianginal agents, diuretics, analgesics, and sedatives.

7. *Is hypotension a manifestation of an allergic or anaphylactoid reaction?* Rash, swelling, and airway compromise are helpful when present, but are not always apparent. Review of the medication list and allergic history are mandatory.

8. *Does endocrinologic dysfunction account for or contribute to hypotension?* Hypothyroidism, diabetes mellitus, and adrenal insufficiency require consideration. Exogenous corticosteroid administration may not result in clinical stigmata and often requires careful questioning for historical documentation.

The patient's history, examination, and clinical course provide information needed to narrow the differential diagnosis of postoperative hypotension. Laboratory data required to complete this evaluation should include a hemoglobin or hematocrit level, white blood cell count and differential, serum electrolyte levels, arterial blood gas measurements, a 12-lead electrocardiogram, and appropriate cultures.

Monitoring

Monitoring is a central issue in following patients with hypotension. Clinical experience, judgment, and common sense as well as knowledge of the resources available at a given institution are required. Invasive monitoring techniques carry substantial morbidity that must be critically weighed against the potential value of the information obtained.[3,4]

All hypotensive patients require electrocardiographic monitoring to follow heart rate continuously and detect arrhythmias, ischemia, and conduction blocks. Abnormalities should be confirmed by 12-lead ECG. If the clinical situation warrants beat-to-beat measurement of blood pressure and frequent sampling of arterial blood, an indwelling arterial catheter may be placed. This allows display of the actual pressure wave and numeric values of systolic, mean, and diastolic pressures. Decisions regarding placement of a central venous or pulmonary artery line should be made on an individual basis. Pulmonary artery monitoring lines allow determination of preload by direct measurement of cardiac filling pressures, contractility by thermodilution, and afterload by derivation from the above measurements. They also allow for collection of data to calculate other hemodynamic variables[5] and sampling of blood for mixed venous gas determinations. Indications for placement of a pulmonary artery catheter are listed in Table 53–1. Central venous access is useful when otherwise irritating vasoactive or cardioactive agents must be given.

Therapeutic Considerations

The threshold level of blood pressure at which intervention is necessary is not absolute, especially in unconscious or anesthetized patients unable to provide important information. Patients can be asymptomatic with a systolic pressure of 70 torr, while others manifest signs of hypotension at much higher pressures if they have been chronically hypertensive in the past. Nevertheless, a decrease of 20% from the usual measured blood pressure as ascertained from the clinical record is frequently used as an empiric threshold for therapeutic intervention.

TABLE 53–1. Indications for Placement of a Pulmonary Artery Catheter

1. Cardiac dysfunction
   a. myocardial ischemia
   b. valvular heart disease
   c. cardiomyopathy
2. Management of intravascular volume replacement
3. Administration of vasoactive drugs
4. Specialized indications
   a. mixed venous oximetry
   b. cardiac pacing
   c. determination of cardiac output by thermodilution
5. Diagnostic problems
   a. cardiogenic versus noncardiogenic pulmonary edema
   b. right ventricular infarction
   c. pericardial tamponade

HYPOTENSION DUE TO DECREASED PRELOAD (HYPOVOLEMIA)

Decrease in circulating volume after surgery can result from blood loss, fluid shift to extravascular compartments, or vasodilation. Hemorrhage is an ever-present concern in the surgical setting. Its consequences depend on the patient's preoperative condition, the degree and rate of blood loss, and the site of the procedure. An expanding hematoma in the neck of a 75-year-old man after carotid endarterectomy and a bleeding tonsillar bed in an 8-year-old child after tonsillectomy are similar in terms of airway management but quite different in the ability to tolerate hypotension and decreased cerebral blood flow.

Fluid shifts from the intravascular to the interstitial compartment are the result of imbalance in the components of the Starling equation:

$$Q = K \left[(P_{MV} - P_{PMV}) - \sigma (\pi_{MV} - \pi_{PMV}) \right]$$

where Q is the net transvascular fluid filtration rate; K is the fluid conductance of the microvascular barrier; P is the hydrostatic pressure in the microvascular (mv) lumen and in the perimicrovascular (pmv) interstitial fluid space, respectively; σ is the reflection coefficient representing the resistance of the microvascular barrier to protein leakage; and π_{MV} and π_{PMV} are the osmotic pressure of protein in the microvascular and perimicrovascular fluids, respectively. These factors are influenced by nutritional status and underlying disorders affecting protein synthesis as well as by pathologic processes affecting cell membranes like peritonitis or ARDS.

Vasodilation leads to increases in the volume of the intravascular compartment, rendering the patient relatively hypovolemic. Changes in vascular tone are usually due to pharmacologic interventions, changes in core temperature, and allergic reactions. Sodium nitroprusside, nitroglycerin preparations, and trimethaphan camsylate are often used to lower blood pressure in the treatment of cardiac ischemia or congestive failure and can often overshoot target blood pressures. This is especially common in those who are relatively hypovolemic. Many oral antihypertensive agents, including calcium channel blockers, alpha-adrenergic blockers, and angiotensin-converting enzyme inhibitors, can cause significant

vasodilation. Opiates, especially morphine, are well-known venodilators and frequently require concurrent fluid therapy. Morphine causes histamine-medicated venodilation, thereby decreasing cardiac preload. When coupled with decreased endogenous catecholamine release, it can result in significant hypotension.[6] This effect can be exacerbated if a benzodiazepine sedative is administered simultaneously.[7]

Hypothermia is common in patients who have sustained trauma in cold environments, in those who have undergone major procedures in cold operating rooms, and in those undergoing open-heart procedures in whom it is deliberately induced. These patients usually require volume replacement over and above ongoing losses. Hypothermia due to myxedema should not be overlooked.

Allergic reactions and certainly anaphylaxis can cause life-threatening hypotension due to vascular dilation. Discontinuation of the offending agent; protection of the airway; oxygen administration; repletion of intravascular volume; and administration of epinephrine, alpha-adrenergic agents, antihistamines, and steroids are the mainstays of therapy.[8]

Positive pressure ventilation, especially when positive end-expiratory pressure (PEEP) is utilized, lowers blood pressure by decreasing venous return to the right heart, thereby reducing preload and cardiac output. This has been well studied in animal models and humans.[9,10] Fluid administration augments ventricular filling and normalizes cardiac output.[11] However, other mechanisms have been implicated in PEEP-induced hypotension. PEEP increases right ventricular afterload and limits stroke volume by causing a leftward shift of the intraventricular septum.[9] In addition, PEEP is associated with decreased subendocardial blood flow in dogs.[12] Cross-circulation studies also show that humoral agents liberated from the lung mediate decreased cardiovascular function.[13]

Cardiac tamponade can be considered a special subset of hemorrhage, and is seen in four percent of cardiac procedures.[14] It can occur in the first few hours after surgery or several days later, especially after anticoagulant therapy has been initiated.[15] It can also be a consequence of chest trauma, aortic dissection, or acute myocardial infarction. Cardiac tamponade is characterized by elevated central venous pressure, equalization of right- and left-sided diastolic filling pressures, and prominent systolic x descent and an attenuated y descent on the pulmonary artery catheter tracing. Pulsus paradoxus is variably present. Electrical alternans and decreased voltages may be seen on the ECG. Echocardiography is usually diagnostic. Therapy consists of increasing preload with fluid administration and pericardiocentesis if necessary.

Fluid Replacement Therapy

The best fluid to use to treat hypovolemia remains controversial.[16–18] Some clinical studies support the use of colloid;[19–21] others champion the use of crystalloid;[22] and several state that there is no real difference in terms of morbidity and mortality.[18,23,24] A favorable outcome depends more on the timeliness of fluid administration than on the composition of the fluid.[16,17]

The advantages of crystalloid solutions include modest cost, ready availability, compatibility with most pharmacologic agents, lack of allergic reactions, and low risk of transmission of infection. Current practice dictates that crystalloid and colloid solutions should be given in a ratio of 3:1 in order to maintain the integrity of the intravascular compartment in the face of ongoing hemorrhage.[16,18,23] Equilibration between intravascular and extravascular compartments occurs within 20 to 30 minutes after infusion of an isotonic crystalloid solution.[16] Less than 20% of the original volume infused remains in the intravascular compartment one to two hours later.[25]

Albumin in 5% and 25% solutions, 6% hetastarch, and low-molecular-weight dextran (Dextran 40) are commonly used colloidal solutions. Albumin solutions have been used as volume expanders for over 50 years. The plasma half-life of albumin is 16 hours and is similar to that of endogenously produced albumin.[26] Hydroxyethyl starch or hetastarch is a synthetic starch with an average molecular weight of 69,000, closely resembling glycogen. It is available for infusion in a 6% solution and has plasma-expanding properties similar to those of albumin.[27] There have been reports of mild coagulopathies when more than 1500 ml have been administered in a 24-hour period. The risk of anaphylactic reactions is less than .085 percent per unit infused.[28] Hetastarch acts as an osmotic diuretic and is excreted by the kidneys.[27]

Dextran is a branched-chain polysaccharide available in a number of molecular weights. In the United States, low-molecular-weight dextran (MW = 40,000) is most commonly used. Like hydroxyethyl starch, it is osmotically active and remains in the intravascular compartment for a prolonged period of time. The use of dextran has been greatly hindered by early reports of anaphylaxis usually associated with the high-molecular-weight form. Anaphylaxis is related to the presence of dextran antibodies of the IgG class. Difficulty in cross-matching blood after use of high-molecular-weight dextran solution has also been noted.

The incidence of severe dextran-induced allergic reactions in two large retrospective studies was found to be in the range of 0.002 to 0.013 percent per unit infused for Dextran-40 and 0.017 to 0.025 percent for Dextran-60/75.[28,29] In a smaller prospective study of low-dose heparin and Dextran-70 administered as prophylaxis against thromboembolic complications, the incidence of severe reactions was 0.25 percent per patient treated.[30] Anaphylaxis due to hetastarch and albumin is only slightly less common than similar reactions to low-molecular-weight dextran.[28] However, reactions to albumin are usually mild and limited to urticaria, fever, and chills.

A very-low-molecular-weight dextran (MW = 1000), marketed under the name Promit-R, reduces the risk of anaphylactic reactions when given before higher-molecular-weight dextrans. It acts as a hapten and occupies the majority of the binding sites on the dextran-reactive antibodies in the serum, thereby preventing antigen-antibody crosslinking, complement activation, and amplification of the allergic reaction. It should be administered intravenously 2 to 20 minutes before antigenic challenge. Allergic reactions to this low-molecular-weight product are rare.[31]

Colloidal solutions are usually available in most institutions and act more quickly to replete the intravascular compartment, because they do not cross the normal capillary-endothelial barrier. However, they are more expensive.[26] Theoretically, they can escape into the interstitial space when capillary permeability is increased. They should therefore be avoided in disease states such as ARDS, sepsis, intestinal obstruction, and burns.[32,33]

In summary, either isotonic crystalloid or colloid solutions can be used for fluid replacement. However, this author prefers crystalloids in routine clinical situations and a colloid, usually 6% hetastarch, when rapid repletion of the intravascular compartment is desired.

Blood Product Transfusions

The decision to transfuse packed red blood cells or other blood products requires careful consideration. Patients who have lost 10 percent of their blood volume, or about 500 ml, can usually be replaced with full-strength crystalloid or colloidal solutions.[34] Those who sustain acute blood losses of 20 to 30 percent usually exhibit tachycardia, decreased systolic blood pressure, decreased stroke volume as shown by a narrow pulse pressure, blanching of cutaneous capillary beds, and oliguria, and require blood transfusion. Losses in excess of 40 percent are life-threatening and are accompanied by worsening oliguria, decreased cerebral perfusion, respiratory failure, and lactic acidosis. Acute, unreplaced losses of 50 percent or more are usually fatal. Factors in the decision to transfuse include the degree of anemia, its duration, the surgical procedure, the probability of continued blood loss, and coexisting cardiopulmonary, cerebrovascular, and peripheral vascular disease.

There are no carefully controlled randomized trials providing definitive guidelines for perioperative transfusion.[35] The traditional transfusion threshold level of a hemoglobin of 10 g is no longer universally accepted. Transfusing patients with levels between 7 and 10 g is a matter of clinical judgment in the individual patient. Hemodilution studies have helped to define morbidity and mortality rates in these situations.[36–39] The use of a hemoglobin level of 7 g as a threshold is based on studies showing that below this level cardiac output rises dramatically to compensate for decreased oxygen-carrying capacity. The advantages of decreased blood viscosity and increased capillary flow produced by hemodilution are offset by decreased oxygen-carrying capacity.[40] However, in cases of major trauma or extensive surgical bleeding, repletion of intravascular volume is paramount, and clinical judgment should guide decisions to initiate transfusion.

In view of current concerns regarding the transmission of infection, alternatives such as autotransfusion have become popular. Devices to scavenge and reinfuse a patient's own blood have found wide application.[41–43]

HYPOTENSION DUE TO DECREASED CARDIAC INOTROPY

Surgery, anesthesia, and complications of underlying disease decrease myocardial function in the perioperative period in patients with coronary artery disease. Dysfunction is due to an imbalance between myocardial oxygen supply and demand. When volume replacement is unsuccessful or contraindicated, a number of inotropic agents can be used to improve cardiac function, depending on the pathophysiology of the underlying situation.[44,45] This discussion excludes antianginal agents and digoxin, which may be required in particular situations.

Pharmacologic Interventions

Phenylephrine

Some practitioners administer small amounts of alpha-adrenergic agents like phenylephrine to patients with a high likelihood of having underlying cardiac disease who have undergone surgical procedures. Phenylephrine contracts the vascular space, facilitates fluid replacement, and rapidly raises the mean arterial pressure to improve coronary artery and cerebral perfusion. It is usually administered in boluses of 25 to 100 μg through a central venous line and may be repeated. It should be emphasized that the use of phenylephrine is only a temporizing measure until more definitive therapy is initiated. Concern is frequently expressed regarding the effect of alpha-adrenergic stimulation on arterioles in the kidney. However, transient use of phenylephrine to support blood pressure does little to affect renal function.

Calcium

Low serum concentrations of ionized calcium are associated with left ventricular depression and decreased peripheral vascular resistance. In the postoperative setting, hypocalcemia can result from administration of heparin[46] and albumin[47,48] and transfusion of blood preserved with citrate.[49] It is also frequently seen during and after cardiac surgery.[50]

Calcium ions increase myocardial contractility and have a variable effect on systemic vascular resistance. Intravenous administration of calcium produces a predictable but transient rise in systemic arterial pressure.[51] However, its use in cardiac resuscitation has been deemphasized because of concern that it can induce cardiac reperfusion injury as well as coronary and cerebral vasospasm.[52] The use of calcium chloride is probably best confined to the treatment of acute hyperkalemia or hypotension in hypocalcemic patients receiving calcium channel blockers.

Dopamine

Dopamine is useful in a wide range of clinical situations,[53] including cardiogenic shock,[54] congestive heart failure,[55] and following cardiac surgery. The hemodynamic effects of dopamine are modulated by release of norepinephrine from sympathetic nerve endings and direct stimulation of alpha, beta, and dopaminergic receptors. Dopamine has three pharmacologic dose ranges.[56] At doses of 0.5 to 2.0 μg/kg/min, renal blood flow and urine output increases while total peripheral resistance decreases. At 3 to 10 μg/kg/min, beta-adrenergic effects predominate with an increase in inotropy and chronotropy that augment cardiac output. At 10 μg/kg/min and above, alpha-adrenergic effects increase total peripheral resistance.

Dopamine is used widely in a variety of clinical situations, particularly when an increase in renal blood flow is desired. Disadvantages include the risk of developing tachyarrhythmias and extrasystoles in susceptible patients.

Dobutamine

Like isoproterenol, dobutamine decreases peripheral vascular resistance and has powerful inotropic properties without the tendency to cause the tachycardia seen with dopamine.[57] Because of this, it is useful in low cardiac output states when increases in left ventricular end-diastolic volume and pulmonary vascular resistance are not desirable.[57] In a study comparing dopamine and dobutamine in patients with heart failure, Leier et al. noted that dobutamine increases cardiac output by augmenting stroke volume when used at doses up to 10 μg/kg/min. However, dopamine in doses over 4 μg/kg/min no longer does so and increases heart rate, pulmonary wedge pressure, and the number of ventricular ectopic beats.[58] Dobutamine does not affect renal blood flow or promote diuresis other than by increasing cardiac output.[58]

Dobutamine is most useful when cardiac output is low because of decreased inotropy accompanied by increased filling pressures or afterload. Since it lacks significant vasoconstrictive properties,

it may not be appropriate in many hypotensive patients. It may in fact decrease blood pressure even while improving other hemodynamic indices.[58]

Epinephrine

Epinephrine is a naturally occurring catecholamine found in the adrenal medulla. Because of its beta$_1$, beta$_2$, and alpha-adrenergic properties, it increases cardiac contractility, augments systolic and mean blood pressures, and serves as an effective bronchodilator. It is usually administered as an infusion beginning at a dose of 0.005 to 0.02 μg/kg/min, and titrating up or down to achieve desired cardiac output and blood pressure. In cardiopulmonary resuscitation, it is effective when instilled through an endotracheal tube. However, the plasma concentration and hemodynamic effects of the drug after tracheal administration are about 10 percent of those observed after a similar intravenous dose.[44]

Amrinone

Amrinone is a noncatecholamine inotropic agent with hemodynamic properties similar to those of dobutamine. It increases cardiac inotropy and slightly decreases total peripheral resistance, thereby improving cardiac output.[59] Amrinone inhibits phosphodiesterase to increase cyclic AMP in the sarcomere. This results in increased uptake, storage, and release of calcium by the sarcoplasmic reticulum during excitation-contraction coupling.

The use of amrinone in clinical medicine has not been defined, and experience with it is limited. It may increase myocardial oxygen consumption less than other inotropes. The mean half-life of amrinone is 3.6 hours in normal subjects but is prolonged in patients with congestive heart failure to five to eight hours.[60] It should be prepared in saline solutions because it is inactivated by those containing glucose.

Norepinephrine

Norepinephrine (levarterenol bitartrate) is identical to that found in the adrenal medulla and postganglionic sympathetic nerve endings. It exhibits beta-adrenergic properties at infusion rates under 5 μg/min, but has intense alpha-adrenergic effects at higher doses which modulate increases in peripheral vascular resistance.

Norepinephrine is used when hypotension is refractory to less potent agents and adequate fluid replacement. In such cases, it may raise diastolic pressure to 70 to 80 torr, enough to ensure adequate coronary artery blood flow. It can also be used to increase peripheral vascular resistance in septic states. However, administration of norepinephrine is potentially risky because it produces intense vasoconstriction, increases afterload enough to increase myocardial oxygen demand, and can compromise renal blood flow.

HYPOTENSION DUE TO DECREASED TOTAL PERIPHERAL RESISTANCE

Decreases in peripheral vascular resistance are less common than decreases in preload or inotropy. Some reduction in total peripheral resistance is seen in patients during corporeal rewarming, but it is usually the result of pharmacologic agents such as hydralazine and nitroprusside. Anaphylaxis also produces a profound decrease in total peripheral resistance. Hypotension in sepsis is due to a decrease in total peripheral resistance and probably to depression of myocardial function as well.[61,62] Fluid and vasopressors are frequently required, but measures to treat underlying infection including appropriate antibiotics are crucial.

HYPOTENSION AFTER CARDIAC SURGERY

Patients undergoing coronary artery bypass grafting (CABG), correction of congenital anomalies, and valvular replacement present unique challenges in the postoperative period. However, nearly all have undergone preoperative cardiac catheterization and come to surgery with a large data base regarding their coronary anatomy and ventricular function. In addition, any difficulty in weaning from cardiopulmonary bypass provides important information in anticipating difficulties in the postoperative period. Invasive monitoring allows measurement of all hemodynamic parameters with pulmonary artery and central venous pressure catheters or dedicated lines in specific cardiac chambers.

Virtually all patients undergoing open-heart surgery have biventricular dysfunction for at least 24 hours after the procedure.[63] Corporeal rewarming in the first few hours causes vasodilation requiring volume repletion with crystalloid, colloid, or blood products. Since hypothermia itself increases systemic venous tone and thereby decreases venous capacity, venodilators like nitroglycerin and nitroprusside may reverse these effects and enhance rewarming. However, if vasodilator therapy is inadequate, hypothermic patients may initially display normal blood pressure but will have high SVR, decreased intravascular volume, low cardiac output, and reduced mixed-venous oxygen saturation. In such cases, interventions such as rapid rewarming that cause sudden decreases in SVR and increases in venous capacity produce more severe hypotension in the face of decreased cardiac output. Such patients commonly have preexisting left ventricular dysfunction that, when compounded by hypothermia, cardioplegic arrest, or any myocardial damage, produces the so-called "stunned myocardium." Many require inotropic support with dopamine, dobutamine, epinephrine, or amrinone. Other causes of hypotension peculiar to these patients include medications like protamine or other vasoactive drugs such as nitroprusside, nitroglycerin, nifedipine, and hydralazine. In hypotensive patients with postoperative cardiac dysfunction, the intra-aortic balloon pump may provide inotropic support with no increase in myocardial oxygen consumption, but this is not without risk.[64-66]

Pericardial tamponade commonly occurs after cardiac surgery despite adequately functioning pleural or mediastinal chest tubes. Even leaving open the pericardium at the time of chest closure does not completely protect against tamponade. The diagnosis of cardiac tamponade can be difficult to make. Widening of the mediastinum on chest x-ray is a rather nonspecific finding because it is seen in essentially all postoperative heart patients. Equalization of left and right heart pressures as determined by the pulmonary arterial catheter is suggestive of tamponade. Bedside echocardiography is most helpful but may not be absolutely diagnostic. Surgical exploration may be needed when cardiac tamponade is suspected. Other hypotensive patients who may require reoperation include those with postoperative ischemia after CABG and those with valvular leak or dysfunction after placement of a prosthesis.

SUMMARY

1. Effective diagnosis of postoperative hypotension requires understanding the physiologic parameters of preload, inotropy, afterload, and heart rate and systematically considering a wide and complex differential diagnosis.

2. Overall treatment rests on careful monitoring, specific therapy of the underlying disease, and a careful balance of fluid and appropriate vasopressors when necessary.

3. Either isotonic crystalloid or colloid solutions are acceptable alternatives for fluid replacement.

4. Phenylephrine and cardiac inotropic agents such as calcium, dopamine, dobutamine, epinephrine, and amrinone should be chosen on the basis of their specific hemodynamic effects.

REFERENCES

1. Guyton AC: *Arterial Pressure and Hypertension.* Philadelphia, Saunders, 1980, pp 276–283.
2. Braunwald E: *Mechanisms of Contraction of the Normal and Failing Heart,* 2d ed. Boston, Little Brown, 1976.
3. Paulson DM, Scott SM, Sethi GK: Pulmonary hemorrhage associated with balloon flotation catheters: A report of a case and review of the literature. *J Thorac Cardiovasc Surg* 80:453, 1980.
4. Sprung CL, Jacobs LJ, Caralis PV et al: Ventricular arrhythmias during Swan-Ganz catheterization of the critically ill. *Chest* 79:413, 1981.
5. Sonnenblick EH, Strobeck JE: Current concepts in cardiology: Derived indexes of ventricular and myocardial function. *N Engl J Med* 296:978, 1977.
6. Lowenstein E, Hallowell P, Levine FH et al: Cardiovascular response to large doses of intravenous morphine in man. *N Engl J Med* 281: 1389–1393, 1969.
7. Hoar PF, Nelson NT, Mangano DT et al: Adrenergic response to morphine-diazepam anesthesia for myocardial revascularization. *Anesth Analg* 60:406–411, 1981.
8. Giansiracusa DF, Upchurch KS: Anaphylactic and anaphylactoid reactions. *Intens Care Med* 16:1102–1112, 1985.
9. Scharff SM, Caldini P, Ingram RH Jr: Cardiovascular effects of increasing airway pressure in the dog. *Am J Physiol* 232:H35, 1977.
10. Jardin F, Farcot JC, Boisante L et al: Influence of positive end-expiratory pressure on left ventricular performance. *N Engl J Med* 304:387, 1981.
11. Walkinshaw M, Shoemaker WC: Use of volume loading to obtain preferred levels of PEEP: A preliminary study. *Crit Care Med* 8:81, 1980.
12. Manny J, Justice R, Hechtman HB: Abnormalities in organ blood flow and its distribution during positive end-expiratory pressure. *Surgery* 85:425, 1979.
13. Piper DJ, Vane JR: The release of prostaglandins from lung and other tissues. *Ann NY Acad Sci* 180:363, 1971.
14. Reddy PS, Curtiss EI, O'Toole JD et al: Cardiac tamponade: Hemodynamic observations in man. *Circulation* 58:265, 1978.
15. Borken AM, Schaff HV, Gardner TJ et al: Diagnosis and management of postoperative pericardial effusions and late cardiac tamponade following open-heart surgery. *Ann Thorac Surg* 31:512, 1981.
16. Hauser CJ, Shoemaker WC, Turpin I: Oxygen transport responses to colloids and crystalloids in critically ill surgical patients. *Surg Gynecol Obstet* 150:811–816, 1980.
17. Moss GS, Siegel DC, Cochin A et al: Effects of saline and colloid

solutions on pulmonary function in hemorrhagic shock. *Surg Gynecol Obstet* 133:53–58, 1971.

18. Virgilio RW, Rice CL, Smith DE et al: Crystalloid versus colloid resuscitation: Is one better? A randomized clinical study. *Surgery* 85:129–139, 1979.

19. Boutros AR, Reuss R, Olson L: Comparison of hemodynamic, pulmonary, and renal effects of use of three types of fluid after major surgical procedures on abdominal aorta. *Crit Care Med* 7:9–13, 1979.

20. Jelenko C III, Williams JB, Wheeler ML et al: Studies in shock and resuscitation: I. Use of a hypertonic, albumin-containing, fluid demand regimen (HALFD) in resuscitation: A physiologically appropriate method. *Crit Care Med* 7:157, 1979.

21. Skillman JJ, Restall DS, Salzman EW: Randomized trial of albumin versus electrolyte solutions during abdominal aortic operations. *Surgery* 78:291–303, 1975.

22. Granger DN, Gabel JC, Drahe RE, Taylor AD: Physiologic basis for the clinical use of albumin solutions. *Surg Gynecol Obstet* 146:97–104, 1978.

23. Metildi LA, Shackford SR, Virgilio RW et al: Crystalloid versus colloid in fluid resuscitation of patients with severe pulmonary insufficiency. *Surg Gynecol Obstet* 158:207–212, 1984.

24. Lowe RJ, Moss GS, Jilek J et al: Crystalloid versus colloid in the etiology of pulmonary failure after trauma: A randomized trial in man. *Surgery* 81:676–683, 1977.

25. Carey JS, Scharschmidt BF, Cuillford AT: Hemodynamic effectiveness of colloid and electrolyte solutions for replacement of stimulated operative blood loss. *Surg Gynecol Obstet* 131:679–686, 1970.

26. Tullis JL: Albumin: I. Background and use. *JAMA* 237:355–360, 1977.

27. Metcalf W, Papdopoulos A, Talano R: Clinical physiologic study of hydroxyethyl starch. *Surg Gynecol Obstet* 131:255–267, 1970.

28. Ring J, Messmer K: Incidence and severity of anaphylactoid reactions of colloid volume substitutes. *Lancet* 1:466–469, 1977.

29. Ljungstroem KG, Renck H, Strandberg K et al: Adverse reactions to dextran in Sweden 1970–1979. *Acta Chir Scand* 149:253–262, 1983.

30. Gaggiano V: Red blood cell transfusions, in Silver H (ed): *Blood, Blood Components and Derivatives in Transfusion Therapy*. Washington DC, American Association of Blood Banks, 1980, pp 1–28.

31. Renck H, Ljungstroem KG, Hedin H et al: Prevention of dextran-induced–anaphylactic reactions by hapten inhibition. A Scandinavian multicenter study of the effects of 20 ml Dextran 1, 15%, administered before Dextran 70 or Dextran 40. *Acta Chir Scand* 149:355–360, 1983.

32. Esrig BC, Fulton RL: Sepsis, resuscitated hemorrhagic shock and "shock lung." An experimental correlation. *Ann Surg* 182:218–227, 1975.

33. Rowe MI, Arango A: Colloid versus crystalloid resuscitation in experimental bowel obstruction. *J Pediatr Surg* 11:635–643, 1976.

34. Shoemaker WC, Schluchter M, Hopkins JA: Fluid therapy in emergency resuscitation: Clinical evaluation of colloid and crystalloid regimens. *Crit Care Med* 9:367–368, 1981.

35. National Institutes of Health Consensus Development Conference Statement: *Perioperative Red Cell Transfusion*. Bethesda, US Department of Health and Human Services, 1988, no 7, p 4.

36. Chapler CK, Cain SM: The physiologic reserve in oxygen-carrying capacity: Studies in experimental hemodilution. *Can J Physiol Pharmacol* 64:7–12, 1986.

37. Crystal GJ, Salem MR: Myocardial oxygen consumption and segmental shortening during selective coronary hemodilution in dogs. *Anesth Analg* 67:500–508, 1988.

38. Czer LSC, Shoemaker WC: Optimal hematocrit value in critically ill postoperative patients. *Surg Gynecol Obstet* 147:363, 1978.

39. Martin E, Hansen E, Peter K: Acute limited normovolemic hemodilution: A method for avoiding homologous transfusion. *World J Surg* 11:53, 1987.

40. Most AS, Ruocco NA Jr, Gerwirtz H: Effect of a reduction in blood viscosity on maximal myocardial oxygen delivery distal to a moderate coronary stenosis. *Circulation* 74:1085–1092, 1986.

41. Cutler BS: Avoidance of homologous transfusion in aortic operations: The role of autotransfusion, hemodilution, and surgical technique. *Surgery* 95:717–723, 1984.

42. Hallet JW Jr, Popovsky M, Ilstrup D: Minimizing blood transfusions during abdominal aortic surgery: Recent advancements in rapid autotransfusion. *J Vasc Surg* 5:601–606, 1987.

43. Stanton PE Jr, Shannon J, Rosenthal D et al: Intraoperative autologous transfusion during major aortic reconstructive procedures. *South Med J* 80:315–319, 1987.

44. Chernow B, Rainey TG, Lake CR: Endogenous and exogenous catecholamines. *Crit Care Med* 10:409, 1982.

45. Colucci WS, Wright RF, Braunwald E: New positive inotropic agents in the treatment of congestive heart failure: Mechanisms of action and recent clinical developments. *N Engl J Med* 314:290–349, 1986.

46. Urban P, Scheidegger D, Buchmann B, Skarvan K: The hemodynamic effects of heparin and their relation to ionized calcium levels. *J Thorac Cardiovasc Surg* 91:303, 1986.

47. Dahn MS, Lucas CE, Ledgerwood AM et al: Negative inotropic effect of albumin resuscitation for shock. *Surgery* 86:235, 1979.

48. Kovalik SG, Ledgerwood AM, Lucas CE et al: The cardiac effect of altered calcium homeostasis after albumin resuscitation. *J Trauma* 21:275, 1981.

49. Kahn RC, Jascott D, Carlon GC et al: Massive blood replacement: Correlation of ionized calcium, citrate, and hydrogen ion concentration. *Anesth Analg* 58:274–278, 1979.

50. Catinella FP, Cunningham JN, Strauss ED et al: Variations in total and ionized calcium during cardiac surgery. *J Cardiovasc Surg* 24:593–602, 1983.

51. Gallagher JD, Geller EA, Moore RA et al: Hemodynamic effects of calcium chloride in adults with regurgitant valve lesions. *Anesth Analg* 63:723, 1984.

52. Dembo DH: Calcium in advanced life support. *Crit Care Med* 9:358, 1981.

53. Goldberg LI: Dopamine—clinical uses of an endogenous catecholamine. *N Engl J Med* 291:707, 1974.

54. Sturm JT, Fuhrman TM, Sterling R et al: Combined use of dopamine and nitroprusside therapy in conjunction with intraaortic balloon pumping for the treatment of postcardiotomy low-output syndrome. *J Thorac Cardiovasc Surg* 82:13, 1981.

55. Loeb HS, Ostrenga JP, Gaul W et al: Beneficial effects of dopamine combined with intravenous nitroglycerin on hemodynamics in patients with severe left ventricular failure. *Circulation* 68:813, 1983.

56. Goldberg LI, Rajfer SI: Dopamine receptors: Applications in clinical cardiology. *Circulation* 72:245, 1985.

57. Sonnenblick EH, Frishman WH, LeJemtel TH: Dobutamine, a new synthetic cardioactive sympathetic amine. *N Engl J Med* 300:17, 1979.

58. Leier CV, Heban PT, Huss P et al: Comparative systemic and regional effects of dopamine and dobutamine in patients with cardiomyopathic heart failure. *Circulation* 58:466, 1978.

59. Konstam MA, Cohen SR, Weiland DS et al: Relative contribution of inotropic and vasodilator effects to amrinone-induced hemodynamic improvement in congestive heart failure. *Am J Cardiol* 57:242, 1986.

60. Goldstein RA: Clinical effects of intravenous amrinone in patients with congestive heart failure. *Circulation* 73:111–191, 1986.

61. Parillo JE, Burch C, Shelhammer J et al: A circulating myocardial depressant substance in humans with septic shock: Septic shock patients with a reduced ejection fraction have a circulating factor that depresses myocardial cell performance. *J Clin Invest* 76:1539, 1985.

62. Parker MM, Shelhammer JH, Bacharach SL et al: Profound but reversible myocardial depression in patients with septic shock. *Ann Intern Med* 100:483, 1984.

63. Mangano DT: Biventricular function after myocardial revascularization in humans: Deterioration and recovery patterns during the first 24 hours. *Anesthesiology* 62(5):571, 1985.

64. Bergman D, Nichols AB, Weiss MB et al: Percutaneous intraaortic balloon insertion. *Am J Cardiol* 46:261, 1980.

65. Dunkman WB, Leinbach RC, Buckley MJ et al: Clinical and hemody-namic results of intraaortic balloon pumping and surgery for cardio-genic shock. *Circulation* 46:465, 1972.

66. LeFemine AA, Kosowsky B, Madoff I: Results and complications of intraaortic balloon pumping in surgical and medical patients. *Am J Cardiol* 40:416, 1977.

54 POSTOPERATIVE HYPERTENSION

Constance F. Neely

Hypertension is common after surgery and, when defined as a systolic blood pressure over 200 mmHg or a diastolic blood pressure over 100 mmHg, occurs in 3 to 73 percent of patients.[1–5] This chapter reviews the causes of postoperative hypertension and emphasizes contributing factors and their mechanisms. Hypertension following certain procedures is explored in detail. Guidelines on indications for treatment and available antihypertensive regimens are offered with a final section on the choice of agents in the immediate postoperative period.

INCIDENCE AND MECHANISMS

Except for patients undergoing coronary artery bypass surgery (CABG) or valve replacement, a history of hypertension before surgery is the single most important contributing factor in the development of hypertension thereafter.[1–3,5–7] In a series of 1844 patients, Gal and Cooperman reported the incidence of postoperative hypertension to be 3.25 percent, of whom 50 percent had a history of hypertension.[1] Other contributing factors included pain (36 percent), excitement on emergence from anesthesia (17 percent), reaction to the endotracheal tube (15 percent), hypercarbia (2 percent), hypothermia (7 percent), hypoxia (17 percent), and hypervolemia (7 percent). Eighty percent of hypertensive events occurred within 30 minutes of admission to the recovery room and resolved within three hours. Goldman and Caldera reported that hypertensive events occurred during or after 57 percent of abdominal aortic aneurysm resections, 29 percent of peripheral vascular procedures, 8 percent of intraabdominal or intrathoracic operations, and only 4 percent of other surgical procedures.[2] The only predictors of perioperative hypertension in this series were the type of operation and a history of previous hypertension with a diastolic blood pressure over 111 mmHg. Adequacy of blood pressure control before surgery and anesthetic technique were not significant predictors.[2] The data suggest that the incidence of postoperative hypertension is highest in patients following cardiac, aortic, and carotid artery surgery.[2,5,6,8] These procedures are reviewed in more detail to illustrate the mechanisms underlying postoperative hypertension.

Hypertension Following Carotid Artery Surgery

The incidence of sustained increase in systolic blood pressure above 200 mmHg is about 20 percent after carotid endarterectomy[5,9,10] and is as high as 79.6 percent in those with a history of hypertension in one series.[5] The maximal hypertensive response occurred at 2.3 hours after surgery with an average time of onset of 1.4 hours and persisted from 1 to 15 or an average of 5.6 hours.[5] The incidence of neurologic deficit was 10.2 percent in patients with sustained hypertension but only 3.4 percent in those who remained normotensive. Death occurred only in those with postoperative hypertension. However, it was not always clear whether postoperative hypertension followed a cerebrovascular event or caused it.[5]

In addition to preoperative hypertension, pain, agitation, new neurologic deficit, and alterations in baroreceptor function immediately following surgery can mediate changes in blood pressure and heart rate in patients undergoing carotid endarterectomy.[9] Baroreceptors lie in the adventitial tissue of the carotid sinus slightly above the bifurcation.[11] They carry afferent impulses to the vasomotor center in the lower brain stem and are affected by pulse pressure, carotid sinus diameter, and distensibility of the arterial wall. Baroreceptor impulses act on the vasomotor center to inhibit vasoconstriction and increase vagal activity. Excitation therefore causes a decrease in arterial pressure and heart rate.

During mobilization of the carotid bifurcation, intercarotid nerves may be damaged resulting in interruption of baroreceptor function and postoperative hypertension.[12] Surgical techniques to avoid dissection in this area have been advocated. However, in one series, nerve-sparing did not affect the incidence of postoperative hypertension.[5] Moreover, baroreceptor sensitivity decreases with advancing age, especially after age 40, and in chronic congestive heart failure, cerebrovascular disease, and diabetes mellitus,[5,13–15] but the contribution of these changes in baroreceptor sensitivity to the development of postoperative hypertension after carotid endarterectomy is difficult to ascertain. Patients undergoing staged bilateral carotid endarterectomies have a higher risk of postoperative hypertension, especially if the operations are performed more than 60 days apart.[16] Changes in baroreceptor sensitivity after stripping tumors from the carotid artery during radical neck surgery do not contribute to postoperative hypertension. The incidence of this complication in these patients is only 9.6 percent.[17]

Other causes of hypertension after carotid endarterectomy include cerebral or myocardial ischemia; withdrawal from drugs such as clonidine, propranolol, and nitroprusside; or abrupt discontinuation of inhalational anesthetics like isoflurane that act as potent systemic vasodilators. In one study, the use of isoflurane was correlated with postoperative hypertension,[18] and the authors suggested that inhalational anesthetics may contribute to postoperative hypertension by altering cerebral autoregulation. The hallmark of hypertension after carotid endarterectomy is increased sympathetic activity. This is supported by dog studies in which total epidural anesthesia blocked the hypertensive response following bilateral carotid occlusion.[19]

Hypertension Following Cardiac Surgery

The incidence of hypertension after cardiac surgery varies from 30 to 80 percent for coronary artery bypass grafting (CABG) and from 8 to 37 percent for valve replacement.[3,4,6,20,21] Estafanous et al. reported that hypertension after valve replacement, occurring in 8.1 percent, and myocardial revascularization, occurring in 33 percent, was associated with a decrease in central venous pressure and a mild increase in left atrial pressure.[3] Hypertension after mitral valve replacement, occurring in 5.9 percent, was noted within one hour and persisted for up to six hours. The incidence was slightly higher in patients with mitral stenosis, but none of the patients with mixed mitral valve disease developed it. The incidence was 12.1 percent after aortic valve replacement, occurring within five hours and lasting 6 to 12 hours. The incidence was similar in those with aortic stenosis or aortic regurgitation but was rare in those with mixed aortic valve disease.

In both CABG and valve replacement, preoperative hypertension was not a significant contributing factor in the development of postoperative hypertension. Improvement in ventricular function after surgery may play an important role, especially in the development of systolic hypertension. Cooper et al. reported hypertension in 37 percent after valve replacement and 62 percent after CABG. Patients receiving beta-blockers preoperatively and those with higher left ventricular ejection fractions had a greater risk of developing it.[6] The type of anesthetic, duration of cardiopulmonary bypass, and number of grafts do not affect the incidence of hypertension after CABG.[20]

Systemic vascular resistance is increased and cardiac output is normal in patients with systemic hypertension after cardiopulmonary bypass. Systemic vasoconstriction may be due to sympatho-adrenal-mediated responses, renin and angiotensin release, and other cardiac reflexes.[4,7,20-24] Elevated serum levels of epinephrine and norepinephrine have been documented after CABG.[4,7] The role of renin in mediating hypertension after CABG is controversial. Cardiac and great vessel pressor reflexes have been implicated in the mechanism of hypertension following cardiac surgery.[20,22] Sympathetic afferent impulses mediate increases in systemic vascular resistance, and unilateral stellate ganglion block reduces blood pressure and systemic vascular resistance without affecting cardiac output.[24]

Hypertension Following Aortic Surgery

Hypertension following repair of aortic coarctation was first described by Sealy in 1957.[25] Early postoperative hypertension is primarily systolic and occurs within 8 to 12 hours after surgery in 17 to 56 percent of patients.[20,25] As in CABG, it is associated with increases in serum norepinephrine levels. Intermediate postoperative hypertension begins 36 to 48 hours after surgery in 1 to 12 percent and is proportional to the degree of coarctation and the age of the patient.[20] It is characterized by a rise in diastolic blood pressure and tachycardia and may be accompanied by symptoms of an acute abdomen due to mesenteric arteritis. Mesenteric vessels, accustomed to a lower arterial pressure, are subjected to severe hypertension resulting in an endarteritis, vascular necrosis, and intestinal ischemia and infarction.[26] Release of norepinephrine, mediated by spinal sympathetic afferent impulses and subsequent release of renin, may play a role in the development of hypertension frequently seen after surgery on the ascending and descending aorta.

Hypertension Following Renal Transplantation

Hypertension following renal transplantation may be due to rejection, renin release from the diseased native kidney, hypervolemia, drugs such as methylprednisolone and cyclosporine, primary hypertension in the donor or recipient, and renal artery stenosis.[27] Methylprednisolone increases salt and water retention. Cyclosporine causes a dose-dependent decrease in renal blood flow that can be reversed by phenoxybenzamine, suggesting that cyclosporine-induced hypertension due to renal vasoconstriction is mediated by sympathetic activity.[28]

Other Etiologies

Postoperative hypertension can be the result of the intense sympathetic response to cerebral ischemia, intracerebral hemorrhage, increased intracranial pressure, myocardial ischemia, hypervolemia, alcohol withdrawal, or undiagnosed pheochromocytoma. In addition, sympathomimetic drug administration; rebound hypertension following withdrawal of drugs such as clonidine, propranolol, or nitroprusside; and inhalational anesthetics may contribute. Hypertension associated with toxemia of pregnancy usually abates with removal of the placenta but may persist into the postpartum period.

The incidence of withdrawal syndrome after cessation of beta-blockers is difficult to estimate. In an early prospective controlled trial, 10 of 20 patients experienced unstable angina, ventricular tachycardia, myocardial infarction, or sudden death.[29] Withdrawal symptoms usually began 12 to 72 hours after discontinuing the drug.[30]

Clonidine withdrawal, characterized by tremulousness, anxiety, headache, insomnia, nausea, and vomiting, occurs in 5 to 20 percent of patients.[31] These symptoms can occur as early as eight but more often 18 to 24, hours after stopping this drug and are more common in those who have taken higher doses.[31] Rebound hypertension is seen less frequently than other symptoms.

A blood pressure of 140/90 mmHg taken on two separate occa

sions is diagnostic of hypertension in pregnancy.[32] The mechanism of hypertension in the toxemia of pregnancy is unknown. Although it usually abates after delivery, it can continue for up to 48 hours.

Hypertension associated with pheochromocytoma is paroxysmal in 50 percent of patients and may therefore be overlooked. One review of the literature documented 50 cases of undiagnosed pheochromocytomas in the perioperative period, with a mortality rate of 80 percent.[33]

ASSESSMENT OF RISK: WHEN TO TREAT

In its 1984 report, the Joint National Committee on Detection, Evaluation, and Treatment of High Blood Pressure defined a hypertensive emergency as one in which blood pressure must be lowered within an hour to reduce patient risk. A hypertensive urgency is one in which severe elevation in blood pressure is not causing immediate end-organ damage but requires control within 24 hours for the same reason.[34] Although the committee defined severe hypertension in adults as a diastolic pressure of 115 mmHg or greater, the rate of change in blood pressure may be more important than the absolute level. A diastolic blood pressure over 100 mmHg is considered a hypertensive emergency in pregnant patients. However, many other patients with longstanding hypertension tolerate higher blood pressures without evidence of end-organ damage and are not in immediate danger.[35] However, it must be emphasized that hypertension in the postoperative period associated with encephalopathy, acute left ventricular failure, myocardial ischemia or infarction, dissecting aortic aneurysm, stroke or head trauma, progressing renal insufficiency, eclampsia with convulsions, or postoperative bleeding constitutes a hypertensive emergency requiring immediate treatment.[35]

Although hypertension, defined as a systolic blood pressure more than 50 mmHg higher than preoperative levels or greater than 200 mmHg, is not an independent variable in predicting postoperative cardiac complications,[2] an increase in incidence of myocardial ischemia and infarction, hemorrhagic cerebral infarction, anastomotic bleeding, and progressive renal failure are associated with systolic blood pressures greater than 200 to 225 mmHg after vascular surgery.[36] Severe systemic hypertension increases myocardial oxygen consumption and left ventricular wall tension, and can induce myocardial ischemia and arrhythmias in patients with coronary artery disease or congestive heart failure. As noted above, Towne et al. noted an increased incidence of fixed neurologic deficits in 10.2 percent of patients with sustained systolic blood pressures over 200 mmHg after carotid endarterectomy.[5]

Hypertensive encephalopathy may occur with sudden increases in pressure above the limits of autoregulation in chronically hypertensive patients and is characterized by severe headache, nausea, vomiting, apprehension, confusion, seizures, stupor, and coma if not reversed by blood pressure control.[32] This syndrome is rarely seen unless the diastolic blood pressure exceeds 140 mmHg, but in patients with toxemia of pregnancy encephalopathic symptoms may occur at pressures as low as 160/100 mmHg.[32]

The mechanism of hypertensive encephalopathy is poorly understood. In patients with chronic hypertension, cerebral vascular resistance changes to maintain blood flow over a wider range in mean arterial pressure. This range is 60 to 160 mmHg (60 to 110 mmHg in those with toxemia of pregnancy), but it narrows after control is achieved with treatment. Hypertensive encephalopathy may be due to an abnormality in cerebral autoregulation with arteriolar spasm or to a breakthrough in cerebral autoregulation with an increase in capillary hydrostatic pressure, transudation of protein, cerebral edema, petechial hemorrhage, and microinfarction.[32] If untreated, intracerebral hemorrhage and infarction may result. When it occurs in the hypothalamus or brain stem, it can produce severe refractory hypertension with increased morbidity and mortality. After acute infarction, cerebral autoregulation in the area surrounding the infarction fails, and perfusion becomes wholly pressure-dependent.

Postoperative hypertension may increase the incidence of bleeding and produce disruption of suture lines, especially in vascular graft anastomoses. Patients with previous renal insufficiency may progress to irreversible renal failure if severe hypertension is not controlled.

Thus, except in pregnant patients who develop encephalopathy at lower blood pressures of 160/100 mmHg, morbidity and mortality do not increase after noncardiac surgery until the diastolic blood pressure exceeds 110 mmHg.[2] This level therefore serves as a useful criterion for considering therapy. It is important to verify the accuracy of the measurement by taking at least two readings three minutes apart in both arms and to exclude other treatable contributing factors before instituting antihypertensive therapy. It is equally important to monitor organ perfusion during therapy. Because the lumens of small arterial vessels are reduced in size and resistance to blood flow is increased in hypertensive patients, perfusion of vital organs may be compromised when pressure falls below the lower limit of autoregulation. Rapid or excessive reduction in blood pressure may therefore cause significant myocardial, cerebral, or renal ischemia.

Antihypertensive drugs should be considered only when other remediable causes have been excluded or treated. These include pain, agitation, hypoxia, hypercarbia, and hypothermia. The choice of drug depends on (1) the urgency of therapy as indicated by the presence or absence of cardiac or cerebral dysfunction or the risk of disruption in a suture line; (2) the level of nursing care and monitoring available; (3) the physiological mechanisms underlying blood pressure elevation; and (4) the contributions of associated medical conditions such as aortic stenosis and increased intracranial pressure.

In those hypertensive emergencies listed above, blood pressure should be reduced within one hour using parenteral antihypertensives such as sodium nitroprusside, nitroglycerin, trimethaphan camsylate, diazoxide, labetalol, or hydralazine.[35] Hypertensive urgencies in which end-organ dysfunction is not immediately compromised are usually treated with agents such as clonidine, nifedipine, captopril, or labetalol. Most often, hypertensive urgencies in the early postoperative period can be treated with drugs similar to those used before surgery. These include beta-blockers, calcium channel blockers, sublingual nifedipine, angiotensin-converting enzyme inhibitors, or diuretics. With the exception of nifedipine, these drugs are available for intravenous use until the patient is able to take oral medications. Antihypertensive drugs should be titrated to the patient's "normal" preoperative blood pressure or a diastolic blood pressure of 100 to 110 mmHg with careful monitoring.

DRUGS USED TO TREAT POSTOPERATIVE HYPERTENSION (TABLE 54–1)

Direct-Acting Vascular Smooth Muscle Vasodilators

Sodium Nitroprusside

Sodium nitroprusside is a potent direct-acting vasodilator that acts on both arteries and veins but has more effect on arteriolar vascular smooth muscle than on venous capacitance.[37] It is most often used to treat hypertension after cardiac and major vascular surgery. Its onset of action is one to two minutes, and its effects dissipate as soon as it is discontinued, making it especially useful when the patient's condition is changing rapidly. However, because of its potency and the risk of overshoot, careful administration by infusion pump and intraarterial blood pressure monitoring are recommended. Since it decreases afterload, it can be used to treat low cardiac output states in which left ventricular end-diastolic volume is elevated.[37–39] Unlike nitroglycerin, which improves coronary collateral blood flow to ischemic areas of myocardium, nitroprusside reduces coronary perfusion pressure and blood flow to ischemic areas without augmenting intercoronary collateral flow, thus creating a "steal effect" during periods of ischemia.[40–42]

Ferrous ions found in nitroprusside react with sulfhydryl compounds in red blood cells and release cyanide.[43] Cyanide is then reduced to thiocyanate in the liver, has a half-life of three to four days, and is excreted in the urine. The risk of cyanide toxicity with nitroprusside increases with the dose and duration of therapy and is higher in patients with liver disease and renal insufficiency. Symptoms seen when cyanide levels exceed 500 μg/liter include nausea, vomiting, restlessness, air hunger, tachypnea, irregular pulse, dry skin, partial paralysis, confusion, convulsions, and somnolence. Cyanide interferes with electron transport in cellular oxidative phosphorylation, resulting in acidosis with elevated serum lactate levels and increased mixed-venous oxygen tension. Thiocyanate levels over 10 mg/dl are associated with psychosis, hypotension, coma, and death.[43–45]

In one series of patients undergoing CABG, tachyphylaxis to the drug and loss of consciousness were the predominant signs of cyanide toxicity.[45] In addition, all of these patients exhibited abnormal breathing patterns, none had an elevated mixed-venous oxygen tension, and only one demonstrated an acidosis. Although they all had increased cyanide levels over 500 μg/liter, none had elevated thiocyanate levels. Of seven who developed signs of cyanide toxicity, only five responded to treatment with thiosulfate, and the other three died with multiorgan failure. The authors suggested that patients undergoing CABG may have reduced thiosulfate pools or compromised enzyme systems responsible for metabolizing cyanide to thiocyanate. The dose and duration of sodium nitroprusside therapy should therefore be minimized in this setting.[45]

Kaplan et al. have observed that nitroprusside infusion rates of under 1 μg/kg/min and total doses under 1.5 to 2 mg/kg in 24 hours in patients with normal hepatic and renal function are not associated with thiocyanate toxicity, methemoglobinemia, or metabolic acidosis.[40] If larger doses are required, adding another drug like nitroglycerin is suggested. Others have recommended that the dose of nitroprusside not exceed 0.5 mg/kg/hr[46] or 8 μg/kg/min, and that the duration of the infusion not exceed 72 hours[47] to avoid cyanide toxicity. Alternate treatments of cyanide toxicity with thiosulfate include hydroxocobalamin and sodium nitrites.[44] Sodium nitrites oxidize hemoglobin to methemoglobin, which combines with the cyanide ion to yield cyanomethemoglobin. Hydroxocobalamin combines with cyanide to form cyanocobalamin or

TABLE 54–1. Intravenous Antihypertensives for the Treatment of Postoperative Hypertension

Drug	Initial Dose	Maintenance Dose	Onset	Duration	Important Side Effects
Direct Acting Vasodilators					
Nitroprusside	0.3–0.5 μg/kg/min	3–8 μg/kg/min	1–2 min	3–5 min	Reflex tachycardia; cyanide and thiocyanate toxicity; intrapulmonary shunting; increased intracranial pressure
Nitroglycerin	3–5 μg/min	5–100 μg/min	1–2 min	3–5 min	Reflex tachycardia; increased intracranial pressure
Hydralazine	5–10 mg	—	10–20 min	2–4 hrs	Reflex tachycardia; increased intracranial pressure
Diazoxide	50–100 mg	15–30 mg/min	1–5 min	6–12 hrs	Reflex tachycardia; increased intracranial pressure
Adrenergic Blockers					
Trimethaphan	0.3–3 mg/min	0.3–3 mg/min	1–5 min	10 min	Histamine release; mydriasis, cycloplegia; ileus; urinary retention
Esmolol	300–500 μg/kg	25–300 μg/kg/min	2–5 min	9 min	Myocardial depression
Labetalol	5–20 mg	0.05–0.75 mg/kg/hr	2–5 min	3.5–4.5 hrs	Increase in liver transaminases; postural hypotension
Calcium Channel Blockers					
Nicardipine	5–15 mg/hr	3–15 mg/hr	5–20 min	10–40 min	Reflex tachycardia; increased intracranial pressure
ACE Inhibitors					
Enalaprilat	1.25 mg	—	5 min	6–12 hrs	

vitamin B_{12}. In patients with renal insufficiency, thiocyanate can be removed with dialysis.[43]

Other side effects of nitroprusside include reflex tachycardia and inhibition of hypoxic pulmonary vasoconstriction, leading to increased intrapulmonary shunting and decreased arterial oxygen tension (PaO_2), particularly in patients undergoing CABG.[48–50] Nitroprusside crosses the placenta and can cause fetal cyanide poisoning.[44] Because it dilates cerebral vessels and increases cerebral blood flow, it should be used with caution in patients with increased intracranial pressure.[51] Baroreceptor-mediated increases in heart rate and cardiac output increase myocardial oxygen consumption and, when combined with reduction in coronary perfusion, may result in myocardial ischemia. Increases in heart rate also reduce the time available for left ventricular filling and coronary artery perfusion and threaten the myocardium especially in patients with critical aortic stenosis. The usual starting dose of nitroprusside is 0.3 to 0.5 μg/kg/min. Average doses of 3 μg/kg/min reduce diastolic pressure by 30 to 40 percent.[43]

Nitroglycerin

Like nitroprusside, nitroglycerin produces relaxation of vascular smooth muscle. In lower doses, nitroglycerin predominantly relaxes veins to reduce preload. At higher doses, it is a potent arterial vasodilator.[40] Nitroglycerin is metabolized in the liver to water soluble dinitrated metabolites and inorganic nitrite, which are less-potent vasodilators.[52] There are no known toxic metabolites, but at high doses nitroglycerin may produce methemoglobinemia. It is a potent coronary vasodilator and, unlike nitroprusside, improves coronary blood flow to ischemic areas.[40–42] Nitroglycerin is therefore the drug of choice for treatment of postoperative hypertension in patients with coronary artery disease. In those with elevated left ventricular end-diastolic volume, nitroglycerin improves cardiac output by reducing afterload.[48] In those with left ventricular failure, it improves blood flow to potentially ischemic areas of myocardium by reducing preload and wall tension.[52] However, in those without left ventricular failure, it may decrease stroke volume because of its predominant effect in reducing preload.

Following CABG, both nitroprusside and nitroglycerin are effective in controlling hypertension.[40,48] Approximately 80 percent of patients undergoing CABG respond with comparable blood pressure reductions to either agent. Both also decrease right atrial pressure and increase heart rate. Nitroglycerin increases the alveolar-to-arterial oxygen gradient slightly less than nitroprusside.[48] Both increase cerebral blood flow and should be used cautiously in patients with increased intracranial pressure.[53]

When mixed in plastic bags, nitroglycerin loses about 60 percent of its potency due to absorption by the polyvinyl chloride bag and tubing after eight hours and should therefore be made up in glass bottles.[40] The recommended starting dose of intravenous nitroglycerin is 5 μg/min, and it can be increased in increments of 5 to 10 μg/min every three to five minutes.[52]

Hydralazine

Hydralazine is another direct-acting arteriolar vascular smooth muscle relaxant, but it has little effect on venous capacitance.[43] Baroreceptor-mediated increases in stroke volume increase cardiac output. This hyperdynamic cardiac response partially offsets the antihypertensive effect of the drug. The reflex tachycardia may precipitate angina in patients with coronary artery disease. Small intravenous doses of propranolol (0.25 to 0.5 mg) have been used to prevent the increase in heart rate, myocardial contractility, and cardiac output produced by hydralazine.[54] An intravenous bolus of hydralazine in a dose of 5 to 10 mg has an onset of action of about 15 minutes, and its effect lasts two to four hours.[43]

Hydralazine is used by obstetricians to treat hypertension in toxemia of pregnancy, but is used less often by other physicians in the postoperative period because of its unpredictable onset of action and reflex tachycardia.[55] It does not cross the blood-brain barrier and cause sedation or somnolence,[55] and in the past it has been used to treat hypertension after craniotomy. Hydralazine does not cause postural hypotension[54] and may therefore be useful in treating hypertension in ambulatory surgical patients.

Diazoxide

Diazoxide is another direct-acting vasodilator used to treat hypertensive emergencies. Large boluses of 300 mg produce uncontrolled reductions in blood pressure within three to five minutes, lasting up to 24 hours, and sometimes resulting in myocardial infarction and stroke.[55] It produces reflex tachycardia that may precipitate angina in patients with coronary artery disease. Smaller boluses of diazoxide containing 50 to 100 mg reduce blood pressure within 30 seconds and can be repeated in 10 to 15 minutes. Reflex tachycardia may require small doses of intravenous propranolol in doses of 0.25 to 0.5 mg. Slow continuous infusion of diazoxide at a rate of 15 to 30 mg/min may produce safe effective treatment without the need for intraarterial line monitoring.[56] Side effects include angina, nausea, vomiting, and hyperglycemia.[43]

Ganglionic Blocking Drugs

Trimethaphan

Trimethaphan lowers blood pressure through ganglionic blockade and reduction of sympathetic tone in arterioles and veins, resulting in peripheral vasodilation, venous pooling, decreased venous return, and decreased cardiac output, which are potentiated in the erect position.[57] Trimethaphan also has a lesser direct effect on arteriolar smooth muscle and histamine release. It is primarily used to lower blood pressure in patients with dissecting aortic aneurysms,[35] especially when involving the descending aorta, since its sympathetic blockade reduces contractility and velocity of left ventricular ejection.[55] Its effects on heart rate depend on the initial resting pulse rate and vagal tone.[57] Ganglionic blockade usually produces mild tachycardia; however, baseline tachycardia may be slowed by the drug.

The initial intravenous dose of trimethaphan is 0.3 to 3.0 mg/min, and intraarterial monitoring is recommended. Side effects of ganglionic blockade include mydriasis, cycloplegia, ileus, urinary retention, xerostomia, and anhidrosis. Trimethaphan can also potentiate neuromuscular blocking drugs and histamine release and should be used cautiously in patients with a history of asthma. Peripheral pooling and reduction in cardiac output reduce cerebral blood volume and intracranial pressure.[58] During controlled hypotension in animals, trimethaphan produces an increase in intrapulmonary shunting.[59] Tolerance to trimethaphan may develop, but it can be used successfully with other drugs like nitroprusside, allowing reduced doses of both.

Peripheral Alpha-Adrenergic Blockers

Phentolamine

Phentolamine is a nonselective alpha-blocking drug used primarily in hypertensive emergencies associated with high circulating levels of catecholamines in pheochromocytoma or rebound hypertension after withdrawal of central alpha$_2$ agonists like clonidine.[55] Phentolamine is usually administered as a bolus of 1 to 5 mg.[60]

Prazosin

Prazosin is a selective postsynaptic alpha$_1$ receptor antagonist that reduces arterial blood pressure with little or no increase in heart rate.[43] The usual oral dose is 1 mg two to three times daily, and its peak effect occurs one to three hours after oral administration. Its plasma half-life is two to three hours but is prolonged in patients with renal failure and congestive heart failure. Because it can cause postural hypotension, syncope may occur in as many as one percent of patients who receive 2 mg or more, so the initial dose should be limited to 1 mg and given just before bedtime.[43]

Central Alpha-Adrenergic Agonist Drugs

Methyldopa

Methyldopa is a central alpha$_2$ agonist that produces a decrease in sympathetic outflow from the central nervous system after metabolism to alpha-methylnorepinephrine.[43] This metabolite is taken up by peripheral presynaptic adrenergic nerve terminals and then released as a false transmitter, producing a weaker contractile response in arterial smooth muscle than norepinephrine.[61] However, the peripheral effect of methyldopa plays only a minor role in the antihypertensive effect of the drug.[43]

Although not suitable for hypertensive emergencies, it may be used parenterally in patients unable to take oral medications for several days. It can produce sedation and somnolence,[43] and should not be used in patients with changing mental status or in those undergoing intracranial procedures. The usual parenteral dose is 250 to 500 mg every six hours. Peak serum concentrations are reached in two to three hours. The dose should be reduced in patients with hepatic or renal dysfunction. Abrupt withdrawal may rarely result in rebound hypertension.[30]

Clonidine

Clonidine is a centrally acting antihypertensive that also acts on alpha$_2$ adrenergic receptors in the central nervous system and decreases sympathetic outflow from the brain.[43] Its antihypertensive effect correlates with reduction in the concentration of circulating norepinephrine. It reduces heart rate and stroke volume acutely in supine individuals and can produce postural hypotension.

The dose of clonidine is 0.1 to 0.3 mg twice daily orally. It peaks in two hours after administration and has a half-life of nine hours.[43] Its effect on blood pressure correlates with plasma concentration.[62] There is also a transdermal system of administration in which plasma levels increase for two days and remain stable in the range of those achieved with equivalent doses of oral clonidine for five days.[63] Transdermal clonidine used once weekly lowers diastolic blood pressure to 90 mmHg or less in 65 percent of patients[64] and can be used in patients with renal failure.[43]

Sedation and dry mouth are the most frequent side effects.

Severe rebound hypertension may follow abrupt discontinuation of the drug.[30] The sympathetic overactivity associated with withdrawal can be treated with a combination of alpha- and beta-blockers like phentolamine and propranolol or the combined adrenergic blocking drug labetalol.[65] Treatment with beta-blockers alone may exaggerate hypertension due to unopposed alpha-adrenergic activity. Use of transdermal clonidine or crushed tablets suspended in saline or sorbitol and given rectally usually obviates the need for other agents.[66] Patients already taking oral or transdermal clonidine therapy should receive their regular doses until the time of surgery.

Beta-Adrenergic Blockers

Beta-blockers reduce blood pressure by decreasing cardiac output and renin release[60] through their effects on beta$_1$ receptors. They differ in their cardiac selectivity, lipid solubility, ability to penetrate the central nervous system, membrane-stabilizing activity, and intrinsic sympathomimetic activity.[67] Cardioselective beta-blockers include metoprolol, atenolol, acebutolol, and esmolol.[67,68] Their beta$_1$ receptor blockade activity produces a decrease in heart rate, contractility, and cardiac output, achieved at doses lower than those required to block beta$_2$ receptors in bronchi and peripheral blood vessels.[60] At higher doses, these drugs are no longer cardioselective. Other beta-blockers such as propranolol are nonselective and affect both beta$_1$ and beta$_2$ receptors.

Beta-blockers with high lipid solubility include propranolol, metoprolol, and pindolol. They are absorbed rapidly and completely from the gastrointestinal tract and after metabolism in the liver cross the blood-brain barrier.[67] Those with lower lipid solubility include atenolol, nadolol, and an active metabolite of acebutolol; these are not appreciably further metabolized, tend to be more water-soluble, and have longer half-lives and fewer central nervous system effects. Pindolol and acebutolol possess partial agonist activity and produce less bradycardia than the others.[67]

Withdrawal symptoms occur in 5 percent of patients following abrupt discontinuation of short-acting beta-blockers like propranolol.[30] Intravenous beta-blockers like propranolol and esmolol can be used to treat excessive tachycardia and especially supraventricular tachyarrhythmias.[68] Propranolol and esmolol are equally effective, but the very short half-life of esmolol allows it to be easily titrated for control of these arrhythmias.[69,70] Relative contraindications include a history of congestive heart failure, reactive airways disease in asthma or chronic obstructive pulmonary disease, atrioventricular conduction defects, and bradycardia.[60]

Esmolol is a newer cardioselective intravenous beta-blocker with a rapid onset of action and short half-life of about nine minutes.[70] It is metabolized by esterases in red blood cells. After CABG, sodium nitroprusside and esmolol both produce rapid titratable control of blood pressure in about the same time.[49] However, unlike nitroprusside, esmolol decreases heart rate, cardiac index, and stroke volume index; increases right atrial pressure; and has no effect on arterial PaO$_2$. In one study of 20 patients receiving esmolol after CABG, one developed severe left ventricular dysfunction, and another developed wheezing, both of which resolved within 30 minutes after discontinuing the drug.[49] However, because beta-blockers depress the myocardium, most physicians are reluctant to give them in this setting.

Esmolol has also been used successfully to treat hypertension after neurologic surgery.[71,72] Unlike direct-acting vasodilators such as nitroprusside, nitroglycerin, and hydralazine,[73] alpha- and beta-blockers do not increase cerebral blood flow and intracranial pressure. Esmolol has also been used to treat beta-blocker withdrawal and aortic dissection. In combination with direct-acting vasodilators, it is effective in the treatment of postoperative hypertension in patients who have an increased risk of myocardial ischemia.[69]

Combined Alpha- and Beta-Blockers

Labetalol

Labetalol is a unique antihypertensive drug with both competitive nonselective beta-blocking and selective alpha$_1$-blocking properties.[70] Its antihypertensive effect is due to alpha$_1$ blockade and beta$_2$ agonist activity. It lowers blood pressure by reducing systemic vascular resistance, and reflex tachycardia is inhibited by simultaneous beta-blockade. Labetalol is 25 to 35 percent less potent than propranolol in its beta$_1$ and beta$_2$ blockade and 10 to 20 percent as potent as phentolamine in its alpha$_1$ blockade. Its ratio of beta- to alpha-blockade is 3:1 after oral and 7:1 after intravenous administration.

The mechanism by which intravenous labetalol lowers blood pressure depends upon the characteristics of the patient and the dose of the drug. In patients with less severe hypertension, lower doses of labetalol decreases peripheral vascular resistance without significantly affecting heart rate. In those with more severe hypertension, it decreases peripheral vascular resistance but also slightly lowers heart rate and cardiac index. Labetalol effectively lowers blood pressure in hypertensive patients with coronary artery disease and acute myocardial infarction, but its effects on heart rate, cardiac index, and other hemodynamic parameters are variable and sometimes dose-dependent.[74]

The onset of action after an intravenous dose is one to two minutes with a peak effect within 5 to 10 minutes and a plasma half-life of 3.5 to 4.5 hours.[70] Using an initial bolus of 20 mg followed by incremental doses of 20 to 80 mg given at 10-minute intervals, 90 percent of medical patients with hypertensive emergencies experience satisfactory reduction in blood pressure with no significant adverse effects.[75] However, it is now recommended to give a bolus of 10 to 20 mg and to double the dose every 10 minutes up to a total of 300 mg with no single dose exceeding 80 mg.[65] Labetalol can be used orally in doses up to 2400 mg daily to maintain blood pressure control.

Studies using this dose range have documented that labetalol controls blood pressure in patients who develop hypertension after a variety of surgical procedures.[76-82] After cerebrovascular surgery, it is useful in reducing required doses of nitroprusside.[78] Both labetalol and esmolol are equally effective in controlling blood pressure on emergence from anesthesia after intracranial surgery, but labetalol more often decreases the heart rate.[72]

Labetalol is equally effective as nitroprusside in treating hypertension after CABG.[83] A continuous infusion of labetalol lowers blood pressure in patients with good left ventricular function with little of the decrease in systemic vascular resistance and reflex tachycardia seen with nitroprusside. Labetalol may therefore enable a better balance between oxygen supply and demand in the myocardium and decrease requirements for nitroprusside with its attendant danger of cyanide toxicity.[83] Labetalol should be used in lower doses in patients with a cardiac index under 2.5 liters/min/m^2.[80,81]

Labetalol has been used to lower blood pressure in acute aortic dissection,[84] toxemia of pregnancy, and rebound hypertension following clonidine withdrawal. It has been used in pheochromocytoma[65] but may produce paradoxical increases in blood pressure.[55] It is effective in renovascular hypertension and hypertension associated with renal parenchymal disease, and has also been used in the treatment of acute myocardial ischemia and infarction and a variety of dysrhythmias.[75] It has been used safely in patients with known reactive airways disease.[74,85]

The side effects of labetalol include postural hypotension due to alpha$_1$ blockade when higher doses are used.[86] Contraindications are the same as those of other beta-blockers and include known hypersensitivity, history of asthma, active bronchospasm, congestive heart failure, cardiogenic shock, heart block, and sinus bradycardia. Labetalol is metabolized in the liver, and its excretion is not affected by renal insufficiency.[65] When renal function is abnormal and the use of nitroprusside is limited by thiocyanate toxicity, labetalol is an effective alternative.[87] Transient rises in liver function tests have been noted with the drug.[88,89] Although these usually return to normal when the drug is stopped, there are reported deaths from severe hepatocellular injury.[90] It should therefore be avoided in patients with liver disease or jaundice and discontinued immediately if liver function tests become abnormal.

Diuretics

Loop Diuretics

Loop diuretics such as furosemide, bumetanide, and ethacrynic acid are used to treat postoperative hypertension due to increased intravascular volume.[91] Before effecting diuresis, they increase venous capacitance and decrease left ventricular filling pressure. The effect on venous capacitance is thought to be prostaglandin-mediated.[91] In addition, loop diuretics enhance renal blood flow, and furosemide redistributes blood flow from the medulla to the cortex.[91] The usual intravenous doses are 20 to 80 mg for furosemide, 0.5 to 1.0 mg for bumetanide, and 25 to 50 mg for ethacrynic acid. Side effects include metabolic alkalosis due to contraction of the extracellular volume and excretion of titratable acid, hypokalemia, hyponatremia, hypocalcemia, hyperglycemia, and hyperuricemia.[91]

Calcium Channel Blockers

Calcium channel blockers include verapamil, diltiazem, nifedipine, and nicardipine. They block voltage-sensitive calcium channels, preventing entry of calcium into vascular smooth muscle and cardiac muscle.[92] They decrease renal vascular resistance, increase renal perfusion and glomerular filtration, and produce a natriuresis.[92,93] Because of their effect on renal vascular resistance, they are particularly useful in cyclosporine-induced hypertension.[94] All calcium channel blockers improve coronary blood flow and reduce myocardial oxygen demand.[93] Nifedipine and nicardipine decrease systemic vascular resistance without affecting preload and produce a mild reflex tachycardia.[93] Verapamil has a greater effect on sinoatrial and atrioventricular impulse formation and on conduction and is recommended for treatment of supraventricular tachyarrhythmias. Nifedipine has been shown to be an effective antihypertensive in the postoperative period and to decrease the requirement for nitroprusside in patients undergoing CABG.[95]

However, intravenous diltiazem and intranasal nifedipine may depress myocardial performance in this setting.[96]

The absorption of nifedipine is greater when given orally than sublingually. However, if the drug is removed from the capsule, it can be administered sublingually and intranasally with better absorption. Because it is lipid-soluble, intranasal nifedipine begins to act in two to five minutes compared to 15 to 30 minutes after oral or sublingual administration.[95,96] However, mixing the contents of the capsule with saline causes immediate precipitation of most of the drug.[97] The antihypertensive effect lasts for three to five hours.[98] Nifedipine, verapamil, and nicardipine cross the blood-brain barrier and increase cerebral blood flow.[93,98] They should therefore be used cautiously in patients with increased intracranial pressure. Nifedipine is susceptible to photodegradation.

Nicardipine is a newer, short-acting, water-soluble, light-stable calcium channel blocker similar to nifedipine and is available in parenteral form for intravenous administration.[93] Because it does not affect conduction or depress the myocardium, it has been used with beta-blockers in the treatment of patients with hypertension and ischemic heart disease.[93] Although it is a peripheral vasodilator, both animal and human studies have demonstrated that it is more selective for the coronary and cerebral vasculature and has been shown to protect the heart and brain during periods of ischemia.[93] However, there are reports that intravenous nicardipine can precipitate or worsen congestive failure in some patients with severe left ventricular dysfunction.[99–101] Moreover, less than one percent of patients with coronary artery disease may experience an exacerbation of angina after nicardipine is begun.[102] This may be due to a reduction in coronary perfusion pressure and reflex tachycardia. Intravenous nicardipine is not approved for prevention or treatment of angina pectoris.

Nicardipine is effective in the treatment of hypertensive emergencies,[103] postoperative hypertension,[101,104–107] coronary vasospasm and myocardial ischemia,[93] and cerebral vasospasm following subarachnoid hemorrhage.[108] Like nitroprusside, nicardipine acts rapidly and is equally effective in treating postoperative hypertension. Nicardipine requires fewer dose adjustments and causes fewer adverse effects, including ischemic changes on electrocardiogram, tachycardia, and hypotension.[101,105,107]

Nicardipine lowers blood pressure by producing a dose-dependent decrease in systemic vascular resistance. This decrease in afterload allows increases in ejection fraction, stroke work, and cardiac output in patients with normal and markedly reduced left ventricular function or in those with acute uncomplicated myocardial infarction.[109] However, unlike nitroglycerin, it does not affect preload by decreasing venous capacitance, pulmonary artery pressure, or left ventricular end-diastolic pressure. Intravenous nicardipine directly augments coronary blood flow[110] but has a negligible effect on heart rate.[101,103,105,107,109]

An initial intravenous infusion of 5 mg/hr, titrated 2.5 mg/hr every 15 minutes without exceeding 15 mg/hr, usually achieves smooth blood pressure control within an hour.[111] Higher doses of 10 mg/hr initially titrated 2.5 mg/hr every five minutes will control the pressure within minutes.[106] The half-life of the drug is short, and its effect dissipates within 20 to 30 minutes.[112] Nicardipine is metabolized in the liver, and patients with hepatic dysfunction may require lower doses. Although few drug interactions have been reported with the parenteral form, oral nicardipine interacts with cimetidine and cyclosporine. Cimetidine increases plasma levels of nicardipine, and nicardipine increases plasma levels of cyclospor-ine.[113,114] Nicardipine is not compatible with sodium bicarbonate or lactated Ringer's solutions. Local phlebitis may occur at peripheral infusion sites after prolonged administration.[103]

Angiotensin-Converting Enzyme Inhibitors

Angiotensin-converting enzyme (ACE) inhibitors such as captopril, enalapril, and lisinopril are used to treat systemic hypertension and congestive heart failure. By inhibiting the conversion of inactive angiotensin I to active angiotensin II, they decrease the pressure response to angiotensin II and the secretion of aldosterone.[115] ACE inhibitors produce a decrease in systemic vascular resistance with no baroreceptor-mediated increase in heart rate or postural hypotension. The initial reduction in blood pressure correlates with a decrease in plasma renin activity and angiotensin II levels. In patients with chronic congestive heart failure, oral ACE inhibitors decrease systemic and pulmonary vascular resistance; reduce right atrial, mean arterial, and pulmonary capillary wedge pressures; and increase cardiac output.[116] Although they decrease myocardial oxygen demand, cerebral and coronary blood flow is maintained even with reduction in systemic blood pressure.[115]

ACE inhibitors also decrease renovascular resistance, improve renal blood flow, and induce a natriuresis.[115] Captopril and enalapril may induce renal insufficiency in patients with bilateral renal artery stenosis or renal artery stenosis of a single or transplanted kidney.[115,117] Increased levels of angiotensin II in renal artery stenosis produce vasoconstriction of efferent renal arterioles, thereby supporting glomerular filtration. ACE inhibitors decrease angiotensin II levels and exacerbate renal insufficiency in patients with stenosis.

Of the three commonly used ACE inhibitors—captopril, lisinopril, and enalapril—only enalapril (enalaprilat) is available for intravenous use.[118] The recommended dose is 1.25 mg every six hours intravenously. ACE inhibitors are effective in treating postoperative hypertension after CABG in patients with elevated plasma renin activity.[119] Enalaprilat is also useful in stable patients who have taken ACE inhibitors before surgery but who cannot take oral medications in the perioperative period. However, because ACE inhibitors have long half-lives, they may not be good choices in postoperative patients with an increased risk of hypotension from blood loss, arrhythmias, or pericardial tamponade. Because the renin-angiotensin system may play a protective role in maintaining blood pressure and renal perfusion, they should be particularly avoided in those with a high risk of hemorrhagic shock.[118]

Choice of Antihypertensives in the Immediate Postoperative Period

The choice of antihypertensive in the immediate postoperative period depends on the presence of life-threatening complications, the underlying mechanisms of hypertension, associated medical conditions, and the level of nursing care and monitoring available. Because of its potency and ability to be titrated, nitroprusside remains the drug of choice for treatment of hypertensive emergencies in the immediate postoperative period. The side effects of reflex tachycardia, increased intrapulmonary shunt, increase in intracranial pressure, cyanide toxicity, methemoglobinemia, intracoronary steal, and risk of overshoot can be reduced with concomitant therapy with other agents such as nitroglycerin, trimethaphan, labetalol, nifedipine, and captopril. The use of nitroprusside requires intraarterial monitoring and continuous observation.

The choice of drug, whether intravenous or oral, used to wean patients from sodium nitroprusside depends on the underlying pathophysiology and treatment prior to surgery. After cardiac and noncardiac surgery, intravenous nicardipine is as effective as nitroprusside with fewer adverse experiences. Systemic hypertension associated with a hyperdynamic state and increased catecholamine effects is best treated with beta-blockers. Propranolol or esmolol may be used acutely, but unopposed alpha-adrenergic activity may contribute to systemic vasoconstriction. A combined alpha- and beta-adrenergic blocker like labetalol may be preferable. When systemic hypertension is associated with an increase in plasma renin activity, beta-blockers or ACE inhibitors are particularly useful.

Because of their beneficial effects on coronary collateral circulation, nitroglycerin and nicardipine are the drugs of choice for postoperative hypertension in patients with coronary artery disease, especially in those with evidence of myocardial ischemia. All direct-acting vasodilators, including nitroprusside, nitroglycerin, diazoxide, and hydralazine, produce reflex tachycardia that may partially offset their antihypertensive effects. Low doses of a beta-blocker may be required to counteract this response. Calcium channel blockers, especially nifedipine or nicardipine, remain the best choices for small-vessel vasospasm. Sublingual nifedipine and intravenous nicardipine are excellent choices for hypertension after peripheral vascular surgery. Diuretics are useful when hypertension is due to hypervolemia.

Antihypertensive therapy should be titrated to a defined endpoint while organ perfusion is carefully monitored. Initially, low doses of intravenous drugs should be used to avoid overshoot. It is important to wait for the peak effect of the drug before giving more. Combinations of drugs may be efficacious and produce fewer side effects than higher doses of an individual agent.

SUMMARY

1. Except in patients undergoing coronary artery bypass surgery or valve replacement, preoperative hypertension is the most important predictor of hypertension following surgery.

2. Postoperative hypertension is frequently the result of sympathetic stimulation and an increase in systemic vascular resistance due to a variety of stimuli, including pain, hypoxia, drug withdrawal, hypervolemia, and increased intracranial pressure.

3. Postoperative hypertension should be treated emergently with parenteral agents in the presence of encephalopathy, severe congestive failure, myocardial ischemia, dissecting aneurysm, progressive renal failure, stroke, preeclampsia with seizures, or bleeding. In other cases, treatment with oral or parenteral antihypertensives is recommended when diastolic blood pressure exceeds 110 mmHg and other contributing factors have been excluded or treated.

4. Available drugs include direct vasodilators; ganglionic blockers; alpha-, beta-, and combined adrenergic blockers; calcium channel antagonists; angiotensin-converting enzyme inhibitors; and diuretics. Choice depends upon the urgency of the situation, the mechanism of the hypertension, the nature of the surgery, the presence of complicating underlying diseases, and the availability of appropriate monitoring.

5. In the immediate postoperative period, nitroprusside is the drug of choice in most hypertensive emergencies because of its immediate action, potency, and ability to be titrated. Reflex tachycardia, intrapulmonary shunting, increase in intracranial pressure, cyanide toxicity, intracoronary steal, and risk of overshoot can be avoided by using lower doses in combination with other agents, depending upon the underlying pathophysiology. Alternatively, intravenous nicardipine is equally effective with fewer side effects.

6. Hyperdynamic states can be treated with combined sympathetic antagonists like labetalol. Patients with coronary artery disease or active ischemia should receive nitroglycerin or nicardipine. Those with peripheral vascular disease or vasospasm may benefit from sublingual nifedipine or intravenous nicardipine. Volume overload requires the addition of diuretics.

7. The goal of therapy after noncardiac surgery should be to reduce blood pressure to preoperative levels or to a diastolic pressure between 100 and 110 mmHg.

8. In all cases during therapy, the accuracy of blood pressure measurements should be verified, perfusion of critical organs assured, and appropriate monitoring carried out.

REFERENCES

1. Gal TJ, Cooperman LH: Hypertension in the immediate postoperative period. *Br J Anaesth* 47:70–74, 1975.
2. Goldman L, Caldera DL: Risks of general anesthesia and elective operation in the hypertensive patient. *Anesthesiology* 50:285–292, 1979.
3. Estafanous FG, Tarazi RC, Brickley S et al: Arterial hypertension in immediate postoperative period after valve replacement. *Br Heart J* 40:718–724, 1978.
4. Landmore RW, Murphy DA, Kinley CE: Hypertension following myocardial revascularization: Its prevalence and etiology. *Can J Surgery* 23:468–470, 1980.
5. Towne JB, Bernhard VM: The relationship of postoperative hypertension to complications following carotid endarterectomy. *Surgery* 88:575–580, 1980.
6. Cooper TJ, Clutton-Brock TH, Jones SN et al: Factors relating to the development of hypertension after cardiopulmonary bypass. *Br Heart J* 54:91–95, 1985.
7. Wallach R, Karp RB, Reves JG et al: Pathogenesis of paroxysmal hypertension developing during and after coronary bypass surgery: A study of hemodynamic and humoral factors. *Am J Cardiol* 46:559–565, 1980.
8. Goldman L, Caldera DL, Southwick FS et al: Cardiac risk factors and complications in noncardiac surgery. *Medicine* 57:357–370, 1978.
9. Bove EL, Fry WJ, Gross WS et al: Hypotension and hypertension as consequences of baroreceptor dysfunction following carotid endarterectomy. *Surgery* 85:633–637, 1979.
10. Corson JD, Chang BB, Leopold PW et al: Perioperative hypertension in patients undergoing carotid endarterectomy: Shorter duration under regional block anesthesia. *Circ* 74(Suppl 1):1–4, 1986.
11. Guyton AC: *Textbook of Medical Physiology*, 6th ed. Philadelphia, Saunders, 1981, pp 249–250.
12. Cafferata HT, Merchant RF, DePalma RG: Avoidance of postcarotid endarterectomy hypertension. *Ann Surg* 196:465–472, 1982.

13. Appenzeller O, Descarries L: Loss of baroreceptor reflexes in patients with cerebrovascular disease. *Trans Am Neurol Assoc* 89:177–178, 1964.

14. Appenzeller O, Descarries L: Circulatory reflexes in patients with cerebrovascular disease. *N Engl J Med* 274:820–823, 1964.

15. Braunwald E: *Heart Disease: A Textbook of Cardiovascular Medicine*, 3d ed. Philadelphia, Saunders, 1988, p 442.

16. Satiani B, Vasko JS, Evans WE: Hypertension following carotid endarterectomy. *Surg Neurol* 11:357–359, 1979.

17. McGuirt WF, May JS: Postoperative hypertension associated with radical neck dissection. *Arch Otolaryngol Head Neck Surg* 113:1098–1100, 1987.

18. Skydell JL, Machleder HI, Baker D et al: Incidence and mechanism of postcarotid endarterectomy hypertension. *Arch Surg* 122:1153–1155, 1987.

19. Moore WS, Hall AD: Pathogenesis of arterial hypertension after occlusion of cerebral arteries. *Surg Gynecol Obstet* 131:855–893, 1970.

20. Estafanous FG, Tarazi RC: Systemic arterial hypertension associated with cardiac surgery. *Am J Cardiol* 46:685–694, 1980.

21. Landymore RW, Murphy DA, Kinley CE et al: Does pulsatile flow influence the incidence of postoperative hypertension? *Ann Thorac Surg* 28:261–266, 1978.

22. James TN, Hageman GR, Urthaler F: Anatomic and physiologic considerations a cardiogenic hypertensive chemoreflex. *Am J Cardiol* 44:852–859, 1979.

23. Brown AM: Coronary pressor reflexes. *Am J Cardiol* 44:849–851, 1979.

24. Tarazi RC, Estafanous FG, Fouad FM: Unilateral stellate block in the treatment of hypertension after coronary bypass surgery. *Am J Cardiol* 42:1013–1018, 1978.

25. Sealy WC, Harris JS, Young WG et al: Paradoxical hypertension following resection of coarctation of aorta. *Surgery* 42:135–147, 1957.

26. Goodall McC, Sealy WC: Increased sympathetic nerve activity following resection of coarctation of the thoracic aorta. *Circ* 39:245–251, 1969.

27. Steinmuller DR: Refractory hypertension after renal transplantation. *Clev Clin J Med* 56:377–383, 1989.

28. Murray BM, Puller MS, Ferris TF: Effect of cyclosporine administration on renal hemodynamics in conscious rats. *Kidney Int* 28:764–774, 1985.

29. Miller RR, Olson HG, Amsterdam EA et al: Propranolol: Withdrawal rebound phenomenon. *N Engl J Med* 82:431, 1975.

30. Hart GR, Anderson RJ: Withdrawal syndromes and cessation of antihypertensive therapy. *Arch Inter Med* 141:1125–1127, 1981.

31. Reid JL, Durgie HJ, Davies DS et al: Clonidine withdrawal in hypertension. *Lancet* 1:1171, 1977.

32. Alpert MA, Bauer JH: Hypertensive emergencies: Recognition and pathogenesis. *CV Rev and Reports* 6:407–426, 1985.

33. Sellevold OFM, Raeder J, Stenseth R: Undiagnosed pheochromocytoma in the perioperative period. *Acta Anesth Scand* 29:474–479, 1985.

34. Joint National Committee on Detection, Evaluation, and Treatment of High Blood Pressure: The 1984 Report of the Joint National Committee. *Arch Intern Med* 144:1045–1057, 1984.

35. Ferguson RK, Vlasses PH: Hypertensive emergencies and urgencies. *JAMA* 255:1607–1613, 1986.

36. Martin DE, Kammerer WS: The hypertensive surgical patient. *Surg Clin N Am* 63:1017–1032, 1983.

37. Miller RRI, Vismara LA, Zelis R et al: Clinical use of sodium nitroprusside in chronic ischemic heart disease: Effects on peripheral vascular resistance and venous tone and on ventricular volume pump and mechanical performance. *Circ* 51:328–336, 1975.

38. Stinson EB, Halloway EL, Derby GC et al: Control of myocardial performance early after open-heart operations by vasodilator treatment. *J Thorac Cardiovasc Surg* 73:523–530, 1976.

39. Miller RR, Vismara LA, Williams DO et al: Pharmacological mecha-

nism for left ventricular unloading in clinical congestive heart failure: Differential effects of nitroprusside, phentolamine, and nitroglycerin on cardiac function and peripheral circulation. *Circ Res* 39:127, 1976.

40. Kaplan JA, Finlayson DC, Woodward S: Vasodilator therapy after cardiac surgery: A review of the efficacy and toxicity of nitroglycerin and nitroprusside. *Can Anesth Soc J* 27:254–259, 1980.

41. Chiariello M, Gold H, Leinbach RC et al: Comparison between the effects of nitroprusside and nitroglycerin on ischemic injury during acute myocardial infarction. *Circ* 54:766, 1976.

42. Capurro NL, Kent KM, Epstein SE: Comparison of nitroglycerin, nitroprusside, and phentolamine induced changes in coronary collateral function in dogs. *J Clin Invest* 60:295, 1977.

43. Rudd P, Blaschke TF: Antihypertensive agents and the drug therapy of hypertension, in Gilman AG, Goodman LS, Rall TW (eds): *The Pharmacological Basis of Therapeutics*, 7th ed. New York, Macmillan, 1985, pp 784–805.

44. Adams AP, Hewitt PB: Clinical pharmacology of hypotensive agents. *Int Anaesth Clin* 20:95–109, 1982.

45. Patel CB, Laboy V, Venus B et al: Uses of sodium nitroprusside in postcoronary bypass surgery: A plea for conservatism. *Chest* 89:663–667, 1986.

46. Michenfelder JD, Tinker JH: Cyanide toxicity and thiosulfate protection during chronic administration of sodium nitroprusside in the dog: Correlation with a human case. *Anesthesiology* 47:441–448, 1971.

47. Cohn JN, Burke LP: Nitroprusside. *Ann Intern Med* 91:752–757, 1979.

48. Flaherty JT, Magee PA, Gardner TL et al: Comparison of intravenous nitroglycerin and sodium nitroprusside for treatment of acute hypertension developing after coronary artery bypass surgery. *Circ* 65:1072–1077, 1982.

49. Gray RJ, Bateman TM, Czer LSC et al: Comparison of esmolol and nitroprusside for acute postcardiac surgical hypertension. *Am J Cardiol* 59:887–891, 1987.

50. Naeije R, Melot C, Mols P et al: Effects of vasodilators on hypoxic pulmonary vasoconstriction in normal man. *Chest* 82:404–410, 1982.

51. Turner JM, Powell D, Gibson RM et al: Intracranial pressure changes in neurosurgical patients during hypotension induced with sodium nitroprusside or trimethaphan. *Br J Anaesth* 49:419–424, 1977.

52. Needleman P, Corr PB, Johnson EM Jr: Drugs used for the treatment of angina: Organic nitrates, calcium channel blockers, and beta-adrenergic antagonists, in Gilman AG, Goodman LS, Rall TW, Murad F (eds): *The Pharmacological Basis of Therapeutics*, 7th ed. New York, Macmillan, 1985, pp 806–826.

53. Shapiro HM: Anesthesia effects upon cerebral blood flow, cerebral metabolism, electroencephalogram, and evoked potentials, in Miller RD (ed): *Anesthesia*, 2d ed. New York, Churchill Livingstone, 1986, pp 1249–1288.

54. Albrecht RF, Toyooka ET, Polk SLH et al: Hydralazine therapy for hypertension during the anesthetic and postanesthetic periods. *Int Anesthesiol Clin* 16:299–312, 1978.

55. Vidt DG: Current concepts in treatment of hypertensive emergencies. *Am Heart J* 111:220–225, 1986.

56. Garrett BN, Kaplan NM: Efficacy of slow infusion of diazoxide in the treatment of severe hypertension without organ hypoperfusion. *Am Heart J* 103:390–394, 1982.

57. Taylor P: Ganglionic stimulating and blocking agents, in Gilman AG, Goodman LS, Rall TW, Murad F (eds): *The Pharmacological Basis of Therapeutics*, 7th ed. New York, Macmillan, 1985, pp 215–221.

58. Turner JM, Powell D, Gibson RM et al: Intracranial pressure changes in neurosurgical patients during hypotension induced with sodium nitroprusside or trimethaphan. *Br J Anaesth* 49:419–424, 1977.

59. Skene DS, Sullivan FS, Patterson RW: Pulmonary shunting and lung volumes during hypotension induced with trimethaphan. *Br J Anaesth* 50:339–344, 1978.

60. Weiner N: Drugs that inhibit adrenergic nerves and block adrenergic

receptors, in Gilman AG, Goodman LS, Rall TW (eds): *The Pharmacological Basis of Therapeutics*, 7th ed. New York, Macmillan, 1985, pp 181–214.

61. Weber MA, Drayer JM: Centrally acting antihypertensive agents: A brief overview. *J Cardiovasc Pharmacol* 6(Suppl):5803–5807, 1984.

62. Hogan MJ, Wallin JD, Chu L: Plasma clonidine concentration and pharmacologic effects. *Clin Pharmacol Ther* 30:729–734, 1981.

63. Arndts D, Arndts K: Pharmacokinetics and pharmacodynamics of transdermally administered clonidine. *Eur J Clin Pharmacol* 26:79–85, 1984.

64. Weber MA, Drayer JM, McMahon G et al: Transdermal administration of clonidine for treatment of high blood pressure. *Arch Intern Med* 144:1211–1213, 1984.

65. Wallin JD, O'Neill WM: Labetalol: Current research and therapeutic status. *Arch Intern Med* 143:485–490, 1983.

66. Johnston RY, Nicholas DA, Lawson NW et al: The use of rectal clonidine in the perioperative period. *Anesthesiology* 64:288–290, 1986.

67. *Medical Letter* 28:20–22, February 14, 1986.

68. Morganroth J, Horowitz LN, Anderson J et al: Comparative efficacy and tolerance of esmolol to propranolol for control of supraventricular tachyarrhythmia. *Am J Cardiol* 56:33F–39F, 1985.

69. Kaplan JA: Dupon critical care lectures: Role of ultrashort-acting beta-blockers in the perioperative period. *J Cardiothorac Anesth* 2:683–691, 1988.

70. Lowenthal DT, Porter S, Saris SD et al: Clinical pharmacology, pharmacodynamics and interactions with esmolol. *Am J Cardiol* 56:14F–17F, 1985.

71. Gibson BE, Black S, Maass L et al: Esmolol for the control of hypertension after neurologic surgery. *Clin Pharmacol Ther* 44:650–653, 1988.

72. Muzzi DA, Black S, Lossasso TJ et al: Labetalol and esmolol in the control of hypertension after intracranial surgery. *Anesth Analg* 70:68–71, 1990.

73. Van Alan H, Cottrell JE, Anger C et al: Treatment of intraoperative hypertensive emergencies in patients with intracranial disease. *Am J Cardiol* 63:43C–47C, 1989.

74. Goa K, Benfield P, Sorken EM: Labetalol: a reappraisal of its pharmacology, pharmacokinetics and therapeutic use in hypertension and ischemic heart disease. *Drugs* 37:583–627, 1989.

75. Wilson DJ, Wallin DJ, Vlachakis ND et al: Intravenous labetalol in the treatment of severe hypertension and hypertensive emergencies. *Am J Med* 75:95–102, 1983.

76. Leslie JB, Kalayjian RW, Singo MA et al: Intravenous labetalol for the treatment of postoperative hypertension. *Anesthesiology* 67:413–416, 1987.

77. Goldberg ME, Seltzer JL, Azad S et al: Postcarotid endarterectomy hypertension: The role of epinephrine (E) norepinephrine (NE) and renin (R) and treatment with labetalol (LAB). *Anesthesiology* 67:A569, 1987.

78. Orlowski JP, Shiesley D, Vidt DG et al: Labetalol to control blood pressure after cerebrovascular surgery. *Crit Care Med* 16:765–768, 1988.

79. Costantino F, Vidt DG, Orlowski JP et al: The safety of cumulative doses of labetalol in perioperative hypertension. *Clev Clin J Med* 56:371–376, 1989.

80. Morel DR, Forster A, Suter PM: IV labetalol in the treatment of hypertension following coronary artery surgery. *Br J Anaesth* 54:1191–1195, 1982.

81. Sladen R, Klamerus K, Mann H et al: Labetalol for the control of elevated blood pressure following coronary bypass grafting. *Anesthesiology* 69:A151, 1988.

82. Chauvin M, Deriaz H, Viars P: Continuous IV infusion of labetalol for postoperative hypertension. *Br J Anaesth* 59:1250–1256, 1987.

83. Cruise CJ, Skrobik Y, Webster RE et al: Intravenous labetalol versus sodium nitroprusside for treatment of hypertension postcoronary bypass surgery. *Anesthesiology* 71:835–839, 1989.

84. Grubb BP, Sirio C, Zelis R: Intravenous labetalol in acute aortic dissection. *JAMA* 258:78–79, 1987.

85. Michelson EL, Frishman WH: Labetalol: An alpha- and beta-adrenoceptor blocking drug. *Ann Int Med* 99:553–554, 1983.

86. Vlachakis ND, Maronde RF, Maloy JW, Medakovic M, Kassem N: Pharmacodynamics of intravenous labetalol and follow-up therapy with oral labetalol. *Clin Pharmacol Ther* 38:503–508, 1985.

87. Graves JW: Prolonged continuous infusion labetalol: A new alternative for parenteral antihypertensive therapy. *Crit Care Med* 17:759–761, 1989.

88. Frishman WH, Michelson EL, Johnson BF et al: Multiclinic comparison of labetalol to metoprolol in treatment of hypertension. *Am J Med* 75:54–67, 1983.

89. Michelson EL, Frishman WH, Lewis JE et al: Multicenter clinical evaluation of long-term efficacy and safety of labetalol in treatment of hypertension. *Am J Med* 75:68–80, 1983.

90. Douglas D, Yang R, Jansen P et al: Fatal labetalol-induced hepatic injury. *Am J Cardiol* 87:235–236, 1987.

91. Weiner IM, Mudge GH: Diuretics and other agents employed in the mobilization of edema fluid, in Gilman AG, Goodman LS, Rall TW, Murad F (eds): *The Pharmacological Basis of Therapeutics*, 7th ed. New York, Macmillan, 1985, pp 896–900.

92. Kaplan NM: Calcium entry blockers in the treatment of hypertension: Current status and future prospects. *JAMA* 262:817–823, 1989.

93. Sorkin EM, Clissold SP: Nicardipine: A review of its pharmacodynamic and pharmacokinetic properties and therapeutic efficacy in the treatment of angina pectoris, hypertension and related cardiovascular disorders. *Drugs* 33:296–345, 1987.

94. Jessup M, Cavarocchi N, Narins B et al: Antihypertensive therapy in patients after cardiac transplantation: A step-care approach. *Transplant Proc* 20(Suppl 1):801–802, 1988.

95. Iyer VS, Russell WJ: Nifedipine for postoperative blood pressure control following coronary artery vein grafts. *J Royal Coll Surg Engl* 68:3–6, 1986.

96. Mullen JC, Miller DR, Weisel RD et al: Postoperative hypertension: A comparison of diltiazen, nifedipine and nitroprusside. *J Thorac Cardiovasc Surg* 96:122–132, 1988.

97. Rietbrock, Kausch M, Englehardt M et al: Non-bioequivalence of sublingual nifedipine. *Br J Clin Pharmacol* 23:589, 1987.

98. Bauer JH, Reams GP: The role of calcium entry blockers in hypertensive emergencies. *Circ* 75(Suppl V):V174–V180, 1987.

99. Tondi S, Zennaro RG, Mascioco L et al: Acute hemodynamic effects of nicardipine in patients with chronic congestive heart failure. *Cardiologia* 34:1013–1019, 1989.

100. Aroney CN, Semigras MJ, Dee GW et al: Inotropic effect of nicardipine in patients with heart failure. Assessment by left ventricular end-systolic pressure–volume analysis. *J Am Coll Cardiol* 14:1331–1338, 1989.

101. Van Wezel HB, Koolen JJ, Visser CA et al: Antihypertensive and anti-ischemic effects of nicardipine and nitroprusside in patients undergoing coronary artery bypass grafting. *Am J Cardiol* 64:22–27H, 1989.

102. Silke B, Verma SP, Hafizullah M et al: Hemodynamic effects of nicardipine in acute myocardial infarction. *Postgrad Med J* 60(Suppl 4):29–34, 1984.

103. Wallin JD, Cook ME, Blanski L et al: Intravenous nicardipine for the treatment of severe hypertension. *Am J Med* 85:331–338, 1988.

104. Kaplan JA: Clinical considerations for the use of intravenous nicardipine in the treatment of postoperative hypertension. *Am Heart J* 119:443–446, 1990.

105. David D, Dubois C, Loria Y: Comparison of nicardipine and sodium nitroprusside in the treatment of paroxysmal hypertension following aorto-coronary bypass surgery. *J Cardiothorac Vasc Anesth* 5:357–361, 1991.

106. IV Nicardipine Group: Efficacy and safety of intravenous nicardipine in the control of postoperative hypertension. *Chest* 99:393–398, 1991.

107. Halpern NA, Goldberg M, Neely C et al: Postoperative hypertension: A multicenter prospective randomized comparison between intravenous nicardipine HCl and sodium nitroprusside. *Crit Care Med* 20:1637–1643, 1992.

108. Flamm ES, Adams HP Jr, Beck DW et al: Dose escalation study of intravenous nicardipine in patients with aneurysmal subarachnoid hemorrhage. *J Neurosurg* 68:393–400, 1988.

109. Singh BN, Josephson MA: Clinical pharmacology, pharmacokinetics and hemodynamic effects of nicardipine. *Am Heart J* 119:427–443, 1990.

110. Lambert CR, Hill JA, Nichols WW et al: Coronary and systemic hemodynamic effects of nicardipine. *Am J Cardiol* 55:652–656, 1985.

111. Wallin JD, Fletcher E, Ram VS et al: Intravenous nicardipine for the treatment of severe hypertension. *Arch Int Med* 149:2662–2669, 1989.

112. Cook E, Clifton GG, Vargas R et al: Pharmacokinetics, pharmacodynamics and minimum effective clinical dose of intravenous nicardipine. *Clin Pharmacol Ther* 47:706–718, 1990.

113. Cantarovech M, Hiesse C, Lockiec F et al: Confirmation of the interaction between cyclosporine and the calcium channel blocker nicardipine in renal transplant patients. *Clin Nephrol* 28:190–193, 1987.

114. Bourbigot B, Guiserix J, Airiau J et al: Nicardipine increases cyclosporine blood levels. *Lancet* 1:1447, 1986.

115. Douglas WW: Polypeptides—angiotenin, plasmakinins and others, in Gilman AG, Goodman LS, Rall TW, Murad F (eds): *The Pharmacological Basis of Therapeutics*, 7th ed. New York, Macmillan, 1985, pp 647–653.

116. Gavras H: Cardioprotective effects of angiotensin-converting enzyme inhibitors in hypertension. *Prac Cardiol* 15:25–31, 1989.

117. Hricik DE: Antihypertensive and renal effects of enalapril in post-transplant hypertension. *Clin Nephrol* 27:250–259, 1987.

118. Mirenda JV, Grisom TE: Anesthetic implications of the renin-angiotensin system and angiotensin-converting enzyme inhibitors. *Anesth Analg* 72:667–683, 1991.

119. Roberts AJ, Niaechos AP, Subramanian VA et al: Hypertension following coronary artery bypass graft surgery. *Circ* 58(Suppl): 1–43, 1978.

55

CHEST PAIN AND DYSPNEA IN THE SURGICAL PATIENT

Joseph S. Savino

Stuart J. Weiss

CHEST PAIN

The diagnostic challenge of postoperative chest pain is distinguishing trivial disorders from myocardial ischemia and other serious problems. This can be especially difficult in the postoperative period, in which the severity of pain may correlate poorly with the seriousness of its cause.[1] Life-threatening disorders requiring immediate recognition include myocardial ischemia and infarction, arrhythmias, pulmonary edema, pneumothorax, and pulmonary embolism. These and the other causes of chest pain are discussed in this chapter. Perioperative arrhythmias are reviewed in Chap. 56.

Myocardial Ischemia and Infarction

Primary cardiac dysfunction is the leading cause of death following anesthesia and surgery, especially in patients with coronary artery disease. Preoperative cardiac risk factors predicting significant morbidity and mortality are uncompensated congestive heart failure, unstable angina, ventricular dysrhythmias, hypertension, peripheral vascular disease, aortic stenosis, age over 70, and recent myocardial infarction.[2] Unstable angina, congestive heart failure, and previous myocardial infarction carry the highest risk.

The risk of reinfarction in these patients is related to the interval between the previous myocardial infarction and surgery. It is approximately 6 to 30 percent if the myocardial infarction occurred less than three months before surgery, 2 to 16 percent if between three and six months, and 5 to 6 percent if longer than six months.[3–5,12] When reinfarction occurs, operative mortality is approximately 50 percent. It occurs most commonly within 24 to 72 hours after surgery and has an overall incidence of 0.1 to 0.7 percent in the general population.[6,7]

The risk of perioperative myocardial ischemia and cardiac death in patients with stable controlled angina is unclear,[8,9] but management is aimed at optimizing the determinants of myocardial oxygen balance. Patients with peripheral vascular disease usually have concurrent ischemic heart disease. Over 45 percent of those undergoing repair of abdominal aortic aneurysms have severe coronary artery disease on arteriography.[10] Claudication may limit exercise and mask the symptoms of underlying ischemic heart disease until the stress of surgery creates an imbalance of myocardial oxygen supply and demand.

Intraoperative factors associated with the greatest risk of perioperative cardiac morbidity are: (1) surgery involving the great vessels, thorax, or upper abdomen; (2) emergency surgery; and (3) the degree and duration of intraoperative hypotension.[12] Aggressive monitoring and early detection and treatment of cardiovascular instability may decrease the risk of reinfarction.[13]

The postoperative period poses the greatest risk for patients with coronary artery disease undergoing noncardiac surgery. Significant changes in fluid balance, body temperature, pulmonary function, autonomic activity, and somatic stimulation create physiologic instability. Moreover, the symptoms of postoperative myocardial ischemia are frequently masked or silent. Residual anesthetic, postoperative analgesics, incisional pain, regional blocks, and the expectation that postoperative pain is normal may explain why myocardial ischemia and infarction frequently occur without documented symptoms.[13] Postoperative myocardial ischemia occurs in over 40 percent of high-risk patients undergoing noncardiac surgery and, when it arises in the early postoperative period, is associated with a threefold increase in the risk of an adverse cardiac event.[14]

Diagnosis

Differentiating myocardial ischemia from other causes of chest discomfort after surgery requires careful review of the past medical history and current medications, presenting symptoms, physical examination and laboratory data, and intraoperative anesthetic and surgical management. Patients with risk factors for coronary atherosclerosis should be questioned about symptoms of ischemic heart disease before surgery. A history of angina, previous myocardial infarction, or exercise intolerance is especially important.

The preoperative electrocardiogram (ECG) should be examined

for ST-segment abnormalities and Q waves and compared to earlier ones if they are obtainable. The lead(s) that demonstrate such changes should be monitored perioperatively. Medications used before surgery to treat ischemic heart disease should be reviewed. These include beta-blockers to decrease myocardial oxygen demand, calcium channel blockers to increase supply, or nitrates to do both. Chronic antianginal therapy should be administered up to and including the day of surgery and continued into the postoperative period. Parenteral forms of medication should be substituted as needed.

Accurate assessment of chest pain may be difficult after surgery. A sedated patient may be unable to convey his symptoms, or important symptoms may be disregarded or assumed to be normal or expected by the patient. Interpretation of chest pain may be complicated by the specific procedure or type of anesthetic. Upper-abdominal, thoracic, shoulder, or neck surgery may cause incisional pain mimicking angina pectoris. Irritation from placement of esophageal monitors may cause precordial discomfort. Difficult laryngoscopy and intubation may lead to airway and pharyngeal trauma producing neck and jaw discomfort similar to the radiating pain of myocardial ischemia.

The cardiovascular effects of myocardial ischemia are predictable and progressive (see Fig. 55–1). Findings include tachycardia, electrocardiographic ST-segment abnormalities, segmental wall-motion abnormalities, arrhythmias, hypoxemia, tachypnea, increases in pulmonary artery wedge or central venous pressures, and hypotension. Changes in blood pressure and heart rate are nonspecific but serve as important prognostic indices. Hypotension, a new holosystolic murmur of mitral regurgitation, an S_3 gallop, and pulmonary rales suggest significant left ventricular

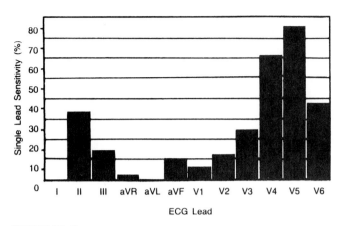

FIGURE 55–2.

Distribution of ischemic ST-segment changes in each of the 12 leads. The estimated sensitivity was calculated from the number of changes in a single lead as a percentage of the total number of episodes. Sensitivity was highest in lead V_5 (75%).

Source: From London.[27]

dysfunction. Cool, pale, or cyanotic extremities suggest low cardiac output with peripheral vasoconstriction.

The ECG remains the most important diagnostic study, and comparison with preoperative tracings may reveal subtle changes suggestive of myocardial ischemia. Modern intraoperative ECG monitors have automated ST-segment analysis and graphic display of ST-segment displacement. They permit continuous recording of ST-segment trends without the use of a strip-chart recorder.[15-17] The most sensitive lead for detecting perioperative ischemia is often V_5 unless preoperative testing has demonstrated electrocardiographic evidence of ischemia elsewhere (see Fig. 55–2).

Continuous ECG monitoring cannot provide 12-lead recording and can be limited by electrical interference and the lack of specificity of ST–T wave abnormalities. For example, injury to the central nervous system or intracerebral hemorrhage can produce dramatic ECG changes often accompanied by bradycardia. A proposed mechanism is disruption of the sympathetic innervation to the heart by way of the stellate ganglion.[18]

Serum levels of creatine kinase (CK) and its isoenzymes may not be useful because of the high incidence of false positive tests and delay in obtaining results. CK and CK-MB fraction activity are related to specific procedures. Although there is no change in CK-MB activity after cystoscopy, there are marked increases in the majority of patients after cholecystectomy.[19] Skeletal muscle trauma can elevate levels of CK-MB, but the increase should not be more than six percent of the total CK level.[19] Simultaneous determination of lactate dehydrogenase isoenzyme levels may increase the specificity of these tests. If available, technetium pyrophosphate imaging is both sensitive and specific in detecting acute myocardial infarction.[20,21] Magnetic resonance imaging and spectroscopy can also detect infarction but have not been evaluated in surgical patients.[22,23]

Anesthetic and Surgical Management

A full understanding of the anesthetic and operative course is useful in evaluating these patients, and discussion with the anesthesiologist is often illuminating. There are several factors that increase cardiac work in the perioperative period, including anxi-

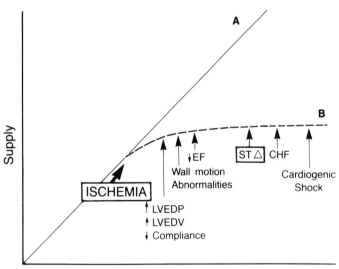

FIGURE 55–1.

The line of identity (A) illustrates the normal relationship between myocardial oxygen demand and supply. In patients with ischemic heart disease, increases in demand may not be matched with appropriate increases in oxygen supply (B). The result is myocardial ischemia and associated cardiac dysfunction.

Source: Adapted from Barash.[104]

LVEDP = left ventricular end-diastolic pressure
LVEDV = left ventricular end-diastolic volume
EF   = ejection fraction
STΔ   = ST segment changes on ECG
CHF   = congestive heart failure

ety, pain, fever, and circulatory instability induced by anesthetics, drugs, and blood loss. Intraoperative myocardial ischemia is clearly associated with postoperative myocardial infarction.[24,25] In addition, the duration and degree of intraoperative hypotension correlate with the risk of infarction.[26]

Intraoperative electrocardiographic monitoring should be extended into the postoperative period. Hemodynamic changes indicated by a pulmonary artery catheter can lead to early recognition of myocardial ischemia but are less sensitive and specific than electrocardiography or transesophageal echocardiography.[27,28] These changes include elevated pulmonary capillary wedge pressure induced by decreases in left ventricular compliance and increases in filling pressures or sudden appearance of V waves on the tracing suggesting mitral regurgitation from papillary muscle ischemia. However, pulmonary artery pressure can be affected by intravascular volume status, vasoactive drugs, circulating catecholamine levels, and sympathetic tone and the mode of ventilation. Transesophageal echocardiography provides qualitative data regarding segmental left ventricular wall-motion abnormalities that occur early and are relatively specific for myocardial ischemia.[29,30]

Most local, regional, and general anesthetics affect the heart. Epinephrine-containing local agents are quickly absorbed and commonly cause hypertension, tachycardia, and arrhythmias. Major neural axis blocks including spinal and epidural anesthesia can produce hypotension when high levels of anesthesia are required or when administered to hypovolemic patients. Volatile anesthetics cause a dose-related depression of myocardial work. Their negative inotropic effects decrease oxygen consumption and actually improve myocardial oxygen balance as long as reductions in coronary blood flow resulting from decreases in blood pressure are not excessive. However, these effects may precipitate heart failure and hypotension in patients with left ventricular dysfunction. Intravenous anesthetics exert variable effects on myocardial oxygen balance. Narcotics have little or no negative inotropic effect and may be useful in patients with ischemic heart disease and heart failure. However, they may cause hypotension if administered too rapidly or in large doses. Morphine does so by facilitating histamine release, and fentanyl and its analogues do so by reducing sympathetic tone. On the other hand, narcotic-based anesthesia may not blunt the sympathetic response to surgical stimulation as effectively as inhalational agents. Barbiturates, etomidate, and benzodiazepines that are used to induce anesthesia have negative inotropic and vasodilating properties that may cause hypotension if administered in large doses or rapidly injected.

The timing, dose, and rate of administration of anesthetics are more important determinants of hemodynamic response than the choice of drug. For example, the hemodynamic responses to airway stimulation and surgery itself are hypertension and tachycardia. These can be attenuated by anticipating them and increasing the depth of anesthesia.

Therapy

Treatment of postoperative myocardial ischemia is multifactorial. Sinus tachycardia due to hypovolemia should be judiciously treated with volume replacement. Hypertension and tachycardia from incisional pain can be alleviated with parenteral analgesics like narcotics or regional blocks. Hypoxemia and hypercarbia decrease myocardial oxygen delivery, increase sympathetic nervous system activity, and increase pulmonary vascular resistance. Establishing a secure airway and providing adequate ventilation are mandatory.

Shivering and nonshivering thermogenesis are common sequelae of hypothermia and recovery from inhalation anesthesia. Concurrent activation of the sympathetic nervous system, increased systemic oxygen consumption, and increased cardiac output can precipitate myocardial ischemia. Prompt use of warm blankets, heated intravenous fluids, and heating lamps facilitates rewarming. Meperidine in low doses is effective for shivering.[31]

The treatment of myocardial ischemia in the postoperative patient is otherwise similar to that in nonsurgical patients except for the relative contraindications to intravenous heparin and thrombolytic therapy. Myocardial oxygen supply can be augmented by administering oxygen, optimizing hematocrit with transfusions, and decreasing coronary vascular resistance while maintaining coronary perfusion pressure with pharmacologic agents. Nitroglycerin is most commonly used and can be titrated to relief of symptoms and blood pressure level. Calcium channel blockers reduce myocardial oxygen demand by decreasing afterload. Beta-blockers can accomplish this by decreasing contractility and heart rate.

Drug therapy is not without risk in the postoperative setting. The desired negative inotropic effect of beta-blockers may precipitate congestive heart failure, especially in patients with preexisting left ventricular dysfunction. Calcium channel blockers and nitroglycerin are potent vasodilators and may cause hypotension. Nonselective beta-blockers may cause bronchospasm in those with concomitant obstructive lung disease. They may also increase the risk of conduction disturbances by decreasing conduction velocity and increasing the effective refractory period in the AV node. Calcium channel blockers like verapamil decrease conduction in the AV node. The development of a major conduction disturbance in the setting of acute myocardial ischemia is an indication for the placement of a temporary transvenous pacemaker (see Chap. 56).

It is unclear why myocardial ischemia and infarction are more likely to occur in the 24 to 72 hours following surgery rather than during or just after the procedure. Mobilization of fluid; decreased monitoring leading to delayed intervention; and suboptimal control of incisional pain, activity, anemia, fever, and atelectasis may be contributing factors. Some advocate extending the stress-free intraoperative environment into the postoperative period for high-risk cardiac patients. In this regard, acute pain services have developed to continue effective pain control into the postoperative period.

Other Common Causes of Chest Pain

The differential diagnosis of chest discomfort in the postoperative period is as exhaustive as it is at any other time. Preexisting esophageal disease, gastritis, or peptic ulcer disease may become symptomatic with the stress of surgery. Preoperative anxiety, fasting, and pain increase gastric volume and acidity and decrease gastric motility. Although prophylactic therapy with H_2 antagonists effectively increases gastric pH, administration of antacid is controversial because it increases gastric volume and may increase the risk of aspiration. Antacids containing aluminum hydroxide are especially toxic to the lung and should be avoided.[32] Sodium citrate is one alternative and is used in patients with a history of peptic ulcer disease or in those with increased gastric acidity due to chronic steroid therapy.

Disease of the gallbladder and biliary system usually causes right-upper quadrant pain but may also cause chest pain. Narcotics increase smooth muscle tone in the sphincter of Oddi and are thought to increase the risk of biliary colic. However, such increases in biliary pressure are small, and their clinical significance is unclear.[33] Narcotic-induced biliary colic can often be reversed with naloxone. Similarly, acute pancreatitis can simulate myocardial infarction clinically and produce ECG abnormalities suggesting subendocardial ischemia. Concomitant abdominal tenderness and appropriate elevations in serum amylase and lipase levels usually establish the diagnosis.

Chest-wall trauma due to preoperative injury or surgical intervention can cause severe chest pain. Intraoperative maneuvers to facilitate surgical exposure or excision of chest-wall tumors may cause rib fractures, and local tenderness and shallow breathing are common findings. Associated findings include pneumo- or hemothorax and pulmonary contusions. Intercostal nerve blocks with long-acting local anesthetics such as bupivacaine or epidural narcotics provide rapid pain relief and improvement in respiratory mechanics.

Anterior chest-wall trauma may cause contusion of the right ventricle or biventricular injury and myocardial rupture if severe. Right ventricular contusion can lead to ischemic ECG changes, heart block, and dysrhythmias as well as right-heart failure. Echocardiogram can be helpful in showing a dilated hypokinetic right ventricle, tricuspid regurgitation, and sometimes hemopericardium. Concomitant pulmonary contusion may exacerbate right-heart failure by increasing pulmonary vascular resistance. Therapeutic modalities include fluids, pacemaker support, inotropic drugs, and mechanical ventilation as needed. Serial ECG's should be performed in all patients with anterior chest-wall trauma.

Diaphragmatic irritation is common during abdominal surgery and can cause upper-abdominal discomfort or chest pain radiating to the shoulders. It can be due to the surgical trauma itself, chemical irritation, or residual gas in the peritoneum. Gas is often insufflated into the peritoneal cavity to facilitate exposure during laparoscopy. Despite attempts to remove it at the end of the procedure, small quantities remain and collect under the diaphragm and can be seen on upright abdominal x-rays. The subsequent abdominal discomfort, bloating, and left shoulder pain often mimic symptoms of myocardial ischemia. Such findings in patients who have not undergone abdominal surgery are diagnostic of bowel perforation.

Pleurodesis with agents like tetracycline is effective in treating recurrent pneumothoraces and malignant pleural effusions. The procedure creates a sterile pleuritis and can be painful enough to require general anesthesia. Postoperative pleuritic pain is nonfocal and severe but can be minimized by adding local anesthetic to the sclerosing agent.

Costochondritis or Teitze's syndrome, caused by inflammation of the cartilaginous joints between the ribs and the sternum, is characterized by local tenderness and chest discomfort aggravated by respiration. Treatment includes nonsteroidal anti-inflammatory drugs, narcotics, and infiltration with local anesthestics.

Chest pain due to pulmonary embolism is variable and may be absent, making diagnosis difficult. Postoperative pulmonary embolism is covered in detail in Chap. 59.

The symptoms of pericardial inflammation are difficult to distinguish from those of pulmonary embolism, pleuritis, and myocardial infarction, and may include chest pain, malaise, and dyspnea. Fever, rales, pericardial rubs, or effusions may be present. Characteristic ECG changes include transient global ST-segment elevations followed by T wave inversion. The etiologies

of pericarditis include trauma, tumor, infection, drug reaction,[34] and myocardial infarction. Pericarditis occurring within 48 hours of an acute myocardial infarction is caused by an immune response to myocardial injury. However, when it develops several weeks or months after the infarction, it is termed Dressler's syndrome.[35]

In the postpericardiotomy syndrome, pericarditis follows cardiac surgery or procedures such as median sternotomy, mediastinoscopy, and even placement of a central venous catheter or cardiac pacemaker that causes bleeding to the pericardium. The incidence of postpericardiotomy syndrome after cardiac surgery is 10 to 18 percent[36,37] and usually develops within one to three weeks of the procedure. Nonsteroidal anti-inflammatory drugs are effective in providing symptomatic relief to patients with pericarditis.[38] Postpericardiotomy syndrome is usually self-limited but may occasionally progress to pericardial tamponade, pulmonary edema,[35] or constrictive pericarditis.

DYSPNEA

Ingram and Braunwald define dyspnea as an "abnormally uncomfortable awareness of breathing."[39] Increased ventilation after strenuous physical activity is not associated with difficulty in breathing, since metabolic demands are matched by appropriate increases in ventilation. Dyspnea occurs when the work of breathing is excessive. Although it may have a single cause, it is more often multifactorial in origin.

Unlike chest pain, the severity of dyspnea usually correlates with the severity of an underlying cardiopulmonary disorder. Evaluation of dyspnea in the postoperative patient includes review of the preoperative history and physical examination with attention to the cardiac and pulmonary systems; current medications; preoperative laboratory data; the operative record detailing the type of surgery and anesthetic management; and postoperative physical examination, laboratory tests, and diagnostic studies.

The dyspneic patient is usually agitated and exhibits labored breathing. Tachypnea, abnormal auscultatory findings, sternal retractions, and the use of accessory muscles may be present. Pallor or cyanosis may also be evident, and hypertension and tachycardia are common.

Results of chest x-rays, arterial blood gas measurements, pulmonary function tests, and ECG are helpful in diagnosis and management. Pulse oximetry has become standard during surgery and immediately thereafter. It provides continuous assessment of arterial oxyhemoglobin saturation to spot dangerous trends in arterial oxygen tension and to judge the effectiveness of therapeutic interventions.

Hypoxemia is common after general anesthesia because ventilatory response to hypoxia is markedly depressed by residual anesthetics.[40,41] In this setting, hypoxia can occur without dyspnea, and patients may experience dangerously low arterial oxygen tensions without an increase in minute ventilation. Supplemental oxygen should therefore be administered to all patients after general anesthesia.

Cardiac Dysfunction

Dyspnea due to heart failure is caused by a decrease in lung compliance from increased lung water, hypoxemia from increased pulmonary shunting, and an increase in physiologic dead space

Decreased lung compliance increases the work of breathing. In low cardiac output states, metabolic acidosis may further stimulate the respiratory center to increase minute ventilation.

The dyspneic patient with postoperative congestive heart failure usually has an identifiable risk factor such as ischemic heart disease, hypertension, aortic stenosis, or hypothyroidism, and therapy is aimed at improving cardiac performance. Left ventricular dysfunction due to myocardial ischemia may respond to decreases in afterload with nitroprusside or hydralazine and in preload with nitroglycerin. Respiratory distress due to hypervolemia often develops 24 to 48 hours after surgery when interstitial fluid is being mobilized into the vascular space. Diuresis is first-line treatment in this situation. Severe volume overload and pulmonary edema may require mechanical ventilation, positive end-expiratory pressure, and vasodilator therapy. Antiarrhythmics or electrical cardioversion may be necessary in patients with new atrial fibrillation after surgery.

It is important to consider compromise of diastolic filling by pericardial fluid as a cause of postoperative cardiac dysfunction. The degree of cardiac decompensation is related to the amount of fluid and the rate of accumulation. Significant pericardial fluid can develop in patients with lung or breast cancer, pericarditis, renal failure, or acute aortic dissection, or in those who have undergone procedures complicated by cardiac perforation, including cardiac catheterization and placement of a central access line. Although elevated venous pressures on examination and an enlarged cardiac silhouette on chest x-ray may be helpful, echocardiogram is the most sensitive test for detecting pericardial fluid.

Airway Obstruction

Upper Airway: Mouth and Pharynx

The most common sites of postoperative airway obstruction are the mouth and pharynx. Risk factors include obesity, a large tongue, trauma to the airway, a history of sleep apnea, abnormal airway anatomy, and residual sedation. Surgical complications that may cause upper-airway obstruction include excessive bleeding, soft-tissue swelling after pharyngeal or cervical surgery, and failure to remove throat packs after airway or dental surgery. Patients with obstruction exhibit snoring, use of respiratory accessory muscles, and increased work of breathing. Despite an increase in respiratory rate, decreased tidal volume and minute ventilation result in hypoventilation. Progressive hypercarbia and hypoxemia lead to obtundation, respiratory failure, and cardiac arrest if untreated. Supplemental oxygen should always be administered while efforts are made to identify and relieve the obstruction.

Physical examination should include inspection for tracheal deviation or swelling. The posterior oropharynx should be cleared of blood, secretions, and other foreign matter, and a stable airway should be established. Alert and responsive patients can assist in relieving obstruction by changing position, expectorating any foreign matter from the airway, and cooperating with placement of an oral or nasopharyngeal airway. Sedated patients have a higher risk of obstruction and aspiration because of decreased pharyngeal muscle tone and a depressed gag reflex. This leads to posterior displacement of the tongue against the posterior pharyngeal wall, requiring therapeutic subluxation of the jaw and placement of an oral airway. Endotracheal intubation is indicated if airway obstruction persists or progresses but may be technically difficult be-cause of inadequate visualization of the glottic opening. Fiberoptic intubation is an alternative to direct laryngoscopy if not limited by lack of patient cooperation or blood and secretions in the airway.

Lower Airway: Larynx, Trachea, and Bronchi

The most common site of obstruction in the larynx is at the level of the vocal cords. It has the smallest cross-sectional area and is most vulnerable to obstruction by an aspirated foreign body. Laryngospasm is a common cause of airway obstruction during emergence from general anesthesia or in response to tracheal irritation and is due to sustained contraction of the adductor muscles of the vocal cords. In the operating room, it is treated with continuous positive airway pressure and 100% oxygen while arterial oxygen saturation is closely monitored by pulse oximetry. If laryngospasm persists or worsens, a hypnotic like sodium thiopental is administered, followed by intravenous succinylcholine in small doses of 10 to 20 mg, to relax the vocal cords and reestablish airway patency. Respiratory efforts in the presence of an obstructed airway generate high negative intrathoracic pressure and may lead to pulmonary edema.[42,43] Controlled ventilation is required after the administration of succinylcholine until neuromuscular function and spontaneous ventilation return.

In parathyroid and thyroid surgery, transient or permanent injury to the recurrent laryngeal nerve can cause unilateral vocal cord paralysis. The vocal cords in patients undergoing these procedures should be inspected by laryngoscopy after reversal of neuromuscular blockade but before emergence from general anesthesia and extubation. Movement of both cords assures that the recurrent laryngeal nerve function in closing the glottis is intact. Recurrent laryngeal nerve injury may necessitate postoperative tracheal intubation.

Obstruction of the trachea or bronchi can be extrinsic or intrinsic. Extrinsic compression is usually due to an anterior mediastinal mass or hematoma compromising the lumen. Large aneurysms of the aortic arch may compress the left main-stem bronchus or stretch the left recurrent laryngeal nerve. Intrinsic obstruction of the large airways of the lung can be due to edema, tracheomalacia, endobronchial or tracheal tumors, tracheal stenosis from previous surgery, or aspiration of a foreign body. Differentiating between extrinsic and intrinsic compression is accomplished with neck and chest x-rays or bronchoscopy. Persistent lower-airway obstruction may prohibit extubation. Treatment may include bronchoscopic removal of an obstructing foreign body, surgical intervention, or the administration of steroids or racemic epinephrine to treat soft-tissue swelling.

Reactive Airway Disease

Bronchospasm is a common cause of dyspnea in the postoperative patient and is characterized by tachypnea, expiratory wheezing that may progress to loss of breath sounds, use of accessory muscles, intercostal retractions, nasal flaring, and increased sympathetic nervous system activity. Chest x-rays demonstrate hyperinflation with air-trapping. Arterial blood gas measurements and serum theophylline levels should be performed as indicated. Hypoxemia and hypocarbia are early findings; hypercarbia and respiratory acidosis supervene as the patient fatigues or bronchospasm worsens.

Asthma may flare in the postoperative period. Precipitating factors include dehydration, instrumentation of the trachea, use of dry gases, viscous secretions, impaired mucociliary function, pain, histamine release, subtherapeutic levels of bronchodilators, and effects of drugs that exacerbate bronchospasm (e.g., beta-blockers).[44] Management should be directed toward treating precipitating factors and administering bronchodilators, humidified oxygen, fluids, and often corticosteroids.

Pulmonary Edema

Pulmonary edema is an increase in lung water resulting in decreased lung compliance, increased work of breathing, and intrapulmonary shunting. Clinical manifestations include dyspnea, tachypnea, agitation, coughing, rales, wheezing, jugular venous distentions if associated with heart failure, cyanosis, and pink frothy sputum. Pertinent laboratory data include chest x-ray, arterial blood gas levels, and pulmonary artery and central venous pressure measurements.

Postoperative pulmonary edema can be cardiac or noncardiac in origin. Cardiac pulmonary edema is the result of left ventricular failure due to hypervolemia or ischemic, hypertensive, or valvular heart disease. Treatment is dictated by the underlying disease. Noncardiac pulmonary edema can occur after reexpansion of a collapsed lung. Examples include chest-tube placement for pneumothorax, evacuation of a pleural effusion, and single-lung ventilation.[45,46] Noncardiac edema can also be the result of inspiratory efforts made against an obstructed airway,[42,43] adult respiratory distress syndrome,[47] sepsis, and hypervolemia. Intravenous administration of naloxone can rarely provoke pulmonary edema and can occur with doses as small as 100 μg.[48–50] Although the mechanism is unknown, it may be due to an increase in sympathetic activity resulting in venoconstriction, pulmonary hypertension, and increased vascular permeability.[50] Therapy includes oxygen administration, proper positioning, diuresis, fluid restriction, vasodilator therapy, and assisted or controlled ventilation with positive end-expiratory pressure.

Retained Secretions

Retained secretions are common after surgery and can cause ventilatory compromise. Increased airway resistance and obstruction can occur at any level of the respiratory tree and lead to atelectasis and air-trapping. If untreated, increases in the work of breathing and physiologic dead space cause shunting, hypoxia, and hypercarbia. Factors predisposing patients to accumulate and retain secretions include preexisting inflammatory disease in the airways, as in pneumonia, bronchitis, and asthma; unopposed parasympathetic tone produced by acetylcholinesterase inhibitors used to reverse muscle relaxants; impaired mucociliary function in smokers and after inhalation anesthesia; and inability to generate an effective cough due to muscle weakness, sedation, or splinting.

Such patients may exhibit dyspnea, agitation, hypercarbia, and hypoxia. Physical examination often reveals viscous secretions in the oropharynx or endotracheal tube. Tracheal rhonchi and decreased breath sounds over areas of atelectasis are common. Chest x-rays frequently confirm atelectasis.

Postural drainage, suctioning, chest physical therapy, pain control, humidified oxygen, and attention to exacerbating factors facilitate clearance of mucus. For example, inability to generate an effective cough because of splinting after a thoracotomy can be treated with intercostal nerve blocks or epidural narcotics. Tracheal

suctioning should be performed every one to three hours when patients cannot cough. Tenacious secretions in those with bronchitis are more effectively cleared after intravenous hydration and humidified oxygen are initiated. Bronchoscopy is occasionally required to remove large mucous plugs refractory to conventional therapy.[51,52]

Restricted Lung Mechanics

The causes of restricted lung mechanics vary but share similar pathophysiology. Lung expansion is impeded by compression due to pleural effusion, hemothorax, and pleural tumors; limited diaphragmatic excursion seen with bowel distention, obesity, ascites, and suboptimal positioning; and restricted chest-wall mobility due to surgical dressings, term pregnancy, chest restraints, positioning, and obesity. All can lead to hypoxia from ventilation-perfusion mismatching and shunting, hypercarbia, and cardiac dysfunction.

The effect of position on pulmonary function should be considered in all patients with respiratory distress. In general, the supine position is poorly tolerated in such patients. Decreased diaphragmatic excursion reduces the functional residual capacity (FRC) and total lung capacity and increases the work of breathing. These changes become more important when considered in relation to the closing volume (CV). The CV is the lung volume at which the elastic recoil of the lung overcomes the passive forces that maintain airway patency. If the CV is greater than the FRC, early airway closure produces air-trapping, atelectasis, and an increased alveolar-arterial (A-a) oxygen gradient.

The pulmonary pathophysiology and management of obesity are applicable to other causes of restricted lung mechanics. In those with body weight greater than 20% above ideal level, abnormal pulmonary function is characterized by decreased lung volumes, increased intraabdominal pressure, decreased chest-wall compliance, hypoxemia, and hypercarbia. These factors increase the work of breathing and systemic oxygen consumption. Although most have a normal arterial carbon dioxide tension, those with hypoventilation and resting hypercarbia are categorized as having the obesity-hypoventilation syndrome.[53] It is associated with biventricular cardiac enlargement, polycythemia, decreased vital capacity, and severe hypoxemia.[54]

Body habitus is a major factor in anesthetic and surgical management. Obese patients are more likely to have traumatic intubations, larger surgical incisions, and longer operations, all of which contribute to pulmonary morbidity. In addition, they are more likely to have hypertension, heart failure, ischemic heart disease, and cerebrovascular disease.[55] Exacerbation of any of these conditions may lead to postoperative ventilatory failure.

There is no ideal anesthetic for obese patients. Potent long-acting respiratory depressants are usually avoided. Although regional anesthesia is an attractive alternative to general anesthesia, spinal or epidural anesthesia is not without risk. The loss of lower abdominal or intercostal muscle function may precipitate dyspnea or respiratory failure in morbidly obese patients.

Obese patients have a higher risk of aspiration.[56] Increased gastric volume, decreased gastric emptying, and difficulty in securing the airway contribute to this risk. Obese patients are more susceptible to the effects of residual neuromuscular weakness, restrictive dressings, retained secretions, incisional pain, and cardiac dysfunction. Avoidance of potent analgesics and central nervous system depressants may be difficult. Epidural or intrathecal narcot ics provide good analgesia with minimal sedation and should be considered in obese patients undergoing thoracic or upper-abdominal procedures.

Atelectasis is a common cause of postoperative dyspnea in obese patients and is more often confirmed on x-rays in this group.[57] Radiologic signs of atelectasis can persist up to 24 hours after surgery in 50 percent. Incentive spirometry, clearance of secretions, and early ambulation may contribute to early resolution. Obese patients are also prone to upper-airway obstruction. Traumatic intubation may cause significant bleeding and soft-tissue swelling. A large tongue or redundant folds of tissue may also cause upper-airway obstruction.

In the absence of excessive sedation or airway trauma, nasopharyngeal or oral airways and changes in body position may be beneficial in obese patients. Upright positioning decreases the effect of increased intraabdominal pressure on diaphragmatic excursion. When this is not feasible, semirecumbent and lateral decubitus positioning should be considered.[55] Continuous monitoring of arterial oxygenation with pulse oximetry is mandatory in the immediate postoperative period. Significant airway obstruction may require reintubation.

Preexisting Pulmonary Dysfunction

Patients with preexisting pulmonary disease obviously have an increased risk of postoperative dyspnea and respiratory complications. They benefit from a thorough preoperative evaluation and efforts to improve pulmonary function as reviewed in Chap. 22.

Muscle Weakness

Postoperative dyspnea may be caused by muscle weakness. The use of muscle relaxants to facilitate intubation, improve operating conditions, and prevent movement is the most common etiology of residual weakness after surgery. The effect of muscle relaxants should be reversed before emergence from general anesthesia. Weakness can be readily evaluated in awake and anesthetized patients. In the latter, neuromuscular function is assessed by determining the response to a presynaptic electrical stimulus. In the former, it is assessed by evaluating the patient's hand grasp, ability to sustain a head lift for more than five seconds, and evaluation of respiratory parameters. The head life maneuver and measurement of vital capacity and inspiratory force are much more sensitive indicators of residual weakness than tidal volume, which can be maintained despite considerable neuromuscular blockade. The diaphragm is also relatively resistant to paralysis and may demonstrate activity in an otherwise flaccid patient. Consequently, spontaneous ventilation returns before the patient is fully able to maintain an adequate airway, clear secretions, and sustain a normal vital capacity. Those with preexisting pulmonary disease or obesity are obviously more vulnerable to the residual effects of muscle relaxants.

The effects of muscle relaxants are potentiated by a variety of drugs, including antibiotics such as aminoglycosides, polymyxins, and lincomycins;[58] residual inhalational anesthetics,[59] magnesium;[60] local anesthetics;[61,62] calcium channel blockers;[63] and quinidine.[64] Delayed recovery and prolonged paralysis may occur with hypokalemia,[65] hypermagnesemia,[60] hypocalcemia,[58] respiratory acidosis,[66] metabolic alkalosis,[67] and hypothermia.[68,69]

Reversal of muscle relaxants need not be done at the end of the procedure in all patients. The decision to do so is dependent on the type of surgery and the degree of neuromuscular blockade, and is influenced by a variety of metabolic and electrolyte disturbances. These patients can be mechanically ventilated until the elimination of the muscle relaxant permits recovery of neuromuscular function or another dose of acetylcholinesterase inhibitor can be administered to reverse the blockade.

Patients with myasthenia gravis,[70] Eaton-Lambert syndrome,[71] and myotonia[72] are more sensitive to muscle relaxants and can experience postoperative weakness even if such agents are not administered during surgery. All patients with neuromuscular disorders should be monitored for weakness in the postoperative period, and provisions should be immediately available if assisted ventilation is required.

Residual muscle weakness occurs in 24 percent of patients in the immediate postoperative period.[72] Loss of muscle tone, floppy movements, difficulty with vocalization, tachypnea, shallow breathing, and severe anxiety are characteristic signs. Decreased vital capacity and negative inspiratory force suggest significant ventilatory compromise and require immediate intervention to avoid hypercarbia and further weakness. Cardiovascular instability characterized by hypertension, tachycardia, and dysrhythmias may result from progressive respiratory acidosis, hypoxemia, and increased autonomic sympathetic activity.

Therapeutic management depends on the etiology. Patients are frequently awake and alert and should be kept informed and reassured. Ventilation with 100% oxygen by face mask should be initiated immediately. Intubation and mechanical ventilation is required if there is risk of aspiration or respiratory failure. Knowledge of preoperative respiratory status and intraoperative course, including the time and dose of all drugs administered, dictate further management. Hypothermia and metabolic and electrolyte disturbances should be corrected.

An uncommon cause of ventilatory failure is paralysis of the diaphragm caused by surgical trauma to the phrenic nerve in head and neck surgery,[73] cardiac surgery,[74] regional nerve block,[75] or certain positions.[76] However, unilateral phrenic nerve dysfunction rarely causes significant respiratory compromise in patients with otherwise normal lung function.[77]

Trauma

Direct trauma to the chest can cause rib fractures, pneumothorax, and pulmonary contusion. Dyspnea is common and may be associated with hypoxemia, airway obstruction, splinting, chest-wall tenderness, flail chest, and multiple organ system injury. Cardiac contusion, aortic dissection, and tracheal or bronchial lacerations should also be considered. Lung contusions usually produce local hemorrhage and pulmonary thrombosis. The severity of hypoxemia produced by pulmonary contusion parallels the extent of parenchymal involvement and airway compromise. Most contusions improve rapidly if the airways are clear of blood.

Chest injury sustained before or during surgery may not be apparent until after the procedure. Traumatic intubation[78,79] or surgical traction creating laryngeal edema, expanding hematoma, or injury to the phrenic or recurrent laryngeal nerves[80] may cause new-onset dyspnea after surgery. Pneumothorax should be considered if anesthetic blocks of the stellate ganglion,[81] brachial plexus,[82] or surgical field[83–85] may have violated the pleura or if central venous access was placed in the subclavian or internal jugular veins.[86,87]

Treatment consists of ventilatory support until pulmonary function is self-supporting. A pneumothorax of more than 20% or associated with respiratory distress requires placement of a chest tube.[88] Blunt injury to the phrenic nerve frequently causes transient dysfunction and does not compromise pulmonary function unless there is bilateral involvement, other pulmonary injury, or preexisting lung disease.

Pain

Pain is a potent respiratory stimulant that increases respiratory rate and minute ventilation and decreases tidal volumes. The breathing pattern changes to minimize pain, frequently resulting in abnormal ventilatory mechanics that increase the work of breathing and total body oxygen consumption. These changes are especially important in patients undergoing thoracic or upper-abdominal procedures. Decreases in vital capacity, expiratory flow rate, residual capacity and lung compliance are common after thoraco-abdominal surgery. Impaired cough and reduced ability to clear secretions predispose the patient to atelectasis, pulmonary shunting, and progressive hypoxemia. Postoperative pain is discussed in Chap. 72.

Adverse Drug Reactions

Adverse drug reactions have been classified as predictable and unpredictable.[89] Predictable reactions account for about 80 percent of such drug responses and are dose-dependent, due to direct drug toxicity, or related to a predictable secondary effect such as drug-induced histamine release.[90–92] Unpredictable reactions are associated with unexpected immunologic responses due to anaphylactic (antibody-mediated) or anaphylactoid mechanisms.[93]

The spectrum of anaphylactic and anaphylactoid reactions ranges from minor cutaneous manifestations like urticaria or flushing to severe respiratory and cardiovascular compromise with pulmonary edema, pulmonary hypertension, hypotension, and arrhythmias.[94] Most drugs administered in the perioperative period have been implicated in producing postoperative dyspnea through an immune-mediated mechanism. These include induction agents (e.g., barbiturates and etomidate), local anesthetics (e.g., procaine, chloroprocaine, and tetracaine), muscle relaxants, opioids, antibiotics, protamine, and contrast dyes.[95–97] Blood products are also associated with immune-mediated bronchospasm and dyspnea.[97]

The universal treatment of drug-induced bronchospasm and pulmonary edema is administration of oxygen and discontinuation of the precipitating agent. The mechanism of the reaction guides additional therapy. Diphenhydramine may prevent exacerbation of a reaction due to drug-induced histamine release. Bronchospasm is managed with beta-adrenergic agonists, aminophylline, and steroids. Treatment of anaphylactic or anaphylactoid reactions may require aggressive pulmonary and hemodynamic support as well as intravenous fluids and epinephrine. Patients should be closely monitored in an intensive care unit.

Aspiration

Residual sedation, nausea, obesity, gastric distention, pregnancy, recent food ingestion, cholinergic agents, or bowel irritation may lead to passive regurgitation or vomiting in the postoperative period. Pregnant or obese patients and those undergoing surgery on the brain or auditory system may experience severe nausea postoperatively.

Precautions should be taken to minimize the risk of aspiration and the extent of pulmonary injury should it occur. Prophylactic therapy is aimed at decreasing gastric volume, increasing gastric pH, and identifying those patients who require airway precautions. Nonparticulate antacids like sodium citrate can be used to increase gastric pH. Gastric volume can be reduced by evacuating the stomach with a nasogastric tube, increasing gastric emptying with metaclopramide,[98] and decreasing acid secretion with H_2 blockers.[99,100] Patients in whom nausea is expected should be extubated only when they are awake and capable of protecting their airways.

The clinical manifestations of aspiration depend on the composition and quantity of the aspirate and underlying pulmonary function. Chunks of food can obstruct large airways and produce atelectasis, ventilation-perfusion mismatch, and hypoxemia. An acidic aspirate with pH under 2.5 inhibits ciliary function and causes a severe chemical pneumonitis.[101,102]

Dyspnea and respiratory distress begin abruptly after aspiration. The mouth and oropharynx should be suctioned immediately with the head down to minimize further aspiration. Oxygen therapy is crucial to treat the increased intrapulmonary shunting and hypoxia. Intubation is indicated if respiratory failure becomes imminent. Steroids are not recommended, and prophylactic antibiotics are controversial.[103] Aspiration is more fully discussed in Chap. 57.

SUMMARY

1. The differential diagnosis of postoperative chest pain is extensive and requires meticulous review of the symptoms, medical history, physical examination, current medications, laboratory data, and intraoperative anesthetic and surgical management.

2. Myocardial ischemia must be differentiated from other causes of chest pain, including preexisting esophageal disease, gastritis, or peptic ulcer; gallbladder and biliary system disease; pancreatitis; pulmonary embolism; pericarditis, including postpericardiotomy syndrome; pneumothorax; chest wall trauma; diaphragmatic irritation resulting from abdominal surgery; and costochondritis.

3. Preoperative cardiac risk factors include uncompensated congestive heart failure, unstable angina, ventricular dysrhythmias, hypertension, peripheral vascular disease, aortic stenosis, age over 70, and a history of a previous myocardial infarction. Intraoperative risk factors include surgery involving the great vessels, thorax or upper abdomen, emergency surgery, and the degree and duration of intraoperative hypotension.

4. The postoperative period poses the greatest risk for patients with underlying coronary artery disease undergoing noncardiac surgery. Postoperative myocardial ischemia occurs in more than 40 percent of high-risk patients and carries a threefold increase in the risk of an adverse cardiac event. Most ischemic events occur within 24 to 72 hours after surgery.

5. The presentation of postoperative myocardial infarction can be atypical, and electrocardiographic and serum enzyme abnormalities can be nonspecific and misleading. Continuous intraoperative and postoperative monitoring is recommended in high-risk patients. The treatment of postoperative myocardial ischemia is the same as in other patients except for the relative contraindications of heparin and thrombolytic therapy.

6. Postoperative dyspnea due to congestive heart failure is most common in patients with an identifiable risk factor (e.g., ischemic heart disease, hypertension, aortic stenosis, or hypothyroidism) and a precipitating cause (e.g., myocardial ischemia, arrhythmia, or overzealous fluid administration). Respiratory distress due to hypervolemia usually develops within 24 to 72 hours after surgery when operative interstitial fluid is mobilized into the vascular space. Management includes diuresis and treatment of the underlying cause.

7. Other causes of postoperative dyspnea include pneumothorax, pleural effusion, pericardial tamponade, upper- and lower-airway obstruction, reactive airway disease, noncardiac pulmonary edema, retained secretions, restricted lung mechanics, preexisting pulmonary dysfunction, muscle weakness, trauma, pain, adverse drug reactions, and aspiration. Careful analysis of the history, physical examination, clinical course, and laboratory data establish the diagnosis and dictate treatment in the individual patient.

REFERENCES

1. Braunwald E: Chest pain and palpitations, in Isselbacher KJ, Adam RD, Braunwald E, Petersdorf RG, Wilson JD (eds): *Harrison's Principles of Internal Medicine*, 9th ed. New York, McGraw-Hill, 1980, pp 28–34.
2. Mangano D: Perioperative cardiac morbidity. *Anesthesiology* 72:153–184, 1990.
3. Tarhan S, Moffitt E, Taylor WF et al: Myocardial infarction after general anesthesia. *JAMA* 220:1451–1454, 1972.
4. Knapp RB, Topkins MJ, Artusio JF Jr: The cerebrovascular accident and coronary occlusion in anesthesia. *JAMA* 182:332–334, 1962.
5. Topkins MJ, Artusio JF: Myocardial infarction and surgery: A five-year study. *Anesth Analg* 43:716–720, 1964.
6. Roberts SL, Tinker JH: Cardiovascular disease, in Brown DL (ed): *Risk and Outcome in Anesthesia*. Philadelphia, Lippincott, 1988, pp 33–49.
7. Plumlee JE, Boettner RB: Myocardial infarction during and following anesthesia and operation. *South Med J* 65:886–889, 1972.
8. Goldman L, Caldera DL, Nussbaum SR et al: Multifactorial index of cardiac risk in noncardiac surgical procedures. *N Engl J Med* 297:845–850, 1977.
9. Foster ED, Davis KB, Carpenter JA et al: Risk of noncardiac operation in patients with defined coronary disease: The coronary artery surgery study (CASS) registry experience. *Ann Thorac Surg* 41:42–50, 1986.
10. Hertzer NR, Beven EG, Young JR et al: Coronary artery disease in peripheral vascular patients. A classification of 1000 coronary angiograms and results of surgical management. *Ann Surg* 199:223–233, 1984.
11. Goldman L: Cardiac risks and complications of noncardiac surgery. *Ann Intern Med* 98:504–513, 1983.
12. Rao TLK, Jacobs KH, El-Etr AA: Reinfarction following anesthesia in patients with myocardial infarctions. *Anesthesiology* 59:499–505, 1983.
13. Dershwitz M, Sherman EP: Acute myocardial infarction symptoms masked by epidural morphine? *J Clin Anesth* 3:146–148, 1991.
14. Mangano DT, Browner WS, Hollenberg M et al: Association of perioperative myocardial ischemia with cardiac morbidity and mortality in men undergoing noncardiac surgery. *N Engl J Med* 323:1781–1788, 1990.
15. Marriott HKL: Myocardial infarction, in *Practical Echocardiography*, 7th ed. Baltimore, Williams & Wilkins, 1983, pp 373–401.
16. Weinfurt PT: Electrocardiographic monitoring: An overview. *J Clin Monit* 6:132–138, 1990.
17. Kotter G, Kotrly K, Kalbfleisch J et al: Myocardial ischemia during cardiovascular surgery as detected by an ST-segment trend monitoring system. *J Cardiothorac Anesth* 1:190–199, 1987.
18. Roger MC, Abildskov JA, Preston JB: Neurogenic ECG changes in critically ill patients: An experimental model. *Crit Care Med* 1:192, 1973.
19. Presswitz W, Neumier D: Creatine-kinase and CK-MB isoenzyme activity in serum of patients after surgical operations, polytrauma and other damage to skeletal muscle. *Clin Biochem* 12:225, 1979.
20. Buja LM, Parkey RW, Dees JH et al: Morphologic correlates of ^{99m}technetium stannous pyrophosphate imaging of acute myocardial infarcts in dogs. *Circulation* 52:596–607, 1975.
21. Holman BL, Wynne J: Infarct avid (hot-spot) myocardial scintigraphy. *Radiol Clin N Am* 18:487–499, 1980.
22. Pflugfelder PW, Wisenberg G, Prato FS et al: Early detection of canine myocardial infarction by magnetic resonance imaging in vivo. *Circulation* 71:587–594, 1985.
23. McNamara MT, Higgins CB, Schectmann N et al: Detection and characterization of acute myocardial infarction in man with use of gated magnetic resonance. *Circulation* 71:717–724, 1985.
24. Lieberman RW, Orkin FK, Jobes DR et al: Hemodynamic predictors of myocardial ischemia during halothane anesthesia for coronary artery revascularization. *Anesthesiology* 59:36–41, 1983.
25. Prys-Roberts C, Meloche R, Foex P: Studies of anaesthesia in relation to hypertension: I. Cardiovascular responses to treated and untreated patients. *Br J Anaesth* 43:122–137, 1971.
26. Steen PA, Tinker JH, Tarhan S: Myocardial reinfarction after anesthesia and surgery. *JAMA* 239:2566–2570, 1978.
27. London MJ, Hollenberg M, Wong WG et al: Intraoperative myocardial ischemia: Localization by continuous 12-lead electrocardiography. *Anesthesiology* 69:232–241, 1988.
28. van Daele ME, Sutherland GR, Mitchell MM et al: Do changes in pulmonary capillary wedge pressure adequately reflect myocardial ischemia during anesthesia: A correlative preoperative hemodynamic, electrocardiographic, and transesophageal echocardiographic study. *Circulation* 81:865–871, 1990.
29. Smith JS, Cahalan MK, Benefiel DJ et al: Intraoperative detection of myocardial ischemia in high-risk patients: Electrocardiography versus two-dimensional transesophageal echocardiography. *Circulation* 72:1015–1021, 1985.
30. Buffington CW, Coyle RJ: Altered load dependence of postischemic myocardium. *Anesthesiology* 75:464–474, 1991.
31. MacIntyre PE, Pavlin EG, Dwersteg JF: Effect of meperidine on oxygen consumption, carbon dioxide production, and respiratory gas exchange in postanesthesia shivering. *Anesth Analg* 66:751–755, 1987.
32. Gibbs CP, Schwartz DJ, Wynne JW et al: Antacid pulmonary aspiration in the dog. *Anesthesiology* 51:380–385, 1979.
33. Radnay PA, Duncalf D, Novakoric M et al: Common bile duct pressure changes after fentanyl, morphine, meperidine, butorphanol and naloxone. *Anesth Analg* 63:441–444, 1984.
34. Engle MA, Gay WA Jr, Kaminsky ME et al: The postpericardiotomy syndrome then and now. *Curr Prob Cardiol* 312:1–40, 1978.
35. Kassanoff AH, Martirossian MG: Postpericardiotomy and postmyocardial infarction syndrome presenting as noncardiac pulmonary edema. *Chest* 99(6):1410–1414, 1991.
36. Walton K, Holt PJ: Rheumatic symptoms after cardiac surgery: A prospective study. *Br Med J* 197(6640):21–24, 1988.
37. Miller RH, Horneffer PJ, Gardner TJ et al: The epidemiology of the postpericardiotomy syndrome: A common complication of cardiac surgery. *Am Heart J* 116(5):1323–1329, 1988.

38. Horneffer PJ, Miller RH, Pearson TA et al: The effective treatment of postpericardiotomy syndrome after cardiac operations. A randomized placebo-controlled trial. *J Thorac Cardiovasc Surg* 100(2):292–296, 1990.

39. Ingram RH Jr, Braunwald E: Dyspnea and pulmonary edema, in Isselbacher KJ, Adams RD, Braunwald E et al: (eds): *Harrison's Principles of Internal Medicine*, 9th ed. New York, McGraw-Hill, 1980, pp 162–166.

40. Hirshman CA, McCullough RE, Cohen PJ et al: Effect of pentobarbitone on hypoxic ventilatory drive in man. *Br J Anaesth* 47:963–968, 1975.

41. Weiskopf RB, Raymond LW, Severinghaus JW: Effects of halothane on canine respiratory responses to hypoxia with and without hypercarbia. *Anesthesiology* 41:350–360, 1974.

42. Lee KW, Downes JJ: Pulmonary edema secondary to laryngospasm in children. *Anesthesiology* 59:347–349, 1983.

43. Lorch DG, Sahn SA: Post-extubation pulmonary edema following anesthesia induced by upper airway obstruction. Are certain patients at increased risk? *Chest* 90:802–805, 1986.

44. Stoelting RK, Dierdorf F, McCammon RL: Obstructive airway diseases, in *Anesthesia and Co-Existing Disease*, 2d ed. New York, Churchill Livingstone, 1988, pp 195–226.

45. Milne B, Spence D, Beverly Lynn R et al: Unilateral reexpansion pulmonary edema during emergence from general anesthesia. *Anesthesiology* 59:244–245, 1983.

46. Gurman G, Collins GI, Fradis M et al: Unilateral pulmonary edema after bilateral pneumothorax. *Anaesthesia* 33:613–616, 1978.

47. Dal Nogare AR: Adult respiratory distress syndrome. *Am J Med Sci* 296:413–430, 1989.

48. Taff RH: Pulmonary edema following naloxone administration in a patient without heart disease. *Anesthesiology* 59:576–577, 1983.

49. Schwartz JA, Koenigsberg MD: Naloxone-induced pulmonary edema. *Ann Emerg Med* 16:1294–1296, 1987.

50. Prough DS, Roy R, Baumgardner J, Shannon G: Acute pulmonary edema in healthy teenager following conservative doses of intravenous naloxone. *Anesthesiology* 60:485–486, 1984.

51. Wanner A, Landa J, Nieman R et al: Bedside bronchofiberoscopy for atelectasis and lung abscess. *JAMA* 224:1281–1283, 1973.

52. Dreisin R, Albert R, Talley P et al: Flexible fiberoptic bronchoscopy in teaching hospital: Yield and complications. *Chest* 74:144–149, 1978.

53. Rochester DF, Enson Y: Current concepts in the pathogenesis of obesity-hypoventilation syndrome. *Am J Med* 57:402–420, 1974.

54. Vaughan RW, Vaughan MS: Unusual patients, pathologic obesity, in Martin JT (ed): *Positioning in Anesthesia and Surgery*. Philadelphia, Saunders, 1987, pp 281–290.

55. Vaughan RW, Vaughan MS: Morbid obesity: Implications for anesthetic care. *Sem Anesth* 3:218–227, 1984.

56. Vaughan RW, Bauer S, Wise L: Volume and pH of gastric juice in obese patients. *Anesthesiology* 43:686–689, 1975.

57. Strandberg A, Tokics L, Brismar B et al: Constitutional factors promoting development of atelectasis during anaesthesia. *Acta Anaesth Scand* 31:21–24, 1987.

58. Bevan DR, Bevan JC, Donati F: Drug interactions, in *Muscle Relaxants in Clinical Anesthesia*. Chicago, Year Book Medical, 1988, pp 389–413.

59. Miller RD, Way WL, Dolan WM et al: Comparative neuromuscular effects of pancuronium, gallamine and succinylcholine during forane and halothane anesthesia in man. *Anesthesiology* 35:509–514, 1971.

60. Ghoneim MM, Long JP: The interaction between magnesium and other neuromuscular blocking agents. *Anesthesiology* 33:23–29, 1970.

61. Zukaitis MG, Hoech GP: Train of four measurement of potentiation of curare by lidocaine. *Anesthesiology* 51:S288, 1979.

62. Usubiaga JF, Wikinsk JA, Morales RL: Interaction of intravenously administered procaine, lidocaine and succinylcholine in anesthetized subjects. *Anesth Analg* 46:39–45, 1967.

63. Durant NN, Ngyugen N, Katz RL: Potentiation of neuromuscular blockade with verapamil. *Anesthesiology* 60:298–303, 1984.

64. Way WL, Katzunoz BS, Lawson CP: Recurarization with quinidine. *JAMA* 200:163–164, 1967.

65. Feldman SA: Effect of changes in electrolytes, hydration and pH upon the reactions to muscle relaxants. *Br J Anaesth* 35:546–550, 1963.

66. Witavouri K, Salmenpera M, Tauristo T: Effect of hypocarbia and hypercarbia on the antagonism of pancuronium-induced neuromuscular blockade with neostigmine in man. *Br J Anaesth* 54:51–61, 1982.

67. Miller RD, Roderick LL: Acid-base balance and neostigmine antagonism of pancuronium neuromuscular blockade. *Br J Anaesth* 50:317–324, 1978.

68. Ham CG, Miller RD, Benet LZ et al: The pharmacokinetics and pharmacodynamics of D-tubocurarine during hypothermia in the cat. *Anesthesiology* 49:324–329, 1978.

69. Miller RD, Agostons, Van der Pol F et al: Hypothermia and pharmacokinetics and pharmacodynamics of pancuronium in the cat. *J Pharmacol Exp Ther* 207:532–535, 1978.

70. Grob D, Namba T: Characteristics and mechanism of neuromuscular block in myasthenia gravis. *Ann NY Acad Sci* 274:143–199, 1976.

71. Bevan DR, Bevan JC, Donati F: Neuromuscular diseases, in *Muscle Relaxants in Clinical Anesthesia*. Chicago, Year Book Medical, 1988, pp 414–430.

72. Viby-Mogensen J, Jorgensen BC, Ording H: Residual curarization in the recovery room. *Anesthesiology* 50:539–541, 1979.

73. Moore WS: Complications of vertebral and subclavian repair, in Bernhard VM, Tawne JD (eds): *Complications in Vascular Surgery*, 2d ed. Orlando, Grune & Stratton, 1985, pp 753–761.

74. Markand ON, Moorthy SS, Mahomed Y et al: Postoperative phrenic nerve palsy in patients with heart surgery. *Ann Thorac Surg* 39:68–73, 1985.

75. Knoblanche GE: Incidence and etiology of phrenic nerve blockade associated with supraclavicular brachial plexus block. *Anaesth Inten Care* 7:346–349, 1979.

76. Barnaka A, Hemady K, Yamut E et al: Postoperative paralysis of phrenic nerve and recurrent laryngeal nerves. *Anesthesiology* 55:78–80, 1981.

77. Murphy TM: Nerve blocks, in Miller RD (ed): *Anesthesia*, 2d ed. New York, Churchill Livingstone, 1986, pp 1015–1060.

78. Hahn FW, Martin JT, Lillie JC: Vocal-cord paralysis with endotracheal intubation. *Arch Otol* 92:226–229, 1970.

79. Halley HS, Gilden JE: Vocal-cord paralysis after tracheal intubation. *JAMA* 215:281–284, 1971.

80. Ellis VF, Tremblay NAG: Recurrent laryngeal nerve palsy and endotracheal intubation. *J Laryngol Otol* 89:823–826, 1975.

81. Paulsen K, Reinhardt M: The blockade of the stellate ganglion and its dangers. *MMW* 112:817, 1970.

82. Hughes TJ, Desgrand DA: Upper limb blocks, in Wildsmith AV, Armitage EN (eds): *Principles and Practice of Regional Anesthesia*. Edinburgh, Churchill Livingstone, 1987, pp 138–154.

83. Doctor NH, Hussain Z: Bilateral pneumothorax associated with laparoscopy. *Anaesthesia* 28:75–81, 1973.

84. Smiler BG, Falick YS: Complications during anesthesia and laparoscopy. *JAMA* 226:676, 1973.

85. Chaix C, Verret J, Girault M et al: Pneumomediastinum, pneumothorax and pneumoperitoneum complicating cervical surgery. *Anes Analg* 33:127–134, 1976.

86. Defalque R, Nord NJ: Supraclavicular technique of subclavian vein puncture for the anesthetist. *Anaesthetist* 19:197, 1970.

87. Mitchell A, Steer HW: Late appearance of pneumothorax after subclavian vein catheterization: An anaesthetic hazard. *Br Med J* 281:133, 1980.

88. Katz S: Spontaneous pneumothorax, in Moser KM, Spragg RG (eds): *Respiratory Emergencies*. St. Louis, Mosby, 1982, pp 176–193.

89. Levy JH: Allergy and anesthesia, in *40th Annual Refresher Cours*

Lectures and Clinical Update Program. American Society of Anesthesia, 1989, p 453.

90. Rosen CE, Moss J, Philbin DM et al: Histamine release during morphine and fentanyl anesthesia. *Anesthesiology* 56:93–96, 1982.

91. Hirshman CA, Edelstein RA, Eastman CL: Histamine release by barbiturates in human mast cells. *Anesthesiology* 63:533–536, 1985.

92. Levy JH, Kettiskamp N, Goertz P et al: Histamine release by vancomycin: A mechanism for hypotension in man. *Anesthesiology* 67:756–766, 1989.

93. Levy JH: Systems that can generate immediate hypersensitivity reactions independent of IgE, in *Anaphylactic Reactions in Anesthesia and Intensive Care*. Boston, Butterworths, 1986, pp 39–50.

94. Mosoioki RA, Sookin SM, Corsello BF et al: Anaphylaxis during induction of anesthesia; subsequent evaluation and management. *J Allergy Clin Immunol* 86:325–332, 1990.

95. Moneret-Vautrin DA, Widmer S, Gueant J et al: Simultaneous anaphylaxis to thiopentone and a neuromuscular blocker: A study of two cases. *Br J Anaesth* 64:743–745, 1990.

96. Watkins J: Anaphylactoid reactions to IV substances. *Br J Anaesth* 51:51–60, 1979.

97. Levy JH: Common anaphylactic and anaphylactoid reactions the anesthesiologist sees, in *Anaphylactic Reactions in Anesthesia and Intensive Care*. Boston, Butterworths, 1986, pp 129–152.

98. Schulze-Delrieu K: Metaclopramide. *Gastroenterol* 77:768–779, 1979.

99. Toung L, Cameron JL: Cimetidine as preoperative medication to reduce the complications of gastric contents. *Surgery* 87:205–208, 1980.

100. Goudsouzidan N, Cote CJ, Linn LMP et al: The dose-response effects of oral cimetidine on gastric pH and volume in children. *Anesthesiology* 55:533–536, 1981.

101. Wynne JW, Modell JH: Respiratory aspiration of stomach contents. *Ann Intern Med* 87:466–474, 1977.

102. Mendelson CL: The aspiration of stomach contents into the lungs during obstetrical anesthesia. *Am J Obstet Gynecol* 52:191–205, 1946.

103. Wynne JW, Demarco FJ, Hood CI: Physiological effects of corticosteroids in foodstuff aspiration. *Arch Surg* 116:46–49, 1981.

104. Barash PG: Monitoring myocardial oxygen balance: Physiologic basis and clinical application, in *American Society of Anesthesiologists Refresher Course in Anesthesiology*. Philadelphia, Lippincott, 1985, vol 8, pp 21–32.

56 PERIOPERATIVE ARRHYTHMIAS AND CARDIAC ARREST

Mark E. Rosenthal

Disturbances of cardiac rhythm are common in the perioperative period and can range from relatively trivial arrhythmias such as premature atrial depolarizations to ventricular fibrillation and cardiac arrest. They may be markers of underlying cardiac disease or the result of disturbances in other organ systems. This chapter reviews the epidemiology, etiology, and management of perioperative arrhythmias and cardiac arrest.

EPIDEMIOLOGY OF PERIOPERATIVE ARRHYTHMIAS

Incidence

Several previous studies have documented the overall incidence of cardiac arrhythmias occurring in a wide range of surgical procedures. With arrhythmia defined as any aberration from normal sinus rhythm, the incidence ranges from 18 to 84 percent in surgical series.[1-3] Methods of detection (e.g., continuous electrocardiographic monitoring or random postoperative electrocardiogram), anesthetic agents used, and types of operative procedure all vary in these studies.

Supraventricular arrhythmias are common and are generally slow in rate.[1,2,4] They include junctional or nodal rhythms, sinus bradycardia, and wandering atrial pacemaker. They occur most commonly during surgery and are usually transient with no particular hemodynamic significance. Premature supraventricular complexes are also commonly noted.[1,2,3]

Supraventricular tachycardia (SVT) was noted in four percent of the patients in Goldman's large series.[4,5] Utilizing a 12-lead electrocardiogram (ECG) on the fifth postoperative day or at a time of change in clinical status, he found that atrial fibrillation was the most common SVT, followed by SVT of undetermined mechanism, atrial flutter, paroxysmal atrial tachycardia, and multifocal atrial tachycardia.[5] In an earlier series, Rogers et al. found the incidence of SVT to be lower at about one percent, but atrial fibrillation and flutter were the most common supraventricular tachyarrhythmias noted.[6]

Serious ventricular arrhythmias are not detected in most surgical patients. While premature ventricular depolarizations occur frequently, there are few cases of nonsustained or sustained ventricular tachyarrhythmias.[1,3,4,7] The incidence of perioperative cardiac arrest is low, occurring in approximately one out of every 500 to 2000 cases.[8-12] It is due to ventricular tachycardia (VT) or fibrillation (VF) in approximately 50 percent and to severe bradyarrhythmias or asystole in the remainder.[8,9]

Timing of Perioperative Arrhythmias

A number of studies have documented the time in the perioperative period at which cardiac arrhythmias are most likely to appear. Bertrand et al. found the highest incidence at the time of anesthesia administration and intubation when 84 of 100 patients experienced aberration from normal sinus rhythm.[3] By comparison, 48 had arrhythmias during recovery from surgery. Similar analyses in patients suffering perioperative cardiac arrest have noted that 25 to 67 percent of episodes occur during induction and intubation, 30 to 60 percent during surgery, and up to 40 percent during recovery.[9,10,12,13]

In the postoperative period there is usually a delay after surgery before arrhythmias emerge. In the series of Rogers et al., the average onset of clinically detected SVT was 4.9 days after surgery, with 45 percent of the episodes occurring after the second postoperative day.[6] In a series of patients undergoing lung resection, Mowry et al. noted that 87 percent of arrhythmias occurred between the second and sixth postoperative day.[14] In Goldman's series, 23 percent of postoperative SVT occurred by the end of the first postoperative day, but 75 percent did so by the end of the third.[5] Analysis of postoperative cardiac arrest reveals that up to 50 percent occur during the postoperative recovery phase.[13]

Type of Operative Procedure

The type of surgical procedure may influence the occurrence of cardiac arrhythmias perioperatively. Goldman found that perioperative SVT is more common in patients undergoing intraabdominal, intrathoracic, or major vascular procedures.[5] Perioperative cardiac arrest is six times as likely to occur during emergency surgery as during elective surgery.[10]

Intrathoracic procedures are associated with a uniquely increased incidence of associated cardiac arrhythmias. Mowry et al. noted the incidence of arrhythmias after lung resection to be 3.8 percent with 73 percent due to atrial fibrillation and 27 percent to atrial flutter.[14] Ghosh et al. documented a 34 percent incidence of arrhythmias in patients undergoing thoracotomy, with atrial fibrillation and flutter accounting for almost one-half of the arrhythmias noted and premature atrial and ventricular depolarizations constituting the remainder.[15] Krowka found a 22 percent incidence of arrhythmias in patients undergoing pneumonectomy with 77 percent of the episodes due to either atrial fibrillation or flutter.[16] Goldman et al. reported a 10 percent incidence of SVT in thoracic surgery.[4] Interestingly, pulmonary malignancy is associated with a higher incidence of arrhythmia in thoracic surgery, possibly due to the extent of the procedure.[15,17]

Coronary artery bypass surgery is also associated with an increased incidence of perioperative cardiac arrhythmias. As might be expected, atrial manipulation at the time cardiopulmonary bypass is initiated leads to a preponderance of supraventricular arrhythmias. The incidence ranges from 15 to 40 percent[18–23] with the majority again being atrial fibrillation or flutter. Premature ventricular depolarizations are also common[24–26] and usually have no hemodynamic significance. New sustained ventricular arrhythmias are uncommon and occurred in only 12 of 1675 patients or 0.7 percent in the series of Topol et al.[27]

ETIOLOGIC FACTORS (TABLE 56–1)

Intraoperative Factors

Agents used for induction and maintenance of anesthesia may play a role in the development of bradycardic rhythms during surgery. Halothane, enflurane, isoflurane, and fentanyl can all decrease the rate of sinus node depolarization,[28,29] leading to sinus bradycardia or wandering atrial or junctional rhythms. Succinylcholine can produce bradycardia or tachycardia but rarely has been shown to cause severe bradycardia or asystole during surgery unless a second intravenous dose is given too soon after the first.[9,28,29]

Anesthetic agents may play a role in the development of intraoperative cardiac tachyarrhythmias. Halothane is known to sensitize the myocardium to circulating catecholamines, decrease the threshold for cell membrane excitability, and increase nonuniformity of myocardial electrical recovery.[28,30] This may account for the increased incidence of arrhythmias with this agent when compared to enflurane[31] or isoflurane.[32] All inhalational general anesthetics can cause myocardial depression.[30] Subsequent worsening of left ventricular function may adversely affect intracardiac filling pressure and precipitate supraventricular and ventricular arrhythmias. Other agents used during induction that may precipitate tachycardia include pancuronium, gallamine, atropine, succinylcholine, and D-tubocurarine.[9,28] In addition, there are anecdotal reports of intra-

TABLE 56–1. Causes of Perioperative Arrhythmias

Intraoperative Factors

Arrhythmogenic effects of anesthetic agents
Endotracheal intubation
Activation of vagal reflexes during surgical manipulation (eye, nasopharynx, lateral rectus muscle, bronchi, peritoneum)
Myocardial irritation from intracardiac catheters
Anesthetic error

Medical Factors

Cardiac
- Myocardial ischemia and infarction
- Congestive heart failure
- Existing substrate for arrhythmias

Pulmonary
- Inadequate ventilation
- Pneumonia
- Pulmonary embolus
- Pneumothorax
- Pleural effusions

Metabolic/Electrolyte Disturbances
- Hypokalemia/hyperkalemia
- Hypomagnesemia
- Hypercalcemia/hypocalcemia
- Hyponatremia/hypernatremia
- Acidemia/alkalemia
- Hypoxemia/hypercarbia

Medications
- Pressor and inotropic agents
- Proarrhythmic effects of antiarrhythmic drugs
- Bronchodilator therapy
- Calcium channel and beta-blocking agents
- Withdrawal from beta-blocking agents, clonidine
- Withdrawal from narcotic analgesics

Miscellaneous
- Fever
- Anemia
- Alcohol withdrawal

operative cardiac arrest due to the presumed inadvertent intravascular administration of local anesthetics.[33,34]

Various anesthetic and surgical manipulations during the procedure may also predispose to aberrations in cardiac rhythm. Endotracheal intubation causes an increase in circulating catecholamines and subsequent cardiac adrenergic stimulation that can lead to tachycardia and an increased frequency of ectopy.[3,28,30] Inadequate anesthesia has similar effects. In contrast, surgical manipulation of the eye, nasopharynx, lateral rectus muscle, bronchi, or peritoneum may activate vagal reflexes with resultant bradycardia and hypotension.[29,35]

The use of intracardiac monitoring with pulmonary artery catheters is becoming increasingly common in patients with more advanced cardiac dysfunction undergoing surgery. These catheters may irritate the surrounding myocardium and cause new supraventricular and ventricular arrhythmias. In addition, direct trauma to the atrioventricular (AV) conduction system may occur during passage of catheters and cause advanced heart block, especially in patients with preexisting left bundle branch block.

Medical Factors

Preexisting cardiac disease is more common in patients who develop perioperative cardiac arrhythmias.[1,3–6] In general, its severity is proportional to the likelihood of developing arrhythmias. Acute cardiac decompensation due to myocardial ischemia or congestive heart failure may account for the sudden emergence of cardiac arrhythmias. Rogers et al. documented acute cardiac problems in 20 percent of 50 patients with postoperative SVT.[6] Goldman identified an acute cardiac event in 46 percent of such patients.[5] Worsening congestive heart failure was the most common precipitating factor, followed by new myocardial ischemia or infarction. The incidence of newly diagnosed myocardial infarction in this series was 11 percent.

Pulmonary complications with hypoxemia may also contribute to new perioperative arrhythmias. In an analysis of patients with postoperative SVT, 16 of 35 patients had respiratory instability. Seven of them had a $PaO_2 < 60$ mmHg, six had pneumonia, but none had documented pulmonary embolus.[5] In contrast, Rogers et al. documented pulmonary embolus in 6 percent of 50 patients with postoperative SVT.[6] Pulmonary compromise due to adult respiratory distress syndrome, large pleural effusions, pneumothorax, or atelectasis can also lead to hypoxemia and hypercarbia and subsequent perioperative arrhythmias.

Metabolic disturbances may precipitate new cardiac rhythm disturbances. Derangements in serum potassium, sodium, magnesium, or calcium concentration can cause supraventricular or ventricular arrhythmias.[28,36] Low levels of potassium and magnesium are associated with ventricular arrhythmias and prolongation of the QT–u interval. The latter abnormality can lead to the potentially fatal form of VT known as torsade de pointes. In addition to sinus tachycardia, fever can precipitate both supraventricular and ventricular tachyarrhythmias.

Other medications may also cause new arrhythmias. Systemic pressors such as dopamine and epinephrine and inotropic agents including dobutamine and amrinone increase the incidence of supraventricular and ventricular ectopic complexes and tachyarrhythmias. Beta-blockers and calcium channel blockers may cause excessive bradycardia or cardiac arrest when used in combination with anesthetics.[37–39] Intravenous antiarrhythmic agents such as procainamide and lidocaine have potential proarrhythmic effects and can exacerbate or produce new ventricular arrhythmias and worsen function of the sinus node and His-Purkinje system. Psychotropic medications used postoperatively in agitated patients can cause tachycardia and the more serious torsade de pointes associated with QT–u interval prolongation. Intravenous aminophylline and inhalational sympathomimetic bronchodilator therapy commonly cause sinus tachycardia and can exacerbate both supraventricular and ventricular tachyarrhythmias. Attention should be paid to drugs associated with a withdrawal syndrome that includes a hyperadrenergic state and a propensity for arrhythmias. These include alcohol, narcotics, certain sedatives, and sympathetic blocking agents such as beta-blockers and clonidine.

MANAGEMENT OF PERIOPERATIVE ARRHYTHMIAS

A general approach to the patient who develops a perioperative cardiac arrhythmia includes assessment of the patient's clinical and hemodynamic status before, during, and after the arrhythmia; diagnosis of the mechanism or type of arrhythmia; a search for possible reversible causative factors; and selection of an appropriate therapeutic strategy based on the preceding evaluation.

In all cases, the clinical status of the patient during the arrhythmia largely determines the therapeutic approach to a specific arrhythmia. Sustained arrhythmias associated with hemodynamic compromise from shock, congestive heart failure, or myocardial ischemia require immediate attempts to stop the rhythm disturbance. Signs of hypoperfusion or congestive heart failure should be looked for on physical examination. The ECG should be reviewed for findings consistent with myocardial ischemia or infarction. If available, hemodynamic data including cardiac output, pulmonary capillary wedge pressure, and calculated systemic vascular resistance should be assessed. Decreased urine output may indicate poor renal perfusion from reduced cardiac output during the arrhythmia.

In all cases, a 12-lead ECG should be obtained during a sus-

TABLE 56–2. An Approach for Analyzing Wide Complex Tachycardias

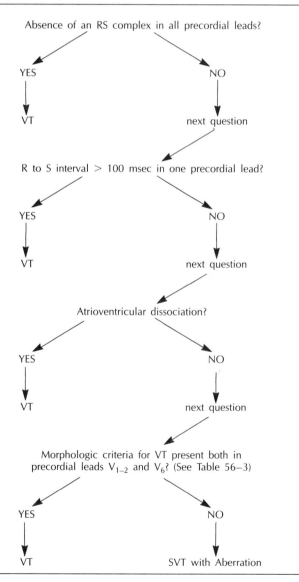

Source: From Brugada P, Brugada J, Mont L et al: A new approach to the differential diagnosis of a regular tachycardia with a wide QRS complex. *Circulation* 83:1649–1659, 1991.

tained arrhythmia. Atrial activity should be identified if present to determine the relationship between atrial and ventricular conduction in order to diagnose AV dissociation or patterns of AV block. Wide-complex tachycardias due to aberrant SVT and VT can be differentiated by using the algorithms in Tables 56–2 and 56–3. When the mechanism of an arrhythmia remains unclear, atrial activity can be recorded with an esophageal electrode.[40] In patients undergoing cardiac surgery, epicardial electrodes placed in atrial and ventricular tissue at the time of the procedure can be used to record unipolar or bipolar atrial and/or ventricular electrograms to facilitate identification of arrhythmias.

A comprehensive search for possible causative factors is essential in the evaluation of perioperative arrhythmias. Possible myocardial ischemia or infarction should be assessed with a careful review of the 12-lead ECG for signs such as ST-segment elevation or depression, new Q waves, or unexplained new conduction disturbances. When increased ventricular ectopic activity and nonsustained or sustained supraventricular or ventricular arrhythmias occur, cardiac enzyme levels, including those of creatine kinase with MB fractions, should be obtained every eight hours over a 24-hour period in patients with possible coronary artery disease. Those with a low risk of coronary disease and no worrisome ECG changes do not require this evaluation.

Serum potassium, magnesium, sodium, and calcium concentrations should be checked emergently. Electrocardiographic changes associated with hypokalemia or hypomagnesemia should be docu-

mented on a 12-lead ECG. Arterial blood gas determination provides information on acid-base balance and possible hypoxemia and hypercarbia. Pulmonary complications leading to metabolic derangements and perioperative arrhythmias may not be evident on physical examination. A chest x-ray can be invaluable in documenting pneumonia, atelectasis, pleural effusions, pneumothorax, or incorrect placement of the endotracheal tube in intubated patients. If present, fever should be treated.

Medications should be carefully reviewed, and any agents possibly contributing to the arrhythmia should be discontinued or reduced in dose. When available, blood concentrations of drugs with cardiac effects should be followed. This is particularly important for digitalis glycosides if signs of toxicity should occur or if medications known to augment blood levels of digitalis such as verapamil, quinidine, and amiodarone are administered simultaneously. Changes in renal function affect elimination of digitalis and require close attention to blood levels.

Deciding when to pursue the diagnosis of pulmonary embolism is often difficult. In conscious patients who develop sudden pleuritic chest pain, hyperventilation, and unexplained hypoxemia with a new perioperative cardiac arrhythmia, the decision is straightforward. However, in less clear situations, other factors must be considered in the decision. These include a previous history of thromboembolic events and the presence of conditions that predispose the patient to the development of deep-venous thrombosis such as prolonged immobilization, orthopedic or urologic surgery, and congestive heart failure. Since anticoagulation increases the risk of bleeding in the immediate postoperative period, the diagnosis should always be confirmed or excluded with a ventilation-perfusion lung scan and if necessary a pulmonary angiogram.

TABLE 56–3. Morphology Criteria Used in Analyzing a Wide QRS Tachycardia

Criteria	Analysis
1. Is QRS width > .14 seconds?	If so, VT is likely, but cannot exclude SVT with preexisting BBB or SVT conducting antegrade over an AV bypass tract.
2. Is the frontal plane QRS axis superiorly directed?	If so, VT is likely, but cannot exclude SVT with preexisting BBB or SVT conducting antegrade over a right-sided or posteroseptal AV bypass tract.
3. What is the QRS configuration in V_1 and V_6?	
In RBBB shaped QRS	A monophasic R or qR in V_1 suggests VT.
	An R:S ratio in V_6 < 1 suggests VT.
In LBBB shaped QRS	R in V_1, V_2 during tachycardia higher than the R in V_1, V_2 during NSR suggests VT.
	Initial positive deflection in V_1 > 30 msec in duration suggests VT.
	A qR in V_6 suggests VT.

Abbreviations: AV—atrioventricular; BBB—bundle branch block; LBBB—left bundle branch block; NSR—normal sinus rhythm; RBBB—right bundle branch block; SVT—supraventricular tachycardia; VT—ventricular tachycardia.
Source: Adapted from Wellens HJJ, Brugada P: The approach to the patient with ventricular tachycardia. *Learning Center Highlights* 4:9, 1989.

THERAPEUTIC STRATEGIES FOR SPECIFIC ARRHYTHMIAS (TABLE 56–4)

Supraventricular Arrhythmias

Premature Atrial Depolarizations

Premature atrial depolarizations are common in the perioperative period and have no hemodynamic significance in most cases. Other than reversing any metabolic or electrolyte disturbance, no specific therapy is required.

Atrial Fibrillation

The most important hemodynamic considerations in atrial fibrillation are loss of effective atrial contraction and rapid ventricular rates. When left ventricular compliance is low in left ventricular hypertrophy due to hypertension, aortic stenosis, or hypertrophic cardiomyopathy, sudden loss of the atrial contribution to left ventricular filling can lead to hypotension, hypoperfusion, and occasionally hemodynamic collapse. In this setting, immediate electrical cardioversion is first-line therapy.

In stable hemodynamic situations, the first goal of therapy is to slow the ventricular rate. Digoxin is commonly given intravenously or orally in an initial dose of 0.25 to 0.50 mg. A total of 0.75 to 1 mg is administered in the first 24 hours in divided doses, and a subsequent daily maintenance dose is chosen on the basis of renal function. The cardiac rate usually begins to slow 3

TABLE 56–4.   Antiarrhythmic Agents

Drug	Class	Dose	Indications
Quinidine	IA	PO: 200–400 mg q 4–6 h	A-fib, A-flutter, SVT, PVC, VT, VF
Procainamide	IA	IV: 12 mg/kg (no more than 100 mg q 5 min) load, then 2–6 mg/min PO: 50 mg/kg/day q 3–4 h (or q 6 h with long-acting)	A-fib, A-flutter, SVT, PVC, VT, VF
Disopyramide	IA	PO: 100–200 mg q 6 h	A-fib, A-flutter, SVT, PVC, VT, VF
Lidocaine	IB	IV: 1 mg/kg over 2 min, then 2 mg/kg over 20 min or 20 mg/min over 10 min Maintenance: 1–4 mg/min	PVC, VT, VF
Mexiletine	IB	PO: 100–200 mg q 8 h initially, with up to 1200 mg/day maximum in divided doses	PVC, VT, VF
Tocainide	IB	PO: 200–400 mg q 8 h up to a maximum of 2400 mg/day in divided doses	PVC, VT, VF
Flecainide	IC	PO: 100 mg q 12 h initially, increased q 4–6 days if needed by 50 mg increments to a maximum of 400 mg/day	SVT in the absence of structural heart disease, sustained VT or VF
Propafenone	IC	PO: 150 mg q 8 h initially, then increased q 4–6 days if needed by 75 mg increments to a maximum of 300 mg q 8 h	SVT in the absence of structural heart disease, sustained VT or VF
Propranolol	II	PO: 10–80 mg q 6 h IV: up to .1 mg/kg (1 mg/min)	Slowing of ventricular response in A-fib, A-flutter, termination of SVT
Esmolol	II	IV: 500 mcg/kg over 1 min followed by 25 mcg/kg/min Increase infusion by 25–50 mcg/kg/min q 4 min as needed Maintenance: 100–300 mcg/kg/min	Slowing of ventricular response in A-fib, A-flutter, termination of SVT
Amiodarone	II	PO: loading 800–1600 mg/day for 1–3 weeks Maintenance: 400–600 mg/day	A-fib, A-flutter, SVT, PVC, VT, VF
Bretylium	III	IV: loading 5 mg/kg with additional doses of 10 mg/kg to maximum of 30 mg/kg	VT, VF

TABLE 56–4.   *(Continued)*

Drug	Class	Dose	Indications
		Maintenance: 5–10 mg/kg q 6 h or 1–2 mg/min.	
Verapamil	IV	IV: 5–10 mg over 2–3 min; repeat in 30 min if needed IV infusion: .375 mg/min after initial dose, then .125 mg/min PO: 40–120 mg tid–qid	Slow ventricular response in A-fib, A-flutter, termination of SVT
Digoxin	—	Load (IV or PO): .5 mg initially, then .25 mg q 6 h to a total of 1 mg Maintenance: .125 mg to .5 mg daily	Slow ventricular response in A-fib, A-flutter, termination of SVT
Adenosine	—	IV: 6 mg rapidly via a central vein if possible as initial dose; if unsuccessful, a second dose of 12 mg may be given	Termination of SVT

Abbreviations: A-fib—atrial fibrillation; A-flutter—atrial flutter; PVC—premature ventricular complex; SVT—supraventricular tachycardia; VT—ventricular tachycardia; VF—ventricular fibrillation.

to 45 minutes after intravenous administration. The presence of elevated catecholamine levels after surgery can counteract the effect of digitalis in slowing AV nodal conduction.

Alternative agents, either alone or in combination with digitalis, can be used to slow ventricular response in atrial fibrillation. Intravenous verapamil can be administered in 2.5 to 5 mg doses as needed, and the arterial hypotension sometimes seen with this agent can be prevented by giving calcium chloride beforehand. If needed, oral verapamil can be continued in a dose of 80 to 120 mg every eight hours to maintain rate control. Beta-blockers can also be administered intravenously. Propranolol in doses of 1 to 2 mg up to 0.1 mg/kg can be repeated every four to six hours as needed. Intravenous beta-blockers should not be given in combination with intravenous verapamil to avoid potential hypotension and severe myocardial depression in patients with preexisting cardiac disease. Hypotension, exacerbation of bronchospasm, and compromise of peripheral arterial flow in patients with severe peripheral vascular disease are side effects of beta-blockers.

Esmolol is an ultrashort-acting cardioselective intravenous beta-blocker with a half-life of only nine minutes. It is as effective as propranolol in controlling ventricular rate in atrial fibrillation but is associated with an increased incidence of systemic hypotension.[41,42] It is given by continuous intravenous infusion and can be titrated to the desired ventricular rate.

Once the ventricular rate is controlled, conversion to normal sinus rhythm should be attempted. In some cases, administration of digoxin, verapamil, or beta-blockers or correction of causative factors like congestive failure result in conversion to sinus rhythm. Therefore, an observation period of 24 to 48 hours is warranted before initiating more definitive therapy. Should atrial fibrillation persist, antiarrhythmic therapy with a type IA agent like oral quinidine or oral or intravenous procainamide should be administered, with special attention paid to the corrected QT–u interval to avoid excessive prolongation and torsade de pointes. If antiarrhythmic therapy is unsuccessful, electrical cardioversion can be performed after appropriate sedation. Systemic anticoagulation is not recommended before electrical or chemical cardioversion of atrial fibrillation of less than three days' duration. In patients with atrial fibrillation lasting four or more days, a three-week course of oral warfarin is recommended by some before attempting electrical or pharmacologic cardioversion.[43]

Atrial Flutter

Atrial flutter may present perioperatively with typical saw-tooth flutter waves seen best in the inferior leads of an ECG or as a supraventricular rhythm with a rate of about 150 beats per minute without obvious flutter waves. The latter represents 2:1 AV block, the most common pattern of AV conduction seen with flutter. Maneuvers to increase the degree of block such as carotid sinus massage or use of intravenous AV-blocking agents can make flutter waves more obvious.

As in atrial fibrillation, excessively rapid ventricular rate should be controlled with digoxin, intravenous verapamil, or beta-blockers. It is often more difficult to keep the ventricular rate under 100 beats per minute in atrial flutter than in atrial fibrillation. Occasionally, in correcting reversible causes or administering AV nodal blocking agents, conversion to normal sinus rhythm or atrial fibrillation occurs.

There are a number of options to convert atrial flutter to sinus rhythm. Pharmacologic therapy with an intravenous or oral type IA agent can be undertaken with continuous electrocardiographic monitoring, or electrical cardioversion can be attempted. Overdrive atrial pacing may also be effective in terminating atrial flutter or converting it to atrial fibrillation. This technique requires insertion of a temporary transvenous electrode catheter into the atrium under fluoroscopic guidance or use of epicardial atrial wires placed at the time of cardiac surgery. Systemic anticoagulation is generally not recommended for cardioversion of atrial flutter.[43]

Junctional Rhythms

Junctional rhythms are usually transient and have no hemodynamic significance in the perioperative period. Excessive vagal tone is often the cause, and intervention is usually not required. However, occasional patients exhibit decreased cardiac output and hypoperfusion with the loss of normal atrioventricular synchrony. In these cases, intravenous administration of atropine in a dose of 0.5 to 1 mg increases the sinus rate and restores normal AV conduction. Agents that suppress sinus node function, such as calcium channel antagonists and beta-blockers, should be withdrawn. Accelerated junctional rhythms with rates over 70 beats per minute suggest digitalis toxicity.

Supraventricular Tachycardia

The most common supraventricular tachycardias are reentrant in mechanism and arise in the atrium, AV node, or AV circuits involving a bypass tract.[44] Automatic atrial rhythms rarely account for clinically observed SVT. The following discussion therefore focuses on the management of presumed reentrant SVT.

Once SVT is diagnosed, the patient should be assessed for signs and symptoms of hemodynamic compromise. In shock, worsening congestive failure, or angina pectoris believed due to the arrhythmia, immediate electrical cardioversion is indicated. If the SVT is well-tolerated, slowing AV nodal conduction with vagal maneuvers should be attempted. If this is unsuccessful, intravenous adenosine or verapamil will convert reentrant SVT confined to the AV nodal region of the right atrium or via a bypass tract to sinus rhythm in 80 to 100 percent of patients with comparable efficacy.[39,45–47] Adenosine offers the benefit of an extremely short-elimination half-life under 10 seconds without the potential for hemodynamic compromise occasionally seen with verapamil. Alternatively, intravenous propranolol can be given in increments of 1 to 2 mg up to a total dose of 0.1 mg/kg. Digoxin may be used, but its onset of action is usually delayed, making it less practical in emergency situations. In patients with automatic or reentrant atrial tachycardia, treatment may increase the degree of AV block without terminating the arrhythmia.

In patients with known AV reentry involving a bypass tract, pharmacologic agents that act to inhibit conduction in the accessory pathway can be used. These include procainamide, quinidine, disopyramide, lidocaine, and amiodarone. The intravenous drug of choice is procainamide. In patients with preexcitation by way of an AV bypass tract, as in the Wolff-Parkinson-White syndrome, the development of atrial fibrillation can cause hemodynamic compromise with degeneration to ventricular fibrillation. In this setting, immediate electrical cardioversion of the atrial arrhythmia is recommended as first-line therapy. Use of AV-blocking agents is contraindicated because they can accelerate the ventricular rate.

Perioperative Prevention of Supraventricular Tachyarrhythmias

Patients undergoing surgery frequently have a history of supraventricular tachyarrhythmia and may be on antiarrhythmic therapy. They should take their morning dose of medication on the day of surgery and resume it as soon as possible after surgery. In prolonged periods without oral intake, an intravenous equivalent should be substituted or a suitable intravenous alternative given (e.g., procainamide for quinidine). Once the patient is eating, preoperative medications can be resumed.

Several studies have examined the efficacy of preoperative prophylactic therapy of supraventricular tachyarrhythmias. Prophylactic digitalis administration has met with mixed results in patients undergoing coronary artery bypass graft surgery[2,18] and thoracic surgery,[48,49] although it has previously been recommended for these procedures.[50] There is evidence to support the prophylactic use of perioperative propranolol[19,20] and verapamil[21] to prevent supraventricular tachyarrhythmias after coronary artery bypass graft surgery.

Ventricular Arrhythmias

Premature Ventricular Depolarizations

Premature ventricular depolarizations are common in patients with and without structural heart disease. In those with no clinical cardiac disease, they are not associated with adverse prognosis.[51]

In those with coronary artery disease and left ventricular dysfunction, premature ventricular complexes may portend a worse prognosis,[52] but there is no evidence to support routinely suppressing them. In the perioperative setting, pharmacologic suppression is not necessary unless there is a decrease in the effective arterial pulse rate leading to inadequate cardiac output.

A sudden increase in ventricular ectopic activity or the new onset of premature ventricular complexes should prompt a thorough search for possible reversible causes, including electrolyte disturbances, hypoxemia, or evidence of myocardial ischemia or infarction. If suppressive therapy is needed, intravenous lidocaine or procainamide can be used during surgery or immediately thereafter. Effective oral agents include procainamide, quinidine, disopyramide, mexilitine, tocainide, and amiodarone. In some patients, beta-blockers provide effective suppression of ventricular premature beats after surgery.

Nonsustained Repetitive Ventricular Ectopy

The management of nonsustained repetitive ventricular arrhythmias like ventricular couplets and nonsustained ventricular tachycardia remains controversial. There is an increasing trend not to treat patients with these arrhythmias when they are asymptomatic, but this approach is not universally accepted. Some institute therapy if arrhythmias occur during surgery or immediately thereafter and eventually discontinue it after observation with continuous electrocardiographic monitoring. Others withhold therapy in the absence of hemodynamic compromise. Nonsustained repetitive ventricular arrhythmias associated with hemodynamic instability should be suppressed in the perioperative period. The decision regarding chronic oral suppression is then made later in the postoperative course. Administration of any antiarrhythmic drug should include careful consideration of its potential proarrhythmic effects.

Sustained Ventricular Tachycardia

Morphologically, sustained ventricular tachycardia (VT) can be classified as uniform or polymorphic. In uniform or monomorphic VT, all of the QRS complexes are identical, and the rate is generally stable. This rhythm is thought to be due to intraventricular reentry[53] and usually occurs in the setting of prior myocardial infarction and other cardiomyopathic processes. Sustained uniform VT may be tolerated without adverse hemodynamic consequences or may cause partial or complete cardiovascular collapse. In polymorphic sustained VT, the QRS morphology constantly changes, and the rate is often rapid and irregular. When this rhythm occurs in conjunction with congenital or acquired QT-interval prolongation, it is termed torsade de pointes. Myocardial ischemia, electrolyte abnormalities, and drug-induced prolongation of the QT interval should be considered in this setting.

The approach to therapy of sustained VT depends upon how it is tolerated. In the setting of hemodynamic compromise, electrical cardioversion should be performed after appropriate sedation. Otherwise, intravenous therapy with lidocaine or procainamide can be initiated with a loading dose. If the VT persists, low-dose electrical cardioversion with 10 to 20 J or overdrive pacing with a transvenous right ventricular electrode catheter should be attempted. Overdrive pacing can also be performed using epicardial wires left in place after cardiac surgery. If it is attempted, equipment for immediate electrical cardioversion should be available

because it can accelerate otherwise well-tolerated VT or convert it to ventricular fibrillation. As soon as normal sinus rhythm is reestablished, reversible etiologic factors should be investigated and corrected, and intravenous lidocaine or procainamide should be given for at least 24 hours to prevent recurrent episodes. In sustained uniform VT, appropriate therapy may be best determined by cardiac electrophysiologic study once the patient is stable. The role of invasive electrophysiologic study in the assessment of polymorphic VT is less clear. When it occurs in this setting, efforts should be made to exclude severe coronary artery disease if no other etiology is found.

Ventricular Fibrillation

Ventricular fibrillation is responsible for approximately 50 percent of the episodes of intraoperative cardiac arrest[8,9] and is associated with an extremely poor prognosis.[8,9,10,12,54] If resuscitation and cardioversion are successful, myocardial ischemia or infarction should be excluded as the likely cause with serial electrocardiograms and serum creatine kinase measurements. If severe myocardial ischemia is suspected, cardiac catheterization may be feasible when the patient is stable. As in the case of sustained ventricular tachycardia, once normal sinus rhythm is restored, a continuous intravenous infusion of lidocaine, procainamide, or bretylium should be initiated to prevent recurrence. If no obvious etiologic factor can be identified, invasive electrophysiologic study should be considered, although its role in the management of perioperative cardiac arrest is unclear.

Disturbances of Conduction

First-Degree Atrioventricular Block

First-degree AV block is seen on the ECG as prolongation of the P-R interval with a duration over 20 msec. It is generally a hemodynamically insignificant finding and requires no therapy.

Second-Degree Atrioventricular Block

Mobitz Type I or Wenckebach AV block refers to progressive prolongation of AV conduction until complete AV block transiently occurs. It is usually due to conduction delay in the AV node. In most cases, it is well-tolerated without prolonged pauses or subsequent development of high-grade AV block and requires no therapy. When it infrequently causes significant bradycardia, drugs that depress AV nodal conduction such as digoxin, beta-blockers, and calcium channel antagonists should be withdrawn. Administration of atropine in a dose of 0.5 to 1 mg intravenously usually reverses excessive vagal tone and facilitates AV conduction. Temporary pacing is rarely necessary.

Mobitz Type II AV block is usually due to sudden loss of AV conduction in the His-Purkinje system. The risk of sudden progression to high-grade or complete AV block is higher, and this form of AV block is therefore considered potentially malignant. If discovered before surgery, elective permanent pacing should be considered before the procedure if no reversible etiologic factor can be identified and corrected. If it arises during or after surgery, temporary pacing should be instituted emergently to guard against sudden development of complete heart block.

Third-Degree Atrioventricular Block

Complete atrioventricular block may be congenital or acquired. Congenital AV block generally occurs at the level of the AV node and is associated with a stable junctional escape rhythm. In contrast, acquired AV block may occur in the AV node or the His-Purkinje system. The latter variety is associated with a potentially unreliable ventricular escape rhythm.

Patients with congenital AV block undergoing surgery may frequently remain relatively asymptomatic without a pacemaker. However, a conservative approach involves placement of a temporary ventricular pacing electrode to prevent excessive bradycardia from intraoperative changes in vagal tone. Patients with acquired third-degree AV block should have a temporary pacemaker placed if they do not already have a permanent pacemaker. Intravenous isoproterenol can be used to increase the ventricular escape rhythm until arrangements for temporary pacing are made.

Bundle Branch Block

Patients with preexisting bundle branch block or intraventricular conduction delays require no special precautions in the perioperative period. If hemodynamic monitoring with a right-heart catheter is planned in patients with preexisting left bundle branch block, a temporary transvenous pacing catheter or an external transthoracic pacemaker can be used to treat inadvertent traumatic complete heart block. Alternatively, intravenous isoproterenol can be available for rapid use.

New bundle branch block is usually not associated with hemodynamic compromise but should prompt a search for an underlying cause. Sinus tachycardia with aberrant conduction may result in rate-related bundle branch block requiring no therapy. However, new left bundle branch block can mask characteristic electrocardiographic changes of ischemia and infarction and should prompt an investigation to exclude these possibilities in appropriate patients with a history of coronary artery disease or in those with symptoms of angina or congestive failure. Other factors including concomitant antiarrhythmic therapy, electrolyte abnormalities, and systemic acid-base disturbances should also be considered.

Bifascicular block consists of the combination of right bundle branch block and either left anterior or left posterior fascicular block. Several investigators have shown that it does not progress to complete heart block more frequently in the perioperative period.[4,55-59] Therefore, prophylactic temporary pacing is not indicated.

Methods of Temporary Pacing

Until recently, the management of bradyarrhythmias unresponsive to pharmacologic therapy required placement of a temporary transvenous pacing catheter, requiring cannulation of a central vein under fluoroscopic guidance to properly position the tip of the catheter in the apex of the right ventricle. Although safe in experienced hands, the procedure has a risk of hemorrhage, venous thrombosis, infection, cardiac perforation, and aggravation of atrial or ventricular arrhythmias.

An alternative is transcutaneous pacing with large externally placed anterior and posterior thoracic pads. This technique is effective in treating bradycardia emergently[60] and can be used in nonthoracic surgical procedures.[61] A recent intraoperative study documented 100 percent ventricular capture using 50 to 200 mA during surgery.[61] However, it can cause painful stimulation of the pectoral muscles and is often poorly tolerated in conscious patients.

Patients with Implanted Arrhythmia Management Devices

Permanent Pacemakers

The use of electrocautery represents a major risk to patients with implanted permanent pacemakers. The electrical signal emitted by electrosurgical devices may inhibit demand pacemakers, cause triggering of pacing in some devices, or lead to pacemaker reprogramming.[61,62] These problems can be avoided by keeping the electrosurgical device at least 6 and preferably 12 inches away from the pacemaker generator. In pacemaker-dependent patients without a reliable underlying rhythm, the pacemaker should be set in the asynchronous or non-sensing mode when electrocautery is used by fixing a magnet over the pacemaker generator or by programming the pacemaker to an asynchronous mode.[63] This provides continued pacing support and eliminates sensing of cardiac and noncardiac signals. All pacemakers should be checked after surgery. This should include interrogation with an appropriate programmer and determination of sensing and pacing thresholds.

Internal Cardioverter Defibrillator

Occasional patients undergoing surgery have survived the occurrence of malignant ventricular arrhythmias and have internal cardioverter-defibrillators. The currently available generator is placed in an abdominal subcutaneous pocket and is connected either to two extracardiac patch electrodes or to one patch and a spring electrode in the superior vena cava. The generator delivers about 30 J to the patches or electrode-patch combination. These devices sense ventricular tachycardia or fibrillation that initiates automatic charging of the device and defibrillation once the sensing algorithm is satisfied. Investigational devices incorporating a totally transvenous system as well as antitachycardia pacing ability are now being utilized.

The major perioperative hazard in patients with automatic implantable cardioverter-defibrillators is electrocautery. In order to prevent sensing of its high-frequency signal as ventricular fibrillation, the cardioverter-defibrillator should be temporarily deactivated before surgery. This should be done by a cardiologist familiar with the device. Electrocautery should be kept at least six inches from the generator to avoid damage to the circuitry. In abdominal surgery, the surgeon should be familiar with the route of the electrodes to avoid inadvertent damage to the leads.

SUMMARY

1. Supraventricular arrhythmias are commonly noted in the perioperative period but are generally slow and well-tolerated. The most common perioperative SVT is atrial fibrillation. Serious ventricular arrhythmias are rarely detected in surgical patients.

2. Perioperative arrhythmias are most commonly noted during induction of anesthesia and intubation.

3. Intrathoracic surgery is associated with a high incidence of atrial tachyarrhythmias, over half of which are atrial fibrillation or flutter.

4. Assessment of patients with perioperative arrhythmias should include determination of hemodynamic status, a 12-lead ECG to exclude myocardial ischemia, and a search for metabolic derangements and other precipitating causes listed in Table 56–1.

5. Asymptomatic nonsustained supraventricular or ventricular arrhythmias do not generally require treatment unless they are accompanied by hemodynamic compromise.

6. Initial therapy of perioperative atrial fibrillation or flutter is directed at control of the ventricular rate with agents that slow AV nodal conduction, such as digoxin, verapamil, or beta-blockers. Conversion to normal sinus rhythm should be considered when the ventricular rate has fallen below 100 beats per minute.

7. Temporary transvenous or transcutaneous pacing is rarely required in the perioperative setting but may be useful during the placement of pulmonary artery catheters in the setting of chronic left bundle branch block. Prophylactic pacing is not required in chronic bundle branch block or bifascicular block.

8. Electrocautery should be minimized in patients with implantable arrhythmia devices such as pacemakers or internal cardioverter-defibrillators. The latter should be programmed off during surgery utilizing electrocautery and reactivated in the immediate postoperative period.

REFERENCES

1. Vanik PE, Davis HS: Cardiac arrhythmias during halothane anesthesia. *Anesth Analg* 47:299–307, 1968.
2. Kuner J, Enescu V, Utsu F et al: Cardiac arrhythmias during anesthesia. *Dis Chest* 52:580–587, 1967.
3. Bertrand CA, Steiner NV, Jameson AG et al: Disturbances of cardiac rhythm during anesthesia and surgery. *JAMA* 216:1615–1617, 1971.
4. Goldman L, Caldera DL, Southwick FS et al: Cardiac risk factors and complications in noncardiac surgery. *Medicine* 57:357–370, 1978.
5. Goldman L: Supraventricular tachyarrhythmias in hospitalized adults after surgery. *Chest* 73:450–454, 1978.
6. Rogers WR, Wroblewski F, LaDue JS: Supraventricular tachycardia complicating surgical procedures. *Circulation* 7:192–199, 1954.
7. Goldman L, Caldera DL, Nussbaum SR et al: Multifunctional index of cardiac risk in noncardiac surgical procedures. *N Engl J Med* 297:845–850, 1977.
8. Pierce JA: Cardiac arrests and deaths associated with anesthesia. *Anesth Analg* 45:407–413, 1966.
9. Foex P: Cardiac arrest during anesthesia. *Am J Emerg Med* 2:241–245, 1989.
10. Keenan RL, Boyan CP: Cardiac arrest due to anesthesia. *JAMA* 253:2373–2377, 1985.
11. Stephen CR: Cardiac arrest is on the decline. *Ann Surg* 155:345–352, 1962.
12. McClure JN, Skarpasis GM, Brown JM: Cardiac arrest in the operating area. *Am Surg* 38:241–246, 1972.
13. Pottecher T, Tiret L, Desmonts JM et al: Cardiac arrest related to anesthesia: A prospective survey in France. *Eur J Anesth* 1:305–308, 1984.
14. Mowry FM, Reynolds EW: Cardiac rhythm disturbances complicating resectional surgery of the lung. *Ann Int Med* 61:688–695, 1964.
15. Ghosh P, Pakrash BC: Cardiac dysrhythmias after thoracotomy. *Br Heart J* 34:374–376, 1972.
16. Krowka MJ, Pairolero PC, Trastek VF et al: Cardiac dysrhythmia following pneumonectomy. *Chest* 91:490–495, 1987.
17. Beck-Nielsen J, Sorenson HR, Alstrap P: Atrial fibrillation following thoracotomy for noncardiac diseases in particular cancer of the lung. *Acta Med Scand* 193:425–429, 1973.
18. Csiesko VF, Schatzlein MH, King RD: Immediate postoperative digitalization in the prophylaxis of supraventricular arrhythmias following coronary artery bypass. *J Thorac Cardiovasc Surg* 81:419–422, 1981.
19. Mohr R, Smolinsky A, Goor DA: Prevention of supraventricular tachyarrhythmias with low-dose propranolol after coronary bypass. *J Thorac Cardiovasc Surg* 81:840–845, 1981.
20. Silverman NA, Wright R, Levitsky S: Efficacy of low-dose propranolol in preventing postoperative supraventricular tachyarrhythmias. *Ann Surg* 196:194–197, 1982.
21. Ferraris VA, Ferraris SP, Gilliam H et al: Verapamil prophylaxis for postoperative atrial dysrhythmias: A prospective randomized, double-blind study using drug level monitoring. *Ann Thorac Surg* 43:530–553, 1987.
22. Tyras DH, Stothert JC, Kaiser GC et al: Supraventricular tachyarrhythmias after myocardial revascularization: A randomized trial of prophylactic digitalization. *J Thorac Cardiovasc Surg* 77:310–314, 1979.
23. Stephenson LW, MacVaugh H, Tomasello D et al: Propranolol for the prevention of postoperative cardiac arrhythmias: A randomized study. *Ann Thorac Surg* 29:113–116, 1980.
24. DeSoyza N, Thenabadu PN, Murphy ML et al: Ventricular arrhythmias before and after aorta-coronary bypass surgery. *Int J Cardiol* 1:123–130, 1981.
25. Michaelson EL, Morganroth J, MacVaugh H: Postoperative arrhythmias after coronary artery and cardiac valvular surgery detected by long-term electrocardiographic monitoring. *Am Heart J* 97:442–448, 1979.
26. Kron JL, DiMarco JP, Harman PK et al: Supraventricular arrhythmias following coronary artery bypass. *J Thorac Cardiovasc Surgery* 86:594–600, 1983.
27. Topol EJ, Lerman BB, Baughman KL, Platia EV, Griffith LSC: De novo ventricular tachyarrhythmias after coronary revascularization. *Am J Cardiol* 57:57–59, 1986.
28. Kumar SM, Zsigmund EK: Practical management aspects of intraoperative arrhythmias: The anesthesiologist's viewpoint. *Int Anesth Clin* 18:171–187, 1980.
29. Rogers MC: Diagnosis and treatment of intraoperative cardiac dysrhythmias, in Miller RD (ed): *Anesthesia*. New York, Churchill Livingstone, 1986, pp 491–521.
30. Dripps RD, Eckerhoff JE, Vandam LD: *Introduction to Anesthesia—The Principles of Safe Practice*. Philadelphia, Saunders, 1988, pp 122–123, 202–203.
31. Williams HD, Sone L: Cardiac arrhythmias during coronary artery operations with halothane or enflurane anesthesia. *Anesthesiology* 50:551–553, 1979.
32. Rodrigo MRC, Moles TM, Lee PK: Comparison of the incidence and nature of cardiac arrhythmias occurring during isoflurane or halothane anesthesia. *Br J Anesth* 58:394–400, 1986.
33. Albright BA: Cardiac arrest following regional anesthesia with etidocaine or bupivacaine. *Anesthesiology* 51:285–287, 1979.
34. Prentiss JE: Cardiac arrest following caudal anesthesia. *Anesthesiology* 50:51–53, 1979.
35. Philbin DM, Hutter AM: Intraoperative cardiac arrhythmias. *Int Anesth Clin* 17:55–65, 1979.
36. Katz RL, Bigger JT: Cardiac arrhythmias during anesthesia and operation. *Anesthesiology* 33:193–212, 1970.
37. Moller IW: Cardiac arrest following IV verapamil combined with halothane anesthesia. *Br J Anesthesia* 59:522–526, 1987.
38. Hartwell BL, Mork JB: Combinations of beta-blockers and calcium

channel blockers: A cause of malignant perioperative conduction disturbances? *Anesth Analg* 65:905–907, 1986.

39. Lowenthal DT, Porter S, Saris SD et al: Clinical pharmacology, pharmacodynamics and interactions with esmolol. *Am J Cardiol* 56:14F–18F, 1985.

40. Kates RA, Zaidon JR, Kaplan JA: Esophageal lead for intraoperative electrocardiographic monitoring. *Anesth Analg* 9:781–785, 1982.

41. Gray RJ, Bateman TM, Czer LSC et al: Esmolol: A new ultrashort-acting beta-adrenergic blocking agent for rapid control of heart rate in postoperative supraventricular tachycardia. *J Amer Coll Cardiol* 5:1451–1456, 1985.

42. Morganroth J, Horowitz LN, Anderson J et al: Comparative efficacy and tolerance of esmolol to propranolol for control of supraventricular tachycardia. *Am J Cardiol* 56:33F–39F, 1985.

43. Dunn M, Alexander J, de Silva R et al: Antithrombotic therapy in atrial fibrillation. *Chest* 95:1185–1275, 1989.

44. Josephson ME, Seides SF: *Clinical Cardiac Electrophysiology*. Philadelphia, Lea & Febiger, 1979, pp 147–190.

45. Sung RJ, Elser B, McAllister RG: Intravenous verapamil for termination of reentrant supraventricular tachycardia: Intracardiac studies correlated with plasma verapamil concentrations. *Int Med* 93:682–689, 1980.

46. Rinkenberger RL, Prystowsky EN, Heger JJ et al: Effects of intravenous and chronic oral verapamil administration in patients with supraventricular tachycardia. *Circulation* 62:996–1010, 1980.

47. DiMarco JP, Miles W, Akhtar M et al: Adenosine for paroxysmal supraventricular tachycardia: Dose ranging and comparison with verapamil. Assessment in placebo-controlled multicenter trials. *Ann Int Med* 113:104–110, 1990.

48. Juler GL, Stemmer EA, Connelly JE: Complications of prophylactic digitalization in thoracic surgical patients. *J Thorac Cardiovasc Surg* 58:352–358, 1962.

49. Shields TW, Ujiki GT: Digitalization for prevention of arrhythmias following pulmonary surgery. *Surg Gynecol Obstet* 126:743–746, 1968.

50. Deutsch S, Dalen JE: Indications for prophylactic digitalization. *Anesthesiology* 30:648–656, 1969.

51. Kennedy HL, Whitlock JA, Sprague MK et al: Long-term follow-up of asymptomatic healthy subjects with frequent and complex ventricular ectopy. *N Engl J Med* 312:193–197, 1985.

52. Schulze RA, Strauss HW, Pitt B: Sudden death in the year following myocardial infarction: Relation to ventricular premature contractions in the late hospital phase and left ventricular ejection fraction. *Am J Med* 62:192–199, 1977.

53. Josephson ME, Horowitz LN, Farshidi A et al: Recurrent sustained ventricular tachycardia. 1. Mechanisms. *Circulation* 57:431–440, 1978.

54. Bomor WE, Thompson WR, Ashmore JD: Preoperative factors in production of cardiac arrest. *JAMA* 92:41–43, 1960.

55. Rooney SM, Goldiner PL, Muss E: Relationship of right bundle branch block and marked left axis deviation to complete heart block to general anesthesia. *Anesthesiology* 44:64–66, 1976.

56. Berg GR, Kotler MN: The significance of bilateral bundle branch block in the preoperative patient. *Chest* 54:62–67, 1971.

57. Venkatarama K, Madias VE: Indications for prophylactic preoperative insertion of pacemakers in patients with right bundle branch block and left anterior hemiblock. *Chest* 68:501–506, 1975.

58. Kunastadt D, Punja M, Cagin N et al: Bifascicular block: A clinical and electrophysiologic study. *Am Heart J* 86:173–181, 1973.

59. Bellocci F, Santarelli P, DiGennaro M et al: The risk of cardiac complications in surgical patients with bifascicular block. *Chest* 77:343–348, 1980.

60. Falk RH, Zoll PM, Zoll RH: Safety and efficacy of noninvasive cardiac pacing: A preliminary report. *N Engl J Med* 309:1166–1168, 1983.

61. Berliner D, Okun M, Peters RW et al: Transcutaneous temporary pacing in the operating room. *JAMA* 254:84–86, 1985.

62. Furman S, Hayes DL, Holmes DR: *A Practice of Cardiac Pacing*. Mt. Kisco NY, Futura, 1986, pp 451–462.

63. Irnich W, Barold SS: Interference protection in cardiac pacemakers, in Barold SS (ed): *Modern Cardiac Pacing*. Mt. Kisco NY, Futura, 1985, pp 839–855.

57 POSTOPERATIVE ATELECTASIS, PNEUMONIA, AND ASPIRATION PNEUMONITIS

Gregory R. Owens

Pulmonary complications constitute the leading cause of postoperative morbidity and mortality. This chapter focuses on management of aspiration, one of the most serious postoperative pulmonary complications, and on atelectasis, one of the most common.

ASPIRATION

Three groups of patients have an increased risk of developing aspiration and its complications: (1) those with an altered level of consciousness; (2) those with motor disorders of the esophagus or hypopharynx; and (3) those with mechanical disruption of glottic closure such as that due to a tracheostomy or of gastroesophageal sphincter function such as that caused by a nasogastric tube.[1]

Aspiration pneumonia and aspiration pneumonitis are different syndromes, each with its own etiology, pathophysiology, clinical course, and treatment. Pneumonitis results from aspiration of normally sterile gastric contents, causing a chemical burn of the tracheobronchial tree and pulmonary parenchyma, and is usually not complicated by bacterial infection. Pneumonia results from aspiration of mouth contents at physiologic pH and subsequent bacterial infection.

Aspiration Pneumonitis

Since the time of Mendelson's first description of pulmonary complications following aspiration of gastric contents, the pH of the aspirated material has been considered the most important determinant of damage to the lung.[2] Numerous experimental studies have shown that the extent of damage correlates with the volume and pH of the aspirate. Traditionally, it has been felt that material with a pH of less than 2.5 causes injury and that increasing destruction correlates with decreasing pH, reaching a maximum when the pH is 1.5.[3,4] Moreover, aspiration of small particles of food creates an inflammatory response comparable to that caused by acid.[3] Even aspiration of saline is associated with transient physiologic changes in the lungs.[5] However, a more recent report casts doubt on the importance of pH and suggests that food particles may be the major cause of pulmonary complications in aspiration.

The pathology of gastric aspiration can be divided into two stages based on the sequence of changes in the lung. Early changes include peribronchial accumulation of neutrophils, separation of basement membranes from epithelial cells, erythrocytes in the alveoli, and pulmonary edema. These changes can be induced by many fluids, including buffered gastric juice, hypertonic saline, and acid. Although aspiration of nonacidic fluids is usually of little significance,[2] acidic fluids cause progressive damage with necrosis of type I alveolar cells, alveolar hemorrhage, bronchial mucosal sloughing, and hyaline membrane formation.[6]

The diagnosis of aspiration pneumonitis is usually readily apparent. Aspiration follows an episode of vomiting or regurgitation and results in the abrupt onset of dyspnea and bronchospasm within one to four hours. Patients often become hypotensive and may produce thin frothy sputum easily mistaken for the fluid of pulmonary edema.[7] Except for significant hypoxemia and usually hypocapnia, laboratory data are nonspecific.[8] A chest x-ray may be helpful since aspiration of oral or gastric contents tends to involve specific lobes of the lung determined by gravity and position. The superior segment of the right lower lobe, the left lower lobe, and the posterior segment of the right upper lobe are most commonly affected, but any area of the lung may be involved. The infiltrates are fluffy, mottled, and alveolar in pattern. In massive aspiration, the adult respiratory distress syndrome may develop with its characteristic diffuse bilateral alveolar infiltrates.[9] The morbidity and mortality of aspiration pneumonitis cannot be underestimated. Recent experience differs from that described in Mendelson's classic monograph. There were no deaths in his series, and all of the patients recovered within 36 hours. However, recent studies document mortality rates of 35 to 60 percent and as high as 100 percent when the gastric pH is under 1.75.[4]

Since damage to the pulmonary parenchyma and airways occurs instantly, there is no reason to attempt to evacuate or neutralize the acid.[10] However, endotracheal suctioning immediately following an observed aspiration is indicated because it may remove enough aspirate to clear the upper airway and stimulate cough. Fiberoptic or rigid bronchoscopy is required if there is evidence of aspiration of food particles in the suctioned material or if segmental or lobar atelectasis or obstructive emphysema is seen on chest x-ray.[11] Neutralization of acid with bronchial lavage is ineffective, and experimental evidence suggests that it may increase the extent of the damage.[12]

Because aspiration pneumonitis represents a chemical burn of the tracheobronchial tree and pulmonary parenchyma, immediate use of antibiotics is not indicated. However, there is no consensus on this point in the literature, and many have strongly advocated their use.[6,8,13] All well-controlled clinical trials suggest that they are of no value and may select for more virulent organisms and expose the patient to possible drug toxicity.[14–16] The most logical approach is to withhold antibiotics until there is clear evidence of bacterial infection.

Controversy surrounding the use of corticosteroids in gastric aspiration has generated much data but few definitive results. Early studies, usually small and poorly-controlled, claimed that steroids decreased pulmonary pathology and improved survival.[17–19] However, more recent data suggest that steroids are of no benefit.[9,20,21] Moreover, one report showed that corticosteroids significantly increased the incidence of gram-negative pneumonias.[22] This is not surprising in view of the adverse effects of corticosteroids on leukocyte function and the documented increased susceptibility to gram-negative infections in steroid-treated animals.[23]

Ventilatory support is the keystone of therapy in aspiration pneumonitis and may determine ultimate outcome. Since hypoxemia and hypocapnia usually occur initially, efforts to improve arterial oxygenation are crucial. Supplementary oxygen given by face mask may suffice in mild aspiration, but positive-pressure ventilation may be required to overcome intrapulmonary shunting and avoid toxic concentrations of inspired oxygen.[24] The three methods of ventilatory support are assist/control ventilation, intermittent mandatory ventilation, and pressure support. While theoretical arguments have been advanced to recommend one modality over another,[25,26] controlled clinical studies have shown no differences in clinical course or outcome when they are directly compared.[27,28]

Uncertainties remain about the role of positive end-expiratory pressure (PEEP) in aspiration pneumonitis. PEEP increases functional residual capacity and improves ventilation-perfusion matching to provide better oxygenation in patients with severe hypoxemia. It may also obviate the use of toxic concentrations of inspired oxygen and support the patient while the damaged lung improves. It is not clear, however, that PEEP itself is therapeutic, and recent studies suggest that it may actually cause lung damage.[29]

Complications of PEEP occur in as many as 25 percent of patients.[30] Depression of cardiac output and systemic hypotension are common and reversible problems. They occur with initiation of or increase in PEEP and are primarily the result of decreased venous return due to constant positive intrathoracic pressure.[31] Patients who develop hypotension on PEEP are usually relatively hypovolemic and respond to increased intravascular volume. PEEP may also cause a decrease in cardiac output because of increased right ventricular afterload and decreased ventricular distensibility. Continuous positive airway pressure (CPAP) with a tightly fitting face mask causes less depression of cardiac output than PEEP and does not require intubation.[32]

Barotrauma is a more serious complication of PEEP and consists of subcutaneous or mediastinal emphysema or pneumothorax. Unfortunately, it is impossible to identify subsets of particularly susceptible patients or to determine the level of PEEP above which barotrauma is likely to occur. However, one study showed that barotrauma is more frequent in patients with aspiration pneumonitis.[33] Lung tissue damaged by acid or other necrotizing processes may be more susceptible to barotrauma because of decreases in its supporting structure. Development of subcutaneous crepitance, abrupt onset of systemic hypotension, and a precipitous rise in the ventilator pressure required to inflate the lungs are the clinical hallmarks of barotrauma. Some have advocated the use of prophylactic chest tubes when high levels of PEEP are used, but this strategy is usually unnecessary.

Aspiration Pneumonia

Aspiration of the contents of the oropharynx occurs commonly in small amounts even in normal persons. Clinical illness is prevented by the defense mechanisms of the tracheobronchial tree, which include the cough reflex, mucociliary transport, and alveolar macrophages. The term aspiration pneumonia is applied to the development of pneumonia caused by organisms inhabiting the oropharynx of patients with compromised upper-airway defenses. It may occur as a primary event or as a complication of the aspiration of gastric contents. Hospitalized patients who develop aspiration pneumonia differ in many respects from those who develop it outside of the hospital.

Inoculation of oropharyngeal contents into the lung with subsequent development of pneumonia occurs commonly in a variety of settings. Predisposing factors include alcoholism, seizure disorders, stroke, drug addiction, anesthesia, nasogastric suction, and head trauma. In addition, the use of H_2 blockers and antacids to neutralize gastric pH is associated with an increased frequency of nosocomial pneumonia[34,35] and may be due to bacterial colonization in the stomach and subsequent aspiration into the lung.

The clinical course of aspiration pneumonia is usually less fulminant than that of aspiration pneumonitis and may be indolent.[36] The episode of aspiration is rarely observed and may only be suspected when pneumonia develops in a dependent segment of the lung. Fever may be the only sign. Sputum is usually purulent but not foul-smelling, and there is no predominant organism on gram stain.[37] Tissue necrosis may develop in 8 to 14 days, and, when a characteristic lung abscess or necrotizing pneumonia develops, the sputum becomes copious and foul-smelling.

The bacteriology of aspiration pneumonia confirms that it is caused by aspiration of oropharyngeal contents. The predominant bacteria in the oropharynx are anaerobic and belong to several different species. They number about 10^8 per milliliter of saliva in normal persons and up to 10^{11} in persons with poor oral hygiene.[38] Peptostreptococci, *Bacteroides melaninogenicus*, and *Fusobacterium nucleatum* account for the majority of isolates, but other organisms may predominate in critically ill patients. The majority of patients who develop aspiration pneumonia outside the hospital have mixed infections with three or four organisms. Anaerobes of the aforementioned species predominate. Aerobic organisms alone are isolated in only 6 percent of patients but make up part of the mixed flora in 30 percent.[30] Those aerobes are usually streptococcal species including *Streptococcus pneumoniae*.

The bacteriologic picture is more complex in hospitalized patients. Within 96 hours of hospitalization, the oropharynx becomes colonized by pathogenic aerobic bacteria including *Staphylococcus aureus*, *Pseudomonas aeruginosa*, *Proteus* species, and *Escherichia coli*.[39] Changes in flora are associated with the use of antibiotics, prolonged hospital stay, and the severity of the underlying illness. About 40 percent of critically ill patients in intensive care units are colonized with pathogenic aerobic organisms, usually gram-negative rods.[40] Upper-airway colonization occurs rapidly in the first 8 to 10 days of hospitalization and then stabilizes.[41] The bacteria isolated from patients with aspiration pneumonia are usually the same as those that have colonized the oropharynx. Anaerobic organisms are recovered less frequently in nosocomial aspiration, and pathogenic aerobic organisms are more often found. Anaerobes are isolated in only 30 percent of such patients and are the sole pathogens in only 10 percent.[42] Sputum is rarely putrid.

In the past decade, there has been a growing recognition of the importance of nosocomial aspiration pneumonia. Approximately 400,000 patients develop nosocomial pneumonia per year, and 20,000 patients die from it.[43] Recent studies have shown that the clinical course of the adult respiratory distress syndrome is primarily determined by the presence of infection. Patients with nosocomial pneumonia are much more likely to develop multiorgan failure and die.[44,45]

The treatment of aspiration pneumonia depends on where the infection was acquired. In community-acquired cases with the predominantly anaerobic organisms, penicillin G was the treatment of choice for many years[46] despite the fact that *B. fragilis*, an organism found in approximately 20 percent of anaerobic pneumonias, is resistant to penicillin. However, patients appeared to do well, and penicillin was thought to alter the milieu of the lung by killing other organisms and thereby eradicating *B. fragilis*. More recently, a multicenter comparison of penicillin G and clindamycin found that patients treated with penicillin more often failed treatment and had fever and purulent sputum for a longer period of time.[47] However, many physicians still rely on penicillin G in a dose of 2 to 5 million units daily in divided doses, and the Medical Letter endorses both agents.

The treatment of nosocomial pneumonia has also changed. In the past, only penicillin was used unless the gram stain showed gram-negative rods. In view of the virulence of nosocomial pneumonias and the relative safety of using broad-spectrum antibiotics until culture results are known, empiric coverage of aerobic organisms is now the standard approach. A combination of an aminoglycoside (gentamicin or tobramycin) and a semisynthetic penicillin (piperacillin or mezlocillin) or a broad-spectrum cephalosporin may be used. When culture results become available, the appropriate antibiotic with the narrowest spectrum and least toxicity should be chosen.

Empiric therapy may vary with local factors. If *Legionella* is known to be a significant pathogen in a hospital, all regimens should contain erythromycin in a dose of four grams daily intravenously. If *Pseudomonas* is not prevalent and the patient has renal insufficiency, the use of monotherapy with ceftazidime or imipenem/cilastatin may be better. Patients who develop nosocomial pneumonia while on antibiotics should be managed in the same way, but fungal pneumonia should be excluded.

There are little data regarding the outcome of aspiration pneumonia, especially in hospitalized patients. One large study found that no deaths occurred in patients who developed aspiration pneumonia in the community but noted a death rate of 20 percent in nosocomial aspiration pneumonia.[37] Other series of patients with nosocomial pneumonia have noted considerably higher death rates with only a minority of patients surviving a nosocomial pneumonia. There are few studies evaluating long-term sequelae of aspiration pneumonitis and pneumonia.[34,48] Although pulmonary fibrosis has been noted in a few survivors, pulmonary function tests and chest radiographs generally return to normal.[49]

ATELECTASIS

Risk and Prevention

Postoperative atelectasis is the most common complication of surgery, with an incidence as high as 70 percent in patients undergoing upper-abdominal and thoracic surgery.[50] The extent of atelectasis may vary from "plate-like" with no associated symptoms or physical findings to lobar involvement with significant respiratory compromise.

Efforts to identify patients with a higher-than-normal risk of developing postoperative pulmonary complications have continued since Stein and Cassara showed that diligent preoperative preparation and postoperative care decreased the complication rate.[51] They found that when high-risk patients were treated with a program of cessation of smoking, bronchodilator therapy, inhalation of humidified air, chest physical therapy, and postural drainage, the incidence of postoperative pulmonary complications dropped from 60 percent to 22 percent. Similarly, Dripps and Deming found that the incidence of significant atelectasis decreased by 50 percent when intensive pre- and postoperative measures including chest physical therapy were instituted.[52] Although factors responsible for atelectasis and pneumonia are similar, no study has shown that atelectasis leads to pneumonia or that postoperative pneumonias develop only in areas of preceding atelectasis.

Numerous additional therapeutic modalities have been proposed for the prevention of postoperative pulmonary complications. Most have attempted to produce periodic hyperinflation to counteract repetitive low tidal-volume ventilation, the typical breathing pattern seen in the postoperative period.[53,54] The most commonly discussed measures are intermittent positive-pressure breathing (IPPB), blow bottles, incentive spirometry, PEEP or CPAP, and assisted coughing with voluntary deep-breathing exercises. A recent survey reveals that prophylactic and postoperative measures are widely used in the United States.[55] Over 90 percent of patients receive incentive spirometry both before and after surgery, but IPPB and chest physical therapy are utilized in less than one-third.

IPPB, the subject of greatest debate, has been used to provide hyperinflation, to promote removal of secretions, and to decrease the work of breathing after surgery.[56] After initial use in patients with chronic obstructive pulmonary disease, IPPB gained rapid acceptance in perioperative care in the early 1950s. IPPB has been studied extensively.[57-62] The majority of recent well-controlled studies fail to show significant benefit when pulmonary function, duration of postoperative fever, atelectasis, other postoperative pulmonary complications, and length of hospital stay are examined.

IPPB may not be effective because of delivery of pressure to inappropriate areas of the lung, inadequacy of the standard regimen of four treatments per day, reliance on delivery of a specific pressure rather than volume, and inability of patients to use the apparatus correctly. The American Thoracic Society concluded, "As routinely applied . . . IPPB does not alter the incidence of postoperative pulmonary complications."[63] In patients undergoing cardiac surgery, it is no more effective in preventing atelectasis than routine ventilatory care.[64]

On the other hand, two recent studies have evaluated the utility of continuous positive airway pressure (CPAP), a variant of PEEP, in preventing postoperative complications.[65,66] Both conclude that postoperative CPAP is more effective than other forms of therapy. Moreover, it requires no patient effort and does not cause discomfort.

Passive hyperinflation of the lungs during surgery correlates with a lower incidence of atelectasis. Several studies have shown that sustained inspiratory maneuvers reduce atelectasis in normal subjects and in those who have undergone surgery.[67,68] All patients should be instructed in deep-breathing exercises before surgery, and assisted coughing should be performed postoperatively. The latter modality is especially effective when the patient is in the lateral decubitus position, and the physician supports the surgical incision with the hand.

Incentive spirometry induces deep sustained inspiration with no emphasis on force or duration of expiration. Spirometric devices provide the patient with a quantitative measure of inspiratory effort. Incentive spirometry is less hazardous than IPPB and may be more effective in preventing postoperative atelectasis.[69,70] However, several recent studies have questioned its efficacy.[71,72] In a comparison study of several commonly used incentive spirometers, no single device was found to be superior.[73]

In summary, the incidence of postoperative atelectasis can be reduced by perioperative care centered around assisted coughing and induction of deep inspiration. Good nursing care, cessation of smoking, and bronchodilator therapy significantly decrease atelectasis.[58] Incentive spirometry, a relatively inexpensive therapeutic modality, may further decrease postoperative pulmonary complications.

Treatment

A critical evaluation of the various modalities currently used in the treatment of established atelectasis has not been performed. This may be due in part to the fact that atelectasis is generally a self-limited process that usually resolves by the fifth to the seventh postoperative day. Studies advocating one therapy over another suffer from lack of control groups and small sample size. Only one small prospective study has evaluated different treatment modalities and found that bronchoscopy was no better than conventional chest physical therapy in relieving acute lobar atelectasis.[74] The presence of an air bronchogram within the atelectatic area was felt to predict slow resolution. A reinterpretation of this study suggested that bronchoscopy actually was effective, especially in patients who were not intubated.[75]

Other studies have suggested the IPPB utilizing increasing pressure until maximal volume is achieved may help alleviate atelectasis.[76] In patients who are intubated, PEEP may lead to its resolution.[77] More recently, the use of nasal continuous positive airway pressure (CPAP) has been shown to promote rapid improvement in patients with atelectasis.[78–80] Therefore, no definitive statements

can be made about the relative advantages of IPPB, bronchoscopy, incentive spirometry, or chest physical therapy in treating atelectasis. For asymptomatic or mildly symptomatic patients, a trial of deep-breathing maneuvers, assisted cough, and chest physical therapy should be undertaken. If the atelectasis does not clear, either nasal CPAP or bronchoscopy may be necessary. In significantly symptomatic patients in whom conservative measures prove ineffective, therapeutic bronchoscopy may quickly alleviate the problem.[81] In most patients with complete atelectasis of a lung who are not intubated, bronchoscopy is probably indicated without a trial of chest physical therapy.

SUMMARY

1. Aspiration pneumonitis resulting from aspiration of gastric contents is characterized by the onset of thin sputum production, significant hypoxemia, hypocapnia, and infiltrates on chest x-ray within four hours of aspiration.

2. Antibiotics are not recommended in the treatment of aspiration pneumonitis.

3. Treatment of hypoxemia with oxygen therapy is mandatory and may obviate intubation. Toxic concentrations of oxygen may be avoided with the use of mechanical ventilation and PEEP. Barotrauma and hypotension often accompany PEEP therapy.

4. Aspiration pneumonia resulting from aspiration of oropharyngeal contents follows a more indolent course characterized by fever and purulent sputum production.

5. Community-acquired aspiration pneumonia should be treated with either penicillin G in a dose of 2 to 5 million units daily intravenously in four divided doses or clindamycin in a dose of 300 mg four times daily orally or intravenously.

6. Hospital-acquired aspiration pneumonia requires broad-spectrum antibiotics until culture results are available. Initial empiric therapy should include an aminoglycoside and either a penicillinase-resistant penicillin or cephalosporin. Local factors may alter the approach.

7. The incidence of postoperative atelectasis is decreased by preoperative preparation consisting of cessation of smoking, bronchodilator therapy, and chest physical therapy, and by postoperative measures centered around assisted coughing and sustained inspiratory maneuvers.

8. If atelectasis develops, conservative measures are generally effective, although bronchoscopy may be needed in more serious cases.

REFERENCES

1. Hughes R, Freilich R, Bytell D et al: Aspiration and occult esophageal disorders. *Chest* 80:489–495, 1981.
2. Mendelson C: Aspiration of stomach contents into the lungs during obstetric anesthesia. *Am J Obstet Gynecol* 52:191, 1946.
3. Teabeaut J: Aspiration of gastric contents: Experimental study. *Am Pathol* 28:51, 1952.
4. Hemelberg W, Bosomworth P: Aspiration pneumonitis: Experimental studies and clinical observations. *Anesth Analg* 43:669, 1964.
5. Jones JG, Grossman R, Berry M et al: Alveolar capillary membrane

permeability: Correlation with functional, radiographic, and postmortem changes after fluid aspiration. *Am Rev Respir Dis* 120:399, 1979.

6. Greenfield L, Singleton R, McCaffree D et al: Pulmonary effects of experimental graded aspiration of hydrochloric acid. *Ann Surg* 170:74, 1969.

7. Dines D, Baker W, Scantland W: Aspiration pneumonitis—Mendelson's syndrome. *JAMA* 176:229, 1961.

8. Dines D, Titus J, Sissler A: Aspiration pneumonitis. *Mayo Clin Proc* 45:347, 1970.

9. Bynum L, Pierce A: Pulmonary aspiration of gastric contents. *Am Rev Respir Dis* 114:1129, 1976.

10. Awe W, Fletcher W, Jacob S: The pathophysiology of aspiration pneumonitis. *Surgery* 50:232, 1966.

11. Kim I, Brummitt W, Humphrey A et al: Foreign body in the airway: A review of 202 cases. *Laryngoscope* 83:347, 1973.

12. Taylor G, Pryse-Davies J: Evaluation of endotracheal steroid therapy in acid pulmonary aspiration syndrome. *Anesthesiology* 29:17, 1968.

13. McCormick P: Immediate care after aspiration of vomit. *Anaesthesia* 30:658, 1975.

14. Petersdorf R, Curtin J, Hoeprich P: A study of antibiotic prophylaxis in unconscious patients. *N Engl J Med* 257:1001, 1957.

15. Aldrete J, Liem S, Carrow D: Pulmonary aerobic bacterial flora after aspiration pneumonitis. *J Trauma* 15:1014, 1975.

16. Murray H: Antimicrobial therapy in pulmonary aspiration. *Am J Med* 66:188, 1979.

17. Bannister W, Sattilaro A: Vomiting and aspiration during anesthesia. *Anesthesiology* 23:251, 1962.

18. Lawson D, Defalco A, Phelps J et al: Corticosteroids as treatment for aspiration of gastric contents: An experimental study. *Surgery* 59:845, 1966.

19. Tinstman T, Dines D, Arms R: Postoperative aspiration pneumonia. *Surg Clin N Am* 53:859, 1973.

20. Cameron J, Mitchell W, Zuidema G: Aspiration pneumonia: Clinical outcome following documented aspiration. *Arch Surg* 106:49, 1973.

21. Downs J, Chapman R, Modell J et al: An evaluation of steroid therapy in aspiration pneumonitis. *Anesthesiology* 40:129, 1974.

22. Wolfe J, Bone R, Ruth W: Effects of corticosteroids in the treatment of patients with gastric aspiration. *Am J Med* 63:719, 1977.

23. Kass E, Finland M: Corticosteroids and infection. *Adv Intern Med* 9:45, 1958.

24. Cameron J, Caldini P, Toung J et al: Aspiration pneumonia: Physiologic data following experimental aspiration. *Surgery* 72:238, 1972.

25. Downs J, Klein E, Desautels D et al: Intermittent mandatory ventilation: A new approach to weaning patients from mechanical ventilation. *Chest* 64:331, 1973.

26. MacIntyre N: Respiratory function during pressure support ventilation. *Chest* 89:677–683, 1986.

27. Schachter EN, Tucker D, Beck GJ: Does intermittent mandatory ventilation accelerate weaning? *JAMA* 246:1210–1214, 1981.

28. Culpepper J, Rinaldo J, Rogers R: Effect of mechanical ventilation mode on tendency to respiratory alkalosis. *ARRD* 132:1075–1078, 1985.

29. Demling R, Staub N, Edmunds L: Effect of end-expiratory airway pressure on accumulation of extravascular lung water. *J Appl Physiol* 38:907, 1975.

30. Zwillich C, Pierson D, Creagh CE et al: Complications of assisted ventilation: A prospective study of 354 consecutive episodes. *Am J Med* 57:161, 1974.

31. Dorinsky PM, Whitcomb ME: The effect of PEEP on cardiac output. *Chest* 84:210–216, 1983.

32. Venus B, Jacobs HK, Lim L: Treatment of the adult respiratory distress syndrome with continuous positive airway pressure. *Chest* 76:257, 1979.

33. DeLatorre F, Tomasa A, Klamburg J et al: Incidence of pneumothorax and pneumomediastinum in patients with aspiration pneumonia requiring ventilatory support. *Chest* 72:141, 1977.

34. Craven D, Kunches L, Kilinsky V et al: Risk factors for pneumonia and fatality in patients receiving mechanical ventilation. *ARRD* 133:792–796, 1986.

35. Driks M, Craven D, Celli B et al: Nosocomial pneumonia in intubated patients given sucralfate as compared with antacids or histamine type 2 blockers: The role of gastric colonization. *N Engl J Med* 317:1376–1382, 1987.

36. Bartlett J, Gorbach S, Finegold S: The bacteriology of aspiration pneumonia. *Am J Med* 56:202, 1974.

37. Bartlett J: Anaerobic bacterial infections of the lung. *Chest* 91:901–909, 1987.

38. Rosebury T: *Microorganisms Indigenous to Man*. New York, McGraw-Hill, 1966, pp 314.

39. Johanson W, Pierce A, Sanford J: Changing pharyngeal bacterial flora of hospitalized patients. *N Engl J Med* 281:1137, 1969.

40. Johanson W, Pierce A, Sanford J et al: Nosocomial respiratory infections with gram-negative bacilli. *Ann Intern Med* 77:701, 1972.

41. Langer M, Mosconi P, Cigada M et al: Long-term respiratory support and risk of pneumonia in critically ill patients. *ARRD* 140:302–305, 1989.

42. Lorber B, Swenson R: Bacteriology of aspiration pneumonia: A prospective study of community- and hospital-acquired cases. *Ann Intern Med* 81:329, 1974.

43. Jay S: Nosocomial pneumonia. *Post Med* 74:221–235, 1983.

44. Bell R, Coalson J, Smith J et al: Multiple organ system failure and infection in adult respiratory distress syndrome. *Ann Int Med* 99:293–298, 1983.

45. Montgomery B, Stager M, Carrico J et al: Cause of mortality in patients with the adult respiratory distress syndrome. *ARRD* 132:485–489, 1985.

46. Bartlett J, Gorbach S: Treatment of aspiration pneumonia and primary lung abscess: Penicillin G versus clindamycin. *JAMA* 234:935, 1975.

47. Levison M, Manigura C, Lorber B et al: Clindamycin compared with penicillin for the treatment of anaerobic lung abscess. *Ann Intern Med* 98:466–471, 1983.

48. Bryan C, Reynolds K: Bacteremic nosocomial pneumonia: Analysis of 172 episodes from a single metropolitan hospital. *ARRD* 129:668–671, 1984.

49. Sladen A, Zanca P, Hadnott W: Aspiration pneumonia—the sequelae. *Chest* 59:448, 1971.

50. Rudnikoff I, Headland C: Pulmonary changes following cholecystectomy. *JAMA* 146:989, 1951.

51. Stein M, Cassara E: Preoperative pulmonary evaluation and therapy for surgery patients. *JAMA* 211:787, 1970.

52. Dripps R, Deming M: Postoperative atelectasis and pneumonia: Diagnosis, etiology, and management based on 1240 cases of upper abdominal surgery. *Ann Surg* 24:94, 1946.

52. Mead J, Collier C: Relation of volume history of lungs to respiratory mechanics in anesthetized dogs. *J Appl Physiol* 14:669, 1959.

54. Bendixen H, Bullwinkel B, Hedley-Whyte J et al: Atelectasis and shunting during spontaneous ventilation in anesthetized patients. *Anesthesiology* 25:297, 1964.

55. O'Donohue W Jr: National survey of the usage of lung expansion modalities for the prevention and treatment of postoperative atelectasis following abdominal and thoracic surgery. *Chest* 87:76–80, 1985.

56. Noehren T, Lasry J, Legters L: Intermittent positive pressure breathing for the prevention and management of postoperative pulmonary complications. *Surgery* 43:658, 1958.

57. Rudy N, Crepeau J: Role of IPPB preoperatively. *JAMA* 167:1093, 1958.

58. Anderson W, Dossett B, Hamilton G: Prevention of postoperative pulmonary problems. *JAMA* 186:763, 1963.

59. Sands J, Cypert C, Armstrong R et al: A controlled study using routine intermittent positive pressure breathing in the post-surgical patient. *Dis Chest* 40:128, 1961.

60. Baxter W, Levine R: An evaluation of intermittent positive pressure

breathing in the prevention of postoperative pulmonary complications. *Arch Surg* 98:795, 1969.

61. Cottrell J, Siker E: Preoperative intermittent positive pressure breathing therapy in patients with COLD: Effect on postoperative complications. *Anesth Analg* 52:258, 1973.

62. Dohi S, Gold M: Comparison of two methods of postoperative respiratory care. *Chest* 73:592, 1978.

63. Pontoppidan H: Mechanical aids to lung expansion. *Am Rev Respir Dis* (Suppl)122:109, 1980.

64. Good J, Wolz J, Anderson J et al: The routine use of positive end-expiratory pressure after open heart surgery. *Chest* 76:397, 1979.

65. Ricksten S, Bengtsson A, Soderberg C et al: Effects of periodic positive airway pressure by mask on postoperative pulmonary function. *Chest* 89:774–781, 1986.

66. Stock M, Downs J, Gauer P et al: Prevention of postoperative pulmonary complications with CPAP, incentive spirometry, and conservative therapy. *Chest* 87:151–157, 1985.

67. Ward R, Danziger F, Bonica J et al: An evaluation of postoperative respiratory maneuvers. *Surg Gynecol Obstet* 123:51, 1966.

68. Bartlett R, Hanson E, Moore F: Physiology of yawning and its application to postoperative care. *Surg Forum* 21:222, 1970.

69. Iverson L, Ecker R, Fox H et al: A comparative study of IPPB, the incentive spirometer and blow bottles: The prevention of atelectasis following cardiac surgery. *Ann Thorac Surg* 25:197, 1978.

70. Pontoppidan H: Mechanical aids to lung expansion. *ARRD* 122:109, 1980.

71. Schwieger I, Gamulin A, Forster A et al: Absence of benefit of incentive spirometry in low-risk patients undergoing elective cholecystectomy. *Chest* 89:652–656, 1986.

72. Jung R, Wight J et al: Comparison of three methods of respiratory care following upper abdominal surgery. *Chest* 78:31–35, 1980.

73. Lederer D, Van De Water J, Indech R: Which deep breathing device should the postoperative patient use? *Chest* 77:610, 1980.

74. Marini JJ, Pierson DJ, Hudson LD: Acute lobar atelectasis; a prospective comparison of fiberoptic bronchoscopy and respiratory therapy. *Am Rev Resp Dis* 119:971–978, 1979.

75. Friedman SA: Comparison of fiberoptic bronchoscopy and respiratory therapy. *Am Rev Respir Dis* 116:367–368, 1982.

76. O'Donohue W: Maximum volume IPPB for the management of pulmonary atelectasis. *Chest* 76:683, 1979.

77. Fowler A, Scoggins W, O'Donohue W: Positive end-expiratory pressure in the management of lobar atelectasis. *Chest* 74:497, 1978.

78. Duncan S, Negrin R, Mihm F et al: Nasal continuous positive airway pressure in atelectasis. *Chest* 92:621–624, 1987.

79. Pinilla JC, Oleniuk FH, Tan L et al: Use of a nasal continuous positive airway pressure mask in the treatment of postoperative atelectasis in aortocoronary bypass surgery. *Chest* 18:836–840, 1990.

80. Thommi G: Nasal CPAP in treatment of persistent atelectasis. *Chest* 99:1551, 1991.

81. Wanner A, Landa J, Nieman R et al: Bedside bronchofiberoscopy for atelectasis and lung abscess. *JAMA* 224:1281, 1973.

58 THE ADULT RESPIRATORY DISTRESS SYNDROME

Paul N. Lanken

The adult respiratory distress syndrome (ARDS) is an acute severe respiratory disorder with three cardinal clinical features: hypoxemia poorly responsive to oxygen therapy; diffuse alveolar infiltrates on chest radiograph; and absence of left-sided congestive heart failure.[1,2,3] Synonyms for ARDS include noncardiogenic pulmonary edema, shock lung, white lung, permeability pulmonary edema, and pulmonary capillary leak syndrome. As the latter two terms imply, pulmonary edema in ARDS develops because of increased permeability of the alveolar-capillary membrane despite normal or only modestly elevated pulmonary capillary hydrostatic pressure. In contrast, pulmonary edema in left-sided congestive heart failure results from excessive filtration of plasma due to high intravascular hydrostatic pressure.

CAUSES

ARDS is the result of direct or indirect injury to the alveolar-capillary membrane and leakage of plasma into pulmonary interstitial and alveolar spaces. It represents a final common pathway in response to a wide variety of injuries. Table 58–1 lists the major clinical conditions that predispose patients to ARDS.[4,5,6] Although certain individual conditions like gastric aspiration are associated with a relatively high incidence of ARDS, the likelihood of developing it increases three- to fourfold when multiple predisposing conditions are present.[4,7] However, there is still no way to prevent ARDS. Controlled clinical trials have demonstrated that prophylactic positive end-expiratory pressure (PEEP)[8] and the use of high-dose corticosteroids in patients with sepsis have no beneficial effect.[9]

PRESENTATION

Patients presenting with ARDS typically experience the acute onset of respiratory distress without other pulmonary symptoms. On physical examination, they have rapid shallow respirations with scattered inspiratory rales but no other signs of congestive heart failure. Chest radiographs characteristically show diffuse alveolar infiltrates without enlargement of the cardiac silhouette. In severe cases, this evolves into a "white out" of the lung fields. Arterial blood gas analysis in early ARDS demonstrates hypoxemia and hypocapnia with a primary respiratory alkalosis. Hypoxemia becomes more marked and does not improve with administration of supplemental oxygen. In severe cases, tachypnea and high spontaneous minute ventilation lead to respiratory muscle fatigue and hypercapnia. Table 58–2 summarizes the diagnostic features of ARDS. The clinical presentation of some patients with ARDS may be dominated by associated injuries or life-threatening conditions such as major trauma with hemorrhagic or septic shock. In these cases, ARDS becomes apparent only after volume resuscitation.

TABLE 58–1. Clinical Conditions Predisposing to ARDS

Conditions with Direct Mechanisms of Injury
Gastric aspiration
Smoke or other toxic gas inhalation
Viral pneumonia
Other diffuse pneumonias (e.g., bacterial, pneumoaptis)
Oxygen toxicity
Near drowning
Thoracic trauma with lung contusion

Conditions with Indirect Mechanisms of Injury
Sepsis and septic shock
Multiple (nonthoracic) trauma
Burns
Acute pancreatitis
Massive emergency blood transfusions
Disseminated intravascular coagulation (DIC)
Severe acute hepatic failure
Neurogenic pulmonary edema, especially due to head trauma.*

*Neurogenic pulmonary edema probably involves a combination of permeability and hydrostatic mechanisms.

TABLE 58–2.   Clinical Diagnosis of ARDS

History
  Acute Dyspnea
  One or more predisposing conditions (see Table 58–1)

Physical Examination
  Respiratory distress (tachypnea, use of accessory muscle
    respiration)
  Cyanosis
  Absence of signs of left-sided congestive heart failure

Chest Radiograph
  Diffuse alveolar infiltrates
  Usually normal cardiac size

Physiologic Measurement
  Hypoxemia refractory to oxygen therapy, e.g., PaO_2/FiO_2 ratio
    < 100–300
  Diminished static compliance of the respiratory system, e.g.,
    < 50 ml/cm H_2O.
  No evidence for left-sided congestive heart failure, e.g.,
    pulmonary wedge pressure < 18 mmHg

DIFFERENTIAL DIAGNOSIS

The differential diagnosis of severe ARDS is limited to cardiogenic pulmonary edema and rarely diffuse pulmonary hemorrhage or aspiration of blood. All of these result in fluid-filled alveoli and similar patterns of physiologic derangements. Evidence favoring congestive heart failure (CHF) can often be obtained from the patient's history, the size of the heart on chest x-ray, and the presence or absence of a third heart sound on auscultation. Rapid clinical response and resolution of radiographic infiltrates after diuretic therapy suggest CHF rather than ARDS. In these patients, left-ventricular filling pressure is greatly elevated with pulmonary capillary wedge pressures typically above 28 mmHg.[10] Wedge pressures below 18 mmHg generally support the diagnosis of ARDS, except in patients with CHF who have been diuresed in the interval between evaluation of a chest radiograph demonstrating pulmonary edema and determination of wedge pressure, and in those with "flash" pulmonary edema due to transient ischemic left ventricular dysfunction that has resolved by the time the wedge pressure is measured.

PATHOPHYSIOLOGY AND CHANGES IN PULMONARY FUNCTION

Altered Lung Fluid Balance

Edema formation in the lung is due to changes in the factors governing net transvascular fluid flow as expressed by the Starling equation:[11]

$$\text{Net fluid flow} = K[(P_{MV} - P_{INT}) - \sigma(\pi_{MV} - \pi_{INT})]$$

where K is the fluid conductance across the microvessels and a property of the alveolar-capillary membrane; P_{MV} is the hydrostatic pressure in pulmonary microvessels; P_{INT} is the hydrostatic pressure in interstitial space of the lung; σ is equal to the protein reflection coefficient, normally about 1.0, indicating that the transvascular membrane restricts entry of albumin permitting establishment of an effective oncotic gradient; π_{MV} is the oncotic pressure of plasma in pulmonary microvessels; and π_{INT} is the oncotic pressure in interstitial space of the lung.

Normally, because conductance is low and the reflection coefficient is close to unity, hydrostatic and oncotic pressures balance each other. Consequently, only a small net amount of fluid flows into the lungs and is removed by lymphatics. In CHF, excessive fluid accumulates because of a rise in Pmv. In ARDS, edema is formed because of an increase in K and a decrease in σ affecting the permeability of the lung to fluid and macromolecules, respectively. These changes result in less restriction to fluid flow and decreased effectiveness of the normal oncotic pressure gradient to facilitate reabsorption of filtered fluid. In this setting, small elevations in the hydrostatic pressure gradient increase lung fluid imbalance even at wedge pressures normally not associated with hydrostatic edema formation, i.e., below 20 mmHg.

Hypoxemia

In ARDS, the most life-threatening problem is severe hypoxemia predominantly due to a high right-to-left intrapulmonary shunt through numerous fluid-filled alveoli. The increase in shunt is proportional to a decrease in functional residual capacity.[12] The magnitude of the shunt can be calculated while the patient is breathing 100% oxygen by estimating a shunt of 5% for every 100 mmHg decrease in PaO_2 below 700. For example, if PaO_2 on 100% oxygen is 200 mmHg, then the shunt is approximately 25%. This estimate is accurate for PaO_2 values above 150 mmHg.[13] Patients with ARDS requiring mechanical ventilation usually develop right-to-left shunts in the range of 20% to 50% (normal up to 5%). Increased shunting underlies the difficulty in improving hypoxemia with simple supplemental oxygen even with concentrations of 100%. Management should be aimed at decreasing the shunt fraction.

Low Compliance

Decreased compliance of the lungs in ARDS is due to widespread alveolar and interstitial edema and collapsed alveoli. Alveolar instability is worsened by decreased alveolar surfactant activity.[14] Increased lung stiffness is reflected by low compliance in both the lungs and chest wall as measured in patients receiving mechanical ventilation. Compliance is normally 50 to 100 ml/cm H_2O. For example, a tidal volume of 1000 ml delivered by a ventilator without the use of positive end-expiratory pressure (PEEP) produces an end-inspiratory pressure change of 10 cm H_2O by the following calculations:

$$\text{C stat (compliance)} = \Delta \text{ volume } / \Delta \text{ pressure}$$

$$100 \text{ ml/cm } H_2O = 1000 \text{ ml } / \text{ pressure}$$

pressure = 10 cm H_2O = end-inspiratory pressure, if PEEP = 0

The peak inspiratory pressure of the ventilator in this example is about 12 cm H_2O if airway resistance and the inspiratory flow rate are normal.

In contrast, a patient with ARDS with a compliance of 20 ml/cm H_2O has an end-inspiratory pressure of 50 cm H_2O when given the same tidal volume of 1000 ml. Moreover, the peak inspiratory pressures produced by the ventilator are much higher because of the high inspiratory flow rates needed to provide adequate minute ventilations in the face of greatly elevated deadspace to tidal volume ratios.[15]

PATHOLOGY

Acute Exudative Phase

There are two major pathologic phases in ARDS. An acute exudative phase associated with the initial injury and onset of edema is followed by a second subacute remodeling phase of lung repair and fibrosis.[15–19] At the beginning of the exudative phase, there may be no morphological changes seen histologically or ultrastructurally other than edema in the interstitium of the alveolar-capillary membrane. Later, alveolar edema forms and may be severe. Lungs from patients with ARDS dying of acute hypoxemia can weigh over 1000 g each, many times the normal weight.

On histologic examination, protein-rich edema fills most of the alveoli. Evidence of acute lung injury and inflammatory cells may be seen, depending on the nature of the injury. Hyaline membranes made up of fibrin strands form a pseudoepithelium over denuded alveolar basement membranes. They indicate excessive leakage of high molecular weight fibrinogen into the alveolar space.

Subacute Reparative/Remodeling Phase

Remodeling of alveolar and interstitial spaces probably begins shortly after initial lung injury in patients who survive the acute exudative phase. Evidence of interstitial and intraalveolar fibrosis can be documented histologically about one to two weeks after the onset of ARDS.[15,17,18] The thin delicate lining of squamous alveolar epithelium composed of type I pneumocytes is replaced by a thicker cuboidal layer of alveolar type II pneumocytes. The type II pneumocytes proliferate after necrosis of the type I cells and eventually differentiate into type I pneumocytes to reconstitute the alveolar epithelium. Alveolar and interstitial edema give way to interstitial fibroblast proliferation and migration with new production of collagen, resulting in alveolar and interstitial fibrosis. Fibrotic changes are marked in patients who die after prolonged ventilator support.[17]

Oxygen toxicity may contribute to the pathologic changes of ARDS, but its exact role is difficult to assess for several reasons. First, patients with ARDS are nearly always exposed to high concentrations of oxygen. Second, oxygen toxicity itself is a well-established cause of ARDS. Finally, safe upper limits of fractional inspired oxygen concentration (FiO_2) for patients with injured lungs are not established.

PATHOGENESIS

Acute Exudative Phase

ARDS Due to Conditions With a Direct Mechanism of Injury

Experimental and clinical observations firmly support the hypothesis that alveolar epithelial injury leading to altered permeability is the mechanism involved in predisposing conditions which act di-

rectly on the lung (see Table 58–1). Injury and lysis of alveolar type I cell pneumocytes has been documented in pneumonias due to *Pneumocystis carinii*[20] and after inhalation of toxic fumes like those from nitrogen dioxide.[21]

Loss of alveolar surfactant activity has also been documented in ARDS[14] and may secondarily contribute to the pathogenesis of ARDS. In contrast, in the respiratory distress syndrome (RDS) of premature infants, inadequate surfactant production due to immaturity of the lung is thought to be the primary mechanism of respiratory failure.[22] In ARDS, at least three different mechanisms may lead to decreased alveolar surfactant activity. First, flooding of the alveolar spaces may simply wash it out. Second, injury to alveolar type II pneumocytes that produce and secrete surfactant may decrease production. Finally, surfactant may be inactivated by contact with plasma proteins. Although loss of surfactant activity probably contributes to the physiologic abnormalities and respiratory failure seen in ARDS, its relative importance remains unclear.

ARDS Due to Conditions With an Indirect Mechanism of Injury

Lung injury may occur in conditions leading to widespread organ failure (see Table 58–1).[23–25] Injury to the lungs and other organs is probably mediated predominantly through activation of endogenous cellular and noncellular mechanisms by the predisposing condition. For example, ARDS occurs in 20 to 40 percent of patients with gram-negative sepsis.[9,26] In this setting, neutrophils are thought to be an important mediator of lung injury. They are first sequestered in pulmonary capillaries by endotoxin-mediated complement activation[27,28] or by cytokine release.[29] Neutrophils then release proteolytic enzymes and produce reactive oxygen species like hydrogen peroxide, which damage endothelial and epithelial cells, their intercellular junctions, and cell-substrate connections to increase permeability. Although this hypothesis is attractive, ARDS has occurred in severely neutropenic patients,[30] indicating the likelihood of alternative mechanisms. Direct injury to endothelium and epithelium by cytokines like tumor necrosis factor (TNF) may be one of these.[29]

Subacute Reparative Phase

The subsequent subacute phase, characterized by continued diffuse alveolar damage, type II cell hyperplasia, interstitial cellular infiltration, and fibrosis, begins within several days of the onset of ARDS. The mechanisms of these changes are unclear. Possible etiologies include effects of severe lung inflammation[18] and those of the original injurious agents or primary mediators. Toxicity from high concentration of oxygen[17] and overdistention of alveoli due to high pressures produced by positive-pressure mechanical ventilation and PEEP may contribute.[31]

MANAGEMENT

Specific Therapy

The first step in the therapy of ARDS is to diagnose and treat any underlying predisposing conditions. The second is to reverse the specific pathogenetic mechanisms discussed above. However, as in the case of prevention,[8,9] effective specific therapy for established

ARDS is still lacking. Controlled clinical trials reveal that high-dose corticosteroids used to suppress diffuse lung inflammation do not affect outcome or mortality rates in patients with ARDS.[32,33] Similarly, prolonged infusion of prostaglandin E_1, a pulmonary and systemic vasodilator with anti-inflammatory properties, does not alter outcome in these patients even though it significantly increases oxygen delivery and consumption and decreases pulmonary and systemic vascular resistance.[34] Other anti-inflammatory agents of various types show promise in experimental studies but require large controlled clinical trials.[35]

Surfactant replacement therapy is effective in improving pulmonary function in established cases of respiratory distress syndrome (RDS) of the newborn.[22] Extension of this therapy to patients with ARDS has been proposed based on experimental support.[14,36,37] Although extracorporeal membrane oxygenation (ECMO)[38] does not improve the survival rate in patients with severe ARDS (PaO_2/FiO_2 ratios of 50 or less), use of an extracorporeal membrane to remove CO_2 rather than to provide oxygen has been reported to be useful in uncontrolled studies.[39] One of its goals is to prevent damage to the lung from overdistention of alveoli by high alveolar pressure required to ventilate patients with ARDS.[31]

Supportive Therapy

Oxygen Therapy

Patients with ARDS and mild-to-moderate shunts of 5 to 15 percent can be managed successfully without endotracheal intubation and mechanical ventilation. Supplemental oxygen is given to achieve an oxygen saturation in the blood of 90% or a PaO_2 of 60 mmHg. Nasal prongs or simple face masks provide a FiO_2 of 0.5 or less. If the arterial PaO_2 remains below 55 mmHg, the FiO_2 can be increased by using masks with rebreathing or nonrebreathing reservoir bags. When tightly fitted, they can provide oxygen concentrations of almost 90 to 100%. Close monitoring of patients requiring a high FiO_2 is best performed in an intensive care unit, since unnoticed removal of the mask by a confused patient in a general care unit can rapidly lead to severe arterial oxygen desaturation.

Mechanical Ventilation and Use of Positive End-Expiratory Pressure (PEEP)

Indications for intubation and mechanical ventilation with positive end-expiratory pressure (PEEP) include inability to keep the PaO_2 above 50 to 55 mmHg with simple supplementary oxygen administration; prolonged exposure to > 90% oxygen concentration for more than a day; and development of respiratory muscle fatigue and hypercapnia. The goal of mechanical ventilation and PEEP is to maintain adequate arterial oxygenation at nontoxic inspired oxygen concentrations in the 50% to 60% range.

Because patients with ARDS have stiff lungs and high deadspace-to-tidal volume ratios (Vd/Vt), they commonly require high peak inflation pressures of 100 cm H_2O or more and high minute ventilations of 25 to 35 liters per minute. Mechanical ventilators with high flow and pressure capabilities are preferred. Narcotic administration, sedation, and paralysis are routinely used to improve synchrony between the ventilator and the patient in order to decrease peak inspiratory pressures, control discomfort and agitation, decrease the work of breathing, and reduce total body oxygen consumption and CO_2 production. Barbiturate-induced

coma, paralysis, and total-body hypothermia to 90 to 91°F to decrease O_2 consumption and lower the range of acceptable PO_2 to 35 to 45 mmHg have been utilized in desperate cases.

Although its mechanism of action is not completely understood, PEEP improves arterial oxygenation and decreases high right-to-left shunting in patients with ARDS.[12,15,40] PEEP is designed to reverse life-threatening levels of hypoxemia acutely and maintain oxygen delivery and tissue oxygenation with the lowest possible FiO_2 in an effort to avoid further injury from toxic concentrations of oxygen. PEEP increases the passive end-expiratory position of the lungs (functional residual capacity) by inflating previously fluid-filled alveoli and expanding those that are partially fluid-filled or collapsed. By decreasing the number of alveoli with low V/Q ratios, PEEP decreases the shunt fraction and improves oxygenation.[12] PEEP also improves lung compliance, making it possible to deliver the same tidal volumes at lower airway pressures.[41]

In severe cases, PEEP is initiated with 100% oxygen. Although increasing PEEP raises the PaO_2 and the oxygen content of arterial blood (CaO_2), it may reduce cardiac output by decreasing venous return to the thorax.[41] The term "best PEEP" refers to that level of PEEP that achieves the best oxygen delivery defined as the product of cardiac output and CaO_2. As shown in Fig. 58–1, PEEP is applied in increments of 3 cm H_2O from 0 up to 15 cm H_2O. After 15 to 20 minutes at each level, PaO_2 and cardiac output calculated by thermodilution are measured, and oxygen saturation (O_2 Sat) is determined directly by co-oximetry or derived from a nomogram from the PaO_2. The product of cardiac output and O_2 Sat is then calculated for each PEEP level, and the highest value indicates the best PEEP.[41] Reduction in cardiac output induced by PEEP can usually be reversed by intravascular volume expansion, although this can cause more lung edema. The best PEEP may change during the course of therapy due to alterations in cardiac output or changes in oxygenation from other causes. In addition, because O_2 consumption is dependent on delivery in some patients with ARDS and especially in those with sepsis,[42] measurement of O_2 saturation in mixed-venous blood and estimation of changes in cardiac output from the Fick equation should not substitute for direct measurement of cardiac output.

In cases of ARDS with refractory hypoxemia with PO_2 < 50 mmHg despite administration of 100% oxygen and PEEP levels above the usual therapeutic range of 0 to 15 cm H_2O, some clinicians use much higher levels of PEEP up to 35 cm H_2O in conjunction with intermittent mandatory ventilation (IMV).[43] IMV is used to reduce mean intrathoracic pleural pressure in order to prevent severe cardiovascular insufficiency.

Hemodynamic and Fluid and Diuretic Therapy

Patients with ARDS develop worsening pulmonary edema with only moderate elevations in intravascular volume. For this reason, diuretics and fluid restriction to decrease mean pulmonary capillary hydrostatic pressure are commonly instituted to lower pulmonary capillary wedge pressure as much as blood pressure, cardiac output, and critical organ perfusion permit. Inotropic agents like dopamine are commonly added to compensate for decreased left-ventricular preload, maintain renal function, and keep pulmonary capillary pressure low.[44] One study documented a relationship between fluid balance and mortality in ARDS in which weight gain and more positive fluid balance after the second day of illness

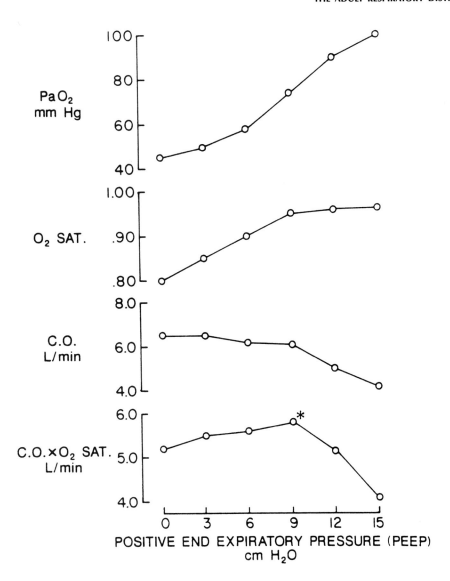

FIGURE 58–1. Schematic representation of typical trial of positive end-expiratory pressure (PEEP), i.e., a "best PEEP" trial, in a patient with ARDS receiving mechanical ventilation. Each point represents the value of each variable at baseline (0 cm H_2O of PEEP) and after 20 minutes at 3 cm H_2 increments of PEEP up to 15 cm H_2O. During this trial, the inspired oxygen concentration remains the same. Note the marked response of arterial PO_2 (PaO_2) and improvement in oxygen saturation (O_2 Sat) to increases in PEEP. Because the cardiac output (C.O.) falls more markedly after 9 cm H_2O of PEEP, oxygen delivery, as represented in this example by the product of C.O. and O_2 Sat (C.O. × O_2 Sat), is maximal at 9 cm of PEEP (asterisk), which would then be considered to be the best PEEP. Reprinted with permission.[61]

correlated with poor outcome.[45] However, weight gain and a more positive fluid balance might be markers rather than causes of a worse prognosis.

These interventions are designed to maintain adequate cardiac output and oxygen delivery and to avoid worsening pulmonary edema. However, in certain situations like ARDS in septic shock, cardiac dysfunction may be more life-threatening than ARDS itself and require higher rather than decreased intravascular volume. Although fluid management in these situations is controversial,[45] both crystalloid and colloid solutions are commonly used for vol-

ume expansion. Some argue that massive infusions of crystalloid should be avoided because they reduce plasma oncotic pressure by diluting plasma proteins, while colloid increases plasma oncotic pressure and draws out pulmonary edema fluid. However, the effects of such infusions also depend on resultant changes in interstitial hydrostatic and oncotic pressures. Furthermore, albumin rapidly equilibrates between plasma and edema fluid in the lung in ARDS, and there is little evidence that dilution of plasma proteins by crystalloid causes significant pulmonary edema except when pulmonary capillary wedge pressure is elevated. Monitoring of intravascular volume by measuring pulmonary capillary wedge pressure is therefore crucial.

Because discontinuation of PEEP in patients with ARDS may cause profound desaturation that improves only slowly after it is reinstituted,[15,41] it is unwise to do so solely to measure pulmonary capillary wedge pressure. Although elevated wedge pressures measured on PEEP reflect PEEP-induced rise in the intrapleural pressure, the elevation is balanced by reduction in left atrial pressure due to decreased venous return. After differentiating cardiogenic from noncardiogenic pulmonary edema, relative rather than absolute changes in wedge pressure are most important in the hemodynamic management of patients with ARDS.

Barotrauma

Mechanical ventilation at high inflation pressures and PEEP levels may induce barotrauma. This term refers to lung injury caused by high alveolar pressures. Tension pneumothorax is the most severe form of barotrauma and causes sudden elevation in inspiratory pressure, hypotension with tachycardia, and subcutaneous emphysema. Absence of chest sounds on the affected side may be difficult to appreciate. Diagnosis is confirmed by a portable chest x-ray showing the pneumothorax with persistent inflation of the ipsilateral lung,[46] requiring immediate insertion of a chest tube. Prophylactic chest tube placement to prevent tension pneumothorax carries excessive risk because the lung in ARDS does not collapse as readily as a normal lung when the pleural space is opened to atmospheric pressure.

Persistent air leaks occur commonly after chest tube placement in ARDS, indicating the presence of a bronchopleural fistula. Leakage of a large fraction of the tidal volume can cause inadequate ventilation and death. Spontaneous closure of a fistula is uncommon while the patient is receiving tidal volumes at high pressures and high levels of PEEP. If possible, inserting multiple chest tubes to expand the lung fully may diminish the leak. Alternatively, high-frequency jet ventilation that lowers peak airway pressures can be used in an attempt to decrease the air leak and may lead to closure of the fistula in difficult cases.[47] Surgical closure of the leak is usually not feasible in unstable patients with extensive parenchymal disease.

General Medical Care

Patients with ARDS on mechanical ventilation require comprehensive medical management, including intensive nursing care, prophylaxis against stress-related gastric erosions,[48] nutritional therapy,[49,50] early detection and treatment of nosocomial infections, and physical and occupational therapy as indicated.[51] ARDS occurs commonly as part of the multiple-systems organ failure syndrome[25] in which nonpulmonary organs are compromised by underlying conditions like sepsis or trauma, the adverse hemodynamic effects of therapy for ARDS itself, or nosocomial pneumonias and other infections. The combination of ARDS and failure of other organ systems greatly increases mortality.[52] ARDS and acute renal failure make management of volume status more difficult. Intravascular volume overload caused by renal failure worsens pulmonary edema unless fluid is removed by dialysis or ultrafiltration. Continuous

arterial-venous hemofiltration is usually reasonably well tolerated and especially useful in hypotensive patients on vasopressors.[53]

PROGNOSIS

ARDS carries a high mortality rate of 50 to 60 percent and up to 90 percent in severe cases.[38] Cause of death varies depending on predisposing conditions. For example, in the ECMO study of 90 patients with ARDS due to viral pneumonia, 40 percent of deaths were attributed to respiratory failure. In other series of patients with ARDS due mainly to sepsis, most died from infection and only 15 percent from respiratory failure.[54,55] The lung in ARDS is unusually susceptible to gram-negative pneumonias. Mortality rate increases significantly with additional organ-system failure. The syndrome of multiple-systems organ failure is uniformly lethal unless a treatable source of sepsis is found.[52]

Patients who survive and can be weaned from mechanical ventilation have a surprisingly good prognosis for continued recovery of lung function.[56,57] Many have minimal or no evidence of residual lung damage.

SUMMARY

1. The diagnosis of ARDS requires documenting hypoxemia and pulmonary edema in the absence of congestive heart failure in the setting of a likely predisposing cause (Table 58–1).

2. Congestive heart failure can be excluded by measuring pulmonary capillary wedge pressure. In ARDS, wedge pressure is < 18 mmHg, and in congestive heart failure it is > 28 mmHg. Wedge pressures between 18 and 28 mmHg should be treated initially as congestive failure and followed closely.

3. The FiO_2 should be increased to maintain the PaO_2 at a minimum of 55 to 60 mmHg but not higher than 70 mmHg when a FiO_2 above 0.6 is required to do so.

4. Patients with severe hypoxemia despite oxygen therapy should be intubated and mechanically ventilated. Initial ventilator settings are as follows:

   a. *Tidal volume:* 8 to 10 ml/kg ideal body weight or less in order to maintain end-inspiratory pressures below 40 to 50 cm H_2O.

   b. *FiO₂:* Begin at $FiO_2 = 1.0$ to estimate the shunt fraction. On 100% oxygen, the shunt is 5% for every 100 mmHg in the PaO_2 below 700 mmHg.

   c. *Respiratory rate:* With the ventilator in the assist mode and the patient triggering it, the $PaCO_2$ can usually be maintained below 40 mmHg. If sedation or paralysis is needed, the machine rate should be adjusted to keep the $PaCO_2$ between 30 and 40 mmHg. If peak inspiratory pressures are > 50 cm H_2O, $PaCO_2$ can be allowed to rise somewhat to lower airway pressure.

   d. *PEEP:* If the patient requires an FiO_2 over 60% to maintain a PaO_2 of 55 mmHg or higher, determine the best PEEP as described above and illustrated in Fig. 58–1.

   e. *Peak flow:* Adjust this parameter to ensure an inspiratory-to-expiratory ratio of less than 1:2 unless using inverse-ratio ventilation described below.

   f. If peak airway pressures remain > 50 cm H_2O, consider using pressure-controlled ventilation to avoid the deleterious ef fects of lung overinflation.[58] If hypoxemia is severe and peak pressures are persistently high, consider use of inverse-ratio pressure-cycled or pressure-controlled ventilation.[59]

5. A radial artery cannula should be inserted for continuous blood pressure and frequent arterial blood gas monitoring. Pulse oximetry is also useful for continuous monitoring of blood oxygen saturation.

6. A Swan-Ganz catheter is required to monitor pulmonary capillary wedge pressure. Wedge pressures should be maintained below 15 mmHg or as low as hemodynamically tolerated.

7. Hypotension should be treated with pressors and volume expansion as indicated by hemodynamic alterations in cardiac output and systemic vascular resistance.

8. Diuretics can be used to decrease pulmonary capillary hydrostatic pressures as long as end-organ perfusion is preserved. If urine output is insufficient despite use of diuretics, ultrafiltration can be initiated to reduce wedge pressure to the desired level.

9. Daily chest roentgenograms should be obtained in anticipation of pneumothorax and nosocomial pneumonia.

10. Tracheostomy can be deferred for two weeks in patients who have undergone nasotracheal or endotracheal intubation. With well-monitored low-pressure cuffed tubes, prolonged translaryngeal intubation for three to four weeks or longer may be safe.

11. Pneumonia, sepsis, and other nosocomial infections such as occult sinusitis due to nasal tubes should be recognized early and treated aggressively.

12. Weaning from the ventilator should be a slow process with emphasis on decreasing FiO_2 to 0.6 or below before reducing levels of PEEP. PEEP should be decreased slowly in 2.5 to 3.0 cm H_2O increments.

REFERENCES

1. Ashbaugh DG, Bigelow DB, Petty TL et al: Acute respiratory distress in adults. *Lancet* 2:319–323, 1967.
2. Petty TL: The adult respiratory distress syndrome. Clinical features, factors influencing prognosis, and principles of management. *Chest* 60:233–239, 1971.
3. Murray JF, Matthay MA, Luce JM et al: An expanded definition of the adult respiratory distress syndrome. *Am Rev Respir Dis* 138:720–733, 1988.
4. Pepe PE, Potkin RT, Reus DH et al: Clinical predictors of the adult respiratory distress syndrome. *Am J Surg* 4:124–130, 1982.
5. Fowler AA, Hamman RF, Good JT et al: Adult respiratory distress syndrome: Risk with common predispositions. *Ann Intern Med* 98:593–597, 1983.
6. Hyers TM, Fowler AA: Adult respiratory distress syndrome: Causes, morbidity, and mortality. *Fed Proced* 45:25–29, 1986.
7. Maunder RJ: Clinical prediction of the adult respiratory distress syndrome. *Clin Chest Med* 6:413–426, 1985.
8. Pepe PE, Hudson LD, Carrico CJ: Early application of positive end-expiratory pressure in patients at risk for the adult respiratory distress syndrome. *N Engl J Med* 311:281–286, 1984.
9. Bone RC, Fisher CJ Jr, Clemmer TP et al: Early methylprednisolone treatment for septic syndrome and the adult respiratory distress syndrome. *Chest* 92:1032–1036, 1987.
10. Forrester JS, Diamond G, McHugh TJ et al: Filling pressures in the right and left sides of the heart in acute myocardial infarction—a reappraisal of central venous pressure monitoring. *N Engl J Med* 285:190–193, 1971.
11. Staub NC: Pulmonary edema. Physiologic approaches to management. *Chest* 74:559–564, 1978.
12. Dantzker DR: Gas exchange in the adult respiratory distress syndrome. *Clin Chest Med* 3:57–68, 1982.
13. Lanken PN: Weaning from mechanical ventilation, in Fishman AP (ed): *Update: Pulmonary Diseases and Disorders.* New York, McGraw-Hill, 1982, pp 366–386.
14. Enhoring G: Surfactant replacement in adult respiratory distress syndrome. *Am Rev Respir Dis* 140:281–283, 1989.
15. Lamy M, Fallat RJ, Koeniger E et al: Pathologic features and mechanisms of hypoxemia in adult respiratory distress syndrome. *Am Rev Respir Dis* 114:267–284, 1976.
16. Kapanci Y, Weibel ER, Kaplan HP et al: Pathogenesis and reversibility of the pulmonary lesions of oxygen toxicity in monkeys. *Lab Invest* 20:101–118, 1969.
17. Pratt PC: Pulmonary morphology in a multi-hospital collaborative extracorporeal membrane oxygenation project: I. Light microscopy. *Am J Pathol* 95:191–214, 1979.
18. Bachofen M, Weibel ER: Alternations of the gas exchange apparatus in adult respiratory insufficiency associated with septicemia. *Am Rev Respir Dis* 116:589–615, 1987.
19. de los Santos R, Seidenfeld JJ, Anzueto A et al: One hundred percent oxygen lung injury in adult baboons. *Am Rev Respir Dis* 136:657–661, 1987.
20. Lanken PN, Minda M, Pietra GG et al: Alveolar response to experimental *Pneumocystis carinii* pneumonia in the rat. *Am J Pathol* 99:561–588, 1980.
21. Evans MJ, Cabral LJ, Stephens RJ et al: Renewal of alveolar epithelium in the rat following exposure to NO_2. *Am J Pathol* 70:175–179, 1973.
22. Horbar JD, Soll RF, Sutherland JM et al: A multicenter, placebo-controlled trial of surfactant therapy for respiratory distress syndrome. *N Engl J Med* 320:959–965, 1989.
23. Bell RC, Coalson JJ, Smith JD et al: Multiple organ system failure and infection in adult respiratory distress syndrome. *Ann Intern Med* 99:293–298, 1983.
24. Kreuzfelder E, Joka T, Keinecke HO et al: Adult respiratory distress syndrome as a specific manifestation of a general permeability defect in trauma patients. *Am Rev Respir Dis* 137:95–99, 1988.
25. Sheagren JN: Mechanism-oriented therapy for multiple systems organ failure. *Crit Care Clin* 5:393–409, 1989.
26. Fein AM, Lippmann M, Holzman H et al: The risk factors, incidence, and prognosis of ARDS following septicemia. *Chest* 83:40–42, 1983.
27. Tate RM, Repine JE: Neutrophils and the adult respiratory distress syndrome. *Am Rev Respir Dis* 128:552–559, 1983.
28. Rinaldo JE, Rogers RM: Adult respiratory distress syndrome: Changing concepts of lung injury and repair. *N Engl J Med* 306:900–909, 1982.
29. Tracey KJ, Lowry SF, Cerami A: Cachetin/TNF in septic shock and septic adult respiratory distress syndrome. *Am Rev Respir Dis* 138:1322–1329, 1988.
30. Ognibene FB, Martin SE, Parker MM et al: Adult respiratory distress syndrome in patients with severe neutropenia. *N Engl J Med* 315:547–555, 1986.
31. Kolobow R, Moretti MP, Gumagalli R et al: Severe impairment in lung function induced by high peak airway pressure during mechanical ventilation. An experimental study. *Am Rev Respir Dis* 135:312–315, 1987.
32. Bernard GR, Luce GM, Spring CL et al: High-dose corticosteroids in patients with the adult respiratory distress syndrome. *N Engl J Med* 317:1565–1570, 1987.

33. Bone C, Fisher CJ Jr, Clemmer TP et al: Early methylprednisolone treatment for septic syndrome and the adult respiratory distress syndrome. *Chest* 92:1032–1036, 1987.

34. Bone RC, Slotman G, Maunder R et al: Randomized double-blind, multicenter study of prostaglandin E_1 in patients with the adult respiratory distress syndrome. *Chest* 96:114–119, 1989.

35. Mandell GL: ARDS, neutrophils, and pentoxifylline. *Am Rev Respir Dis* 138:1103–1105, 1988.

36. Holm BA, Notter RH: Surfactant therapy in adult respiratory distress syndrome and lung injury, in Shapiro DL, Notter RH (eds): *Surfactant Respiratory Therapy*. New York, Liss, 1989, pp 273–304.

37. Harris JD, Jackson F, Moxley MA et al: Effect of exogenous surfactant instillation on experimental acute lung injury. *J Appl Physiol* 66:1846–1851, 1989.

38. Zapol WM, Snider MT, Hill JD et al: Extracorporeal membrane oxygenation in severe acute respiratory failure. A randomized prospective study. *JAMA* 242:2193–2196, 1979.

39. Gattinoni L, Pesenti A, Mascheroni D et al: Low-frequency positive-pressure ventilation with extracorporeal CO_2 removal in severe acute respiratory failure. *JAMA* 256:881–886, 1986.

40. Weisman IM, Rinaldo JE, Rogers RM: Positive end-expiratory pressure in adult respiratory failure. *N Engl J Med* 307:1381–1384, 1982.

41. Suter PM, Fairley HB, Isenberg MD: Optimum end-expiratory airway pressure in patients with acute pulmonary failure. *N Engl J Med* 292:284–289, 1975.

42. Danek SJ, Lynch JP, Weg JF et al: The dependence of oxygen uptake on oxygen delivery in the adult respiratory distress syndrome. *Am Rev Respir Dis* 122:387–395, 1980.

43. Kirby RR, Downs JB, Civetta JM et al: High level positive end-expiratory pressure (PEEP) in acute respiratory insufficiency. *Chest* 67:156–163, 1975.

44. Prewitt RM, Matthay MA, Ghignone M: Hemodynamic management in the adult respiratory distress syndrome. *Clin Chest Med* 4:251–268, 1983.

45. Simmons RS, Berdine GG, Seidenfeld JJ et al: Fluid balance and the adult respiratory distress syndrome. *Am Rev Respir Dis* 135:924–929, 1987.

46. Bitto T, Mannion J, Stephenson LW et al: Pneumothorax during positive pressure mechanical ventilation. *J Cardiovasc Thor Surg* 89:585–591, 1985.

47. Albelda SM, Hansen-Flaschen JH, Taylor E et al: Evaluation of high-frequency jet ventilation in patients with bronchopleural fistulas by quantitation of the airleak. *Anesthesiology* 63:551–554, 1985.

48. Shuman RB, Schuster DP, Zuckerman GR: Prophylactic therapy for stress ulcer bleeding: A reappraisal. *Ann Int Med* 106:562–567, 1987.

49. Berger R, Adams L: Nutritional support in the critical care setting (part 1). *Chest* 96:139–150, 1989.

50. Berger R, Adams L: Nutritional support in the critical care setting (part 2). *Chest* 96:372–380, 1989.

51. Kirkpatrick MB, Bass JB: Quantitative bacterial cultures of bronchoalveolar lavage fluids and protected brush catheter specimens from normal subjects. *Am Rev Respir Dis* 139:546–548, 1989.

52. Knaus WA, Wagner DP: Multiple systems organ failure: Epidemiology and prognosis. *Crit Care Clin* 5:221–232, 1989.

53. Lauer A, Saccaggi A, Ronco C et al: Continuous arteriovenous hemofiltration in the critically ill patient. *Ann Intern Med* 99:455–459, 1983.

54. Montgomery AB, Stager MA, Carrico CJ et al: Causes of mortality in patients with the adult respiratory distress syndrome. *Am Rev Respir Dis* 132:485–489, 1985.

55. Seidenfeld JJ, Pohl DF, Bell RC et al: Incidence, site, and outcome of infections in patients with the adult respiratory distress syndrome. *Am Rev Respir Dis* 134:12–16, 1986.

56. Lakshminarayan S, Stanford RE, Petty TL: Prognosis after recovery from adult respiratory distress syndrome. *Am Rev Respir Dis* 113:7–16, 1976.

57. Elliot CG, Rasmusson BY, Crapo RO et al: Prediction of pulmonary function abnormalities after adult respiratory distress syndrome (ARDS). *Am Rev Respir Dis* 135:634–638, 1987.

58. Dreyfuss D, Saumon G: Lung overinflation; physiologic and anatomic alterations leading to pulmonary edema, in Zapol WM, Lemaire F (eds): *Adult Respiratory Distress Syndrome*. New York, Marcel Dekker, 1991, pp 433–449.

59. Marcy TW, Marini JJ: Inverse ratio ventilation in ARDS. *Chest* 100:495, 1991.

60. Humphrey HJ, Hall J, Sznajder JI et al: Improved survival following pulmonary capillary wedge pressure reduction in patients with ARDS. *Chest* 97:1176, 1990.

61. Lanken PN: Adult respiratory distress syndrome, in Carlson RW, Geheb MA (eds): *The Principles and Practice of Medical Intensive Care*. Philadelphia, Saunders, 1993, pp 826–838.

59 POSTOPERATIVE THROMBOEMBOLIC DISEASE AND FAT EMBOLISM

Mark A. Kelley

Thromboembolic disease is a major cause of complications and death in surgical patients.[1] Clot in the deep venous system of the lower extremities can be documented in over 40 percent of such patients.[2] In patients over age 60 and in those with malignancy, the incidence is 50 percent.[3-5] In those undergoing hip surgery, it is even higher at 70 percent.[4,6]

Over 500,000 cases of pulmonary embolism occur annually in the United States, with surgical patients forming the majority.[9] One large well-controlled prospective study showed that fatal pulmonary emboli occur in one percent of patients undergoing general surgery, but, because of differences in diagnostic criteria, the incidence of nonfatal pulmonary embolism remains uncertain.[10] Another more limited study found that as many as 18 percent of patients demonstrate new perfusion defects on lung scan after surgery.[11] The mortality rate of pulmonary embolism in one large prospective study was 30 percent if untreated[9] but only 2.5 percent in those who received therapy.[12]

Diagnosis of deep vein thrombosis (DVT) and pulmonary embolism is difficult, particularly in the perioperative period when other processes may confuse the clinical picture. Treatment with anticoagulants is also complex because of the risk of bleeding. This chapter discusses the problems of diagnosis and treatment of pulmonary embolism. Prevention of DVT and pulmonary embolism are reviewed in Chap. 48.

PATHOPHYSIOLOGY

Clot formation in the deep venous system is associated with a number of conditions. Except in uncommon coagulation disorders such as protein C deficiency, it is difficult to demonstrate a hypercoagulable state in patients with thromboembolism. Malignancy, trauma, and surgery may activate the clotting system for unclear reasons. Immobility predisposes patients to clot formation, probably because of sluggish venous blood flow and platelet aggregation.[13] Preexisting venous disease may also cause stasis and local inflammation. Other conditions associated with thromboembolism include congestive heart failure, pregnancy, use of oral contraceptives, stroke, and obesity. Oral contraceptives may affect coagulation directly, but most of the other conditions probably predispose patients to thrombosis because they cause immobility.[13] Thrombosis of the upper extremities and superior vena cava, often due to instrumentation, can also cause pulmonary emboli.[14,15]

Fibrinogen scanning reveals ongoing clot formation before, during, and after surgery.[2,16,17] This may be associated in part with a decrease in fibrinolytic activity during and for two days after anesthesia.[18] Except in orthopedic procedures and injuries, direct trauma to veins plays a relatively minor role in the pathogenesis of venous thrombosis.

When clots embolize to the lung, they usually migrate from the large-capacitance veins of the lower extremities or from major vessels in the abdomen.[19] DVT below the knee is clinically significant only if it progresses to involve larger more proximal vessels. However, there is some evidence that even thrombi in calf veins may embolize.[19]

When a clot embolizes to the lung, a series of poorly understood events follow.[20] The patient often becomes acutely dyspneic through reflex stimulation of lung receptors or release of local mediators like serotonin. Arterial P_{O_2} may fall because of ventilation-perfusion mismatch. Pulmonary artery pressure is not usually significantly elevated in otherwise normal patients unless at least 50 percent of the pulmonary circulation becomes occluded by one or more clots.[9] However, a relatively small volume of clot may elevate pulmonary artery pressure in those with preexisting cardiopulmonary disease. In either case, increased pulmonary artery pressure can lead to right-heart failure.

Death from pulmonary embolism occurs for several reasons. A fragile patient with underlying cardiopulmonary disease may not tolerate the additional stress of hypoxemia or the increased work of breathing. However, in most fatal cases, death is due to circulatory failure after a large volume of clot blocks the pulmonary circulation and produces pulmonary hypertension and cor pulmonale. Although this may be due to a single massive clot, it is more often the result of a succession of multiple smaller emboli that have gone unrecognized over a period of days or weeks. Clots usually lyse over days or weeks, but some larger ones may fragment within hours.

DIAGNOSIS

Deep Venous Thrombosis

Although tenderness and swelling of the calf nearly always suggest DVT, only 50 percent of patients with these signs are found to have it on venogram. Conversely, only about 50 percent of patients with documented DVT on venogram display clinical signs.[21] Therefore, the diagnosis must be made with laboratory tests. Since DVT occurs in 40 percent or more of surgical patients, screening and diagnosis may present major logistical problems.[1]

There are four methods for diagnosing venous thrombosis: radioactive fibrinogen scanning, impedance plethysmography (IPG), Doppler ultrasonography, and contrast venography. Fibrinogen scanning has been used extensively to study venous thrombosis in surgical patients, but the limitations of this technique make it impractical in patient management. The technique requires ongoing active clot formation in the leg for injected fibrinogen to be incorporated into the thrombus and localized by an external radiation detector. Accuracy is lost when the method is applied to large vessels in or above the thigh.[21] Overlying soft tissue may shield radioactivity, or radioactive fibrinogen may be deposited in areas of inflammation outside the venous system after procedures in and around the hip. Most pulmonary emboli arise in large veins at or above the knee in areas where fibrinogen scanning is least useful. Moreover, since the risk of pulmonary embolism from calf-vein thrombosis is unknown, indications for anticoagulation are unclear in a patient with a positive fibrinogen scan of the calf.

IPG and Doppler ultrasonography are more clinically useful noninvasive techniques that indirectly measure the patency of the large vessels of the upper leg and abdomen.[21,22] The IPG measures electrical resistance in the leg before and after venous compression. Differences in resistance reflect changes in venous capacitance, and these changes provide an indirect measure of venous blood flow. Compared to venography, IPG has an accuracy of 80 to 90 percent, making it an excellent screening test for DVT. In a large prospective study of ambulatory patients, a negative IPG, when repeated over several days, effectively ruled out proximal DVT.[23] No such study has been performed in hospitalized patients, but the results are probably applicable to this population.

The Doppler technique uses ultrasound to detect flow patterns in large vessels and is less reliable than IPG because it requires experience in interpretation. However, recent reports of B-mode ultrasonography combined with color Doppler imaging claim accuracy approaching that of venography for proximal DVT.[24,25] This technology requires simple but expensive instrumentation and may be easier to perform in immobilized patients, but has not yet been evaluated as rigorously as IPG in large clinical trials. Venous obstruction due to ascites or right-heart failure can lead to false-positive results on ultrasonography or IPG. False-negative results occur when DVT is confined to veins below the knee.

More recently, the Doppler and IPG venous techniques have been shown to be insensitive in detecting asymptomatic DVT. In two different studies of patients undergoing orthopedic procedures, the sensitivity of IPG was 19 percent[26] and that of Doppler only 38 percent.[27] Most errors in diagnosis were due to failure to detect partially occluded veins. These results suggest that noninvasive studies may only be reliable for symptomatic patients in whom clot totally occludes portions of the venous system.

Venography is the most invasive but most reliable method of documenting DVT.[21] Although easy to perform, it requires experience in interpretation, particularly in patients with preexisting venous disease. The volume of contrast injected during venography is considerable and often exceeds the amount administered for a pulmonary arteriogram. The risk of dye-induced phlebitis is variable, but careful technique and reduced dye concentrations have eliminated the problem. The venogram remains the standard against which all other diagnostic tests for venous thrombosis are compared and provides a measure of the extent of thrombosis.

Application of these techniques in diagnosing symptomatic DVT depends on therapeutic strategy. In choosing this approach, the unresolved question of the clinical importance of distal DVT must be considered. Most pulmonary emboli arise from proximal veins, and some clinicians believe that distal DVT therefore does not require treatment. In such cases, serial noninvasive studies may be a good strategy to detect proximal propagation. Others feel compelled to treat distal DVT, particularly when it is deep within the calf. In this situation, they would use noninvasive studies to screen for DVT and proceed to venography if evidence of distal DVT is compelling.

Pulmonary Embolism

Most pulmonary emboli probably are unrecognized because clinical signs and symptoms are easily confused with other conditions. In postoperative patients, pneumonia, atelectasis, bronchospasm, and congestive heart failure can mimic pulmonary embolism. The classic syndrome of sudden shortness of breath, pleuritic chest pain, and acute right-heart failure is rarely seen.[28] The patient may instead appear more dyspneic than usual or experience atypical chest discomfort or a new arrhythmia, problems associated with several different disorders. However, when patients fail to respond to treatment for presumed pneumonia or congestive failure, pulmonary embolism should be suspected. Any type of new chest pain or a sudden unexplained drop in blood pressure strongly suggests pulmonary embolus. Less common manifestations of pulmonary embolism include tachycardia, arrhythmias, and fever. The temperature is almost never above 102°F and is usually accompanied by other signs or symptoms.

Physical examination is often not helpful in diagnosing pulmonary embolism. Signs of right-heart strain, including a right ventricular heave or gallop, elevated jugular venous pressure, and evidence of pulmonary hypertension with accentuation of the pulmonic component of the second heart sound are rarely seen. More often, only a nonspecific increase in respiratory rate and pulmonary rales are the only findings. A pleural rub is present in less than 5 percent of cases.[28] Signs of phlebitis are found in about one-third of these patients but are not specific for DVT.

Routine Laboratory Studies

Conventional laboratory data are not helpful in diagnosing pulmonary embolism. The white blood cell count is normal or slightly elevated. Serum enzyme levels are similarly of little value. The triad of elevated serum lactic dehydrogenase and bilirubin levels and a normal serum transaminase concentration, once thought to be useful in diagnosis, lacks sensitivity and specificity.

Measurement of fibrin degradation products enjoyed brief popularity as an adjunct in detecting pulmonary emboli. However, the test also lacks sensitivity and specificity and has not been well standardized. It is useless in patients who have suffered trauma or undergone surgery in whom active fibrinolysis is ongoing.

The electrocardiogram (ECG) is probably more useful in excluding myocardial ischemia than in diagnosing pulmonary embolism.[29] The most common ECG findings in pulmonary embolism are nonspecific ST-T changes that usually reflect underlying cardiac disease. Atrial fibrillation is an uncommon manifestation of the disease, and premature atrial or ventricular beats are nonspecific. Acute right-heart strain with new right-axis deviation, right bundle branch block, and ST-T changes in the early precordial leads are not common in pulmonary embolism but, if present, strongly suggest the diagnosis.

Arterial blood gas determinations have a limited diagnostic role.[30] Because most emboli cause transient ventilation-perfusion (V/Q) abnormalities, gases measured some time after embolism has occurred may be unimpressive, particularly in otherwise normal patients. Although it is unusual for patients with significant pulmonary emboli to have absolutely normal blood gas measurements, abnormalities may be due to any underlying cardiopulmonary disorder.

The chest radiograph may provide helpful information but is also limited. Pulmonary embolism rarely produces the classic peripheral wedge-shaped infiltrate indicative of pulmonary infarct. The x-ray may show infiltrate, atelectasis, effusion, or some combination thereof[31] which may be due to pneumonia, postoperative effusion, or splinting from pain. About 20 percent of patients with pulmonary embolism have a normal x-ray. A very large embolus may obliterate perfusion of one lung and rarely cause diminished vascular markings on the affected side.

Radionuclide Lung Scanning

The radionuclide ventilation-perfusion lung scan is the most useful test for diagnosing pulmonary embolism. The perfusion scan images the pulmonary arterial bed by detecting infused labeled albumin after it has lodged in the pulmonary capillaries. The ventilation scan detects the distribution of inhaled radioactive xenon. When interpreted together, these two techniques provide a radiographic image of the ventilation and perfusion patterns in the lung.

Much of the controversy about lung scanning has been resolved by the results of the multicenter study entitled "Prospective Investigation of Pulmonary Embolism Diagnosis" or PIOPED.[32] Patients suspected of pulmonary embolism were prospectively recruited and had standardized lung scans and pulmonary angiograms. These studies were interpreted by panels of experts according to predetermined criteria. For lung scans, the widely used criteria of Biello et al. were used, in which scans are read as indicating high, intermediate, low, or very low ("nearly normal") probability for pulmonary embolism.[33] Scan readings were compared to the likelihood of pulmonary embolism determined from clinical information, results of angiograms, and the clinical follow-up.

The PIOPED study showed that the lung scan can only provide estimates of the likelihood of pulmonary embolism. A high probability scan was about 85 percent accurate in establishing the diagnosis of pulmonary embolism. False-positive results occurred most often in patients with previous pulmonary embolism. A low-probability scan result excluded pulmonary embolism with about 85 percent accuracy. Normal scans and those with minimal perfusion defects were almost never associated with pulmonary embolism. Intermediate probability scans were of no diagnostic value.

Several important new findings emerged from PIOPED. First, most patients with pulmonary embolism do not have a high-probability scan, suggesting that the lung scan alone is insufficient in establishing a diagnosis. Second, the predictive value of the scan could be improved when coupled with the clinical likelihood of pulmonary embolism. This improvement was most notable in the case of low-probability scans. When coupled with a low clinical likelihood, pulmonary embolism was present in less than 5 percent of patients.

These findings suggest that the common practice of using the lung scan to confirm a clinical impression is sound, particularly in excluding the diagnosis. Normal lung scans or those with trivial defects make pulmonary embolism extremely unlikely. Low clinical probability supported by a low-probability scan may be enough to exclude the diagnosis but may demand confirmation by other studies if the patient has serious cardiopulmonary disease and no diagnostic error is acceptable. Similarly, a high-probability scan provides strong evidence to support clinical suspicion of pulmonary embolism. However, if treatment for pulmonary embolus may be particularly dangerous in a given patient, additional supportive data may be helpful. Finally, an indeterminate lung scan, commonly seen in patients with and without pulmonary embolism, requires additional diagnostic studies.

Pulmonary Angiography

Pulmonary angiography is the most direct but most invasive means of diagnosing pulmonary embolism. The PIOPED project confirmed previous data about its safety and accuracy. The mortality rate from the procedure was well under one percent. Death occurred almost exclusively in patients who were unstable and in those who had severe underlying cardiopulmonary disease.[34] Morbidity was also low and consisted largely of local problems like wound hematoma. With selective injection and magnification, angiography was confirmed as highly accurate in diagnosing pulmonary embolism. Prospective follow-up for one year demonstrated that the negligible diagnostic error of angiography occurred primarily in patients with chronic thromboembolism. The pulmonary angiogram thus remains the diagnostic gold standard.

The Noninvasive Approach to Diagnosing Pulmonary Embolism

Since pulmonary angiography requires special expertise and is not widely available, some investigators have advocated a noninvasive approach to this diagnosis.[35] This strategy views DVT and pulmonary embolism as different ends of the same process of thromboembolism requiring the same treatment with anticoagulation. Therefore, finding pulmonary embolism and/or proximal DVT has the same therapeutic implications.

In this strategy, lung scan and noninvasive studies of the proximal venous system can be combined to detect thromboembolic disease. The lung scan should be used as the initial screening test for pulmonary embolism. In the PIOPED study, patients with very-low-probability or normal lung scans did not have pulmonary embolism or DVT on follow-up and did not require additional diagnostic studies. Therefore, these scan results effectively rule out thromboembolic disease.

The patient with an intermediate-probability lung scan result is more problematic. A pulmonary angiogram could be performed to document pulmonary embolism, or IPG could be done to confirm proximal vein thrombosis for which treatment would be the same. However, pulmonary embolism and proximal DVT overlap incompletely. At least one-third of patients with pulmonary embolism confirmed on angiography do not have evidence of proximal DVT.[36] Therefore, the absence of proximal DVT on noninvasive studies does not completely exclude the possibility of pulmonary embolism. This noninvasive approach to the diagnosis of pulmonary embolism has been recently summarized and is shown in Fig. 59–1.[37]

TREATMENT

The treatment of thromboembolic disease is based on several important considerations. First, if thromboembolism has been reasonably well tolerated, therapy with anticoagulants is given to prevent further clot formation and allow clot organization and endogenous fibrinolysis to occur. Most patients with DVT and pulmonary embolism fall into this category. Second, if significant clot formation and migration occur when anticoagulation is adequate or if anticoagulation is contraindicated, venous interruption should be considered to prevent massive pulmonary embolism. Third, if massive clot has already filled the pulmonary circulation, thrombolytic therapy may be used to dissolve the clot rapidly and reduce right-heart strain.

Anticoagulation

Only one controlled trial has examined the influence of anticoagulation on the mortality of pulmonary embolism.[38] Despite technical limitations, it strongly suggests that anticoagulation is beneficial. Subsequent clinical experience has confirmed this conclusion.

The two drugs that are available for anticoagulation are heparin and warfarin. Although it requires parenteral administration, heparin has the advantage of rapid onset. It has direct effects on antithrombin, blocks factor IX activation, and inhibits activated factor X. Warfarin alters the biologic activity of several clotting factors synthesized by the liver but requires several days to work and is less predictable than heparin.

For all practical purposes, DVT and pulmonary embolism are treated identically with heparin in order to prevent further thrombus formation.[39] There is indirect evidence to support a recommended optimal range of heparin anticoagulation. The activated partial thromboplastin time (PTT) should be 1.5 to 2 times or the whole-blood clotting time should be two to three times the control values. Patients with lower values have a higher recurrence rate of thromboembolic disease.[39,40] While higher values could be associated with more bleeding complications, inadequate anticoagulation poses a much greater risk.[41]

The risk of bleeding on heparin is a major problem in surgical patients. Significant hemorrhage occurs in approximately 20 percent of those who have undergone recent surgery; have received intramuscular injections or platelet-suppressive drugs; or suffer from thrombocytopenia, uremia, or an underlying bleeding disorder. However, bleeding is a major concern in surgical patients receiving heparin even in the absence of these conditions. The risk of bleeding must therefore be weighed against that of life-threatening thromboembolism.

Continuous infusion of heparin is associated with fewer hemorrhagic complications.[39] Its anticoagulant effect is more predictable than that of bolus therapy, which transiently produces an anticoagulant effect well beyond the therapeutic range. In addition, the total daily dose of heparin required may be higher when the bolus method is used. Heparin may also be given in adjusted doses subcutaneously. This method has been shown to be as effective and safe as continuous intravenous infusion.[42]

The recommended starting dose of continuous heparin for uncomplicated patients is an intravenous bolus of 5000 units followed by a continuous infusion of 25,000 to 30,000 units over 24 hours. The intermittent infusion consists of 5000 to 7000 units every six hours. The PTT or whole-blood clotting time is measured four to six and again 24 hours after therapy is initiated and then daily thereafter. Patients with a high risk of bleeding should be started and maintained on lower doses. They can be given a bolus of 2000 to 4000 units and a maintenance dose of 15,000 to 20,000 units over 24 hours. This dose avoids anticoagulant effect beyond the therapeutic range and allows for appropriate adjustment to maintain the PTT in the lower part of the range. Adjusted-dose heparin is given subcutaneously every 12 hours and adjusted to achieve a PTT of 1.5 to 2 times the control value when measured four hours after the last dose. In all cases, heparin requirements may fall after several days of treatment. Initially large doses may be needed because of consumption of heparin by active thrombosis.

If bleeding occurs during heparin therapy, the dose can be lowered or the drug discontinued. If bleeding is life-threatening, anticoagulation can be rapidly reversed with protamine. The source of bleeding should be investigated and treated. For example, gastrointestinal bleeding from stress ulceration may respond to antacids or H_2 antagonists. Other common sources of bleeding are cutdown sites, surgical wounds, and recent fractures. It may therefore be possible to control bleeding with transfusions and temporary discontinuation of heparin while the primary source of bleeding is treated. Heparin can often be carefully reinstituted in low doses in several days.

Thrombocytopenia and thrombosis are incompletely understood complications of heparin therapy and may be due to immune-mediated endothelial injury induced by the drug. They can occur most commonly about five days after heparin is started but may be seen earlier in patients who have been previously treated with heparin. The initial manifestation is a rapid decline in the platelet count. Arterial thrombosis may also occur in severe cases. Heparin should be discontinued and warfarin or vena cava blockade substituted.

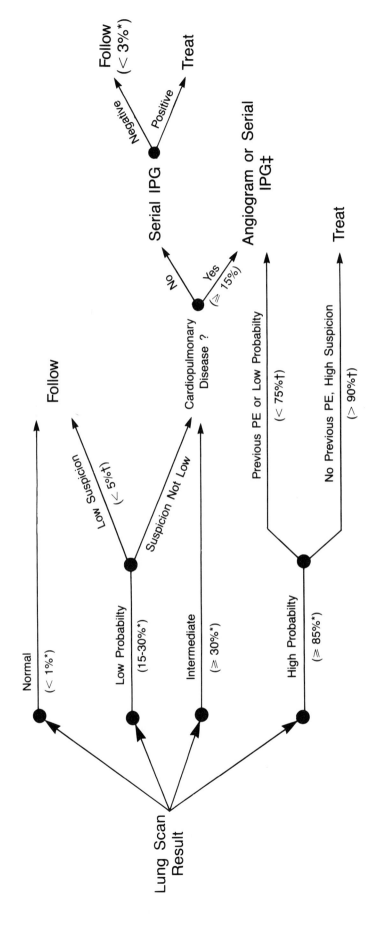

FIGURE 59–1. Diagnostic algorithm. A normal scan effectively rules out PE. A high probability scan supports the diagnosis of PE except in the presence of previous PE or low clinical suspicion. Other scan results were less helpful except the combination of low probability and low clinical suspicion. A positive IPG supports the diagnosis of thromboembolism. A negative result reliably excludes this disorder only in patients with nondiagnostic scans and no cardiopulmonary disease.

Abbreviations:

PE = pulmonary embolism
IPG = impedance plethysmography
( ) = likelihood of PE
*   = strongly supported by clinical studies
†   = suggested by clinical studies, needs confirmation
‡   = a single negative IPG may not be sufficient to rule out thromboembolism

Source: From Kelley MA, Carson JL, Palevsky HI, Schwartz JS: Diagnosing pulmonary embolism: New facts and strategies. *Ann Int Med* 114:304, 1991.

Oral anticoagulants are used for long-term treatment of thromboembolic disease. Heparin is usually given for 7 to 10 days, and anticoagulation is continued with warfarin. Animal studies show that endothelialization of clot is complete after 10 days. However, in one large study, patients adequately anticoagulated with heparin were given warfarin immediately.[43] When therapeutic levels of anticoagulation were achieved with warfarin in three to five days, heparin was discontinued. Hospitalization stay was shortened, and there was no increase in recurrence of thromboembolism. However, in another study, treating venous thromboembolism with coumadin alone was associated with excessively high rates of recurrent thrombosis.[44]

Oral anticoagulation can be initiated with maintenance doses without a loading dose. For patients who are not already anticoagulated, warfarin can be given in a dose of 10 mg daily for the first two days. Lower doses should be used in patients weighing less than 90 pounds, those older than 80 years, those with congestive heart failure and liver disease, and those with poor nourishment. On the third day of treatment, if the prothrombin time (PT) is two seconds above the baseline value, 15 mg of warfarin are given. If it is two to four seconds above the control value, 10 mg are given. If it is four to eight seconds above, five mg are given. If more than eight seconds, the dose is omitted. By the fourth day, the PT should reflect steady state at which time a dose of 5 to 7.5 mg per day is usually required. Heparin should be continued until the PT becomes adequately prolonged.

It is important to continue both heparin and warfarin until full anticoagulation is achieved with the latter, because warfarin alone can theoretically produce a transient hypercoagulable state. It interferes with the production of clotting factors II, VII, IX, and X and synthesis of protein C, a naturally occurring inhibitor of the clotting. The decline in protein C level occurs before the other clotting factors are reduced, rendering the patient more prone to thrombosis. This is a particular problem in those with protein C deficiency.

The recommended dose of warfarin for thromboembolism has been changed. The PT suffers from considerable variability among laboratories, depending on the type of tissue thromboplastin used to initiate in vitro coagulation. Previous therapeutic recommendations were based on less sensitive measurements of the PT and often resulted in excessive anticoagulation. An effort is being made to standardize the test by reporting results in relation to an international standard. Based on this information, the current recommendation is to adjust the coumadin dose to achieve a PT of 1.25 to 1.5 times the patient's control value.[45]

Anticoagulation is customarily continued for at least three months. This recommendation is based on retrospective studies and therapeutic trials demonstrating that recurrent thromboembolism is most frequent in the first six weeks. Anticoagulation for more than three months is probably unnecessary in most patients. If a patient experiences a recurrence months or years after anticoagulation has been discontinued, long-term anticoagulation should be considered.

Oral anticoagulants carry significant risk. Bleeding occurs in 5 to 20 percent of patients and is more common in patients who are elderly or unreliable with medications and in those with a potential bleeding site. The risk of complications also increases with the duration of therapy.[46] The PT must be monitored frequently, especially because the effect of warfarin is influenced by many common drugs.

An alternative to chronic anticoagulation with warfarin is adjusted-dose heparin as described above. It is equally effective as warfarin in preventing recurrence of thromboembolism and does not require frequent monitoring. Chronic heparin therapy is expensive but is useful when warfarin is contraindicated in pregnancy or when other factors such as drug-drug interactions complicate therapy.

Venous Blockade

Some patients do not respond to anticoagulation therapy and continue to have pulmonary emboli despite adequate anticoagulation. Others cannot tolerate anticoagulation either because of complications or anticipated problems with compliance and drug monitoring. Therefore, some mechanical means of blocking migration of clot to the lungs must then be considered. Although venous blockade is widely accepted, no controlled studies have indicated when or how such blockade should be performed.

The three methods of venous blockade are vena cava ligation, plication, and insertion of a filter.[47] Both ligation and plication of the vena cava require abdominal surgery. Ligation rapidly produces lower-extremity edema that can become chronic and disabling, and collateral vessels large enough to transmit clot can develop over weeks or months. Plication by clipping or suturing is designed to allow blood flow through fenestrations small enough to block clot. However, the fenestrations may become occluded with clot and cause caval interruption. The most widely used mechanical device to prevent clot migration is a wire filter placed intravenously into the vena cava. In experienced hands, the filter can usually be inserted under fluoroscopic guidance without surgery. The most popular device is the Greenfield filter, which has an excellent record of efficacy and patency.[48] Other caval filter devices include the wire-mesh "bird's nest" filter that may be easier to insert than the Greenfield filter. No controlled studies have been performed comparing the efficacy of these devices.

The best method of caval blockade depends on the experience of the institution and the underlying condition of the patient. In most patients, the safety and convenience of the filter far outweigh any disadvantages. More recent devices like the Greenfield filter have rarely presented technical problems and have worked well for many years. Chronic anticoagulation is unnecessary, especially with the Greenfield filter.

The decision to perform caval blockade should be based on several considerations. Continuing thromboembolism despite effective anticoagulation is one clear indication. If recurrent emboli are suspected, several steps should be taken. Anticoagulation therapy should be reviewed and, if inadequate, adjusted appropriately. A repeat perfusion lung scan should be obtained. A scan with no new defects compared to previous scans argues strongly against recurrent emboli. If new defects are present and other disease processes are excluded, the size of the clot burden should be estimated. If 20 percent or less of the vasculature is obliterated, patients without cardiopulmonary disease may be able to tolerate additional small clots. Noninvasive studies of the proximal vein may then be used to assess the clot burden in the large-capacitance vessels of the lower extremities. In uncertain cases, venography and/or pulmonary angiography may be necessary to confirm ongoing thromboembolism. A large clot burden in the lung and new emboli, particularly in the setting of ongoing proximal DVT, argue strongly for venous blockade.

Patients with bleeding complications of anticoagulation therapy present a slightly different set of problems. If lower doses of heparin and attention to the primary bleeding site fail, venous blockade should be considered. If pulmonary emboli are present, the decision to perform caval blockade should be approached in the same way as it is in the setting of recurrent emboli. If there is little clot in the lung, low-dose heparin can be used before caval blockade is performed.

Finally, a filter may be inserted when conventional therapy is too risky. For example, patients with poor cardiopulmonary reserve who cannot tolerate even a small recurrent embolus may benefit from a filter. Those who are not compliant with medications or have ongoing reasons for thrombosis like malignancy may be better protected by a mechanical device.

Thrombolytic Therapy

The widespread use of thrombolytic agents in the coronary circulation has generated some enthusiasm for expanding their role in the treatment of thromboembolism. The indications for thrombolytic therapy in surgical patients are necessarily limited since recent surgery is most often a contraindication to its use.

The multicenter Urokinase Pulmonary Embolism Trial (UPET) showed that urokinase did not decrease mortality more than heparin.[49] This may be due to the fact that few patients die of pulmonary embolism when it is recognized and treated with anticoagulants.[12] Because of natural fibrinolysis and the reserve of the pulmonary vascular bed, even fragile patients who initially present with severe cardiopulmonary compromise may respond to anticoagulation and supportive therapy alone.

All thrombolytic drugs activate plasminogen and accelerate clot lysis. They effectively reduce clot burden in the pulmonary circulation and decrease pulmonary artery pressure and right-heart strain.[50] However, since most patients with pulmonary embolism do not present with right-heart failure, it is not surprising that thrombolytic therapy has not improved survival rates. Despite the lack of data from controlled studies, some investigators favor the use of thrombolytic therapy, particularly when clot obliterates at least 40 percent of the pulmonary circulation. There is some indirect evidence that the pulmonary microcirculation may improve more with thrombolytics than with conventional anticoagulation.[51]

The use of thrombolytic agents in DVT is even less certain. There have been anecdotal reports showing that lytic agents accelerate clot resolution and reduce long-term sequelae such as venous stasis. However, no large clinical trials have confirmed their efficacy in the treatment for DVT.

The three most widely used and available thrombolytic agents are streptokinase, urokinase, and tissue-type plasminogen activator (TPA). A detailed discussion of these drugs can be found in a number of reviews.[52-54] None is clearly superior in treating pulmonary embolism and reducing clot burden. The major side effect is bleeding. Although often used as a local lytic agent, TPA causes clot lysis only in doses that produce some systemic fibrinolytic effect. Because it is a foreign protein, streptokinase more commonly produces febrile and allergic reactions.

To reduce total dose, some investigators have infused these drugs directly into the pulmonary circulation. Unfortunately, this method still produces a systemic lytic effect and can result in bleeding complications.[55] Therefore, local infusion into the pulmonary artery cannot be recommended.

Any active bleeding process or a history of a central nervous system event within the preceding three months is an absolute contraindication to thrombolytic therapy. Lytic agents should not be given immediately after invasive diagnostic procedures or surgery. The appropriate interval of time after such procedures is controversial but should span at least several days. It is wise to wait 7 to 10 days after surgery to initiate such therapy.

Embolectomy

Embolectomy should be considered in patients who have large clot burden with hemodynamic compromise and in whom lytic therapy is contraindicated or ineffective. Surgical embolectomy was previously associated with dismal outcome.[56,57] However, more recently, data are emerging suggesting that this approach may be beneficial in patients who have central clot that can be mechanically retrieved from the pulmonary artery.[58,59] Long-term survival may be as high as 70 percent in such patients provided they have not sustained a cardiac arrest.

One alternative is embolectomy with a specially designed suction catheter placed in the pulmonary circulation.[60] Experience with this technique has been limited, but, in successful cases, large collections of clot have been removed with immediate improvement in clinical status. This method and surgical embolectomy should be considered only if thrombolytic therapy cannot be used. All patients undergoing embolectomy should have an IVC filter placed thereafter.

The therapeutic approach to pulmonary embolism is summarized in Fig. 59–2. Most patients suffer submassive embolism and can be treated with conventional anticoagulation. Those with massive pulmonary embolism should be considered for thrombolytic therapy. If this is not feasible, an IVC filter should be placed, and in severe cases surgical or catheter embolectomy should be considered.

THE FAT EMBOLISM SYNDROME

Patients who have suffered serious trauma may develop neurologic and respiratory abnormalities attributed to the fat embolism syndrome (FES).[61] Such patients have usually sustained multiple fractures or a major fracture of a long bone. Less commonly, fat embolism is associated with complex orthopedic procedures like total hip replacement and has even been described in patients with sickle-cell crisis[62] and after liposuction.[63] FES occurs in about 5 percent of trauma patients and carries an estimated mortality of 10 to 20 percent, usually due to irreversible respiratory failure. At autopsy, fat deposits are found in multiple organs, particularly in the lung and brain.[64]

Within 12 to 72 hours after trauma or surgery, the patient develops fever, unexplained respiratory distress, mental confusion, and often a petechial rash. Frank respiratory failure and coma, sometimes accompanied by renal failure, may supervene.[61,65] The respiratory process resembles the adult respiratory distress syndrome (ARDS) with noncardiac pulmonary edema, a high alveolar-arterial oxygen gradient, and stiff lungs. The neurologic picture may begin with mild confusion and progress to stupor and coma, and occasionally includes focal neurologic signs.

The source of fat deposition remains controversial.[61,65] The

THERAPEUTIC
STRATEGY

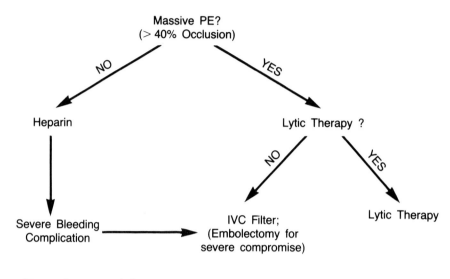

PE = pulmonary embolism
IVC = inferior vena cava

FIGURE 59–2.   Therapeutic algorithm for treating pulmonary embolism.

most popular theory, supported by a large body of experimental evidence, proposes that the fracture of long bones disrupts the adipose architecture of the marrow. Adipose tissue is extruded into the circulation and gives rise to fat emboli. A similar phenomenon may occur when there is trauma to fat stores as in rapid decompression from a hyperbaric environment. A second, less popular theory hypothesizes that the stress of trauma induces biochemical changes in the circulation, causing aggregation of circulating chylomicrons into fat droplets that are deposited in various organs. Neither pathogenetic theory offers practical information for treating or preventing FES.

Deposition of fat in the microcirculation can derange organ function in several ways. Intravascular fat deposits may cause circulatory sludging and ischemia. In the lung, the fat load may be high enough to elevate pulmonary artery pressure and produce acute cor pulmonale. More commonly, diffuse leakage from alveolar capillaries develops and causes ARDS. The capillary leak in FES may have a biochemical basis. Since the lung is rich in lipases, fat deposits may be readily degraded into free fatty acids that are toxic to the lung. Circulating fat may also cause platelet aggregation, leading to thrombocytopenia and petechiae. Platelet collections may also release serotonin which can exacerbate ventilation-perfusion abnormalities in the lung.[61,65]

Clinical Features

The diagnosis of FES should be considered in any patient with fractures who develops respiratory distress, neurologic signs, or petechial hemorrhage, particularly within the first three days after injury. Respiratory distress appears as mild tachypnea and may

rapidly progress to respiratory failure. Neurologic manifestations range from restlessness and mild disorientation to stupor and coma. The petechial rash occurs exclusively on the upper part of the body and sometimes affects the conjunctiva and soft palate. Sometimes fat can be seen in retinal vessels. Fever and tachycardia are common.

Laboratory data may reveal mild to severe thrombocytopenia and mild anemia. Elevations in serum lipase levels and lipiduria occur, but these can also be seen in trauma patients without FES.[61,65] An ECG may reveal ischemia or right-heart strain with cor pulmonale. The chest x-ray may be normal early in the course, but a pattern of pulmonary edema is usually seen if respiratory failure develops. Arterial blood gas measurements are essential for documenting progression of respiratory impairment.

The patient with confusion, respiratory distress, and petechiae poses little diagnostic problem. However, FES can also present with isolated neurologic or pulmonary findings easily confused with other conditions. Disoriented trauma patients may have suffered cerebral injury that may not be evident for hours or days. Elderly patients receiving analgesics may become easily confused if metabolic derangements like hypoxia develop. Respiratory failure has multiple causes, including lung contusion, pneumonia, congestive heart failure, and pulmonary embolism.

Treatment and Prevention

The treatment of FES is supportive. Respiratory failure should be treated with supplemental oxygen and artificial ventilation if necessary. If oxygen concentrations over 50% are required, positive end-expiratory pressure may improve the alveolar-arterial oxygen gradient and reduce the oxygen requirement. Measurement of pulmonary capillary wedge pressure can be used to assess intravascular volume. The patient should be rigorously monitored for nosocomial infection and barotrauma.

A number of drugs have been used to treat fat embolism. The role of corticosteroids in FES is controversial. Many investigators believe that massive doses of corticosteroids (e.g., methylprednisolone in a dose of 10 to 15 mg/kg per day intravenously for four to five days) are beneficial in FES.[61,65-67] Theoretically, corticosteroids should be effective because they reduce inflammation, stabilize lysosomes, reverse bronchospasm, and decrease cerebral edema. However, these benefits have not been demonstrated in controlled studies. Heparin and intravenous alcohol are not effective. Diuretics are used in the treatment of respiratory failure to lower left atrial pressure and minimize fluid leak into the lungs, but their use should be guided by measurements of pulmonary capillary wedge pressure.

Beside early immobilization of fractures, there are no known measures to prevent FES. Prophylactic administration of corticosteroids to high-risk patients may reduce clinical severity,[68] but it is uncertain if early intervention affects outcome. FES can develop in patients undergoing total hip replacement. Forceful insertion of the femoral component of the prosthesis can traumatize the medulla and release marrow fat. This can be minimized by venting the femoral intramedullary canal during the procedure.

AIR EMBOLISM

The introduction of air into the circulation can occur in the intensive care unit or the operating room. Air usually enters through a venous access site like a central catheter or a wound above the level of the heart like those produced in neurosurgical procedures. Prompt recognition and treatment of air embolism is essential to avoid permanent neurologic sequelae and death.

Intravenous instrumentation and injection are common events in hospitalized patients. Small clinically insignificant volumes of air are often introduced into the venous circulation. Routine procedures such as injection of radiographic contrast or insertion of pacemaker wires can result in clinically silent air embolism.[69,70] Even intraarterial injection can result in retrograde embolization to the cerebral circulation.[71]

The hemodynamic results of air embolism are due to the introduction of a large volume of air into the right side of the circulation. The air bolus becomes trapped in the pulmonary outflow tract and produces acute right-heart failure.[72,73] Volumes of at least 100 ml or injection rates of 70 to 150 ml per second are lethal. Volume and rate depend on the diameter and length of the venous access instrument. For example, a 14-gauge needle can transmit 100 ml of air per second. Smaller gauge needles or long catheters require much longer periods of time to transmit the same volume of air.

Small volumes of air introduced directly into the arterial circulation can produce serious consequences. Air injected into the venous circulation may cross into the arterial system in two ways.[72-74] It may traverse a patent foramen ovale, particularly when it has been opened by acute right-heart failure, or pass directly through the pulmonary microcirculation and aggregate in the pulmonary veins to form larger emboli. In the latter case, such

volumes of air may be too small to cause hemodynamic compromise to the right side of the heart.

Clinical Features

Sudden hemodynamic collapse or new neurologic signs or symptoms are the most common manifestations of air embolism. However, the differential diagnosis is broad in the surgical setting. Complaints of chest pain, dyspnea, or cough during intravenous instrumentation, particularly with central venous line insertion, are suggestive of air embolism. Although sudden hypotension could be due to tension pneumothorax, arrhythmia, or bleeding, the presence of a loud churning or "mill wheel" murmur may be a clue to air trapped in the pulmonary outflow tract.[72,73] Aspirating a pulmonary artery catheter already in place may reveal air. In patients with massive air embolism, noncardiac pulmonary edema may develop for unclear reasons.

Neurologic manifestations of air embolism may take minutes to hours to develop. While focal signs and symptoms are most common, patients may also develop nonfocal findings such as confusion, stupor, and coma.

Treatment and Prevention

Treatment of air embolism must be initiated rapidly and based largely on clinical suspicion. Cardiovascular collapse can be avoided by preventing the air bolus from reaching the pulmonary outflow tract.[72,73] This can be accomplished by keeping the right heart in a superior position by placing the patient on the left side in Trendelenberg position, a maneuver that also prevents any arterial air from entering the cerebral circulation. In desperate circumstances, aspiration of air through a central catheter or transthoracic puncture of the right heart has been advocated. Cardiopulmonary bypass may be used if other resuscitative efforts are unsuccessful.

The next step is to reduce the volume of air in the circulation and minimize blockade of the venous or arterial circulation.[73,74] Administration of 100% oxygen saturates the air bubbles with oxygen and makes them more amenable to reabsorption. If available, the use of hyperbaric oxygen should be considered, particularly if the patient has neurologic deficits.[74]

Prevention of air embolism should focus mainly on techniques of central venous line insertion.[72] The head should be down so that central venous pressure is positive. Uncooperative patients should be sedated to avoid trauma at the insertion site or sudden upright movement. When a large-bore needle is introduced, the hub should always be occluded except when the central catheter is being threaded. All catheters and central venous lines should be taped securely to avoid disconnection. Moisture or staining of the dressing should be investigated in case lines have become disconnected. Whenever central lines are removed, they should be compressed and dressed with occlusive dressing to prevent air from entering along the catheter track.

SUMMARY

1. Pulmonary embolism should be considered in any surgical patient with dyspnea, chest pain, or unexplained drop in blood pressure. Physical findings, except for signs of acute cor pulmonale or a pleural rub, are not helpful in diagnosis.

2. Conventional laboratory tests are usually of little help in the diagnosis of pulmonary embolism. Normal arterial blood gas measurements are unusual in pulmonary embolism, but abnormal values are nonspecific. Electrocardiographic changes of acute right-heart strain strongly suggest the diagnosis but are rare. Chest x-ray often reveals nonspecific findings of infiltrate, effusion, or atelectasis. Lung scanning provides probabilities of pulmonary embolism based on patterns of V/Q abnormalities. In experienced hands, a low- or high-probability scan has an accuracy of 85 percent. A normal perfusion scan with no defects excludes pulmonary embolism. The pulmonary angiogram is the most accurate but technically most complex study for diagnosis of pulmonary embolism and should be used if other laboratory tests are equivocal.

3. All patients with thromboembolic disease should be treated with anticoagulants unless there is substantial risk of serious bleeding. Heparin should be used for at least three days before initiating warfarin. Anticoagulant effect should be monitored to produce a PTT of 1.5 to 2 times or a whole-blood clotting time of two to three times the control values. Bleeding complications should be treated by discontinuing or reducing the dose of anticoagulant and correcting the underlying disorder. Oral anticoagulation can be started within several days and should continue for three months. The dose of warfarin should be adjusted to maintain the PT at 1.25 to 1.5 times the control value.

4. Blockade of the inferior vena cava may be indicated in patients with recurrent pulmonary emboli on therapeutic doses of heparin; those with substantial thromboembolic disease who have serious bleeding complications on anticoagulation; and those with massive emboli. The choice of technique for venous interruption depends on the condition of the patient and local experience with these techniques.

5. Thrombolytic therapy may be dangerous in surgical patients because of the risk of bleeding and should be reserved for desperately ill patients who have not responded to conventional treatment. Pulmonary embolectomy either by surgery or catheter suction may have a role in treating certain patients with massive pulmonary emboli.

6. The fat embolism syndrome should be considered in any patient with confusion, respiratory distress, and petechiae occurring within three days of trauma. Corticosteroids like methylprednisolone in doses of 10 to 15 mg/kg per day for five days may be beneficial. Heparin and intravenous alcohol should not be used.

7. Air embolism most often results from venous or arterial instrumentation and can have dramatic hemodynamic and neurologic consequences. Immediate therapy consists of cardiovascular stabilization and high doses of oxygen, including hyperbaric treatment if available. Meticulous technique in the insertion and care of central venous lines is necessary to prevent this complication.

REFERENCES

1. Rose SD: Prophylaxis of thromboembolic disease. *Med Clin N Am* 63:1205, 1979.

2. Flanc C, Kakkar VV, Clarke MB: The detection of venous thrombosis of the legs using 125I-labelled fibrinogen. *Br J Surg* 55:742, 1968.

3. Kakkar VV, Howe CT, Nicolaides AN et al: Deep vein thrombosis of the leg. Is there a high risk group? *Am J Surg* 120:527, 1970.

4. Gallus AS, Hirsh J, Tuttle RJ et al: Small subcutaneous doses of heparin in prevention of postoperative deep vein thrombosis. *N Engl J Med* 293:1296, 1975.

5. Gordon-Smith IC, LeQuesne LP, Grundy DJ et al: Controlled trial of two regimens of subcutaneous heparin in prevention of postoperative deep vein thrombosis. *Lancet* 1:1133, 1972.

6. Harris WH, Salzman LW, Athanasoulis C et al: Comparison of warfarin, low molecular weight dextran, aspirin and subcutaneous heparin in prevention of venous thromboembolism following total hip replacement. *Am J Bone Joint Surg* 56:1552, 1974.

7. Kumowski M, Vandendris M, Steinberger R et al: Prevention of postoperative deep vein thrombosis by low dose heparin in urological surgery. *Urol Res* 5:123, 1977.

8. Nicholaides AN, Field CS, Kakkar VV et al: Prostatectomy and deep vein thrombosis. *Br J Surg* 59:487, 1972.

9. Dalen JE, Alpert JS: Natural history of pulmonary embolism. *Prog Cardiovasc Dis* 517:259, 1979.

10. International Multi-center Trial: Prevention of fatal postoperative pulmonary embolism by low doses of heparin. *Lancet* 2:45, 1975.

11. Browse NC, Clemenson G, Croft DN: Fibrinogen detectable thrombosis in the legs and pulmonary embolism. *Br Med J* 1:603, 1974.

12. Carson JL, Kelley MA, Duff A et al: The clinical course of pulmonary embolism. *N Engl J Med* 326:1240–1245, 1992.

13. Colman RW, Rubin RN: Prophylaxis and treatment of thromboembolism based on pathophysiology of clotting mechanisms, in Fishman AP (ed): *Pulmonary Diseases and Disorders*. New York, McGraw-Hill, 1988, p 1049.

14. Adelstein DJ, Hiknes JD, Carter SG et al: Thromboembolic events in patients with malignant superior vena cava syndrome and the role of anticoagulation. *Cancer* 62:2258, 1988.

15. Wanscher B, Frifelt JJ, Smith-Silverstein C et al: Thrombosis caused by polyurethane double-lumen subclavian superior vena cava catheter and hemodialysis. *Crit Care Med* 16:624, 1988.

16. Heatley RV, Morgan A, Hughes LB et al: Preoperative or postoperative deep vein thrombosis? *Lancet* 1:437, 1976.

17. Kakkar VV: The 125I-labelled fibrinogen test and phlebography in the diagnosis of deep vein thrombosis. *Milbank Mem Fund Q* 50:206, 1972.

18. Mansfield AO: Altered fibrinolysis associated with surgery and venous thrombosis. *Br J Surg* 59:754, 1972.

19. Havig O: Deep vein thrombosis and pulmonary embolism. *Acta Chir Scand* 478(Suppl):1, 1977.

20. McIntyre KM, Sasahara AA: Hemodynamic and ventricular responses to pulmonary embolism. *Prog Cardiovasc Dis* 17:175, 1979.

21. Hull, RD, Raskob GE, Leclere JR et al: The diagnosis of clinically suspected venous thrombosis. *Clin Chest Med* 5:439, 1984.

22. Wheeler HB, Anderson FA Jr: Diagnostic approaches for deep vein thrombosis. *Chest* 89:4075, 1986.

23. Huisman MV, Buller HR, ten Cate JW et al: Serial impedance plethysmography for suspected deep venous thrombosis in outpatients. *N Engl J Med* 314:823, 1986.

24. Lensing WA, Prandoni P, Brandjes D et al: Detection of deep vein thrombosis by real-time B-mode ultrasonography. *N Engl J Med* 320:342, 1989.

25. White RH, McGahan JP, Daschback MM et al: Diagnosis of deep vein thrombosis using duplex ultrasound. *Ann Int Med* 111:297, 1989.

26. Agnelli G, Cosmi B, Ranucci V et al: Impedance plethysmography and asymptomatic deep-vein thrombosis. *Arch Intern Med* 151:2167, 2171, 1991.

27. Davidson BL, Elliott CG, Lensing AWA et al: Low accuracy of color doppler ultrasound in the detection of proximal leg vein thrombosis in asymptomatic high-risk patients. *Ann Int Med* 117:735, 1992.

28. Bell WR, Simon TL: The clinical features of submassive and massive pulmonary emboli. *Am J Med* 62:355, 1977.

29. Stein PD, Dalen J, McIntyre KM et al: The electrocardiogram in acute pulmonary embolism. *Prog Cardiovasc Dis* 17:247, 1975.

30. Wilson JE, Pierce AK, Johnson RL Jr et al: Hypoxemia in pulmonary embolism. A clinical study. *J Clin Invest* 50:481, 1971.

31. Bynum LJ, Wilson JE: Radiographic features of pleural effusions in pulmonary embolism. *Am Rev Respir Dis* 117:829, 1978.

32. The PIOPED Investigators: Value of the ventilation/perfusion scan in acute pulmonary embolism: Results of the prospective investigation of pulmonary embolism diagnosis (PIOPED). *JAMA* 263:2753, 1990.

33. Biello DR, Mattar AG, McKnight RC et al: Ventilation-perfusion studies in suspected pulmonary embolism. *Am J Roentgenol* 133:1033, 1979.

34. Stein PD, Athanasoulis C, Alavi A et al: Complications and validity of pulmonary angiography in acute pulmonary embolism. *Circulation* 85:462, 1992.

35. Hull RD, Raskob GE, Hirsh J: The diagnosis of clinically suspected pulmonary embolism: Practical approaches. *Chest* 89:417, 1986.

36. Hull RD, Hirsh J, Carter CJ et al: Pulmonary angiography, ventilation lung scanning and venography for clinically suspected pulmonary embolism with abnormal perfusion lung scan. *Ann Intern Med* 98:891, 1983.

37. Kelley MA, Carson JL, Palevsky HI et al: Diagnosing pulmonary embolism: New facts and strategies. *Ann Int Med* 114:300, 1991.

38. Barrit DW, Jordan SC: Anticoagulant drugs in the treatment of pulmonary embolism. A controlled trial. *Lancet* 1:1309, 1960.

39. Hyers TM, Hull RD, Weg JG: Antithrombotic therapy for venous thromboembolic disease. *Chest* 85:375, 1989.

40. Wheeler AP, Jaquiss RDB, Newman JH: Physician practices in the treatment of pulmonary embolism and deep venous thrombosis. *Arch Intern Med* 148:1321, 1988.

41. Hull RD, Raskob GE, Rosenbloom D et al: Optimal therapeutic level of heparin therapy in patients with venous thrombosis. *Arch Intern Med* 152:1589, 1992.

42. Doyle DJ, Turpie AGG, Hirsh J et al: Adjusted subcutaneous heparin or continuous intravenous heparin in patients with acute deep vein thrombosis. *Ann Int Med* 107:441, 1987.

43. Gallus A, Jackaman J, Tillett J et al: Safety and efficacy of warfarin started early after submassive venous thrombosis or pulmonary embolism. *Lancet* 2:1293, 1986.

44. Brandjes DPM, Heijboer H, Buller HR et al: Acenocoumarol and heparin compared with acenocoumarol alone in the initial treatment of proximal-vein thrombosis. *N Engl J Med* 327:1485, 1992.

45. Hirsh J, Poller L, Deykin D et al: Optimal therapeutic range for oral anticoagulants. *Chest* 95:55, 1989.

46. Petitti DB, Strom BL, Melmon KL: Duration of warfarin anticoagulant therapy and the probabilities of recurrent thromboembolism and hemorrhage. *Am J Med* 81:255, 1986.

47. Kinasewitz GT, George RB: Management of thromboembolism. Anticoagulants, thrombolytics, or surgical intervention? *Chest* 86:106, 1984.

48. Kanter B, Moser KM: The Greenfield vena cava filter: *Chest* 93:170, 1988.

49. Pulmonary Embolism Trial Study Group: Urokinase-streptokinase embolism trial and phase 2 results. A cooperative study. *JAMA* 229:1606, 1974.

50. Goldhaber SZ: Tissue plasminogen activator in acute pulmonary embolism. *Chest* 95:282S, 1989.

51. Sharma GVK, Burleson VA, Sasahara AA: Effect of thrombolytic therapy on pulmonary capillary blood volume in patients with pulmonary embolism. *N Engl J Med* 303:842, 1980.

52. Volgesang GB, Bell WR: Treatment of pulmonary embolism and deep vein thrombosis with thrombolytic therapy. *Clin Chest Med* 5:487, 1984.

53. Marder VJ, Sherry S: Thrombolytic therapy: Current status. *N Engl J Med* 318:1512, 1585, 1988.

54. Sharma GVRK, Cella G, Parisi AF et al: Thrombolytic therapy. *N Engl J Med* 306:1268, 1982.

55. Leeper KV, Popovich J, Lesser BA et al: Treatment of massive acute pulmonary embolism: The use of low doses of intrapulmonary arterial streptokinase combined with full doses of systemic heparin. *Chest* 93:234, 1988.

56. Alpert JS, Smith RE, Ockene IS et al: Treatment of massive pulmonary embolism: The role of pulmonary embolectomy. *Am Heart J* 89:413, 1975.

57. Miller GAH, Hall RJC, Paneth M: Pulmonary embolectomy, heparin, and streptokinase: Their place in the treatment of acute massive pulmonary embolism. *Am Heart J* 93:568, 1977.

58. Gray HH, Morgan JM, Paneth M et al: Pulmonary embolectomy for acute massive pulmonary embolism: An analysis of 71 cases. *Br Heart J* 60:196, 1988.

59. Meyer G, Tamisier D, Sors H et al: Pulmonary embolectomy: a 20-year experience at one center. *Ann Thorac Surg* 51:232, 1991.

60. Greenfield LJ: Vena caval interruption and pulmonary embolectomy. *Clin Chest Med* 5:494, 1984.

61. Oh WH, Mital MA: Fat embolism: Current concepts of pathogenesis, diagnosis and treatment. *Orthop Clin N Am* 9:769, 1978.

62. Shapiro MP, Hayes JA: Fat embolism in sickle cell disease. *Arch Intern Med* 144:181, 1984.

63. Laub DR Jr, Laub DR: Fat embolism syndrome after liposuction: A case report and review of the literature. *Ann Plast Surg* 25:48, 1990.

64. Dines DE, Burgher LW, Okazaki H: The clinical and pathologic correlation of fat embolism. *Arch Surg* 109:12, 1974.

65. Levy D: Fat embolism: A review. *Clin Orthop and Related Res* 261:281, 1990.

66. Fischer JE, Turner RH, Herndon HH et al: Massive steroid therapy in severe fat embolism. *Surg Gynecol Obstet* 132:493, 1966.

67. Ashbaugh DG, Petty TL: The use of corticosteroids in the treatment of respiratory failure associated with massive fat embolism. *Surg Gynecol Obstet* 123:493, 1966.

68. Schonfeld SA, Yongyudh P, DiLisio R et al: Fat embolism prophylaxis with corticosteroids: A prospective study in high-risk patients. *Ann Int Med* 99:438, 1983.

69. Woodring John H, Fried AM: Nonfatal venous air embolism after contrast-enhanced CT. *Radiology* 167:405, 1988.

70. Gottdiener JS, Papademetriou V, Notargiacomo A et al: Incidence and cardiac effects of systemic venous air embolism: Echocardiographic evidence of arterial embolization via noncardiac shunt. *Arch Intern Med* 148:795, 1988.

71. Chang C, Dughi J, Shitabata P et al: Air embolism and the radial arterial line. *Crit Care Med* 16:141, 1988.

72. Kashuck JL, Penn I: Air embolism after central venous catheterization. *Surg Obstet Gyn* 159:249, 1984.

73. O'Quin RJ, Lakshminarayan S: Venous air embolism. *Arch Intern Med* 142:2173, 1982.

74. Murphy BP, Harford FJ, Cramer FS: Cerebral air embolism resulting from invasive medical procedures. *Ann Surg* 201:242, 1985.

60 DISORDERS OF VOLUME AND TONICITY IN THE SURGICAL PATIENT

Harold Szerlip

Paul M. Palevsky

Malcolm Cox

Several homeostatic mechanisms are involved in maintaining optimal perfusion of vital organs and ensuring the stability of body fluid tonicity. In normal individuals, these physiologic control systems enable regulation of extracellular fluid volume and body fluid tonicity within narrow ranges despite wide variations in sodium and water intake. Surgical patients commonly develop problems with volume and tonicity after surgery, and even otherwise healthy patients may retain sodium and water during the postoperative period. In those with underlying systemic diseases, the ability to maintain normal extracellular fluid volume and body fluid tonicity may be even more significantly impaired. Although the regulation of extracellular fluid volume and body fluid tonicity are interrelated, this chapter considers each separately and offers an ordered approach to diagnosis and management.

DISORDERS OF VOLUME HOMEOSTASIS

Adequate tissue perfusion depends on maintaining the "fullness" of the arterial circulation, or the "effective arterial blood volume" (EABV). EABV depends not only on actual arterial blood volume but also on cardiac output and vascular capacitance. Intricate homeostatic controls monitor EABV and regulate intravascular fluid volume, cardiac output, and vascular capacitance in an integrated fashion. Although all of these variables are important in determining EABV, regulation of intravascular fluid volume is most important to this discussion. However, the neurohumoral mechanisms active in volume regulation have marked effects on the cardiovascular system, and volume regulation should not be viewed as a separate phenomenon.

Normal Response to Surgery

Regardless of the nature of the surgery or the type of anesthesia used, most patients retain sodium in the postoperative period.[1-10] Although all of the factors responsible for sodium retention have not been well delineated, they include decreases in absolute or effective arterial blood volume and activation of one or more of the different effector systems involved in sodium homeostasis by stimuli that are not directly related to alterations in volume.[7-10]

Many studies have documented decreased intravascular fluid (IVF) volume following surgery.[1,2,4-6] The decrement is usually greater than that attributable to blood loss alone and is probably due to sequestration of fluid in traumatized tissue where it is no longer in equilibrium with the extracellular fluid (ECF) compartment. This phenomenon is known as "third-space" sequestration.[1,2,11]

The stress of surgery is also known to increase the release of antinatriuretic hormones.[7-10] Circulating catecholamine and aldosterone levels are elevated in the immediate postoperative period and may play a role in sodium retention. Hyperaldosteronism is due to stimulation of the renin-angiotensin system by decreased intravascular volume and a stress-related increase in adrenocorticotrophic hormone (ACTH) secretion.[7-9] However, since the ACTH-mediated increase in aldosterone secretion is short-lived, volume depletion is probably the dominant influence on aldosterone secretion in surgical patients.

Because of their tendency to retain sodium, postoperative patients frequently become sodium overloaded, and those with underlying heart disease easily develop congestive heart failure. Redistribution of sodium from "third spaces" into the vascular space results in a brisk diuresis if cardiac and renal function are normal, but signs and symptoms of intravascular volume overload can develop if this is not the case.

Approach to the Patient

Disorders of volume homeostasis are best classified on the basis of changes in IVF rather than ECF volume. The distinction between intravascular volume depletion or expansion is usually made easily by history and physical examination. Intravascular volume depletion is characterized by tachycardia, hypotension, and enhanced reabsorption of sodium and water by the kidney. Chronic intravascular volume depletion is generally well tolerated, and blood pressure, cardiac output, and pulse remain near normal despite losses of up to 25 percent of total body sodium.[12,13] More rapid losses are much less well tolerated. Acute decreases in ECF or IVF volume of only 5 to 10 percent are associated with resting tachycardia. As losses approach 15 percent, orthostatic hypotension develops. At 20 percent, cardiac output declines, and supine hypotension is common. At 25 percent, tissue perfusion becomes compromised and vascular collapse supervenes.[14] Dry axillae and mucous membranes and decreased skin turgor are less reliable signs of volume depletion. Patients may also complain of thirst and crave salt.[15,16]

Volume depletion is associated with oliguria (urine volume < 20 ml/hr), sodium retention (urine sodium concentration < 10 meq/liter), and water retention (urine osmolality > 700 mOsm/kg). The serum uric acid level may also be elevated, and prerenal azotemia is common.[17] Because the serum sodium concentration reflects water balance and not volume status, it can be high, low, or normal.

The hallmark of intravascular volume expansion is pulmonary vascular congestion manifested by dyspnea. Although intravascular volume expansion is always associated with expansion of the entire ECF compartment, pulmonary function can become compromised well before sufficient sodium has accumulated to cause peripheral edema. Increases in total body sodium reflect either a primary or secondary decrease in renal sodium excretion. Regardless of the underlying cause of renal sodium retention, volume-overloaded patients are often oliguric with a low urine sodium concentration and a high urine osmolality. Hyperuricemia and prerenal azotemia may also be present. As in the case of volume depletion, because the serum sodium concentration reflects water balance and not volume status, it can be high, low, or normal.

Volume Depletion

The presence of hypotension, the principal clinical sign of significant intravascular volume depletion, in a patient without edema or ascites generally indicates the coexistence of IVF and ECF volume depletion. This may result from relatively selective contraction of the intravascular compartment as seen in hemorrhage, from third-space sequestration of fluid, or from a proportional contraction of both the intravascular and interstitial fluid compartment as seen in sodium depletion (see Table 60–1). On the other hand, the presence of peripheral edema, the principal clinical sign of ECF volume expansion, in a patient with hypotension usually indicates the coexistence of IVF volume depletion and ECF volume expansion. This occurs in patients with capillary leak syndrome but not, as was once thought, in those with hypoalbuminemia.

Although albumin is the major contributor to plasma colloid osmotic (oncotic) pressure,[37] and hypoalbuminemia is associated with a shift of fluid from the intravascular to the interstitial fluid compartment, the resulting decrement in intravascular volume is generally not sustained.[38] Countermanding influences include a rise in interstitial fluid hydrostatic pressure, a fall in intravascular hydrostatic pressure, accelerated return of fluid to the intravascular space by the lymphatic system, and renal sodium and water retention. Thus, children with congenital analbuminemia do not have edema,[39] intravascular volume does not change when plasma oncotic pressure is acutely lowered by plasmaphereis,[38,40] and intravascular volume in patients with hepatic cirrhosis and nephrotic syndrome is increased rather than decreased.[41–45]

TABLE 60–1. Disorders of Volume Homeostasis

Causes of IVF Volume Depletion with Decreased ECF Volume
- Hemorrhage
- Third-space sequestration[11,17–20]
- Sodium depletion
  Cutaneous losses[17,18]
    sensible perspiration[29]
    burns
    open wounds
    toxic epidermal necrolysis
  Renal losses[21]
    diuretics[22]
    osmotic diuresis[23]
      diabetes mellitus
      mannitol
    chronic renal failure[24,25]
    medullary cystic disease[26]
    diuretic phase of ATN[27]
    postobstructive diuresis[28]
    primary adrenal insufficiency
  Gastrointestinal losses (see Table 60–2)[30]
    vomiting[31,32]
    nasogastric suction
    bile or pancreatic drainage
    diarrhea[33]

Causes of IVF Volume Depletion with Increased ECF Volume
- Capillary leak syndrome
  Snake bites[106]
  Interleukin-2 therapy[34]
  Lung reexpansion in treatment of pleural effusion or pneumothorax[35,36]
  Bacterial toxins (e.g., sepsis)

Causes of IVF Volume Expansion with Increased ECF Volume
- Isotonic saline infusion
- Renal failure
  Advanced chronic
  Acute oliguric
- Congestive heart failure[48–51]
- Hepatic cirrhosis[41,42,50]
- Nephrotic syndrome[41–45,52]

Therapy of Volume Depletion

The primary goal in treating volume depletion is to restore blood pressure and tissue perfusion by administering intravenous fluids.[46,47] The quantity and composition of the replacement fluid should be guided by the patient's hemodynamic status and the underlying cause of the volume depletion. When it is the result of hemorrhage, the ideal replacement fluid is blood. If blood is not immediately available, therapy should be initiated with either a colloid in the form of albumin, plasmanate, or hydroxyethylstarch, or isotonic crystalloid as 0.9% saline or Ringer's lactate.[47] Colloid remains exclusively within the intravascular space, while isotonic crystalloid solutions are distributed throughout the ECF compartment with only one-fourth of the volume remaining within the intravascular space. Five percent dextrose in water is not a useful intravascular volume expander because only one-twelfth of its volume remains within the intravascular space. Moreover, it may cause significant hyponatremia in volume-depleted patients.

Volume depletion from external loss or sequestration of sodium-rich fluid within the body (third-spacing) should be treated by replacing these losses in kind. Therapy is guided by the magnitude and nature of the accumulated deficit, the magnitude and composition of ongoing losses, the presence of any associated

TABLE 60–2. Gastrointestinal Secretions: Normal Volume and Composition

	Volume (liters/day)	Concentration (meq/liter)			
		$Na+$	$K+$	$Cl-$	HCO_3-
Saliva	~ 1	20–80	10–20	20–40	20–160
Gastric juice	1–2	20–100	5–10	120–160	—
Bile	~ 1	150–250	5–10	40–60	20–60
Pancreatic juice	1–2	120	5–10	10–60	80–120
Succus entericus	1–2	140	5	Variable	Variable

Source: After Phillips SF, in Maxwell MH, Kleeman CR (eds): *Clinical Disorders of Fluid and Electrolyte Metabolism*, 3d ed. New York, McGraw-Hill, 1980.

disturbances in acid-base and potassium homeostasis, and the availability of therapy for the underlying disorder.

The magnitude of the initial sodium deficit is often difficult to estimate clinically. Hypotension due to sodium depletion usually indicates a loss of more than 15 percent of the ECF volume or more than two liters of isotonic saline in a 70 kg patient. However, regardless of such estimates, enough fluid should be given to stabilize the blood pressure. When hypotension is severe, colloid solutions should be used initially, and isotonic crystalloid can be used to correct the sodium deficit thereafter. Continued infusion of colloid once blood pressure has normalized is unnecessary and may lead to rapid intravascular volume expansion and pulmonary edema, especially in patients with underlying heart disease. If the patient is more stable, isotonic crystalloid can be used from the outset.

Whenever possible, the replacement solution should reflect the composition of the fluid lost. In most circumstances, 0.9% NaCl is the isotonic crystalloid solution of choice. Although rapid infusion of isotonic saline may produce dilutional metabolic acidosis, it is usually insignificant unless the patient is already acidemic. In patients with shock and associated lactic acidosis, half-isotonic saline (0.45% NaCl) can be made approximately isotonic by the addition of one to two ampules of sodium bicarbonate, each containing 50 meq of sodium.

Ringer's lactate is a widely used alternative but has several disadvantages. Organic anions like lactate are normally rapidly converted to bicarbonate by the liver, but this conversion may be compromised by decreased hepatic perfusion in patients with severe hypotension. Therefore, in situations complicated by acidemia, it is advisable to use bicarbonate-containing solutions. In addition, Ringer's lactate contains small amounts of potassium and calcium, which the patient may not require. It is always preferable to tailor fluid replacement therapy to the specific situation.

Once existing deficits have been repleted, ongoing losses should be addressed, and attempts should be made to eliminate or reduce them. If this is not possible, ongoing fluid replacement is best accomplished by determining the volume and electrolyte composition of the fluid being lost. This is particularly important in seriously ill patients, patients expected to experience long-term ongoing losses, and patients with compromised renal function.

The adequacy of fluid replacement must be monitored by physical examination to keep the blood pressure and pulse normal and avoid volume overload. Frequent blood pressure determinations, chest auscultation, and examination of the jugular venous pulse are mandatory. In seriously ill patients, continuous monitoring of the blood pressure, central venous pressure, and pulmonary capillary wedge pressure may be indicated. In the absence of renal disease, a urine sodium concentration over 20 meq/liter is considered a good marker of adequate intravascular volume.

The therapy of intravascular volume depletion in patients with increased ECF volume is problematic. Patients suffering from the diffuse capillary leak syndrome quickly lose both colloid and crystalloid across the capillary endothelium. Because further accumulation of colloid in the interstitial space favors movement of fluid from the intravascular space, colloid-containing solutions are not recommended as ongoing replacement therapy. Treatment is best aimed at the underlying disorder. Blood pressure support should include the infusion of packed red blood cells and crystalloid and the judicious use of pressor agents.

Volume Expansion

Volume-expanded patients are characterized by pulmonary vascular congestion, the principal sign of intravascular volume expansion, as well as peripheral edema and/or ascites, the hallmarks of ECF volume overload. Volume expansion may be associated with proportional increases in the intravascular and interstitial fluid compartments, as in renal failure, or with maldistribution of fluid between the two compartments, as in congestive heart failure, hepatic cirrhosis, and nephrotic syndrome (see Table 60–1).

Therapy of Volume Expansion

The treatment of volume expansion is aimed at removing excess sodium and water from the ECF space without compromising hemodynamic status. This can be accomplished with diuretics or, if necessary, by ultrafiltration or hemofiltration. Edema alone is not an indication for treatment. It is more important to determine intravascular volume status, whether pulmonary vascular congestion is present, and whether edema is adversely affecting vital functions like respiration, cutaneous integrity, or wound healing.

Diuretics

Diuretics inhibit renal tubular sodium reabsorption. The magnitude of the resulting natriuresis depends on adequate delivery of the drug to its site of action, the amount of sodium normally reabsorbed at that site, and the overall adaptive response of the kidney to diuretic-induced intravascular volume depletion. All diuretics, with the exception of the aldosterone antagonist spironolactone, act from the luminal side of the tubular epithelium and are therefore dependent on glomerular filtration for their delivery.[53]

By reducing pulmonary congestion, diuretics improve oxygenation and myocardial function in congestive heart failure. Because they do not enhance cardiac contractility and may reduce cardiac output by decreasing venous return or preload, they are best used in conjunction with agents that have direct inotropic effects, like digoxin, or with agents that improve myocardial function by reducing afterload, like angiotensin-converting enzyme inhibitors.

Since mild diuretics may be ineffective, those acting in the loop of Henle such as furosemide, ethacrynic acid, and bumetanide are more commonly used in treating congestive heart failure. However, whenever possible, treatment should be initiated with a less potent agent like a thiazide diuretic. Both thiazide and loop diuretics produce significant potassium and magnesium depletion, and blood chemistries should be carefully monitored during therapy.

The initial therapy of patients with hepatic cirrhosis should be dietary sodium restriction and bed rest. Significant edema can often be mobilized over a period of days to weeks with this approach. Diuretics should be used with caution since natriuresis often leads to intravascular volume depletion and decreased tissue perfusion, especially in patients with ascites who are not edematous. Unlike peripheral edema, ascitic fluid is not in rapid equilibrium with intravascular fluid and cannot be rapidly mobilized. The maximal rate at which ascites can be reduced is about one liter per day.[54] Consequently, diuretic-induced weight loss of about 0.5 to 1.0 kg/day is more than adequate in nonedematous cirrhotic patients. When edema is present, about twice this amount can be safely removed. Slow diuresis allows time for reequilibration among the intravascular, interstitial, and peritoneal spaces.

Although intravascular volume may be increased in patients with decompensated cirrhosis, an increase in circulatory capacitance always leads to a decrease in effective arterial blood volume.[42] Consequently, aggressive diuresis reduces renal blood flow further and worsens prerenal azotemia. In contrast, recent evidence suggests that paracentesis of large volumes of ascites can be performed without compromising intravascular volume and may even improve cardiac output.[55,56] However, patients should be carefully observed after paracentesis. Diagnostic small-volume paracentesis can be safely done at any time.

Spironolactone is the initial diuretic of choice in patients with cirrhosis. This otherwise mild agent often promotes a greater natriuresis than loop diuretics in cirrhotic patients.[57] In addition, it does not produce hypokalemia, which can precipitate hepatic encephalopathy.[58] However, it does inhibit hydrogen ion secretion and may produce hyperchloremic metabolic acidosis in some patients. Acid-base status should be monitored whenever spironolactone is used. In patients unresponsive to conventional therapy, peritoneal-venous shunts have sometimes proven helpful in controlling ascites.

The treatment of choice for volume-overloaded patients with nephrotic syndrome is dietary sodium restriction, and diuretics can be judiciously added if needed. Thiazides are rarely effective, and loop diuretics are usually chosen. Because of associated hypoalbuminemia, overly aggressive diuresis can result in intravascular volume depletion, hypotension, and worsening prerenal azotemia. It is advisable to restrict diuretic therapy to patients in whom marked peripheral edema inhibits normal activities or interferes with cutaneous integrity or wound healing. Intermittent administration of diuretics is often best, allowing time for reequilibration of the intravascular and interstitial fluid compartments.

In patients with edema due to renal insufficiency, therapy depends on the glomerular filtration rate. When the glomerular filtration rate is only mildly decreased, restriction of sodium intake is often adequate. As renal insufficiency progresses, diuretics can be added to the regimen. In the severely oliguric or anuric patient, dialysis may be necessary. The indiscriminate use of potent diuretics in patients with renal insufficiency should be avoided to prevent intravascular volume depletion, hypotension, and prerenal azotemia. Potent diuretics may also produce a variety of electrolyte and acid-base disturbances that complicate any preexisting derangements related to the renal insufficiency itself.

Although many edematous patients can be controlled using only a single diuretic, some develop resistance that may be due to increased sodium intake, a further decline in glomerular filtration rate, or progression of the underlying renal disease. As the glomerular filtration rate decreases, less diuretic reaches its site of action. Progression of the renal disease may result in increased sodium avidity at uninhibited sites of reabsorption. Diuretic resistance can be managed by increasing the dose of the diuretic, switching to a more potent diuretic, or using a combination of diuretics that act at different sites along the nephron. Since all of these approaches can result in serious volume depletion and electrolyte disturbances, frequent monitoring of the urinary output, weight, and serum electrolyte levels is mandatory.

Ultrafiltration and Hemofiltration

Severely volume-overloaded patients refractory to diuretic therapy often benefit from fluid removal by ultrafiltration or hemofiltration. Ultrafiltration is similar to hemodialysis except that dialysate does not have to be used. Access to the venous circulation is obtained by means of a large-bore catheter placed in a central vein and connected to a hemodialysis machine. Negative pressure is applied to the outside of the membrane, resulting in ultrafiltration of plasma. Ultrafiltration can be used alone, at any time before or after hemodialysis, or at the same time as hemodialysis. Depending on the pressure gradient applied across the membrane and the ultrafiltration coefficient of the membrane, large volumes of fluid can be removed. However, ultrafiltration requires a hemodialysis machine and careful monitoring and can only be used for several hours at a time. In addition, it cannot always be performed in hemodynamically unstable patients who may develop hypotension and shock.

More recently, continuous renal replacement therapies, including continuous arteriovenous hemofiltration (CAVH) and continuous venovenous hemofiltration (CVVH), have been used in patients with multiorgan failure who require daily removal of large quantities of fluids,[59,60] and are gaining acceptance in the treatment of those who are critically ill. These continuous renal replacement therapies are well tolerated by hemodynamically unstable patients and can be continued for several days. Cardiac index remains unchanged or increases, even in patients with poor myocardial function.[61] Patients undergoing these continuous extracorporeal therapies should be monitored in an intensive care unit to avoid excessive fluid removal.

DISORDERS OF TONICITY HOMEOSTASIS

Total body water (TBW) is distributed between the extracellular fluid (ECF) and intracellular fluid (ICF) compartments. While ECF volume is determined by sodium balance, ICF volume is determined by body fluid tonicity. Hypotonicity leads to expansion, and hypertonicity to contraction, of the ICF compartment.

Body fluid tonicity is precisely regulated. Although plasma osmolality may range from 280 to 295 mOsm/kg in normal humans, it does not vary over time by more than one to two percent in a given individual. Precise defense of body fluid tonicity depends on changes in total body water achieved by appropriate adjustments in water balance. Two interrelated physiologic feedback systems regulate water balance and thereby body fluid tonicity: (1) thirst and variable water ingestion; and (2) antidiuretic hormone (ADH) and variable renal water excretion (see Fig. 60–1). Disorders of tonicity homeostasis are always caused by derangements in one or both of these regulatory systems.[62–77]

Normal Response to Surgery

Most patients retain water in the postoperative period regardless of the nature of the surgery or the type of anesthesia used. Some of the factors responsible for postoperative water retention include decreases in absolute or effective arterial blood volume resulting in decreased delivery of fluid to the renal diluting sites and volume-related ADH release; relative or absolute hypotension resulting in decreased delivery and baroreceptor-mediated ADH release; positive-pressure ventilation causing decreased central blood volume; and narcotics, general anesthetics, nausea, pain, and stress, all of which directly or indirectly affect ADH release.

The relative importance of these factors in limiting electrolyte-free water excretion during and after surgery is unknown. Circumstantial evidence suggests that increased ADH release plays a major role. When patients are volume-expanded postoperatively, their urine often remains concentrated as body fluid tonicity falls. Antidiuresis thus persists despite correction of hypovolemia. In addition, postoperative patients with no evidence of intravascular volume depletion commonly become severely hypotonic if water is administered indiscriminately. It is therefore mandatory to closely monitor fluid intake and output and the serum sodium concentration following all but trivial surgical procedures. Routine prescription of hypotonic fluids in the postoperative period should be avoided.

Approach to the Patient

Because body fluids are in osmotic equilibrium, plasma osmolality reflects the osmolality of all body fluids. Osmolality can be measured directly using an osmometer or calculated as follows when [Glucose] and [BUN] are reported in mg/dl: 2 [Na] + [Glucose]/18 + [BUN]/2.8.

In calculating plasma tonicity, the urea term is excluded because urea is freely permeable across cell membranes. In the absence of azotemia, the calculated osmolality and tonicity differ by less than 10 mOsm/kg. However, in azotemic patients, body fluid osmolality may be higher than body fluid tonicity. Ethanol and methanol likewise contribute to osmolality but not to tonicity, because they readily traverse cell membranes and distribute throughout total body water. In contrast, mannitol, sorbitol, and glycerol are relatively restricted to the ECF compartment and contribute to both osmolality and tonicity.

The symptoms of hypo- and hypertonicity are nonspecific, and disturbances of tonicity homeostasis are usually detected by alterations in the serum sodium concentration. However, there is not always a direct correlation between the serum sodium concentration and body fluid tonicity. Since symptoms relate to abnormal tonicity and not to abnormalities in the serum sodium concentration per se, it is important to realize that hyponatremia may be associated not only with hypotonicity (hypotonic hyponatremia), but also with isotonicity (isotonic hyponatremia) and hypertonicity (hypertonic hyponatremia). In contrast, hypernatremia always implies concomitant hypertonicity.

Isotonic hyponatremia or "pseudohyponatremia" is a laboratory artifact that has largely been eliminated by changing analytical techniques.[78] Marked hyperlipidemia and hyperproteinemia distort the normal relationship between plasma volume and plasma water content, but have negligible effects on osmolality. Analytical techniques that utilize diluted specimens or flame photometry therefore underestimate the true sodium concentration in the aqueous phase of plasma. Pseudohyponatremia should be suspected in asymptomatic patients with severe hyponatremia, especially if the serum is grossly lipemic or viscous. Diagnosis can be confirmed by measuring plasma osmolality, which will be normal. Newer techniques utilizing ion-specific electrodes and undiluted specimens avoid this artifact.[78]

Hypertonic hyponatremia occurs when the ECF contains increased concentrations of a nonelectrolyte solute like glucose. Water shifts from the ICF to the ECF to maintain osmotic equilibrium between the two body-fluid compartments. The result is ICF volume contraction, ECF volume expansion, dilution of ECF sodium concentration (hyponatremia), and hypertonicity due to the prevailing hyperglycemia.

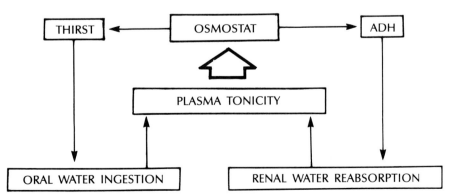

FIGURE 60–1.   Homeostatic control of body fluid tonicity.
Source: From Geheb M, Singer I, Cox M: in McDonald FD (ed): *Progress in Clinical Kidney Disease and Hypertension.* New York, Thieme-Stratton, 1980.

Hypotonicity

Hyponatremia, defined as a serum sodium concentration below 135 meq/liter, occurs frequently in hospitalized patients. The incidence and prevalence are about one percent and 2.5 percent, respectively, in patients on general medical and surgical wards.[79] In postoperative patients, the incidence is 4.4 percent, and most have hypotonic hyponatremia.[80] Hypotonicity is associated with significant morbidity and mortality. Patients with hyponatremia have a seven- to sixtyfold increase in mortality,[79-81] most of which reflects progression of underlying disease processes.[73,79-81] However, severe hyponatremia itself can be life-threatening.[82]

Hypotonic hyponatremia always reflects inability of the kidney to excrete sufficient electrolyte-free water to match water intake. The normal response to ingestion of enough water to produce hypotonicity is excretion of maximally dilute urine with an osmolality (Uosm) below 100 mOsm/kg. The finding of such a dilute urine in a patient with hypotonic hyponatremia implicates excessive water intake as the cause of the hypotonicity. In contrast, the finding of a less than maximally dilute urine in the face of hypotonicity signifies impaired renal electrolyte-free water excretion. In most patients excessive water intake and impaired renal water excretion occur concurrently. In the surgical setting, administration of hypotonic intravenous fluids is a prominent cause of hypotonicity,[80] and impairment of renal diluting ability resulting from the nonosmotic release of ADH has been demonstrated in most hypotonic surgical patients.[79]

Hypotonicity can arise from an isolated increase in total body water (TBW); a greater relative deficit in total body effective solute (TBES) than in TBW; and a greater relative increase in TBW than in TBES. In constructing a differential diagnosis, it is helpful to relate the different causes of hypotonic hyponatremia to ECF volume status. Hypotonic hyponatremia can be associated with normal, decreased, or increased ECF volume (total body sodium) (see Table 60–3).

Euvolemic Hypotonicity

Euvolemic hypotonicity results from an increase in total body water with only minimal, if any, change in body sodium content. Euvolemic hypotonicity can be attributed to excessive water intake, impaired electrolyte-free water excretion, or a combination of both. Hyponatremia due solely to excessive water intake is uncommon in view of the ability of the normal kidney to excrete 15 to 20 liters of electrolyte-free water daily. The diagnosis of primary (psychogenic) polydipsia should be suspected whenever hyponatremia, polyuria, and maximally dilute urine coexist. Such patients require psychiatric evaluation. Hypotonicity resolves once water intake returns to more reasonable levels.

Acute water intoxication may occur after urologic surgery. Vigorous bladder irrigation using hypotonic glycine-containing fluids is frequently done during transurethral prostate surgery. Absorption of this fluid can produce severe hyponatremia and alterations in mental status in the so-called "post-TURP syndrome."[83] Although hyponatremia resolves with water restriction, hypertonic saline infusions may be required in severely symptomatic patients.

More commonly euvolemic hypotonicity is due to impaired renal electrolyte-free water excretion resulting from the nonosmotic release of ADH and is often exacerbated by excessive water intake. A variety of disorders have been associated with the syndrome of inappropriate ADH (SIADH), including CNS disorders (trauma, tumor, meningitis, subarachnoid hemorrhage), pulmonary diseases (tuberculosis, pneumonia, asthma, bronchiectasis, hypoxia, hypercarbia), positive-pressure ventilation, intestinal traction, nausea, malignancies, and stress. In addition, a large number of medications including general anesthetics, narcotics, phenothiazines, tricyclic antidepressants, thiazides, chlorpropamide, vinca alkaloids, and cytoxan have been associated with SIADH. In the immediate postoperative period, circulating ADH levels are elevated and may remain high for three to five days.[80]

The diagnosis of SIADH rests on several criteria. First, abso-

TABLE 60–3. Hypotonic States

TBES	TBW	$\frac{\text{TBES}}{\text{TBW}}$	ECF Volume	EABV	Pathophysiology		Conditions
↔	↑	↓	↔	↔	↑ H₂O intake		Psychogenic polydipsia
					↓ Renal diluting ability		Syndrome of inappropriate ADH Reset osmostat Glucocorticoid insufficiency Hypothyroidism
↓↓	↓	↓	↓	↓	Hypotonic fluid loss, continued H₂O intake, ↓ renal diluting ability	Renal	Diuretics Osmotic diuresis Adrenal insufficiency Postobstructive diuresis Diuretic phase ATN
						Extrarenal	GI losses: diarrhea, vomiting, NG drainage Cutaneous losses: sensible perspiration, burns Third-space sequestration: peritonitis, ileus, etc.
↑	↑↑	↓	↑	↓	Renal Na+ and H₂O retention, continued H₂O intake, ↓ renal diluting ability		Renal insufficiency Congestive heart failure Hepatic cirrhosis Nephrotic syndrome

TBES = total body osmotically effective solute; TBW = total body water; ECF = extracellular fluid; EABV = effective arterial blood volume; ATN = acute tubular necrosis; GI = gastrointestinal; NG = nasogastric; ↔ = normal; ↓ = decreased; ↑ = increased.

lute or effective hypovolemia are potent stimuli to ADH release and must be excluded before SIADH is invoked. However, they are often difficult to recognize in patients who are acutely ill or have just returned from surgery. In patients who are not sodium-restricted and have normal renal function, hypovolemia can be excluded if the urine sodium concentration is over 20 meq/liter. Second, the urine must be inappropriately concentrated. When plasma osmolality is below 280 mOsm/kg, a urine osmolality above 100 mOsm/kg is inappropriate. Third, renal, cardiac, hepatic, adrenal, and thyroid function must be normal. Cardiac and hepatic disease can cause volume-mediated alterations in ADH secretion and renal water handling. Cortisol deficiency is associated with release of ADH despite hypotonicity[74,75] and may also increase the water permeability of the collecting duct.[84] Profound hypothyroidism has also been associated with incomplete suppression of ADH release.[85]

The syndrome of the reset osmostat is an important variant of SIADH. Patients have mild hyponatremia with serum sodium concentrations usually above 125 meq/liter. They defend body fluid concentration at a lower tonicity than normal, diluting the urine if given a water load and concentrating it if water is restricted. Most are elderly and suffer from chronic debilitating diseases. Since hyponatremia is mild and usually asymptomatic, no specific therapy is required.[86]

Water restriction remains the cornerstone of therapy for asymptomatic or minimally symptomatic patients with SIADH. In patients with postoperative SIADH, the abnormality in ADH secretion is generally short-lived, and water restriction is usually sufficient to correct the hyponatremia. If the SIADH is chronic or if water restriction is ineffective or poorly tolerated, demeclocycline may be helpful. Demeclocycline blocks ADH-mediated water reabsorption in the collecting duct, thereby promoting the excretion of a dilute urine.[87,88] Providing that thirst sensation is intact, such treatment rarely leads to hypernatremia. Demeclocycline is contraindicated in patients with renal disease, hepatic cirrhosis, or congestive heart failure because acute renal failure has been described in these situations.[88,89]

Hypovolemic Hypotonicity

Patients with hypovolemic hypotonicity have both sodium and water deficits, but the sodium deficit is greater. Negative sodium balance from excessive renal, gastrointestinal, or cutaneous sodium losses leads to a reduction in ECF volume. In surgical patients, volume depletion may also result from excessive gastric or biliary drainage, third-spacing, and inadequate replacement of intraoperative fluid losses.

Hypovolemia enhances fluid reabsorption in the proximal nephron, decreasing fluid delivery to the renal diluting sites and limiting generation of electrolyte-free water. In addition, volume depletion increases ADH secretion, increasing reabsorption of water in the collecting duct. These processes limit the capacity of the kidney to excrete a water load. Consequently, water given to sodium-depleted patients cannot be excreted in sufficient quantities and progressive hypotonicity ensues.

The treatment of hypovolemic hypotonicity should be directed at correcting the sodium deficit. Restoration of ECF and IVF volume will restore renal water excretion to normal. Since hypovolemic hypotonicity is usually mild, correction of the sodium deficit

with isotonic saline or a high-sodium diet is usually sufficient to produce a water diuresis and restore body fluid tonicity to normal.

Hypervolemic Hypotonicity

Hypervolemic hypotonicity results from increases in both total body sodium and water with a greater increase in total body water. Positive sodium balance implies diminished renal sodium excretion due to a reduction in glomerular filtration rate, as in renal insufficiency, or to enhanced renal tubular sodium reabsorption, as in the pathologic edema-forming states. ECF volume expansion may be associated with increased or decreased effective arterial blood volume (EABV). EABV and intravascular volume are usually normal or increased in hyponatremic patients with renal insufficiency, but EABV is decreased in the edematous disorders.

Renal failure is commonly associated with hyponatremia. In acute renal failure, the underlying disease directly impairs electrolyte-free water generation, and the low glomerular filtration rate prevents the excretion of sufficient electrolyte-free water to match even a modest water intake. However, electrolyte-free water generation is normal in most patients with chronic renal failure,[90] and hyponatremia is primarily due to reduction in glomerular filtration rate. Although the healthy kidney can excrete 15 to 20 liters of electrolyte-free water daily,[90] a reduction in glomerular filtration rate to 10 ml/min reduces electrolyte-free water excretion to less than two liters per day. If water intake exceeds the sum of renal and insensible electrolyte-free water excretion, hypotonicity is the predictable result. Parenteral fluid management of patients with renal insufficiency therefore requires careful monitoring in the perioperative period.

The pathophysiologic processes contributing to the development of hyponatremia in edematous patients are similar to those in hypovolemic hypotonicity. Decreased EABV results in enhanced proximal tubular fluid reabsorption, decreased distal delivery, and decreased electrolyte-free water generation. ADH levels are elevated because of the reduced EABV, and water reabsorption in the collecting duct is increased. The net result is often a marked impairment in electrolyte-free water excretion. When electrolyte-free water excretion drops below the level of water intake, ingested water is retained and body fluids are progressively diluted. Early in the course of congestive heart failure and cirrhosis, the decrement in EABV is generally not great enough to produce hypotonicity, but as the underlying disease progresses EABV declines further, progressively limiting electrolyte-free water excretion.

Although the mechanisms underlying water retention in hypovolemic and hypervolemic hypotonicity are similar, the treatment of the two states differs markedly. The mainstay of therapy in edematous hypotonic patients is water and sodium restriction, and resolution of hypotonicity is ultimately dependent on the control of the underlying disease process. The use of isotonic or hypertonic saline in these patients is usually counterproductive. Although saline may improve plasma tonicity, it rapidly equilibrates throughout the entire ECF space, worsens the peripheral edema, and may precipitate pulmonary edema. In rare situations in which hypertonic saline must be used emergently in the treatment of symptomatic hypotonicity in edematous patients, potent diuretics should be administered concurrently.

Diuretic therapy is a double-edged sword in edematous hypotonic patients. Although diuretics control peripheral edema and forestall pulmonary edema, they may further reduce EABV and limit electrolyte-free water excretion. Diuretics that act in the proximal tubule such as acetazolamide and metolazone may be more helpful because they inhibit proximal reabsorption and increase the delivery of fluid to the distal diluting sites.[91] However, these agents are relatively ineffective in sustaining a diuresis when used alone and are usually used with more potent loop diuretics.[91]

Diuretic-Induced Hypotonicity

Hyponatremia due to diuretic therapy is common in outpatients. It can be associated with either low or normal total body sodium. When diuretics produce overt volume depletion, they cause hyponatremia by decreasing delivery to the diluting sites and increasing circulating ADH levels. Thiazides and loop diuretics also directly inhibit electrolyte-free water generation by blocking sodium reabsorption in the renal diluting segments. This may contribute to hyponatremia in some patients.

Thiazide diuretics have also been associated with severe symptomatic hyponatremia in the absence of overt volume depletion. The cause of this alarming syndrome remains uncertain, but subclinical volume depletion, inhibition of diluting site function, primary polydipsia despite impaired renal electrolyte-free water excretion, SIADH, and severe potassium depletion have all been implicated. Withdrawal of the diuretic usually restores normal water balance, but the syndrome may recur when the diuretic is reinstituted.

Clinical Manifestations of Hypotonicity

The cardinal feature of hypotonicity is cellular overhydration manifested as cerebral edema. Most cells, including those of the brain, can adapt to tonicity-related volume changes. Increases in intracellular water peak within one or two hours after hypotonicity develops. Thereafter, solute is lost, causing water efflux and reestablishment of normal cell volume. Solute loss is initially rapid and consists largely of electrolytes in the first 6 to 12 hours. Over the next 24 to 72 hours, organic solutes consisting mainly of amino acids follow.

The clinical manifestations of hypotonicity depend on the magnitude and duration of the disturbance, the age of the patient, and the nature and severity of the underlying disease. Mild or moderate degrees of hypotonicity, especially if chronic, are usually asymptomatic and should be treated conservatively with water restriction. More severe hypotonicity with serum sodium concentrations below 120 meq/liter, especially if relatively acute in onset, is more often symptomatic and associated with significant morbidity and mortality.[82,92-94]

The signs and symptoms of hypotonicity are nonspecific and may be obscured in the acutely ill patient. When body fluid tonicity falls below 250 mOsm/kg or a serum sodium concentration of 125 meq/liter, patients may complain of anorexia, nausea, and malaise. At serum sodium levels of 110 to 120 meq/liter, headache, lethargy, confusion, agitation, and obtundation develop. More severe symptoms, including seizures and coma, may occur at levels below 110 meq/liter. Focal neurologic findings are unusual but can occur, and transtentorial cerebral herniation has been described in severe cases. Although symptoms generally resolve with correction of the hypotonicity, there may be permanent neurologic deficits.

The cause of irreversible neurologic deficits in patients with severe hyponatremia remains controversial. Hypoxic encephalopathy may contribute in patients with seizures or in those who vomit and aspirate. However, permanent neurologic sequelae have also been described in those with otherwise uncomplicated hyponatremia. Recently, rapid correction of hyponatremia, rather than hyponatremia itself, has been implicated in producing central pontine myelinolysis,[92,94] a disorder associated with a variety of fixed neurologic deficits.

Emergency Therapy of Symptomatic Hypotonicity

Emergency therapy of severe symptomatic hypotonicity, irrespective of etiology, is directed at raising ECF tonicity, thereby shifting water from the ICF to the ECF and ameliorating cerebral edema. There is considerable controversy about how rapidly the serum sodium concentration should be corrected.[82,92-94] Most feel that the time course over which therapy is given should reflect both the magnitude and chronicity of water intoxication.[93] Asymptomatic hyponatremia, unless profound, is best treated conservatively with water restriction. In hyponatremia that has developed over many days or weeks, the serum sodium concentration should not be raised more than 0.5 meq/liter/hr. In contrast, severe symptomatic hypotonicity that has developed over hours to a few days, or asymptomatic profound hypotonicity with serum sodium concentrations below 110 meq/liter, requires more aggressive treatment. The serum sodium concentration should be raised by about 10%, but to a level not more than 120 meq/liter, at a rate of 1.0 to 2.0 meq/liter/hr. Thereafter, the remainder of the correction can be made over several days.

When aggressive therapy is indicated, the treatment of choice is hypertonic (3%) saline in combination with a loop-acting diuretic like furosemide. In general, an infusion of 1 to 2 ml/kg/hr of 3% saline will usually increase the serum sodium concentration by approximately 1 to 2 meq/liter/hr.[93,94] Because hypertonic saline can produce rapid intravascular volume expansion and can precipitate pulmonary edema, combination therapy with a loop diuretic is usually necessary. Patients receiving hypertonic saline should be monitored closely for evidence of volume overload and must have frequent determinations of serum sodium concentration to ensure that the rate of correction of hypotonicity is not excessively rapid.

Hypertonicity

Because sodium is the predominant cation in the ECF, hypernatremia, defined by a serum sodium concentration above 145 meq/liter, always implies coexistent hypertonicity.[95] However, the converse is not always true, and hypertonicity can occur in the absence of hypernatremia. High concentrations of nonelectrolyte solutes like glucose can cause hypertonicity with a normal, decreased, or increased serum sodium concentration. Hypernatremic hypertonicity is emphasized in this section; hyperglycemia-related hypertonicity is discussed later.

Because hypernatremia is a potent stimulus to thirst and ADH release,[77] it usually develops only in patients with insufficient water intake. Such patients may not have access to water or lack the ability to respond to thirst as a result of illness, medications, altered mental status, or surgery. Water intake rather than renal water conservation is thus the primary defense against progressive dehydration. It is important to determine why water intake has failed to keep pace with ongoing losses in all hypertonic patients. Hypernatremia due to the administration of hypertonic sodium-containing solutions is the only exception to the otherwise invariable association of hypernatremia with insufficient water intake.

Like hypotonicity, hypertonicity can be classified on the basis of relative alterations in TBES and TBW. Hypertonicity can be due to an isolated decrease in TBW; decreases in both TBW and TBES with a greater decrease in TBW; and increases in both TBW and TBES with a greater increase in TBES. In constructing a differential diagnosis, it is helpful to relate the different causes of hypertonicity to ECF volume (total body sodium), which can be normal, decreased, or increased (see Table 60–4).

Euvolemic Hypertonicity

Isolated decreases in TBW, unless very large, do not cause clinically significant ECF and intravascular volume depletion. This is due to the fact that only one-third and one-twelfth of pure water deficits are derived from the ECF and intravascular compartments, respectively. Patients with such deficits usually appear euvolemic, with elevations in BUN and serum uric acid levels as the only evidence of the decreased TBW.

Pure water deficits arise from inadequate water intake in the face of normal or increased insensible and renal electrolyte-free water losses. In patients with normal renal function who are hypernatremic due to decreased water intake and/or increased insensible losses, oliguria, a low urine sodium concentration (below 10 meq/liter), and a high Uosm (above 700 mOsm/kg) are usually found. In contrast, if hypernatremia is the result of excessive renal electrolyte-free water losses, a less than appropriately concentrated urine is the rule.

Euvolemic hypernatremia is common in surgical patients, usually resulting from inadequate water intake in the face of ongoing or increased cutaneous and pulmonary insensible water losses (e.g., due to fever and hyperventilation) rather than from excessive renal electrolyte-free water losses (e.g., due to diabetes insipidus). However, it is not uncommon for hospitalized patients to exhibit

modest urinary concentrating defects when they are chronically ill or protein-malnourished as in the postoperative period.[96,97] After surgery, patients may be unable to obtain water voluntarily or sense thirst normally because of changes in mental status, medications, or underlying diseases. Such patients are often dependent on intravenous fluids and require meticulous attention to replacement of ongoing water losses.

Elderly patients may exhibit the more uncommon primary or "pure" hypodipsia, a defect in thirst without associated abnormal ADH release.[98] Often called "geriatric hypodipsia," such patients present with hypernatremia despite free access to water and normal renal concentrating ability for age. Adequate water intake may have to be prescribed to prevent recurrent episodes of hypernatremia.

Essential hypernatremia is a variant of primary hypodipsia characterized by euvolemia and chronic nonprogressive hypernatremia. Patients with this disorder defend body fluid tonicity at a higher-than-normal osmolality. Geriatric hypodipsia and essential hypernatremia should be kept in mind when evaluating otherwise unexplained and usually asymptomatic hypernatremia in preoperative patients.

Diabetes insipidus may be due to deficiency of ADH (hypothalamic diabetes insipidus) or end-organ hyporesponsiveness to the hormone (nephrogenic diabetes insipidus). Diabetes insipidus need not be associated with hypertonicity unless there is a concomitant defect in thirst or lack of access to water. Complete diabetes insipidus, whether hypothalamic or nephrogenic, is characterized by marked polyuria, secondary polydipsia, and excretion of dilute urine. Although most have urine osmolalities under 150 mOsm/kg, volume-depleted patients with diabetes insipidus may be able to concentrate urine to 300 to 400 mOsm/kg as a result of decreased distal tubular flow and ADH-independent water reabsorption. Patients with partial diabetes insipidus have more modest degrees of polyuria and polydipsia and less impairment of renal concentrating ability but cannot maximally concentrate in response to water

TABLE 60–4. Hypertonic States

TBES	TBW	TBES/TBW	ECF Volume	EABV	Pathophysiology		Conditions
↔	↓	↑	↔	↔	↓ H$_2$O intake		Obtundation Primary hypodipsia Essential hypernatremia
					↑ H$_2$O loss ± ↓ H$_2$O intake	Insensible	Hyperthermia Hyperventilation
						Renal	Diabetes insipidus
↓	↓↓	↑	↓	↓	Hypotonic fluid loss, ± ↓ H$_2$O intake	Renal	Diuretics Osmotic diuresis Adrenal insufficiency Postobstructive diuresis Diuretic phase ATN
						Extrarenal	GI losses: diarrhea, vomiting, NG drainage Cutaneous losses: sensible perspiration, burns Third-space sequestration: peritonitis, ileus, etc.
↑↑	↑	↑	↑	↑	Hypertonic fluid administration		Usually iatrogenic (see Table 60–5)

TBES = total body osmotically effective solute; TBW = total body water; ECF = extracellular fluid; EABV = effective arterial blood volume; ATN = acute tubular necrosis; GI = gastrointestinal; NG = nasogastric; ↔ = normal; ↓ = decreased; ↑ = increased.

deprivation.[97] Diabetes insipidus should be suspected in any hypernatremic polyuric patient with relatively solute-free urine. The diagnosis is confirmed by a standard dehydration test. Hypothalamic and nephrogenic varieties can be differentiated on the basis of responsiveness to exogenous ADH.[97,99]

Hypothalamic diabetes insipidus results from damage to the neurons that synthesize and secrete ADH.[100] Causes include surgical hypophysectomy, head trauma, tumors (craniopharyngioma, pinealoma, metastatic breast cancer, leukemia), infections (meningitis, encephalitis, tuberculosis, syphilis), vascular disorders (aneurysms, cavernous sinus thrombosis, stroke, postpartum pituitary infarction), sarcoidosis, and eosinophilic granuloma. There are also familial and idiopathic forms.

Nephrogenic diabetes insipidus can be due to loss of the normal corticomedullary osmotic gradient or hyporesponsiveness of the collecting duct to ADH.[101] It can be congenital or the result of drug therapy (lithium, demeclocycline, methoxyflurane, amphotericin B), electrolyte disorders (hypercalcemia), obstructive uropathy, or chronic tubulo-interstitial renal disease (associated with analgesic abuse, multiple myeloma, amyloid, sarcoidosis, Sjogren's syndrome, sickle cell disease, or polycystic disease). Nephrogenic diabetes insipidus is usually multifactorial in etiology, especially in hospitalized patients.

The treatment of euvolemic hypernatremia consists of repleting total body water, matching losses with increased oral water intake or intravenous infusion of 5% dextrose solutions, and eliminating excessive insensible and renal water losses. Normalization of body temperature, controlling ambient temperature, and ensuring that mechanical ventilators deliver appropriately humidified air are important in patients with hypertonicity. Adequate water intake for hypodipsia and specific therapy for diabetes insipidus should be initiated as appropriate. Replacing water deficits orally is always preferable. However, if the magnitude of the deficit or the patient's condition prohibit oral replacement, intravenous therapy with 5% dextrose in water should be instituted.

Ongoing renal water losses in patients with hypothalamic diabetes insipidus are easily controlled by hormone replacement. ADH (arginine vasopressin) can be administered as aqueous vasopressin in a dose of 5 to 10 units every two to six hours intramuscularly as required. The synthetic analog, 1-desamino-8-D-arginine vasopressin (DDAVP), has a longer duration of action and can be administered in a dose of 1 to 2 μg subcutaneously or intravenously, or 5 to 20 μg intranasally, every 12 to 24 hours as required. Oral chlorpropamide in a dose of 250 to 500 mg daily, or clofibrate in a dose of 1 to 2 g daily in divided doses every six to eight hours, can sometimes be beneficial in partial hypothalamic diabetes insipidus.[102] Chlorpropamide enhances the effect of ADH on the collecting duct and may also increase ADH release,[102] but hypoglycemia may limit its use. Clofibrate increases ADH release.[102]

Therapy for reversible forms of nephrogenic diabetes insipidus consists of treating the underlying disorder or discontinuing the offending drug. Although patients with this disorder are unresponsive to hormone therapy, polyuria can be attenuated by restricting dietary protein and sodium, thereby reducing obligate urinary solute excretion. Thiazide diuretics may also be helpful by producing ECF volume depletion and increasing proximal tubular fluid reabsorption.

Hypovolemic Hypertonicity

The coexistence of hypernatremia and ECF volume depletion indicates unequal losses of both sodium and water with a greater deficit in total body water than in sodium. The coexistence of hypotension and hypernatremia almost always implies significant concomitant sodium losses. Hypotension is rarely a manifestation of pure water loss.

Hypotonic fluid losses can occur through the skin, gastrointestinal tract, or kidney. Sensible, as opposed to insensible, perspiration and most gastrointestinal secretions, with the exception of biliary and pancreatic drainage, contain significant amounts of sodium but are hypotonic (see Table 60–2). Prolonged vomiting, nasogastric drainage, or diarrhea can thus cause hypovolemic hypernatremia. Diuretics and osmotic diuresis due to glucose, mannitol, or urea cause similar hypotonic fluid losses through the kidney. Osmotic diuresis is especially important in surgical patients receiving hyperalimentation, in which large carbohydrate and protein loads often lead to impressive polyuria. Hypovolemic hypernatremia can also be the result of redistribution of isotonic fluid from the ECF to a third space in the face of water intake insufficient to match ongoing electrolyte-free water losses.

Tachycardia, hypotension, decreased central venous pressure, and prerenal azotemia are common in patients with hypovolemic hypernatremia. If hypotonic losses are extrarenal in origin and renal function is normal, oliguria, low urine sodium concentration, and high urine osmolality result. In contrast, if losses are renal in origin, urine sodium concentration will be high, and urine osmolality will be inappropriately low.

The first priority in the treatment of hypovolemic hypernatremia is to restore intravascular volume. Isotonic saline or, if hemodynamic collapse is imminent, colloid should be administered. In many patients, volume resuscitation and restoration of adequate oral water intake correct the hypertonicity. When oral intake is not possible, intravenous 5% dextrose can be given once sodium and potassium deficits have been replaced. Correction of hypertonicity should be gradual to avoid cerebral edema.

Hypervolemic Hypertonicity

In surgical patients, hypervolemic hypertonicity is primarily an iatrogenic complication resulting from intravenous administration of hypertonic solutions (see Table 60–5). Hypertonic sodium bicarbonate is frequently administered for severe metabolic acidosis or in cardiopulmonary resuscitation. Hypertonic mannitol is used to treat cerebral edema, establish a diuresis in patients with oliguric acute renal failure, and facilitate excretion of nephrotoxic radiological contrast agents. Hypertonic solutions are occasionally given inadvertently, as in accidental intravenous instead of intra-amniotic infusion of hypertonic saline in therapeutic abortions. Hypervolemic hypernatremia may also result from the overcorrection of hypotonicity with 3% saline.

As in any hypertonic state, development of cerebral dehydration can be life-threatening. However, in this setting, it can develop rapidly and overwhelm compensatory mechanisms that defend cerebral cell volume. Concomitant ECF volume expansion can also lead to rapid development of pulmonary edema. Therapy for acute hypertonicity and cerebral dehydration requires prompt and rapid

TABLE 60–5. Therapeutic Hypertonic Solutions

Solute	Molecular Weight (g)	Concentration (%)	Water (mOsm/kg)	Usual Container Size (ml)	Use
Sodium chloride	58.5	3	1026	500	Emergency treatment
		5	1711	500	of hypotonic states
		20	6845	250	Intraamniotic instillation for therapeutic abortion
Sodium bicarbonate	84	5	1190	500	Metabolic acidosis,
		7.5	1786	50	hyperkalemia, and cardiopulmonary arrest
Dextrose	198	10	505	500, 1000	Caloric agent
		20	1010	500	Treatment of
		50	2525	50, 500	hypoglycemia
Mannitol	182	10	549	500, 1000	Osmotic diuresis,
		20	1099	250, 500	acute renal failure,
		25	1374	50	cerebral edema, and acute glaucoma
Glycerol	92	50	5435	120	Cerebral edema and
		75	8152	120	acute glaucoma

Source: From Feig PU, McCurdy DK: *N Engl J Med* 297:1444, 1977.

administration of large amounts of electrolyte-free water. The volume of water needed to correct hypertonicity can be estimated from the serum osmolality, as discussed below. To prevent further ECF volume expansion, therapy must also include solute removal with potent diuretics like furosemide. In patients with massive volume overload or oliguric renal failure, hemodialysis or hemofiltration may be required.

Clinical Manifestations of Hypertonicity

The most significant effects of hypertonicity are the neurologic manifestations associated with cerebral dehydration. These include lethargy, muscle weakness, fasciculations, seizures, coma, and death. Reduction in brain volume may lead to rupture of cerebral veins, causing intracerebral and subarachnoid hemorrhage and irreversible neurologic deficits. The severity of symptoms is related not only to the magnitude of the hypertonicity but also to the rapidity with which it develops and the duration of the hypertonic state.

When hypertonicity develops rapidly, all cells shrink. With chronic hypertonicity, most tissues dehydrate, but some cells (e.g., red blood cells) regain volume by taking up ECF solute.[95,103] However, the response of the central nervous system to hypertonicity is different from that of most other tissues. The brain defends cell volume not only by accumulating ECF electrolyte but also by generating new intracellular solute or "idiogenic" osmoles in the form of amino acids, polyols, and methylamines.[104] Gradual development of hypertonicity allows time for production of idiogenic osmoles to limit cerebral dehydration. This response also depends on the nature of the offending solute.[95,103] For example, the generation of idiogenic osmoles in response to hyperglycemia is more rapid than in response to hypernatremia.

Repletion of Water Deficits

Although idiogenic osmoles in the brain protect against cellular dehydration, they predispose to cerebral edema if water deficits are corrected too rapidly. Consequently, gradual correction of hypertonicity is always advisable. No more than half of the calculated water deficit should be replaced in the first 12 to 24 hours. The remainder of the deficit can then be replaced over the next 24 to 48 hours. Neurologic status should be closely monitored. If it initially improves but then deteriorates, cerebral edema should be suspected and water replacement discontinued. Hypertonic mannitol can be used to reverse the cerebral edema.

Calculation of the water deficit is based on the assumption that total body solute (TBW × Posm) has remained constant. The serum sodium concentration (SNa) is used in the calculation rather than Posm because it better reflects plasma tonicity in the presence of azotemia. Thus:

$$\text{(Normal TBW)} \times \text{(Normal SNa)} = \text{(Present TBW)} \times \text{(Present SNa)}$$

or

$$\text{Present TBW} = \frac{\text{(Normal TBW)} \times \text{(Normal SNa)}}{\text{(Present SNa)}}$$

The water deficit is then equal to normal TBW minus present TBW. For example, if a patient who weighs 70 kg has a serum sodium concentration of 170 meq/liter, present TBW = (0.6 × 70) × (140/170) = 34.6, and the water deficit is 42 − 34.6 or 7.4 liters. Despite inherent inaccuracies in this formula, it provides a useful estimate of the water deficit in guiding initial therapy of hypertonicity.

Diabetes Mellitus and Tonicity Homeostasis

Hypertonicity due to hyperglycemia is frequent in surgical patients. The stress of surgery and anesthesia, use of intravenous glucose solutions, and hyperalimentation all contribute to the development of hyperglycemia. Approximately 40 percent of postoperative patients with marked hyperglycemia have no preceding history of diabetes mellitus.[80]

Glucose is an osmotically active solute and permeates cell membranes poorly. At high plasma concentrations, it is also a potent osmotic diuretic. Hyperglycemia produces hypertonicity both through its presence in the ECF and indirectly as a result of hypotonic fluid losses induced by glycosuria. Although patients with hyperglycemic hypertonicity are usually volume-depleted, the effects of sodium depletion may be masked by water shifts from the ICF to the ECF in response to the hyperglycemia. Significant potassium depletion also usually accompanies glycosuria.

By drawing water from the ICF to the ECF, hyperglycemia tends to lower the serum sodium concentration and may even produce hyponatremia in the setting of hypertonicity. The relationship between serum glucose and sodium concentrations depends on the degree of hyperglycemia and volume depletion. In euvolemic patients, the serum sodium concentration falls by 1.6 meq/liter for each increase of 100 mg/dl in the serum glucose concentration above normal.[105] In volume-depleted patients, sodium concentration falls 2.0 meq/liter for each 100 mg/dl rise in glucose concentration.[105] Under these circumstances, a "normal" serum sodium concentration of 140 meq/liter indicates a substantial water deficit.

The serum sodium concentration in patients with hyperglycemia can be low, normal, or high. In any given situation, it is dependent on the extent of the associated osmotic diuresis, the magnitude of the glucose-related shift of water from the ICF to the ECF, and the level of water intake. If the osmotic diuresis predominates, hypernatremia usually results. If water intake is substantial, the serum sodium concentration may be normal or low even in the face of hypertonicity.

Volume deficits should be promptly replaced with intravenous isotonic saline. Volume repletion increases renal glucose clearance and thus helps to correct the hyperglycemia. In the absence of severe ketoacidosis, it is advisable to delay insulin therapy until the blood pressure is stable. Early administration of large doses of insulin may cause circulatory collapse as glucose and water move rapidly into cells. Low doses of intravenous insulin should be given after volume repletion is underway in an effort to normalize the serum glucose concentration over approximately 24 hours. Hypotonic saline or 5% dextrose in water can be substituted for isotonic saline over the next 24 to 48 hours to reverse any residual hypertonicity. The treatment of diabetic ketoacidosis is discussed in more detail in Chap. 24.

SUMMARY

Volume

1. Tissue perfusion depends on the effective arterial blood volume. Effective arterial blood volume is a function not only of actual intravascular volume but also of cardiac output and vascular capacitance.

2. The renal response to surgery or trauma is sodium and water retention.

3. The principal clinical sign of intravascular volume depletion is hypotension. The principal clinical signs of intravascular and extracellular fluid expansion are pulmonary edema and peripheral edema, respectively.

4. Intravascular volume depletion can be associated with decreased extracellular fluid volume, as in hemorrhage, third-space sequestration, and sodium depletion, or with increased extracellular fluid volume, as in the capillary leak syndrome.

5. Sodium depletion can result from renal, gastrointestinal, or cutaneous sodium losses.

6. Diuretics and the osmotic diuresis of uncontrolled diabetes mellitus are common causes of renal sodium loss.

7. Surgical patients may suffer extensive sodium losses from the gastrointestinal tract or in serous drainage from open wounds or burns.

8. The primary goal in treating volume depletion is to restore blood pressure and tissue perfusion.

9. Therapy of the volume-depleted patient depends on the magnitude and type of deficit, the rapidity of its development, the nature and severity of ongoing losses, and the presence of associated disturbances in potassium and acid-base homeostasis.

10. Volume expansion can be associated with proportional increases in the intravascular and interstitial fluid compartments, as in renal failure, or with maldistribution of fluid between the two compartments, as in congestive heart failure, hepatic cirrhosis, and nephrotic syndrome.

11. The primary goal in treating volume expansion is to remove excess sodium and water without compromising hemodynamic status. This can be accomplished with diuretics, ultrafiltration, or continuous arteriovenous (or venovenous) hemofiltration. Attention must always be given to ameliorating the underlying cause of the sodium retention as well.

12. In order to avoid intravascular volume expansion, dietary and intravenous fluid management should be closely monitored in patients with cardiac, renal, or liver disease.

Tonicity

1. Intracellular volume is largely determined by body fluid tonicity. Hypotonicity leads to cell volume expansion, and hypertonicity leads to cell volume contraction.

2. The cardinal feature of hypotonicity is cerebral edema. The most significant effects of hypertonicity are the neurologic consequences of cerebral dehydration.

3. Disturbances of tonicity homeostasis are usually detected by alterations in the serum sodium concentration. Hypotonicity usually accompanies hyponatremia. However, if the extracellular fluid contains large amounts of glucose, mannitol, lipids, or protein, hyponatremia can exist without hypotonicity. In contrast, hypertonicity always accompanies hypernatremia.

4. Hypotonicity always reflects on inability of the kidney to excrete sufficient electrolyte-free water to match water intake.

5. Hypotonicity can occur in association with normal, decreased, or increased total body sodium content (extracellular fluid volume).

6. Euvolemic hypotonicity can be attributed to excessive water intake, as in primary polydipsia, or to impaired electrolyte-free water excretion resulting from the nonosmotic release of antidiuretic hormone, as in the syndrome of inappropriate antidiuretic hormone (SIADH).

7. Water restriction is the cornerstone of therapy for asymptomatic patients with SIADH.

8. The treatment of hypovolemic hypotonicity should be directed at correcting the sodium deficit.

9. The mainstay of therapy of hypervolemic hypotonicity is sodium and water restriction. Resolution of hypotonicity is ultimately dependent on control of the underlying disease process.

10. Emergency therapy of severe symptomatic hypotonicity, irrespective of etiology, should be directed at raising extracellular fluid tonicity, thereby shifting water from the intracellular to the extracellular compartment and ameliorating cerebral edema. The treatment of choice is judicious use of hypertonic (3%) saline with or without a potent diuretic like furosemide.

11. Hypertonicity usually reflects inadequate water intake in the face of normal or increased insensible, renal, or gastrointestinal fluid losses.

12. Hypertonicity can occur in association with normal, decreased, or increased total body sodium content (extracellular fluid volume).

13. Euvolemic hypertonicity can be attributed to decreased water intake alone (primary hypodipsia) or to inadequate water intake in the face of excessive insensible losses or excessive renal electrolyte-free water loss (diabetes insipidus).

14. Water repletion is the cornerstone of therapy of euvolemic hypertonicity. Specific therapy for diabetes insipidus should be initiated when indicated.

15. The first priority in the treatment of hypovolemic hypertonicity is to restore intravascular volume with isotonic (0.9%) saline or colloid as appropriate. Correction of the hypertonicity and any associated electrolyte or acid-base disturbances can be addressed thereafter.

16. Hypervolemic hypertonicity is usually iatrogenic in origin. The compensatory mechanisms that defend cerebral volume may be overwhelmed, and pulmonary edema can develop. Treatment should be directed at correcting the acute hypertonicity with intravenous electrolyte-free water and the extracellular volume expansion with potent diuretics like furosemide.

REFERENCES

1. Shires T, Williams J, Brown F: Acute changes in extracellular fluids associated with major surgical procedures. *Ann Surg* 154:803–810, 1961.
2. Irvin TT, Modgil VK, Hayter CJ et al: Plasma-volume deficits and salt and water excretion after surgery. *Lancet* 2:1159–1162, 1972.
3. Bevan BR: The sodium story: Effects of anaesthesia and surgery on intrarenal mechanisms concerned with sodium homeostasis. *Proc Roy Soc Med* 66:1215–1220, 1973.
4. Maddox DA, Price DC, Rector FC: Effects of surgery on plasma volume and salt and water excretion in rats. *Am J Physiol* 233:F600–F606, 1977.
5. Robarts WM: Nature of the disturbance in the body fluid compartments during and after surgical operations. *Br J Surg* 66:691–695, 1979.
6. Roberts JP, Roberts JD, Skinner C et al: Extracellular fluid deficit following operation and its correction with Ringer's lactate. *Ann Surg* 202:1–8, 1985.
7. Cochrane JPS: The aldosterone response to surgery and the relationship of this response to postoperative sodium retention. *Br J Surg* 65:744–747, 1978.
8. Chernow B, Alexander R, Smallridge RC et al: Hormonal responses to graded surgical stress. *Arch Intern Med* 147:1273–1278, 1987.
9. Udelsman R, Chrousos GP: Hormonal response to surgical stress. *Adv Exp Med Biol* 245:265–272, 1988.
10. Cross JS, Gruber DP, Gann DS et al: Hypertonic saline attenuates the hormonal response to injury. *Ann Surg* 209:684–692, 1989.
11. Blalock A: Trauma to the intestines. The importance of local loss of fluid in the production of low blood pressure. *Arch Surg* 22:314–324, 1931.
12. McCance RA: Experimental sodium chloride deficiency in man. *Proc Roy Soc* 119:245–267, 1936.
13. Coleman TG, Cowley AW, Guyton AC: Angiotensin and the hemodynamics of chronic salt deprivation. *Am J Physiol* 229:167–171, 1975.
14. Elkington JR, Danowski TS, Winkler AW: Hemodynamic changes in salt depletion and in dehydration. *J Clin Invest* 25:120–129, 1946.
15. Denton DA: The brain and sodium homeostasis conditions. *Reflex* 8:125–146, 1973.
16. Fitzsimons JT: The physiologic basis of thirst. *Kidney Int* 10:3–11, 1976.
17. Dossetor JB: Diagnosis and treatment, creatinemia versus azotemia—the relative contribution of blood urea nitrogen and serum creatinine concentrations in azotemia. *Ann Intern Med* 65:1287, 1966.
18. Demling RH: Burns. Fluid and electrolyte management. *Crit Care Clin* 1:27–45, 1985.
19. Chan STF, Kapadia CR, Johnson AW et al: Extracellular fluid volume expansion and third space sequestration at the site of small bowel anastomoses. *Br J Surg* 70:36–39, 1983.
20. Sauven P, Playforth MJ, Evans M et al: Fluid sequestration: An early indicator of mortality in acute pancreatitis. *Br J Surg* 73:799–800, 1986.
21. Shapiro JI, Anderson RJ: Sodium depletion states, in Brenner BM, Stein JH (eds): *Body Fluid Homeostasis.* New York, Churchill Livingstone, 1987, pp 245–276.
22. Jamison RL, Ross JC, Kempson RL et al: Surreptitious diuretic ingestion and pseudo-Bartter's syndrome. *Am J Med* 73:142–147, 1982.
23. Gennari JF, Kassirer JP: Osmotic diuresis. *N Engl J Med* 291:714–720, 1974.
24. Coleman AJ, Aria M, Carter NW et al: The mechanism of salt-wasting in chronic renal disease. *J Clin Invest* 45:1116–1125, 1966.
25. Danovitch GM, Bourgoignie J, Bricker NS: Reversibility of the "salt losing" tendency of chronic renal failure. *N Engl J Med* 296:14–19, 1977.
26. Uribarri J, Oh MS, Carroll HJ: Salt-losing nephropathy: Clinical presentation and mechanisms. *Am J Nephrol* 3:193–198, 1983.
27. Anderson RJ, Linas SL, Berns AS et al: Nonoliguric acute renal failure. *N Engl J Med* 296:1134–1138, 1977.
28. Howards S: Postobstructive diuresis: A misunderstood phenomenon. *J Urol* 110:537–540, 1973.
29. Conn JW: The mechanism of acclimatization to heat. *Adv Intern Med* 3:373–393, 1949.
30. Phillips SF: Water and electrolytes in gastrointestinal diseases, in

Maxwell MH, Kleeman CH (eds): *Clinical Disorders of Fluids and Electrolyte Metabolism*. New York, McGraw-Hill, 1980, pp 1267–1290.

31. Kassirer JP, Schwartz WB: The response of normal man to elective depletion of hydrochloric acid. *Am J Med* 40:10–18, 1966.

32. Ziyadeh FH, Badr KF: Fractional excretion of chloride in prerenal axotemia. *Arch Intern Med* 145:1929, 1985.

33. Perez GO, Oster JR, Rogers A: Acid-base disturbances in gastrointestinal disease. *Dig Dis Sci* 32:1033–1043, 1987.

34. Chang AE, Rosenberg SA: Overview of interleukin-2 as an immunotherapeutic agent. *Sem Surg Oncol* 5:385–390, 1989.

35. Sprung CL, Elser B: Reexpansion pulmonary edema. *Chest* 84:788, 1983.

36. Mahfood S, Hix WR, Aaron BL et al: Reexpansion pulmonary edema. *Ann Thor Surg* 45:340–345, 1988.

37. Tullis JL: Albumin. *JAMA* 237:355–360, 1977.

38. Reineck HJ: Mechanisms of edema formation in nephrotic syndrome, in Brenner BM, Stein JH (eds): *Contemporary Issues in Nephrology*. 9:31–46, 1982.

39. Buehler BA: Hereditary disorders of albumin synthesis. *Ann Clin Lab Sci* 8:283–286, 1978.

40. Joles JA, Koomans HA, Kortlandt W et al: Hypoproteinemia and recovery from edema in dogs. *Am J Physiol* 254:F887–F894, 1988.

41. Rocco VK, Ware AJ: Cirrhotic ascites: Pathophysiology, diagnosis and management. *Ann Intern Med* 105:573–585, 1986.

42. Schrier RW, Arroyo V, Bernardi M et al: Peripheral arterial vasodilation hypothesis: A proposal for the initiation of renal sodium and water retention in cirrhosis. *Hepatology* 8:1151–1157, 1988.

43. Brown EA, Markandu N, Sagnella GA et al: Sodium retention in nephrotic syndrome is due to an intrarenal defect: Evidence from steroid-induced remission. *Nephron* 39:290–295, 1985.

44. Meltzer JL, Keim HJ, Laragh JH et al: Nephrotic syndrome: Vasoconstriction and hypervolemic types indicated by renin profiling. *Ann Intern Med* 91:688–696, 1979.

45. Dorhout Mees EJ, Geers HA, Koomans HA: Blood volume and sodium retention in the nephrotic syndrome: Controversial pathophysiological concepts. *Nephron* 36:201–211, 1984.

46. Latta T: Relative to the treatment of cholera by the copious injection of aqueous and saline fluids into the veins (letter). *Lancet* 2:274, 1932.

47. Falk JL, Rackow EC, Weil MH: Colloid and crystalloid fluid resuscitation, in Shoemaker WC, Ayres S, Grenvik A et al (eds): *Textbook of Critical Care*. Philadelphia, Saunders, 1989, pp 1055–1073.

48. Mettauer B, Rouleau JL, Bichet D et al: Sodium and water excretion abnormalities in congestive heart failure. *Ann Intern Med* 105:161–167, 1986.

49. Dzau VJ: Renal and circulatory mechanisms in congestive heart failure. *Kidney Int* 31:1402–1415, 1987.

50. Schrier RW: Pathogenesis of sodium and water retention in high-output and low-output cardiac failure, nephrotic syndrome, cirrhosis, and pregnancy. *N Engl J Med* 319:1065–1072, 1127–1134, 1988.

51. Kubo SH: Neurohormonal activity in congestive heart failure. *Crit Care Med* 18:S39–S44, 1990.

52. Ichikawa I, Rennke HG, Hoyer JR et al: Role of intrarenal mechanisms in the impaired salt excretion of experimental nephrotic syndrome. *J Clin Invest* 71:91–103, 1983.

53. Laski ME: Diuretics: Mechanism of action and therapy. *Sem Nephrol* 6:210–223, 1986.

54. Shear L, Ching S, Gabuzda GJ: Compartmentalization of ascites and edema in patients with hepatic cirrhosis. *N Engl J Med* 282:1391–1396, 1970.

55. Pinto PC, Amerian J, Reynolds TB: Large-volume paracentesis in nonedematous patients with tense ascites: Its effect on intravascular volume. *Hepatology* 8:207–210, 1988.

56. Gines P, Arroyo V, Quintero E et al: Comparison of paracentesis and diuretics in the treatment of cirrhotics with tense ascites. *Gastroenterology* 93:234–241, 1987.

57. Perez-Ayuso RM, Arroyo V, Planas R et al: Randomized comparative study of efficacy of furosemide versus spironolactone in nonazotemic cirrhosis with ascites. *Gastroenterology* 84:961–968, 1983.

58. Gabuzda GS, Hall PW: Relation of potassium depletion to renal ammonium metabolism and hepatic coma. *Medicine* 45:481–490, 1966.

59. Macias WL, Mueller BA, Scarin SK et al: Continuous venovenous hemofiltration: An alternative to arteriovenous hemodialfiltration and hemodiafiltration in acute renal failure. *Am J Kidney Dis* 18:451–458, 1991.

60. Sigler MH, Teehan BP: Continuous arteriovenous hemodialysis (CAVHD), in Nissenson AR, Fine RN, Gentile DE (eds): *Clinical Dialysis*. Norwalk, CT, Appleton & Lange, 1989, pp 720–734.

61. Rimondini A, Cipolla CM, Bella DP et al: Hemofiltration as short-term treatment for refractory congestive heart failure. *Am J Med* 83:43–48, 1987.

62. Baumber CD, Clark RG: Insensible water loss in surgical patients. *Br J Surg* 61:53–56, 1974.

63. Binder HJ, Sandleg GI: Electrolyte absorption and secretion in the mammalian colon, in Johnson LR (ed): *Physiology of the Gastrointestinal Tract*, 2d ed. New York, Raven Press, 1987, pp 1389–1418.

64. Lassiter WE, Gottschalk CW: Regulation of water balance: Urine concentration and dilution, in Schrier RW, Gottschald CW (eds): *Diseases of the Kidney*. Boston, Little Brown, 1988, pp 119–142.

65. Ramsay DJ: Osmoreceptors subserving vasopressin secretion and drinking—an overview, in Schrier RW (ed): *Vasopressin*. New York, Raven Press, 1985, pp 291–298.

66. Robertson GL, Shelton RL, Athar S: The osmoregulation of vasopressin. *Kidney Int* 10:25–37, 1976.

67. Vokes T, Robertson GL: Effect of insulin in the osmoregulation of thirst and vasopressin, in Schrier RW (ed): *Vasopressin*. New York, Raven Press, 1985, pp 271–279.

68. Wang BC, Goetz KL: Volume influences on the plasma osmolality—plasma vasopressin relationship mediated by cardiac receptors, in Schrier RW (ed): *Vasopressin*. New York, Raven Press, 1985, pp 221–228.

69. Kamoi K, Robertson GL: Opiates and vasopressin secretion, in Schrier RW (ed): *Vasopressin*. New York, Raven Press, 1985, pp 259–264.

70. Robertson GL: The regulation of vasopressin function in health and disease. *Recent Progr Horm Res* 33:333–385, 1987.

71. Kendler KS, Weitzman RF, Fisher DA: The effect of pain on plasma arginine vasopressin concentrations in man. *Clin Endocrinol* 8:89–94, 1978.

72. Rose CE, Dixon BS, Anderson RJ: Effects of hypoxemia and hypercapnic acidosis on renal water excretion on vasopressin secretion, in Schrier RW (ed): *Vasopressin*. New York, Raven Press, 1985, pp 517–523.

73. Anderson RJ: Hospital-associated hyponatremia. *Kidney Int* 29:1237–1247, 1986.

74. Linas SL, Berl T, Robertson GL et al: Role of vasopressin in the impaired water excretion of glucocorticoid deficiency in the rat. *Kidney Int* 18:58–67, 1980.

75. Mandell IN, DeFronzo RA, Robertson GL et al: Role of plasma arginine vasopressin in the impaired water diuresis of isolated glucocorticoid deficiency in the rat. *Kidney Int* 17:186–195, 1980.

76. Robinson AG: Neurohypophyseal function in hypothyroidism, in Schrier RW (ed): *Vasopressin*. New York, Raven Press, 1985, pp 507–515.

77. Robertson GL: Osmoregulation of thirst and vasopressin secretion: Functional properties and their relationship to water balance, in Schrier RW (ed): *Vasopressin*. New York, Raven Press, 1985, pp 203–212.

78. Weisberg LS: Pseudohyponatremia: A reappraisal. *Am J Med* 86:315–318, 1989.

79. Anderson RJ, Chung H-M, Kluge R et al: Hyponatremia: A prospective analysis of its epidemiology and the pathogenetic role of vasopressin. *Ann Intern Med* 102:164–168, 1985.

80. Chung H-M, Kluge R, Schrier RW et al: Postoperative hyponatremia. *Arch Int Med* 146:333–336, 1986.

81. Tierney WM, Martin DK, Greenlee MC et al: The prognosis of hyponatremia at hospital admission. *J Gen Intern Med* 1:380–385, 1986.

82. Arieff AI: Hyponatremia, convulsions, respiratory arrest and permanent brain damage after elective surgery in healthy women. *N Engl J Med* 314:1529–1535, 1986.

83. Rhymer JC, Bell TJ, Perry RC et al: Hyponatremia following transurethral resection of the prostate. *Br J Urol* 57:450–452, 1985.

84. Schwartz MJ, Kokko JP: Urinary concentrating defect of adrenal insufficiency. *J Clin Invest* 66:234–242, 1980.

85. Derubertis FR, Michelis M, Blood ME et al: Impaired water excretion in myxedema. *Am J Med* 51:41–53, 1971.

86. DeFronzo RA, Goldberg M, Agus AS: Normal diluting capacity in hyponatremia patients. *Ann Int Med* 84:538–542, 1976.

87. Forrest JN, Cox M, Hong C et al: Superiority of demeclocycline over lithium in the treatment of chronic syndrome of inappropriate secretion of antidiuretic hormone. *N Engl J Med* 298:173–177, 1978.

88. Geheb M, Cox M: Renal effects of demeclocycline. *JAMA* 243:2519–2520, 1980.

89. Braden G, Geheb M, Shook A et al: Demeclocycline-induced natriuresis and renal failure: In-vivo and in-vitro studies. *Am J Kid Dis* 5:270–277, 1985.

90. Bricker NS, Fine LG: The renal response to progressive nephron loss, in Brenner BM, Rector FC (eds): *The Kidney*, 2d ed. Philadelphia, Saunders, 1981, pp 1056–1096.

91. Fernandez PC, Weisberg LS, Palevsky PM: Physiologic basis for the use of sequential nephron blockade in patients with resistant edema, in Puschett JB, Greenberg A (eds): *Diuretics II: Chemistry, Pharmacology and Clinical Applications*. New York, Elsevier, 1987, pp 301–307.

92. Sterns RH, Riggs JE, Schochet SS: Osmotic demyelination syndrome following correction of hyponatremia. *N Engl J Med* 314:1535–1542, 1986.

93. Berl T: Treating hyponatremia: What is all the controversy about? *Ann Int Med* 113:417–419, 1990.

94. Sterns RH: The management of symptomatic hyponatremia. *Sem Nephrol* 10:503–514, 1990.

95. Feig PU, McCurdy DK: The hypertonic state. *N Engl J Med* 297:1444–1454, 1977.

96. Klahr S, Tripathy K, Garcia FJ et al: On the nature of the concentrating defect in malnutrition. *Am J Med* 43:84–96, 1967.

97. Miller M, Dalakos T, Moses AM et al: Recognition of partial defects in antidiuretic hormone secretion. *Ann Intern Med* 73:721–729, 1970.

98. Miller PD, Krebs RA, Neal BJ et al: Hypodipsia in geriatric patients. *Am J Physiol* 73:354–356, 1982.

99. Zerbe RL, Robertson GL: A comparison of plasma vasopressin measurements with a standard indirect test in the differential diagnosis of polyuria. *N Engl J Med* 305:1539–1546, 1981.

100. Robinson AG: Disorders of antidiuretic hormone secretion. *Clin Endocrinol Metab* 14:55–88, 1985.

101. Singer I: Differential diagnosis of polyuria and diabetes insipidus. *Med Clin N America* 65:303–320, 1981.

102. Moses AM, Miller M: Drug-induced dilutional hyponatremia. *N Engl J Med* 291:1234–1239, 1974.

103. Arieff AI, Guisado R: Effects on the central nervous system of hypernatremic and hyponatremic states. *Kidney Int* 10:104–116, 1976.

104. Helig CW, Steomski ME, Blumenfeld JD et al: Characterization of the major brain osmolytes that accumulate in salt-loaded rats. *Am J Physiol* 257:F1108–F1116, 1989.

105. Moran SM, Jamison RL: The variable hyponatremia response to hyperglycemia. *West J Med* 142:49–53, 1985.

106. Nelson BK: Snake evenomation. Incidence, clinical presentation and management. *Med Toxicol Adverse Drug Exp* 4:17–31, 1989.

61 ELECTROLYTE DISORDERS IN THE SURGICAL PATIENT

James A. Kruse

Tusar K. Desai

Michael A. Geheb

Electrolyte disorders arising in the perioperative period may be manifestations of underlying disease or complications of acute illness, surgery itself, or postoperative therapy. Although there are few if any data to guide clinicians in determining when a specific electrolyte disturbance may increase the risk of surgery, the literature does provide enough information to allow them to predict which derangements are most likely to arise in seriously ill surgical patients and to treat them expectantly. This chapter discusses disturbances in potassium, calcium, phosphate, and magnesium homeostasis in the context of the perioperative period. The reader is referred to standard textbooks of medicine for a more comprehensive review of etiologies and pathophysiology.

POTASSIUM

The majority of the 3500 meq of potassium in the body of a 70-kg individual is found in skeletal muscle.[1,2] Total body potassium content is regulated by external potassium balance or the difference between potassium intake and excretion. The extracellular concentration of potassium is approximately but inconsistently proportional to potassium stores in the body. Internal potassium balance or the relationship between intracellular and extracellular potassium concentration is influenced by a variety of physiologic, hormonal, and pharmacologic factors. These factors most often affect extracellular potassium concentration without altering total body potassium level. Hyperkalemia can be seen in the presence of normal or even decreased total body potassium content, but hypokalemia is more reliably associated with decreased potassium stores. Although 98 percent of potassium is intracellular, the extracellular potassium concentration is critically important in maintaining normal cardiac rhythm and neuromuscular function. Disorders of extracellular potassium concentration caused by disease, trauma, surgery, drugs, and other therapies are common in surgical patients.

Hypokalemia

Hypokalemia is probably the most common electrolyte disturbance in surgical patients[3–10] and is associated with significant hospital mortality.[8,11] In most cases, hypokalemia reflects a deficiency in total body potassium due to decreased potassium intake, increased excretion, or both. Normal dietary potassium intake ranges from 50 to 120 meq/day. The kidneys regulate total body potassium content and can efficiently conserve potassium when intake is decreased. Therefore, dietary potassium restriction results in hypokalemia only after prolonged deprivation in patients who are starved or suffer from chronic alcoholism. In such cases, the urine potassium concentration can decrease to 10 meq/liter or less.

On the other hand, significant renal potassium wasting may occur following injury or surgery even in the face of potassium depletion.[4,12–14] Fasting patients on prolonged infusions of potassium-free intravenous fluids and those receiving inadequate replacement of potassium losses in the perioperative period have an increased risk of developing hypokalemia. Persistent kaliuresis despite hypokalemia may also indicate renal potassium wasting due to diuretic administration, mineralocorticoid excess, renal tubular acidosis, or excess solute losses after administration of intravenous fluids. Urine potassium concentration may also be increased in the presence of nonrenal potassium losses due to vomiting, nasogastric suction, or diarrhea if there has been insufficient time for renal conservation to occur or if associated volume depletion has stimulated aldosterone secretion. The hypokalemia seen with vomiting or nasogastric suction is predominantly due to aldosterone stimulation of renal potassium secretion and direct potassium loss in gastric fluid accounts for a much smaller portion of the deficit. The metabolic alkalosis resulting from gastric fluid loss may also play a role in hypokalemia by affecting internal potassium distribution. Direct potassium losses occur in diarrheal fluid. Like the kidney, the colon increases potassium secretion in response to increased mineralocorticoid levels induced by volume depletion.

Table 61–1 lists the many causes of hypokalemia. Inadequate

TABLE 61–1. Causes of Hypokalemia

Hypokalemia related to altered internal potassium balance

Acid-base disorders
  Metabolic alkalosis
  Respiratory alkalosis (mild hypokalemia)

Pharmacologic agents
  Insulin
  Sodium bicarbonate
  Beta-adrenergic agonists

Acute cellular proliferation
  Treatment of megaloblastic anemia with B_{12} or folate
  Total parenteral nutrition

Other
  Hypokalemic periodic paralysis

Hypokalemia related to altered external potassium balance

Dermal losses
  Sweat
  Burns

Gastrointestinal losses
  Diarrhea
  Villous adenoma
  Noninsulin-secreting islet-cell tumor
  Ureterosigmoidostomy
  Obstructed ileal loop
  Fistulas
  Biliary drainage
  Laxative abuse

Renal potassium wasting
  Vomiting or nasogastric suction
  Renal tubular acidosis
  Diuretics
  Osmotic diuresis
    Osmotic diuretics
    Uncontrolled diabetes mellitus
    Sodium bicarbonate administration
    Saline loading
    Diuretic phase of acute tubular necrosis
    Postobstructive diuresis
    Nonreabsorbable anion administration (e.g., carbenicillin)

Mineralocorticoid excess
  Primary hyperaldosteronism (Conn's syndrome)
  Secondary hyperaldosteronism
    Volume depletion (including third-spacing)
    Diuretics
    Osmotic diuresis
    Cirrhosis
    Nephrotic syndrome
    Congestive heart failure
    Malignant hypertension
    Renal artery stenosis
    Renin-secreting tumors
  Exogenous corticosteroids
  Cushing's syndrome
  Bartter's syndrome
  ACTH-producing tumors
  Reninoma
  Licorice abuse (due to glycyrrhizic acid)
  Carbenoxolone
  Congenital adrenal hyperplasia

intake, gastrointestinal losses, renal losses due to diuretic therapy, and hormonal changes induced by the stress of surgery or trauma are among the most common etiologies in surgical patients.[3,13] Induction of anesthesia itself is generally accompanied by a decrease in serum potassium.[15] Like metabolic alkalosis, respiratory alkalosis causes a net shift of potassium into the intracellular space and can produce mild hypokalemia. Alkalemia induced by hyper-

ventilation during general anesthesia has been correlated with serum potassium decreases of up to 0.05 meq for every one torr change in carbon dioxide tension.[16,17] Patients undergoing cardiac surgery experience fluctuation in serum potassium levels during surgery and can become hypokalemic thereafter. This may be related to the use of extracorporeal circulatory bypass and hypothermia.[18] The association between hypokalemia and hypothermia has also been noted during and after other types of surgery, and is likely due to an intracellular shift of potassium ions.[19] Epinephrine, used frequently in the surgical setting, has long been known to lower serum potassium concentration.[20] Recent studies show that this is due to internal potassium redistribution mediated by $beta_2$ adrenergic agonist activity.[21–23] Thus, sympathetic and adrenal responses to the stress of anesthesia, surgery, and disease most likely play a role in mediating internal shifts in potassium during the perioperative period.

Inadequate extracellular potassium concentration impairs skeletal, cardiac, and smooth muscle function. Potassium deficiency may cause or potentiate metabolic alkalosis, commonly seen in critically ill surgical patients.[24] Hypokalemia increases renal ammoniagenesis and results in increased circulating ammonia levels that may precipitate or exacerbate hepatic encephalopathy in patients with severe liver disease and in those undergoing portal-systemic shunt surgery. Severe hypokalemia can cause skeletal muscle weakness or even frank paralysis, which can result in respiratory failure and death. In experimental settings, hypokalemia augments the paralytic effects of pancuronium bromide and blunts the antagonist effect of neostigmine,[25] but these effects are probably clinically insignificant.[26] Rhabdomyolysis resulting in myoglobinuric renal failure has been attributed to severe potassium depletion.[27] Impaired smooth-muscle function due to hypokalemia may cause gastroparesis or intestinal ileus.

Hypokalemia has several important effects on cardiac function. Severe potassium depletion can cause orthostatic hypotension and exert a negative inotropic effect on the myocardium.[15,28–30] Characteristic electrocardiographic manifestations of hypokalemia include low T-wave amplitude and the development of U waves. The Q-T interval does not lengthen, but the appearance of large U waves and absence of T waves can be easily mistaken for an increased Q-T interval. Experimental and clinical studies in hospitalized patients have demonstrated that hypokalemia may precipitate ventricular arrhythmias. Patients with acute myocardial infarction and those who have undergone cardiac surgery are particularly vulnerable to these arrhythmias.[11,31–37] Even mild-to-moderate hypokalemia can markedly exacerbate the cardiac toxicity of digitalis.

Hypokalemia therefore represents a major cardiac risk factor in general anesthesia and surgery. Because potassium concentrations below 3.0 meq/liter have been shown to be associated with an increased risk of life-threatening complications and death,[38] hypokalemia should be corrected before surgery. Some investigators feel that elective surgery should be postponed until the serum potassium concentration is at least 4.0 meq/liter.[39] However, it is difficult to make strict recommendations applicable to all patients because underlying disease and the chronicity of the electrolyte disturbance are important factors in relating the severity of hypokalemia to operative risk.[3]

The treatment of hypokalemia should begin with determination of the likely cause. Hypokalemia due solely to a shift from the extracellular to the intracellular compartment can be corrected by effectively addressing the cause of redistribution. However, distributional hypokalemia is usually associated with potassium depletion as well. Because of the many factors influencing serum potassium concentration, it is impossible to estimate the extent of potassium depletion accurately. However, potassium levels of 3.0 meq/liter are often associated with a total body deficiency in the range of 100 to 300 meq, and levels of 2.0 meq/liter may indicate a 400 to 700 meq deficit. Hypokalemia associated with ongoing potassium losses requires higher-than-normal replacement and maintenance doses.

Potassium replacement and maintenance are frequently required in preparing patients for surgery and in the postoperative period. Although oral replacement is safest, parenteral therapy may be the only option. Because intravenous potassium can cause substantial morbidity and mortality when used indiscriminately or without careful attention to detail,[40] the dose and rate of infusion should be carefully selected. Recommendations for parenteral replacement vary. If necessary, up to 20 meq of potassium diluted in 100 ml of saline can be safely administered if infused over at least one hour in a closely monitored setting such as an intensive care unit.[41] The dose may be repeated, but the serum potassium level should be monitored frequently to avoid hyperkalemia. Higher infusion rates are rarely indicated. Much lower concentrations and infusion rates should be used in less urgent situations or when continuous electrocardiographic monitoring is not available. Concentrations greater than 40 meq/liter have been associated with pain and phlebitis at the infusion site, but infusion into a large peripheral or central vein or using lower concentrations usually obviates this complication.

The replacement dose and infusion rate are determined by the severity of the potassium deficit, level of renal function, extent of any ongoing renal or gastrointestinal losses, concomitant use of drugs affecting potassium distribution or excretion, and intake of potassium from other sources such as hyperalimentation formulas. Particular caution should be exercised in administering potassium to patients with impaired renal function. The administration of agents that cause redistribution of potassium to the intracellular compartment, such as sodium bicarbonate, insulin, or glucose, can exacerbate hypokalemia. For this reason, it is preferable to administer parenteral potassium in saline rather than in dextrose-containing solutions. If sodium bicarbonate or insulin are necessary to treat concomitant problems, they should be used with caution or withheld if possible until hypokalemia is at least partially treated. In patients with hypokalemia and significant hypoglycemia, administration of glucose cannot be postponed, but this may cause transient exacerbation of hypokalemia if enough potassium is not given expeditiously.

Parenteral potassium is usually administered as the chloride salt. Potassium citrate, acetate, lactate, or gluconate should be considered in hypokalemic patients with metabolic acidosis because these anions are metabolized to bicarbonate. However, if administered to patients with metabolic alkalosis, these alkaline salts exacerbate the acid-base disturbance and lead to further urinary potassium loss. Since hypokalemia is frequently accompanied by metabolic alkalosis, the chloride salt is usually preferred and facilitates correction of the alkalosis.

Hyperkalemia

Hyperkalemia has many causes but is not commonly seen after surgery (see Table 61–2). Metabolic acidosis, intravascular hemolysis, massive erythrocyte transfusions, reabsorption of large hematomas, and severe trauma or tissue destruction cause hyperkalemia

TABLE 61–2. Causes of Hyperkalemia

Hyperkalemia related to altered internal potassium balance

Acid-base disorders
    Metabolic (inorganic) acidosis
    Respiratory acidosis (mild hyperkalemia)

Pharmacologic agents
    Beta-adrenergic antagonists
    Digitalis (severe intoxication)
    Succinylcholine
    Arginine and lysine hydrochloride

Acute cell necrosis
    Rhabdomyolysis; trauma; crush injury
    Hemolysis, including from transfused erythrocytes
    Reabsorption of hematoma
    Burn injury
    Chemotherapy of myelo- and lymphoproliferative disorders

Hormonal deficiency
    Diabetic ketoacidosis
    Hyporenin–hypoaldosterone syndrome

Other
    Hypertonicity
    Hyperkalemic periodic paralysis
    Gastrointestinal hemorrhage
    Malignant hyperthermia

Hyperkalemia related to altered external potassium balance

Potassium administration
    Enteral
        Dietary
        Salt substitutes
        Medicinal oral potassium supplements
    Parenteral
        Maintenance intravenous fluid infusions
        Total parenteral nutrition solutions
        Drugs (e.g., potassium penicillin)
        Transfusion of stored blood

Renal failure (impaired renal filtration)
    Acute renal failure
    Chronic oliguric renal failure

Impaired renal potassium secretion
    Chronic interstitial nephritis (sickle cell disease,
        amyloid, postrenal transplant, lupus)
    Drugs (spironolactone, triamterene, amiloride, angiotensin-
        converting enzyme inhibitors, digitalis)

Aldosterone deficiency
    Addison's disease
    Selective hypoaldosteronism
        Diabetes mellitus
        Chronic interstitial nephritis
        Prostaglandin inhibitors

Tubular unresponsiveness to aldosterone
    Spironolactone
    Chronic interstitial nephritis
    Amyloidosis
    Systemic lupus erythematosis
    Postrenal transplant

Pseudohyperkalemia

Prolonged tourniquet application
In vitro hemolysis
Thrombocytosis
Leukocytosis

by altering internal potassium balance. However, external imbalance due to renal insufficiency or excessive potassium intake is more common. Renal dysfunction is the most frequent reason for hyperkalemia in the perioperative setting.[42]

Pseudohyperkalemia is caused by in vitro hemolysis and release of potassium in a blood specimen. In vitro release of potassium from platelets or leukocytes is rarely seen in patients with severe thrombocytosis or leukemia.[43,44] Analyzing potassium from promptly separated plasma most often resolves the issue. Prolonged tourniquet application combined with fist-clenching may result in spurious elevation of potassium levels in both serum and plasma due to potassium release from ischemic exercising muscle.

Acidemia can cause an increase in serum potassium concentration, sometimes to frankly hyperkalemic levels. Animal studies examining the effects of inorganic acids like hydrochloric acid have demonstrated that potassium levels increase from 0.2 to 1.7 meq/liter for every change of 0.1 unit in pH.[17] Accumulation of sulfuric and phosphoric acids probably plays a role in the development of hyperkalemia in patients with renal failure. On the other hand, experimental infusions of organic acids like lactic or keto-acids do not cause significant changes in potassium levels, and patients with severe lactic acidosis or alcoholic ketoacidosis generally show no change in serum potassium concentration. The nature of the anion therefore appears to be a more important determinant of changes in potassium level than pH itself. The effects of respiratory acidosis are negligible.[17,45]

Although organic acidosis does not elevate serum potassium concentration, hyperkalemia is commonly observed in untreated patients with diabetic ketoacidosis even though they almost invariably have a substantial deficit in total body potassium. This suggests that factors other than pH play a role in determining serum potassium levels. Current evidence implicates several of the effects of insulin deficiency. Insulin is necessary for optimal potassium uptake by hepatic and skeletal muscle tissue, and lack of insulin results in accelerated catabolism and release of intracellular potassium into the serum.[46] The osmotic diuresis resulting from hyperglycemia can eventually lead to renal hypoperfusion and impairment of potassium excretion. In addition, many diabetics have preexisting renal insufficiency. Hypertonicity, whether due to hyperglycemia or infusion of hypertonic saline or mannitol, results in a redistribution of potassium from the intracellular to the extracellular compartment when insulin and aldosterone are deficient.[47–50] Autonomic neuropathy is common in diabetics and may also play a role by interfering with catecholamine release.

Hyperkalemia can be caused by a variety of disorders involving the renin-aldosterone axis, including Addison's disease, congenital adrenal enzyme deficiencies, and corticosteroid withdrawal. The syndrome of hyporeninemic hypoaldosteronism is not uncommon in patients with mild-to-moderate renal insufficiency or diabetes mellitus, and they have a greater risk of developing hyperkalemia if treated with potassium supplements, potassium-sparing diuretics, or angiotensin-converting enzyme inhibitors.[51] Heparin interferes with aldosterone synthesis and has been reported to cause hyperkalemia.[52]

Several other pharmacologic agents can cause hyperkalemia. Succinylcholine has variable effects on serum potassium levels, ranging from none to severe hyperkalemia, with a usual increase of up to 10 percent. However, in patients with major trauma or certain central nervous system disorders, increases of over 80 percent have been observed.[15,53,54] Just as beta-adrenergic agonists may induce hypokalemia, beta-blockers have been reported to cause hyperkalemia.[55] Massive overdoses of digitalis can cause severe hyperkalemia by inhibiting the Na^+K^+-ATPase pump, resulting in efflux of intracellular potassium. Treatment of myeloproliferative and lymphoproliferative disorders with chemotherapeutic agents can lead to substantial tumor necrosis and enough release of intracellular potassium to cause hyperkalemia.[56] The opposite phenomenon has been observed in patients with severe megaloblastic anemia treated with vitamin B_{12} or folic acid in whom rapid increases in blood cell production can result in dangerously low levels of serum potassium.[57,58]

The predominant effects of hyperkalemia are neuromuscular and cardiac. The initial electrocardiographic findings include tall peaked T waves followed by widening of the QRS complex and finally ventricular tachycardia, fibrillation, and/or asystole. Direct inhibition of conduction from the sinus node to the atrioventricular node can result in atrial standstill and absent P waves despite underlying sinus activity. When accompanied by QRS widening, this phenomenon may be indistinguishable from idioventricular rhythm. Acute hyperkalemia is more likely to cause severe cardiac dysfunction than chronic hyperkalemia. Mild-to-moderate hyperkalemia may occur without electrocardiographic changes, but it is distinctly unusual for severe hyperkalemia to occur without significant ECG manifestations.[59] In any case, moderate-to-severe hyperkalemia with levels above 6.0 meq/liter should always be treated as an emergency.[60] Concomitant hypocalcemia, acid-base disturbances, digitalis or catecholamine administration, and underlying cardiac disease are all likely to lower the threshold of cardiac sensitivity to hyperkalemia.

An understanding of the causes of hyperkalemia and appropriate monitoring of the serum potassium concentration minimize the development of serious hyperkalemia in hospitalized patients. Intraoperative potassium measurements may be helpful during prolonged procedures involving substantial muscle trauma or massive blood transfusion.[42] Patients with renal failure require vigilant monitoring in the perioperative period.

Severe hyperkalemia demands immediate institution of therapy to prevent potentially fatal cardiac arrhythmias (see Table 61–3). Intravenous calcium is most rapidly effective and should be the first line of therapy for hyperkalemia associated with ECG changes or severe hyperkalemia with or without ECG manifestations. One-gram ampules of calcium chloride or calcium gluconate provide 13.6 and 4.6 meq of calcium, respectively. An ampule should be infused or injected over at least two minutes, and the dose may be repeated in five minutes if necessary. Calcium does not alter total body potassium stores or affect potassium distribution but directly antagonizes the cardiac effects of hyperkalemia. Its effects are immediate following intravenous administration, but its duration of action is only about 30 minutes. Therapy to redistribute potassium from the extracellular to the intracellular compartment should therefore be instituted immediately after intravenous calcium is given.

Sodium bicarbonate in a dose of 50 to 100 meq, or a combination of insulin and glucose in a dose of 10 units of regular insulin in 500 ml of 10% dextrose given intravenously, lowers the serum potassium concentration within 15 to 30 minutes and acts for up to several hours. Either regimen can be used as first-line therapy for less severe degrees of hyperkalemia without ECG changes. Increasing the extracellular bicarbonate concentration, independent of any change in extracellular pH, results in redistribution of potassium to the intracellular compartment.[61] Sodium bicarbonate is preferred in patients with metabolic acidosis but should be avoided in those with significant alkalemia and metabolic alkalosis. In the presence of alkalemia, calcium followed by glucose and

TABLE 61–3. Treatment of Hyperkalemia

Treatment	Mechanism	Effects on Ks	Effects on TBK	Onset	Duration
Calcium	Direct antagonism	None	None	Seconds	~ 30 min
NaHCO$_3$	Direct antagonism Redistribution	↓	None	15–30 min	Few hours
Glucose and insulin	Redistribution	↓	None	15–30 min	Few hours
Kayexalate	GI excretion	↓	↓	Few hours	Few hours
Peritoneal dialysis	Direct removal	↓	↓	Few hours	Hours–days
Hemodialysis	Direct removal	↓	↓	Few min	Hours–days

Abbreviations: Ks = serum potassium concentration; TBK = total body potassium content.

insulin is the preferred initial treatment of severe hyperkalemia. Intravenous infusions of calcium and bicarbonate are incompatible and result in precipitation of calcium carbonate.

Epinephrine and other beta$_2$ agonists lower serum potassium concentration by causing internal redistribution. Albuterol has also been reported to lower potassium in patients with renal failure.[62] Sodium polystyrene sulfonate (Kayexalate) is an ion-exchange resin that binds approximately one meq of potassium per gram, and can be administered orally or by retention enema in doses of 20 to 50 g with enough sorbitol to effect an osmotic catharsis. However, significant elimination of potassium requires repeated doses and several hours. Hemodialysis is a rapid and highly effective means of removing potassium from the body but may require substantial time to arrange. Peritoneal dialysis is simpler to implement but slower and less effective. The ECG should be monitored continuously during acute therapy of hyperkalemia. Potassium supplements, potassium-sparing diuretics and potassium-containing drugs, and infusions like potassium penicillin and parenteral nutrition formulas should be discontinued.

CALCIUM

Calcium is a key component in a "universal messenger system," mediating muscle contraction; secretion of exocrine, endocrine, and neurocrine products; transport and secretion of fluids and electrolytes; and cell growth.[63,64] There are approximately 1200 grams of calcium in a 70-kg adult, of which 99 percent is found in bones and teeth. Hydroxyapatite, noncrystalline calcium phosphates and carbonates, and small amounts of other calcium salts are found in bone. Body fluids and cells contain only about 10 grams of calcium.[65]

Circulating calcium is found in three forms: protein-bound (40 percent); diffusible and nonionized calcium chelated with phosphate, sulfate, and citrate (15 percent); and physiologically active ionized calcium (45 percent). Most protein-bound calcium is bound to albumin, while 10 to 29 percent is bound to alpha- and beta-globulins. Alterations in serum albumin levels cause marked differences in the circulating concentration of total calcium. In addition, changes in pH affect the fraction of calcium bound to albumin, causing variation in ionized calcium concentration without changes in total calcium levels. Acidemia increases the ionized calcium concentration by decreasing protein-binding, and alkalemia has the opposite effect.[65] Therefore, measurement of ionized calcium levels is necessary to determine the physiologically active fraction. This can now be accomplished rapidly and reliably using ion-selective electrodes. The ionized calcium value is usually corrected to a standard pH of 7.4, although correction to an individual patient's arterial pH may have more physiologic relevance. Proper handling of the blood specimen with minimal delay in measurement and anaerobic precautions similar to those required for blood gas analysis is necessary to obtain accurate data.[66]

The circulating calcium level is closely regulated by parathormone (PTH) and various vitamin D hormones through their effects on bone, kidney, and the gut. A decrease in circulating calcium level elicits an increase in PTH, which stimulates osteoclastic-mediated mobilization of calcium from bone and renal tubular reabsorption of calcium. PTH also stimulates 1-alpha-hydroxylation of 25-hydroxycalciferol in the kidney, leading to the formation of the active vitamin D metabolite 1,25-dihydroxycalciferol.[67] This metabolite stimulates absorption of dietary calcium in the duodenum and colon. The 1,25-dihydroxy form of vitamin D is also necessary for acute mobilization of calcium from bone in response to PTH.[68,69] Although vitamin D deficiency impairs acute mobilization, chronic mobilization in response to increased levels of PTH does not depend on vitamin D.[68] Hypocalcemia may therefore result from inadequate PTH response, vitamin D deficiency, or skeletal resistance to either hormone. The influence of severe acute systemic illness on this homeostatic system is unclear.

Hypocalcemia

Several recent reports suggest that hypocalcemia may occur commonly in acutely ill patients, but there is a wide range in its incidence. Low total and calculated ionized calcium concentrations are found in as many as two-thirds of patients in intensive care units.[70,71] However, calculating ionized calcium levels from total calcium and protein measurements is much less accurate than direct measurement of the physiologically active ionized fraction. Even when direct measurement is performed, the prevalence of ionized hypocalcemia varies between 10 percent and 60 percent among studies.[70–74] This wide variation is probably due to differences in underlying nutritional status, severity of illness, and baseline health status in the patients studied. For example, the prevalence of ionized hypocalcemia in a surgical intensive care unit of a naval hospital was 10 percent, but in medical intensive care units caring for medically indigent populations or patients with cancer it was as high as 60 percent. In our experience, the underlying causes of hypocalcemia cannot be clinically identified in over half of the patients.

The etiologies of hypocalcemia in critically ill patients are shown in Table 61–4. Magnesium (Mg) deficiency is rarely seen alone and is usually part of a complex syndrome of multiple mineral/vitamin deficiencies. Table 61–5 summarizes clinical settings in which hypomagnesemia is most often encountered. Over 20 percent of patients receiving aminoglycosides develop hypomagnesemia, and approximately 10 percent of those develop hypocalcemia. Those with poor oral intake and relative low-normal magnesium levels before therapy are particularly susceptible to hypomagnesemia.[75] Severe hypomagnesemia with levels below 1.2 mg/dl may inhibit parathyroid hormone secretion in response to hypocalcemia.[76] In addition, resistance of bone to the action of PTH also plays a role in the development of hypocalcemia in these patients.[78] Paradoxically, mild hypomagnesemia in the range of 1.2 to 1.8 mg/dl stimulates secretion of PTH.[77] Therefore, hypocalcemia should not be attributed to hypomagnesemia if the serum magnesium concentration is above 1.2 mg/dl. Magnesium is primarily an intracellular cation, and the serum levels can only be used as a rough guide to total body magnesium. In our experience, hypomagnesemia is commonly associated with hypocalcemia in acutely ill patients, and hypocalcemia cannot be corrected until magnesium stores are repleted.[79]

Several mechanisms contribute to hypocalcemia in renal insufficiency, including loss of 1-alpha-hydroxylase activity and skeletal resistance to PTH because of 1,25-dihydroxy vitamin D deficiency.[80] Intestinal absorption of calcium is also impaired even with supplementation of 1,25-dihydroxycalciferol. In addition, hyperphosphatemia, commonly found in renal insufficiency, directly suppresses 1-alpha-hydroxylase activity.[81] These derangements do not usually develop until glomerular filtration is severely compromised. Even then, less than half of the patients with a glomerular filtration rate below 25 ml/min become hypocalcemic.[82] However, severe hypocalcemia develops in patients with oliguric renal failure due to rhabdomyolysis. These patients have marked hyperphosphatemia, hyperuricemia, and elevated creatine phosphokinase levels.[83] Hypocalcemia in these patients may be related to elevation in serum phosphate concentrations and depression of 1,25-dihydroxycalciferol levels. Although renal failure is common in

TABLE 61–4. Etiologies of Hypocalcemia in Critically Ill Patients

Hypomagnesemia (Mg < 1.2 mg/dl)
Vitamin D deficiency
Renal insufficiency (GFR < 25 ml/min)
Alkalemia
Chelation
Citrate (blood transfusion)
Edetate (contrast dyes)
Acute pancreatitis
Trauma to or surgery of the neck
Sepsis
Anticonvulsant therapy
Phenytoin (Dilantin)
Phenobarbital

TABLE 61–5. Etiologies of Hypomagnesemia

Dietary deficiency
Alcoholism
Malabsorption
Malnutrition
Excess loss
Renal
Diabetic ketoacidosis
Renal tubular disorders
Drugs (diuretics, aminoglycosides, cisplatin, amphotericin)
Hyperaldosteronism
Gastrointestinal
Vomiting
Nasogastric suction
Diarrhea
Gastrointestinal fistulae

intensive care units, hypocalcemia should not be assumed to be the result of renal insufficiency unless the glomerular filtration rate is below 25 ml/min.

Alkalemia leads to a fall in the ionized calcium level by increasing binding to calcium.[84] Acidemic patients with borderline low-ionized calcium concentrations can develop tetany after the acidemia is corrected with rapid bicarbonate infusion. Ionized calcium levels decrease by approximately 0.05 mmol/liter for each increase of 0.1 unit in pH. This effect is blunted in the presence of severe hypoalbuminemia.[85]

Massive transfusions of citrate-containing blood may result in chelation of calcium by citrate and a drop in serum ionized calcium levels. Citrate is metabolized primarily by the liver and kidneys, and patients with compromised hepatic or renal function may be particularly susceptible to hypocalcemia after multiple transfusions.[86] Hypothermia and shock also impair citrate clearance. Most patients who develop transfusion-related hypocalcemia do not suffer hemodynamic compromise, and complications such as hypotension and heart failure occur primarily in those with underlying heart disease.[87] Radiographic contrast media also contain calcium chelators, including citrate and edetate. The amount of contrast used for routine cranial computed tomography can lower ionized calcium levels by 0.1 to 0.2 mmol/liter for up to 30 minutes.[88] This may be clinically significant in critically ill patients who may already have relatively low blood pressure. Other less-widely appreciated chelating agents that may induce hypocalcemia include albumin, phosphate, and lipid emulsion solutions used in total parenteral nutrition.

Profound ionized hypocalcemia may develop in acute pancreatitis and is associated with a poor prognosis.[89] Hypocalcemia has been attributed to formation of calcium and fatty-acid complexes in the peripancreatic areas. Hypocalcemia is particularly likely to occur in patients who have very high serum triglyceride levels.[90] These patients have extremely high plasma free fatty-acid levels that may play a role in inducing hypocalcemia.[91] Fatty acids may do this through several mechanisms, including increasing calcium binding to albumin. Plasma free fatty-acid levels may be markedly elevated in other settings like myocardial infarction and diabetic ketoacidosis which are not associated with hypocalcemia.

In addition, these mechanisms cannot entirely explain the prolonged duration of hypocalcemia in patients with acute pancreatitis. Sharp decreases in serum calcium levels should lead to increased PTH secretion with subsequent mobilization of calcium from bone and readjustment of the serum ionized calcium level toward normal. Protracted hypocalcemia in pancreatitis suggests that the PTH-vitamin D axis responsible for maintaining calcium homeostasis may be impaired. Numerous investigators have studied the parathyroid response to hypocalcemia in acute pancreatitis, but the results are conflicting and it is unclear if end-organ responsiveness to PTH remains normal. The vitamin D system has received less attention in pancreatitis, but a single report documents appropriate elevation in serum levels of 1,25-dihydroxycalciferol.[92] Alcoholics have a higher incidence of hypocalcemia when they develop pancreatitis.[93] This may be explained by the vitamin D deficiency and impaired skeletal response to PTH often found in alcoholism.[94]

The hypocalcemia associated with various forms of circulatory shock is difficult to characterize. Animal experiments have documented a decrease in ionized calcium from 1.4 to 1.1 mmol/liter in septic shock. Fluid resuscitation of these animals with lactated Ringer's solution further decreases ionized calcium levels. The same is true in experimental hemorrhagic shock, but the decreases in ionized calcium concentration are smaller.[95] Multiple factors may underlie hypocalcemia in this setting. The PTH response to hypocalcemia appears to be blunted.[96] Although sepsis primarily has been thought to induce hypocalcemia, hypocalcemia may actually predispose patients to sepsis.[70,71,86,96] The role of calcium and vitamin D in modulating activity of the immune system has attracted considerable attention. The active vitamin D metabolite 1,25-dihydroxycalciferol stimulates peroxide secretion in macrophages,[97] modulates monocyte adherence, and stimulates fibronectin secretion.[98] In addition, 1,25-dihydroxycalciferol stimulates synthesis of heat shock proteins that aid in cellular resistance to oxidative and thermal injury.[99]

Chronic therapy with the anticonvulsants phenytoin and phenobarbital can lead to hypocalcemia. Both drugs induce microsomal enzymes in the liver, which may increase metabolism of the active metabolites of vitamin D. They may also directly interfere with absorption of calcium in the gut. However, hypocalcemia does not develop until at least six weeks of treatment have elapsed.[100] Patients on long-term anticonvulsant therapy are particularly prone to the development of hypocalcemia after surgery.

Patients who sustain trauma to the neck or undergo surgery in that area can develop hypocalcemia from damage to or removal of parathyroid tissue. The diagnosis of hypocalcemia in this group of patients is usually straightforward. In other patients, the diagnosis of hypoparathyroidism is usually apparent from the history before surgery or suspected because of low serum calcium and high phosphate levels in the absence of renal insufficiency.

Of the clinical signs of hypocalcemia listed in Table 61–6, neuromuscular irritability, manifested in its more severe forms as

TABLE 61–6. Clinical Manifestations of Hypocalcemia

Neuromuscular
Seizures
Tetany
Trousseau's sign
Chvostek's sign
Cardiovascular
Hypotension
Congestive Heart Failure
Electrophysiologic
Prolonged Q-T interval

seizures and tetany, is the most notable. Trousseau's and Chvostek's signs are early indicators of neuromuscular irritability. Trousseau's sign is seen most frequently, appears earlier, and is often the only clinical sign of hypocalcemia. The blood pressure cuff should be inflated above the systolic pressure for two to three minutes. Ipsilateral carpal spasm should then appear with relaxation following within 5 to 10 seconds of deflation. Immediate relaxation on deflation should arouse suspicion regarding the veracity of the spasm. Chvostek's sign is elicited by tapping the preauricular area. Twitching of the nasal alae and orbital muscles constitutes a truly positive sign.[100–102] Twitching of the corners of the mouth in itself is not specific and occurs in 25 percent of normal subjects.

Experimental animal studies have demonstrated a direct correlation between the concentration of calcium in the extracellular fluid and the contractile state of the heart and vascular smooth muscle.[103,104] Various types of muscle show differences in the extent of their network of sarcoplasmic reticulum. Skeletal muscle has the most extensive network, cardiac muscle is intermediate, and vascular smooth muscle has the least.[105] Calcium ions required to initiate muscle contraction in skeletal muscle are derived almost entirely from the extensive sarcoplasmic reticulum, but cardiac muscle is more dependent upon extracellular calcium. Vascular smooth muscle depends almost entirely on extracellular calcium to initiate contraction. Acute decreases in extracellular calcium concentration have been reported to precipitate hypotension and left ventricular dysfunction.[106–108] Chronic congestive heart failure may be refractory to therapy with digitalis, diuretics, or sympathomimetic agents in the presence of hypocalcemia.[108] Ionized hypocalcemia may make patients with cardiomyopathy particularly prone to hypotension or ventricular failure.

Patients with end-stage renal failure also demonstrate clinically significant alterations in blood pressure and left ventricular function with changes in circulatory calcium levels. Hypotension and ventricular dysfunction have been correlated with decreases in ionized calcium levels that occur with dialysis, and dialysis against high calcium concentrations may prevent these complications.[109,110] Infusion of calcium increases mean arterial pressure, cardiac index, stroke work index, and stroke volume in acutely ill hypocalcemic patients.[73]

The clinical significance of hypocalcemia in acutely ill patients with otherwise normal cardiac and renal function remains unclear. The increase in circulating calcium after infusion with calcium is temporary, as are the vasopressor and hemodynamic effects. It remains to be seen if calcium supplementation reduces the mortality rate in severely ill hypocalcemic patients in intensive care units.

Ionized hypocalcemia prolongs the Q-T interval by prolonging the S-T interval.[111] However, Q-T prolongation, even if corrected for rate, is neither a specific nor sensitive indicator of hypocalcemia because other factors can cause Q-T prolongation. Moreover, Q-T intervals are often normal in patients with ionized hypocalcemia.[111]

The treatment of ionized hypocalcemia should begin with an assessment of its time course and severity. An extremely low level of ionized calcium associated with symptoms obviously requires rapid intravenous calcium replacement. However, the clinician should attempt to identify the underlying causes of hypocalcemia (see Table 61–4) to develop a rational approach to management.

Measurement of serum magnesium levels is important in patients with ionized hypocalcemia because magnesium replacement may be all that is needed to correct the hypocalcemia, often within

24 hours. Calcium infusion should be avoided until magnesium stores are repleted. Calcium accumulates within muscle cells of animals with experimentally induced hypomagnesemic hypocalcemia, and calcium infusion may lead to further increases in intracellular calcium and subsequent cell injury.[112–114] Patients with magnesium levels under 1.0 mg/dl should be assumed to have a total body magnesium deficit between 1 to 4 meq/kg and should receive parenteral magnesium replacement of about 1 mmol/kg over 24 hours. Since 1 g of magnesium sulfate ($MgSO_4$) contains 98 mg of elemental magnesium, equivalent to 8.1 meq or 4 mmol, a 70-kg patient might require 9 g of $MgSO_4$ in the first day. Further therapy should be guided by serum magnesium levels. If tetany or convulsions are present, 2 to 3 g may be given rapidly over five minutes in 30 ml of 5% dextrose in water, and 4 to 6 g may be given over the next two to three hours. The renal tubular threshold for magnesium reabsorption is relatively low, and half of parenterally administered magnesium is excreted into the urine. In the presence of severe renal dysfunction, the dose should be decreased. Patients with hypomagnesemic hypocalcemia often have hypokalemia due to renal potassium wasting, and potassium deficits should be replaced concomitantly.[115] In severe renal failure when creatinine clearance is below 25 to 30 ml/min, phosphate-binding antacids should be used as well to lower serum phosphate and increase serum calcium levels. Vitamin D supplementation can be initiated if the serum ionized calcium level remains low after correction of the serum phosphate concentration.[100,101]

In the large proportion of critically ill patients with hypocalcemia with no readily identifiable cause, calcium infusion raises the serum calcium level only transiently. Within 24 hours, the calcium concentration returns to a depressed level, presumably because the underlying abnormality has not been addressed. In the presence of sustained hypotension, infusion of elemental calcium in a dose of 5 to 10 mg/kg/hr can temporarily improve myocardial function and blood pressure. The patient with hypocalcemic tetany should be treated with 10% calcium gluconate in a dose of 10 to 30 ml over 10 to 15 minutes. A continuous drip of calcium gluconate may then be initiated with close monitoring of serum ionized calcium levels. Vitamin D and calcium supplementation are the treatments of choice in the hypocalcemia found in 20 percent of patients on chronic phenytoin therapy.

Hypercalcemia

In acutely ill patients, hypercalcemia is found much less frequently than hypocalcemia.[101,116] Malignancy and hyperparathyroidism are by far the two most common etiologies of hypercalcemia, and the most common cause of hypercalcemia among hospitalized patients is carcinoma with bony metastases. Other endocrinopathies rarely cause hypercalcemia, and laboratory investigation of these disorders should be pursued only if clinical findings suggest the diagnosis.

Clinical features suggestive of hyperparathyroidism include a history of kidney stones, idiopathic pancreatitis, or refractory peptic ulcer disease in patients who do not smoke. Hypercalcemia documented for more than one year is unlikely to be due to malignancy.[117] A ratio of serum chloride-to-phosphate concentration above 33 and a hematocrit level over 37% suggest hyperparathyroidism. In one series, only 10 percent of patients with hyperparathyroidism and 51 percent of those with nonparathyroid causes of hypercalcemia were anemic.[118] Calcium levels above 14 mg/dl also suggest nonparathyroid etiologies. Only 4 percent of

patients with hyperparathyroidism develop calcium levels above 14 mg/dl as compared to 65 percent of those with hypercalcemia attributable to other causes.[118] The presence of renal insufficiency and hypercalcemia strongly suggests multiple myeloma. Clinical manifestations of hypercalcemia include anorexia, nausea, vomiting, constipation, somnolence, and polyuria due to nephrogenic diabetes insipidus.

Patients with hypercalcemia may have profound volume deficits, and volume repletion with normal saline is the mainstay of treatment. Because hypercalcemia increases vascular tone, blood pressure may be relatively preserved in the presence of severe volume depletion. Saline loading stimulates renal excretion of calcium, and patients may require between four and six, and occasionally up to 12, liters of normal saline per day. Intravenous furosemide should be used to maintain urine output once volume is repleted. Aggressive volume therapy may exacerbate depletion of potassium and magnesium. Hypokalemia and hypomagnesemia may induce cardiac arrhythmias, and hypercalcemia potentiates the arrhythmic effect of these deficiencies. Intravenous use of diphosphonates is effective after saline diuresis has lowered the serum calcium level below 12 mg/dl. The effect of calcitonin may be only transient, and mithramycin should be reserved as the last treatment.

PHOSPHATE

As the major intracellular anion, phosphate is required for many cellular reactions and serves as a component of phospholipids, phosphoproteins, and phosphosugars. The extracellular fluid contains about 1 percent of total body phosphorus, and 80 to 85 percent is found in bone. Gastrointestinal absorption of phosphorus is determined primarily by the amount ingested and is regulated to some extent by 1,25-dihydroxycalciferol. Excess phosphorus is excreted by the kidney. In general, diuretics tend to increase phosphorus excretion.

Hypophosphatemia

Depletion of intracellular phosphate results in hypophosphatemia, but the serum phosphorus level provides only an approximate gauge of the degree of depletion. Clinical signs are not apparent until serum levels fall below 1 mg/dl. Markedly reduced levels of inorganic phosphate, ATP, and ADP have been found in erythrocytes and muscle cells of patients with clinically apparent hypophosphatemia.[119,120]

Of the causes of severe hypophosphatemia listed in Table 61–7, chronic alcoholism is the most common. Multiple factors contribute to phosphate depletion and hypophosphatemia in alcoholic patients. Feeding alcohol to experimental animals causes cellular phosphate depletion, even when they receive nutritionally balanced diets containing phosphate.[121] Protein malnutrition is common in alcoholics and contributes to phosphate depletion. Respiratory alkalosis, a feature of alcoholic withdrawal, causes a shift of phosphate from the extracellular to the intracellular space and further depresses serum phosphate concentration.[122] Alcoholics frequently have coexisting hypomagnesemia that induces a renal tubular phosphate leak,[123] and vitamin D and calcium deficiency with secondary hyperparathyroidism may also contribute to phosphaturia.

TABLE 61–7. Causes of Severe Hypophosphatemia in Critically Ill Patients

Chronic alcoholism
Recovery from diabetic ketoacidosis
Respiratory alkalosis
Hyperalimentation
Recovery from severe malnutrition

TABLE 61–8. Clinical Consequences of Severe Hypophosphatemia

Rhabdomyolysis
Erythrocyte dysfunction and hemolysis
Leukocyte dysfunction
Platelet dysfunction
Myocardial dysfunction
Respiratory muscle weakness and acute respiratory failure

Phosphate depletion can be particularly difficult to identify in alcoholics because of several factors that exert conflicting effects on serum phosphate concentration. Alcohol directly injures muscle cells and can predispose patients to rhabdomyolysis and release of phosphate into the extracellular compartment. Alcoholic ketoacidosis can also shift phosphate from the intracellular to the extracellular space. Therefore, an initially borderline serum phosphate level may fall to a very low level a day or two later as nutritional repletion, correction of acidosis, and development of the alkalosis that frequently accompanies alcohol withdrawal all shift extracellular phosphate into the cell.[119]

Phosphate depletion in diabetic ketoacidosis is partially due to urinary phosphate losses caused by the osmotic diuresis induced by glucosuria. Ketoacidosis also inhibits phosphorylation and thereby shifts phosphates from the intracellular to the extracellular compartment. Phosphate supplementation in patients with diabetic ketoacidosis is controversial. Phosphate levels are usually normal or high on presentation and decrease after treatment with insulin and correction of the acidosis shifts phosphate into cells by the second or third hospital day. Depressed levels of serum phosphate usually correct spontaneously thereafter without treatment, and phosphate supplementation has not been shown to reduce mortality or alter clinical outcome. However, hypophosphatemia in patients with diabetic ketoacidosis may indicate significant phosphate depletion. These patients should be observed for signs of phosphate depletion and may require therapy.[119]

Respiratory alkalosis can lead to hypophosphatemia by shifting phosphate from the extracellular to the intracellular space. Urine phosphate declines to virtually unmeasurable levels. In contrast, metabolic alkalosis induced by the infusion of sodium bicarbonate causes only a slight fall in serum phosphate levels and may actually increase urinary phosphate concentration.[124] Hypophosphatemia has also been reported after recovery from respiratory acidosis.[125]

The hypophosphatemia associated with hyperalimentation has been attributed to a shift of phosphate into the cell due to caloric loading. It characteristically appears five to six days after total parenteral nutrition is initiated. Most patients developing symptoms are severely malnourished and are given large caloric loads of more than 3500 kcal per day.[126] Urinary phosphate levels are usually low, suggesting cellular accumulation of phosphate.[120,126] The hypophosphatemic effect of a caloric load is also observed in a standard glucose tolerance test, and antecedent starvation potentiates the effect.[127] Concurrent cirrhosis and diabetes mellitus also potentiate the effect,[128] while sepsis and beta-blockers blunt it.[65,129]

The clinical features of hypophosphatemia are listed in Table 61–8. Rhabdomyolysis is usually clinically mild and asymptomatic, and occurs in patients receiving caloric loads or in those with diabetic ketoacidosis. Hypophosphatemia has been reported to impair myocardial function.[130] Hemolysis is rare and occurs only when the erythrocyte is exposed to an additional stress like metabolic acidosis. Depletion of 1,2-diphosphoglycerate decreases the ability of hemoglobin to unload oxygen to the tissues.[119,122]

White blood cell function is also compromised by hypophosphatemia. Intracellular levels of ATP, chemotaxis, phagocytosis, and bactericidal activity of granulocytes are impaired in animals made hypophosphatemic after hyperalimentation, and correction of hypophosphatemia reverses these defects. Hypophosphatemia has also been associated with a variety of reversible platelet abnormalities in the experimental setting, including thrombocytopenia, depressed ATP levels, and shortened platelet survival. Although there are few data in humans, these effects have significant clinical implications.

A neurologic picture of areflexic paralysis resembling Guillain-Barré syndrome has been described in patients with hypophosphatemia. A characteristic sequence of neurologic abnormalities develops in those with hypophosphatemia induced by hyperalimentation within about one week of initiating therapy. Tingling of the hands and feet may progress to hypesthesia and weakness, and mental status changes and grand mal seizures have been reported. Respiratory failure has been seen in patients with hypophosphatemia and underlying lung disease.[66,131,132] A strong positive correlation between maximal inspiratory pressure and the serum phosphate level has been documented.[133]

Urgent treatment of hypophosphatemia is indicated only when the serum phosphate level is less than 1 mg/dl and clinical signs or symptoms appear. Intravenous infusion of 0.25 mmol/kg over six hours is a reasonable starting dose. However, infusion rates of 2 to 15 mmol/hr have been used.[119,134–138]

Administering phosphorus to patients with hypercalcemia can result in metastatic calcification. To avoid causing hyperphosphatemia and hypocalcemia, serial serum phosphorus and calcium concentrations should be performed during parenteral phosphate administration. Hypomagnesemia may predispose patients to hypocalcemia after phosphate infusion because it may inhibit the response of PTH to a falling serum calcium level.

When the serum phosphate level is greater than 1 mg/dl, phosphate can be administered orally by increasing phosphorus in the diet or by prescribing neutral sodium phosphate in a dose of 250 mg twice or three times daily. However, oral therapy is often limited by diarrhea. Phosphorus can also be added to hyperalimentation fluid as needed.

Hyperphosphatemia

Hyperphosphatemia is most commonly caused by impaired renal function. Other causes include increased intake, vitamin D intoxication, hypoparathyroidism, and release of intracellular phosphate stores as seen in acidosis, rhabdomyolysis, hemolysis, malignant hyperthermia, and tumor lysis syndrome. Hyperphosphatemia has rarely been reported following the use of phosphate-containing enemas.[139,140]

There is usually a reciprocal relationship between serum levels of phosphate and calcium, and clinical manifestations of hyperphosphatemia are generally related to the concomitant hypocalcemia. Extreme elevations in serum phosphate concentrations, particularly when the serum calcium level is normal or elevated, can lead to metastatic calcification of calcium phosphate in various tissues including the heart, blood vessels, lungs, kidneys, and cornea.

Treatment of hyperphosphatemia is aimed at controlling phosphate intake and enhancing renal and gastrointestinal excretion. Dietary restriction alone is usually ineffective in patients with significant renal insufficiency. Volume expansion and diuretic administration are effective in severe acute hyperphosphatemia like that seen in tumor lysis syndrome or rhabdomyolysis if renal function is normal, but these measures may not be feasible in patients with severe renal failure. Aluminum hydroxide and aluminum carbonate antacids effectively bind phosphate in the intestinal tract, resulting in the formation of nonabsorbable complexes.

MAGNESIUM

Magnesium is a required cofactor in hundreds of intracellular enzymatic reactions necessary for normal biochemical and physiologic function. Approximately 99 percent of total body magnesium is found in the intracellular space. Dietary magnesium is absorbed in the small intestine and excreted by the kidney. Serum levels poorly reflect intracellular concentration.

Hypomagnesemia

Hypomagnesemia is the most common electrolyte disturbance seen in hospitalized patients, particularly in the critically ill, and severe hypomagnesemia is associated with increased mortality.[141-145] The causes of hypomagnesemia are listed in Table 61–5. Clinical manifestations, usually not apparent unless the serum magnesium level is extremely depressed, include alterations in mental status, nystagmus, muscle twitching, weakness, and tremor.[146]

Hypomagnesemia can provoke ventricular and supraventricular arrhythmias, and case reports have demonstrated that rapid correction of hypomagnesemia is beneficial in patients with a variety of rhythm disturbances including ventricular tachycardia.[147] Several studies have shown that magnesium supplementation decreases the incidence of arrhythmias following acute myocardial infarction and may improve survival.[148-152] It is therefore routine practice to administer magnesium to hospitalized patients with hypomagnesemia, particularly those with a high risk of arrhythmias.

Because intracellular magnesium deficiency is not uncommon in patients with normal serum magnesium concentrations,[153,154] parenteral magnesium should also be considered in patients with normal levels who have serious or life-threatening arrhythmias. Parenteral magnesium administration is generally safe in patients with normal renal function. However, the ion has vasodilator properties and can cause transient hypotension, especially if given by rapid intravenous injection.

Hypermagnesemia

Although uncommon, hypermagnesemia has been reported in as many as 5 percent of postoperative patients and 9 percent of medical patients admitted to intensive care units.[144,145] It develops primarily in patients with abnormal renal function who ingest increased magnesium and is usually seen in those with renal failure who are taking large doses of magnesium-containing antacids. Severe elevations are associated with respiratory paralysis, hypotension, bradycardia, and cardiac arrest. Treatment begins with ensuring that magnesium intake is curtailed. In extreme cases, calcium should be administered as an antagonist, and dialysis should be seriously considered.

SUMMARY

1. Disorders of potassium, calcium, phosphate and magnesium homeostasis arising in the perioperative period may be manifestations of underlying disease or complications of acute illness, surgery itself, or postoperative therapy. These disorders are best treated by understanding and addressing the underlying cause.

2. Hypokalemia is most often due to depletion from inadequate intake, gastrointestinal losses, renal losses due to diuretic therapy and hormonal changes induced by the stress of surgery and anesthesia. Inadequate extracellular potassium concentrations impair skeletal, cardiac and smooth muscle function. Although serum concentrations may not accurately reflect tissue levels, subnormal concentrations should be treated with oral or parenteral replacement.

3. Although less common that hypokalemia, hyperkalemia in the perioperative period is most frequently caused by renal insufficiency and is often exacerbated by administration of potassium and certain pharmacologic agents. In hyperkalemic patients, electrocardiographic monitoring is essential to avoid cardiac complications. Depending on the urgency of the situation, treatment consists of discontinuing all potassium-containing fluids; administering calcium, sodium bicarbonate, insulin and glucose, and/or sodium polystyrene sulfonate; or instituting dialysis.

4. The treatment of hypocalcemia is dictated by its etiology (see Table 61–4), time course, and severity. In cases of ionized hypocalcemia, underlying hypomagnesemia should be documented and treated before calcium replacement is instituted. However, severe symptomatic hypocalcemia manifested by neuromuscular irritability should be treated with parenteral calcium gluconate. Hypocalcemia can contribute to hypotension and left ventricular dysfunction in seriously ill surgical patients.

5. Hypercalcemia is less common than hypocalcemia in surgical patients, is usually due to underlying malignancy or hyperparathyroidism, and can cause anorexia, vomiting, constipation, somnolence and polyuria. Hypercalcemic patients can maintain relatively normal blood pressure in the presence of severe hypovolemia. Initial treatment consists of volume repletion with saline followed by diuresis with furosemide.

6. Severe hypophosphatemia can develop in malnourished surgical patients with chronic alcoholism when they are nutritionally repleted or in those receiving hyperalimentation. When feasible oral phosphate can be administered, but more rapid parenteral therapy is required when the serum phosphate level falls below one mg/dl and clinical signs or symptoms as enumerated in Table 61–8 appear.

7. Hyperphosphatemia is most often the result of impaired renal function but in the surgical setting can be the result of rhabdomyolysis, hemolysis or malignant hyperthermia. Symptoms are usually due to concomitant hypocalcemia. Treatment consists of limiting phosphate intake and enhancing renal and gastrointestinal excretion with volume expansion, diuretics and aluminum-containing antacids.

8. Hypomagnesemia is the most common electrolyte disturbance seen in hospitalized patients. Severe hypomagnesemia is associated with cardiac arrhythmias and increased mortality. Magnesium should therefore be replaced expectantly in all surgical patients with decreased serum levels.

9. Hypermagnesemia is almost always encountered in patients with renal insufficiency who ingest excess magnesium or take large doses of magnesium-containing antacids. Magnesium intake should be curtailed, and in extreme cases calcium should be administered and dialysis seriously considered.

REFERENCES

1. DeFronzo RA, Bia M: Extrarenal potassium homeostasis, in Seldin DW, Giebish G (eds): *The Kidney: Physiology and Pathophysiology.* New York, Raven Press, 1985, pp 1179–1206.

2. Horton R, Zipser RD: Hypokalemia and hyperkalemia, in Massry SG, Glassock RJ (eds): *Textbook of Nephrology.* Baltimore, Williams & Wilkins, 1983, vol 3, pp 40–48.

3. Sack RA, Kroener WF Jr: Hypokalemia of various etiologies complicating elective surgical procedures. *Am J Obstet Gynec* 149:74–78, 1984.

4. Miller TA, Duke JH Jr: Fluid and electrolyte management, in Dudrick SJ, Baue AE, Eiseman B et al (eds): *Manual of Preoperative and Postoperative Care.* Philadelphia, Saunders, 1983, pp 51–61.

5. Wharton RS, Masse RI: Fluid and electrolyte problems, in Orkin FK, Cooperman LH (eds): *Complications in Anesthesiology.* Philadelphia, Lippincott, 1983, pp 396–399.

6. Richardson RMA, Kunau RT Jr: Potassium deficiency and intoxication, in Seldon DW, Giebisch G (eds): *The Kidney: Physiology and Pathophysiology.* New York, Raven Press, 1985, pp 1251–1267.

7. Newmark SR, Dluhy RG: Hyperkalemia and hypokalemia. *JAMA* 231:631–633, 1975.

8. Paice BJ, Paterson KR, Onyanga-Omara F et al: Record linkage study of hypokalemia in hospitalized patients. *Postgrad Med J* 62:187–191, 1986.

9. McCarron D: Correcting potassium depletion. *Drug Therapy* 4:65–72, 1979.

10. Ferguson CM, Sherman R, Lubin MF: Metabolic disturbances, in Lubin MF, Walker HK, Smith RB III (eds): *Medical Management of the Surgical Patient,* 2d ed. Boston, Butterworths, 1988, pp 463–464.

11. Nordrehaug JE, von der Lippe G: Hypokalemia and ventricular fibrillation in acute myocardial infarction. *Br Heart J* 50:525–529, 1983.

12. Tweedle DEF: Electrolyte disorders in the surgical patient. *Clin Endocrinol Metab* 13:351–365, 1984.

13. Bevan DR: Acute biochemical disorders, in Vickers MD (ed): *Medicine for Anaesthetists,* 2d ed. Boston, Blackwell, 1982, pp 322–325.

14. Schaber DE, Uden DL, Stone FM et al: Intravenous KCl supplementation in pediatric cardiac surgical patients. *Pediatr Cardiol* 6:25–28, 1985.

15. Vaughan RS, Lunn JN: Potassium and the anaesthetist. *Anaesthesia* 28:118–131, 1973.

16. Edwards R, Winnie AP, Remamurthy S: Acute hypocapneic hypokalemia: An iatrogenic anesthetic complication. *Anesth Analg* 56:786–792, 1977.

17. Adrogue HJ, Madias NE: Changes in plasma potassium concentration during acute acid-base disturbances. *Am J Med* 71:456–467, 1981.

18. Drake HF, Treasure T, Smith B: Continuous display of plasma potassium during cardiac surgery. *Anaesthesia* 42:23–29, 1987.

19. Boelhouwer RU, Bruining HA, Ong GL: Correlations of serum potassium fluctuations with body temperature after major surgery. *Crit Care Med* 15:310–312, 1987.

20. D'Silva JL: The action of adrenaline on serum potassium. *J Physiol* 82:393–398, 1934.

21. Brown MJ, Brown DC, Murphy MB: Hypokalemia from beta$_2$ receptor stimulation by circulating epinephrine. *N Engl J Med* 309:1414–1419, 1983.

22. Rohr AS, Spector SL, Rachelefsky GS et al: Efficacy of parenteral albuterol in the treatment of asthma. Comparison of its metabolic side effects. *Chest* 89:348–351, 1986.

23. Struthers AD, Whitesmith R, Ried JL: Prior thiazide diuretic treatment increases adrenaline-induced hypokalemia. *Lancet* 1:1358–1361, 1983.

24. Wilson RF, Gibson D, Percinel AK et al: Severe alkalosis in critically ill surgical patients. *Arch Surg* 105:197, 1972.

25. Miller RD, Roderick LL: Diuretic-induced hypokalemia, pancuronium neuromuscular blockade, and its antagonism by neostigmine. *Br J Anaesth* 50:541–544, 1978.

26. Stoelting RK, Dierdorf SF, McCammon RL: *Anesthesia and Coexisting Disease,* 2d ed. New York, Churchill Livingstone, 1988, pp 456–465.

27. Knochel JP, Schlein EM: On the mechanism of rhabdomyolysis in potassium depletion. *J Clin Invest* 51:1750–1758, 1972.

28. Abbrecht PH: Cardiovascular effects of chronic potassium deficiency in the dog. *Am J Physiol* 223:555–559, 1972.

29. Gelbart A, Hall RJ, Goldman R: Effects of hypokalemia on the cardiotropic actions of digoxin in dogs. *Circ Res* 46(Suppl):I173–I174, 1980.

30. Biglieri EG, McIlroy MB: Abnormalities of renal function and circulatory reflexes in primary aldosteronism. *Circulation* 33:78–86, 1966.

31. Hulting J: In-hospital ventricular fibrillation and its relation to serum potassium. *Acta Med Scand* 647(Suppl):101–107, 1981.

32. Fisch C: Relation of electrolyte disturbances to cardiac arrhythmias. *Circulation* 47:408–419, 1973.

33. Poole-Wilson PA: Potassium and the heart. *Clin Endocrinol Metab* 13:249–268, 1984.

34. Helfant RH: Hypokalemia and arrhythmias. *Am J Med* 80(Suppl 4A):13–22, 1986.

35. Manning SH, Angaran DM, Arom KV et al: Intermittent intravenous potassium therapy in cardiopulmonary bypass patients. *Clin Pharm* 1:234–238, 1982.

36. Kafka H, Langevin L, Armstrong PW: Serum magnesium and potassium in acute myocardial infarction. Influence on ventricular arrhythmias. *Arch Intern Med* 147:465–469, 1987.

37. Hohnloser SH, Verrier RL, Lown B et al: Effect of hypokalemia on susceptibility to ventricular fibrillation in the normal and ischemic canine heart. *Am Heart J* 112:32–35, 1986.

38. Goldman L, Caldera DL, Nussbaum SR et al: Multifactorial index of cardiac risk in noncardiac surgical procedures. *N Engl J Med* 297:845–850, 1977.

39. Narins RG, Lazarus JM: Renal system, in Vandam LD (ed): *To Make the Patient Ready for Anesthesia: Medical Care of the Surgical Patient,* 2d ed. Menlo Park, CA, Addison-Wesley, 1984, pp 94–101.

40. Lawson DH: Adverse reaction to potassium chloride. *Quart J Med* 43:433–440, 1974.

41. Kruse JA, Carlson RW: Rapid correction of hypokalemia using concentrated intravenous potassium chloride infusions. *Arch Intern Med* 150:613–617, 1990.

42. Yim CW: Maintaining renal function of surgical patients, in Bolt RJ (ed): *Medical Evaluation of the Surgical Patient*. Mt. Kisco, NY, Futura, 1987, pp 301–306.

43. Bronson WR, Devita VT, Carbone PK: Pseudohyperkalemia due to release of potassium from white blood cells during clotting. *N Engl J Med* 274:369–375, 1966.

44. Ingram RH, Seki M: Pseudohyperkalemia with thrombocytosis. *N Engl J Med* 267:895–900, 1962.

45. Magner PO, Robinson L, Halperin RM et al: The plasma potassium concentration in metabolic acidosis: A reevaluation. *Am J Kidney Dis* 11:220–224, 1988.

46. Perez GO, Oster JR, Vaamonde CA: Serum potassium concentration in academic states. *Nephron* 27:233–243, 1981.

47. Makoff DL, Dasilva JA, Rosenbaum BJ: On the mechanism of hyperkalemia due to hyperosmotic expansion with saline and mannitol. *Clin Sci* 42:383, 1971.

48. Goldfarb S, Cox M, Singer I et al: Acute hyperkalemia induced by hyperglycemia: Hormonal mechanisms. *Ann Intern Med* 84:426–432, 1976.

49. Viberti GC: Glucose-induced hyperkalemia: A hazard for diabetics. *Lancet* 1:690, 1978.

50. Nicolis GL, Kahn T, Sanchez A, Gabrilove JL: Glucose-induced hyperkalemia in diabetic subjects. *Arch Intern Med* 141:49–53, 1981.

51. Hollenberg NK, Michiewicz C: Hyperkalemia in diabetes mellitus. *Arch Intern Med* 149:1327–1330, 1989.

52. O'Kelly R, Magee F, McKenna J: Routine heparin therapy inhibits adrenal aldosterone production. *J Clin Endocrinol Metab* 56:108–112, 1983.

53. Inaba H, Ohwada T, Sato J et al: Effects of salbutamol and hyperventilation on the rise in serum potassium after succinylcholine administration. *Acta Anaesth Scand* 31:524–528, 1987.

54. Minton MD, Stirt JA, Bedford RF: Serum potassium following succinylcholine in patients with brain tumors. *Can Anaesth Soc J* 33:328–331, 1986.

55. Clausen T: Adrenergic control of Na+-K+-homeostasis. *Acta Med Scand* 672(Suppl):111–115, 1983.

56. Arseneau JC, Bagley CL, Anderson T et al: Hyperkalemia, a sequel to chemotherapy of Burkitt's lymphoma. *Lancet* 1:10, 1973.

57. Lawson DH, Murray RM, Parker JLW: Early mortality in the megaloblastic anaemias. *West J Med* 41:1–14, 1972.

58. Hesp R, Chanarin I, Tait CE: Potassium changes in megaloblastic anemia. *Clin Sci Molec Med* 49:77, 1975.

59. Szerlip HM, Weiss J, Singer I: Profound hyperkalemia without electrocardiographic manifestations. *Am J Kidney Dis* 7:461–465, 1986.

60. Weisberg LS, Szerlip HM, Cox M: Disorders of potassium homeostasis in critically ill patients. *Crit Care Clin* 5:835–854, 1987.

61. Fraley DS, Adler S: Isohydric regulation of plasma potassium by bicarbonate in the rat. *Kidney Int* 9:333, 1976.

62. Montoliu J, Lens XM, Revert L: Potassium-lowering effect of albuterol for hyperkalemia in renal failure. *Arch Intern Med* 147:713–717, 1987.

63. Rasmussen H: The calcium messenger system (part 1). *N Engl J Med* 314:1194–1201, 1986.

64. Rasmussen H: The calcium messenger system (part 2). *N Engl J Med* 314:1164–1170, 1986.

65. Massry SG, Kaptein EM: Hypercalcemia and hypocalcemic states, in Seldin DW, Geibisch G (eds): *The Kidney*. New York, Raven Press, 1985, pp 1337–1364.

66. Agusti A, Torres A, Agustividal A: Hypophosphatemia as a cause of failed weaning: The importance of metabolic factors. *Crit Care Med* 12:142–152, 1984.

67. Booth BE, Tsai HC, Morris RD: Parathyroidectomy reduces 25-hydroxy-vitamin D_3-1-alpha-hydroxylase activity in the hypocalcemic vitamin D-deficient chick. *J Clin Invest* 60:1314–1320, 1977.

68. Breslau NA, Pak CYC: Hypoparathyroidism. *Metabolism* 28:1261–1276, 1979.

69. Holick MD, DeLuca HF: The role of vitamin D metabolites in nephric resorption. *Calcif Tissue Res* 12:295–301, 1973.

70. Chernow B, Zaloga GP, McFadden E et al: Hypocalcemia in critically ill patients. *Crit Care Med* 10:848–851, 1982.

71. Zaloga GP, Chernow B, Cook D et al: Assessment of calcium homeostasis in the critically ill patient. The diagnostic pitfalls of the McLean-Hastings nomogram. *Ann Surg* 202:587–594, 1985.

72. Desai TK, Carlson RW, Geheb MA: The parathyroid-vitamin D axis in critically ill patients with unexplained hypocalcemia. *Kidney Int* 32(Suppl 22):S225–S228, 1987.

73. Desai TK, Geheb MA, Haupt MT et al: Hypocalcemia in critically ill patients. *Am J Med* 84:209–214, 1988.

74. Szyfelbein SK, Drop LJ, Martyn J: Persistent ionized hypocalcemia in patients during resuscitation and recovery phases of body burns. *Crit Care Med* 9:454–458, 1981.

75. Zaloga GP, Chernow B, Pock A et al: Hypomagnesemia is a common complication of aminoglycoside therapy. *Surg Gynecol Obstet* 158:561–565, 1984.

76. Anast CS, Mohs JM, Kaplan S et al: Evidence for parathyroid failure in magnesium deficiency. *Science* 177:606–660, 1972.

77. Buckle RM, Care AD, Cooper CW et al: The influence of plasma magnesium concentration on parathyroid secretion. *J Endocrinol* 42:529–534, 1968.

78. Estep H, Shaw WA, Watlington C et al: Hypocalcemia due to hypomagnesemia and reversible parathyroid unresponsiveness. *J Clin Endocrinol Metab* 29:842–848, 1969.

79. Shils ME: Experimental human magnesium depletion. *Medicine* 48:61–85, 1969.

80. Coburn JW, Slatopolsky E: Vitamin D, parathyroid hormone and renal osteodystrophy, in Brenner BM, Rector FC (eds): *The Kidney*. Philadelphia, Saunders, 1986, pp 1657–1729.

81. Tanaka Y, DeLuca HF: The control of 25-hydroxyvitamin D metabolism by inorganic phosphorus. *Arch Biochem Biophys* 154:566–574, 1973.

82. Coburn J, Popovitzer M, Massry SG et al: The physiochemical state and renal handling of divalent ions in chronic renal failure. *Arch Intern Med* 124:302–311, 1969.

83. Grossman RA, Hamilton RW, Morse BM et al: Nontraumatic rhabdomyolysis and acute renal failure. *N Engl J Med* 291:807–811, 1974.

84. Moore E: Ionized calcium in normal serum, ultrafiltrates and whole blood determined by ion-exchange electrode. *Clin Invest* 49:318–334, 1970.

85. Wybenga DR, Ibbot FA, Cannon DC: Determination of ionized calcium in serum that has been exposed to air. *Clin Chem* 22:1009–1011, 1976.

86. Zaloga GP, Chernow B: Hypocalcemia in critical illness. *JAMA* 256:1924–1929, 1986.

87. Olinger GN, Hottenrot C, Mulder DG et al: Acute clinical hypocalcemic myocardial depression during rapid blood transfusion and postoperative hemodialysis. *J Thorac Cardiovasc Surg* 72:503–511, 1976.

88. Berger RE, Gomez LD, Mallette LE: Acute hypocalcemic effects of clinical contrast media injections. *Am J Radiol* 138:283–288, 1982.

89. Ranson JHC, Rifkind KM, Turner JW: Prognostic signs and nonoperative peritoneal lavage in acute pancreatitis. *Surg Gynecol Obstet* 143:209–219, 1976.

90. Cameron JL, Crisler C, Margolis S et al: Acute pancreatitis with hyperlipemia. *Surgery* 70:53–61, 1971.

91. Warshaw AL, Lee KH, Napier TW et al: Depression of serum calcium by increased plasma free fatty acids in the rat: A mechanism for hypocalcemia in acute pancreatitis. *Gastroenterology* 89:814–820, 1985.

92. Hauser CJ, Kamrath RW, Sparks J et al: Calcium homeostasis in

patients with acute pancreatitis. *Surgery* 94:830–835, 1983.

93. Decaux G, Hallemans R, Mockel J et al: Chronic alcoholism: A predisposing factor for hypocalcemia in acute pancreatitis. *Digestion* 20:175–179, 1980.

94. Bikle DD, Genant HK, Cann C et al: Bone disease in alcohol abuse. *Ann Intern Med* 103:42–48, 1985.

95. Trunkey D, Carpenter MA, Holcroft J: Ionized calcium and magnesium: The effect of septic shock in the baboon. *J Trauma* 18:166–172, 1978.

96. Taylor B, Sibbalb WJ, Edmonds MW et al: Ionized hypocalcemia in critically ill patients with sepsis. *Can J Surg* 21:429–433, 1978.

97. Cohen MS, Mesler DE, Snipes RG et al: 1,25(OH$_2$) D$_3$ activates H$_2$O$_2$ secretion by human monocyte derived macrophages. *Clin Res* 33:397A, 1985.

98. Palmiere GMA, Bertorini TE, Nutting DS et al: Muscle accumulation in muscular dystrophy and acute pancreatitis: A common pathogenic mechanism. *Acta Endocrinol Suppl* 256:103, 1983.

99. Polla BS, Healy AM, Amento EP et al: 1,25(OH$_2$) D$_3$ maintains adherence of human monocytes and protects them from thermal injury. *J Clin Invest* 77:1332–1338, 1986.

100. Benabe V, Martinez-Maldonado M: Disorders of calcium metabolism, in Maxwell MH, Kleeman CR, Narins RG (eds): *Clinical Disorders of Fluid and Electrolyte Metabolism.* New York, McGraw-Hill, 1987, pp 759–788.

101. Massry SG, Kaptein EM: Hypercalcemia and hypocalcemic states, in Seldin DW, Giebisch G (eds): *The Kidney: Physiology and Pathophysiology.* New York, Raven Press, 1985, vol 2, pp 1337–1364.

102. Duboise GD, Arieff AI: Clinical manifestations of electrolyte disorders, in Arieff AI, DeFronzo RA (eds): *Fluid, Electrolyte, and Acid-Base Disorders.* New York, Churchill Livingstone, 1985, pp 1087–1144.

103. Bristow MR, Schwartz HD, Binetti G et al: Ionized calcium and the heart. *Circ Res* 41:565–573, 1977.

104. Dillon PF, Murphy RA: Tonic force maintenance with reduced shortening velocity in arterial smooth muscle. *Am J Physiol* 242:102–209, 1982.

105. Franzini-Armstrong C: Fine structure of sarcoplasmic reticulum and transverse tubular system in muscle fibers. *Fed Proc* 23:887–895, 1964.

106. Bashour T, Basha HS, Cheng TO: Hypocalcemic cardiomyopathy. *Chest* 78:663–665, 1980.

107. Connor TB, Rosen BL, Blaustein MP et al: Hypocalcemia precipitating congestive heart failure. *N Engl J Med* 307:869–872, 1982.

108. Ginsberg R, Esserman LJ, Bristow MR: Myocardial performance and extra-cellular ionized calcium in a severely failing human heart. *Ann Intern Med* 98:603–606, 1983.

109. Henrich WL, Hunt JM, Nixon JV: Increased ionized calcium and left ventricular contractility during hemodialysis. *N Engl J Med* 310:19–23, 1984.

110. Maynard JC, Cruz C, Kleerekoper M et al: Blood pressure response to changes in serum ionized calcium during hemodialysis. *Ann Intern Med* 104:358–361, 1986.

111. Rumancik WM, Denlinger JK, Nahrwold ML et al: The QT interval and serum ionized calcium. *JAMA* 240:366–368, 1978.

112. Knochel JM: Neuromuscular manifestations of electrolyte disorders. *Am J Med* 72:521–535, 1982.

113. Okuno F, Orrego H, Israel Y: Calcium requirement for anoxic liver cell injury. *Res Commun Chem Pharmacol* 39:437–443, 1983.

114. Schane FA, Kane AB, Young EE: Calcium dependence of toxic cell death: A common pathway. *Science* 206:770–772, 1979.

115. Brautbar N, Massry SG: Hypomagnesemia and hypermagnesemia, in Maxwell MH, Kleeman CR, Narins RG (eds): *Clinical Disorders of Fluid and Electrolyte Metabolism.* New York, McGraw-Hill, 1987, pp 31–49.

116. Skrabanek P, McParth J, Powell D: Tumor hypercalcemia and "ectopic hyperparathyroidism." *Medicine* 59:262–280, 1980.

117. Wong ET, Freier EF: The differential diagnosis of hypercalcemia: An algorithm for more effective use of laboratory tests. *JAMA* 247:75–80, 1982.

118. Lafferty FW: Primary hyperparathyroidism: Changing clinical spectrum, prevalence of hypertension, and discriminant analysis of laboratory tests. *Arch Intern Med* 89:1761–1766, 1981.

119. Knochel JP: Hypophosphatemia. *West J Med* 134:15–26, 1981.

120. Lichtman MA, Miller DK, Cohen J et al: Reduced red-cell glycolysis, 2,3-DPG, and ATP concentration and increased hemoglobin oxygen affinity caused by hypophosphatemia. *Ann Intern Med* 74:562–568, 1971.

121. Blachley J, Ferguson E, Carter N et al: Chronic alcohol ingestion induces phosphorus deficiency and myopathy in the dog. *Trans Assoc Am Physicians* 93:110–122, 1980.

122. Brautbar N, Kleeman CR: Hypomagnesemia and hypermagnesemia, in Maxwell MH, Kleeman CR, Narins RG (eds): *Clinical Disorders of Fluid and Electrolyte Metabolism.* New York, McGraw-Hill, 1979, pp 31–49.

123. Cronin RE, Ferguson ER, Shannon WA et al: Skeletal muscle injury after magnesium depletion in the dog. *Am J Physiol* 243:F113–F120, 1982.

124. Mostellat ME, Tuttle EP: The effects of alkalosis on plasma concentration and urinary excretion of inorganic phosphate in man. *J Clin Invest* 43:138–149, 1964.

125. Storm TL: Severe hypophosphatemia during recovery from acute respiratory acidosis. *Br Med J* 289:456–457, 1984.

126. Silvis SE, Paragas PD: Paresthesias, weakness, seizures, and hypophosphatemia in patients receiving hyperalimentation. *Gastroenterology* 62:413–420, 1972.

127. Corredor DG, Sabeh G, Mendelsohn LV et al: Enhanced postglucose hypophosphatemia during starvation therapy of obesity. *Metabolism* 1:754–763, 1969.

128. Danowski TS, Gillespie HK, Fergus EB et al: Significance of blood sugar and serum electrolyte changes in cirrhosis following insulin, glucagon or epinephrine. *Yale J Biol Med* 29:361–375, 1956.

129. Riedler GF, Scheitlon WA: Hypophosphatemia in septicemia: Higher incidence in gram-negative than in gram-positive infections. *Br J Med* 1:753–756, 1969.

130. O'Connor LR, Wheeler WS, Bethune JS: Effect of hypophosphatemia on myocardial performance in man. *N Engl J Med* 297:901–903, 1977.

131. Newman JH, Neff TA, Ziporin P: Acute respiratory failure associated with hypophosphatemia. *N Engl J Med* 296:1101–1103, 1977.

132. Varsano S, Shapiro M, Taragan R et al: Hypophosphatemia as a reversible cause of refractory ventilatory failure. *Crit Care Med* 11:908–909, 1983.

133. Aubier M, Murciano D, Lecocquic Y et al: Effect of hypophosphatemia on diaphragmatic contractility in patients with acute respiratory failure. *N Engl J Med* 313:420–424, 1985.

134. Kingston M, Al-Siba'l MB: Treatment of severe hypophosphatemia. *Crit Care Med* 13:16–18, 1985.

135. Lentz RD, Brown DM, Kjellstrand CM: Treatment of severe hypophosphatemia. *Ann Intern Med* 9:941–944, 1978.

136. Lloyd CW, Johnson CE: Management of hypophosphatemia. *Clin Pharm* 7:123–128, 1988.

137. Zaloga GP: Hypophosphatemia in COPD: How serious—and what to do? *J Crit Illness* 7:364–375, 1992.

138. Kruse JA, Al-Douahji M, Carlson RW: Rapid intravenous phosphorus replacement in critically ill patients. *Crit Care Med* 20:S104, 1992.

139. Reedy JC, Zwiren GT: Enema-induced hypocalcemia and hyperphosphatemia leading to cardiac arrest during induction of anesthesia in an outpatient surgery center. *Anesthesiology* 59:578–579, 1983.

140. Biberstein M, Parker BA: Enema-induced hyperphosphatemia. *Am J Med* 79:645–646, 1985.

141. Whang R, Ryder KW: Frequency of hypomagnesemia and hypermagnesemia. Requested versus routine. *JAMA* 263:3063–3064, 1990.

142. Ryzen E, Wagers PW, Signer FR et al: Magnesium deficiency in a medical ICU population. *Crit Care Med* 13:19–21, 1985.

143. Rubeiz GJ, Thill-Baharozian M, Hardie D et al: Association of hypomagnesemia and mortality in acutely ill medical patients. *Crit Care Med* 21:203–209, 1993.

144. Reinhart RA, Desbiens NA: Hypomagnesemia in patients entering the ICU. *Crit Care Med* 13:506–507, 1985.

145. Chernow B, Bamberger S, Stoiko M et al: Hypomagnesemia in patients in postoperative intensive care. *Chest* 95:391–397, 1989.

146. Kingston ME, Al-Siba'l MB, Skooge WC: Clinical manifestations of hypomagnesemia. *Crit Care Med* 14:950–954, 1986.

147. Perticone F, Adinolfi L, Bonaduce D: Efficacy of magnesium sulfate in the treatment of torsade de pointes. *Am Heart J* 112:847–849, 1986.

148. Teo KK, Yusuf S, Collins R et al: Effects of intravenous magnesium in suspected acute myocardial infarction: Overview of randomized trials. *Br Med J* 303:1499–1503, 1991.

149. Smith LF, Heagerty AM, Bing RF et al: Intravenous infusions of magnesium sulfate after acute myocardial infarction: Effects on arrhythmias and mortality. *Int J Cardiol* 12:175–183, 1986.

150. Rasmussen HS, Suenson M, McNair P et al: Magnesium infusion reduces the incidence of arrhythmias in acute myocardial infarction. A double-blind placebo-controlled study. *Clin Cardiol* 10:351–356, 1987.

151. Woods KL, Fletcher S, Roffe C et al: Intravenous magnesium sulphate in suspected acute myocardial infarction: Results of the second Leicester Intravenous Magnesium Intervention Trial (LIMIT-2). *Lancet* 339:1553–1558, 1992.

152. Horner SM: Efficacy of intravenous magnesium in acute myocardial infarction in reducing arrhythmias and mortality. *Circulation* 86:774–779, 1992.

153. Ryzen E, Nelson TA, Rude RK: Low blood mononuclear cell magnesium content and hypocalcemia in normomagnesemic patients. *West J Med* 147:549–553, 1987.

154. Reinhart RA: Magnesium metabolism. A review with special reference to the relationship between intracellular content and serum levels. *Arch Intern Med* 148:2415–2420, 1988.

62 ACID-BASE DISTURBANCES IN THE SURGICAL PATIENT

Arthur Greenberg

Acid-base disorders commonly arise in the perioperative period. Proper diagnosis and therapy require a thorough understanding of the underlying pathophysiology. After a pertinent review of basic acid-base terminology and physiology, this chapter covers specific acid-base disturbances as they relate to the surgical patient.

ACID-BASE TERMINOLOGY

Blood pH is closely regulated between 7.38 and 7.42. Although there are a number of intracellular and extracellular buffer systems, including hemoglobin, cellular proteins, and bone, the principal extracellular fluid buffer system is the carbonic acid–bicarbonate system:

$$H^+ + HCO_3^- \rightleftharpoons H_2CO_3 \rightleftharpoons CO_2 + H_2O$$

The Henderson-Hasselbach equation describes the role of this system in regulating blood pH and maintaining it around 7.4. When the $[HCO_3^-]$ is normal at 24 mmol/liter and the P_{CO_2} is similarly normal at 40 torr:

$$pH = 6.1 + \log \frac{[HCO_3^-]}{0.03 \times P_{CO_2}}$$

$$pH = 6.1 + \log \frac{(24 \text{ mmol/l})}{1.2 \text{ mmol/l}}$$

$$pH = 6.1 + \log 20 = 7.4$$

The ratio of bicarbonate to dissolved CO_2 must remain 20:1 to ensure normal blood pH. Conditions that alter pH by affecting bicarbonate concentration are metabolic disturbances and those that affect P_{CO_2} are respiratory disturbances. Factors that lower pH lead to acidosis, and those that raise pH result in alkalosis. The terms acidemia and alkalemia refer to the measured arterial pH and reflect the sum of the effects of acidosis or alkalosis either alone or in combination.

Because it is an open system, carbonic acid–bicarbonate buffer-

ing is particularly effective. New CO_2 formed by titration of bicarbonate during metabolic acidosis is rapidly excreted by the lungs, thereby minimizing changes in the $HCO_3^-:CO_2$ ratio. The system allows for respiratory compensation for metabolic disturbances and metabolic compensation for respiratory disturbances. For example, reduced blood pH and bicarbonate concentration in metabolic acidosis lead to hyperventilation. The P_{CO_2} decreases and the pH rises toward normal to help reestablish the $HCO_3^-:CO_2$ ratio. Similarly, when respiratory failure causes a rise in P_{CO_2} and respiratory acidosis, the kidney compensates by generating more bicarbonate.

In a simple acid-base disturbance, only the primary process, whether metabolic or respiratory, and its expected compensation are operating. Since compensation is incomplete, the pH is never normal in a simple disturbance except in chronic respiratory alkalosis, and the pH generally reflects the nature of the primary process. In a mixed acid-base disturbance, two or more primary processes are ongoing simultaneously. The pH may be increased, decreased, or normal depending on the magnitude of each individual disturbance.

The physician should attempt to identify each acid-base disturbance separately to guide appropriate therapy. There are several comprehensive reviews of methods used to accurately diagnose mixed acid-base disturbances.[1-3] These methods can be confirmed by using one of the published acid-base nomograms like that shown in Figure 62–1.[4] If values fall within a shaded zone, a simple disturbance is likely. If they lie outside these zones, there is a 95 percent chance that the disturbance is mixed.

The physician should be aware of the possible laboratory error that can confound diagnosis of acid-base disturbances. The laboratory parameter reported with the electrolytes is in fact the total CO_2 (tCO_2), which represents the total of bicarbonate, carbonic acid, and dissolved CO_2. The contribution of carbonic acid to the total is negligible, and the dissolved CO_2 is also a small number equal to the solubility coefficient multiplied by the P_{CO_2} (0.03 × 40 torr, or 1.2 mmol/liter). The tCO_2 is thus only slightly higher than the bicarbonate concentration $[HCO_3^-]$. The bicarbonate level cannot be measured directly and is calculated from the pH and

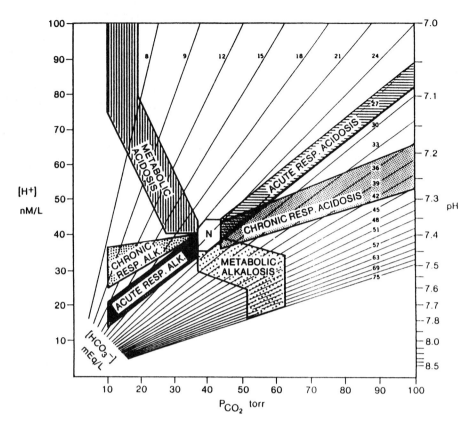

FIGURE 62–1. This-acid base nomogram is used to ascertain whether a given set of values, determined by arterial blood gas analysis, represents a simple or a mixed acid-base disturbance. Values for pH, P_{CO_2} and HCO_3^- are provided by the laboratory. The point at which any two values intersect is then evaluated in relation to the shaded areas. These areas represent the confidence limits, as determined by review of the literature, for the predicted response of a group of persons to a given perturbation in P_{CO_2} (respiratory disturbances) or HCO_3^- (metabolic disturbances). If a value falls outside a shaded area, a mixed disturbance is likely. The nomogram may also be used to verify that the laboratory has properly calculated the HCO_3^- value from the directly measured pH and P_{CO_2} values. See Goldberg et al.[4] for details regarding the use of the nomogram.

P_{CO_2} measurements made with ion-selective electrodes from arterial blood. If the simultaneously measured tCO_2 level reported with the electrolytes is not a few mmol higher than the $[HCO_3^-]$ calculated from the blood sample, the values are inconsistent. In addition, too much heparin in the syringe can dilute the arterial blood gas specimen and lower the P_{CO_2} without changing the pH, resulting in a falsely low calculated $[HCO_3^-]$ result.[5]

Cardiovascular Effects of Acidemia and Alkalemia

Mild acidemia and alkalemia are well tolerated, but marked deviation in the blood pH can profoundly affect cardiovascular function and cellular metabolism.[6,7] Acidemia reduces myocardial contractility when the pH falls below 7.2. Acidemia also induces release of catecholamines that mitigate the direct depressant effect of mild acidemia. However, when the pH is below 7.1, the inotropic response of the heart to catecholamines is diminished. Patients treated with beta-blockers are especially sensitive to mild degrees of acidemia.

Low pH increases vagal tone by inhibiting acetylcholinesterase, and, when the pH falls below 7.1, the risk of bradycardia and

cardiac arrest rises. Hyperkalemia induced by acidosis further increases the likelihood of these complications. In addition, acidemia causes venoconstriction that may further compromise cardiac function in patients with increased ventricular preload. This effect is partly offset by a decrease in ventricular afterload due to systemic arterial vasodilation induced by the acidemia.

The direct effects of alkalemia on cardiac contractility are less striking. Decreases in serum potassium and ionized calcium induced by alkalemia increase myocardial irritability. This is especially important in digitalized patients since the effects of digitalis and hypokalemia in producing arrhythmias are additive.

Central Nervous System Effects of Acid-Base Disturbances

Intracerebral blood flow and intracerebral or cerebrospinal fluid (CSF) pH affect central nervous system (CNS) function and are sensitive to metabolic changes induced by acidosis or alkalosis. Low intracerebral pH decreases cerebrovascular resistance and increases cerebral blood flow, and elevated intracerebral pH has the opposite effect.[6] The blood-brain barrier permits free diffusion of dissolved CO_2 but retards passage of bicarbonate. During periods of rapid systemic acid-base changes, PCO_2 rather than systemic pH or bicarbonate concentration is the principal determinant of the pH of the CSF and cerebral interstitium. For example, when PCO_2 falls, pH and vascular resistance rise and cerebral blood flow decreases. Impaired oxygen delivery and CNS dysfunction may result from rapidly developing respiratory alkalosis or rapid respiratory compensation for acute metabolic acidosis. Decrease in the pH of the CSF can also cause cerebral dysfunction independent of changes in cerebral blood flow. Acute respiratory acidosis can thus affect CNS function despite an increase in cerebral blood flow and cause decreased mentation, personality changes, asterixis, lethargy, and coma.

Bicarbonate equilibrates across the blood-brain barrier with time. Cerebrovascular tone and CSF pH then reflect systemic bicarbonate concentration and PCO_2. Although blood flow is increased by chronic respiratory or metabolic acidosis, the low pH alone may depress brain function. In severe chronic respiratory or metabolic alkalosis, diminished blood flow and elevated pH may lead to CNS dysfunction.

METABOLIC ALKALOSIS

Metabolic alkalosis develops from a net loss of acid or a net gain of bicarbonate. The factors responsible for generation of metabolic alkalosis are listed in Table 62–1A.

Oral or parenteral administration of alkali in the form of bicarbonate, or of organic anions like acetate, citrate, and lactate that are readily metabolized to bicarbonate, raises the serum bicarbonate level. Because one mmol bicarbonate is produced for each mmol gastric acid secreted, loss of gastric acid by vomiting or gastric aspiration has a similar effect.

New bicarbonate is also produced in the kidney. When sodium is reabsorbed in the distal nephron, potassium or hydrogen ions are secreted. Since intraluminal hydrogen ion is buffered by phosphate as titratable acid or ammonia as ammonium ion, one mmol of bicarbonate is retained for each mmol of hydrogen ion secreted. In stimulating sodium reabsorption in the distal nephron, aldosterone promotes secretion of hydrogen ions and generation of bicarbonate. This is seen in primary hyperaldosteronism and secondary hyperaldosteronism due to volume depletion or hyperreninism, or when exogenous mineralocorticoid or glucocorticoid is administered.

The kidney is normally easily able to excrete the excess bicarbonate accumulated in these conditions, and maintenance of metabolic alkalosis requires the failure of these homeostatic mechanisms.[8] Factors contributing to the maintenance of metabolic alkalosis are listed in Table 62–1B.

Volume, chloride, and potassium depletion as well as reduced glomerular filtration rate (GFR) are most important in maintaining a metabolic alkalosis.[9-12] In the proximal nephron, sodium is reabsorbed in parallel with chloride or in exchange for hydrogen ions. In the latter case, bicarbonate is generated and absorbed. Volume depletion decreases the GFR, reduces the amount of sodium and chloride available for reabsorption, and thereby stimulates the proximal tubule to reabsorb sodium. If less chloride is available in the tubule, sodium-hydrogen exchange is stimulated, and more bicarbonate is generated and absorbed. Chloride depletion may also promote the renal retention of bicarbonate in the distal tubule. Potassium depletion leads to a shift of potassium out of cells and of hydrogen ion into cells, causing an intracellular acidosis. This increases hydrogen ion secretion in the kidney and augments bicarbonate reabsorption. Hypercapnia has a similar effect. The relative importance of these factors in maintaining metabolic alkalosis is controversial. However, in any case, if volume depletion, chloride depletion, hypokalemia, or hypercapnia are present, the kidney may be unable to excrete enough excess bicarbonate.

The decrease in effective arterial volume seen in congestive heart failure or liver disease affects proximal tubular reabsorption in the same way as true extracellular volume depletion. When patients with severe renal failure receive excessive amounts of bicarbonate or lose significant quantities of acid through vomiting or nasogastric suction, the profound decrease in glomerular filtration rate and associated reduction in the filtered load of bicarbonate may render them unable to excrete the increased bicarbonate, thereby producing a metabolic alkalosis.

Clinical Presentations

Metabolic alkalosis is the most common acid-base disorder[13] and is frequently seen in the postoperative period.[14,15] In one report, it developed as an isolated disturbance in 15 percent and in combination with respiratory alkalosis in 51 percent of patients with organ trauma admitted to a surgical service.[16] It is an adverse prognostic sign in critically ill patients.[17]

The diagnosis of metabolic alkalosis is made when the tCO_2 or serum bicarbonate concentration is elevated in the absence of a primary respiratory acidosis. Chronic metabolic alkalosis induces

TABLE 62–1A. Factors Responsible for Generation of Metabolic Alkalosis

Gain of Alkali
  $NaHCO_3$ (oral or parenteral)
  Lactate (lactated Ringer's solution)
  Citrate (citrate-phosphate-dextrose anticoagulated blood)
  Acetate (intravenous hyperalimentation, purified protein fraction)
  Rapid correction of hypercapnia

Loss of Acid
  Gastrointestinal
    Vomiting
    Nasogastric suction
  Renal
    Primary hyperaldosteronism (Conn's syndrome)
    Secondary hyperaldosteronism
    Cushing's syndrome or disease
    Diuretic therapy
    Bartter's syndrome
    Urinary diversion with gastrocystoplasty

TABLE 62–1B. Factors Contributing to Maintenance of Metabolic Alkalosis

Decreased filtration of bicarbonate
  Renal failure
Increased reabsorption of bicarbonate
  Volume depletion
  Potassium depletion
  Chloride depletion
  Hypercapnia

an incomplete respiratory compensation in which P_{CO_2} rises by 3 to 4 torr for each 10 mmol/liter rise in serum bicarbonate level. Formulas estimating the expected degree of respiratory compensation for a primary metabolic alkalosis are unfortunately inaccurate.[2] Compensatory hypoventilation results in a fall in Pa_{O_2} as required by the alveolar air equation. Hypoxia limits the rise in P_{CO_2} to approximately 55 torr, and a higher P_{CO_2} suggests a concomitant respiratory acidosis. However, the P_{CO_2} may rise above 60 torr in patients with metabolic alkalosis alone if they are receiving supplemental oxygen.[18]

The frequent use of nasogastric suction after surgery makes metabolic alkalosis a common problem. The electrolyte content of normal gastric fluid is shown in Table 62–2.[19] Gastric suction can produce hydrogen ion losses of up to 400 to 500 mmol per day. Concurrent losses of chloride and sodium in the fluid and increased renal bicarbonate reabsorption due to secondary hyperaldosteronism and potassium-wasting sustain the alkalosis. In patients with renal failure, prolonged gastric acid aspiration invariably results in alkalosis unless the accumulated bicarbonate is removed by dialysis or neutralized by endogenous acid production or exogenous acid infusion. H_2-receptor blockers may be useful in reducing gastric acid secretion.[20]

Excessive bicarbonate administration during cardiopulmonary resuscitation or treatment of lactic acidosis may lead to rebound alkalosis once tissue perfusion is restored and accumulated organic anions are metabolized to bicarbonate. Similarly, metabolic alkalosis can be caused by administering bicarbonate to patients receiving rapid transfusions of stored blood containing lactic as well as citric acids.[21,22] More recent studies have shown that the clinical acidosis in this situation is insignificant and need not be treated with bicarbonate.[23,24] In addition, several commercially available plasma protein fractions are relatively hypochloremic and contain more than 40 mmol/liter of acetate. Infusion of large volumes has caused significant alkalosis in patients with renal failure.[25]

A mild, clinically insignificant metabolic alkalosis frequently occurs after cardiopulmonary bypass and has been attributed to infusion of citrate in blood used to prime the membrane oxygenator or infused during transfusion.[26] In one prospective study, the degree of alkalosis was decreased by administration of the carbonic anhydrase inhibitor acetazolamide.[27] However, if renal function is normal and neither volume nor potassium depletion is present, the accumulated bicarbonate is promptly excreted.

A significant amount of acid may be lost in the urine in patients who undergo creation of a new bladder or bladder augmentation with a gastric segment. In these cases, the gastric mucosa continues to secrete acid that is excreted in the urine.[28] Omeprazole may be a useful therapeutic adjunct in such patients.[29]

Volume depletion is a principal mechanism for the maintenance of metabolic alkalosis in surgical patients. Common causes include hemorrhage, loss of gastrointestinal fluid through aspiration, administration of diuretics, diarrhea, and accumulation of extracellular fluid in the third space created by adynamic ileus. Measurement of urinary electrolytes may be helpful in confirming the presence of volume depletion. A urine chloride concentration of less than 20 mmol/liter is indicative of the avid chloride retention underlying the chloride-sensitive alkalosis of volume depletion. The urine sodium concentration is less reliable because a rapid rise in serum bicarbonate concentration may transiently overwhelm the capacity to reabsorb bicarbonate and result in excretion of sodium even when the patient is volume-depleted.[30] The urine chloride concentration cannot be used in patients receiving diuretics that cause volume depletion by enhancing renal sodium and chloride excretion. Injudicious use of diuretics can itself cause metabolic alkalosis in the perioperative period.

Potassium depletion is a frequent accompaniment of volume depletion and should be anticipated in patients with vomiting or diarrhea and in those requiring nasogastric aspiration, diuretics, or mineralocorticoid therapy. Although volume and chloride depletion are the main factors responsible for maintaining metabolic alkalosis, it may be impossible to induce renal excretion of bicarbonate with sodium chloride alone in some patients with profound potassium deficits of 400 to 500 mmol. In such "chloride-resistant" alkalotic patients, urinary chloride concentrations above 40 mmol/liter are not unusual. Inducing bicarbonate excretion and correcting the alkalosis may not be possible until potassium is repleted.[31]

Primary hyperaldosteronism (Conn's syndrome) and secondary hyperaldosteronism due to hyperreninemia associated with renovascular disease or Bartter's syndrome also cause increased distal tubular acid excretion and metabolic alkalosis. Exogenous mineralocorticoid or high-dose glucocorticoid administration may have the same effect. The extracellular fluid volume in these conditions is usually increased, urinary chloride and sodium excretion are typically high, and expansion with sodium chloride does not correct the alkalosis. Chloride resistance may thus provide important diagnostic clues.

Treatment

In the surgical setting, the etiology of metabolic alkalosis is often multifactorial and requires understanding before effective therapy can be given. For example, in patients undergoing cardiac surgery, it may be generated by transfusion of citrate-phosphate-dextrose (CPD) anticoagulated blood and gastric aspiration. Diminished GFR due to low cardiac output and diuretic-induced volume and

TABLE 62–2. Composition of Gastrointestinal Fluids

	Na (mmol/l)	K (mmol/l)	Cl (mmol/l)	HCO_3^- (mmol/l)	pH
Gastric Fluid	20–100	5–10	120–160	—	1–7
Bile	150–250	5–10	40–80	20–40	7–8
Pancreatic Fluid	120	5–10	10–60	80–120	7–8
Enteric Fluid	140	5	variable	variable	7–8

Source: After Phillips SF, in Maxwell MH, Kleeman CR, Narins RG (eds): *Clinical Disorders of Fluid and Electrolyte Metabolism*, 4th ed. New York, McGraw-Hill, 1987.

potassium depletion maintain the alkalosis. Concomitant renal failure may further delay recovery.[32]

In patients with normal renal function, metabolic alkalosis is usually mild, with a blood pH below 7.5 and a serum bicarbonate concentration below 38 mmol/liter. Correction of extracellular fluid volume and potassium deficits leads to increased bicarbonate excretion and correction of blood pH within 36 to 48 hours. In rare instances, when more rapid correction is necessary because of severe alkalemia and compensatory hypoventilation that compromise respiratory or neurological function, hydrogen ion may be administered in the form of dilute hydrochloric acid. Because peripheral administration may cause venous sclerosis, a central venous catheter is required. Although concentrated 1 N hydrochloric acid (HCl) has been used, most authorities recommend 0.1 or 0.25 N HCl prepared by mixing 1 N HCl with 5% dextrose in water. Acid should be infused at a rate of about 0.2 mmol/kg/hr.[33-36] Since chloride space equals 20 to 25 percent of total body weight (TBW), the required dose of acid in mmol is:

$$TBW \times 0.2 \times (103 \text{ mmol/liter} - \text{present } [Cl^-])$$

If the GFR is near normal, excess renal bicarbonate reabsorption may be decreased by infusing acetazolamide in a dose of 250 to 500 mg intravenously every four to six hours. This therapy is particularly useful in metabolic alkalosis induced by hypercapnia. Oral therapy is an acceptable alternative.[37] In patients with severe renal dysfunction, bicarbonate excretion is significantly impaired, and correction of the alkalosis requires infusion of hydrochloric acid and dialysis against a dialysate of reduced base content.[38,39]

METABOLIC ACIDOSIS

Daily nonvolatile acid production from dietary precursors such as methionine-containing proteins and phosphoproteins and from incomplete metabolism of neutral food stuffs approximates one mmol of hydrogen ion per kilogram of body weight. This acid load is excreted through renal secretion of hydrogen ions which are buffered by compounds such as phosphate to produce titratable acid or are combined with ammonia to form ammonium. The normal kidney can increase total acid excretion significantly, but its capacity can be impaired or overwhelmed, leading to metabolic acidosis.

Clinical Presentations

Metabolic acidosis is characterized by a fall in the serum bicarbonate concentration and pH, and hypocapnia usually provides respiratory compensation. In addition to the fall in pH, several conditions underlying metabolic acidosis may independently stimulate ventilation and sometimes produce an accompanying primary respiratory alkalosis. It is essential to distinguish such a mixed acid-base disturbance from simple metabolic acidosis with respiratory compensation. From a series of patients with pure metabolic acidosis due to diarrhea, Winters et al. developed a regression formula to predict the expected degree of respiratory compensation as expressed by the P_{CO_2}:[40]

$$\text{Expected } P_{CO_2} = (1.5 \times [HCO_3^-]) + 8 \pm 2$$

If the P_{CO_2} is less than the calculated value, a primary respiratory alkalosis is present. If the P_{CO_2} exceeds this predicted value, the

diagnosis of respiratory acidosis may be inferred even if the P_{CO_2} is at or below the normal value of 40 torr.

Calculation of the undetermined serum anion concentration or "anion gap" is invaluable in the diagnosis of metabolic acidosis:[41,42]

$$\text{anion gap (mmol/l)} = [Na^+] \text{ mmol/l} - ([Cl^-] \text{ mmol/l} + [HCO_3^-] \text{ mmol/l})$$

The normal anion gap is 12 ± 4 and is comprised of proteins, phosphate, sulfate, and other unmeasured organic or inorganic acid anions that are buffered by bicarbonate. Increases in the concentrations of these acids decrease the serum bicarbonate level and increase the anion gap, thereby defining a high-anion-gap metabolic acidosis. In contrast, hyperchloremic metabolic acidosis due to retention of hydrochloric acid or loss of bicarbonate depresses the serum bicarbonate concentration as chloride rises but does not increase the anion gap. Once the distinction between high- and normal-anion-gap acidosis is made, the specific etiology is usually apparent from the clinical presentation. Causes of metabolic acidoses with normal and high anion gaps are summarized in Tables 62–3A and 62–3B.

Metabolic Acidosis with a Normal Anion Gap (Hyperchloremic Acidosis)

Proximal or type 2 renal tubular acidosis (RTA) is characterized by a decreased proximal tubular threshold for bicarbonate reabsorption. Classic distal or type 1 RTA is characterized by a failure to lower urine pH despite acidemia. These uncommon disorders are associated with normal glomerular filtration rate and hypokalemia.[43]

Impairment of urinary acid excretion is an early finding in mild chronic renal failure[44,45] and is the result of impaired renal ammonia production due to diminished renal mass. In addition, several forms of RTA with hyperkalemia may occur in patients with mild chronic renal failure. Patients with a higher risk include those with diabetes mellitus, lupus erythematosus, sickle cell nephropathy, lead nephropathy, and obstructive uropathy.[46-48] The most widely

TABLE 62–3A. Common Causes of Metabolic Acidosis with a Normal Anion Gap

Bicarbonate Loss
  Renal disease (tubulointerstitial disease, renal tubular acidosis)
  Drugs (acetazolamide, mafenide, cholestyramine, spironolactone)
  Urinary diversion (ureterosigmoidostomy, ileal loop with stasis, continent ileal pouch)
  Gastrointestinal (diarrhea, pancreatic drainage or transplant, jejunoileal bypass)

Acid Gain
  Acid administration: NH_4Cl, cationic amino acids

TABLE 62–3B. Causes of Metabolic Acidosis with an Increased Anion Gap

  Diabetic or alcoholic ketoacidosis
  Uremia
  Lactic acidosis
  Toxin ingestion: salicylate, methanol, ethylene glycol, iron

recognized is type 4 RTA, characterized by impaired production of ammonia, hyporeninemic hypoaldosteronism, and normal ability to lower the urine pH during acidemia. Spironolactone may induce a type 4 RTA in cirrhotics.[49] In another type of hyperkalemic distal RTA, urine pH remains elevated even during acidemia, and aldosterone deficiency may or may not be present.

Specialized testing is required to define the tubular defects underlying these hyperkalemic acidoses but is seldom necessary. Since they are most often seen in patients with mildly impaired renal function, excretion of fixed acid anions is normal and an anion gap does not develop. All of these disorders are characterized by tubulointerstitial renal disease and produce a mild acidosis with serum bicarbonate concentrations in the range of 18 to 22 mmol/liter requiring no specific treatment. However, affected patients cannot increase acid excretion much beyond the basal level, and severe acidosis can result from even a minimal increase in acid generation. They also have an increased risk of developing hyperkalemia.

High-capacity bicarbonate reabsorption in the proximal tubule is dependent on the enzyme carbonic anhydrase. Its inhibition results in bicarbonaturia and hyperchloremic acidosis. The carbonic anhydrase inhibitor acetazolamide is helpful in correcting posthypercapnic metabolic alkalosis but can cause metabolic acidosis as an unwanted side effect in the treatment of glaucoma. The topical antibiotic mafenide (Sulfamylon) is absorbed systemically when used extensively in the treatment of burns and may produce a hyperchloremic acidosis because of its carbonic anhydrase effect. Cholestyramine, a cationic resin that binds bile salts in the gut, also binds bicarbonate and may cause metabolic acidosis by inducing gastrointestinal bicarbonate loss.

The intestinal lumen, particularly that of the colon, can secrete bicarbonate in exchange for chloride. Hyperchloremic acidosis was a frequent complication of ureterosigmoidostomy and led to abandonment of the procedure in favor of the ileal conduit. Metabolic acidosis is less frequent in patients with ileal conduits but may develop if stasis occurs in an ileal segment that is too large or strictured or if a continent ileal pouch has been created.[50,51]

The electrolyte content of pancreatic fluid, bile, and enteric fluid are listed in Table 62–2. Pancreatic or biliary tract drainage, diarrhea, and even excessive preoperative bowel cleansing may cause loss of bicarbonate and severe metabolic acidosis.[52] This may also occur after jejunoileal bypass, in which case up to 300 mmol/day of bicarbonate or even reanastomosis may be required to treat the acidosis.[53] Drainage of exocrine secretions from a whole pancreas transplant into the bladder by way of a duodenocystostomy may also lead to a metabolic acidosis.[54]

The two types of amino acid mixtures currently used in intravenous hyperalimentation are casein or fibrin hydrolysates and synthetic mixtures of amino acids. Early synthetic mixtures contained a high percentage of cationic amino acids such as lysine, arginine, and histidine as hydrochloride salts. When metabolized, these amino acids yield one mmol of hydrogen ion for each mmol administered and can produce a metabolic acidosis.[55] Protein hydrolysates contain fewer cationic amino acids, and modification of synthetic mixtures has essentially obviated the problem. However, modern synthetic mixtures and hydrolysates may produce acidosis in patients unable to increase acid excretion[56] or in those in whom acid excretion is blocked by a potassium-sparing diuretic.[57] Acidosis can be readily detected if serum electrolyte concentrations are followed closely in patients receiving intravenous hyperalimentation.

Substitution of sodium acetate for sodium chloride in the electrolyte mixture provides a rapid and simple means of correction.

Although the cause of hyperchloremic acidosis is usually evident from the clinical setting, the urinary anion gap has recently been proposed as a helpful diagnostic clue. The urinary anion gap is the sum of the urinary sodium and potassium concentrations minus the chloride concentration and provides a quick estimate of urinary ammonium content. A negative value indicates the presence of significant ammonium in the urine and suggests that renal acidification is normal, as in patients with diarrhea or other gastrointestinal losses of bicarbonate. In contrast, when the urine anion gap is positive, ammonia excretion is low, suggesting inadequate renal acidification. This calculation appears useful but has not been widely validated.[58]

Metabolic Acidosis with a High Anion Gap

Diagnosis of high-anion-gap acidosis depends upon identification of the retained anion. This is most easily accomplished when the anion gap exceeds 30 mmol/liter.[59] High-anion-gap acidosis carries significant morbidity. With the exception of stable chronic renal failure, the conditions underlying it are usually more severe than those causing hyperchloremic acidosis. Early recognition and treatment are mandatory.[60]

The high-anion-gap acidosis of renal failure results from accumulation of anions of strong acids like sulfate and phosphate. The serum bicarbonate concentration usually remains above 15 mmol/liter with an anion gap of less than 25 mmol/liter. Acidosis developing in postoperative acute renal failure is poorly tolerated because of the hemodynamic problems induced by the acidosis itself and the hypercatabolism and hyperkalemia accompanying it. Although the acidosis of acute renal failure may be managed conservatively, early dialysis should be considered (see Chap. 63). Acidosis developing in chronic renal failure is well tolerated and does not increase operative risk if the blood pH is above 7.3. Attempts to correct acidosis rapidly with sodium bicarbonate can result in volume overload.

Free fatty acids and their ketoacid metabolites accumulate during states of insulin lack. Ketoacidosis is a frequent complication of diabetes mellitus, and a combined ketoacidosis and lactic acidosis can occur in starvation and alcoholism. Bedside determination of serum or urine ketoacids by the nitroprusside test is easy and rapidly confirmatory. In severe ketoacidosis, a low intracellular redox state and a high mitochondrial NADH:NAD$^+$ ratio favor reduction of acetoacetate to betahydroxybutyrate, a nonketoacid that does not react with nitroprusside. In this case, the nitroprusside test may be negative or only weakly positive.

Alcoholic ketoacidosis is usually seen on admission but rarely develops de novo in hospitalized patients. In contrast, diabetic ketoacidosis can be a complication of perioperative stress. Treatment of alcoholic ketoacidosis includes volume repletion and administration of bicarbonate and glucose as needed. Although administration of insulin has been proposed in alcoholic ketoacidosis, it is usually unnecessary and may produce hypoglycemia.[61,62] Treatment of diabetic ketoacidosis is discussed in Chap. 24.

A history of drug or toxin ingestion should be obtained in any patient with a high-anion-gap acidosis. Ingestion of methanol or ethylene glycol produces a metabolic acidosis but can also cause abdominal pain with or without pancreatitis leading to admission to surgical services. The diagnosis is suggested by a discrepancy of more than 15 mOsm/kg between the measured and calculated serum osmolality called the osmolal gap. For example, methanol in a concentration of 100 mg/dl increases the measured serum osmolality 31 mOsm/kg above the osmolality calculated from serum sodium, urea, and glucose concentrations. Like urea, relatively low-molecular-weight alcohols readily diffuse across cell membranes and contribute to the measured but not to the "effective" osmolality. Consequently, neither a change in tonicity nor serum sodium concentration results. Although less specific, the osmolal gap can be determined more rapidly than individual plasma toxin assays.

Clinical findings may suggest a specific toxin. Blindness with retinal edema and optic nerve hyperemia point to methanol ingestion. Ethylene glycol ingestion is associated with acute renal failure induced by oxalate, its principal metabolite, and bipyramidal oxalate crystals may be found on urinalysis. Dialysis is required to remove these two toxins. In addition, ethanol infusion is useful because it competes for metabolism with ethylene glycol or methanol and reduces production of their toxic metabolites.[63,64] 4-methylpyrazole may be used in the same way.[65]

Salicylate intoxication may occur in hospitalized patients receiving aspirin for rheumatologic disorders or topical methyl salicylate as a keratolytic. The diagnosis can be easily missed. In one series of 73 consecutive patients with salicylate intoxication, delay in diagnosis of up to 72 hours was documented in 27 percent. The mortality rate was 25 percent, and severe morbidity occurred in 30 percent.[66] Salicylates stimulate respiration and produce coexistent respiratory alkalosis and high-anion-gap metabolic acidosis. The diagnosis can be confirmed by review of medication records and determination of blood salicylate levels. Dialysis may be required in patients with renal failure or in those with blood salicylate levels above 80 mg/dl, but forced alkaline diuresis is usually adequate in patients with less severe intoxication.[67] Acetazolamide should be avoided because acidemia augments salicylate toxicity.[68]

Lactic acidosis is the most severe form of high-anion-gap acidosis. Morbidity and mortality depend upon the severity and reversibility of the underlying cause. In spontaneous lactic acidosis, mortality can be as high as 100 percent. Shock induced by hemorrhage, low cardiac output, or sepsis is the most frequent cause of lactic acidosis. Generation of lactate increases when hypoperfusion and inadequate oxygen delivery to tissues lead to increased anaerobic metabolism and impaired hepatic uptake and utilization of lactate. The more unusual D-lactic acidosis may result from production of D-lactic acid by bacteria in patients who have undergone jejunoileal bypass or have short-bowel syndrome or other gastrointestinal abnormalities.[69,70]

The pathophysiologic mechanism underlying lactic acidosis has been extensively reviewed.[71–73] Its clinical presentation is variable. It may develop as a prominent feature in established shock or herald developing sepsis. It is frequently associated with primary respiratory alkalosis, particularly when sepsis is the underlying cause. It may also occur in states of localized hypoperfusion, burns, tumors, and arterial occlusion.[74–77]

The diagnosis of lactic acidosis is suggested by the clinical setting and a high-anion-gap acidosis without concurrent uremia, diabetes, or ingestion of alcohol or toxin. Diagnosis can be confirmed by measuring the blood lactate level, which is normally 0.5 to 1.5 mmol/liter.[6] Exercise and catecholamines can transiently increase lactate levels, and alkalosis can stimulate glycolysis and lactate production.[73] Levels below 5 mmol/liter are usually not clinically significant, but in shock levels above 4 mmol/liter, are associated with increased mortality. Clinically insignificant lactic acidosis occurring after cardiopulmonary bypass may not be associated with an increased anion gap, perhaps because the gap is lowered by hemodilution. The causes of lactic acidosis are listed in Table 62–4.

Treatment

Treatment of metabolic acidosis requires attention to the underlying pathophysiologic process and correction of the acidemia. Renal disease is usually not remediable, but in chronic renal failure with hyperchloremic acidosis, serum bicarbonate levels should be corrected to 20 mmol/liter. Once the bicarbonate deficit is corrected, daily bicarbonate requirements are relatively modest and amount to one mmol/kg except in patients with type 2 renal tubular acidosis. Parenteral or oral sodium bicarbonate can be given. Each 325 mg tablet is equivalent to 3.9 mmol. In patients who experience bicarbonate-induced gastrointestinal discomfort, Shohl's solution, a mixture of sodium citrate and citric acid, can be substituted. One ml of solution is equivalent to one mmol of bicarbonate. Modified Shohl's solution containing potassium citrate or potassium citrate tablets is useful in patients with hypokalemic renal tubular acidosis. Hyperchloremic acidosis due to bicarbonate loss from the gastrointestinal tract may be severe. In this case, bicarbonate losses may vary, and daily replacement doses must be individualized.

Severe high-anion-gap acidosis is a medical emergency, and specific treatment must be initiated immediately. Insulin rapidly blocks acid production in diabetic ketoacidosis. Dialysis is specific therapy for uremia and some toxin ingestions. Treatment for lactic acidosis is largely supportive and depends upon the underlying condition. Inadequate tissue perfusion should be corrected with volume repletion and transfusions. Infections should be treated with appropriate antibiotics. Low cardiac output should be augmented. Early revascularization or debridement may be required when limb or mesenteric ischemia is the cause.

Optimizing perfusion requires careful clinical assessment of intravascular volume and usually measurement of central venous or

TABLE 62–4. Causes of Lactic Acidosis

Lactic Acidosis Associated with a Modest or Transient Elevation in Anion Gap

    Alkalemia
    Carbohydrate infusion
    Exercise or seizures[79]
    Catecholamines
    Diabetic ketosis
    Ethanol

Lactic Acidosis with a Marked Elevation of Anion Gap

    Impaired tissue oxygenation
        Hypotension
        Severe anemia
        Arterial occlusion
        Hypoxia
    Glycogen storage diseases
    Malignancies
    D-lactic acidosis
    Spontaneous

pulmonary wedge pressure. Volume deficits should be rapidly corrected with blood and crystalloid. Blood pressure maintenance may require catecholamine infusion. Nitroprusside[80,81] or other unloading agents may also be useful in improving cardiac output. When volume overload and renal failure coexist, dialysis is indicated to improve hemodynamic status and to allow further administration of alkali.

There is no currently approved specific therapy for lactic acidosis. Dichloroacetate stimulates pyruvate dehydrogenase, increases cardiac output, and lowers lactate concentrations in some patients but has not significantly improved survival.[82] The use of bicarbonate to correct high-anion-gap acidosis, and particularly lactic acidosis, has become controversial. It can depress the myocardium and actually increase lactate production in some patients with no improvement in survival.[83] The role of bicarbonate administration in patients with cardiac disease and in those suffering cardiopulmonary arrest has also been questioned.[84] In states of profound hypoperfusion, arterial blood gas measurements may not accurately reflect tissue pH.[85-87] Despite this controversy, most authorities endorse the use of sodium bicarbonate as the alkaline salt of choice for severe acidosis.[88]

The goal of alkali therapy is to maintain the serum bicarbonate concentration above 10 mmol/liter and the blood pH between 7.15 and 7.20. When the pH is below 7.1, myocardial irritability increases markedly, and contractility decreases. When the bicarbonate concentration falls below 5 mmol/liter, maintenance of pH is exquisitely dependent upon hyperventilation. A small increase in Pco_2 or drop in bicarbonate level may lead to profound acidemia, making resuscitation impossible.

The serum bicarbonate concentration should not be corrected to normal. Because treatment of the underlying process itself facilitates rapid metabolism of accumulated ketoacids or lactate to bicarbonate, overly vigorous administration of bicarbonate can result in severe alkalemia. Assuming a bicarbonate space of 50 percent to total body weight (TBW), bicarbonate deficit can be estimated as follows:

$$\text{Bicarbonate deficit (mmol/l)} = 0.5 \times \text{total body weight (kg)} \times (\text{desired } [HCO_3^-] - \text{actual } [HCO_3^-])$$

In practice, therapy must be individualized with frequent determinations of blood pH and bicarbonate concentration. In severe acidosis, continuing acid production and the role of intracellular buffers may increase the bicarbonate space unpredictably to levels far exceeding 50 percent.[89] In lactic acidosis, several hundred millimoles of bicarbonate may be required in the first hour. Hy-

perosmolar bicarbonate can be given in intravenous bolus infusion of 44 or 50 mmol per ampule. Alternatively, a continuous drip can be made up with three ampules of bicarbonate in one liter of 5% dextrose in water to yield a bicarbonate concentration near 140 mmol/liter. Since lactic acidosis is frequently complicated by oliguric renal failure or congestive heart failure, the high sodium and osmolar load of bicarbonate may be poorly tolerated. Early initiation of hemodialysis with bicarbonate-buffered dialysate should be considered. Although its effect on outcome is unclear, continuous ultrafiltration may be useful in patients who are too hypotensive to tolerate hemodialysis.[90]

RESPIRATORY ALKALOSIS

Respiratory alkalosis is the result of abnormal stimulation of ventilation and results in reduction in Pco_2 and increase in blood pH. Simultaneous metabolic acidosis and respiratory alkalosis should be suspected whenever the Pco_2 is lower than predicted by Winters's formula for a given decrease in bicarbonate concentration. Some of the causes of respiratory alkalosis are listed in Table 62–5.

Respiratory alkalosis occurs frequently after surgery. In one series, it occurred as an isolated disturbance in 34 percent of patients with severe trauma and together with metabolic alkalosis in 51 percent.[14] Underlying causes like pneumonia and pulmonary emboli are often obvious, but respiratory alkalosis may be the only clue to early sepsis or hepatic encephalopathy. It is therefore imperative that every effort be made to identify and treat the underlying cause as soon as possible.

Respiratory alkalosis can produce a rapid rise in blood pH and profound clinical deterioration. A sudden fall in Pco_2 from 40 torr to 20 torr in a patient with a serum bicarbonate concentration of 24 mmol/liter results in a pH in excess of 7.7. Paresthesias, tetany, and seizures may occur. Although rebreathing CO_2 or mild sedation may be useful in anxiety-induced hyperventilation, treatment of the alkalosis itself is usually unrewarding. Reports that intermittent mandatory ventilation is less likely to cause respiratory alkalosis than other forms of mechanical ventilation have not been borne out.[91,92] When pulmonary disease, CNS abnormalities, hepatic dysfunction, or sepsis lead to respiratory alkalosis, treatment with opiates or other respiratory depressants is clearly contraindicated if the patient is not intubated and ventilated. Hypophosphatemia due to intracellular shifts of phosphate is a frequent complication of respiratory alkalosis and may necessitate phosphate administration.[93]

RESPIRATORY ACIDOSIS

Respiratory acidosis is caused only by alveolar hypoventilation and CO_2 accumulation. Clinically relevant causes are shown in Table 62–6. Respiratory acidosis is recognized by a rise in Pco_2 and a fall in blood pH. Compensatory retention of bicarbonate causes its level to rise four to five mmol/liter for every increase of 10 torr in the Pco_2. However, the serum bicarbonate concentration seldom exceeds 38 mmol/liter in pure respiratory acidosis, and higher levels suggest concomitant metabolic alkalosis. In such cases, a low serum potassium level may suggest that metabolic alkalosis is due to vomiting or diuretics. The combination of respiratory acido-

TABLE 62–5.   Causes of Respiratory Alkalosis

Anxiety
Fever
Salicylism
CNS disease (cerebrovascular accident, infection, trauma, tumor)
Congestive heart failure
Pneumonia
Pulmonary embolus
Hypoxemia
Hepatic insufficiency
Sepsis
Mechanical ventilation

TABLE 62–6. Causes of Respiratory Acidosis

Causes of Acute Respiratory Acidosis
General anesthesia
Sedation or drug overdose
Cardiac arrest
Pneumothorax
Pulmonary edema
Severe pneumonia
Bronchospasm
Laryngospasm
Upper-airway obstruction from trauma or foreign body
Aspiration
Mechanical ventilation
Respiratory nerve damage
Guillain-Barré syndrome
Hypophosphatemia
Hypokalemia

Causes of Chronic Respiratory Acidosis
Chronic obstructive pulmonary disease
Primary alveolar hypoventilation
Brain tumor
Neurologic diseases of respiratory muscles (polio, myasthenia gravis)
Primary myopathy of respiratory muscles
Restrictive disease of the thorax
Burns
Scleroderma
Severe pneumonia

---

sis and metabolic alkalosis is frequently seen in patients with chronic obstructive lung disease who receive diuretics as treatment for cor pulmonale.

Treatment is directed at the underlying cause of respiratory failure. Although narcotic antagonists such as naloxone are useful in reversing respiratory depression due to opiate administration, respiratory stimulants and analeptics are not useful. Progressive hypercapnia requires emergent endotracheal intubation and control of ventilation.

MIXED ACID-BASE DISTURBANCES

Severely ill patients, often with multisystem disease, may have mixed acid-base disturbances in which two or more primary acid-base disorders are present simultaneously. They may have a concurrent metabolic acidosis and a metabolic alkalosis or any combination of metabolic and respiratory disturbances. By definition, a simultaneous respiratory acidosis and respiratory alkalosis is impossible. Successful management of these patients depends on distinguishing between a single disorder with appropriate compensation and a mixed disorder. The specific clinical setting often suggests etiologies of complex mixed disturbances. Selected mixed acid-base disorders seen most commonly in surgical patients are listed in Table 62–7.

Correct diagnosis of mixed acid-base disturbances depends on accurately interpreting the serum bicarbonate level, anion gap, and blood gas measurements in light of the specific pathophysiologic

TABLE 62–7. Selected Mixed Acid-Base Disturbances

Metabolic Acidosis with Respiratory Alkalosis
  Salicylate intoxication
  Sepsis
  Hepatic failure

Metabolic Alkalosis with Respiratory Acidosis
  Cor pulmonale treated with diuretics
  Nasogastric suction with respiratory failure

Metabolic Alkalosis with Metabolic Acidosis
  Vomiting or nasogastric suction with sepsis or profound volume depletion
  Vomiting or nasogastric suction with renal failure

---

processes going on in the patient.[1-3] Plotting two of the three variables required on the nomogram in Figure 62–1 yields a point outside one of the shaded areas defining simple disorders and confirms suspicion of a mixed disorder. In patients with metabolic acidosis, a discrepancy between the change in bicarbonate level and that in the anion gap[94] or a pH or PCO_2 different from that expected from application of Winters's formula provides valuable information about the nature of the acid-base disorder. For example, an inappropriately high serum bicarbonate level in a patient with a high anion gap from lactic acidosis may indicate a concurrent primary metabolic alkalosis from nasogastric suction. In another instance, an unexpectedly high PCO_2 in such a patient may be the sign of impending respiratory failure.

SUMMARY

1. To determine optimal therapy, each acid-base disturbance should be identified separately. In difficult cases, an acid-base nomogram may provide helpful confirmation of a simple or mixed disorder.

2. Both severe acidemia and alkalemia have deleterious cardiovascular and CNS effects.

3. Metabolic alkalosis is the most common acid-base disturbance in surgical patients and is usually multifactorial in origin.

4. Volume, chloride, and potassium deficits usually underlie metabolic alkalosis, and bicarbonate will not be excreted until these deficits are corrected.

5. Urinary chloride concentrations are useful in differentiating volume depletion, in which the level is less than 20 mmol/liter from diuretic use, from profound potassium depletion or mineralocorticoid excess, in which the level is greater than 30 mmol/liter.

6. Acid administration is rarely required in the treatment of metabolic alkalosis except when severe alkalemia results in compensatory hypoventilation or CNS depression.

7. Severe high-anion-gap metabolic acidosis is a medical emergency. Treatment should focus on the underlying pathology. When the pH falls below 7.2, most authorities recommend administering bicarbonate.

8. Respiratory alkalosis is common after surgery and may be accompanied by hypophosphatemia. Respiratory acidosis is caused by alveolar hypoventilation. Progressive hypercapnia is an indication for emergency intubation.

9. Mixed acid-base disturbances are usually suggested by the clinical situation and can be confirmed by careful interpretation of the serum electrolyte levels and blood gas measurements. Accurate characterization of such disorders may provide early diagnosis of serious postoperative complications like sepsis and respiratory failure.

REFERENCES

1. McCurdy DK: Mixed metabolic and respiratory acid-base disturbances: Diagnosis and treatment. *Chest* 62(Suppl):35–43, 1972.
2. Narins RG, Emmett M: Simple and mixed acid-base disorders: A practical approach. *Medicine* 59:161–187, 1980.
3. Narins RG, Jones ER, Stom MC et al: Diagnostic strategies in disorders of fluid, electrolyte and acid-base homeostasis. *Am J Med* 72:496–520, 1982.
4. Goldberg M, Green SB, Moss ML et al: Computer-based instruction and diagnosis of acid-base disorders. *JAMA* 223:269–275, 1973.
5. Bloom SA, Canzanello VJ, Strom JA et al: Spurious assessment of acid-base status due to dilutional effect of heparin. *Am J Med* 79:528–530, 1985.
6. Mitchell JH, Wildenthal K, Johnson RL Jr: The effects of acid-base disturbances on cardiovascular and pulmonary function. *Kidney Int* 1:375–389, 1972.
7. Relman AS: Metabolic consequences of acid-base disorders. *Kidney Int* 1:347–359, 1972.
8. Seldin DW, Rector FC Jr: The generation and maintenance of metabolic alkalosis. *Kidney Int* 1:306–321, 1972.
9. Jacobson HR, Seldin DW: On the generation, maintenance, and correction of metabolic alkalosis. *Am J Physiol* 245:F425–F432, 1983.
10. Kassirer JP, Schwartz WB: Correction of metabolic alkalosis in man without repair of potassium deficiency. *Am J Med* 40:19–26, 1966.
11. Cogan M, Alpern RJ: Regulation of proximal bicarbonate reabsorption. *Am J Physiol* 247:F387–F395, 1984.
12. Rosen RA, Julian BA, Dubovsky EV et al: On the mechanism by which chloride corrects metabolic alkalosis in man. *Am J Med* 84:449–458, 1988.
13. Hodgkin JE, Soeprono FF, Chan DM: Incidence of metabolic alkalemia in hospitalized patients. *Crit Care Med* 18:725–728, 1980.
14. Berman IR, Moseley RV, Doty DB et al: Post-traumatic alkalosis in young men with combat injuries. *Surg Gynecol Obstet* 133:15, 1971.
15. Lyons JH Jr, Moore FD: Post-traumatic alkalosis: Incidence and pathophysiology. *Surgery* 60:93–106, 1966.
16. Wilson RF, Gibson D, Percinel AK et al: Severe alkalosis in critically ill surgical patients. *Arch Surg* 105:197–203, 1972.
17. Cullen DJ, Ferrara LC, Gilbert J et al: Indicators of intensive care in critically ill patients. *Crit Care Med* 5:173–179, 1977.
18. Webb J: Severe hypercapnia associated with non-respiratory alkalosis. *Br J Dis Chest* 72:62–66, 1978.
19. Phillips SF: Small and large intestinal disorders and associated fluid and electrolyte complications, in Maxwell MH, Cleeman CR, Narins RG (eds): *Clinical Disorders of Fluid and Electrolyte Metabolism*, 4th ed. New York, McGraw-Hill, 1987, pp 865–878.
20. Barton CH, Vaziri ND, Ness RL et al: Cimetidine in the management of metabolic alkalosis induced by nasogastric drainage. *Arch Surg* 14:70–74, 1979.
21. Schweizer O, Howland WS: Significance of lactate and pyruvate according to volume of blood transfusion in man. *Ann Surg* 162:1017–1027, 1965.
22. Committee on Pre- and Post-operative Care, American College of Surgeons: *Manual of Pre-operative and Post-operative Care*. Philadelphia, Saunders, 1967, p 84.
23. Collins JA, Simmons RL, James PM et al: Acid-base status of seriously wounded combat casualties: II. Resuscitation with stored blood. *Ann Surg* 73:6–18, 1971.
24. Collins JA: Blood and blood products, in Committee on Pre- and Postoperative Care, American College of Surgeons: *Manual of Pre-operative and Post-operative Care*. Philadelphia, Saunders, 1983, pp 137–152.
25. Rahilly GT, Berl T: Severe metabolic alkalosis caused by administration of plasma protein fraction in end-stage renal failure. *N Engl J Med* 301:824–826, 1979.
26. Weygandt GR, Roos A: The effects of citrated blood and hypothermia on acid-base balance during cardiopulmonary bypass. *Anesthesiology* 36:268–277, 1972.
27. Grigor KC, Blair JI, Hutchison JRS: The effect of acetazolamide on post-perfusion metabolic alkalosis. *Br J Anaesth* 43:352–361, 1971.
28. Nguyen DH, Mitchell ME: Gastric bladder reconstruction. *Urol Clin N Am* 18:649–657, 1991.
29. Kinahan TJ, Khoury AE, McLorie GA et al: Omeprazole in post-gastrocystoplasty metabolic alkalosis and acidura. *J Urol* 147:435–437, 1992.
30. Harrington JT, Cohen JJ: Measurement of urinary electrolytes—indications and limitations. *N Engl J Med* 293:1241–1243, 1975.
31. Garella S, Chazan JA, Cohen JJ: Saline-resistant metabolic alkalosis or "chloride-wasting nephropathy." *Ann Int Med* 73:31–38, 1970.
32. Heimann T, Brau S, Sakurai H et al: Acid-base changes in renal dysfunction following open heart surgery. *Mount Sinai J Med* 45:471–475, 1978.
33. Kwun KB, Boucherit T, Wong J et al: Treatment of metabolic alkalosis with intravenous infusion of concentrated hydrochloric acid. *Ann J Surg* 146:328–330, 1983.
34. Wagner CW, Nesbit RR, Mansberger AR: The use of intravenous hydrochloric acid in treatment of 34 patients with metabolic alkalosis. *Am Surg* 46:140–146, 1980.
35. Brimioulle S, Vincent JL, Dufaye P et al: Hydrochloric acid infusion for treatment of metabolic alkalosis: Effects on acid-base balance and oxygenation. *Crit Care Med* 13:738–742, 1985.
36. Worthley LIG: The rational use of IV hydrochloric acid in the treatment of metabolic alkalosis. *Br J Anaesth* 49:811–817, 1977.
37. Dickinson GE, Myers ML, Goldbach M, Sibbald W: Acetazolamide in the treatment of ventilatory failure complicating acute metabolic alkalosis. *Anesth Analg* 60:608–610, 1981.
38. Ayus JC, Olivero JJ, Adrogue HJ: Alkalemia associated with renal failure. Correction by hemodialysis with low bicarbonate dialysate. *Arch Intern Med* 140:513–515, 1980.
39. Barcenas CG, Fuller TJ, Knochel JP: Metabolic alkalosis after massive blood transfusion. Correction by hemodialysis. *JAMA* 236:953–954, 1976.
40. Albert MD, Dell RB, Winters RW: Quantitative displacement of acid-base equilibrium in metabolic acidosis. *Ann Intern Med* 66:312–322, 1967.
41. Emmett ME, Narins RG: Clinical use of the anion gap. *Medicine* 56:38–54, 1977.
42. Gabow PA: Disorders associated with an altered anion gap. *Kidney Int* 27:472–483, 1985.
43. Narins RG, Goldberg M: Renal tubular acidosis: Pathophysiology, diagnosis and treatment. *DM* 23(6):1–66, 1977.
44. Widmer B, Gerhardt RE, Harrington JT et al: Serum electrolyte and acid-base composition. The influence of graded degrees of chronic renal failure. *Arch Intern Med* 139:1099–1102, 1979.
45. Warnock DG: Uremic acidosis. *Kidney Int* 34:278–287, 1988.
46. Battle DC, Arruda JAL, Kurtzman NA: Hyperkalemic distal renal tubular acidosis associated with obstructive uropathy. *N Engl J Med* 304:373–380, 1981.
47. Battle D, Itsarayoungyuen K, Arruda JAL et al: Hyperkalemic hyperchloremic metabolic acidosis in sickle cell hemoglobinopathies. *Am J Med* 72:188–192, 1982.

48. Kurtzman NA: Acquired distal renal tubular acidosis. *Kidney Int* 24: 807–819, 1983.
49. Gabow PA, Moore S, Schrier RW: Spironolactone-induced hyperchloremic acidosis in cirrhosis. *Ann Int Med* 90:338–340, 1979.
50. Wagstaff KE, Woodhouse CRF, Rose GA et al: Blood and urine analysis in patients with intestinal bladders. *Br J Urol* 68:311–316, 1991.
51. Boyd SD, Schiff WM, Skinner DG et al: Prospective study of metabolic abnormalities in patients with continent Koch pouch urinary diversion. *Urol* 33:85–88, 1989.
52. Hurdley J: Unexpected metabolic acidosis during rectal surgery. *Anaesthesia* 33:478–480, 1978.
53. Fuller TJ, Garg LC, Harty RF et al: Severe hyperchloremic acidosis complicating jejunoileal bypass. *Surg Gyn Obst* 146:567–571, 1978.
54. Burke GW, Gruessner R, Dunn DL et al: Conversion of whole pancreaticoduodenal transplants from bladder to enteric draining for metabolic acidosis or dysuria. *Transpl Proc* 22:651–652, 1990.
55. Heird WC, Dell RB, Driscoll JM Jr et al: Metabolic acidosis resulting from intravenous alimentation mixtures containing synthetic amino acids. *N Engl J Med* 287:943–948, 1972.
56. Fraley DS, Adler S, Bruns F et al: Metabolic acidosis after hyperalimentation with casein hydrolysate. Occurrence in a starved patient. *Ann Intern Med* 88:352–354, 1978.
57. Kushner RF, Sitrin MD: Metabolic acidosis. Development in two patients receiving a potassium-sparing diuretic and total parenteral nutrition. *Arch Intern Med* 146:343–345, 1986.
58. Battle DC, Hizon M, Cohen E et al: The use of the urinary anion gap in the diagnosis of hyperchloremic metabolic acidosis. *N Engl J Med* 318:594–599, 1988.
59. Gabow PA, Kaehny WD, Fennessey PY et al: Diagnostic importance of an increased serum anion gap. *N Engl J Med* 303:854–858, 1980.
60. Brenner BE: Clinical significance of the elevated anion gap. *Am J Med* 79:289–296, 1985.
61. Levy LJ, Duga J, Girgis M et al: Ketoacidosis associated with alcoholism in nondiabetic subjects. *Ann Intern Med* 78:213–219, 1973.
62. Fulop M, Hoberman HD: Alcoholic ketosis. *Diabetes* 24:785–790, 1975.
63. McCoy HG, Cipolle RJ, Ehlers SM et al: Severe methanol poisoning: Application of a pharmacokinetic model for ethanol therapy and hemodialysis. *Am J Med* 67:804–807, 1979.
64. Peterson CD, Collins AJ, Himes JM et al: Ethylene glycol poisoning: Pharmacokinetics during therapy with ethanol and hemodialysis. *N Engl J Med* 304:21–23, 1981.
65. Baud FJ, Galliot M, Astier A et al: Treatment of ethylene glycol poisoning with intravenous 4-methylpyrazole. *N Engl J Med* 319:97–100, 1988.
66. Anderson RJ, Potts DE, Gabow PA et al: Unrecognized adult salicylate intoxication. *Ann Intern Med* 85:745–748, 1976.
67. Winchester JF, Gelfand MC, Helliwell M et al: Extracorporeal treatment of salicylate or acetaminophen poisoning. Is there a role? *Arch Intern Med* 141:370–374, 1981.
68. Hill JB: Salicylate intoxication. *N Engl J Med* 288:1110–1113, 1973.
69. Stolberg L, Rolfe R, Gitlin N et al: D-lactic acidosis due to abnormal gut flora. *N Engl J Med* 306:1344–1348, 1982.
70. Thurn JR, Pierpont GL, Ludvigsen CW et al: D-lactate encephalopathy. *Am J Med* 79:717–721, 1985.
71. Kreisberg RA: Lactate homeostasis and lactic acidosis. *Ann Intern Med* 92:227–237, 1980.
72. Mizock BA: Controversies in lactic acidosis: Implications in critically ill patients. *JAMA* 258:497–501, 1987.
73. Madias NE: Lactic acidosis. *Kidney Int* 29:752–774, 1986.
74. Eggleston FC, Feierabend TC: The early acidosis of burns: Its relationship to extent of burn and management. *Surgery* 77:641–647, 1975.
75. Spechler SJ, Esposito AL, Koff RS et al: Lactic acidosis in oat cell carcinoma with extensive hepatic metastases. *Arch Intern Med* 138:1663–1664, 1978.
76. Wainer RA, Wiernik PH, Thompson WL: Metabolic and therapeutic studies of a patient with acute leukemia and severe lactic acidosis of prolonged duration. *Am J Med* 55:255–260, 1973.
77. Brooks H, Carey LC: Base deficit in superior mesenteric artery occlusion. An aid to early diagnosis. *Ann Surg* 177:352–356, 1973.
78. Ernest D, Herkes RG, Raper RF et al: Alterations in anion gap following cardiopulmonary bypass. *Crit Care Med* 20:52–56, 1992.
79. Orringer CE, Eustace JC, Wunsch CD et al: Natural history of lactic acidosis after grand-mal seizures. *N Engl J Med* 297:796–799, 1977.
80. Taradash MR, Jacobson LB: Vasodilator therapy of idiopathic lactic acidosis. *N Engl J Med* 293:468, 1975.
81. Brezis M, Rowe M, Shalev O: Reversal of lactic acidosis associated with heart failure by nitroprusside administration. *Br Med J* 2:1399–1400, 1979.
82. Stacpoole PW, Lorenz AC, Thomas GR et al: Dichloroacetate in the treatment of lactic acidosis. *Ann Intern Med* 108:58–63, 1988.
83. Stacpoole PW: Lactic acidosis: The case against bicarbonate therapy. *Ann Int Med* 105:276–279, 1986.
84. Bersin RM, Chatterjee K, Arieff AI: Metabolic and hemodynamic consequences of sodium bicarbonate administration in patients with heart disease. *Am J Med* 87:7–14, 1989.
85. Weil MH, Rackow EC, Trevino R et al: Difference in acid-base state between venous and arterial blood during cardiopulmonary resuscitation. *N Engl J Med* 315:153–156, 1986.
86. Androgue HJ, Rashad MN, Gorin AB et al: Assessing acid-base status in circulatory failure. Differences between arterial and central venous blood. *N Engl J Med* 320:1312–1316, 1989.
87. Bleich HL: The clinical implications of venous carbon dioxide tension. *N Engl J Med* 320:1345–1346, 1989.
88. Narins RG, Cohen JJ: Bicarbonate therapy for organic acidosis: The case for its continued use. *Ann Intern Med* 106:615–618, 1987.
89. Garella S, Dana CL, Chazan JA: Severity of metabolic acidosis as a determinant of bicarbonate requirements. *N Engl J Med* 289:121–126, 1973.
90. Palevsky PM, Relton S, Greenberg A: Slow continuous ultrafiltration and dialysis (SCUD): Experience in 22 ICU patients. *Am Soc Artific Intern Org J*, 1992 Abstracts, p 80.
91. Hudson LE, Hurlow RS, Craig KC et al: Does intermittent mandatory ventilation correct respiratory alkalosis in patients receiving assisted mechanical ventilation? *Am Rev Respir Dis* 132:1071–1074, 1985.
92. Culpepper JA, Rinaldo JE, Rogers RM: Effect of mechanical ventilator mode on tendency towards respiratory alkalosis. *Am Rev Resp Dis* 132:1075–1077, 1985.
93. Knochel JP: The pathophysiology and clinical characteristics of severe hypophosphatemia. *Arch Intern Med* 137:203, 1977.
94. Rose BD: *Clinical Physiology of Acid-Base and Electrolyte Disorders*, 3d ed. New York, McGraw-Hill, 1989, pp 509–510.

63 POSTOPERATIVE ACUTE RENAL FAILURE

Laurence H. Beck

Acute renal failure remains an ominous complication of surgery with a mortality of 40 to 80 percent, depending on the setting. Although there has been little change in the survival rate over the last 40 years, a better understanding of the factors that contribute to the development of acute renal failure can help to prevent it. In this chapter, the term acute renal failure (ARF) will be used inclusively, indicating any abrupt reduction in excretion of nitrogenous wastes with subsequent azotemia and usually oliguria. This definition is useful because it forces the clinician to clarify the diagnosis further and determine whether the ARF is due to prerenal, postrenal, or intrinsic renal factors. The traditional term acute tubular necrosis (ATN) will not be used because it implies a histologic lesion that may or may not be present.[1,2] Instead, the somewhat awkward but more precise term acute reversible intrinsic renal failure (ARIRF) will be employed. Other authors have chosen to use terms like acute ischemic failure, vasomotor nephropathy, and nephrotoxic renal failure, emphasizing the common etiologies of ARIRF.

The clinical picture of ARIRF was first described in traumatized and surgical patients in 1944 during the bombing of London.[3] At that time, mortality was in excess of 90 percent. With the advent of hemodialysis, the mortality of patients with ARIRF in the Korean conflict fell to 53 percent, and in the Vietnam conflict rose slightly to 64 percent.[4,5] Modern reviews of ARIRF in surgical patients yield mortality figures between 56 percent and 70 percent, similar to those from battlefield casualties.[6–13]

Certain factors predict a better or worse prognosis for patients with postoperative ARIRF. Those associated with a worse prognosis include age, extent of extrarenal disease, congestive heart failure or previous myocardial infarction, septicemia, peritonitis, and central nervous system dysfunction.[4,9,14–16] Those predicting a better prognosis are the occurrence of nonoliguric rather than oliguric renal failure and perhaps the use of total parenteral nutrition.[7,9,17–19]

RENAL RESPONSE TO SURGERY

Major changes in renal hemodynamics occur in normal humans undergoing general anesthesia, with decreases in renal blood flow and glomerular filtration rate and increases in renal vascular resistance and filtration fraction.[20] Part of these effects are indirect and mediated by increases in catecholamine secretion or depression of myocardial function. In addition, most general anesthetics exert a dose-related direct effect on renal hemodynamics that can be minimized by adequate extracellular fluid repletion.[21] Regional anesthesia has no direct effect on renal function but may interfere with renal autoregulation, particularly in states of hypovolemia or low cardiac output.[22]

Urinary concentration as measured by osmolality increases during surgery, while urine flow and osmolar clearance decrease. Vasopressin release is stimulated directly by opioids and general anesthesia.[21] In addition, surgery itself and postoperative stress stimulate vasopressin secretion.[23] Therefore, most patients emerge from surgery and general anesthesia with a low flow of concentrated urine. So predictable is this response that a decrease in urinary concentrating ability may serve as a clue to ARIRF in the early postoperative period.

EVALUATION OF ACUTE RENAL FAILURE

In the initial evaluation of a patient with oliguria and a rising blood urea nitrogen (BUN) or serum creatinine concentration, it is important to distinguish among prerenal, postrenal, and intrinsic renal causes. Postrenal failure or obstructive uropathy should be considered in every patient. Bladder outlet obstruction induced by drugs, bed rest, or urinary tract infection is easily diagnosed by physical examination and straight catheterization of the bladder. Obstruction higher in the urinary tract is usually due to extrinsic ureteral compression by hematoma, abscess, or inadvertent suturing. Obstructive uropathy need not be manifested by anuria or persistent oliguria. Although an intravenous urogram was the traditional method for making the diagnosis of upper-tract obstruction, renal ultrasound is currently the method of choice. A normal sonogram virtually excludes obstructive uropathy as the cause of acute renal insufficiency, except in the unusual case where the ureters and/or renal pelvis are encased with tumor or fibrosis.[24]

A more critical task for determining prognosis is differentiating between failure due to renal hypoperfusion and ARIRF. One method involves the use of a test dose of a potent loop diuretic like furosemide or ethacrynic acid.[25] Induced diuresis is thought to indicate that the kidney tubules are intact and that prerenal factors underlie the oliguria, while the absence of diuresis indicates established ARIRF. This hypothesis is based primarily on experimental studies in dogs and has not been tested critically in humans in a prospective manner.[26-28] Experience indicates that the test is poorly predictive, since false-positive and false-negative results occur.

In prerenal azotemia, the kidney is underperfused but otherwise normal and should conserve sodium and water. In ARIRF, it loses its ability to do so and to concentrate the urine maximally.[29] Prerenal azotemia is usually characterized by a urinary sodium concentration (UNa) of less than 20 meq/liter and a urine osmolality (Uosm) of more than 500 mOsm/liter. In ARIRF, the UNa is more than 40 meq/liter and the Uosm is less than 350 mOsm/liter. These parameters do not provide perfect separation, but an index combining measurements of both functions has proven to be better in doing so. Miller et al. described two functions, the fractional excretion of sodium (FEna) and the renal failure index, which are easily calculated from plasma and spot urine measurements:[30]

$$FEna = \frac{UNa/PNa}{Ucreat/Pcreat}$$

$$Renal\ Failure\ Index = \frac{UNa}{Ucreat/Pcreat}$$

In a prospective series of 102 patients with ARF, a renal failure index of less than 1 was found in 84 percent of patients with prerenal azotemia but in no patients with ARIRF. An FEna of less than 1 was found in 90 percent of prerenal cases but in only 1 of 25 patients with ARIRF. These indices also proved useful, but not as specific, in nonoliguric ARIRF.

Although these indices help to categorize patients with ARF, there are two important provisos. First, since mannitol and diuretics block tubular sodium reabsorption even in prerenal patients, these diagnostic indices are useless after such agents have been given. Potent diuretics should therefore be withheld until urine and serum samples have been obtained. Second, distinguishing between ARIRF and prerenal azotemia does not obviate the necessity for attempting to improve renal perfusion in every patient with ARF. Although prerenal indices indicate that azotemia and oliguria can be reversed if renal perfusion is improved, the same hemodynamic factors may be operating in patients with ARIRF and may have even caused the ARIRF. Failure to recognize and correct these factors may prolong and complicate the course of the renal failure.

Because of the serious prognostic implications of postoperative ARIRF, investigators have attempted to develop tests to identify patients with an increased risk of ARIRF early in the postoperative course before oliguria or azotemia develops. Measurement of free water clearance (CH$_2$O) or serial creatinine clearances during the first postoperative days may be helpful in doing so. Normal individuals have a concentrated urine just after surgery, and CH$_2$O should be correspondingly negative. Those with ARIRF have impaired concentrating ability and should have a higher CH$_2$O. In three published series,[31-33] a CH$_2$O more positive than -20 ml/min measured in the early postoperative period predicted the subsequent development of ARIRF. When an abnormal CH$_2$O was accompanied by a creatinine clearance of 25 ml/min or less, development of ARIRF was almost certain. Using these criteria, one group of investigators detected ARIRF at a mean of 1.6 days after surgery, or one to six days earlier than would have been the case if routine criteria had been used.[32]

CH$_2$O and creatinine clearance can be reliably measured during relatively brief urine collection periods of 4 to 12 hours. For patients with a high risk of developing postoperative ARIRF, repeated measurements over the first 24 to 48 hours may allow early detection of ARIRF so that appropriate therapeutic measures can be taken.

ETIOLOGIES OF ACUTE REVERSIBLE INTRINSIC RENAL FAILURE

There are multiple potential etiologies of ARIRF in surgical patients. Although early studies separated nephrotoxic from ischemic causes of ARIRF on a histologic basis, clinical presentation is sufficiently similar in all categories of ARIRF that careful review of the history, medication regimen, and operative record is crucial in diagnosing the underlying etiologic disorder.[34] In this section, two general types of ARIRF, hemodynamic and nephrotoxic, are reviewed, and several specific causes of ARIRF seen most commonly in the surgical patient are discussed. In each case, distinctive clinical features, predisposing factors, and methods of prevention are highlighted.

Ischemic (Hemodynamic)

The most dramatic and easily recognized cause of ARIRF is sustained hypotension due to blood loss, anesthesia, drugs, heart failure, or sepsis. In all cases, hypotension decreases blood flow to the kidney, and active renal vasoconstriction in response to systemic hypotension further compromises renal blood flow and the glomerular filtration rate (GFR). The resultant oliguria prevents additional extracellular fluid loss. Rapid correction of hypotension or volume loss reverses the situation without damage to the kidney. However, if the duration of hypotension is significant and the previous level of renal function is abnormal, the patient may rapidly develop ARIRF despite treatment.

The patient with ischemic ARIRF is usually oliguric from the time of the hypotensive episode and remains so throughout the course of the renal failure until diuresis occurs. Occasionally, several hours of continued urine flow can be documented between the causative event and the onset of oliguria. In some patients, hypotension lasts only minutes and leads to ARIRF, while in others hypotension can continue for hours with no adverse effects. Although it is difficult to predict who will develop ARIRF, patients who are elderly, have underlying renal insufficiency, or are volume-contracted at the time of the hemodynamic insult have the greatest risk. Ischemic ARIRF usually results in 7 to 10 days of oliguria followed by diuresis.[35] Dialysis obviously alters the time course and commonly blunts the diuresis normally seen during the recovery phase.

Septicemia, often due to gram-negative organisms, is a common cause of ischemic ARIRF in surgical patients.[9,36,37] Although frank hypotension can often be identified as the initiating event, septicemia without systemic hypotension can cause oliguric ARIRF that is mediated by intense splanchnic and renal vasoconstriction.[38]

Nephrotoxic

Studies of patients with ARIRF identify nephrotoxins as common etiologic agents even in surgical patients.[9,18] Many drugs and chemicals can cause ARIRF, but aminoglycoside antibiotics, most commonly gentamicin, account for the majority of cases.[39] The clinical course of gentamicin-induced renal failure is usually predictable.[40] After use of the drug for at least two to three days, often in combination with other antibiotics, the BUN and creatinine levels begin to rise usually without oliguria. The rate of rise is less rapid than in ischemic ARIRF, in which the serum creatinine level increases 1.0 to 1.5 mg/dl per day and the duration of renal failure is variable. Some patients recover in a few days after the drug is stopped, and others experience prolonged azotemia with slow improvement in renal function over several weeks.

Predisposing factors in aminoglycoside nephrotoxicity include preexistent renal insufficiency, advanced age, volume depletion, and excessive doses of the drug.[40,41] If serum gentamicin levels are measured, elevated peak or trough levels are usually found in patients with nephrotoxicity.[42] Unfortunately, elevated serum levels probably occur as a result of renal failure, obviating their utility in predicting or preventing ARIRF.[43] Newer methods of assessing early tubular toxicity, including measurement of urinary excretion of lysozyme or beta$_2$-microglobulin, appear promising but have not yet proved clinically useful.[41,44-46]

The relative toxicities of newer aminoglycosides have not been well established. Gentamicin, tobramycin, and amikacin are all potentially nephrotoxic, but recent prospective studies suggest that tobramycin may be less so than gentamicin.[47-49]

Renal Failure After Cardiac Bypass Surgery

Patients undergoing cardiac surgery have a particularly high risk of developing postoperative ARIRF, a complication with a dismal prognosis. Cardiopulmonary bypass has been described as "a form of controlled clinical shock."[50] In addition to variable periods of low flow in the initial stages of bypass, hemolysis, hemagglutination, and redistribution of circulating blood volume may occur. Nonpulsatile blood flow may be particularly deleterious to renal function,[51] but this is controversial.[52]

Several studies document the incidence and course of acute renal failure after cardiac surgery,[53-57] and combined results are remarkably uniform. The incidence of postoperative renal dysfunction defined by a creatinine level of 1.6 mg/dl or higher is 25 to 30 percent. Within this group, there are three distinct categories of increasing severity. In a study of 490 patients undergoing cardiopulmonary bypass, 14 percent developed nonoliguric mild renal insufficiency with creatinine levels below 2 mg/dl.[56] Renal function returned to normal by the fourth postoperative day. A second group, representing 12 percent of the total, developed more severe renal failure with peak creatinine levels of 2 to 5 mg/dl. None experienced oliguria or required dialysis. Renal function recovered after a mean of seven days. The mortality rate in these two groups was 7 percent and 8 percent respectively, but the rate was only 0.5 percent in those who did not develop postoperative renal failure.

The worst prognosis was seen in the smallest group, representing 4 percent of the total. These patients developed oliguric renal failure with creatinine levels rising above 5 mg/dl. Most required dialysis, and the mortality rate was 66 percent. In another study, the mortality rate was 89 percent among the 4 percent of patients who developed severe renal failure with creatinine levels over 5 mg/dl, and all those who required dialysis died.[57] Although one recent series reported a lower incidence of renal failure of 1.5 percent and a lower mortality rate of 27 percent in oliguric patients who received early dialysis,[58] the combination of postbypass oliguria and creatinine levels of 5 mg/dl or greater is an ominous sign.

Factors predicting postoperative renal failure in these patients are old age and preexistent renal dysfunction. Operative risk factors include prolonged bypass time, aortic crossclamping, and hemoglobinemia. However, the strongest predictor of postpump renal failure is profound sustained depression of cardiac function.[59] Maintenance of cardiac performance should therefore be the most important goal in preventing renal failure.[60] None of the studies demonstrated a protective effect of preoperative or intraoperative mannitol or furosemide, although these agents continue to be widely used and recommended to "protect" renal hemodynamics.[60]

Radiocontrast Dye–Induced

Until recently, iodinated radiocontrast materials were thought to carry little or no risk of producing renal failure.[61] However, over the last several years, numerous reports have documented ARIRF following radiocontrast studies, and several predisposing factors have been identified.[62-68] Within 12 to 24 hours of a dye study, oliguria develops. It is usually brief, lasting only hours to a few days, but the serum creatinine level continues to rise and peaks about seven days after the exposure. The majority of patients fully recover renal function, and dialysis is usually not required. Since oliguria is brief, hyperkalemia is rare. A small proportion of patients with preexisting renal disease may progress immediately to irreversible chronic renal failure.[67,69] The mortality rate in dye-induced ARIRF is 5 to 10 percent in most centers.

Oral cholecystographic dyes rarely cause ARIRF, but the incidence of ARIRF after intravenous or intraarterial administration of radiocontrast material is high in some groups of patients,[70-74] including those with previous renal insufficiency, diabetes mellitus, advanced age, dehydration, and multiple myeloma.[68] Some studies report that the incidence of nephrotoxicity rises with increased doses of the contrast material.[75] The major risk factor is probably preexisting renal insufficiency with or without diabetes mellitus.[65] The combination of diabetes and renal insufficiency is thus a contraindication to a dye study. In one study, only 1 of 23 diabetics with a creatinine level under 2 mg/dl developed ARIRF after intravenous pyelography, but 22 of 29 or 76 percent with a creatinine level above 2 mg/dl did.[69] The incidence was 93 percent in those with serum creatinine levels greater than 5 mg/dl. Other investigators reported an incidence of 92 percent in 13 diabetics with nephropathy and a mean serum creatinine level of 6.8 mg/dl in whom coronary arteriograms had been performed.[63]

Although other studies suggest that the incidence of dye-induced ARIRF is low or nonexistent, the consensus of published reports suggests that this complication occurs commonly in the high-risk groups identified above.[62,76] Many surgical patients have dye studies performed before operation. Since the oliguric period is often brief in dye-induced ARIRF, it may not be recognized unless serial creatinine levels are obtained.

Dye-induced ARIRF can be prevented if alternative imaging techniques such as radioisotopic scans, ultrasound, and computerized tomographic (CT) scans without contrast are used instead of dye studies in high-risk patients. If dye studies must be performed, using the smallest possible dose of contrast agent and avoiding dehydration are recommended. Intravenous mannitol infused within an hour of intravenous radiocontrast agents may provide protection against acute renal insufficiency.[77] There is some indication that newer nonionized radiocontrast agents have fewer deleterious effects on renal function,[78] but definitive trials have not yet been reported.

Acute Interstitial Nephritis

Acute (allergic) interstitial nephritis (AIN) is a condition that is increasingly recognized as a common cause of ARF. In one renal biopsy series, AIN accounted for 11 percent of the cases with ARIRF.[79] Because the course of AIN mimics that of ARIRF in many ways, it often goes unrecognized clinically. The histologic hallmark of AIN is an intense diffuse inflammatory infiltrate in the interstitium of the kidney, usually with mononuclear and plasma cells. In some cases, polymorphonuclear leukocytes and eosinophils predominate.[80]

AIN is most often caused by drugs or infection. Although many drugs have been implicated, penicillins, sulfonamide-containing drugs, and methicillin have been the most common offenders.[81,82] More recently, nonsteroidal anti-inflammatory drugs (NSAID's) have been implicated in AIN and often cause a concomitant drug-induced lipoid nephrosis.[83]

The clinical picture of AIN is not distinctive and can vary from transient renal insufficiency to acute oliguric renal failure.[84] Clinical features that may distinguish AIN from ARIRF are unilateral or bilateral flank tenderness and systemic "allergic" signs including fever, skin rash, and eosinophilia, but these signs are absent in most cases. The urinary sediment usually reveals white blood cells, and sometimes eosinophils can be seen on a Wright's stained preparation.[82] However, this latter finding is nonspecific and occurs in several other renal conditions.[85] Urinary indices are usually indistinguishable from those of ARIRF.[80]

The clinical course is that of ARF with oliguria in about 50 percent of patients. Renal insufficiency varies in severity and occasionally requires dialysis. Discontinuation of the responsible drug is followed by recovery of renal function in days or weeks. There is some evidence that the administration of steroids may hasten the recovery of renal function, but the prognosis for complete recovery is excellent without steroids.[80,82]

Other Causes of ARF

Pigment nephropathy, the reversible ARF caused by the heme pigments hemoglobin and myoglobin, is often accompanied by volume depletion, metabolic acidosis, or other serious illness. In surgical patients, hemoglobinuria usually results from serious blood transfusion reactions, and myoglobinuria follows crush injuries to muscles. A clue to the presence of these pigments is a positive urine dipstick test for blood or a positive benzidine reaction when there are no red blood cells in the sediment. In significant amounts, they color the urine red. Because myoglobin is rapidly cleared, patients with myoglobinuria almost never have red serum, but those with hemoglobinuria usually do. In either case, red-orange granular casts are often seen in the urinary sediment.

Although hemoglobinuric ARIRF follows the usual course of ARF, certain features of myoglobinuria renal failure are distinctive.[86,87] Serum creatine kinase levels are usually elevated and, because the contents of muscle cells are released into the extracellular fluid, there is often a rapid rise in the serum potassium and creatinine concentrations. In most types of ARIRF, serum creatinine concentration rises about 1.0 to 1.5 mg/dl per day, but, in myoglobinuric renal failure, it may rise by as much as 2 to 4 mg/dl per day. In the absence of traumatic injury, rhabdomyolysis has been associated with prolonged operating time and the lateral decubitus position[88] and has been reported most commonly following total hip arthroplasty.[89]

Both experimental and clinical evidence suggest that mannitol diuresis can abort pigment nephropathy if administered before ARIRF fully develops.[90,91] Patients with acute hemolysis or muscle injury should be given 12.5 to 25 grams of 25% mannitol to initiate a diuresis of two to three liters per day. This urine volume should be maintained until there is clinical evidence that the pigment load has been reduced.

Approximately 10 percent of patients undergoing surgery for obstructive jaundice develop postoperative ARIRF for unclear reasons.[92] Some cases are clearly related to bacteremia and endotoxemia, but others remain unexplained. Some have suggested that the incidence can be markedly reduced by administering oral bile salts before surgery,[93] but it is premature to recommend this routinely. A small randomized trial has recently shown equivalent protection using either mannitol or bile salts.[94]

Renal atheroembolism, also called the renal microembolization syndrome, can cause ARF, particularly following reconstructive procedures of the aorta in patients with atherosclerosis.[95,96] Atheromatous debris is dislodged from plaques by catheters or manipulation, resulting in a shower of material that may become lodged in small arteries of the kidney and cause ischemia and necrosis. Clinical signs include petechial and subungual infarcts in the toes, livedo reticularis of the abdomen and thighs, and elevated serum amylase levels. The development of new hypertension may suggest this syndrome in the appropriate setting. The course of renal failure may be abrupt in onset with virtual anuria and only rare recovery or more insidious with progressive renal insufficiency developing over days to weeks with some recovery possible.[97] There is no effective therapy once the insult has occurred.

The more common renal complication of aortic surgery is "ischemic" ARIRF, occurring in nearly 60 percent of patients when aortic crossclamping is performed above the renal arteries and in about 20 percent when clamping is infrarenal.[98] Preoperative renal insufficiency is the only significant predictor of postoperative ARIRF in this setting.[99] Renal hypothermia and administration of nitroprusside, mannitol, dopamine, furosemide, and ACE inhibitors have been tried as preventive measures, but most investigators conclude that prevention of volume depletion and optimization of systemic hemodynamics are most important.[100,101]

Drug-related reversible ARF occurs most frequently in older

individuals and those receiving NSAID's or angiotensin-converting enzyme (ACE) inhibitors during the postoperative period. Although the mechanisms are different, most of these drugs alter glomerular hemodynamics, resulting in a functional decrease in GFR. This is particularly likely in patients with congestive heart failure, volume depletion, preexistent renal insufficiency,[102] or, in the case of ACE inhibitors, bilateral renal artery stenosis.[103] Hyperkalemia is common even if renal failure is not severe. These drug effects are completely and rapidly reversible when the offending medications are discontinued.

As discussed earlier, obstructive uropathy should always be considered early in the evaluation of ARIRF because it is usually correctable. Bladder outlet obstruction can be exacerbated by anesthesia, bed rest, and pain. Determination of the residual volume by catheterizing the bladder should always precede more extensive evaluation of postoperative renal failure. Although ureteral injury is a potential complication of gynecologic and other pelvic surgery, bilateral obstruction with renal failure is unusual.[104] It has been reported as a rare complication of aortobifemoral bypass surgery.[105]

The inhalational anesthetic methoxyflurane, now rarely used, was responsible for a large number of cases of vasopressin-resistant nephrogenic diabetes insipidus.[106-108] The acute nephrotoxicity is related to the level of blood fluoride, a metabolite of methoxyflurane.[109] The other fluorinated inhalational anesthetics—halothane, isoflurane, and enflurane—have rarely been implicated in ARF and are clearly much less nephrotoxic.[110,111]

TREATMENT OF ACUTE REVERSIBLE INTRINSIC RENAL FAILURE

The management of ARIRF is similar in surgical and nonsurgical patients. The major concerns are salt and water balance, potassium homeostasis, acid-base problems, and uremic manifestations. Infection and progression of the underlying primary disease are the major threats to survival even in well-managed patients with ARIRF.

All medications must be reviewed. Potentially nephrotoxic drugs should be totally avoided if possible, and those cleared predominantly by the kidney should be given in adjusted doses. Excellent tables of revised drug dosages in renal failure are published regularly.[112] When the serum creatinine level is rising, the GFR should be considered close to zero, and dose modifications for anephric patients should be used. During recovery from ARIRF, the serum creatinine can be used to estimate GFR. Serum levels of potentially nephrotoxic drugs should be followed carefully.

Certain characteristics of ARF may be exaggerated and require a more aggressive approach in surgical patients. Because of trauma and accelerated catabolism, the serum creatinine and BUN concentrations may rise more rapidly, and uremic signs and symptoms may appear earlier. Large endogenous potassium loads make hyperkalemia common. Third-space accumulation of extracellular fluid in the lumen of the bowel or at operative sites and extrarenal fluid losses make assessment of intravascular volume difficult. Swan-Ganz catheter placement is useful and often necessary in critically ill patients.[113]

Most nephrologists institute dialysis in nonsurgical patients with ARIRF only when hyperkalemia, uremic symptoms, or volume overload develop. However, several investigators recommend prophylactic dialysis in ARIRF and suggest that it improves survival.[114-116] These older studies are difficult to interpret because they use historical controls. In view of the continuing improvement in intensive care of critically ill patients, it may not be justifiable to attribute improved survival solely to early dialysis.

There have been two prospective controlled trials comparing intensive prophylactic dialysis to conventional dialysis in seriously ill patients. Conger randomly assigned posttraumatic patients to intensive prophylactic or conventional dialysis therapy.[117] The former group received hemodialysis early and frequently to maintain the serum creatinine level below five mg/dl and the BUN level under 70 mg/dl. The latter group was dialyzed for the usual clinical indications and when the serum creatinine concentration reached 10 mg/dl. In this small study of 18 patients, the mortality was 80 percent in the intensively dialyzed group and 36 percent in the conventionally managed group. Gram-negative septicemia was more frequent in the conventionally dialyzed group. However, in a more recent larger study of 26 patients paired on the basis of similar etiologies of ARF,[118] Conger found no significant difference in mortality between the two dialysis regimens. A more conservative approach to dialysis can therefore be safely recommended, one in which dialysis is carried out when clinically indicated or when the serum creatinine level rises to 10 to 11 mg/dl.

The choice between peritoneal and hemodialysis depends upon the type of surgery performed and the availability of resources. Although peritoneal dialysis requires fewer personnel and avoids the risk of anticoagulation, hemodialysis is more often preferred in the surgical setting because of the risks posed by peritoneal dialysis in patients who have undergone recent abdominal surgery, have prosthetic vascular grafts, or suffer from pulmonary insufficiency. Moreover, the rate of catabolism in surgical patients is often so high that peritoneal dialysis cannot keep pace with the production of nitrogenous wastes.

Malnutrition probably underlies much of the morbidity and mortality in ARF, particularly in patients with high rates of catabolism. The traditional approach to nutrition in ARF was to restrict protein intake to minimize azotemia and provide calories as "protein-sparing" carbohydrate.[35] The availability of dialysis now allows nitrogen and fluid loads to be given safely even in oliguric patients. Many such patients experience enormous nitrogen-wasting and often cannot eat postoperatively. Dudrick et al. demonstrated that positive nitrogen balance could be achieved by supplying total parenteral nutrition (TPN) with solutions of essential amino acids, hypertonic glucose, and other nutrients.[119] Parenteral hyperalimentation has become accepted practice in most surgical intensive care units, but it is unclear whether TPN or other forms of nutritional supplementation affect morbidity and mortality in ARIRF.

Abel et al. compared "renal failure fluid" containing essential amino acids and hypertonic glucose with hypertonic glucose alone in two groups of well-matched patients with ARIRF.[120] Of those receiving renal failure fluid, 75 percent survived, and of those receiving glucose alone, 44 percent survived. The duration of renal failure, number of required dialyses, and incidence of fatal and nonfatal sepsis were all lower in those given renal failure fluid. However, the results of this study have been questioned, and more recent studies comparing various types of mixtures of essential and nonessential amino acids with hypertonic glucose have shown no difference in morbidity or mortality rates.[121-124] Although hyperalimentation has not clearly been shown to improve outcome, it consistently improves nitrogen balance in highly stressed patients.

It therefore seems reasonable to recommend that parenteral hyperalimentation be initiated early in the course of postoperative ARF, particularly in those patients who are expected to have high rates of catabolism.[125]

PREVENTION OF ACUTE REVERSIBLE INTRINSIC RENAL FAILURE AND "CONVERSION" TO THE NONOLIGURIC STATE

Meticulous attention to intraoperative fluid balance and hemodynamics, avoidance of radiocontrast dyes and nephrotoxic drugs, and rapid treatment of systemic infections will certainly prevent some cases of ARIRF. Because decompensated congestive heart failure is a strong predictor of postoperative ARIRF,[126] elective surgery should be postponed until heart failure is under control.

Preoperative mannitol has been recommended for prevention of ARF in high-risk procedures such as abdominal aortic surgery,[127–129] but is no better than saline. Most nephrologists recommend careful volume repletion with saline in preoperative patients who have a high risk of developing ARIRF.[130,131]

The use of mannitol or potent loop diuretics in incipient or established ARIRF is more controversial.[132] Since ARIRF is associated with decreased total renal blood flow and redistribution of flow away from the renal cortex, these agents have become widely used to reverse early ARIRF or establish a diuresis, in part because they increase cortical blood flow.[133,134] The evidence that mannitol can reverse oliguria and alter the clinical course of ARIRF is scant. The best study, although not randomized, suggests that some patients with established ARIRF respond to mannitol with diuresis and have a shorter period of azotemia. A favorable response can be predicted by a urine-to-plasma osmolality ratio of more than 1.05.[125] Although the patients were carefully volume-repleted before they received mannitol, it is possible that the responders were still in a prerenal state. Because mannitol causes marked vascular volume expansion, it cannot be recommended routinely in oliguric patients, especially in those who have already been volume repleted. Intravenous furosemide and a more ototoxic diuretic, ethacrynic acid, have been widely recommended in oliguric patients.[136,137] Although furosemide has been effective in certain animal models, it has no significant effect in established renal failure in man.[138–140] Some investigators believe that furosemide may actually cause renal failure in patients who otherwise would not have developed it.[57,141]

Although furosemide may not reverse established ARIRF, many nephrologists feel that it is useful in early ARF when oliguria may still be converted to nonoliguria.[142] Nonoliguric patients are easier to manage and have less hyperkalemia, fewer dialyses, and better survival rates.[18] The standard approach is to infuse 200 mg of furosemide intravenously over 20 to 30 minutes and to double the dose if there is no diuresis. Lack of response to 400 to 500 mg of furosemide suggests that further efforts at diuresis are probably futile. If diuresis does occur, the dose should be repeated every 6 to 12 hours to maintain a high urine output.

An alternative approach has been suggested by Shin et al.[143] Employing careful invasive hemodynamic monitoring in 18 consecutive trauma patients with ARIRF, they found that cardiac output could be maximized by increasing preload with plasma protein fractions and by decreasing afterload with nitroprusside. They continued to increase preload despite an elevated pulmonary capillary wedge pressure as long as cardiac output increased and pulmonary edema did not develop. This aggressive approach resulted in maintenance of a mean urine output of 100 ml/hr in all 18 patients for the duration of ARIRF and contrasted sharply with the outcome in 17 other patients who were treated more conservatively. These impressive results deserve confirmation in a prospective controlled trial. The ability to "convert" a sizable fraction of patients with postoperative ARIRF to a nonoliguric state may have a beneficial impact on survival.

SUMMARY

1. *Prevention of ARF*
    a. Avoid nephrotoxic drugs if possible. If they are necessary, observe recommended doses, especially in patients undergoing surgery.
    b. Consider alternatives to radiocontrast dye studies for patients with diabetes mellitus and renal impairment. If dye studies are necessary, avoid dehydration, infuse saline for 24 hours beforehand, and consider mannitol infusion at the time of the study. Check serum creatinine levels daily in high-risk patients after the study to avoid proceeding with surgery in the face of undetected ARIRF.
    c. Replete intravascular volume before surgery.
    d. Replace intraoperative fluid losses rapidly to avoid prolonged hypotension.
    e. If a hemolytic transfusion reaction occurs, administer mannitol.

2. *Diagnosis in the acutely azotemic or oliguric patient*
    a. Before administering diuretics or fluids, send a spot urine sample for measurement of sodium and creatinine concentrations and osmolality, and a serum sample for measurement of creatinine concentration. Calculate the Renal Failure Index (RFI):

$$RFI = \frac{UNa}{Ucreat/Pcreat}$$

If RFI is < 1, azotemia is probably prerenal; if RFI is > 1, azotemia is probably due to ARIRF.
    b. Immediately assess volume status. If there is evidence of volume depletion, administer a fluid challenge until hemodynamics are normal. Look for manifestations of congestive heart failure and, if present, optimize cardiac output.
    c. Always consider postrenal (obstructive) failure. Bladder catheterization and renal ultrasound study can rule out obstruction. Obstruction need not cause anuria or oliguria.
    d. Discontinue drugs known to cause acute interstitial nephritis (e.g., semisynthetic penicillins and sulfonamides). Look for accompanying fever, rash, and eosinophilia. Examine the urinary sediment for pyuria and eosinophiluria by using Wright's stain.
    e. If azotemia persists after volume repletion and exclusion of obstruction and interstitial nephritis, treat the patient for ARIRF.

3. *Management of ARIRF*
    a. Attempt to determine from the history, physical examination, anesthesia record, and medication list the most likely cause of ARIRF and correct it if possible.
    b. If the patient has oliguric ARIRF, a trial of up to 500 mg of intravenous furosemide in the first 24 to 48 hours is occasionally useful in "converting" oliguric to nonoliguric ARIRF.

c. Management is the same as in the nonsurgical patient. Because catabolism is increased, BUN, creatinine, and potassium levels rise more rapidly.

d. Early "prophylactic" dialysis is not recommended. Attempt to keep the BUN level below 100 to 120 mg/dl and the creatinine level below 10 mg/dl.

e. Parenteral nutrition with essential amino acids and hypertonic glucose should be administered to highly catabolic patients, unless the course of ARIRF is expected to be brief or the patient can obtain adequate nutrients by oral or enteral feeding.

f. Adjust all drug dosages appropriately. Consider the patient with ARIRF to be anephric until serum creatinine has peaked. Serum drug levels are often helpful.

REFERENCES

1. Finckh ES, Jeremy D, Whyte HM: Structural renal damage and its relation to clinical features in acute oliguric renal failure. *Q J Med* 31:429, 1962.
2. Bohle A, Jahnecke J, Meyer D et al: Morphology of acute renal failure: Comparative data from biopsy and autopsy. *Kidney Int* 10:S9, 1976.
3. Bywaters EGL: Ischemic muscle necrosis. *JAMA* 124:1103, 1944.
4. Griffith GL, Maull KI, Coleman CC et al: Acute reversible intrinsic renal failure. *Surg Gynecol Obstet* 146:631, 1978.
5. Smith LH, Post RS, Teschan PE et al: Posttraumatic renal insufficiency in military casualties. *Am J Med* 18:187, 1955.
6. Kennedy AC, Burton JA, Luke RG et al: Factors affecting the prognosis in acute renal failure. *Q J Med* 42(165):73, 1973.
7. Baek SM, Makabali GG, Shoemaker WC: Clinical determinants of survival from postoperative renal failure. *Surg Gynecol Obstet* 140: 685, 1975.
8. Merino GE, Buselmeier TJ, Kjellstrand CM: Postoperative chronic renal failure: A new syndrome? *Ann Surg* 182:37, 1975.
9. McMurray SD, Luft FC, Maxwell DR et al: Prevailing patterns and predictor variables in patients with acute tubular necrosis. *Arch Intern Med* 138:950, 1978.
10. Kjellstrand CM, Berkseth RO, Klinkmann H: Treatment of acute renal failure, in Schrier RW, Gottschalk CW (eds): *Diseases of the Kidney*. Boston, Little Brown, 1988, pp 150–154.
11. Cameron JS: Acute renal failure in the intensive care unit today. *Intens Care Med* 12:64–70, 1986.
12. Mentzer SJ, Fryd DS, Kjellstrand CM: Why do patients with post-surgical acute tubular necrosis die? *Arch Surg* 120:907–910, 1985.
13. Berisa F, Beaman M, Adu D et al: Prognostic factors in acute renal failure following aortic aneurysm surgery. *Q J Med* 76:689–698, 1990.
14. Gornick CC, Kjellstrand CM: Acute renal failure complicating aortic aneurysm surgery. *Nephron* 35:145–157, 1983.
15. Cioffi WG, Ashikaga T, Gamelli RL: Probability of surviving postoperative acute renal failure. *Ann Surg* 200:205–211, 1984.
16. Lange HW, Aeppli DM, Brown DC: Survival of patients with acute renal failure requiring dialysis after open heart surgery: Early prognostic indicators. *Am Heart J* 113:1138–1143, 1987.
17. Brooks HB, Schulhoff JW: Acute nonoliguric renal failure in the postoperative patient. *Crit Care Med* 4:193, 1976.
18. Anderson RJ, Linas SL, Berns AS et al: Nonoliguric acute renal failure. *N Engl J Med* 296:1134, 1977.
19. Feinstein EI: Parenteral nutrition in acute renal failure. *Am J Nephrol* 5:145–149, 1985.
20. Ngai SH: Current concepts in anesthesiology: Effects of anesthetics on various organs. *N Engl J Med* 302:564, 1980.
21. Cousins MHJ, Skowronski G, Plummer JL: Anesthesia and the kidney. *Anesth Intens Care* 11:292–320, 1983.
22. Halperin BD, Feeley TW: The effect of anesthesia and surgery on renal function. *Int Anesth Clinic* 22:157–168, 1984.
23. Philbin DM, Coggins CH: Plasma antidiuretic hormone levels in cardiac surgical patients during morphine and halothane anesthesia. *Anesthesiology* 49:95, 1978.
24. Ellenbogen PH, Scheible FW, Talner LB et al: Sensitivity of gray scale ultrasound in detecting urinary tract obstruction. *Am J Roentgenol* 130:731, 1978.
25. Whelton A: Posttraumatic acute renal failure. *Bull NY Acad Med* 55:150, 1979.
26. Stone AM, Stahl WM: Effect of ethacrynic acid and furosemide on renal function in hypovolemia. *Ann Surg* 174:1, 1971.
27. Eng K, Stahl WM: Correction of the renal hemodynamic changes produced by surgical trauma. *Ann Surg* 174:19, 1971.
28. Baek SM, Brown RS, Shoemaker WC: Early prediction of acute renal failure and recovery: II. Renal function response to furosemide. *Ann Surg* 178:605, 1973.
29. Schrier RW: Acute renal failure. *Kidney Int* 15:205, 1979.
30. Miller TR, Anderson RJ, Linas SL et al: Urinary diagnostic indices in acute renal failure. *Ann Intern Med* 89:47, 1978.
31. Shin B, Isenhower NN, McAslan C et al: Early recognition of renal insufficiency in postanesthetic trauma victims. *Anesthesiology* 50: 262–265, 1979.
32. Holper K, Struck E, Sebening F: The diagnosis of acute renal failure (ARF) following cardiac surgery with cardiopulmonary bypass. *Thorac Cardiovasc Surg* 27:231–237, 1979.
33. Shin B, Mackenzie CF, Helrich M: Creatinine clearance for early detection of posttraumatic renal dysfunction. *Anesthesiology* 64:605–609, 1986.
34. Oliver J, MacDowell M, Tracy A: The pathogenesis of acute renal failure associated with traumatic and toxic injury. Renal ischemia, nephrotoxic damage and the ischemic episode. *J Clin Invest* 30:1305, 1951.
35. Franklin SS, Merrill JP: Acute renal failure. *N Engl J Med* 262:711–761, 1960.
36. Elmgren DT, Cheung LY, Bloomer A et al: Acute renal failure after abdominal surgery. *Am J Surg* 128:743, 1974.
37. Fischer RP, Polk HC: Changing etiologic patterns of renal insufficiency in surgical patients. *Surg Gynecol Obstet* 140:85, 1975.
38. Levinsky N: Pathophysiology of acute renal failure. *N Engl J Med* 296:1453, 1977.
39. Hou SH, Bushinsky DA, Wish JB et al: Hospital-acquired renal insufficiency: A prospective study. *Am J Med* 74:243–248, 1983.
40. Appel GB, Neu HC: Gentamicin in 1978. *Ann Intern Med* 89:528, 1978.
41. Cronin RE: Aminoglycoside nephrotoxicity: Pathogenesis and prevention. *Clin Nephrol* 5:251–256, 1979.
42. Bennett WM, Plamp C, Porter GA: Drug-related syndromes in clinical nephrology. *Ann Intern Med* 87:582, 1977.
43. Bennett WM, Gilbert DN, Houghton D et al: Gentamicin nephrotoxicity: Morphologic and pharmacologic features. *West J Med* 126:65, 1977.
44. Schentag JJ, Plaut ME: Patterns of urinary beta-microglobulin excretion by patients treated with aminoglycosides. *Kidney Int* 17:654–661, 1980.
45. Wellwood JM, Lovell D, Thompson AE et al: Renal damage caused by gentamicin: A study of the effects on renal morphology and urinary enzyme excretion. *J Pathol* 118:171, 1976.
46. Luft FC, Patel V, Yum MN et al: Experimental aminoglycoside nephrotoxicity. *J Lab Clin Med* 86:213, 1975.
47. Modsen PO, Kjaer TB, Mosegard A: Comparison of tobramycin and gentamicin in the treatment of complicated urinary tract infections. *J Infect Dis* 134(Suppl):S150, 1976.
48. Smith CR, Lipsky JJ, Laskin OL et al: Double-blind comparison of

the nephrotoxicity and auditory toxicity of gentamicin and tobramycin. *N Engl J Med* 302:1106, 1980.

49. Feig PU, Mitchell PP, Abrutyn E et al: Aminoglycoside nephrotoxicity: A double-blind prospective randomized study of gentamicin and tobramycin. *J Antimicrob Chemother* 10:217–226, 1982.
50. Norman JC: Renal complications of cardiopulmonary bypass. *Dis Chest* 54:50, 1968.
51. Wilkens H, Regelson W, Hoffmeister FS: The physiologic importance of pulsatile blood flow. *N Engl J Med* 267:443, 1962.
52. Hickey PR, Buckley MJ, Philbin DM: Pulsatile and nonpulsatile cardiopulmonary bypass: Review of a counterproductive controversy (collective review). *Ann Thorac Surg* 36:720, 1983.
53. Doberneck RC, Reiser MP, Lillebei CW: Acute renal failure after open heart surgery utilizing extracorporeal circulation and total body perfusion. *J Thorac Cardiovasc Surg* 43:441, 1962.
54. Yeboah ED, Petrie A, Pead JL: Acute renal failure and open heart surgery. *Br Med J* 1:415, 1972.
55. Abel RM, Wick J, Beck CH et al: Renal dysfunction following open heart operations. *Arch Surg* 108:175, 1974.
56. Bhat JG, Gluck MC, Lowenstein J et al: Renal failure after open heart surgery. *Ann Intern Med* 84:677, 1976.
57. Abel RM, Buckley MJ, Austen WG et al: Etiology, incidence, and prognosis of renal failure following cardiac operations. *J Thorac Cardiovasc Surg* 71:323, 1976.
58. Gailiunas P, Chawla R, Lazarus JM et al: Acute renal failure following cardiac operations. *J Thorac Cardiovasc Surg* 79:241–243, 1980.
59. Hilberman M, Derby GC, Spencer RJ et al: Sequential pathophysiological changes characterizing the progression from renal dysfunction to acute renal failure following cardiac operation. *J Thorac Cardiovasc Surg* 79:838–844, 1980.
60. Kron IL, Joob AW, Meter CV: Acute renal failure in the cardiovascular surgical patient. *Ann Thorac Surg* 6:590–598, 1985.
61. Ansell G: Adverse reactions to contrast agents. *Invest Radiol* 5:374, 1970.
62. Diaz-Buxo JA, Wagoner RD, Hattery RR et al: Acute renal failure after excretory urography in diabetic patients. *Ann Intern Med* 83:155, 1975.
63. Weinrauch LA, Healy RW, Leland OS et al: Coronary angiography and acute renal failure in diabetic azotemic nephropathy. *Ann Intern Med* 86:56, 1977.
64. Alexander RD, Berkes SL, Abuelo JG: Contrast media–induced oliguric renal failure. *Arch Intern Med* 138:381, 1978.
65. Carvallo A, Rakowski TA, Argy WP et al: Acute renal failure following drip infusion pyelography. *Am J Med* 65:38, 1978.
66. Swartz RD, Ribom KE, Leeming BW et al: Renal failure following major angiography. *Am J Med* 65:31, 1978.
67. VanZee BE, Hoy WE, Talley TE et al: Renal injury associated with intravenous pyelography in nondiabetic and diabetic patients. *Ann Intern Med* 89:51, 1978.
68. Byrd L, Sherman RL: Radiocontrast-induced acute renal failure: A clinical and pathophysiologic review. *Medicine* 58:270, 1979.
69. Harkonen S, Kjellstrand CM: Exacerbation of diabetic renal failure following intravenous pyelography. *Am J Med* 63:939, 1977.
70. Rene RM, Mellinkoff SM: Renal insufficiency after oral administration of a double dose of a cholecystrographic medium. *N Engl J Med* 261:589, 1959.
71. Blythe WB, Woods JW: Acute renal insufficiency after ingestion of a gallbladder dye. *N Engl J Med* 264:1045, 1961.
72. Gottlieb A, Spiera H, Gordis E: Fatal renal insufficiency after oral cholecystography. *N Engl J Med* 267:389, 1962.
73. Seaman WB, Cosgriff S, Wells J: Renal insufficiency following cholecystography. *Am J Roentgenol* 90:859, 1963.
74. Canales CO, Smith GH, Robinson JC et al: Acute renal failure after the administration of iopanoic acid as a cholecystographic agent. *N Engl J Med* 281:89, 1969.
75. Taliercio CP, Vlietstra RE, Fisher LD et al: Risks for renal dysfunction with cardiac angiography. *Ann Int Med* 104:501–504, 1986.
76. Eisenberg RL, Bank WO, Hedgcock MW: Renal failure after major angiography. *Am J Med* 68:43, 1980.
77. Old CW, Lehrner LM: Prevention of radiocontrast-induced acute renal failure with mannitol. *Lancet* 1:885, 1980.
78. Davidson CJ, Hlatky M, Morris KG et al: Cardiovascular and renal toxicity of a nonionic radiographic contrast agent after cardiac catheterization. *Ann Intern Med* 110:119–124, 1989.
79. Wilson DM, Turner DR, Cameron JS et al: Value of renal biopsy in acute intrinsic renal failure. *Br Med J* 2:459, 1976.
80. Van Ypersele de Strihou C: Acute oliguric interstitial nephritis. *Kidney Int* 26:751, 1979.
81. Ditlove J, Weidmann P, Bernstein M et al: Methicillin nephritis. *Medicine* 56:483, 1977.
82. Galpin JE, Shinaberger JH, Stanley TM et al: Acute interstitial nephritis due to methicillin. *Am J Med* 65:756, 1978.
83. Carmichael J, Shakel SW: Effects of nonsteroidal anti-inflammatory drugs on prostaglandins and renal function. *Am J Med* 78:992–1000, 1985.
84. Ooi BS, Jao W, First MR et al: Acute interstitial nephritis: A clinical and pathologic study based on renal biopsies. *Am J Med* 59:614, 1975.
85. Corwin HL, Korbet SM, Schwartz MM: Clinical correlates of eosinophiluria. *Arch Intern Med* 145:1097–1099, 1985.
86. Grossman RA, Hamilton RW, Morse BM et al: Nontraumatic rhabdomyolysis and acute renal failure. *N Engl J Med* 291:807, 1974.
87. Koffler A, Friedler RM, Massry SG: Acute renal failure due to nontraumatic rhabdomyolysis. *Ann Intern Med* 85:23, 1976.
88. Targa L, Droghetti L, Caggese G et al: Rhabdomyolysis and operating position. *Anesthesia* 46(2):141–143, 1991.
89. Lachiewicz PF, Latimer HA: Rhabdomyolysis following total hip arthroplasty. *J Bone Joint Surg* 73B:576–579, 1991.
90. Teschan PE, Lawson NL: Studies in acute renal failure. *Nephron* 3:1, 1966.
91. Wilson DR, Thiel G, Acre ML et al: Glycerol-induced hemoglobinuric acute renal failure in the rat. *Nephron* 4:337, 1967.
92. Cahill CJ, Pain JA: Obstructive jaundice: Renal failure and other endotoxin-related complications. *Surg Ann* 20:17–37, 1988.
93. Cahill CJ: Prevention of postoperative renal failure in patients with obstructive jaundice—the role of bile salts. *Br J Surg* 70:590–595, 1983.
94. Plusa SM, Clark NW: Prevention of postoperative renal dysfunction in patients with obstructive jaundice: A comparison of mannitol-induced diuresis and oral sodium taurocholate. *J Roy Coll Surg Endinb* 36:303–305, 1991.
95. Illiopoulos JI, Zdon MJ, Crawford BG et al: Renal microembolization syndrome: A cause for renal dysfunction after abdominal aortic reconstruction. *Am J Surg* 146:779–783, 1983.
96. Mashiah A, Pasik S, Hurwitz N: Massive atheromatous emboli to both kidneys: A fatal complication following aortic surgery. *J Cardiovasc Surg* 29:60–62, 1988.
97. Smith MC: The clinical spectrum of renal cholesterol embolization. *Am J Med* 71:174–180, 1981.
98. Noirhomme P, Buche M, Louagie Y et al: Ischemic complications of abdominal aortic surgery. *J Cardiovasc Surg* 32:451–455, 1991.
99. Miller DC, Myers BD: Pathophysiology and prevention of acute renal failure associated with thoracoabdominal or abdominal aortic surgery. *J Vasc Surg* 5(3):518–523, 1987.
100. Graziani G, Carabellese G, Lorenzano E et al: Prevention of acute renal failure after aortic surgery. *Nephrol* 70:148–152, 1989.
101. Awad RW, Barham WJ, Taylor DN et al: Technical and operative factors in infrarenal aortic reconstruction and their effect on the glomerular filtration in the immediate postoperative period and six months later. *Eur J Vasc Surg* 4:239–245, 1990.

102. Garella S, Matarese RA: Renal effects of prostaglandins and clinical adverse effects of nonsteroidal anti-inflammatory agents. *Medicine* 63:165–198, 1984.

103. Williams GH: Converting-enzyme inhibitors in the treatment of hypertension. *N Engl J Med* 23:1517–1544, 1988.

104. Mann WJ: Intentional and unintentional ureteral surgical treatment in gynecologic procedures. *Surg Gynecol Obstet* 172(6):453–456, 1991.

105. Sieurarine K, Goodman M, Barry PR: Bilateral ureteral obstruction following aortobifemoral bypass graft. *J Cardiovasc Surg* 32(2):209–211, 1991.

106. Hollenberg NK, McDonald FD, Cotran R et al: Irreversible acute oliguric renal failure. *N Engl J Med* 286:877, 1972.

107. Churchill D, Knaack J, Chirito E et al: Persisting renal insufficiency after methoxyflurane anesthesia. *Am J Med* 56:575, 1974.

108. Singer I, Forrest JN: Drug-induced states of nephrogenic diabetes insipidus. *Kidney Int* 10:82, 1976.

109. Cousins MJ, Mazze RI: Methoxyflurane nephrotoxicity: A study of dose response in man. *JAMA* 225:1611, 1973.

110. Gelman ML, Lichtenstein NS: Halothane-induced nephrotoxicity. *Urology* 17:323–327, 1981.

111. Mazze RI: Fluorinated anaesthetic nephrotoxicity: An update. *Can Anaesth Soc J* 31:S16–S22, 1984.

112. Bennett WM, Aronoff GR, Morrison G et al: Drug prescribing in renal failure. Dosing guidelines for adults. *Am J Kidney Dis* 3:155, 1983.

113. Hesdorffer CS, Milne JF, Meyers AM et al: The value of Swan-Ganz catheterization and volume loading in preventing renal failure in patients undergoing abdominal aneurysmectomy. *Clin Nephrol* 28:272–276, 1987.

114. Kleinknecht D, Jungers P, Chanard J et al: Uremic and nonuremic complications in acute renal failure: Evaluation of early and frequent dialysis on prognosis. *Kidney Int* 1:190, 1972.

115. Teschan PE, Bacter CR, O'Brien TF et al: Prophylactic hemodialysis in the treatment of acute renal failure. *Ann Intern Med* 53:992, 1960.

116. Fischer RP, Griffen WO, Clark DS: Early dialysis in the treatment of acute renal failure. *Surg Gynecol Obstet* 123:1019, 1966.

117. Conger JD: A controlled evaluation of prophylactic dialysis in post-traumatic acute renal failure. *J Trauma* 15:1056, 1975.

118. Teschan PE, Abel RM, Conger JD et al: Acute renal failure versus nutrition: No free lunch in the ICU. *Am Soc Artif Intern Org* 29:764–769, 1983.

119. Dudrick SJ, Steiger E, Long JM: Renal failure in surgical patients. Treatment with intravenous essential amino acids and hypertonic glucose. *Surgery* 68:180, 1970.

120. Abel RM, Beck CH, Abbott WM et al: Improved survival from acute renal failure after treatment with intravenous essential L-amino acids and glucose. *N Engl J Med* 288:695, 1973.

121. Baek SM, Makabali GG, Bryan-Brown CW et al: The influence of parenteral nutrition on the course of acute renal failure. *Surg Gynecol Obstet* 141:405, 1975.

122. Leonard DC, Luke RG, Siegel RR: Parenteral essential amino acids in acute renal failure. *Urology* 6:154, 1975.

123. Knochel JP: Complications of total parenteral nutrition. *Kidney Int* 27:489–496, 1985.

124. Thompson M: Use of essential amino acid/dextrose solutions in the nutritional management of patients with acute renal failure. *Drug Intell Clin Pharm* 19:106–111, 1985.

125. Corwin HL, Bonventre JV: Acute renal failure in the intensive care unit (part 2). *Intens Care Med* 14:86–96, 1988.

126. Charlson ME, MacKenzie R, Gold JP et al: Postoperative renal dysfunction can be predicted. *Surg Gynecol Obstet* 169:303–309, 1989.

127. Barry KG, Cohen A, Knochel JP et al: Mannitol infusion: II. The prevention of acute functional renal failure during resection of an aneurysm of the abdominal aorta. *N Engl J Med* 264:967, 1961.

128. Seitzman DM, Mazze RI, Schwartz FD et al: Mannitol diuresis. A method of renal protection during surgery. *J Urol* 90:139, 1963.

129. Abbott WM, Austen WG: The reversal of renal cortical ischemia during aortic occlusion by mannitol. *J Surg Res* 16:482, 1974.

130. Barry KG, Mazze RI, Schwartz FD: Prevention of surgical oliguria and renal-hemodynamic suppression by sustained hydration. *N Engl J Med* 270:1371, 1964.

131. Blythe WB: The management of intercurrent medical and surgical problems in the patient with chronic renal failure, in Early LE, Gottschalk CW (eds): *Disease of the Kidney*. Boston, Little Brown, 1979, p 517.

132. Whiteside-Yim C, Fitzgerald FT: Preserving renal function in surgical patients. *West J Med* 146:316–321, 1987.

133. Hollenberg NK, Epstein M, Rosen SM et al: Acute oliguric renal failure in man: Evidence for preferential renal cortical ischemia. *Medicine* 47:455, 1968.

134. Mudge GH: Diuretics and other agents employed in the mobilization of edema fluid, in Goodman LS, Gilman A (eds): *The Pharmacological Basis of Therapeutics*. New York, Macmillan, 1975, p 817.

135. Luke RG, Briggs JD, Allison MEM et al: Factors determining response to mannitol in acute renal failure. *Am J Med Sci* 259:168, 1970.

136. Stahl WM, Stone AM: Prophylactic diuresis with ethacrynic acid for prevention of postoperative renal failure. *Ann Surg* 172:361, 1970.

137. Cantarovich F, Galli C, Benedetti L et al: High-dose furosemide in established acute renal failure. *Br Med J* 4:449, 1973.

138. Bailey RR, Natale R, Turnbull DI et al: Protective effect of furosemide in acute tubular necrosis and acute renal failure. *Clin Sci* 45:1, 1973.

139. Kramer JH, Schurmann J, Wassermann C et al: Prostaglandin-independent protection by furosemide from oliguric ischemic renal failure in conscious rats. *Kidney Int* 17:455, 1980.

140. Kleinknecht D, Ganeval D, Gonzalez-Duque LA et al: Furosemide in acute oliguric renal failure: A controlled trial. *Nephron* 17:51, 1976.

141. Lucas CE, Zito JG, Carter KM et al: Questionable value of furosemide in preventing renal failure. *Surgery* 82:314, 1977.

142. Minuth AN, Terrell JB, Suki WN: Acute renal failure: A study of the course and prognosis of 104 patients and of the role of furosemide. *Am J Med Sci* 271:317, 1976.

143. Shin B, Mackenzie CF, McAslan TC et al: Postoperative renal failure in trauma patients. *Anesthesiology* 51:218, 1979.

64 POSTOPERATIVE HEMATOLOGIC ABNORMALITIES

Keith T. Kanel

The postoperative hemogram is almost always obtained to assess surgical blood loss, and serial blood counts are used to detect perioperative bleeding and infection. Trends in the counts can alert the clinician to problems long before the patient becomes symptomatic, and allow monitoring of the functions of the blood in providing tissue oxygenation, immune defense, and hemostasis. Although the hemogram is easily obtained, it is often nonspecific. The clinician must be able to separate insignificant variations from serious medical conditions and act accordingly. This chapter deals with postoperative hematologic problems in adults having no previously detected blood disorders.

POSTOPERATIVE ANEMIA

Anemia is strictly defined as a hemoglobin level below 12.5 g/dl in males and 11.5 g/dl in females, corresponding to hematocrit levels of 40% and 36%, respectively. The decline in the first postoperative hematocrit from preoperative levels can be explained by net surgical blood. However, over the ensuing days the blood count shows considerable variation. The clinician must assess the impact of anemia and determine whether fluctuations in hematocrit are due to benign processes such as intravascular equilibration, phlebotomy, and hemodilution, or to bleeding and hemolysis.

Tolerance of a given level of acute anemia must be carefully weighed against the risk of transfusion. Although a hemoglobin level of 10 g/dl has been cited as the level at which the improved rheology of hemodiluted blood maximizes tissue oxygen delivery,[1,2] in many patients recovery is unaffected at even lower levels. In studies of patients refusing perioperative transfusions for religious reasons, hemoglobin levels as low as six g/dl have posed no significant independent risk.[3,4] In 1988, the National Institutes of Health Consensus Conference on Perioperative Blood Transfusion reviewed all available data and set a hemoglobin level of seven g/dl as the cut-off point below which patients with acute anemia should be transfused.[5,6] In those with levels between 7 and 10 g/dl, the risk of anemia should include consideration of cardio-

pulmonary and nutritional status, the length of the surgical procedure, anticipated perioperative stresses like infection and hypoxemia, and the state of the marrow.

Intolerance of anemia is usually manifested by myocardial dysfunction. The heart not only extracts the most oxygen from the blood but also increases output to meet tissue oxygen demand. Patients with overt or suspected organic heart disease may therefore tolerate anemia poorly. The elderly often fail to increase cardiac output in response to normovolemic anemia even when no cardiac disease has been documented before surgery.[7] Animal studies have shown that noncritical coronary lesions may significantly raise the ischemic threshold for anemia.[8] Therefore, in those with known coronary artery disease, baseline electrocardiographic abnormalities, cardiac risk factors, advanced age, or prior stroke, maintaining the hemoglobin level closer to 10 g/dl may be advisable.

Postoperative anemia does not impair wound healing or increase susceptibility to infection until it becomes marked. Animal studies have shown that incision tensile strength[9,10] and healing of fractures[11] are normal with hematocrits of 30% as long as isovolemia and tissue perfusion are maintained. Human studies have likewise confirmed normal histopathological healing with hemoglobin levels below six g/dl.[12] By using subcutaneous oxygen sensors, tissue oxygenation is acceptable at normovolemic hematocrits of 20% or greater.[13,14]

In the clinical context, postoperative anemia is defined by a hemoglobin level that either continues to fall or fails to rise. Since the life span of the erythrocyte is 120 days, red cell mass should not decrease significantly in the immediate postoperative period unless there is loss or destruction of mature cells. Impairment of erythropoiesis alone does not explain worsening anemia. Therefore, in patients who are not bleeding, a rapid and sustained fall in hemoglobin levels indicates hemolysis until proven otherwise. Hemolytic anemia can result from a myriad of mechanisms driven by immunologic, chemical, and toxic stresses on the erythrocyte (see Table 64–1). Intravascular hemolysis involves destruction of circulating erythrocytes within the vascular space and is easily detected by the presence of significant amounts of hemoglobin, bilirubin,

TABLE 64–1.   Differential Diagnosis of Postoperative Anemia

Hemodilution and physiological variation
Diagnostic phlebotomy
Hemorrhage
Hemolytic anemia
  Drug-induced hemolysis
  Glucose-6-phosphate dehydrogenase (G-6-PD) deficiency
  Unstable hemoglobin disease
  Paroxysmal nocturnal hemoglobinuria
  Autoimmune (warm-antibody) hemolysis
  Infection
  Cold-agglutinin disease
  Transfusion-associated hemolysis
  Microangiopathic hemolysis
  Organ transplantation
  Prosthetic valve hemolysis
  Hypersplenism
  Water-dilution hemolysis
Reticulocytopenic anemia

---

and lactic dehydrogenase in the serum. Such processes can be sudden and fulminant and predispose patients to the nephrotoxic effects of filtered hemoglobin on renal tubular cells. Extravascular hemolysis occurs when cells are rendered abnormal by a biochemical stress or immunoglobin binding and then consumed by the reticuloendothelial system. Although this kind of hemolysis can be massive, it is more often a slower process with only minimal spillage of cellular byproducts into the circulation. Diagnostic markers and toxic effects may therefore be less pronounced.

A hemoglobin that fails to rise after surgery in the absence of blood loss or hemolysis suggests impaired marrow response to anemia and defines a reticulocytopenic anemia. When well tolerated and nonprogressive, the anemia itself may pose little threat to the patient. However, reticulocytopenia itself may be an important clue to underlying medical conditions that may significantly affect patient outcome.

Differential Diagnosis

Hemodilution due to mobilization of fluid from the extravascular space may influence the hematocrit significantly in the first few days after surgery, but it is not known how great a fall in hematocrit may be ascribed solely to hemodilution. Controlled saline infusions of 30 ml/kg in normovolemic volunteers cause decreases in hematocrit in excess of six points with no change in the red cell mass.[15] Operations involving extensive fluid administration are most likely to result in hemodilution. Drawing blood at different times of the day, position during phlebotomy, and sampling technique may alter the hematocrit by more than five points.[16]

The amount of blood drawn for diagnostic phlebotomy should not be underestimated. One study documented a mean loss of 300 ml among surgical intensive care unit patients in the first postoperative day.[17] Decreases in hematocrit of almost six points can be attributed to routine blood work performed in these specialized units.[18]

Postoperative bleeding, most commonly from the surgical site or from stress-related gastric mucosal disease, is the first concern in any patient with a falling hemoglobin level after surgery. Although loss of whole blood usually results in only small changes

in hemoglobin concentration, postoperative patients commonly receive enough intravenous fluids to produce anemia almost immediately. Postoperative bleeding is discussed more fully in Chap. 65.

When hemolysis is suspected, all medications should be reviewed. The majority of routine drugs—anesthetics, heparin, analgesics, and sedatives—are rarely associated with hemolysis. Agents implicated in hemolytic reactions are listed in Table 64–2. There are an increasing number of reports of hemolysis induced by standard prophylactic agents used in perioperative care, such as antibiotics and H_2 antagonists. Cephalosporins have long been known to convert the direct antiglobulin test to positive, but some newer agents have been reported to induce massive intravascular hemolysis.[19] At least two cases of profound hemolysis have been reported following the administration of cefoxitin used in preparing the bowel for surgery.[20,21] Fatal hemolysis has also occurred during ceftriaxone therapy of a healed surgical wound infection.[19] In each case, there was antecedent exposure to the offending drug, but it is still unclear whether prior sensitization is necessary for hemolysis to occur. Immune hemolysis has also occurred after exposure to ranitidine[22] and omeprazole.[23]

Drugs can trigger hemolysis by a variety of immune and nonimmune means. Three immune mechanisms have been identified. In haptenic immune hemolysis, small-molecule drugs like penicillin are recognized by the immune system only after binding to erythrocytes, and the IgG response results in extravascular destruction. Hemolysis ceases upon withdrawal of the drug. Immune complex or "innocent bystander" hemolysis occurs when antibody already present from prior sensitization binds free drug and the complex fixes complement to the erythrocyte membrane before diffusing away. In this case, intravascular hemolysis can be rapid, massive, and potentially fatal.[19] The circulating immune complexes can cause renal failure in 50 percent of patients.[19,24] Thirdly, medications like methyldopa and procainamide can trigger incidental autoantibody induction. Since the drug itself is not thereafter involved, hemolysis may not subside when it is discontinued. More than three months of exposure may be required in this form of hemolysis, and it is unlikely to occur in the postoperative period. In all cases, although it is unclear if all drugs within a class are crossreactive, related agents should be avoided unless clinical alternatives are unavailable.

Drug-induced hemolysis may be induced by nonimmune mechanisms in such disorders as (G-6-PD) deficiency, paroxysmal nocturnal hemoglobinuria, and unstable hemoglobin disease. Individuals congenitally deficient in glucose-6-phosphate dehydrogenase G-6-PD, an enzyme responsible for protecting hemoglobin from oxidant injury, can experience hemolysis in response to stress, infection, and certain drugs. Many agents once thought to induce hemolysis such as aspirin, acetaminophen, procainamide, phenytoin, quinine, and quinidine have since been found to be safe when given in therapeutic doses.[25] Drugs that should be avoided are listed in Table 64–2. Controversy surrounds the use of trimethoprim-sulfamethoxazole in this population. Although sulfamethoxazole is listed among agents known to induce hemolysis, the combination preparation has been used in patients with G-6-PD deficiency.[26] Infection is a much more common stimulus of hemolysis in this disorder than most drugs.

Hemolysis in G-6-PD deficiency is extravascular. Denatured hemoglobin forms Heinz bodies visible on peripheral blood smear. Hemolytic episodes are rarely severe and usually last about a week, since only older erythrocytes experience premature loss of

TABLE 64–2.   Mechanisms of Drug-Induced Hemolytic Reactions

Mechanism	Drugs	Onset	Hemolysis	Course	Diagnosis	Comments
Immune Hemolysis (Haptenic)	Penicillin Cephalosporins Tetracycline Erythromycin	7–10 days	Extravascular	Mild– moderate	+ DAT (Anti-IgG)	Resolves upon drug withdrawal Dose dependent
Immune Hemolysis (Immune Complex)	Cephalosporins Quinidine Sulfonamides Phenacetin Rifampin Ranitidine	Days	Intravascular	Severe	+ DAT (Anti-complement)	Resolves upon drug withdrawal Risk of ensuing renal failure approaches 50%
Immune Hemolysis (Autoantibody Induction)	Methyldopa Procainamide	3–6 months	Extravascular	Mild– moderate	+ DAT (Anti-IgG)	Persists despite drug withdrawal Consider steroids
G-6-PD Deficiency	Certain sulfonamides Nitrofurantoin Methylene blue Doxorubicin Phenazopyridine	Days	Extravascular	Mild– severe	+ Heinz body prep Low G-6-PD level Negative DAT	Often self-limited Risk groups include black and Asian males
Paroxysmal Nocturnal Hemoglobinuria (PNH)	Radiographic contrast Magnesium Acetazolamide	Days	Intravascular	Mild– severe	+ Acid hemolysis test + Sucrose hemolysis test Negative DAT	Associated with thrombosis, thrombocytopenia, leukopenia Consider heparin or dextran
Unstable Hemoglobin Disease	(see G-6-PD deficiency)	Days	Extravascular	Mild– severe	+ Heinz body prep + Isopropanol stability test Abnormal hemoglobin electrophoresis	Often evidence of chronic hemolysis Inheritance usually autosomal dominant

DAT = Direct Antiglobulin Test

enzyme activity and become susceptible.[27] Inheritance is sex-linked. G-6-PD deficiency is seen in males of Middle Eastern and Asian extraction, but in the United States the disorder is most commonly seen in African-Americans, in whom the genetic prevalence is 11 percent.[25]

Extravascular hemolysis in response to infectious or oxidant stress in the absence of G-6-PD deficiency may be attributable to congenital hemoglobin variants. Such conditions are generally inherited in an autosomal dominant pattern and are rarely detected preoperatively. Several dozen variants have been described and are listed in standard textbooks of hematology.[28] Some involve such subtle alpha-chain hemoglobin amino acid substitutions that hemoglobin electrophoresis will be unremarkable. Patients may exhibit jaundice, splenomegaly, "bite cells" on peripheral smear, and Heinz bodies following exposure to some of the same stresses affecting patients with G-6-PD deficiency.[29] However, hemolysis may not abate on removal of the triggering factor. Some dysfunctional variants may also cause cyanosis without anemia when methemoglobin levels rise above 10% in response to oxidizing stresses.

Hemolytic anemia with thrombocytopenia, leukopenia, and thrombotic episodes should raise the possibility of paroxysmal nocturnal hemoglobinuria (PNH). This stem-cell membrane defect is characterized by an enhanced sensitivity of all marrow lines to complement fixation and intravascular destruction. The process can be initiated by hypoxemia, dehydration, and acid-base abnormalities. Drugs known to enhance complement activation include radiographic contrast media, magnesium, and acetazolamide.[30] Hemolysis can be chronic and subclinical or fulminant with severe anemia and hemoglobinuria. Episodes of venous thrombosis due to complement-activated platelet aggregation can involve abdominal viscera and cause pain, ileus, and congestive hepatomegaly. In a series of 10 carefully managed patients with known PNH undergoing elective surgery, only two had significant hemolysis and none experienced clinical thrombosis.[30]

Autoimmune production of antierythrocyte IgG can occur as a primary phenomenon or in the presence of connective tissue diseases, lymphoid neoplasia, and certain drugs. Antibodies bind optimally at body temperature and usually target the Rh locus on the red cell, causing spherocytic transformation and extravascular hemolysis. Although these "Coombs'-positive" anemias represent the most common form of hemolysis in the general patient population, they are not exacerbated by perioperative stress.

Infections can induce hemolysis by a number of diverse mechanisms.[27] Most devastating is the microangiopathic hemolysis of diffuse intravascular coagulation (DIC) in patients with sepsis (see Chap. 65). Intravascular hemolysis can be caused by a specific alpha-hemolysin elaborated by *Clostridium perfringens* and can complicate anaerobic infections.[31]

Intravascular destruction due to T-antigen polyagglutination has been reported in patients with postoperative septicemia.[32] The T-antigen, or Thomsen-Friedenreich cryptantigen, usually hidden in the erythrocyte membrane, is exposed in the presence of neuramidase produced by some bacteria. Immunohemolysis is then mediated by complement-fixing anti-T antibodies present in all individuals. Pathogens that produce neuramidase include pseudomonas, bacteroides, klebsiella, and staphylococcus species. Extravascular and rarely warm-antibody immune hemolysis can also occur in the setting of infection.

Immune hemolysis has been observed in patients exposed to hypothermia in clinical situations ranging from the cold cardioplegia of cardiac surgery[33] to the use of simple cooling mattresses.[34] Cold agglutinins are IgM antibodies that cause hemagglutination, complement fixation, and intravascular hemolysis only below a critical temperature, usually less than 32°C. They may arise de novo or in the presence of certain conditions like mycoplasma pneumonia, mononucleosis, or lymphoproliferative diseases. Patients present with acrocyanosis, vasoocclusive phenomenon of the extremities, and hemolysis ranging from mild extravascular to massive intravascular destruction associated with hemoglobinuria and renal failure. The degree of hemolysis is dependent upon the critical temperature of the antibody, its avidity to complement, and the nature of the hypothermia. In cold cardiopulmonary bypass, erythrocyte clumping may be seen in the extracorporeal pump tubing.[35] The most severe form of cold agglutinin disease is paroxysmal cold hemoglobinuria, a unique variant mediated by an IgG immunoglobin known as the Donath-Landsteiner antibody and directed against the erythrocyte P antigen. Massive intravascular hemolysis can occur at temperatures below 15°C. Although warming halts further antibody-binding, hemolysis continues and can even accelerate in already complexed erythrocytes. Preoperative plasmapheresis has been advocated in known carriers of these antibodies when hypothermia is unavoidable.[33]

Transfusion-associated hemolysis is rarely seen with appropriate crossmatching but can be seen up to two weeks later as a low-grade breakdown of donor cells due to alloantibodies to minor antigens like Kell, Kidd, Duffy, or Rh. Antibodies from prior transfusions or pregnancy may be present in such low titers that they escape detection on crossmatching.[36]

Intravascular shearing and distortion of erythrocytes can occur in settings of intravascular fibrin deposition such as disseminated intravascular coagulation or with the widespread arteriolar damage seen in vasculitis, thrombotic thrombocytopenic purpura, pre-eclampsia, carcinomatosis, and organ transplant rejection. Otherwise uncomplicated surgery on plasminogen-activator-rich tissues such as myomectomy for uterine fibroids has also been associated with microangiopathic hemolysis.[37] The bizarre pattern of schistocytosis is usually diagnostic. Interruption of erythrocyte destruction is dependent upon removal of the inciting factor.

Immunohemolysis following organ transplantation can be the result of a graft (lymphocyte)–versus–host (erythrocyte) or a mild host (lymphocyte)–versus–graft (erythrocyte) reaction. It is most common when an O-group donor is transplanted into an A-, B-, or AB-positive recipient.[38] Significant hemolysis has recently been reported involving non-ABO antigens in patients seroconverted by prior transfusions, pregnancy, or transplantation.[39] Hemolysis occurs within the first two weeks after transplantation surgery. Hemolysis due to microangiopathy[40] and aplastic anemia[41] has also been reported. Immunosuppression induced by cyclosporine may actually contribute to the hemolytic process.[42,43]

Hemolysis from prosthetic heart valves is generally mild and often subclinical[44] but can be severe. Hemolysis is most marked in patients with caged-disk and caged-ball valves and minimal in those with tilting-disk and bioprosthetic devices.[45] Hemolysis is also more common in those with perivalvular leaks, prostheses in the aortic position, and cloth-covered valves. Patients with well-compensated chronic hemolysis may become anemic after a non-cardiac procedure if the stress of surgery briefly interrupts reticulocytosis.

Sequestrational hemolysis due to hypersplenism may occur in patients with diseases ranging from neoplastic infiltration to congestive heart failure. Postoperative anemia has also been attributed to water dilution hemolysis after high-volume irrigation with free water in urological procedures.[46] Hemolysis is presumed to be due to osmotic stresses on the erythrocytes from water absorbed into prostatic and bladder veins. Many urologists now use isotonic fluid for irrigation.

Studies of postoperative anemia in baboons have shown that increased erythropoiesis is not evident for the first few days while the erythroid component of the marrow expands. This "marrow lag" is followed by a brisk reticulocytosis during which the hematocrit may increase by greater than one point per day.[47] However, significant surgical inflammation suppresses marrow iron kinetic and may delay the response for over a week.[48] Absence of reticulocytosis beyond a week should prompt consideration of an impaired marrow.

Nutritional deficiencies of folate, trace elements, and vitamin are rare, but should be considered in selected patients. Iron deficiency is likewise uncommon just after surgery unless it has been present beforehand, but marrow stores become exhausted if subsequent blood loss is excessive. In most patients, a net blood loss of two liters is necessary to deplete marrow iron by one gram, but in menstruating women the loss can be as little as 600 ml.[49] The marrow also remains sluggish in various chronic disease states such as hypothyroidism, renal failure, connective tissue disorders, osteomyelitis, and in alcoholism.[49] Occasionally, marrow damage induced by radiation, tumor infiltration, infection, or chemotherapy escapes preoperative identification.

Drug-induced red cell aplasia has been reported after administration of a variety of agents including chloramphenicol, penicillin, cephalosporins, cimetidine, pentoxifylline, gold, and acetazolamide.[50] Some agents, specifically ranitidine[22] and procainamide,[5] have induced a mixed form of anemia with immune reticulocytopenia and DAT-positive hemolysis. Drug-induced red cell aplasia uniformly resolves upon discontinuation of the offending agent.

Diagnostic Evaluation

Failure of the hemoglobin level to rise within the first week after surgery should prompt a diagnostic evaluation. Exclusion of bleeding is the first concern. If the physical examination reveals no evidence of hematoma and the surgical drainage is not bloody, imaging of the surgical site should be considered. Urine, stool, and gastric aspirate should be tested for heme products. When possible, all diagnostic laboratory work should be obtained before transfusion.

In patients who are not bleeding with a stable anemia that does not improve, either marrow response is impaired or appropriate reticulocytosis is being counteracted by erythrocyte destruction. In such cases, reticulocyte count, serum B_{12} level, and red blood cell folate level should be measured. The reticulocyte count is used to calculate the reticulocyte production index (RPI) as follows:

$$RPI = (\text{reticulocyte count}) (Hct/0.45) (0.5)$$

where Hct is the hematocrit and 0.5 the correction factor for the two-day circulating life of reticulocytes before they mature into erythrocytes. A normal RPI is approximately 1%. Lower values are seen in cases of marrow insufficiency, and those over 3% suggest compensation for hemolysis. A low index does not exclude hemolysis and is found in as many as 37 percent of patients with hemolytic anemia. This may represent a lag in marrow response, and a repeat index a few days later is usually elevated.[52] Serum B_{12} and red cell folate levels should be obtained even if macrocytosis is absent. Serum iron studies are of limited usefulness in the postoperative period, because serum iron levels[48] and transferrin saturation[53] may be factitiously decreased for weeks following surgery. Similarly, ferritin is an acute phase reactant, and its serum level is elevated in 90 percent of postoperative patients.[54] Inadequate iron stores before surgery may be suggested by the preoperative red cell distribution width (RDW), which is often recorded automatically by most modern cell counters. RDW values over 15% may be seen long before abnormalities in the hemoglobin level or mean corpuscular volume are evident.[55,56] If all of the studies are inconclusive, the patient must be evaluated for intercurrent infection, renal failure, malnutrition, and other factors that might impair reticulocytosis. A bone marrow biopsy is appropriate if these studies are not diagnostic.

If the hemoglobin level progressively falls or if the RPI is over 3%, an evaluation for hemolysis should be promptly initiated. The peripheral blood smear may reveal polychromatic macrocytes and nucleated red cells within 12 hours, and the etiologic diagnosis may be evident by identifying erythrocyte "bite cells" seen in G-6-PD deficiency and unstable hemoglobin disease, schistocytes seen in microangiopathic hemolysis, or microspherocytes seen in immune hemolysis. Hemolysis is confirmed by finding elevated levels of free hemoglobin, unconjugated bilirubin, and lactic dehydrogenase, as well as urinary free hemoglobin and renal tubular cells for hemosiderin. Most specific is disappearance of the hemoglobin scavenger proteins haptoglobin and hemopexin. These markers may be only moderately abnormal in extravascular hemolysis but are usually markedly so in intravascular destruction.

Several tests are useful in determining the etiology of hemolytic anemia. The direct antiglobulin test (DAT), also known as the direct Coombs' test, is a polyvalent antibody preparation applied to patient erythrocytes to detect bound IgG, IgM, or complement and is diagnostic in over 90 percent of immune hemolytic anemias.[57] Certain forms of hemolysis such as cold agglutinin disease and innocent bystander drug reactions are diagnosed by unique binding of anticomplement antibody. The DAT is sensitive but not specific. It will be positive in up to 80 percent of patients on cephalosporins in the absence of hemolysis.[20] The indirect antiglobulin test (IAT), formerly the indirect Coombs' test, confirms the presence of free high-titer antierythrocyte antibody by mixing the patient's serum with control red cells and performing a standard DAT. In G-6-PD deficiency and unstable hemoglobin disease, Heinz bodies may not be seen in red cells if they are rapidly removed from the circulation. A Heinz-body preparation is then done by applying supravital stain to cells exposed to in vitro oxidant stress. Other studies ordered to evaluate hemolysis include quantitative G-6-PD level, hemoglobin electrophoresis, acid hemol-

ysis test (Ham's test) for PNH, antinuclear antibody (ANA), and immune complex and complement levels. A normal G-6-PD level during hemolysis does not preclude deficiency because enzyme is depleted from older cells that may have already been destroyed. Lastly, most hematology laboratories can also perform specific drug hemolysis testing by varying the IAT assay in the presence of the drug in question.

Treatment

Patients with postoperative anemia should be kept hydrated and normothermic and should be appropriately monitored for evidence of cardiopulmonary compromise. If hemolysis is suspected, hyperkalemia, acute tubular necrosis, and renal failure should be excluded. Oxygen may be administered, but pulse oximetry and arterial blood gas measurements detect only hemoglobin saturation and dissolved oxygen content and may be normal despite marked reductions in blood oxygen-carrying capacity. Phlebotomy should be minimized, and some advocate use of pediatric phlebotomy tubes for diagnostic studies.[58,59] Medications should be reviewed and appropriately substituted or withdrawn as needed. Folate should be administered empirically.

Blood transfusions should be administered according to the criteria set forth in Chapter 51. In hemolysis due to G-6-PD deficiency, PNH, and unstable hemoglobin disease, transfusion suppresses reticulocytosis and reduces entrance of susceptible cells into the circulation.[60] Crossmatching is occasionally difficult in immune drug-induced or warm-antibody hemolysis because autoantibodies may obscure proper detection of native alloantibodies. Most blood banks therefore screen serum only after autoabsorption of antierythrocyte antibody by expendable red cells. Donor cells may also be rapidly hemolyzed in autoantibody syndromes in which antibody binding is nonspecifically directed against the Rh locus. If compatible blood cannot be found, transfusions should be undertaken carefully with the least incompatible blood.

Recombinant human erythropoietin (rHuEPO) may augment red cell production, but its role in postoperative patients remains unclear. Primate studies reveal that high doses of erythropoietin administered from the first day of marked anemia after surgery accelerate red cell production but produce no significant effects in the first week.[47] The role of perioperative erythropoietin is presently limited to supporting autologous blood donation programs,[61] preparing anemic patients for surgery several weeks in advance,[62] and certain chronic illnesses characterized by erythropoietin deficiency such as renal failure and solid tumors.[63] Since recombinant erythropoietin is usually prepared with an albumin stabilizer, it may not be acceptable for use in those who object to transfusion for religious reasons.

Iron is often administered to anemic patients after surgery, but is useful only in those with true iron deficiency whether present before surgery or due to extensive perioperative blood loss. Such patients are few in number. The transfer of monocyte-macrophage ferritin stores to marrow precursors is blocked by the inflammatory response of surgery during the first postoperative week[48] and cannot be circumvented by iron replacement. In patients with adequate iron stores, restoration of the hematocrit level to normal cannot be accelerated by iron supplements.[53,64] If iron deficiency is confirmed, the patient should be placed on enteral iron. Those unable to tolerate it may be treated with intravenous iron dextran.

There is no evidence that parenteral replacement is superior if gastrointestinal absorption is intact.

Management of reticulocytopenic patients should be directed toward detection and control of erythrosuppressive factors like infection, malignancy, and renal failure. Aside from nutritional support, no particular therapy is necessary pending the results of diagnostic tests. Erythropoietin therapy may be planned for select patients as discussed above.

In the face of a positive DAT, rapidly falling hemoglobin levels, or strong clinical suspicion of immune hemolysis, systemic steroids should be administered pending the results of confirmatory studies. The decision to use them empirically should be tempered by the possibility of underlying infection, the risk of masking other diagnoses, and the likelihood of alternative processes that do not respond to steroids, like G-6-PD deficiency, microangiopathic hemolysis, and PNH. Steroids may suppress extravascular red cell clearance or antibody production. They are not always effective in controlling immune hemolysis. Up to 60 percent of patients with autoantibody syndromes like warm-antibody hemolysis or methyldopa-induced drug hemolysis improve.[60] In those with "innocent bystander" immune hemolysis induced by cephalosporins, the response is far less encouraging, and prompt withdrawal of the medication is more important.[19–21]

Treatment should be initiated with prednisone in a dose of 60 to 100 mg daily orally or methylprednisolone in a dose of 40 to 60 mg every eight hours intravenously. The median time of response is seven days, although many show improvement in 72 hours. Maintenance therapy with prednisone in a dose of 20 mg daily should be administered for two to three months. A positive response to treatment is partly diagnostic, but if testing suggests another diagnosis, steroids should be tapered more rapidly. If immune hemolysis is suspected despite a lack of response to steroids, splenectomy should be considered. Larger doses of steroids, intravenous immunogloubin,[65] or cyclosporine[66] can be tried before splenectomy but are more commonly used in those who do not respond to the procedure.

In nonimmune hemolysis, treatment is directed at removing the hemolytic stimulus. This may mean withdrawing an offending drug; warming the patient in cold antibody disease; administering antibiotic therapy; or preventing osmolar, oxidant, or acid-base stresses. Most nonimmune processes are self-limited. Since thromboembolic complications may occur in confirmed PNH, prophylactic therapy with heparin or dextran should be considered.[30]

Occasionally, patients must be supported through periods of profound anemia because they cannot be crossmatched or refuse transfused blood. Postoperative hematocrits as low as 4% have been tolerated in anecdotal younger patients subjected to the extraordinary measures like skeletal muscle paralysis, hypothermia, and pressor-controlled hypovolemia.[67,68] Synthetic blood substitutes such as Fluosol-DA, a perfluorochemical emulsion with the ability to reversibly bind oxygen, have only minimal oxygen-carrying capacity and do not prevent the morbidity associated with profound anemia.[69]

POSTOPERATIVE ERYTHROCYTOSIS

Erythrocytosis, defined by a hemoglobin level over 17.5 g/dl in men and over 16 g/dl in women, is a rare occurrence after surgery. There are no extravascular erythrocyte stores to increase the circulating red cell mass. Therefore, in the absence of excessive perioperative blood transfusions, an abnormally high hematocrit can only result from a contraction in plasma volume. This relative polycythemia may be related to insufficient crystalloid replacement, diuretic therapy, capillary leak, or significant insensible postoperative fluid losses. A supranormal hematocrit represents no known physiological advantage and can be deleterious. Cerebral blood flow is impaired at hematocrit levels above 50%,[70] and myocardial ischemia and spontaneous thrombosis may occur when blood viscosity is increased.

Postoperative erythrocytosis has been reported following renal transplantation but does not develop for up to 12 months.[71] Postoperative erythrocytosis should alert the clinician to the possibility of volume depletion. Therapeutic phlebotomy should be withheld unless the patient becomes symptomatic despite volume replacement.

POSTOPERATIVE THROMBOCYTOPENIA

Thrombocytopenia is defined as a platelet count under 150,000/μl. Unlike erythrocytes, platelets are rapidly turned over within the circulation and communicate with extravascular stores. Therefore, serial counts are subject to wide variation after surgical procedures. Although older studies reported decreases of up to 50% in platelet counts after surgery,[72] more recent investigations cite decreases in uncomplicated patients of no more than 15 to 20% and rarely to levels below 150,000/μl.[73,74] The etiology of this physiological variation is not known, but may be related to entrapment in the pulmonary microcirculation, catecholamine-activated aggregation, and consumption at the surgical site.[75] After the fourth postoperative day, the platelet count recovers and occasionally rebounds to levels in excess of 500,000/μl.[72,75,76] Reactive thrombocytosis represents accelerated thrombopoiesis as suggested by the appearance of megakaryocytes in the peripheral blood.[76] The biphasic platelet count response usually resolves within two weeks.

The major clinical concern in thrombocytopenia is the risk of bleeding. Anecdotal data suggest that postoperative bleeding is uncommon with counts in excess of 50,000/μl if platelet function is normal.[77–79] This threshold must be considered in light of the particular surgical procedure, blood pressure control, intercurrent coagulopathies, and vascular integrity. The clinician's perception of the morbidity of local bleeding is often a major determinant of this threshold. In a small group of postcraniotomy patients, serious hematoma formation was associated with platelet counts as high as 100,000/μl, particularly in procedures for tumors or vascular lesions.[80] The risk of bleeding and platelet transfusion thresholds must therefore be assessed in the individual patient.

Thrombocytopenia may also serve as a harbinger of other life threatening postoperative complications, including sepsis and thromboembolic events. The etiology of a platelet disorder must be promptly determined. Causes of postoperative thrombocytopenia are listed in Table 64–3. In general, the differential diagnosis can be divided into the categories of increased peripheral destruction, decreased marrow production, or conditions of sequestration and aggregation. In many cases, platelets are affected by the same immunologic phenomena that cause hemolytic anemia and neutropenia. However, such reactions rarely target more than one mature cell line simultaneously,[81] and the presence of multiple cytopenias is more often indicative of a stem-cell disorder.

Clinically, thrombocytopenia may present with petechiae, ec

TABLE 64–3. Differential Diagnosis of Postoperative Thrombocytopenia

Heparin-associated thrombocytopenia (HAT)
Drug-induced thrombocytopenia
Sepsis
Red cell transfusions
Autoimmune thrombocytopenia (AITP)
Amegakaryocytic thrombocytopenia
Cardiopulmonary bypass
Pulmonary artery catheters
Aortic aneurysm
Pulmonary embolism
Acute respiratory failure
Organ transplantation
Type IIB von Willebrand's disease
Splenomegaly
Fat emboli syndrome
Cholesterol emboli syndrome
Paroxysmal nocturnal hemoglobinuria
HELLP syndrome
Pseudothrombocytopenia

chymoses, hematoma formation, and overt mucosal and incisional bleeding. Purpura out of proportion to the thrombocytopenia suggests an immune mechanism, as in immune complex vasculitis, as do the presence of arthralgias, fevers, chills, and urticaria.[82] The most ominous bleeding complication is intracranial hemorrhage.

Differential Diagnosis

Thrombocytopenia due to heparin exposure should be a major consideration in any surgical patient because of the ubiquitous use of the drug in the postoperative period. Heparin-associated thrombocytopenia (HAT) can be the result of any continuous exposure, including the small amount of heparin used to maintain pulmonary artery[83–85] and peripheral intravenous[86–88] catheters. Even the subcutaneous heparin used in standard deep venous thrombosis prophylaxis regimens has been associated with the syndrome.[89]

HAT is an idiosyncratic immune reaction that occurs within 3 to 15 but usually 10 days of therapy, causing decreases in platelet counts to 40,000 to 60,000/μl.[89] Antiheparin IgG and possibly IgM antibody first binds the drug and then attaches to platelet membranes. Platelets become activated and initiate intense local aggregation, thereby depleting the circulating platelet population. Aggregation abates upon withdrawal of the drug despite persistence of the antibody. Thrombocytopenia can recur within minutes of reexposure if antibody titers have not fallen sufficiently. Some have also noted nonimmune thrombocytopenia occurring in the first few days of therapy that is related to the proaggregatory effects of heparin. This form of HAT is benign, short-lived, and rarely associated with platelet counts below 100,000/μl.[90,91]

The incidence of HAT has been reported to be as high as 30 percent.[92] However, in a recent metaanalysis of all prospective studies, the incidence of platelet counts under 100,000/μl was 2.4 percent with porcine heparin and 9.1 percent with bovine lung heparin.[89] Some comparative studies have found no significant difference between heparin from different sources.[93] Most medical centers use porcine heparin as their standard stock anticoagulant.

In a prospective multicenter cohort from which critically ill patients with shock, malignancy, or disseminated intravascular coagulation were excluded, the incidence of thrombocytopenia to levels below 100,000/μl due to porcine heparin was zero.[94] HAT may also vary with lot and route of administration. Pooled prospective studies of low-dose subcutaneous heparin have found the incidence of platelet counts under 100,000/μl to be 0.3 percent, one-eighth that seen after intravascular exposure.[89]

Clinically, HAT should be considered in any patient exhibiting coincident thrombocytopenia and heparin resistance within the first two weeks of continuous exposure. Heparin resistance arises from lost efficacy of complexed drug and causes normalization of the partial thromboplastin time (PTT) on therapy or failure to respond to escalating doses.

HAT can cause spontaneous intravascular thromboemboli as part of the heparin-associated thrombocytopenia with thrombosis (HATT) syndrome. Since thrombi in HATT are composed predominantly of aggregated platelets, it is also known as "the white clot syndrome." In pooled prospective trials, the incidence of HATT is less than 0.5 percent in those exposed to heparin,[89] but as many as half of patients with HAT exhibit the complication. Thrombi in HATT most commonly involve the arterial system and cause ischemic limbs, thrombotic cerebrovascular accidents, and myocardial infarction. Venous involvement is far less frequent. However, its true incidence is clouded by the intrinsic risk of deep venous thrombosis (DVT) in hospitalized patients, inadequate prophylaxis in heparin-resistant patients with HAT, and reduced need for thrombectomy to confirm the presence of "white clot." Cumulative mortality of HATT is as high as 29 percent,[95,96] and the risk of limb loss is approximately 20 percent.[96] Although many consider the onset of thrombocytopenia to be a valuable warning of impending HATT, some have reported thrombotic events before the development of abnormal platelet counts.[97] It is not known why some patients develop HAT and HATT and others do not, but the idiosyncratic roles of variably expressed platelet antigens[98] and endothelial injury[99] are probably significant.

Other medications used in the perioperative period may be responsible for a fall in the platelet count. Drug-induced thrombocytopenia is usually due to immune-mediated peripheral destruction of platelets. However, toxic effects on the megakaryocytes by drugs like thiazides and chemical triggers of intravascular aggregation like ristocetin have also been implicated. Immune destruction of platelets is generally rapid in onset, particularly in patients previously exposed to the same drug. The three mechanisms of immune thrombocytopenia are similar to those listed in Table 64–2 for immune hemolysis.[82] Immune-complex thrombocytopenia causes a precipitous and profound drop in platelet count, seems to require complement, and is mediated by a drug-dependent antibody which may silently persist in the serum long after the drug is withdrawn. Prototypical drugs include quinidine, quinine, sulfisoxazole, penicillin, and cimetidine. Autoimmune thrombocytopenia develops gradually over weeks and is mediated by a nondrug-dependent antiplatelet IgG antibody rise after exposure to agents like methyldopa or gold, resulting in extravascular removal of platelets by the spleen. Finally, a haptenic mechanism has also been proposed.

It is unclear why a given drug triggers immune hemolysis in one patient and thrombocytopenia in another. Recent work has focused on the role of individually expressed neoantigens in these syndromes.[81] There is also evidence that complement may not be involved in immune-complex thrombocytopenia and that antidrug antibody attaches to platelets differently than in autoimmune thrombocytopenia.[100] Some agents may cause thrombocytopenia by more than one mechanism. Ranitidine has been associated with both megakaryocyte arrest and peripheral immune destruction in the same patient.[101]

Thrombocytopenia associated with serious postoperative infections is not uncommon. In a controlled study of patients with culture-positive peritonitis following laparotomy for bowel perforation, 85 percent incurred thrombocytopenia with platelet counts under 100,000/µl with the nadir occurring on about the fourth postoperative day.[73] Even though platelet counts fell to as low as 15,000/µl, no patient exhibited abnormal bleeding, platelet function remained normal as assessed by bleeding time, and spontaneous recovery occurred by the end of the second week. Of greatest concern is the possibility of impending disseminated intravascular coagulation (DIC) and sepsis, which may be heralded by an abrupt fall in the platelet count.[102] Several mechanisms for septic thrombocytopenia have been proposed, including direct endotoxic effects, megakaryocyte suppression, microangiopathic destruction, and sequestration at the site of infection. Recently, an immune mechanism has been described in septic patients with elevated levels of platelet-associated antibody. They were treated successfully with empiric intravenous immunoglobin.[103]

Patients develop thrombocytopenia from transfusions by both dilutional and immune mechanisms. In a study of trauma patients receiving over 20 units of blood, 63 percent developed platelet counts of under 100,000/µl, although many also had evidence of DIC.[104] Some have advocated empiric platelet transfusions after administration of every 10 to 15 units of packed red cells,[105] but others have criticized the practice.[78] Following one replacement of the total blood volume, 35 to 40 percent of platelets remained,[78] reflecting the availability of noncirculating extravascular stores.

In posttransfusion purpura, profound thrombocytopenia occurs one to two weeks after red cell transfusion and is caused by incidental activation of specific antiplatelet alloantibodies directed toward the P1 surface antigen. Patients generally relate a history of low-grade transfusion reactions with fevers, chills, and urticaria. If untreated, platelet counts may remain suppressed for several weeks.

Autoimmune thrombocytopenia (AITP) may be a primary phenomenon as in idiopathic thrombocytopenia (ITP) or may be seen in patients with connective tissue diseases, lymphoproliferative disorders, and certain carcinomas.[106] It is analogous to autoimmune hemolytic anemia (AIHA) in its pathogenesis and management. Platelets are bound by IgG and occasionally IgA or IgM and removed by the splenic reticuloendothelial system.[107] Coincident AITP and AIHA is known as Evan's syndrome. Like AIHA, AITP is not peculiar to the perioperative period, and alternative diagnoses should always be considered.

Because of the short circulating life of platelets, inadequate thrombocytopoiesis in an impaired marrow causes early development of thrombocytopenia. Marrow megakaryocytes may be damaged by immune reactions, viral infections, radiation, alcohol, drugs, or chemotherapy; replaced by tumor infiltration; or rendered dysfunctional by vitamin B_{12}, folate, or iron deficiency.

Many other causes of postoperative thrombocytopenia merit mention, including cardiopulmonary bypass,[108] the use of pulmonary artery catheters,[109] aortic aneurysm,[110] pulmonary embolism,[111] acute respiratory failure,[112] kidney[113] and liver[114]

transplantation, type IIB von Willebrand's disease,[115] splenomegaly, cholesterol emboli syndrome, fat emboli syndrome, and paroxysmal nocturnal hemoglobinuria. Pregnant patients may exhibit the HELLP (hemolysis, elevated liver enzymes, and low platelets) syndrome, an entity distinct from preeclampsia. Pseudothrombocytopenia is a factitious fall in counts due to in vitro clumping in EDTA-containing phlebotomy tubes.[116]

Diagnostic Evaluation

Specific evaluation of postoperative thrombocytopenia can be deferred unless it is severe with platelet counts under 50,000/µl, associated with bleeding or infection, or persistent beyond the fifth postoperative day. Hemostatic integrity should be confirmed by a prothrombin time (PT), partial thromboplastin time (PTT), and bleeding time (BT). The BT may be abnormal if platelets are activated, as in HAT, or if the platelet count falls progressively below 100,000/µl.[117] If the PT or PTT are inexplicably prolonged or the patient is clinically infected, further screening tests for disseminated intravascular coagulation and blood cultures should be drawn. The peripheral blood smear should be examined to exclude pseudothrombocytopenic clumping. An elevated mean platelet volume (MPV) suggests that younger platelets are emerging from an active intact marrow.

Immune thrombocytopenias can be diagnosed by the platelet-associated immunoglobin (PAIg) assay. This radioimmune monoclonal anti-IgG method identifies 90 percent of immune thrombocytopenias and is analogous to the DAT test used in hemolytic anemia. However, it cannot discriminate between various forms of immune thrombocytopenia.[118,119] The PAIg may normalize after 48 hours of glucocorticoid therapy and should therefore be sent promptly.

To confirm HAT, the diagnostic tests of choice are platelet aggregometry and two-point (C^{14}) serotonin release.[89,90] Both tests are commonly available and assess whether donor platelets can be activated by the patient's serum in the presence of heparin, either by aggregating within a spectrophotometric beam or by releasing radiolabeled serotonin granules, respectively. Both tests are more than 90 percent specific for HAT. The PAIg assay is not useful in HAT because the antibody is directed against heparin and not against platelets.

Drug-induced thrombocytopenia is usually confirmed by a rise in the platelet count when the drug is discontinued. In certain situations, confirmation of the immunogenicity of the drug is required, particularly when multiple agents are withdrawn simultaneously or no reasonable alternative medication is available. In vivo challenge with the drug should be avoided. Specialized in vitro drug testing can be carried out by most platelet laboratories using either aggregometry, serotonin release, or other tests of platelet activation using donor platelets, patient serum, and the drug in question.[82] Bone marrow biopsy and aspirate are required only when all other testing is nondiagnostic, amegakaryocytic thrombocytopenia is suspected, or abnormalities of other blood cell lines are evident.

Treatment

Thrombocytopenic postoperative patients must be carefully monitored for bleeding and the development of dangerously low platelet counts. Invasive procedures should be limited and protection against stress-related gastric mucosal damage instituted with antacids or sucralfate. Unless a clinically obvious cause is apparent, all nonessential heparin should be discontinued pending HAT screening studies, including heparin flushes used for intravenous catheter maintenance[120] and low-dose heparin prophylaxis against DVT. Other drugs may be withdrawn at the discretion of the clinician. Most prefer a step-wise revision of the patient's regimen rather than replacement of all first-line medications.

Platelet transfusions should be considered in patients with counts under 50,000/μl, bleeding time prolongation of at least twice normal, active bleeding, or before surgical procedures. Normally one unit per 10 kg of body weight is administered.[78] A repeat platelet count is recommended one hour after transfusion to exclude immune destruction of transfused cells. An increase in count of 5000 to 10,000/μl per unit administered is the expected response. Platelet transfusions and subsequent immune destruction can be associated with anaphylactoid reactions. A suboptimal platelet response may necessitate the need for single-donor or HLA-matched cells. Platelet transfusions should be avoided in HAT due to the risk of enhancing in situ thrombus formation.[89]

If HAT is confirmed by appropriate assays, heparin must be unconditionally discontinued. The practice of switching sources or lots is not recommended. If continued anticoagulation is essential, warfarin should be initiated while short-term alternatives are considered. Most investigators favor the use of ancrod, a defibrinogenating agent derived from snake venom capable of depleting systemic fibrinogen within 12 hours.[89,121,122] Since it is inactive against established fibrin clots, it carries a low risk of hemorrhage even in profoundly thrombocytopenic patients. The drug can be administered by continuous infusion, and serum fibrinogen levels should be monitored every 12 to 24 hours to maintain a level of 20 to 40 mg/dl.[122]

The role of low-molecular-weight heparin (LMWH) and associated heparinoids like dextran-40 in HAT is unclear because of the in vitro demonstration of crossreacting antiheparin antibodies.[89,123] Patients in whom their use is contemplated should be screened with aggregometry beforehand. However, in the absence of additional study, these agents should not be considered as first-line alternatives. An investigational heparinoid, Org 10172, has been used with success in HAT.[124] Antiplatelet agents like aspirin and dipyridamole are often used to prevent some of the thromboembolic complications of HAT but do not affect the thrombocytopenia.[125]

Aside from the need to discontinue heparin, treatment of HAT is similar to that of other forms of thromboembolic disease. Because the majority of thrombi occur within the arterial system, surgical thrombectomy is often required. Thrombolytic therapy has been used with success,[126] including as an adjunct to coronary balloon angioplasty in patients incurring HATT-related myocardial ischemia.[127] Vena caval interruption or Greenfield filter placement should be considered in patients with known lower extremity thrombus[95,128] and even empirically in those with an especially high risk. Plasmapheresis has been used to prevent progression of thrombus and has proven effective in limb ischemia.[129]

Occasionally, patients with a history of HAT will require heparin reexposure as in elective cardiopulmonary bypass. Brief courses of heparin may be tolerated but should be deferred until HAT assays have become negative. For open-heart procedures that cannot be delayed, morbidity has been minimized by pretreatment with aspirin, dipyridamole,[125] and Iloprost, a prostacyclin-like inhibitor of platelet aggregation.[130]

In the absence of a clear nonimmune etiology or evidence of HAT, patients with severe thrombocytopenia should be empirically treated with steroids while diagnostic testing and drug withdrawal are initiated. As in immune hemolysis, steroids are effective in autoimmune thrombocytopenia but are of uncertain value in many drug-induced forms.[82] For this reason, a rapid taper of steroids should be considered if in vitro testing implicates a withdrawn medication or the PAIg is negative. Almost any steroid preparation can be used in doses equivalent to 1 to 2 mg/kg/day of methylprednisolone.[131]

Although previously reserved for patients who fail steroids, intravenous immunoglobin (IVIg) can be used as initial therapy in immune thrombocytopenia. The antiglobulin blocks the Fc receptors of platelet-bound IgG, preventing extravascular recognition and clearance by the reticuloendothelial system. Platelet counts may recover in five days,[132] and the response can last up to three weeks.[131] Treatment failures may indicate heterogeneous immune binding. Failure of these modalities warrants consideration of splenectomy. Cyclophosphamide, vincristine, plasmapheresis, cyclosporine, and danazol have been tried but are more useful in more chronic forms of AITP.[131]

Detection of septic thrombocytopenia represents a rare opportunity to prevent progression to DIC and full-blown septic shock. Broad-spectrum antibiotics should be initiated promptly pending identification of the source of the infection. A recent study has documented enhanced recovery of platelet counts in septic thrombocytopenia without DIC using three-day infusions of IVIg.[103] Amegakaryocytic thrombocytopenia must be managed by medication withdrawal, nutritional support, and efforts to identify known stem-cell disorders. Most nonimmune forms of thrombocytopenia are self-limited and may resolve as perioperative stress abates.

POSTOPERATIVE THROMBOCYTOSIS

A rebound in circulating platelets commonly occurs between the fifth and thirteenth postoperative day, often exceeding the 400,000/μl ceiling defining thrombocytosis.[72,75,76] A prospective study of patients on a general orthopedic service noted thrombocytosis in 65 percent, peaking at the fourteenth day following surgery or injury.[133] Thrombocytosis extending well beyond the second postoperative week is atypical and may suggest other potentially comorbid conditions.

The term reactive thrombocytosis defines increased platelet production as either a nonspecific response to inflammation (e.g., infection, connective tissue disease, or neoplasia), an overcompensation following withdrawal of a thrombocytopenic stimulus (e.g., discontinuing alcohol or treating AITP or B_{12} deficiency), or a bystander response of megakaryocytes in a stimulated marrow (e.g., due to iron deficiency or hemolytic anemia). Even among nonsurgical patients the lag time for reactive thrombocytosis to appear can be deceiving. Hospitalized alcoholic patients may not exhibit platelet increases until after the second week of abstinence.[134] Primary thrombocytosis, a myeloproliferative disease, would be unlikely to develop in the postoperative period, but it may be unmasked by splenectomy.[135]

Postoperative platelet counts may rarely exceed 1,000,000/μl and merit the term extreme thrombocytosis. Such conditions have traditionally raised concern about platelet sludging in the microvasculature, but in reactive disorders the risks of thrombosis and bleeding are not increased.[136] Perhaps the most striking surgical platelet phenomenon is postsplenectomy thrombocytosis, in which 23 percent of patients develop levels above 1,000,000/μl.[137] Although not completely understood, it appears to result from a reactive thrombocytosis exacerbated by absence of splenic filtration of senescent platelets. Platelet counts peak in one to three weeks and may persist for over a month.[138] Prospective ^{125}I-fibrinogen screening in this population documents no increased risk of deep venous thrombosis,[139] confirming larger clinical observations that thromboembolic complications are uncommon.[137]

Aside from addressing the cause of reactive thrombocytosis, no specific treatment is necessary. The role of prophylactic antiplatelet therapy is unclear. Some advocate the use of cytoreductive agents when counts approach 2,000,000/μl, when thrombotic and bleeding risks are less well defined.[136] Patients who do develop thrombosis must be treated promptly, preferably with platelet pheresis.

POSTOPERATIVE LEUKOCYTE ABNORMALITIES

While postoperative increases in circulating erythrocytes and platelets are dependent on marrow production, leukocytes are maintained in dynamic balance among circulating, marginal, and extravascular pools. Quantitative changes in response to a variety of physiologic stresses during and after surgery can occur within hours.[72,140–143] The number of neutrophils, and to a lesser degree monocytes, rises dramatically within two hours of surgery, attaining levels up to twice preoperative baseline levels but rarely exceeding 20,000/μl (see Fig. 64–1). In uncomplicated cases, numbers may then fall precipitously over the next 24 hours, returning to baseline by the sixth postoperative day. This trend parallels changes in serum cortisol levels associated with operative

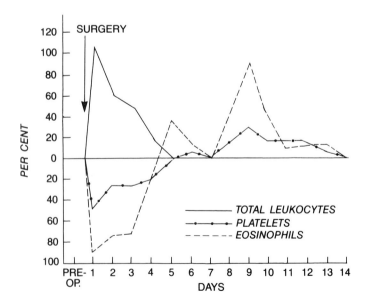

FIGURE 64–1.   Expected Postoperative Changes in Leukocyte, Platelet, and Eosinophil Counts

Source: From Pepper: *Surg Gynecol Obstet* 110:319–326, 1960.

stress and is thought to be due to demargination of peripheral neutrophils.[72,75,142] Lymphocyte levels fluctuate in the opposite direction, reaching overtly lymphocytopenic levels during the first day before normalizing several days later.[140–142] Eosinophil levels display a biphasic pattern in which they virtually disappear from the serum for three days before rebounding to supranormal levels that persist for up to two weeks. Most quantitative leukocyte responses represent redistribution of mature peripheral cells, and the absence of immature forms in the blood smear indicates that marrow reserves are minimally involved.

The magnitude of these changes is influenced by several factors. Surgical procedures of shorter duration and those involving less tissue destruction like corneal transplantation exert fewer effects on the hemogram.[143,144] Epidural[142] and regional[144] anesthesia influence white cell counts less than general. Elderly patients exhibit fewer leukocyte changes after hip surgery than premenopausal women do following hysterectomy.[142,143] Deviations from these patterns deserve evaluation.

Neutropenia

An absolute neutrophil count (ANC) below 1800/μl defines neutropenia. Severe neutropenia with an ANC below 500/μl is sometimes referred to as agranulocytosis. Risk of infection is the major clinical concern in the postoperative period, related not only to the extent of decrease in ANC but also to the surgical procedure, nutritional status, bacterial colonization, and compromise of other host defenses created by bladder catheters, skin breakdown, and open wounds. Neutropenic patients may mount meager inflammatory responses and fail to develop pulmonary infiltrates, pyuria, or purulence. The mortality of drug-induced immune neutropenia exceeds 20 percent in nonsurgical patients.[81,145] How much the postoperative state influences this rate is unknown. In a review of perioperative neutropenia in patients with malignancy, the complication rate was 50 percent.[146]

Neutropenia is the result of destruction of circulating leukocytes or suppression of marrow precursors. Since peripheral neutrophils are normally replaced every 10 hours, either process can result in a precipitous fall in the peripheral white count. Many of the same immunologic and toxic factors implicated in other cytopenias affect white cells and often target both mature cells and myeloid precursors.[147] Other cell lines are often involved, and simultaneous occurrence of a leukocyte count under 3500/μl, platelet count under 50,000/μl, and hematocrit under 30% defines aplastic anemia.[148]

Differential Diagnosis

Drug-induced neutropenia is perhaps the most common cause of postoperative leukopenia. Frequent offenders include penicillin, cephalosporins, gentamicin, captopril, procainamide, quinidine, quinine, propranolol, acetazolamide, thiazide diuretics, and cimetidine.[145] However, the list is so lengthy and ever-expanding that virtually any agent should be suspected. Neutropenia may result from toxic effects on the stem-cell (e.g., chloramphenicol, antithyroid drugs, and chemotherapeutic agents) or immune mechanisms. Because of problems in standardizing antineutrophil antibody assays, the mechanisms of drug-mediated immune destruction in erythrocytes and platelets are only theoretically applicable to neutrophils. Nonetheless, both complement-fixing[149] and complement-free[150] drug-dependent immunoglobins have been identified, but no drug-independent antibodies have yet been described.[81] Medication withdrawal is the mainstay of therapy. Coincident neutropenia, thrombocytopenia, and hemolytic anemia due to quinine has been ascribed to completely different immunoglobins.[149] Drug-dependent antineutrophil antibodies have been reported to persist for up to five months following withdrawal of medication.[151]

Neutropenia can also occur in acute infections, either in the first phase of endotoxemia in bacterial sepsis or in viral infections due to hepatitis viruses, cytomegalovirus, or HIV. Other causes include coincidental autoimmune neutropenia,[152] alcoholism,[134] malnutrition, and marrow disease due to infiltration or a primary preleukemic process. Previously unrecognized benign cyclic neutropenia may also surface in the perioperative period.

Diagnostic Evaluation

The peripheral blood smear should be examined for atypical lymphocytes suggesting a viral process, toxic granulations, and Dohle bodies indicating infection and immature which cell forms. Many laboratories can now perform monoclonal antineutrophil antibody assays that are both sensitive and specific for immune neutropenia.[153] In vitro drug assays have recently been developed[81] but are not widely available. A bone marrow biopsy and aspirate should be considered if recovery from drug withdrawal is sluggish or a preleukemic process is suggested by the blood smear. Viral testing for HIV, CMV, and hepatitis should be performed in appropriate circumstances.

Treatment

Patients with postoperative neutropenia should be kept well hydrated and carefully monitored for signs of infection while drug withdrawal and diagnostic testing are carried out. Infections must be promptly treated with broad-spectrum antibiotics that also cover skin and bowel pathogens. Agranulocytic patients should be subject to the same precautions used on oncology wards, including isolation, avoidance of rectal temperatures, diets restricting fresh vegetables, and empiric antibiotics.

In the absence of significant bacterial infection, drug withdrawal may be all that is required in most cases of neutropenia. Counts generally respond within days, but, if the bone marrow shows maturational arrest, recovery may require weeks. Steroids are not recommended even in confirmed immune neutropenia due to the risk of further immunosuppression. Intravenous immunoglobin (IVIg) has yielded dramatic but inconsistent results in pooled case reports of neutropenic adults.[154] At present, IVIg should only be used in cases of refractory infection or in agranulocytic patients undergoing procedures that carry a high risk of infectious complications like bowel surgery.

The role of granulocyte-colony stimulating factor (G-CSF) in postoperative patients is unknown but is theoretically useful in refractory nonimmune neutropenia. Improved wound healing has been reported in congenitally neutropenic patients treated with G-CSF.[155] Granulocyte transfusions are rarely indicated except in life-threatening infection and should be avoided particularly in cases of immune white cell destruction.

Neutrophilia

Neutrophilia is defined as an absolute neutrophil count of above 7500/μl and is considered abnormal if it extends beyond the first week after surgery. Since neutrophils represent the major circulating leukocyte, neutrophilia is usually detected when the total white blood count exceeds 11,000/μl.

Patients with late postoperative neutrophilia should be regarded as infected until proven otherwise. More than 6% band forms in the differential count and the presence of intracellular toxic granulations and Dohle bodies are highly suggestive of infection.[156] Patients should be carefully screened for wound, pulmonary, soft tissue, gastrointestinal, and urinary tract infections even in the absence of fever. Empiric antibiotics may be withheld in stable patients pending identification of a pathogen. Failure of antibiotics to normalize postoperative neutrophilia in afebrile patients does not exclude bacterial infection and may be a poor prognostic sign.[157]

Neutrophilia can be stimulated by other factors in the perioperative period. Hypoxemia, atelectasis, phlebitis, acidosis, tissue necrosis, pain, gout, alcohol, and drug withdrawal and shock can cause rapid and sustained demargination of mature neutrophils induced by increases in catecholamine and glucocorticoid levels. Exogenous steroids can also induce dose-related leukocytosis with counts as high as 20,000/μl.[156] Accelerated marrow activity associated with hemolytic anemia or recovery from drug-induced neutropenia may cause immature band forms to appear in the peripheral blood. Sustained leukocytosis with counts over 50,000/μl defines a leukemoid reaction. Leukemoid reactions are usually associated with infection or advanced malignancy[158] but have also been documented in conditions such as diabetic ketoacidosis,[159] ulcerative colitis,[160] and alcoholic hepatitis.[161] Acute leukemia arising in the postoperative period would be an extraordinary coincidence. However, if it is a consideration, it can be reasonably excluded by an elevated serum leukocyte alkaline phosphatase (LAP) level.

Lymphocytopenia

Lymphocytopenia with absolute lymphocyte counts under 1000/μl is frequently noted in postoperative patients,[141] but rarely after the first few days after surgery. Variations in counts represent redistribution of circulating lymphocytes and are inversely proportional to cortisol levels induced by surgical stress.[142] Persistent lymphocytopenia may be related to glucocorticoid administration, acute viral illness, malnutrition, marrow aplasia, chemotherapy, or autoimmune disease. In pediatric patients, lymphocytes have been lost through thoracostomy tubes placed for postoperative chylothorax.[162] Lymphocytopenia may also be prolonged after exposure to extracorporeal bypass.[163] Although lymphocytopenia has been associated with increased perioperative mortality even in the absence of infection,[141] other studies refute this finding in patients with normal preoperative counts.[162,164]

Lymphocytosis

Lymphocytosis with absolute lymphocyte counts above 4000/μl is uncommon in the postoperative period and is usually attributable to an intercurrent viral syndrome. Cytomegalovirus (CMV) infection from red cell transfusions[165,166] or extracorporeal bypass[167] is of particular concern. Lymphocyte counts can exceed 12,000/μl approximately three weeks following exposure and are associated with spiking fevers, splenomegaly, abnormal liver tests, and atypical lymphocyte forms on peripheral smear. This syndrome can also be seen in HIV, Epstein-Barr, and hepatitis infections. CMV seroconversion following unscreened blood transfusion occurs in less than one percent of patients. Since the condition is usually benign, most blood banks do not test for the virus except in immunosuppressed and newborn recipients.[168]

The mononucleosis syndrome may also be seen in human immunodeficiency virus (HIV), Epstein-Barr virus, and hepatitis infections. Noninfectious causes of sudden lymphocytosis include acute medical conditions like myocardial infarction, status epilepticus, and trauma,[169] and emerging lymphoreticular neoplasms.

The evaluation of postoperative lymphocytosis should include serum IgM antibody to CMV, appropriate cultures, and HIV antibody testing. These studies may obviate the need for repetitive bacterial cultures and imaging and identify beneficiaries of early antiviral therapy.

Eosinophilia

Postoperative eosinophilia with absolute eosinophil counts above $400/\mu l$ or over five percent of the number of circulating leukocytes is most often due to a hypersensitivity reaction and warrants careful review of new medications. Eosinophilia also accompanies the cholesterol emboli syndrome complicating vascular procedures, also characterized by leukocytosis, thrombocytopenia, livedo reticularis, renal failure, and eosinophiluria.[170–172] Miscellaneous causes of eosinophilia include adrenal insufficiency, malignancy, hypoxemia, connective tissue disorders, and parasitic infections.

Pulmonary infiltrates with eosinophilia (the PIE syndrome) can be the result of a drug reaction, particularly from antibiotics, cytotoxic agents, and nonsteroidal anti-inflammatory medications,[173] or acute eosinophilic pneumonia, which has been reported after major vascular surgery.[174] These steroid-responsive lung processes must be differentiated from the fat emboli syndrome seen after trauma[175] and high-pressure cementing in total hip arthroplasty.[176]

SUMMARY

1. Normovolemic anemia with hemoglobin levels as low as seven g/dl is not associated with increased postoperative morbidity in many patients. However, higher hematocrits should be maintained in those with organic heart disease, advanced age, or significant comorbid disease. Some markedly anemic patients may warrant cardiac monitoring.

2. Progressive anemia in the absence of bleeding should be attributed to hemolysis until proven otherwise. Since drug-induced red cell destruction is a major concern, all medications should be considered for withdrawal or substitution pending the results of a direct antiglobulin test, G-6-PD screen, Heinz-body preparation, reticulocyte production index and serologic markers of erythrocyte breakdown. If unexplained hemolysis persists, glucocorticoid therapy can be administered pending characterization of the hemolytic process.

3. Platelet counts under $50,000/\mu l$ increase the risk of perioperative bleeding and may signal impending sepsis or thromboembolic events. Patients should be immediately screened for infection and antiheparin antibodies to prevent such complications. Management also includes review of newly administered medications and assay for platelet-associated immunoglobin. Patients may

be supported with platelet transfusions and steroids and/or intravenous immunoglobin if an immune etiology is suspected.

4. Heparin-associated thrombocytopenia (HAT) develops in fewer than 10 percent of treated patients but can occur even with minimal exposure. It should be considered in any patient with a sudden fall in platelet count and heparin resistance after 10 days of therapy. Because half of affected patients may develop spontaneous arterial thrombosis, heparin should be discontinued in all suspected cases pending the results of antiheparin antibody assays. Anticoagulation alternatives include ancrod and warfarin. Recovery is prompt after heparin is discontinued, and platelet transfusions should be withheld to avoid the risk of promoting thrombosis.

5. Postoperative thrombocytosis with counts as high as $1,000,000/\mu l$ may occur as an acute phase phenomenon weeks following surgery, particularly after splenectomy, but is not associated with thrombosis or bleeding.

6. Neutropenia extending beyond the first week after surgery is uncommon and carries high morbidity. Drug-induced neutropenia and sepsis are prime concerns, and empiric antibiotics are warranted while the situation is investigated. Intravenous immunoglobin may be beneficial.

7. Quantitative lymphocyte abnormalities are common after surgery but rarely significant. Elevated counts may suggest intercurrent viral infection with EBV, CMV, or HIV, usually weeks after exposure to transfused blood products or extracorporeal bypass.

8. Eosinophilia usually represents a mild hypersensitivity reaction but has been noted in the perioperative setting in the pulmonary infiltrates with eosinophilia (PIE) syndrome and the cholesterol and fat emboli syndromes.

REFERENCES

1. Carpenter RL, Cullen BF: Hematologic and immune function, in Brown DL (ed): *Risk and Outcome in Anesthesia.* Philadelphia, Lippincott, 1988, pp 74–100.
2. Czer LSC, Shoemaker WC: Optimal hematocrit value in critically ill postoperative patients. *Surg Gynecol Obstet* 147:363–368, 1978.
3. Carson JL, Spence RK, Poses RM, Bonavita G: Severity of anemia and operative mortality and morbidity. *Lancet* 1:727–729, 1988.
4. Spence RK, Carson JA, Poses R et al: Elective surgery without transfusion: Influence of preoperative hemoglobin and blood loss on mortality. *Am J Surg* 159:320–324, 1990.
5. NIH Consensus Conference: Perioperative red blood cell transfusion. *JAMA* 260:2700–2703, 1988.
6. Welch HG, Meehan KR, Goodnough LT: Prudent strategies for elective red blood cell transfusion. *Ann Intern Med* 116:393–402, 1992.
7. Rosberg B, Wulff K: Hemodynamics following normovolemic hemodilution in elderly patients. *Acta Anaesth Scand* 25:402–406, 1981.
8. Geha AS, Baue AE: Graded coronary stenosis and coronary flow during acute normovolemic anemia. *World J Surg* 2:645–652, 1978.
9. Fong TP, Ko ST, Streczyn M et al: Chronic anemia, wound healing, and red cell 2,3-diphosphoglycerate. *Surgery* 79:218–223, 1976.
10. Heughan C, Grislis G, Hunt TK: The effect of anemia on wound healing. *Ann Surg* 179:163–167, 1974.
11. Heppenstall RB, Brighton CT: Fracture healing in the presence of anemia. *Clin Orthop* 123:253–258, 1977.
12. Chaudary VK, Sarkar SK: A study of wound healing in iron deficiency anaemia. *J Indian MA* 79:160–163, 1986.

13. Jensen JA, Goodson WH, Vasconez LO et al: Wound healing in anemia. *Western J Med* 144:465–467, 1986.
14. Hunt TK, Rabkin J, von Smitten K: Effects of edema and anemia on wound healing and infection. *Curr Stud Hematol Blood Transf* 53:101–111, 1986.
15. Greenfield RH, Bessen HA, Henneman PL: Effect of crystalloid infusion on hematocrit and intravascular volume in healthy, nonbleeding subjects. *Ann Emerg Med* 18:51–55, 1989.
16. Simmons A: *Hematology: A Combined Theoretical and Technical Approach.* Philadelphia, Saunders, 1989, p 177.
17. Henry ML, Garner WL, Fabri PJ: Iatrogenic anemia. *Am J Surg* 151:362–363, 1986.
18. Eyster E, Bernene J: Nosocomial anemia. *JAMA* 223:73–74, 1973.
19. Garratty G, Postoway N, Schwellenbach J, McMahill PC: A fatal case of ceftriaxone (Rocephin)–induced hemolytic anemia associated with intravascular immune hemolysis. *Transfusion* 31:176–179, 1991.
20. Ehmann WC: Cephalosporin-induced hemolysis: A case report and review of the literature. *Am J Hematol* 40:121–125, 1992.
21. Wagner BKJ, Heaton AH, Flink JR: Cefotetan disodium-induced hemolytic anemia. *Ann Pharmacol* 26:199–200, 1992.
22. Pixley JS, MacKintosh FR, Sahr EA et al: Mechanism of ranitidine associated anemia. *Am J Med Sci* 297:369–371, 1989.
23. Marks DR, Joy JV, Bonheim NA: Hemolytic anemia associated with the use of omeprazole. *Am J Gastroenterol* 86:217–218, 1991.
24. Garratty G, Petz LD: Drug-induced immune hemolytic anemia. *Am J Med* 58:398–407, 1975.
25. Beutler E: Glucose-6-phosphate dehydrogenase deficiency. *N Engl J Med* 324:169–174, 1991.
26. Markowitz N, Saravolatz LD: Use of trimethoprim-sulfamethoxazole in a glucose-6-phosphate dehydrogenase–deficient population. *Rev Inf Dis* 9(Suppl 2):S218–S253, 1987.
27. Berkowitz FE: Hemolysis and infection: Categories and mechanisms of their interrelationship. *Rev Inf Dis* 13:1151–1162, 1991.
28. Beutler E: Hemoglobinopathies associated with unstable hemoglobin, in Williams WJ, Beutler E, Erslev AJ et al: (eds): *Hematology.* New York, McGraw-Hill, 1990, pp 644–652.
29. Yoo D, Lessin LS: Drug-associated "bite cell" hemolytic anemia. *Am J Med* 92:243–248, 1992.
30. Braren V, Jenkins DE, Phythyon JM et al: Perioperative management of patients with paroxysmal nocturnal hemoglobinuria. *Surg Gynecol Obstet* 153:515–520, 1981.
31. Terebelo HR, McCue RL, Lenneville MS: Implication of plasma free hemoglobin in massive clostridial hemolysis. *JAMA* 248:2028–2029, 1982.
32. Lenz G, Goes U, Baron D et al: Red blood cell T-activation and hemolysis in surgical intensive care patients with severe infections. *Blut* 54:89–96, 1987.
33. Diaz JH, Cooper ES, Ochsner JL: Cold hemagglutination pathophysiology: Evaluation and management of patients undergoing cardiac surgery with induced hypothermia. *Arch Intern Med* 144:1639–1641, 1984.
34. Niejadlik DC, Lozner EL: Cooling mattress–induced acute hemolytic anemia. *Transfusion* 14:145–147, 1974.
35. Dake SB, Johnston MF, Brueggeman P et al: Detection of cold hemagglutination in a blood cardioplegia unit before systemic cooling of a patient with unsuspected cold agglutinin disease. *Ann Thorac Surg* 47:915–915, 1989.
36. Soper DE: Delayed hemolytic transfusion reaction: A cause of late postoperative fever. *Am J Obstet Gynecol* 153:227–228, 1985.
37. Sacks PC, Hoyne PM: Disseminated intravascular coagulation, hemolytic anemia, and acute renal failure associated with extensive multiple myomectomy. *Obstet Gynecol* 79:835–838, 1992.
38. Bevan PC, Seaman M, Tolliday B et al: ABO haemolytic anemia in transplanted patients. *Vox Sang* 49:42–48, 1985.
39. Hyma BA, Moore SB, Grande JP et al: Delayed immune hemolysis in a patient receiving cyclosporine after orthotopic liver transplantation. *Transfusion* 28:276–279, 1988.
40. Yoshimura N, Oka T, Ohmori Y et al: Cyclosporine-associated microangiopathic hemolytic anemia in a renal transplant recipient. *Jpn J Surg* 19:223–228, 1989.
41. Tzakis AG, Arditi M, Whitington PF et al: Aplastic anemia complicating orthotopic liver transplantation for non-A, non-B hepatitis. *N Engl J Med* 319:393–396, 1988.
42. Bonser RS, Adu D, Franklin I et al: Cyclosporin-induced haemolytic uraemic syndrome in liver allograft recipient (letter). *Lancet* 2:1337, 1984.
43. Faure JL, Causse X, Bergeret A et al: Cyclosporine–induced hemolytic anemia in a liver transplant patient. *Transplant Proc* 21:2242–2243, 1989.
44. Carrier M, Martineau JP, Bonan R et al: Clinical and hemodynamic assessment of the Omniscience prosthetic heart valve. *J Thorac Cardiovasc Surg* 93:300–307, 1987.
45. McClung JA, Stein JH, Ambrose JA et al: Prosthetic heart valves: A review. *Prog Cardiovasc Dis* 26:237–270, 1983.
46. Lavie CJ, Thomas MA: Intravascular hemolysis secondary to irrigation fluid absorption during an internal urethrotomy. *J Louisiana State Med Soc* 136:14–16, 1984.
47. Levine EA, Rosen AL, Sehgal LR et al: Treatment of acute postoperative anemia with recombinant human erythropoietin. *J Trauma* 29:1134–1139, 1989.
48. Feldthusen U, Larsen V, Lassen NA: Serum iron and operative stress. *Acta Med Scand* 147:311, 1953.
49. Conrad ME, Barton JC: Anemia and iron kinetics in alcoholism. *Sem Hematol* 17:149–163, 1980.
50. Erslev AJ: Erythrocyte disorders: Anemias related to disturbance of erythroid precursor cell proliferation or maturation, in Williams WJ, Beutler E, Erslev AJ et al: (eds): *Hematology.* New York, McGraw-Hill, 1990, pp 430–438.
51. Schifman RB, Garewal H, Shillington D: Reticulocytopenic Coombs' positive anemia induced by procainamide. *Am J Clin Pathol* 80:66–68, 1983.
52. Liesveld JL, Rowe JM, Lichtman MA: Variability of the erythropoietic response in autoimmune hemolytic anemia: Analysis of 109 cases. *Blood* 69:820–826, 1987.
53. DelCampo C, Lukman H, Mehta H et al: Iron therapy after cardiac operation: One prescription less? *J Thorac Cardiovasc Surg* 84:631–635, 1982.
54. Bobbio-Pallavicini F, Verde G, Spriano P et al: Body iron status in critically ill patients: Significance of serum ferritin. *Intens Care Med* 15:171–178, 1989.
55. Thompson WG, Meola T, Lipkin M et al: Red cell distribution width, mean corpuscular volume, and transferrin saturation in the diagnosis of iron deficiency. *Arch Intern Med* 148:2128–2130, 1988.
56. McClure S, Custer E, Bessman JD: Improved detection of early iron deficiency in nonanemic subjects. *JAMA* 253:1021–1023, 1985.
57. Axelson JA, LoBuglio AF: Immune hemolytic anemia. *Med Clinics* 64:597–606, 1980.
58. Smoller BR, Kruskall MS, Horowitz GL: Reducing adult phlebotomy blood loss with the use of pediatric-sized blood collection tubes. *Am J Clin Pathol* 91:701–703, 1989.
59. Smoller BR, Kruskall MS: Phlebotomy for diagnostic laboratory tests in adults. Pattern of use and effect on transfusion requirements. *N Engl J Med* 314:1233–1235, 1986.
60. Tabbara IA: Hemolytic anemias: Diagnosis and management. *Med Clin N Am* 76:649–668, 1992.
61. Goodnough LT, Rudnick S, Price TH et al: Increased preoperative collection of autologous blood with recombinant human erythropoietin therapy. *N Engl J Med* 321:1163–1168, 1989.
62. Green D, Handley E: Erythropoietin for anemia in Jehovah's Witnesses (letter). *Ann Intern Med* 113:720–721, 1990.
63. Miller CB, Jones RJ, Piantadosi S et al: Decreased erythropoietin response in patients with the anemia of cancer. *N Engl J Med* 322:1689–1692, 1990.

64. Zauber NP, Zauber AG, Gordon FJ et al: Iron supplementation after femoral head replacement for patients with normal iron stores. *JAMA* 267:525–527, 1992.

65. MacIntyre EA, Linc DC, Macey MG et al: Successful response to intravenous immunoglobin in autoimmune haemolytic anaemia. *Br J Haematol* 60:387–388, 1985.

66. Hershko C, Sonnenblick M, Ashkenazi J: Control of steroid-resistant autoimmune haemolytic anaemia by cyclosporine. *Br J Haematol* 76:436–437, 1990.

67. Lichtenstein A, Eckhart WF, Swanson KJ et al: Unplanned intra-operative and postoperative hemodilution: Oxygen transport and consumption during severe anemia. *Anesthesiology* 69:119–122, 1988.

68. Nearman HS, Echauser ML: Postoperative management of a severely anemic Jehovah's Witness. *Crit Care Med* 11:142–143, 1983.

69. Gould SA, Rosen AL, Sehgal LR et al: Fluosol-DA as a red-cell substitute in acute anemia. *N Engl J Med* 314:1653–1656, 1986.

70. Humphrey PR, Michael J, Pearson TC: Management of relative poly-cythaemia: Studies of cerebral blood flow and viscosity. *Br J Haematol* 46:427–433, 1980.

71. Bakris GL, Sauter ER, Hussey JL et al: Effects of theophylline on erythropoietin production in normal subjects and in patients with eryth-rocytosis after renal transplantation. *N Engl J Med* 323:86–90, 1990.

72. Pepper H, Lindsay S: Responses of platelets, eosinophils, and total leukocytes during and following surgical procedures. *Surg Gynecol Obstet* 110:319–326, 1960.

73. Iberti TJ, Rand JH, Benjamin E et al: Thrombocytopenia following peritonitis in surgical patients. *Ann Surg* 204:341–345, 1986.

74. O'Brien JR, Etherington MD, Shuttleworth RD, Davison S: Platelet and other tests followed for 14 days after operation. *Clin Lab Haematol* 6:239–245, 1984.

75. Naesh O, Friis JT, Hindberg I et al: Platelet function in surgical stress. *Thromb Hemost* 54:849–852, 1985.

76. Breslow A, Kaufman RM, Lawsky AR: The effect of surgery on the concentration of circulating megakaryocytes and platelets. *Blood* 32:393–401, 1968.

77. Hay A, Olsen KR, Nicholson DH: Bleeding complications in throm-bocytopenic patients undergoing ophthalmic surgery. *Am J Ophthal* 109:482–483, 1990.

78. NIH Consensus Development Summaries: Platelet transfusion therapy. *Conn Med* 51:105–109, 1987.

79. Cote CJ, Letty MPL, Szyfelbein SK et al: Changes in serial platelet counts following massive blood transfusion in pediatric patients. *Anesthesiology* 62:197–201, 1985.

80. Chan KH, Mann KS, Chan TK: The significance of thrombocytope-nia in the development of postoperative intracranial hematoma. *J Neurosurg* 71:38–41, 1989.

81. Salama A, Mueller-Eckhardt C: Immune-mediated blood cell dyscra-sias related to drugs. *Sem Hematol* 29:54–63, 1992.

82. Hackett T, Kelton JG, Powers P: Drug-induced platelet destruction. *Sem Thromb Hemost* 8:116–137, 1982.

83. Moberg PQ, Geary VM, Sheikh FM: Heparin-induced thrombocyto-penia: A possible complication of heparin-coated pulmonary artery catheters. *J Cardiothorac Anesth* 4:226–228, 1990.

84. Laster JL, Nichols WK, Silver D: Thrombocytopenia associated with heparin-coated catheters in patients with heparin-associated antiplatelet antibodies. *Arch Intern Med* 149:2285–2287, 1989.

85. Laster J, Silver D: Heparin-coated catheters and heparin-induced thrombocytopenia. *J Vasc Surg* 7:667–672, 1988.

86. Rizzoni WE, Miller K, Rick M et al: Heparin-induced thrombocyto-penia and thromboembolism in the postoperative period. *Surgery* 103:470–476, 1988.

87. Heeger PS, Backstrom JT: Heparin flushes and thrombocytopenia (letter). *Ann Intern Med* 105:143, 1986.

88. Doty JR, Alving BM, McDonnell DE et al: Heparin-associated thrombocytopenia in the neurosurgical patient. *Neurosurgery* 19:69–72, 1986.

89. Warkentin TE, Kelton JG: Heparin-induced thrombocytopenia. *Prog Hemost Thromb* 10:1–34, 1991.

90. Chong BH, Berndt MC: Heparin-induced thrombocytopenia. *Blut* 58:53–57, 1989.

91. Shojania AM, Turnbull G: Effect of heparin on platelet count and platelet aggregation. *Am J Hematol* 26:255–262, 1987.

92. Nelson JC, Lerner RG, Goldstein R et al: Heparin-induced thrombo-cytopenia. *Arch Intern Med* 138:548–552, 1978.

93. Ansell JE, Price JM, Shah S et al: Heparin-induced thrombocytope-nia: What is the real frequency? *Chest* 88:878–882, 1985.

94. Rao AK, White GC, Sherman L et al: Low incidence of thrombocy-topenia with porcine mucosal heparin. A prospective multicenter study. *Arch Intern Med* 149:1285–1288, 1989.

95. AbuRahma AF, Boland JP, Witsberger T: Diagnostic and therapeutic strategies of white clot syndrome. *Am J Surg* 162:175–179, 1991.

96. King DJ, Kelton JG: Heparin-associated thrombocytopenia. *Ann Intern Med* 100:535–540, 1984.

97. Phelan BK: Heparin-associated thrombosis without thrombocytopenia. *Ann Intern Med* 99:637–638, 1983.

98. Pfueller SL, David R: Different platelet specificities of heparin-dependent platelet aggregating factors in heparin-associated immune thrombocytopenia. *Br J Haematol* 64:149–159, 1986.

99. Cines DB, Tomaski A, Tannenbaum S: Immune endothelial injury in heparin-associated thrombocytopenia. *N Engl J Med* 316:581–589, 1987.

100. Lerner W, Caruso R, Faig D et al: Drug-dependent and non-drug-dependent antiplatelet antibody in drug-induced immunologic throm-bocytopenia purpura. *Blood* 66:306–311, 1985.

101. Spychal RT, Wickham NWR: Thrombocytopenia associated with ranitidine. *Br J Med* 291:1687, 1985.

102. Stone HH, Bourneuf AA, Stinson LD: Reliability of criteria for pre-dicting persistent or recurrent sepsis. *Arch Surg* 120:17–20, 1985.

103. Burns ER, Lee V, Rubinstein A: Treatment of septic thrombocytope-nia with immune globulin. *J Clin Immunol* 11:363–368, 1991.

104. Riska EB, Bostman O, von Bonsdorff H et al: Outcome of closed injuries exceeding 20-unit blood transfusion need. *Injury* 19:273–276, 1988.

105. Reed RL, Claverella D, Heimbach DM et al: Prophylactic platelet administration during massive transfusion. A prospective, random-ized, double-blind clinical study. *Ann Surg* 203:40–48, 1986.

106. Bellone JD, Kunicki TJ, Aster RH: Immune thrombocytopenia associ-ated with carcinoma. *Ann Intern Med* 99:470–472, 1983.

107. Waters AH: Autoimmune thrombocytopenia: Clinical aspects. *Sem Hematol* 29:18–25, 1992.

108. Harding SA, Shakoor MA, Grindon AJ: Platelet support for cardio-pulmonary bypass surgery. *J Thoracic Cardiovasc Surg* 70:350–?, 1975.

109. Kim YL, Richman KA, Marshall BE: Thrombocytopenia associated with Swan-Ganz catheterization in patients. *Anesthesiol* 53:261–262, 1980.

110. Micallef-Eynaud PD, Ludlam CA: Aortic aneurysms and consumptive coagulopathy. *Blood Coag Fibrinol* 2:477–481, 1991.

111. Mustafa MH, Mispireta LA, Pierce LE: Occult pulmonary embolism presenting with thrombocytopenia and elevated fibrin split products. *Am J Med* 86:490–491, 1989.

112. Schneider RC, Zapol WM, Carvalho AC: Platelet consumption and sequestration in severe acute respiratory failure. *Am Rev Resp Dis* 122:445–451, 1990.

113. Bapat AR, Schuster SJ, Dahlke M et al: Thrombocytopenia and autoimmune hemolytic anemia following renal transplantation. *Trans-plantation* 44:157–159, 1987.

114. Munoz SJ, Carabasi AR, Moritz MJ et al: Postoperative thrombocyto-penia in liver transplant recipients: Prognostic implications and treat-ment with high dose of gamma globulin. *Transplant Proc* 21:3545–3546, 1989.

115. Hultin MB, Sussman II: Postoperative thrombocytopenia in type IIB

von Willebrand's disease. *Am J Hematol* 33:64–68, 1990.

116. Pestana D, Marcote C, deCastro MF: EDTA-dependent pseudothrombocytopenia in a postoperative patient. *Acta Anesth Scand* 36:328–330, 1992.

117. Burns ER, Lawrence C: Bleeding time. A guide to its diagnostic and clinical utility. *Arch Pathol Lab Med* 113:1219–1224, 1989.

118. Court WS, Bozeman JM, Soong S et al: Platelet surface-bound IgG in patients with immune and nonimmune thrombocytopenia. *Blood* 69:278–283, 1987.

119. LoBuglio AF, Court WS, Vincour L et al: Immune thrombocytopenic purpura. *N Engl J Med* 309:459–463, 1983.

120. Garrelts JC, LaRocca J, Ast D et al: Comparison of heparin and 0.9% sodium chloride injection in the maintenance of indwelling intermittent IV devices. *Clin Pharm* 8:34–39, 1989.

121. Cole CW, Fournier LM, Bormanis J: Heparin-associated thrombocytopenia and thrombosis: Optimal therapy with ancrod. *Can J Surg* 33:207–210, 1990.

122. Cole CW, Bourmanis J: Ancrod: A practical alternative to heparin. *J Vasc Surg* 8:59–63, 1988.

123. Messmore HL, Griffin B, Koza M et al: Interaction of heparinoids with platelets: Comparison with heparin and low molecular weight heparins. *Sem Thromb Hemost* 17:57–59, 1991.

124. Chong BH, Ismail F, Cade J et al: Heparin-induced thrombocytopenia: Studies with a new low molecular weight heparinoid, Org 10172. *Blood* 73:1592–1596, 1989.

125. Laster J, Elfrink R, Silver D: Re-exposure to heparin of patients with heparin-associated antibodies. *J Vasc Surg* 9:677–682, 1989.

126. Krueger SK, Andres E, Weinand E: Thrombolysis in heparin-induced thrombocytopenia with thrombosis (letter). *Ann Intern Med* 103:159, 1985.

127. Dieck JA, Rizo-Patron C, Unisa A et al: A new manifestation and treatment alternative for heparin-induced thrombosis. *Chest* 98:1524–1526, 1990.

128. Sobel M, Adelman B, Szentpetery S et al: Surgical management of heparin-associated thrombocytopenia. *J Vasc Surg* 8:395–401, 1988.

129. Nand S, Robinson JA: Plasmapheresis in the management of heparin-associated thrombocytopenia with thrombosis. *Am J Hematol* 28:204–206, 1988.

130. Kraenzler EJ, Starr NJ: Heparin-associated thrombocytopenia: Management of patients for open heart surgery. Case reports describing the use of Iloprost. *Anesthesiology* 69:964–967, 1988.

131. Collins PW, Newland AC: Treatment modalities of autoimmune blood disorders. *Sem Hematol* 29:64–74, 1992.

132. Fehr J, Hoffman V, Kappeler U: Transient reversal of thrombocytopenia in idiopathic thrombocytopenic purpura by high-dose intravenous gamma globulin. *N Engl J Med* 306:1254–1258, 1982.

133. Bunting R, Doppelt SH, Lavine LS: Extreme thrombocytosis after orthopaedic surgery. *J Bone Joint Surg* 73B:687–688, 1991.

134. Lindenbaum J, Hargrove RL: Thrombocytopenia in alcoholics. *Ann Intern Med* 68:526–532, 1968.

135. Jamshidi K, Ansari A, Garcia MC, Swaim WE: Postsplenectomy thrombocythemia: An unmasked myeloproliferative disorder. *J Amer Geriatr Soc* 21:419–424, 1973.

136. Buss DH, Stuart JJ, Lipscomb GE: The incidence of thrombotic and hemorrhagic disorders in association with extreme thrombocytosis: An analysis of 129 cases. *Am J Hematol* 20:365–372, 1985.

137. Boxer MA, Braun J, Ellman L: Thromboembolic risk of postsplenectomy thrombocytosis. *Arch Surg* 113:808–809, 1978.

138. Robbins G, Barnard DL: Thrombocytosis and microthrombocytosis: A clinical evaluation of 372 cases. *Acta Haematol* 70:175–182, 1983.

139. Coon WW, Penner J, Clagett GP et al: Deep venous thrombosis and postsplenectomy thrombocytosis. *Arch Surg* 113:429–431, 1978.

140. Jakobson BW, Pedersen J, Egeberg BB: Postoperative lymphocytopenia and leucocytosis after epidural and general anaesthesia. *Acta Anaesth Scand* 30:668–671, 1986.

141. Grossbard LJ, Desai MH, Lemeshow S et al: Lymphocytopenia in the

142. Rem J, Brandt MR, Kehlet H: Prevention of postoperative lymphopenia and granulocytosis by epidural analgesia. *Lancet* 1:283–285, 1980.

143. Ryhanen P: Effects of anesthesia and operative surgery on the immune response of patients of different age. *Ann Clin Res* 9(Suppl):7–75, 1977.

144. Cullen BF, vanBelle G: Lymphocyte transformation and changes in leukocyte count: Effects of anesthesia and operation. *Anesthesiology* 43:563–569, 1975.

145. Vincent PC: Drug-induced aplastic anemia and agranulocytosis. *Drugs* 31:52–63, 1986.

146. Glenn J, Funkhouser WK, Schneider PS: Acute illnesses necessitating urgent abdominal surgery in neutropenic cancer patients: Description of 14 cases and review of the literature. *Surgery* 105:778–789, 1989.

147. Harmon DC, Weitzman SA, Stossel TP: The severity of immune neutropenia correlates with the maturational specificity of antineutrophil antibodies. *Br J Hematol* 58:209–215, 1989.

148. Anti-infective drug use in relation to the risk of agranulocytosis and aplastic anemia. A report from the International Agranulocytosis and Aplastic Anemia Study. *Arch Intern Med* 149:1036–1040, 1989.

149. Stroncek DF, Vercellotti GM, Hammerschmidt DE et al: Characterization of multiple quinidine-dependent antibodies in a patient with episodic hemolytic uremic syndrome and immune agranulocytosis. *Blood* 80:241–248, 1992.

150. Rouveix B, Coulombel L, Aymard JP et al: Amodiaquine-induced immune agranulocytosis. *Br J Hematol* 71:7–11, 1989.

151. Samlowski WE, Frame RN, Logue GL: Flecanide-induced immune neutropenia. Documentation of a hapten-mediated mechanism of cell destruction. *Arch Intern Med* 147:383–384, 1987.

152. Bux J, Mueller-Eckhardt C: Autoimmune neutropenia. *Sem Hematol* 29:45–53, 1992.

153. Sears D, Kickler TS, Johnson RJ et al: The diagnostic usefulness of measuring antineutrophil antibodies in neutropenic patients. *Acta Haematol* 75:65–69, 1986.

154. Blanchette VS, Kirby MA, Turner C: Role of intravenous immunoglobin G in autoimmune hematologic disorders. *Sem Hematol* 29:72–82, 1992.

155. Besner GE, Glick PL, Karp MP et al: Recombinant human granulocyte colony-stimulating factor promotes wound healing in a patient with congenital neutropenia. *J Pediatr Surg* 27:288–290, 1992.

156. Shoenfeld Y, Gurewich Y, Gallant LA et al: Prednisone-induced leukocytosis. *Am J Med* 71:773–778, 1981.

157. Lennard ES, Dellinger EP, Wertz MJ et al: Implications of leukocytosis and fever at conclusion of antibiotic therapy for intra-abdominal sepsis. *Ann Surg* 195:19–24, 1982.

158. McKee LC: Excess leukocytosis (leukemoid reactions) associated with malignant diseases. *South Med J* 78:1475–1482, 1985.

159. Burris AS: Leukemoid reaction associated with severe diabetic ketoacidosis. *South Med J* 79:647–648, 1986.

160. Merrin P, Lancaster-Smith MJ: Leukemoid reaction and ulcerative colitis. *Gut* 30:1154–1155, 1989.

161. Mitchell RG, Michael M, Sandidge D: High mortality among patients with the leukemoid reaction and alcoholic hepatitis. *South Med J* 84:281–282, 1991.

162. Allen EM, vanHeeckeren DW, Spector ML, Blumer JL: Management of nutritional and infectious complications of postoperative chylothorax in children. *J Pediatr Surg* 26:1169–1174, 1991.

163. Ide H, Kakiuchi T, Furuta N et al: The effect of cardiopulmonary bypass on T cells and their subpopulations. *Ann Thorac Surg* 44:277–282, 1987.

164. Lewis RT, Klein H: Risk factors in postoperative sepsis: Significance of preoperative lymphocytopenia. *J Surg Res* 26:365–371, 1979.

165. Rader DL, Mucha P, Moore SB et al: Cytomegalovirus infection in patients undergoing noncardiac surgical procedures. *Surg Gynecol Obstet* 160:13–16, 1985.

166. Baumgartner JD, Glauser MP, Burgo-Black AL et al: Severe cyto-

megalovirus infection in multiply transfused, splenectomised, trauma patients. *Lancet* 2:63–66, 1982.

167. Kantor GL, Goldberg LS: Cytomegalovirus-induced postperfusion syndrome. *Sem Hematol* 8:261–266, 1971.

168. Wilhelm JA, Matter L, Schopfer K: The risk of transmitting cytomegalovirus to patients receiving blood transfusions. *J Infect Dis* 154:169–171, 1986.

169. Teggatz JR, Parkin J, Peterson L: Transient atypical lymphocytosis in patients with emergency medical conditions. *Arch Pathol Lab Med* 111:712–714, 1987.

170. Wilson DM, Salazer TL, Farkouh ME: Eosinophiluria in atheroembolic renal disease. *Am J Med* 91:186–189, 1991.

171. Kasinath BS, Corwin HL, Bidani AK et al: Eosinophilia in the diagnosis of atheroembolic renal disease. *Am J Nephrol* 9:87–88, 1988.

172. Young DK, Burton MF, Herman JH: Multiple cholesterol emboli syndrome simulating systemic necrotizing vasculitis. *J Rheumatol* 13:423–426, 1986.

173. Goodwin SD, Glenny RW: Nonsteroidal anti-inflammatory drug-associated pulmonary infiltrates with eosinophilia. *Arch Intern Med* 152:1521–1524, 1992.

174. St. John RC, Allen JN, Pacht ER: Postoperative respiratory failure due to acute eosinophilic pneumonia. *Intens Care Med* 16:408–410, 1990.

175. Reid CB, Hill DA: Acute cor pulmonale and death due to massive fat embolism. *Aust NZ J Surg* 62:320–322, 1992.

176. Marshall PD, Douglas DL, Henry L: Fatal pulmonary fat embolism during total hip replacement due to high-pressure cementing techniques in an osteoporotic femur. *Br J Clin Pract* 45:148–149, 1991.

65 POSTOPERATIVE BLEEDING

David H. Henry

Postoperative bleeding is due to a breach in the anatomic integrity of a vessel at the operative site or to an underlying coagulopathy that may predispose the patient to bleeding either at that site or elsewhere. In the former case, clinical bleeding may not be obvious and may only be suggested by a falling hemoglobin level or excessive bloody drainage. The decision of whether and when to reoperate can be difficult and is left to the surgeon. In the latter instance, the presence of a coagulopathy can be documented by obtaining four simple blood tests—the prothrombin time (PT), activated partial thromboplastin time (aPTT), platelet count, and bleeding time. This chapter outlines the normal changes in coagulation parameters that occur after surgery and reviews the etiologies and management of postoperative bleeding with emphasis on disseminated intravascular coagulation.

Coagulation requires normal function of clotting factors and platelets. The PT and aPTT measure the clotting factors in the extrinsic and intrinsic pathways, respectively, with the exception of factor XIII which, when deficient, is a rare cause of bleeding. The level of each clotting factor must be at least 25% of normal to assure a normal PT and aPTT and obviate clinical bleeding. Therefore, patients with bleeding due to a coagulopathy should exhibit an abnormally prolonged PT or aPTT. However, a normal clotting test in patients without apparent bleeding may mask an underlying coagulopathy. For example, a patient with factor XI deficiency may have a factor level of 31%, normal clotting studies, and no evidence of bleeding before surgery but may develop abnormal clotting studies and clinical bleeding during or after surgery when factor levels fall.

Clotting also requires an adequate number of normally functioning platelets. Significant bleeding usually does not occur when the platelet count is above 100,000/mm³, and counts above 50,000/mm³ should be adequate for normal hemostasis except in major surgery or trauma. Despite adequate numbers of platelets, bleeding can occur if platelet function is abnormal. Function is evaluated by the standard Ivy bleeding time. The bleeding time will be prolonged above 10 minutes if the platelet count, platelet function, or vascular integrity is abnormal. However, while bleed-

ing times correlate with bleeding tendencies in large population studies, there is significant overlap between both normal and abnormal bleeding times and clinical outcomes. Therefore, an isolated normal or abnormal bleeding time in an individual patient may not correlate with bleeding tendency.[1] Etiologies of thrombocytopenia and abnormal platelet function are discussed below. Abnormal vascular integrity can be the result of aging or disorders like scurvy and amyloid.

If vascular endothelium is injured or diseased, underlying collagen is exposed to the circulation. Platelets adhere to the exposed surface and aggregate to form a platelet plug. Both the intrinsic and extrinsic arms of the clotting cascade are activated. Several anti-clotting mechanisms are simultaneously activated to keep the clot localized. The precursor plasminogen is cleaved to become the active thrombolytic enzyme plasmin, a process accelerated by thrombin, factor XII, and plasmin itself. Plasmin slows or reverses clotting by cleaving fibrinogen and fibrin to yield fibrin and fibrinogen degradation products (FDP). Excess FDP interfere with fibrin polymerization and platelet function. Other systems that prevent excessive clotting include protein C; antithrombin III; and alpha$_2$ globulins, which bind activated clotting factors and prevent them from diffusing away from the clotting surface.

POSTOPERATIVE CLOTTING ABNORMALITIES

It is not unusual to find transient abnormalities in one or more clotting parameters after surgery. The incidence of these abnormalities varies among particular procedures and may be dependent upon the anatomic site of surgery or the presence of prosthetic material. Sometimes it may be difficult to differentiate these abnormalities from low-level disseminated intravascular coagulation (DIC).

Egan studied coagulation parameters in 39 patients before and after surgery and found significant abnormalities in almost all of them.[2] The serum level of fibrin degradation products (FDP) was

659

increased above the normal range in 91 percent of the patients 24 hours after surgery, and values of over 46 μg/ml were found in 90 percent sometime in the postoperative period. Peak values were noted three to four days after surgery. The PT was abnormal sometime after surgery in 82 percent but was never prolonged for more than two seconds above the preoperative control value. Only 21 percent had a significant postoperative decline in platelet count, but no count fell below 125,000/mm³. In 95 percent of the patients, the plasma fibrinogen level rose steadily after surgery, and no patient had a fibrinogen level under 375 mg/dl three to four days after surgery. All surgical procedures were elective, and no patient had a malignancy. These predictable postoperative coagulation changes do not usually lead to clinical bleeding or thrombosis. Therefore, postoperative patients with a PT of more than two seconds above the control value, a platelet count of less than 125,000/mm³, a plasma fibrinogen level below 375 mg/dl three to four days after surgery, and a plasma level of FDP above 120 μg/ml are outside the usual range of postoperative changes in coagulation and may indicate the presence of a coagulopathy.

Changes in coagulation profile are particularly common after certain procedures. Because the brain is rich in thromboplastic substance, consumption of clotting factors and platelets is common after brain injury from head trauma or neurosurgery. In one study evaluating 26 patients with severe head trauma,[3] 50 percent sustained significant brain tissue destruction, and the remainder did not. All 13 patients in the first group exhibited increased systemic fibrinolysis and lower-than-normal plasma fibrinogen levels. Platelet counts were significantly depressed in 4 of the 13. Several patients had significant bleeding from sites unrelated to their primary injury. In the second group, 12 of 13 had normal fibrinogen and platelet levels, three had systemic fibrinolysis, and only one had clinical bleeding. Serial tests after admission revealed that the abnormal coagulation parameters returned to normal after 24 hours without specific treatment. In a later series of 150 patients undergoing brain surgery or sustaining head trauma, 60 showed clinical or laboratory evidence of a brief episode of DIC lasting 24 hours.[4]

Coagulopathies have also been reported after abdominal aortic replacement, orthopedic procedures, prostate surgery, and cardiopulmonary bypass.[5–8] Sustained changes in coagulation parameters are uncommon in these situations. Insertion of a LeVeen or Denver shunt is associated with change in clotting parameters.[9] One study documented changes in PT, plasma FDP levels, and platelet counts indicative of a chronic compensated DIC.[10] These findings are presumably related to the entry of thromboplastic tissues from the peritoneum into the venous circulation. Typical abnormalities included a platelet count of about 100,000/mm³, PT prolongation of four seconds above the control value, and a serum FDP level of 200 μg/ml. These abnormalities correlated with good shunt function and disappeared when the shunt clotted. Clinical bleeding or thrombosis did not occur. Heparin treatment has not been prospectively evaluated in these patients.

COMMON CAUSES OF POSTOPERATIVE BLEEDING

Clotting Factors

Isolated prolongation of the PT indicates the presence of factor VII deficiency (see Fig. 65–1). This is almost always an acquired deficiency due to insufficient vitamin K. The vitamin K–dependent factors—II, VII, IX, and X—eventually decrease enough to prolong the aPTT, but factor VII has the shortest half-life and its level is always the first to fall. If liver function is normal, subcutaneous vitamin K should correct the PT in hours. In polycythemia, the PT or aPTT may be artificially increased by a disproportionately high ratio of anticoagulant to plasma in the collection tube.

Deficiencies of intrinsic pathway factors VIII, IX, XI, or XII prolong the aPTT. Factor XII deficiency usually prolongs the aPTT for more than 90 seconds but is not associated with clinical bleeding. Factor XI deficiency is usually a congenital deficiency, common in northern European Jews with an autosomal recessive inheritance pattern. Therapy consists of fresh frozen plasma (FFP) in a dose of 10 ml/kg daily intravenously. Factor IX deficiency (hemophilia B) is a rare sex-linked recessive disorder occurring only in males. Factor VIII deficiency (hemophilia A), a more common sex-linked recessive disorder, is usually classified as mild (> 5% factor VIII), moderate (1–5%) or severe (< 1%). Patients with mild disease may not even know they have hemophilia until they undergo major surgery or suffer trauma. Therapy of hemophilia A and B is discussed in Chap. 30. Anti-factor VIII antibodies are an uncommon cause of aPTT prolongation but do occur.

The aPTT may be prolonged in von Willebrand's disease (VWD) or by heparin therapy. In VWD, preoperative coagulation studies may all be normal because factor VIII or von Willebrand factor levels may not be low enough to make the aPTT abnormal. Factor consumption during surgery can prolong the aPTT and/or bleeding time and cause postoperative bleeding. If only one of these tests is abnormal, a ristocetin aggregation and factor VIII antigen assay should be performed for confirmation. Heparin given during or after a procedure may also explain an increased aPTT. Blood specimens drawn from an arterial line, central line, or heparin lock contain a small amount of heparin that can prolong the aPTT no matter how much blood is discarded first before drawing the specimen. In such cases, the aPTT should be repeated on blood from a venipuncture for confirmation.

Distinguishing among the various etiologies of a prolonged aPTT begins with a 1:1 mix test, also known as an inhibitor screening test. Equal volumes of the patient's plasma and normal plasma are mixed, and the aPTT is repeated. Complete correction indicates a factor deficiency. Failure to correct completely suggests the presence of an inhibitor. Specific factor assays can be performed to diagnose a specific deficiency. It is helpful to know that an aPTT above 90 sec suggests factor XII deficiency and that hemophilia A and B are exceptionally rare in women. If treatment of a factor deficiency is necessary before a specific diagnosis can be made, fresh frozen plasma in a dose of 15 to 20 ml/kg followed by 3 to 6 ml/kg every 12 hours can be administered. Diagnosis and treatment of inhibitors is discussed in Chap. 30.

If both the PT and aPTT are prolonged, several possibilities should be considered. Vitamin K deficiency can occur relatively rapidly in patients with no oral source of vitamin K or in those receiving intravenous antibiotics that decrease absorption of vitamin K in the bowel. Ten mg of parenteral vitamin K significantly improves the PT and aPTT in 8 to 12 hours if liver function is normal. Although liver disease may be known before surgery, significant factor deficiency may only be appreciated postoperatively when hemostasis is poor. Replacement of factors with fresh frozen plasma (FFP) should attempt to decrease the PT to less than 15 seconds and the aPTT to less than 45 seconds. Repeated infusion of FFP may be necessary every six to eight hours in actively bleeding patients. DIC, seen in sepsis, hypotension, or organ is-

Intrinsic system   Extrinsic system

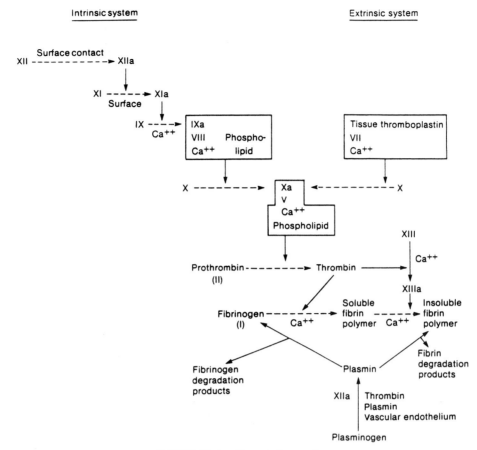

FIGURE 65–1. Coagulation pathway.

chemia, can increase both the PT and aPTT by consuming clotting factors.

Platelets

Platelet number and function should be evaluated in patients who are bleeding after surgery. If the platelet count is normal, the bleeding time provides a measure of platelet function. If the platelet count is significantly below 100,000/mm³, the bleeding time will usually be prolonged by the decrease and need not be performed.

Thrombocytopenia may cause postoperative bleeding if the count is below 80,000/mm³. Most often, drugs, sepsis, or DIC are responsible for thrombocytopenia. The most frequent medications implicated include diuretics, quinidine, nonsteroidal anti-inflammatory agents, sulfonamides, and heparin. Drugs like cimetidine and diuretics exert a direct suppressive effect on bone marrow production, and others like quinidine and heparin initiate immune-mediated peripheral destruction of platelets. Thrombocytopenia can be caused by heparin in any dose administered by any route,[11] but usually develops 7 to 10 days after starting therapeutic intravenous doses (see Chap. 64).[12]

Platelet transfusion may be needed in the interim if bleeding is due to thrombocytopenia. However, platelet transfusion is contraindicated in heparin-induced thrombocytopenia because transfused platelets may be consumed and lead to pathologic clotting. Discontinuing the offending medication allows platelet counts to rise

over a period of days. When thrombocytopenia develops, it is wise to try to discontinue or substitute as many medications as possible since any drug can cause thrombocytopenia.

Infection or full-blown sepsis commonly causes increased platelet consumption and thrombocytopenia. Early diagnosis and prompt therapy with antibiotics can abort platelet consumption, but platelet transfusions may be necessary to restore hemostasis. DIC induced by sepsis is discussed more fully below.

If the platelet count is normal and the bleeding time is prolonged, platelet dysfunction is more likely than abnormal vascular integrity to be the cause of bleeding. Platelet dysfunction with or without thrombocytopenia occurs in several postoperative settings. Intentional or unintentional aspirin administration before or after surgery can alter platelet function enough to require DDAVP or platelet transfusion (see Chap. 30).[13] Many other drugs can cause platelet dysfunction or a prolonged bleeding time, but an association between these defects and clinical bleeding has only been established for aspirin. These include NSAID's, beta-lactam antibiotics, nitroglycerin, propranolol, calcium channel blockers, tricyclic antidepressants, phenothiazines, antihistamines, and radiographic contrast dyes.

Platelet dysfunction also occurs in patients after coronary artery bypass grafting (CABG) and other procedures wherein blood is diverted to an extracorporeal circulating pump. Platelets are activated and damaged during repeated passage through the pump. DDAVP may decrease the bleeding in this setting if it is excessive but does little if bleeding is minimal or moderate.[14,15] In such cases, platelet transfusion is necessary to correct the bleeding time.

Preexisting or acute renal failure with uremia may cause platelet dysfunction and prolongation of the bleeding time, which frequently respond to DDAVP or cryoprecipitate. Congenital platelet abnormalities like von Willebrand's disease (VWD) may be overlooked preoperatively and cause postoperative bleeding. An increased bleeding time, positive ristocetin aggregation test, decreased factor VIII antigen level, and decreased factor VIII coagulant activity are demonstrable in classic VWD and respond to DDAVP or cryoprecipitate.

DISSEMINATED INTRAVASCULAR COAGULATION (DIC)

Under normal conditions, there is an adequate supply of platelets, clotting factors, and inhibitors of coagulation to control clotting and the fibrinolytic process. However, if clotting occurs at a large number of sites simultaneously, these processes can be overwhelmed. In several pathologic states listed in Table 65–1, massive endothelial damage or exposure of tissue to the circulation activates and exhausts these systems and results in the clinical manifestations of DIC. The process can consume more clotting or anticlotting factors at different sites, unbalancing the system and leading to clotting at some locations and bleeding at others.

Acute DIC

In acute DIC, coagulation factors are depressed to abnormally low levels, fibrinolytic activity is increased, and platelets are widely consumed. There is no single laboratory test to confirm or exclude the diagnosis of DIC. Colman retrospectively studied 60 patients with DIC confirmed by the presence of thrombi in the microcirculation.[16] He found that the PT was greater than 15 sec in 90 percent of the patients, the plasma fibrinogen level was less than

TABLE 65–1. Causes of DIC

Infection
Gram-negative sepsis
Gram-positive sepsis
Rickettsial infection, especially Rocky Mountain spotted fever
Viral infection
Obstetrical emergencies
Septic abortion
Abruptio placentae
Retained dead fetus
Toxemia
Malignancies
Tumors, especially carcinoma of the lung, prostate, stomach, and pancreas, and promyelocytic leukemia
Shock of any cause
Miscellaneous
Snake bite
Heat stroke
Burns
Hemolytic transfusion reaction
Vasculitis

160 mg/dl in 70 percent, and the platelet count less than 150,000/mm^3 in 90 percent (see Table 65–2). If all three criteria were met, the diagnosis of DIC could be established with certainty. If two of the three were fulfilled, determination of the plasma fibrin degradation products (FDP) level could be performed for confirmation. Plasma FDP concentrations were increased above five μg/ml in 90 percent of the patients.

Other confirmatory tests are currently being developed. Levels of fibrinopeptide A, resulting from the action of plasmin on fibrinogen, are increased in almost all cases of DIC. However, the test produces false positive results and may therefore be too sensitive.[17] Theoretically, antithrombin III levels should fall in DIC, and the concentration of antithrombin III–thrombin complexes should rise.

Laboratory criteria for DIC presuppose a previously normal coagulation system. However, patients with liver disease may have

TABLE 65–2. Criteria for Diagnosis of DIC

Test	Normal Value (mean ± 1 SD)	Criteria for DIC*	DIC (% abnormal)	DIC Values (mean ± 2 SD)
			Screening	(60 patients, 69 episodes)‡
Prothrombin time (sec)	12 ± 1	≥ 15	91	18 (14.5 − 48)†
Platelets (mg/μl)	250,000 ± 50,000	≤ 150,000	93	52,000 ± 48,000
Fibrinogen (mg/dl)	230 ± 35	≤ 160	77	131 ± 84
			Confirmatory	(45 patients, 54 episodes)§
Fi titer	< 1:8	≥ 1:16	92	1:52 (1:11–1:256)†
Thrombin time (sec)	20 ± 1.6	≥ 25	59	27 (21–36)†
Euglobulin lysis time (min)	> 120	≤ 120	42	

Abnormal Screening Tests	Confirmatory Test	Patients§
3/3	Not required	89%
2/3	Required	20%
0–1/3	Required + fibrin thrombi	9%

*Values greater than 2 SD from normal mean values.
†Range of ± 2 SD.
‡Prospective and retrospective studies combined.
§Prospective study.

abnormal baseline studies because of the role of the liver in the production and metabolism of factors involved in the clotting process. Chronic liver disease affects all coagulation factors except factor VIII and impairs clearance of activated factors, fibrinolytic activators, and FDP's. It also leads to portal hypertension, splenomegaly, and pooling of platelets. In defining DIC in such patients, Colman established a "normal" range for the PT, platelet count, fibrinogen level, and FDP concentration for patients with uncomplicated cirrhosis, and set values two standard deviations outside the mean to indicate DIC.[16] Application of these criteria to 18 patients with uncomplicated cirrhosis allowed separation into two groups. Those with laboratory criteria for DIC had a typical predisposing cause and bled from more than one site, while the others bled only from esophageal varices. Criteria for diagnosing acute DIC in patients with liver disease are shown in Table 65–3.

Bleeding is the hallmark of DIC and is the presenting manifestation in about 80 percent of patients. Bleeding from more than one site occurs in over 50 percent. Petechiae and purpura in the skin are usually counted as one site. Although the risk of bleeding during and after surgery is higher in patients with an established diagnosis of DIC, surgery may be necessary to treat the underlying cause. This is particularly true when DIC is due to obstetrical complications or malignancy. Sepsis and shock are the most common causes of DIC after surgery and require vigorous medical treatment. DIC may develop during surgery and cause diffuse oozing in the surgical field or at venipuncture sites. Ecchymoses ultimately follow if the process is allowed to continue. If mismatched blood is responsible, clumped red blood cells may actually be observed on the scalpel.[18]

Acute DIC after surgery must be differentiated from the expected postoperative changes in coagulation parameters by applying the laboratory criteria described above. All criteria should be met to confirm the diagnosis. However, the plasma FDP concentration is variable after surgery and can be significantly elevated in many patients without DIC.

Management of DIC first requires diagnosis and treatment of the underlying cause. It may be necessary to treat the coagulopathy itself with clotting factors and platelets in the interim. Despite the fear that such therapy may unbalance the coagulation and fibrinolytic systems and promote further bleeding and/or thrombosis, this usually does not occur. Fresh frozen plasma can be administered until the PT is only five seconds or less above the control value, and cryoprecipitate can be given to maintain the blood fibrinogen level above 100 mg/dl.

The literature is divided on the use of heparin in the treatment of DIC.[16,19–21] It can be administered while the primary underlying disease is addressed. However, despite its use in some gynecologic procedures in the past, there are no clear guidelines for administering it in the postoperative setting. Replacement of coagulation factors after heparin is started is theoretically reasonable, but the use of epsilon-aminocaproic acid alone to decrease fibrinolysis is always contraindicated and is only rarely used in conjunction with heparin and clotting factor replacement.

Chronic DIC

Low-grade or chronic DIC may be unsuspected until clotting or bleeding occurs. Cooper studied it extensively in animals by infusing thromboplastin at various rates into dogs and measuring platelet and fibrinogen levels.[22] At high infusion rates, acute DIC developed with significant decreases in platelet count and fibrinogen level. At lower infusion rates, the platelet count fell, but the fibrinogen concentration rose. Cooper postulated that thromboplastin infused at a low infusion rate leads to an increase in fibrinogen

---

TABLE 65–3. Criteria for Diagnosis of DIC when Liver Disease is Present*

Test	Uncomplicated Cirrhosis† (mean ± SD)	Criteria for DIC‡	Mean Value for DIC (9 patients)
Screening			
Prothrombin time (sec)	14 ± 2	> 25	29
Platelets (mg/μl)	176,000 ± 70,000	< 50,000	35,000
Fibrinogen (mg/dl)	204 ± 55	< 125	85
Confirmatory			
Fi titer	≤ 1:16	≥ 1:32	1:84
Thrombin time	92% abnormal	Not used	86%
Euglobulin lysis time	67% abnormal	Not used	57%

When liver disease is present, the diagnosis of DIC requires
1. 3/3 screening criteria for liver disease, or
2. Response to heparin therapy and meeting of regular criteria.

*Patients were considered to have liver disease if any of the following features was manifest: jaundice (bilirubin > 3 mg/dl); cirrhosis suspected clinically (portal hypertension or esophageal varices), histologically, or at laparotomy; recent hepatitis; or centrilobular congestion (serum lactic dehydrogenase (LDH) > 1000 units and glutamic oxaloacetic transaminase (SGOT) > 800 Karmen units) due to congestive heart failure and confirmed by autopsy.

†Source of data: prothrombin time, platelet count, fibrinogen level, and Fi titer. The prothrombin time was originally expressed as the ratio of patient time to control time (average 1.16 ± 0.16). This was converted to seconds for the above comparison with 12 sec as a control time. The average fibrinogen level was 316 ± 73 mg/dl.

‡Values greater than 2 SD from normal mean values.

turnover with a disproportionate rise in hepatic synthesis, resulting in an increased steady-state plasma concentration.

In order to document the presence of ongoing low-grade DIC in which synthesis of clotting factors is sufficient to keep up with consumption, Cooper studied 79 patients with plasma levels of FDP above an arbitrarily chosen normal value.[23] The patients could be separated into three groups on the basis of simultaneously drawn plasma fibrinogen concentrations. Plasma fibrinogen levels of greater than 370 mg/dl were found in 49 or 62 percent. In this group with "overcompensated" fibrinogen production, platelet counts varied widely above and below the normal range. In the absence of liver disease to decrease clearance of FDP or primary fibrinolysis, Cooper postulated the presence of low-grade DIC. The underlying diseases in these patients included vasculitis, primary renal disease, collagen vascular disease, and malignancy. No mention was made of clinical bleeding or clotting abnormalities.

In contrast to the bleeding seen in acute DIC, thrombosis is more common in chronic low-grade DIC. In the nineteenth century, Trousseau recognized an association between cancer and disseminated thrombosis.[24] Sack et al. documented 192 cases of neoplasia associated with some form of arterial or venous coagulation abnormality.[25] The study underscores the variety of abnormalities in coagulation parameters seen in such patients. Platelet counts and plasma fibrinogen levels were increased, decreased, or normal, but plasma FDP concentrations were usually elevated. The most common malignancies observed included carcinoma of the pancreas, lung, prostate, and stomach and acute leukemia. There was evidence of arterial emboli in 42 cases. In 31 or 74 percent, nonbacterial thrombotic endocarditis involving the aortic and mitral valves with equal frequency served as the source of the emboli. Tricuspid valve endocarditis was uncommon.

Sun underscored the frequency of coagulation abnormalities in patients with cancer.[26] Of 61 patients with cancer, only three had no coagulation abnormalities, and 82 percent had increased plasma FDP concentrations. Bleeding was noted in 56 percent, and thrombophlebitis or thromboembolism was seen in 20 percent. Coagulation abnormalities were significantly more common in patients with metastatic disease. An increased frequency of clotting abnormalities in neoplasia was also documented by Hagedorn in 50 patients with inoperable lung cancer.[27] The relationship between chronic DIC and neoplasia has been reviewed extensively.[28]

The clinical significance of chronic DIC in surgical patients is unclear. Mertens studied 42 patients undergoing transurethral resection of the prostate, of whom 50 percent had cancer.[29] Those with malignancy bled more frequently, but the incidence of operative bleeding was highest among those patients with preoperative abnormalities in any coagulation test regardless of their underlying disease. Intervention with preventive treatment such as heparin was not addressed. No controlled therapeutic studies have been performed in patients with chronic DIC.

SUMMARY

1. Postoperative bleeding is the result of a breach in the anatomic integrity of a vessel or a coagulopathy.

2. One of the four coagulation parameters—PT, aPTT, platelet count, and bleeding time—will usually point to a coagulopathy in bleeding patients and help to narrow the differential diagnosis.

3. Minor abnormalities in at least one of these parameters without clinical bleeding occurs in many patients, particularly those who have suffered head trauma or undergone neurosurgery, prostate surgery, orthopedic procedures, cardiopulmonary bypass, or placement of a LeVeen shunt. However, if the PT is prolonged more than two seconds, the platelet count falls below 125,000/mm^3, the plasma fibrinogen level is below 375 mg/dl, or the plasma concentration of fibrin degradation products is above 120 μg/ml three or four days after surgery, an underlying coagulopathy should be suspected and evaluated.

4. After surgery, an isolated prolongation in the PT is almost always due to early vitamin K deficiency. Eventually other vitamin K–dependent factors are affected, and both the PT and aPTT are affected.

5. Both the PT and aPTT are abnormal in patients with vitamin K deficiency, significant liver disease that may have been overlooked before surgery, or DIC. They are also sometimes artificially elevated in patients with polycythemia vera because of a disproportionately high ratio of anticoagulant to plasma in the collection tube. A trial of parenteral vitamin K is warranted if DIC is not documented.

6. Isolated prolongation of the aPTT, if not due to the presence of a lupus anticoagulant detected preoperatively, is most likely the result of postoperative factor depletion in patients with unsuspected von Willebrand's disease or inherited deficiency of one of the factors in the intrinsic coagulation pathway, the inadvertent presence of heparin in the specimen, or an acquired coagulation inhibitor. A 1:1 mix test is the first step in the evaluation.

7. Postoperative thrombocytopenia may cause bleeding when levels are below 80,000/mm^3. The most common causes are sepsis, DIC, and a variety of medications including diuretics, quinidine, NSAID's, sulfonamides, and heparin. Thrombocytopenia resolves with treatment of the underlying cause. Platelet transfusions can be given in the interim except in those with heparin-induced immune thrombocytopenia.

8. Platelet dysfunction without thrombocytopenia is seen in patients undergoing procedures involving diversion of blood to extracorporeal circulating devices, in those with uremia or unsuspected von Willebrand's disease, and in those receiving certain medications. Aside from discontinuation of any offending drugs, DDAVP may be beneficial in improving platelet function.

9. Bleeding is the most common presenting sign of DIC. Of the causes listed in Table 65–1, shock and sepsis are the most common. The criteria for diagnosing DIC are shown in Table 65–2 for patients with previously normal coagulation and in Table 65–3 for those with underlying liver disease. Management of DIC consists of treating the underlying disease process and supporting the patient with platelets and clotting factors in the form of fresh frozen plasma and cryoprecipitate. The use of heparin remains controversial.

10. Chronic DIC is most frequently seen in patients with malignancy and is more often manifested by thrombosis rather than bleeding. Its clinical significance in the surgical setting is unclear.

REFERENCES

1. Rodgers RPG, Levin J: A critical reappraisal of the bleeding time. *Sem Thromb Hemostas* 16:1, 1990.
2. Egan EL, Bowie EJW, Kazmier FJ et al: Effect of surgical operations on certain tests used to diagnose intravascular coagulation and fibrinolysis. *Mayo Clin Proc* 49:658, 1974.
3. Goodnight SH, Kenoyer G, Rapaport S et al: Defibrination after brain tissue destruction. *N Engl J Med* 290:1043, 1974.
4. Van der Sande JJ, Veltkamp JJ, Boekhout-Mussert RJ: Head injury and coagulation disorders. *J Neurosurg* 49:357,365, 1978.
5. Mulcare RJ, Royster TS, Phillips LL: Intravascular coagulation in surgical procedures on the abdominal aorta. *Surg Gynecol Obstet* 143:730, 1976.
6. Demirjian Z, Sara M, Strulbert D et al: Disseminated intravascular coagulation in patients undergoing orthopedic surgery. *Clin Orthop* 102:174, 1974.
7. Friedman NG, Hoag S, Robinson AJ et al: Hemorrhagic syndrome following transurethral prostatic resection for benign adenoma. *Arch Intern Med* 124:341, 1969.
8. Muller N, Popou-Cenic S, Buttner W et al: Studies of fibrinolytic and coagulation factors during open heart surgery: II. Post-op bleeding tendency and changes in the coagulation system. *Thromb Res* 7:589, 1975.
9. LeVeen HH, Christoridian G, Ip M et al: Peritoneovenous shunting for ascites. *Ann Surg* 180:580, 1974.
10. Harman DC, Demirjian Z, Ellman Z et al: Disseminated intravascular coagulation with the peritoneovenous shunt. *Ann Intern Med* 90:774, 1979.
11. Kelton JG: Heparin-induced thrombocytopenia. *Hemostasis* 16(2):123, 1986.
12. Johnson RA, Lazarus KH, Henry DH: Heparin-induced thrombocytopenia: A prospective study. *Am J Hematol* 17(4):349, 1984.
13. Mannucci PM: Desmopressin: A nontransfusional form of treatment for congenital and acquired bleeding disorders. *Blood* 72:1449, 1988.
14. Salzman EW, Weinstein MJ, Weintraub RM et al: Treatment with desmopressin acetate to reduce blood loss after surgery. A double-blind randomized trial. *N Engl J Med* 314(22):1402, 1986.
15. Hackmann T, Gescoyne RD, Naiman SC et al: A trial of desmopressin to reduce blood loss in uncomplicated cardiac surgery. *N Engl J Med* 321(21):1437, 1989.
16. Colman RU, Robboy SJ, Minna JD: Disseminated intravascular coagulation: A reappraisal. *Ann Rev Med* 30:359, 1979.
17. Nossel HL, Younger LR, Wilner GB: Radioimmunoassay of human fibrinopeptide A. *Proc Natl Acad Sci USA* 68:2350, 1971.
18. Owen CA, Bowie EJW: Surgical hemostasis. *J Neurosurg* 51:137, 1979.
19. Heene L: DIC: Evaluation of therapeutic approaches. *Sem Thromb Hemostas* 3:291, 1977.
20. Colman RW, Robboy SJ, Minna JD: Disseminated intravascular coagulation: A reappraisal. *Ann Rev Med* 30:359, 1979.
21. Bowie EJW, Owen CA: Chronic intravascular coagulation and fibrinolysis syndromes. *Sem Thromb Hemostas* 3:268, 1977.
22. Cooper HA, Bowie EJW, Didisheim P et al: Paradoxic changes in platelets and fibrinogen in chemically induced intravascular coagulation. *Mayo Clin Proc* 46:521, 1971.
23. Cooper HA, Bowie EJW, Owen CA: Evaluation of patients with increased fibrinolytic split products (FSP) in their serum. *Mayo Clin Proc* 49:654, 1974.
24. Trousseau A: *Phlegmasia Alba Dolens. Clinique Medicale de L'Hotel Diere de Paris.* London, The New Sydenham Society, 1865, vol 3, p 94.
25. Sack GH, Levin J, Bell WR: Trousseau's syndrome and other manifestations of chronic disseminated intravascular coagulation in patients with neoplasms: Clinical, pathophysiologic and therapeutic features. *Medicine* 1:56, 1977.
26. Sun NJC, Bowie EJW, Kazmier FJ et al: Blood coagulation studies in patients with cancer. *Mayo Clin Proc* 49:636, 1974.
27. Hagedorn AB, Bowie EJU, Elveback LR et al: Coagulation abnormalities in patients with inoperable lung cancer. *Mayo Clin Proc* 49:647, 1974.
28. Weick JK: Intravascular coagulation in cancer. *Sem Oncol* 5:203, 1978.
29. Mertens BF, Greene LF, Bowie EJW et al: Fibrinolytic split products and ethanol gelation test in preoperative evaluation of patients with prostatic disease. *Mayo Clin Proc* 49:642, 1974.

66 COMPLICATIONS OF TRANSFUSION IN SURGICAL PATIENTS

Leslie E. Silberstein
Leigh C. Jefferies

Adverse effects of blood transfusions can be divided into two broad categories as determined by underlying immunologic or nonimmunologic mechanisms (see Table 66–1). Their severity and contribution to morbidity and mortality in the surgical patient are variable. Since many of these complications are unpredictable and cannot be prevented, consideration of the risks and benefits of transfusion should be carefully weighed in every patient. This chapter focuses on recognition and appropriate management of the acute transfusion reactions shown in Table 66–2, key features of major transfusion-transmitted viral diseases, and important problems peculiar to massive blood transfusion.

IMMUNOLOGIC COMPLICATIONS

Acute Hemolytic Transfusion Reactions

Potentially life-threatening acute hemolytic reactions are usually due to transfusion of ABO-incompatible whole blood or packed red blood cells. Mislabeling of a blood sample for ABO determination or transfusion of blood intended for another recipient are usually responsible.[1] The IgM component of naturally occurring anti-A and anti-B antibodies present in the patient's serum agglutinates transfused red blood cells, and activation of complement and acute intravascular hemolysis follow. Infusion of incompatible plasma, usually along with ABO incompatible platelets, rarely causes severe reactions because it is diluted in the large volume of the recipient's plasma. Although the actual incidence of acute hemolytic transfusion reactions is unknown, the mortality rate is low primarily due to appropriate medical intervention.[2]

The onset of symptoms is variable and depends on the characteristics of the antibody involved and the quantity of blood transfused. Signs and symptoms include fever, chills, chest or back pain, nausea, oliguria or anuria, hemoglobinuria, dyspnea, and hypotension. In anesthetized patients, the only clinical signs may be excessive bleeding in the operative field, uncontrolled hypotension, or hemoglobinuria. Serious sequelae may include shock,

TABLE 66–1. Complications of Transfusion

Immunologic
   Hemolytic transfusion reactions, acure and delayed
   Febrile nonhemolytic transfusion reactions
   Noncardiogenic pulmonary edema
   Allergic transfusion reactions
   Alloimmunization
   Graft-versus-host disease

Nonimmunologic
   Infectious disease transmission
      Viral
      Bacterial
      Other
   Complications related to massive transfusion
      Hemostatic abnormalities
      Citrate toxicity
      Hypothermia
      Acid-base imbalance
      Electrolyte abnormalities
   Other Nonimmunologic
      Circulatory overload
      Nonimmune hemolysis

acute renal failure, and disseminated intravascular coagulation. Transfusion should be discontinued immediately if suspicious signs or symptoms develop. Hemoglobinemia can be rapidly confirmed by visual inspection of serum in a sample of clotted blood. Investigation for error should be undertaken promptly.

Laboratory evaluation of a transfusion reaction should include a direct antiglobulin test to detect antibody on the transfused red blood cells. Free hemoglobin in a freshly voided urine sample supports the diagnosis of acute hemolysis. Additional tests include hemoglobin, hematocrit, and lactate dehydrogenase (LDH) levels. Indirect serum bilirubin should peak three to six hours after the hemolytic reaction.

Treating hypotension and promoting adequate renal blood flow are initial priorities. Fluid should be administered to maintain urine flow at or above 100 ml/hr for 18 to 24 hours. Osmotic agents

TABLE 66–2. Acute Complications of Transfusion

Type	Signs and Symptoms	Etiology	Treatment	Prevention
Acute hemolytic reaction	Fever, chills, hemoglobinuria, hemoglobinemia, shock, DIC	Incompatibility due to clerical error (usually ABO)	Stop transfusion, hydrate, support blood pressure and respiration, induce diuresis, treat DIC, shock	Proper identification of patient sample, product, and recipient
Febrile reaction	Fever, chills	Antibodies to leukocyte antigens	Stop transfusion, give antipyretics	Use of leukocyte-poor blood products
Mild allergic reaction	Localized urticaria, pruritis	Antibodies to plasma proteins	Temporarily discontinue transfusion, give antihistamines	Pretransfusion antihistamine
Severe allergic reaction	Anaphylaxis, respiratory distress, hypotension	Antibodies to plasma proteins	Stop transfusion, support blood pressure and respiration, epinephrine, steroids may be necessary	If documented anti-IgA antibodies, transfuse blood from IgA-deficient donors
Noncardiogenic pulmonary edema	Dyspnea, pulmonary edema, normal cardiac pressure	Antibodies to leukocyte antigens	Stop transfusion, support blood pressure and respiration	Use of plasma-depleted blood products
Bacterial sepsis	Shock, fever, chills	Contaminated blood component	Stop transfusion, support blood pressure, antibiotic therapy	Careful blood collection, storage
Hypervolemia	Dyspnea, hypertension, pulmonary edema	Rapid or excessive transfusion	Stop transfusion, induce diuresis, cardiorespiratory support	Avoid rapid or excessive transfusion

like mannitol or diuretics like furosemide[3] may be used. Low-dose dopamine under 5 μg/kg/min promotes dilatation of the renal vasculature and increases cardiac output.[4]

Delayed Hemolytic Transfusion Reactions

Delayed hemolytic transfusion reactions are due to primary or secondary immunization against foreign red cell antigens such as Kell, Duffy, Kidd, E, c, C, or D.[5] Production of alloantibody begins one to two weeks after exposure. As antibodies increase in titer and avidity, they bind transfused red cells in the circulation. The characteristics of the antibody and number of foreign red cells present determine red cell survival and clinical presentation. These reactions are usually subclinical and may only be manifested by a positive direct antiglobulin test, the presence of a new circulating alloantibody, and perhaps an unexplained fall in hemoglobin. A delayed hemolytic transfusion reaction should be considered in a patient who fails to have an expected increase in hemoglobin after transfusion. Secondary anemnestic responses may be accompanied by fever, jaundice, and hemoglobinuria. Some IgG antibodies,

such as anti-Jk^a or anti-Jk^b (Kidd), bind complement and cause intravascular destruction of red blood cells. Patients with these reactions should be monitored for evidence of hemolysis, disseminated intravascular coagulation, and renal dysfunction.[6]

Febrile Nonhemolytic Transfusion Reactions

Febrile nonhemolytic transfusion reactions are characterized by an increase in body temperature of 1°C or more with or without chills during or shortly after transfusion.[7] Acute hemolytic transfusion reaction and other causes of fever must be ruled out. These reactions are due to recipient antibodies directed against antigens on donor lymphocytes, granulocytes, or platelets and lead to activation of complement and/or release of pyrogens. The antibodies may have HLA or granulocyte specificities. Febrile reactions are usually seen in multitransfused or multiparous females.

Management includes discontinuing the transfusion, use of antipyretics, and transfusion-appropriate evaluation as described above. Although usually isolated events, febrile reactions may recur and may warrant prophylactic use of in-line filters to remove contaminating leukocytes from packed red cells, whole blood, or platelets.[8] Laboratory testing to attempt to document the presence of leukoagglutinins in this setting is impractical.

Noncardiogenic Pulmonary Edema

Transfusion recipients may rarely experience acute pulmonary edema accompanied by fever and chills without evidence of left ventricular dysfunction.[9] These reactions may be due to potent leukoagglutinins present in either recipient or donor serum and occur most often in multiparous females. They may be the result of trapping of leukocyte aggregates in the pulmonary microvasculature leading to increased vascular permeability, activation of complement, and generation of anaphylatoxins.[10] In some cases, aggressive supportive measures and intravenous steroids have been beneficial.[11] Following serious reactions, it is prudent to investigate recipient and donor plasma for these leukoagglutinins. If present, patients may require leukocyte-free products and should not be donors.

Urticarial and Other Allergic Reactions

The most common allergic reaction to blood products is urticarial, usually without fever or other adverse effects. These reactions are due to transfused soluble atopens and are more common in patients with a history of allergy. Allergic reactions may follow transfusion of plasma or cellular blood products containing plasma. Symptoms are mediated by histamine released from mast cells coated with IgE and IgG.[12]

It is not necessary to abort the transfusion for simple focal urticarial reactions. Transfusion can be interrupted temporarily while antihistamines are administered. More serious allergic reactions including periorbital or laryngeal edema or diffuse severe urticaria require stopping the transfusion and initiating appropriate supportive measures. If urticarial reactions recur or are not responsive to medication, it may be useful to remove plasma from cellular blood products by plasma reducing or washing.

Anaphylactic Reactions

Severe anaphylactic immediate hypersensitivity reactions with respiratory distress and vascular collapse rarely occur after blood transfusion. Symptoms may develop after only a small volume has been transfused. Many of these reactions occur in patients with IgA deficiency and IgG anti-IgA antibodies in high titer.[13] More recently, IgE anti-IgA antibodies have also been implicated.[14] Although the incidence of IgA deficiency is relatively high at 1 in 700, the occurrence of anaphylactic reactions after transfusion is considerably less common.

Early recognition is essential. Management includes treatment of hypotension, prompt administration of epinephrine, and prevention of hypoxia. Individuals with a class-specific anti-IgA titer of 1:256 or greater, or those who have experienced a previous anaphylactic transfusion reaction due to anti-IgA, should not receive products containing IgA. It may be possible to locate such products in rare donor files at the National Red Cross or other agencies. Alternatively, packed red blood cells may be extensively washed free of plasma. Such patients can be enrolled in autologous donor programs before elective surgery.

Graft-versus-Host Disease

Graft-versus-host disease (GVHD) can occur when immunocompetent allogeneic lymphocytes are transfused or transplanted into a severely immunocompromised host and proliferate in response to host major and minor histocompatibility antigens. GVHD has followed transfusion of whole blood, packed red cells, platelets, granulocytes, or fresh plasma, but not administration of fresh frozen plasma or cryoprecipitate.[15] Clinical manifestations begin within 30 days of transfusion and include fever, liver function abnormalities, diarrhea, and an erythematous skin rash that may progress to generalized erythroderma. Pancytopenia is a hallmark of transfusion-associated GVHD in contrast to GVHD associated with bone marrow transplantation. Despite the use of steroids, antithymocyte globulin, methotrexate, and cyclosporine, the mortality rate is 80 percent and is usually related to infectious disease complications.[16]

Irradiation of all but frozen noncellular plasma products is the most efficient method to prevent transfusion-related GVHD. Absolute indications for blood product irradiation include allogeneic and autologous bone marrow transplantation and congenital immune deficiency syndromes. Relative indications include intrauterine transfusion, neonatal exchange transfusion, Hodgkin's and non-Hodgkin's lymphoma, and acute leukemia. Routine use of irradiated blood is not currently recommended for solid tumors, aplastic anemia, or AIDS.[17] Cases of GVHD have been reported following transfusion of blood from a donor homozygous for an HLA haplotype of the recipient.[18] Therefore, blood donated by family members of the intended recipient should be irradiated before transfusion.

Alloimmunization

Following transfusion or pregnancy, individuals may become immunized against a number of different antigenic components in blood products. These include red blood cell antigens, platelet-specific antigens, granulocyte-specific antigens, HLA antigens on leukocytes and platelets, and plasma proteins. Unexpected alloantibodies against red blood cell antigens, unlike naturally occurring anti-A and anti-B antibodies, are found in 0.3 to 2 percent of the general population.[19] Primary and secondary alloimmune responses can be detected by a rise in titer of specific antibodies. Alloantibodies can cause acute or delayed hemolytic transfusion reactions and therefore require complete characterization to avoid recurrence. It may be difficult to locate compatible blood for those with multiple antibodies or antibodies against antigens of high frequency in the population.

Patients who have received multiple platelet transfusions commonly become refractory to further transfusions because of alloimmunization. Alloimmunization to HLA or platelet-specific antigens occurs commonly in multiply transfused patients with acute leukemia, solid tumors, and aplastic anemia.[20,21] A low platelet count one hour after transfusion usually indicates alloimmunization and distinguishes it from nonimmunologic causes of thrombocytopenia such as bleeding, sepsis, disseminated intravascular coagulation (DIC), or splenomegaly.[22] Patients who are refractory to platelet transfusions may or may not respond to single-donor HLA-matched platelets. Possible explanations for failure of HLA-matched transfusions include unidentified HLA incompatibilities, alloimmunization to platelet-specific antigens, and platelet destruction due to nonimmunologic factors.[23]

Posttransfusion purpura is an uncommon manifestation of alloimmunization to platelet antigens. This syndrome is characterized by sudden development of self-limited thrombocytopenia 5 to 10 days after transfusion and is due to a sudden rise in the titer of a platelet-specific antibody, usually against the Pl^{A1} antigen.[24] It usually occurs in Pl^{A1}-negative females previously sensitized during pregnancy or transfusion and may follow transfusion of any product containing platelet antigens. Differential diagnosis includes autoimmune thrombocytopenic purpura (ITP), sepsis, DIC, bone marrow failure, and drug-induced thrombocytopenia. Although the pathogenesis of this process involves alloimmunization, the recipient's own platelets, although lacking the Pl^{A1} antigen, are also destroyed.[25] Thrombocytopenia is self-limited but may last several days to weeks and is not responsive to platelet transfusions. Steroids have been used during the acute episode, but plasma exchange is the therapy of choice.[26]

NONIMMUNOLOGIC COMPLICATIONS

Transmission of Infectious Disease

Viral Hepatitis

In spite of advances in donor screening over the past decade, viral hepatitis remains the single most common infectious complication of blood transfusion. Most cases are due to hepatitis C, and fewer than two percent are attributable to hepatitis B virus and cytomegalovirus (CMV).[27]

Certain clinical symptoms and laboratory features are common to acute viral hepatitis regardless of etiology. Infection is subclinical in 60 to 80 percent of cases, manifested only by elevated serum transaminases. Symptoms of anicteric hepatitis, including anorexia, nausea, vomiting, diarrhea, arthralgias, myalgias, pharyngitis, and low-grade fever, occur in 20 to 25 percent. More severe symptoms with acholic stools, jaundice, and profound weakness are less common. Fulminant hepatic failure is rare and occurs more often in delta hepatitis than in hepatitis B or C.[28] Therapy rests on supportive care and prevention of transmission. Diagnosis of the particular etiologic agent relies on detection of specific antibodies against viral antigens (see Table 66–3).

Hepatitis B virus is transmitted by sexual contact and direct percutaneous or parenteral inoculation, especially in transplant recipients, health care workers, intravenous drug abusers, and dialysis patients. Newborn infants can acquire the disease from infected mothers. Hepatitis B was a common complication of blood transfusion before routine donor screening for hepatitis B surface antigen (HBsAg).[29] In recent years, screening for antibody to hepatitis B core antigen (anti-HBcAg) has further reduced the incidence of transfusion-related hepatitis.

Two large studies show that the severity of hepatitis B following transfusion has decreased.[27,30] In acute icteric hepatitis B, HBsAg is detected in the blood several weeks after exposure and two to four weeks before clinical manifestations. Serum transaminase levels increase one to four weeks after appearance of HBsAg and usually peak with the onset of symptoms (see Table 66–1). Chronic hepatitis B develops in approximately one to three percent of cases.

Before 1980, the risk of posttransfusion hepatitis C was 7 to 12 percent[31] but has significantly decreased in recent years due to

TABLE 66–3. Three Major Types of Viral Hepatitis

Virus	Cause of Posttransfusion Hepatitis	Incubation Period (range in weeks)	Serologic Markers (antibodies)
Hepatitis A	0%	2–6	Anti-HAV
Hepatitis B	1–2%	4–30	Anti-HBs Anti-HBc Anti-HBe
Hepatitis C	80–95%	2–26	Anti-HCV

implementation of second generation tests for hepatitis C virus and screening for surrogate viral markers.[32] The etiologic agent of hepatitis C has been cloned,[33] and assays have been developed to detect antibody against one of its major gene products.[34] The incubation period in posttransfusion studies is approximately 50 days with a range of 2 to 26 weeks. Infection is usually subclinical, and only about 25 percent develop symptoms or become jaundiced. However, 50 percent of patients with hepatitis C continue to exhibit biochemical evidence of chronic liver disease,[35] and approximately 20 percent of those with chronic hepatitis have histologic evidence of cirrhosis.

The delta agent (HDV) is a defective virus requiring concurrent hepatitis B infection for expression. Infection with HDV may occur simultaneously with acute hepatitis B or constitute a superinfection in a patient with chronic hepatitis B exposed to HBV/HDV-positive blood. HDV causes a severe form of hepatitis and correlates with a greater frequency of cirrhosis. Information concerning transfusion-transmitted delta hepatitis is limited. In areas where delta hepatitis is prevalent, antidelta antibodies occur in 3.5 percent of transfusion recipients who develop hepatitis.[28] Hepatitis A does not produce a carrier state and is an extremely unusual cause of posttransfusion hepatitis.[36]

Herpes Virus Transmission

Among the human herpes viruses, cytomegalovirus (CMV) and Epstein-Barr virus (EBV) may cause transfusion-transmitted disease. Recent prospective studies evaluating CMV transmission document much lower infection rates in the range of 1.2 to 1.5 percent after transfusion in seronegative immunocompetent recipients than in the late 1960s and early 1970s.[37] The majority of transfusion-associated CMV infections as determined by seroconversion are asymptomatic without sequelae. In contrast, CMV infection is seen frequently in patients who are immunocompromised because of prematurity, underlying disease, or immunosuppressive therapy. Infection may present as a mononucleosis syndrome, retinitis, hepatitis, pneumonitis, or disseminated disease.[38] Studies thus support the use of CMV-negative blood products in seronegative infants born to seronegative mothers and in seronegative cardiac and bone marrow transplant recipients with CMV-negative transplants.[39]

In spite of the high number of blood donors capable of transmitting EBV infection, few recipients become infected. Most recipients possess EBV-neutralizing antibodies and are already immune. Seronegative recipients are protected in part by neutralizing antibodies usually present in the infected unit of blood. However, some cases of a posttransfusion infectious mononucleosis–like syndrome may be attributable to EBV rather than CMV.[40] Blood transfusions or donor allografts are the probable

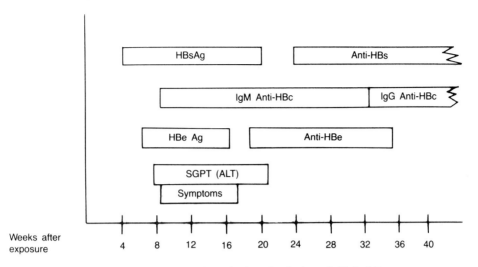

FIGURE 66–1. Acute HBV Infection: Serologic and Clinical Patterns

sources of EBV infection in immunosuppressed recipients of bone marrow, kidney, or heart transplants.[41] Because very few transfusion-acquired infections are symptomatic, there is no need to ensure that all blood components are free of EBV.

Retrovirus Transmission

An uncommon yet potentially devastating complication of transfusion is transmission of the human immunodeficiency virus type 1 (HIV-1). It has been estimated that 12,000 recipients of blood transfusions became infected before HIV-1 antibody testing was initiated in 1985.[42] Improved donor screening, donor self-exclusion, and testing for HIV-1 antibody has reduced the risk of transfusion-associated HIV-1 infection. The estimated risk per unit transfused ranges from 1:60,000 to 1:153,000.[43,44] In adults, the interval between transfusion and diagnosis has ranged from less than a year to more than seven, with a mean latency period of approximately five years.[45] HIV-1 has been transmitted by whole blood, cellular components, and plasma but not by albumin, immunoglobulins, or plasma-derived vaccines.[46] The lipid component of the HIV envelope, unlike that of HBV, allows inactivation of the virus by appropriate heat or chemical treatment. Treatment of clotting factor concentrates has virtually eliminated the risk of transmission.[47]

The human T-lymphotropic virus I (HTLV-I) is another retrovirus not closely related to HIV that can be transmitted by transfusion. The seropositivity rate in the United States is only .01 percent to 1.0 percent in the general population and somewhat higher among intravenous drug users, female prostitutes, and recipients of multiple transfusions. HTLV-I infection is endemic primarily in southwestern Japan, the Caribbean, and some areas of Africa.[48] Transmission of HTLV-I infection by blood transfusion is well documented in Japan, with a seroconversion rate of 63 percent in recipients of whole blood, red blood cells, and platelets.[49] The virus has been etiologically associated with adult T-cell leukemia/lymphoma and the degenerative neurologic disease tropical spastic paraparesis or HTLV-I–associated myelopathy. However, cases of adult T-cell leukemia/lymphoma have not been reported after transfusion partly because of the extremely long latency period of years to decades. Transfusion-associated tropical

spastic paraparesis has been described in Japan[50] but only rarely in the United States.[51] HTLV-II is genetically closely related to HTLV-I and is prevalent among intravenous drug users. Little specific information is available regarding its seroepidemiology, mode of transmission, or association with disease.[52]

Transmission of Nonviral Infectious Disease

Transmission of bacteria and parasites is an uncommon complication of transfusion in the United States. Before World War II, transmission of syphilis was more common, but this problem has been virtually eliminated because of the low prevalence of the organism in donor blood and the current practice of storing blood at 4°C. Although malaria is a worldwide health problem, transfusion-associated malaria is rare in the United States with only 26 cases reported between 1972 and 1981.[53] This low incidence is partly due to routine deferral of donors who have traveled to endemic areas without use of antimalarial drugs and individuals originating from those areas.

Occasionally, bacteria are transmitted by transfusion of blood from an asymptomatic bacteremic donor. Bacterial proliferation is more likely to occur after prolonged storage of platelet concentrates at room temperature. Deaths associated with bacterial contamination of transfused blood have increased in recent years and account for 10 percent of transfusion-related deaths between 1986 and 1988.[54] Evaluation of patients with otherwise unexplained fever associated with transfusion should include culture of both the blood product and the patient's blood. Transfusion of products contaminated with gram-negative bacteria may contain endotoxins that can cause severe shock, DIC, and renal failure. Prompt recognition is essential in the management of severe septic reactions that may necessitate broad-spectrum antibiotics, aggressive fluid replacement, and vasopressors. Other infectious diseases that may be transmitted by transfusion include babesiosis, toxoplasmosis, and trypanosomiasis.

Complications Associated with Massive Transfusion

Massive transfusion is defined as the replacement of at least one blood volume within a 24-hour period. Massive transfusion may be necessary in trauma, complicated vascular surgery, or liver transplantation. Certain complications are seen with massive transfusion that are not usually encountered when smaller volumes of blood components are transfused.

Hemostatic Abnormalities

Coagulation abnormalities and bleeding may be associated with massive transfusion and may be related to several different factors. Whole blood and packed cells do not contain high levels of functioning platelets or the high concentrations of labile coagulation factors found in fresh frozen plasma. Large-volume transfusion may therefore lead to dilution of platelets and coagulation factors. However, coagulopathies and thrombocytopenia are more often related to hypoperfusion, tissue injury, and DIC.[55] In one study, the extent of coagulation abnormalities correlated with the duration of shock rather than the quantity of blood transfused.[56] Prophylactic use of fresh frozen plasma or platelets is not warranted in patients receiving massive transfusion. In one study of 172 patients, 93 percent developed abnormal hemostatic laboratory studies, but prophylactic replacement of platelets and fresh frozen plasma by formula did not prevent the deficiencies.[57] Replacement strategy should be based on assessment of the type and severity of bleeding and laboratory evaluation, including determinations of prothrombin time, partial thromboplastin time, and platelet count.

Although platelet counts would be expected to decline during massive transfusion due to dilution, they do not always do so. This may be partly due to release of sequestered platelets from the splenic pool.[58] In certain cases, qualitative platelet dysfunction should also be considered. The use of aspirin or other medications or exposure to extracorporeal circulation[59] may alter platelet function. In these circumstances, transfusion with random donor platelets may be necessary to correct bleeding even when numbers of circulating platelets appear adequate.

Diffuse bleeding in massively transfused patients may rarely be due to hemolytic transfusion reactions discussed above. Expected signs or symptoms may not be apparent in unconscious patients. Hypotension, tachycardia, DIC, and hemoglobinuria may be erroneously attributed to other processes. Discontinuing the transfusion, institution of supportive measures, and prompt evaluation are necessary in this setting.

Citrate Toxicity

Citrate is a component of anticoagulant solutions used for blood storage. Rapid transfusion of excessive amounts of citrate may have toxic side effects due to binding of circulating calcium. Under normal circumstances, mobilization of calcium from bone and rapid metabolism of citrate by the liver prevent hypocalcemia. Hypocalcemia seen in massively transfused patients does not necessarily correlate with resultant clinical problems.[60] Transfusion of large quantities of citrate have been associated with prolongation of the Q-T interval on the electrocardiogram but not with myocardial depression.[61]

A normothermic adult with a normal liver function can usually tolerate a unit of whole blood every five minutes without requiring supplemental calcium. If this rate is exceeded, particularly in patients with hypothermia, severe liver disease, or acute heart failure, calcium administration may be warranted.[62] Calcium should be given directly to the patient. Adding it to the blood or transfusion tubing can cause clotting. Doses of 10 ml of 10% calcium gluconate or 2.5 ml of 10% calcium chloride for each liter of citrated blood are recommended.[63] Excessive citrate may also cause hypomagnesemia, a potential cause of cardiac arrhythmia,[64] but the incidence of this complication is unknown.

Hypothermia

Hypothermia can be caused by transfusion of massive volumes of refrigerated stored blood. Decrease in body temperature may impair citrate metabolism, cause release of potassium from red cells, increase the affinity of hemoglobin for oxygen, and cause life-threatening cardiac arrhythmias. In one study, patients receiving refrigerated blood at rates greater than 100 ml/min for 30 minutes had an increased incidence of cardiac arrest compared to those receiving blood warmed to 37°C.[65] Although additional studies documenting the beneficial effects are limited,[66] warming should be standard practice when massive transfusion is required. Patients receiving smaller volumes of blood in the range of one to three units over several hours do not have an increased risk of arrhythmias and do not require routine blood warming. The specifically designed devices for warming require careful monitoring because exposure of red cells to temperatures above 37°C may cause hemolysis.

Acid-Base Imbalances

The role of blood transfusion in the development of electrolyte and acid-base abnormalities is difficult to define in massively transfused patients. Metabolic acidosis, due to tissue hypoperfusion or the immediate acid load of citrated blood, is a common early finding that rapidly resolves when normal blood pressure and tissue perfusion are restored.[67] Metabolic alkalosis is a relatively late finding after massive transfusion and is partly due to metabolism of citrate and lactate to bicarbonate. Administration of bicarbonate in an attempt to correct for the presumed acid load has been shown to worsen the alkalosis when perfusion is restored.[68]

Electrolyte Imbalance

Massive transfusion can occasionally cause alterations in blood potassium levels. The concentration of potassium in the plasma of red cell components increases during storage. However, in units stored for several weeks, the total extracellular potassium does not usually exceed 20 meq/liter.[69] The development of significant hyperkalemia is thus relatively uncommon in adults. However, it may be a contributing factor in patients with underlying hyperkalemia and acidosis or in neonates undergoing exchange transfusion. Hypokalemia may occur as part of the metabolic alkalosis due to metabolism of citrate to bicarbonate and can be exacerbated by exogenous bicarbonate.[70] Because potassium abnormalities may affect cardiac function, monitoring potassium levels may be prudent in massively transfused patients.

Other Nonimmunologic Complications

Circulatory Overload

Rapid increases in blood volume may not be well tolerated in patients with chronic anemia, expanded plasma volume, or poor cardiopulmonary function. In susceptible patients, transfusion should be given slowly at a rate of one unit of packed red blood cells over four hours. It may be possible to divide units into aliquots to be given over 24 hours.[71]

Mechanical Trauma to Red Blood Cells

Nonimmune hemolysis can result from excessive heat from faulty in-line blood warmers. Mechanical cell damage may occur with the use of extracorporeal pumps, pressure cuffs, or small-bore needles. Inadvertent exposure of blood to solutions other than isotonic saline during transfusion can cause osmotic hemolysis.[72] Signs of hemolysis associated with transfusion should therefore prompt investigation of both immune and nonimmune causes.

SUMMARY

1. Acute hemolytic transfusion reactions, anaphylactic reactions, endotoxic shock, noncardiogenic pulmonary edema, and acute circulatory overload require immediate discontinuation of the transfusion, complete evaluation, and appropriate therapy. Diagnosis may be difficult in patients who are seriously ill or under general anesthesia.

2. Fever and chills associated with blood transfusion most often represent a reaction to white blood cells or HLA antigens. However, these symptoms may also herald one of the more serious reactions listed above.

3. Other immunologic complications include alloimmunization and graft-versus-host disease. In alloimmunization, patients develop antibodies to red blood cells, HLA, or platelet antigens that can lead to hemolysis or render them refractory to platelet transfusion. Graft-versus-host disease is a grave complication encountered in immunocompromised patients.

4. Although still an important concern, the risk of transfusion-transmitted viral disease has decreased in recent years due to improved methods for detecting hepatitis C and HIV-1 as well as screening for HTLV-I and HTLV-II, testing for surrogate markers of viral disease, and donor self-exclusion.

5. Massive transfusion can be complicated by hypothermia, acid-base imbalance, electrolyte disturbances, citrate toxicity, and hemostatic abnormalities.

REFERENCES

1. Myhre B: Fatalities from blood transfusion. *JAMA* 244:1333–1335, 1980.
2. Holland PV: Risks of red cell transfusion: Overview and perspective, in NIH Consensus Development Conference: *Perioperative Red Cell Transfusion*, 1988, p 83.
3. Greenwalt TJ: Pathogenesis and management of hemolytic transfusion reactions. *Semin Hematol* 18:84–94, 1981.
4. Henderson IS, Beattie TJ, Kennedy AC: Dopamine hydrochloride in oliguric states. *Lancet* 2:827–828, 1980.
5. Goldfinger D: Clinical features of transfusion reactions, in Judd WJ, Bams A (eds): *Clinical and Serologic Aspects of Transfusion Reactions*. Arlington VA, American Association of Blood Banks, 1982, pp 37–49.
6. Pineda AA, Taswell HF, Brzica SM: Delayed hemolytic transfusion

7. Walker RH: Transfusion risks. *Am J Clin Path* 88:374–378, 1987.
8. Wenz B: Microaggregate blood filtration and the febrile transfusion reaction: A cooperative study. *Transfusion* 23:95–98, 1983.
9. Popovsky MA, Moore SB: Diagnostic and pathogenetic considerations in transfusion-related acute lung injury. *Transfusion* 25:573–577, 1985.
10. Seeger W, Schneider U, Kreusler B et al: Reproduction of transfusion-related acute lung injury in an ex vivo model. *Blood* 7:1438–1444, 1990.
11. Hammerschmidt DE, White JG, Craddock PR, Jacob HS: Corticosteroids inhibit complement-induced granulocyte aggregation: A possible mechanism for their efficacy in shock states. *J Clin Invest* 63:798–803, 1979.
12. Roitt I, Brostoff J, Male D: *Immunology*. New York, Gower Medical, 1985, pp 240–241.
13. Mollison PL, Engelfriet CP, Contreras M (eds): *Blood Transfusion in Clinical Medicine*, 8th ed. Oxford, Blackwell, 1988, pp 737–740.
14. Burks AW, Sampson HA, Buckley RH: Anaphylactic reactions after gammaglobulin administration in patients with hypogammaglobulinemia. Detection of IgE antibodies to IgA. *N Engl J Med* 314:560–564, 1986.
15. Holland PV: Transfusion-associated graft-versus-host disease: Prevention using irradiated blood products, in Garratty G (ed): *Current Concepts in Transfusion Therapy*. Arlington VA, American Association of Blood Banks, 1985, pp 295–315.
16. Brubaker DB: Human posttransfusion graft-versus-host disease. *Vox Sang* 45:401–420, 1983.
17. Linden JV, Pisciotto PT: Transfusion-associated graft-versus-host disease and blood irradiation. *Transf Med Rev* 6:116–123, 1992.
18. Thaler M, Shamiss A, Orgad S et al: The role of blood from HLA-homozygous donors in fatal transfusion-associated graft-versus-host disease after open heart surgery. *N Engl J Med* 321:25–28, 1989.
19. Heustis DW, Bove JR, Case J (eds): *Practical Blood Transfusion*, 4th ed. Boston, Little Brown, 1981, pp 76–78.
20. Duffcher JP, Schiffer CA, Aisner J et al: Long-term follow-up of patients with leukemia receiving platelet transfusions: Identification of a large group of patients who do not become alloimmunized. *Blood* 58:1007–1011, 1981.
21. Holohan TV, Terasacki PI, Deisseroth AB: Suppression of transfusion-related alloimmunization in intensively treated cancer patients. *Blood* 58:122–128, 1981.
22. Daly PA, Schiffer CA, Aisner J et al: Platelet transfusion therapy—one hour posttransfusion increments are valuable in predicting the need for HLA matched preparations. *JAMA* 243:435–548, 1980.
23. McCarthy W, Menitove JE (eds): *Immunologic Aspects of Platelet Transfusion*. Arlington VA, American Association of Blood Banks, 1985, pp 1–5.
24. Shulman NR, Jordan JV: Platelet immunology, in Coleman RW, Hirsch J, Marder VJ et al (eds): *Hemostasis and Thrombosis*. Philadelphia, Lippincott, 1982, pp 274–342.
25. Kickler TS, Ness PM, Herman JH et al: Studies on the pathophysiology of posttransfusion purpura. *Blood* 68:347–350, 1986.
26. Lau P, Sholtis CM, Aster RH: Posttransfusion purpura. An enigma of alloimmunization. *Am J Hematol* 9:331–336, 1980.
27. Koziol DE, Holland PV, Alling DW et al: Antibody to hepatitis B core antigen as a paradoxical marker for non-A non-B hepatitis agents in donated blood. *Ann Intern Med* 104:488–495, 1986.
28. Rosina F, Saracco G, Rizzetto M: Risk of posttransfusion infection with the hepatitis delta virus. A multicenter study. *N Engl J Med* 312:1488–1491, 1985.
29. Aach RD, Szmuness W, Mosley JW et al: Serum alanine aminotransferase of donor in relation to the risk of non-A non-B hepatitis in recipients: The transfusion-transmitted viruses study. *N Engl J Med* 304:989–994, 1981.
30. Hollinger FB, Mosley JW, Szmuness W et al: Non-A non-B hepatitis

following blood transfusion: Risk factors associated with donor characteristics, in Szmuness W, Aolter HJ, Maynard JE (eds): *Viral Hepatitis. 1981 International Symposium.* Philadelphia, Franklin Institute Press, 1982, pp 361–376.

31. Deinstag JL: Immunologic mechanisms in chronic viral hepatitis, in Vyas GN, Deinstag JL, Hoofnagle JH (eds): *Viral Hepatitis and Liver Disease.* New York, Grune & Stratton, 1984, pp 135–166.

32. Donahue JG, Munoz A, Ness PM et al: The declining risk of post-transfusion hepatitis C virus infection. *N Engl J Med* 327:369–373, 1992.

33. Choo QL, Kuuo G, Weiner AJ et al: Isolation of a cDNA clone derived from a blood-borne non-A non-B viral hepatitis genome. *Science* 244:359–362, 1989.

34. Aach RD, Stevens CE, Hollinger FB et al: Hepatitis C virus infection in posttransfusion hepatitis. *N Engl J Med* 325:1326–1329, 1991.

35. Alter HJ: Chronic consequences of non-A non-B hepatitis, in Seeff LB, Lewis JH (eds): *Current Perspectives in Hepatology.* New York, Plenum, 1989, pp 83–97.

36. Blum HE, Vyas GN: Non-A non-B hepatitis: A contemporary assessment. *Haematologia* 15:162–183, 1982.

37. Wilheim JA, Matter L, Schopfer K: The risk of transmitting cytomegalovirus to patients receiving blood transfusion. *J Infect Dis* 154:169–171, 1986.

38. Eifenbein GJ, Saral R: Infectioius disease during immune recovery after bone marrow transplantation: A review of ten years experience, in Allen JC (ed): *Infection and the Compromised Host.* Baltimore, Wilkins & Williams, 1981, pp 157–196.

39. Sayers MH, Anderson JC, Goodnaugh LT et al: Reducing the risk for transfusion-transmitted cytomegalovirus infection. *Ann Intern Med* 116:55–62, 1992.

40. Henle W, Henle G, Scriba M et al: Antibody responses to the Epstein-Barr virus and cytomegalovirus after open-heart and other surgery. *N Engl J Med* 28:1068–1074, 1978.

41. Henle W, Henle G: Epstein-Barr virus and blood transfusion, in Dodd RY, Barker LF (eds): *Infection, Immunity and Blood Transfusion.* New York, Liss, 1985, pp 201–209.

42. Peterman TA: What's happening to the epidemic of transfusion-associated AIDS? *Transfusion* 29:659–660, 1989.

43. Busch MP, Eble BE, Khayam-Bashi H et al: Evaluation of screened blood donations for human immunodeficiency virus type 1 infection by culture and DNA amplification of pooled cells. *N Engl J Med* 325:165, 1991.

44. Cumming PD, Wallace EL, Schorr JB, Dodd RY: Exposure of patients to human immunodeficiency virus through the transfusion of blood components that test antibody-positive. *N Engl J Med* 321:941–946, 1989.

45. Lui K-J, Lawrence DN, Morgan WM et al: A model-based estimate of the average incubation and latency period for transfusion-associated acquired immunodeficiency syndrome. *Proc Nat Acad Sci* 83:3051–3055, 1986.

46. Safety of therapeutic immune globulin preparations with respect to transmission of human T-lymphotropic virus III/lymphadenopathy-associated virus infection. *CDC MMWR* 35:231–232, 1986.

47. Gomperts ED: Procedures for the inactivation of viruses in clotting factor concentrates. *Am J Hematol* 23:295–305, 1986.

48. Cuthbertson B, Reid KG, Foster PR: Viral contamination of human plasma and procedures for preventing virus transmission by plasma products, in Harris JR (ed): *Blood Separation and Plasma Fractionation.* New York, Wiley-Liss, 1991, pp 385–435.

49. Okochi K, Sato H, Hinuma Y: A retrospective study on transmission of adult T-cell leukemia virus by blood transfusion: Seroconversion in recipients. *Vox Sang* 56:245–253, 1984.

50. Osarne M, Usuku K, Izumo S: HTLV-I–associated myelopathy, a new clinical entity. *Lancet* 1:1031–1032, 1986.

51. Gout O, Baulac M, Gessain A: Rapid development of myelopathy after HTLV-I infection acquired by transfusion during cardiac transplantation. *N Engl J Med* 322:383–387, 1990.

52. US Department of Health and Human Services Public Health Service: Licensure of screening tests for antibody to human T-lymphotropic virus type I. *MMWR* 387:736–747, 1988.

53. Guerrero IC, Weniger BC, Schultz MG: Transfusion malaria in the United States, 1972–1981. *Ann Intern Med* 9:221–226, 1983.

54. Goldman M, Blajchman MA: Blood product–associated bacterial sepsis. *Transf Med Rev* 5:73–83, 1991.

55. Hewson JR, Neame PB, Kumar N et al: Coagulopathy related to dilution and hypotension during massive transfusion. *Crit Care Med* 13:3897–3901, 1985.

56. Harke H, Rahman S: Haemostatic disorder in massive transfusion. *Br J Haematol* 46:179–188, 1980.

57. Mannucci PM, Federici AB, Sirchia G: Hemostasis testing during massive blood replacement. *Vox Sang* 42:113–123, 1982.

58. Reed DL, Ciavarella D, Heimbach DM et al: Prophylactic platelet administration during massive transfusion. A prospective, randomized double-blind clinical study. *Ann Surg* 203:40–48, 1986.

59. Harker LA, Malpass TW, Branson HE et al: Mechanism of abnormal bleeding in patients undergoing cardiopulmonary bypass–acquired transient platelet dysfunction associated with selective α-granule release. *Blood* 56:824–834, 1980.

60. Kahn RC, Jascott D, Carlton GC et al: Massive blood replacement: Correlation of ionized calcium, citrate, and hydrogen ion concentration. *Anesth Analg* 58:274–278, 1979.

61. Howland WS, Schweizer O, Carlon GC et al: The cardiovascular effects of low levels of ionized calcium during massive transfusion. *Surg Gynecol Obstet* 145:581–586, 1977.

62. Kovalik SG, Ledgerwood AM, Lucas CE et al: The cardiac effects of altered calcium homeostasis after albumin resuscitation. *J Trauma* 21:275–279, 1981.

63. Mollison PL: *Blood Transfusion in Clinical Medicine,* 8th ed. Oxford, Blackwell, 1983, p 751.

64. McLellan BA, Reid SR, Lane PL: Massive blood transfusion causing hypomagnesemia. *Crit Care Med* 12:146–147, 1984.

65. Boyan CP, Howland WS: Cardiac arrest and temperature of bank blood. *JAMA* 183:58–60, 1963.

66. Dybkjaer E, Elkjear P: The use of heated blood in massive blood replacement. *Acta Anaesth Scand* 8:271–278, 1964.

67. Collins JA, Simmons RL, James PM et al: Acid-base status of seriously wounded combat casualties. Resuscitation with stored blood. *Ann Surg* 173:6–18, 1971.

68. Linko K, Saxelin I: Electrolyte and acid-base disturbances caused by blood transfusions. *Acta Anaesth Scand* 30:139–144, 1986.

69. Latham JT, Bove JR, Weirich FL: Clinical and hematologic changes in stored CPDA-1 blood. *Transfusion* 22:158–160, 1982.

70. Carmichael D, Hosty T, Kastl D et al: Hypokalemia and massive transfusion. *South Med J* 77:315–317, 1984.

71. Marriott HL, Kekwick A: Volume and rate in blood transfusion for relief of anemia. *Br Med J* 1:1043–1046, 1940.

72. Walker RH (ed): *Technical Manual.* Arlington VA, American Association of Blood Banks, 1990, no 365, pp 414–415.

67 POSTOPERATIVE GASTROINTESTINAL DYSFUNCTION

Francis J. DuFrayne

Gary W. Crooks

David R. Goldmann

Nausea, vomiting, abdominal pain, and diarrhea, alone or in combination, are common occurrences after surgery and anesthesia and frequently represent physiologic responses to specific procedures and pharmacologic agents. Deciding whether or not these problems are expected "complications" of the postoperative recuperative process or represent more serious underlying disorders can be difficult. This chapter examines the role of surgery and anesthesia in postoperative nausea, vomiting, and ileus; considers the various etiologies of postoperative abdominal pain and diarrhea; and outlines current management strategies.

POSTOPERATIVE NAUSEA AND VOMITING: EPIDEMIOLOGY AND MECHANISMS

Vomiting is a complex physiologic process involving interaction of the central, enteric, and autonomic nervous systems and the musculature of the gastrointestinal tract and abdominal wall. A chemoreceptor trigger zone adjacent to the area postrema in the floor of the fourth ventricle detects circulating emetic agents in both blood and cerebrospinal fluid. It provides input to the emetic center in the lateral reticular formation near the tractus solitarius in the brain stem. The emetic center also responds to stimuli from several other areas, including the pharynx, mediastinum, gastrointestinal tract, vision center, and the vestibular system. After coordinating the complex afferent inputs from these areas and the chemoreceptor trigger zone, the emetic center initiates vomiting.[1-3]

The incidence of postoperative nausea and vomiting is influenced by several factors, including the type of patient, the specific surgical procedure, and the anesthetic agents used.[2] Postoperative emesis occurs more frequently in pediatric patients, reaching a peak incidence in patients between ages 11 and 14.[4] Adult women have a significantly higher rate of postoperative vomiting, particularly if the surgery is performed during the latter half of the menses.[5,6] Patients who suffer from obesity, delayed gastric empty-

ing, motion sickness, previous postoperative nausea, or anxiety also experience postoperative vomiting more frequently.[2,7-9]

The incidence of postoperative emesis is influenced by the type of surgical procedure regardless of the anesthetic technique used. The rate is higher in exploratory laparoscopy; head and neck surgery; extracorporeal shock-wave lithotripsy; procedures involving the stomach, duodenum, and gallbladder; and laparoscopic ovum retrieval in women.[7,10] The effects of individual anesthetic agents on postoperative nausea and vomiting can be difficult to assess when more than one drug is used. However, controlled studies indicate that emesis after a given operative procedure occurs more frequently with some anesthetic agents than with others.[2,8,11]

Without perioperative antiemetics, 20 to 40 percent of patients recovering from general anesthesia develop postoperative vomiting.[7,12,13] Depending on the type and duration of surgery, nausea and vomiting may last 2 to 24 hours. However, most patients experience only one or two bouts of vomiting and are usually asymptomatic by the time they leave the recovery room. For those who remain symptomatic, a variety of effective antiemetic agents are available (see Table 67-1).

POSTOPERATIVE ILEUS

Postoperative ileus, characterized by impaired intestinal motility and the accumulation of bowel gas and fluid, can lead to dilation of the intestine, abdominal distention, nausea, vomiting, and obstipation. Ileus occurs after most abdominal procedures, especially those necessitating entry into the peritoneum. When the peritoneum is penetrated, all myoelectric activity ceases. Animal and human studies show that the duration of postoperative ileus correlates with the type of procedure rather than the length of the operation.[14-16] After surgery, myoelectric activity returns to the intestine and stomach at varying rates. The small bowel usually recovers within 24 hours.[17] Gastric activity is next to resume,

675

TABLE 67–1. Agents Used in the Treatment of Nausea and Vomiting

Prokinetics
  Metoclopramide
  Cisapride
  Domperidone

Phenothiazines
  Prochlorperazine
  Chlorpromazine
  Methotrimeprazine

Butyrophenones
  Haloperidol
  Droperidol

Antihistamines
  Cyclizine
  Promethazine
  Diphenhydramine

Anticholinergics
  Scolpolamine
  Atropine

Serotonin Antagonists
  Ondansetron

TABLE 67–2. Causes of Ileus

Intraabdominal Causes	Extraabdominal Causes
Reflex inhibition	*Reflex inhibition*
Laparotomy	Rib, spine, or
Abdominal trauma	pelvic fractures
	Myocardial infarction
Inflammatory conditions	Pneumonia/pulmonary
Perforated viscus/	embolus
penetrating wounds	Burns
Bile peritonitis	Black widow spider
Chemical peritonitis	bites
Intraperitoneal hemorrhage	
Toxic megacolon	*Drug-induced*
Familial Mediterranean fever	Anticholinergic/
Acute pancreatitis	ganglionic antagonists
Celiac disease	Opiates
	Chemotherapeutic agents
Acute irradiation injury	
Abdominal irradiation	*Metabolic abnormalities*
	Septicemia
Infectious processes	Electrolyte imbalance
Bacterial peritonitis	Heavy metal poisoning
Appendicitis	(lead, mercury)
Cholecystitis	Porphyria
Diverticulitis	Uremia
	Diabetic ketoacidosis
Ischemic processes	Sickle cell disease
Arterial insufficiency	
Venous thrombosis	
Mesenteric arteritis	
Strangulation obstruction	
Retroperitoneal processes	
Ureteropelvic stones	
Pyelonephritis	
Retroperitoneal hemorrhage	
Pheochromocytoma	

Source: Adapted from Summers RW, Lu CC: Approach to the patient with ileus and obstruction, in Yamada T, Alpers DH, Owyang C et al (eds): *Textbook of Gastroenterology.* Philadelphia, Lippincott, 1991, pp 715–731.

followed by recovery of the colon in up to 72 hours. The return of myoelectric activity may precede resumption of normal bowel function. Ileus following extraabdominal procedures is usually brief and may be related more to the anesthetic agent than to interruption of bowel motility.

The lack of effective peristalsis after surgery causes a feeling of fullness and distention that may proceed to nausea, vomiting, and abdominal pain. Although distention can be marked, the abdominal pain is usually mild. The mechanism of nausea in postoperative ileus is poorly understood, but may be associated with sustained contraction of the duodenum and inhibition of gastric tone and motility. Vomiting, if present, is usually mild and bilious in nature.

Treatment for postoperative ileus has changed little since the nasogastric tube was first introduced in the latter part of the nineteenth century. Placement of a tube often relieves symptoms by decompressing the stomach and decreasing intraabdominal pressure and, together with intravenous hydration or total parenteral nutrition, allows the ileus to resolve spontaneously. However, caution is required to prevent the pulmonary and metabolic complications of prolonged nasogastric suction. Although some believe that use of a nasogastric tube decreases the likelihood of aspiration, one study of 300 patients undergoing upper abdominal surgery documented a tenfold greater risk of developing pneumonia, electrolyte disturbances, and metabolic alkalosis in those in whom tubes were placed.[18] Other treatment modalities such as electrical stimulation, pharmacologic adrenergic inhibition with or without cholineric stimulation, and early enteral feeding have failed to reduce the duration of postoperative ileus. Cisapride, a prokinetic agent, has recently been shown to induce early return of propulsive activity in the right colon. It also reduces the period of time until first passage of feces but not of flatus. Further studies with this agent are needed. Metoclopramide, another prokinetic agent, has been reported to both improve and worsen postoperative ileus.[19–24]

Although postoperative ileus usually resolves within three or four days, bowel dysfunction may persist for several days or

weeks. When this occurs, other causes of ileus should be investigated (see Table 67–2). Other etiologies include the use of anticholinergic agents or opiates, electrolyte abnormalities like hypokalemia and hyponatremia, septicemia, uremia, hypotension, myocardial infarction, and diabetic ketoacidosis. Opiates, in particular, are associated with prolonged ileus. Demerol depresses left colonic function, and codeine inhibits both colonic and small bowel activity. Although morphine increases electrical activity in the colon, the activity does not propagate normally. Avoiding narcotics in the immediate postoperative period decreases the duration of postoperative ileus but is often difficult to do.

POSTOPERATIVE BOWEL OBSTRUCTION

Because postoperative ileus and early small-bowel obstruction are often both characterized by bloating, nausea, vomiting, abdominal pain with obstipation, altered bowel sounds, and abdominal tenderness, differentiation can be difficult. In contrast to the mild pain, moderate-to-severe distention, and infrequent episodes of low volume emesis seen in patients with postoperative ileus, those with high small-bowel obstruction usually experience mild pain and less distention but frequent bouts of emesis with copious amounts of bile-stained material. With more distal obstruction, pain and distention become more severe, the frequency and volume of vomiting decreases, and the emesis becomes more feculent in nature.[25]

Radiologic evaluation may be helpful in defining postoperative bowel obstruction. With diffuse ileus, gas and fluid accumulate throughout the gastrointestinal tract and are visible on plain films. In gastrointestinal obstruction, the radiographic findings depend on the degree of obstruction and the level of obstruction. Plain films are not usually helpful in high obstruction above the ligament of Trietz because vomiting decompresses the lumen above the obstruction. As the point of obstruction moves down the length of the bowel, the radiograph is more likely to be abnormal. Complete small-bowel obstruction leads to marked distention and rapid accumulation of gas and fluid proximal to the point of obstruction. If motility is normal, the lumen distal to the obstruction clears gas and feces within 24 hours. Upright films may demonstrate the classic "step-ladder" pattern of multiple air-fluid levels. If the ileocecal valve is competent, colonic obstruction results in gas and fluid accumulation only in the colon. Dilatation and multiple air-fluid levels are seen proximal to the obstruction with decompressed bowel distally. In acute colonic pseudoobstruction (Ogilvie's syndrome), the entire colon becomes dilated, especially in the region of the cecum.

Contrast studies may be needed if a diagnosis cannot not be made with the above studies. A small-bowel study using water-soluble medium may be useful in demonstrating small-bowel lesions. Similarly, a barium enema is useful in patients with suspected colonic obstruction to demonstrate the type and location of obstructing lesion. Computerized tomography may be useful when extrinsic compression of the bowel by fluid collections is suspected.

In a review of postoperative patients with small-bowel obstruction diagnosed within thirty days of surgery, Quatromoni et al. found that only 12 percent of patients had complete obstipation, 39 percent had typical obstructive bowel sounds, and none had abdominal roentgenograms diagnostic of small-bowel obstruction. An oral tracer of barium sulfate was given to half of the patients in the study. Barium passed into the colon in one-third of these patients but was arrested at a presumed site of obstruction in the other two-thirds. Of those requiring surgery, adhesions were the most common cause of obstruction.[26] This study underscores the need for comprehensive evaluation of all patients with prolonged postoperative ileus even when typical radiologic findings of obstruction are absent.

OTHER CAUSES OF ABDOMINAL PAIN, NAUSEA AND VOMITING

When abdominal pain is the predominant postoperative gastrointestinal symptom, is clearly unrelated to the incision, and changes in character or intensity, a number of intraabdominal and extraabdominal etiologies should be considered (see Table 67–3). Acute abdominal pain is usually due to inflammation, ulceration, perforation, or obstruction of an intraabdominal organ.

Acid-Peptic Disease

Acute postoperative erosive gastritis can be asymptomatic or cause nausea, vomiting, abdominal pain, or upper gastrointestinal bleed-

TABLE 67–3. Major Causes of Postoperative Abdominal Pain (with or without nausea or vomiting)

Extraabdominal processes
  Myocardial ischemia or infarction
  Pulmonary embolus or infarct
  Pneumothorax
  Esophagitis
  Esophageal spasm
  Ketoacidosis
  Hyperlipidemia (with or without pancreatitis)
  Sickle cell crisis

Intraabdominal processes
  Gastritis
  Peptic ulcer disease
  Biliary tract disease
    biliary colic
    cholecystitis
    choledocholithiasis
  Pancreatitis
  Intestinal obstruction, partial or complete
  Peritonitis
  Hepatitis
  Abscesses, especially hepatic or splenic
  Pyelonephritis/nephrolithiasis
  Ruptured ovarian follicle
  Acute salpingitis
  Intraabdominal hemorrhage
  Retroperitoneal hemorrhage
  Mesenteric ischemia
  Infectious diarrhea
  Pseudomembranous colitis

ing. Gastric erosions are superficial ulcerations that do not penetrate beyond the mucosal surface. They can be induced by a variety of conditions, including physiologic stress, direct local trauma by nasogastric tubes, prior irradiation, ischemia, bile reflux, or ingestion of caustic agents. Gastritis and gastric erosions are commonly associated with the use of aspirin and other nonsteroidal anti-inflammatory drugs. In addition, the incidence of gastritis correlates with the presence of *Helicobacter pylori* infection.[27-29]

Peptic ulcers, either gastric or duodenal, more often penetrate into the underlying submucosa or beyond. Like gastritis, they are associated with the use of aspirin and nonsteroidal anti-inflammatory agents and the presence of *H. pylori* infection. Approximately 85 to 95 percent of patients with duodenal and 70 to 90 percent of patients with gastric ulcers harbor gastric *H. pylori* infection. Although smokers have an increased risk of developing ulcer disease and impaired rates of ulcer healing, there is little evidence to support an association between alcohol and ulcer disease except in those who develop cirrhosis from chronic consumption.[27-35] Duodenal ulcers are three to five times more prevalent in patients with chronic pulmonary disease, and the death rate in patients with both diseases is five times that in the general population. Patients with gastrinomas, multiple endocrine neoplasia type I, systemic mastocytosis, chronic renal failure, and cirrhosis also have an increased risk of developing duodenal ulcer disease.[36-40]

There is little or no data documenting an association between the use of corticosteroids and ulcer disease. In a review of 42 randomized trials, Conn and Blitzer noted an association between corticosteroid use and peptic ulcer disease only in those who received daily corticosteroids for more than one month at total doses equivalent to one gram of prednisone or more and in those with prior ulcer disease.[36] There is thus no indication for prophylactic antiulcer therapy in patients requiring short-term or low-dose steroids. However, in those patients with a history of ulcer disease who need long-term corticosteroid therapy, the use of antiulcer medication is reasonable.

Perforation and penetration of a peptic ulcer into an adjacent viscus can cause nausea, vomiting, and abdominal pain in the postoperative period. Although the true incidence of penetration is unknown, approximately 15 to 20 percent of intractable ulcers requiring surgery have done so. Gastric ulcers most often penetrate into the left lobe of the liver and less commonly into the transverse colon to create a gastrocolic fistula. Duodenal ulcers most commonly penetrate into the adjacent pancreas. Patients with such ulcers often have pain that radiates to the middle of the back or the region of the first lumbar vertebra and does not respond to standard antiulcer therapy.

Free perforation occurs in approximately seven percent of patients hospitalized for peptic ulcer disease and is the initial presentation of ulcer disease in about two percent of patients with duodenal ulcers.[41,42] Duodenal ulcers perforate more commonly than gastric ulcers. Perforation usually causes sudden sharp and severe pain starting in the epigastrium and spreading over the entire abdomen. Shoulder pain may be the result of diaphragmatic irritation. Nausea is common, but vomiting and hematemesis are unusual. Peritonitis with fever, hypotension, and a surgical abdomen rapidly develop.[43,44]

Acute Pancreatitis

Abdominal surgery is the third most common cause of pancreatitis following gallstones and alcohol. It may occur after any operation but is more frequent after biliary tract surgery, retroperitoneal lymph node dissection, and cardiac and renal transplantation.[45–52]

The diagnosis of pancreatitis can be difficult in the postoperative period because of its wide spectrum of severity. Mild pancreatitis may produce only occasional nausea, vomiting, and abdominal discomfort. However, more severe disease is usually characterized by retching, fever, leukocytosis, and occasionally a left pleural effusion. Severe hemorrhagic pancreatitis can cause lumbar pain accompanied by a blue-gray discoloration of the skin in the flank area (Grey-Turner's sign) or similar changes around the umbilicus (Cullen's sign).

Serum concentrations of amylase usually rise in pancreatitis but may also be elevated in acute cholecystitis, renal insufficiency, intestinal obstruction, perforated ulcer, and inflammatory processes involving the fallopian tubes. Although it has been suggested that a ratio of renal amylase clearance to creatinine clearance above 5:1 supports the diagnosis of pancreatitis, some investigators have shown this to be nonspecific.[53,54] Elevations in serum lipase may be a more sensitive indicator of pancreatitis but must be interpreted cautiously in postoperative patients.

Localized small-bowel ileus in the region of the pancreas, the so-called sentinel loop, may be present on plain film. Computerized tomography may be useful in defining pancreatic fluid collections or abscesses. The treatment of pancreatitis in the postoperative period is similar to the treatment of nonoperative pancreatitis.

Biliary Tract Disease

Acute postoperative nausea, vomiting, and abdominal pain may be due to biliary colic, acute calculus cholecystitis, or acute acalculus cholecystitis. The pain of biliary colic is sudden in onset, most often originates in the epigastrium, and is accompanied by nausea with or without vomiting. It is steady in nature, increases in intensity to a plateau over 15 to 30 minutes, and lasts up to three hours. When symptoms persist for more than three hours, acute cholecystitis is likely. In such cases, pain gradually shifts to the right upper quadrant and often radiates to the back and the right shoulder or intrascapular region. The temperature ranges from 99 to 101°F. Higher fever and rigors suggest possible cholangitis.

Examination of the abdomen reveals mild distention, hypoactive bowel sounds, and right-upper quadrant tenderness. A distended tense gallbladder that moves with respiration is often palpable. Although the white blood cell count is most often 10,000 to 13,000 cells/μl[3], a normal count does not exclude the diagnosis. Mild elevations in serum transaminase, bilirubin, and alkaline phosphatase levels are common, but markedly higher levels are unusual and suggest possible cholangitis. The presence of gallstones can be documented by ultrasound.[55] The need for surgical intervention is determined by the clinical situation.[56,57]

Acute acalculus cholecystitis is a particular concern in the postoperative period. Although it can occur in any setting, it is most common in older males who have suffered trauma, undergo an unrelated surgical procedure, or are otherwise critically ill. Signs and symptoms are similar to those of calculus cholecystitis, but no gallstones are found on ultrasound. In a retrospective review of 40 patients with acalculus cholecystitis, Johnson found that approximately half had normal liver function tests, and only 75 percent had leukocytosis. Important findings on ultrasound included gallbladder enlargement, wall thickening, and pericholecystitic fluid collection. Hepatobiliary scintigraphy may be helpful. Early diagnosis is critical since 40 to 100 percent of patients with acalculus cholecystitis already have gangrene, empyema, or perforation of the gallbladder at surgery. Morbidity and mortality rates are lower in patients undergoing early operative intervention.[58]

Miscellaneous

Many drugs including anesthetic agents, analgesics, aminophylline, cardiac glycosides, and oral antibiotics (e.g., metronidizole or erythromycin) can induce isolated nausea and vomiting in the postoperative period. Although less likely in the perioperative setting, viral infections causing gastroenteritis, postviral gastroparesis, or hepatitis are frequently associated with nausea and vomiting. Patients with underlying diabetic gastroparesis or functional gastric outlet obstruction are especially prone to these symptoms after surgery.

Postoperative abdominal pain, with or without nausea or vomiting, may result from almost any intraabdominal disease process in addition to those discussed above (see Table 67–3). Some of these include appendicitis, nephrolithiasis, pyelonephritis, ruptured ovarian cysts, torsion of an ovary, or pelvic inflammatory disease. Acute mesenteric ischemia due to arterial thrombosis or embolism should always be considered in older patients with perioperative arrhythmias, hypotension, coronary artery disease, or peripheral vascular disease. Mesenteric ischemia can produce manifestations ranging from mild central-abdominal cramping with frequent bowel movements containing occult gross blood to severe pain and toxicity. Fever, leukocytosis, and bowel-wall edema, thumb-printing, and pneumatosis intestinalis on abdominal x-rays are late findings. In addition, extraabdominal etiologies of postoperative abdominal pain include myocardial ischemia or infarction, acute pericarditis pneumonia, pulmonary infarction, esophagitis, diabetic ketoacidosis, and hyperlipidemia.

DIARRHEA

Many of the causes of postoperative intraabdominal pain listed in Table 67–3 are associated with diarrhea. Paramount among these are pseudomembranous colitis, partial small-bowel obstruction, and ischemic bowel. Most causes of postoperative diarrhea are iatrogenic. Many drugs used in the perioperative period can be implicated, including antibiotics, magnesium-containing antacids, cardiac medications, theophylline, laxatives, enteral nutritional formulas, cimetidine, and even some diuretics.

Broad-spectrum antibiotics used in the perioperative period can cause nonspecific diarrhea that usually resolves when they are discontinued. However, all antibiotics, especially clindamycin and more recently amoxicillin/clavulanate, have been associated with the development of pseudomembranous colitis (PMC) due to toxin elaborated by the bacterium *Clostridium difficile*. PMC usually causes watery and sometimes bloody diarrhea, gradually rising temperature, and crampy abdominal pain. Intestinal perforation is a rare but dreaded complication. *C. difficile* has been isolated from hospital personnel and environmental surfaces, interpersonal transmission of *C. difficile* colitis has been documented, and occupants of certain hospital rooms have contracted the disease despite sterilization.[59]

The diagnosis of pseudomembranous colitis is usually established by detecting *C. difficile* cytotoxin in the stool. However, in up to 27 percent of patients with postoperative diarrhea, the assay for toxin is negative, and cultures for the bacterium are positive. If PMC is suspected, empiric treatment can be initiated pending return of culture and toxin assay results. Sigmoidoscopy to look for the typical pseudomembrane overlying the mucosa can be helpful but may not be necessary if the toxin assay is positive.[60]

Oral regimens of vancomycin in a dose of 125 mg every six hours or metronidazole in a dose of 250 mg every eight hours for 10 to 14 days are equally effective. If the patient is unable to tolerate oral feeding or medication through a nasogastric tube, metronidazole but not vancomycin is effective when given intravenously for the same period. However, despite antibiotic treatment, 25 percent of patients relapse and require additional therapy.[61,62]

The evaluation of diarrhea thought to be due to small-bowel obstruction should proceed along the lines outlined in the preceding section and relies primarily on radiologic confirmation of obstruction. Colonic obstruction can also cause diarrhea and is manifested on plain film by air-fluid levels confined to the colon.

Ischemic bowel can cause both abdominal pain and diarrhea containing occult or frank blood. Even in the absence of blood, ischemic bowel should be considered in elderly patients with known diffuse atherosclerotic disease, paroxysmal arrhythmias, or a long history of smoking. The diagnostic test of choice remains a mesenteric arteriogram. However, recent advances in magnetic resonance angiography may allow this newer technology to supersede standard contrast dye studies. Arteriography is essential in determining the need for surgical intervention.[63,64]

Surgical procedures that can be complicated by more chronic diarrhea include vagotomy, ileal resection, pancreatic surgery, cholecystectomy, and partial gastrectomy leading to blind loop syndrome and bacterial overgrowth. In fact, patients undergoing resection of large or small bowel often report their subsequent alteration in bowel habits as "diarrhea." However, looser and more frequent bowel movements following bowel resection need not cause concern unless accompanied by fever, abdominal pain, or leukocytosis. Detailed discussion of long-term gastrointestinal complications of bowel surgery is beyond the scope of this chapter.

Surgery can exacerbate underlying inflammatory bowel disease, sprue, or lactose intolerance, all of which can be managed as they would be in nonsurgical patients. Diarrhea around a fecal impaction is not uncommon and should not be overlooked. Acute gastrointestinal infection is uncommon in the perioperative period.

SUMMARY

1. The diagnostic approach to patients with postoperative nausea, vomiting, or abdominal pain depends on the timing of the symptoms after surgery and the clinical setting. Incisional pain is superficial, localized to the immediate vicinity of the wound, and gradually abates in four to five days. Incisional pain should not be accompanied by hemodynamic instability, fever, or leukocytosis unless infection is present.

2. Symptoms of nausea, vomiting, and diffuse abdominal discomfort within the first few days after surgery are most often due to ileus. Symptoms are often mild and usually respond to nasogastric suction, bowel rest, and intravenous hydration.

3. When symptoms last more than three or four days, further evaluation is warranted. Partial or complete bowel obstruction should be excluded, electrolyte abnormalities should be corrected, and, if possible, all anticholinergic and analgesic medications use should be discontinued. Plain x-rays of the abdomen, including supine and upright views, are required to evaluate intestinal air and fluid patterns. Contrast studies may be required. A chest x-ray should be obtained to exclude pneumonia, pulmonary vascular congestion, and free air under the diaphragm.[64]

4. If postoperative ileus persists beyond several days and no underlying etiology can be determined, intravenous hyperalimentation is recommended. Metoclopramide or cisapride may facilitate the return of bowel motility. If unexplained ileus persists for more than two or three weeks, exploratory laparotomy may be needed.

5. Management of intestinal obstruction depends on the cause of the obstruction, whether it is partial or complete, and the patient's condition. Partial obstruction is often treated with bowel rest, intravenous fluids, and nasogastric suction. Partial obstruction that fails to respond to conservative treatment and complete obstruction frequently requires surgery. A sigmoid volvulus causing a colonic obstruction can sometimes be reduced by either a barium enema or a gentle flexible sigmoidoscopy.

6. Further evaluation of abdominal pain depends on its location, the presence or absence of fever, and other concomitant symptoms and signs. Patients with gastritis, peptic ulcer disease, gastroesophageal reflux, or esophagitis often benefit from a therapeutic trial of intravenous H_2 antagonists, oral antacids, or proton-pump inhibitors. Those with refractory symptoms or occult or gross bleeding may require further evaluation.

7. Patients with right-upper quadrant or epigastric pain require complete blood count and serum levels of liver function tests, amylase, and lipase to determine if biliary tract or pancreatic pathology is present. Patients with suspected cholecystitis should also undergo abdominal ultrasonography. Those with gallstones and evidence of gallbladder inflammation can be treated medically or surgically depending on the clinical situation. Those with equivocal results (e.g., gallstones without gallbladder changes, gallbladder changes without gallstones) and those in whom acalculus cholecystitis is suspected require hepatobiliary scintigraphy. Early intervention in acalculus cholecystitis is essential to reduce morbidity and mortality.

8. The clinical spectrum of postoperative pancreatitis is broad, and accurate diagnosis may require computerized tomography and careful interpretation of serum amylase and lipase levels.

9. Postoperative diarrhea is almost always iatrogenic and is most often due to drug therapy or enteral nutrition formulas. Pseudomembranous colitis, small-bowel obstruction, and ischemic bowel disease are of greatest concern. The diagnosis of PMC rests on identifying *C. difficile* toxin in the stool, that of small-bowel obstruction on appropriate radiologic studies, and that of ischemia on mesenteric arteriography in susceptible elderly patients with atherosclerotic cardiovascular disease. Oral vancomycin or metronidazole and intravenous metronidazole are the drugs of choice in PMC.

REFERENCES

1. Ouyang A: Approach to the patient with nausea and vomiting, in Yamada T, Alpers DH, Owyang C et al: (eds): *Textbook of Gastroenterology*. Philadelphia, Lippincott, 1991, p 647.
2. Watcha MD, White PF: Postoperative nausea and vomiting: Its etiology, treatment and prevention. *Anesthesiology* 77:162, 1992.
3. Allan SG: Antiemetics. *Gastroenterol Clin N Am* 21(3):597, 1992.
4. Cohen MM, Cameron CB, Duncan PG: Pediatric anesthesia. Morbidity and mortality in the perioperative period. *Anesth Analg* 70:160, 1990.
5. Clarke RSJ: Nausea and vomiting. *Br J Anaesth* 56:19, 1984.
6. Beattie WS, Lindblad T, Buckley DN et al: The incidence of postoperative nausea and vomiting in women undergoing laparoscopy is influenced by the day of the menstrual cycle. *Can J Anaesth* 38:298, 1991.
7. Palazzo MGA, Strunin L: Anaesthesia and emesis: I. Etiology. *Can Anaesth Soc J* 31:178, 1984.
8. Bellville JW, Bross IDJ, Howland WS: Postoperative nausea and vomiting: IV. Factors related to postoperative nausea and vomiting. *Anesthesiology* 21:186, 1960.
9. White PF, Shafer A: Nausea and vomiting: Causes and prophylaxis. *Sem Anesth* 6:300, 1988.
10. Dent S, Ramachandra V, Stephen CR: Postoperative vomiting: Incidence, analysis, and therapeutic measures in 3,000 patients. *Anesthesiology* 16:564, 1955.
11. Forrest J, Cahalan MK, Rehder K et al: Multicenter study of general anesthesia: II. Results. *Anesthesiology* 72:262, 1990.
12. Larajani GE, Gratz I, Afshar M et al: Treatment of postoperative nausea and vomiting with ondansetron: A randomized, double-blind comparison with placebo. *Anesth Analg* 73:246, 1991.
13. Palazzo MGA, Strunin L: Anaesthesia and emesis: I. Etiology. *Can Anaesth Soc J* 31:178, 1984.
14. Graber JN, Schulte WJ, Condon RE et al: Relationship of duration of postoperative ileus to extent and site of operative dissection. *Surgery* 92(1):87, 1992.
15. Dabs A, Weise WK, Kopin IJ: Postoperative ileus in the rat: Physiology, etiology and treatment. *Ann Surg* 178:781, 1973.
16. Mishra NK, Appert HE, Howard JM: Studies in paralytic ileus: Effect of intraperitoneal injury on motility of the canine small intestine. *Am J Surg* 129:559, 1975.
17. Livingston EH, Passaro EP: Postoperative ileus. *Dig Dis Sci* 35(1):121, 1990.
18. Argov S, Goldstein I, Barzilai A: Is routine use of the nasogastric tube justified in upper abdominal surgery? *Amer J Surg* 139:849, 1980.
19. Tylosin PO, Cassuto J, Rimback G et al: Treatment of postoperative paralytic ileus with cisapride. *Scand J Gastroenterol* 26:477, 1991.
20. Davidson ED, Hersh T, Brinner RA et al: The effects of metoclopramide on postoperative ileus: A randomized double-blind study. *Ann Surg* 190:27, 1979.
21. Brevick H, Lind B: Anti-emetic and propulsive peristaltic properties of metoclopramide. *Br J Anaesth* 43:400, 1971.
22. Jepsen S, Klaerke A, Nielson PH et al: Negative effect of metoclopramide in postoperative adynamic ileus. A prospective randomized, double blind study. *Br J Surg* 73:290, 1986.
23. Scout AJPN, Bogaard JW, Grade AC et al: Effects of cisapride, a new gastrointestinal prokinetic substance, on interdigestive and postprandial motor activity of the distal oesophagus in man. *Gut* 26:246, 1985.
24. Stature G, Steinringer H, Schneider C et al: Effects of cisapride on jejunal motor activity in fasting healthy humans. *Gastroenterology* 90:1210, 1986.
25. Summers RW, Lu CC: Approach to the patient with ileus and obstruction, in Yamada T, Alpers DH, Owyang C, et al (eds): *Textbook of Gastroenterology*. Philadelphia, Lippincott, 1991, p 715.
26. Quatromoni JC, Rosoff L, Halls JM et al: Early postoperative small bowel obstruction. *Ann Surg* 1:72, 1980.
27. Price A, Levi J, Dolby J et al: *Campylobacter pyloridis* in peptic ulcer disease: Microbiology, pathology, and scanning electron microscopy. *Gut* 26:1183, 1985.
28. Rauws EAJ, Langenberg W, Houthoff HJ et al: *Camphylobacter pyloridis*–associated chronic active antral gastritis. A prospective study of its prevalence and the effects of antibacterial and antiulcer treatment. *Gastroenterology* 94:33, 1988.
29. Dooley CP, McKenna D, Humphreys H et al: Histological gastritis in duodenal ulcer: Relationship to *Campylobacter pylori* and effect of ulcer therapy. *Am J Gastroenterol* 83:278, 1988.
30. Piper DW, Sasiry R, McIntosh J et al: Smoking, alcohol, analgesics, and chronic duodenal ulcer. *Scand J Gastroenterol* 19:1015, 1984.
31. Sonnenberg A, Muller-Lissner SA, Vogel E et al: Predictors of duodenal ulcer healing and relapse. *Gastroenterology* 81:1061, 1981.
32. Doll R, Jones FA, Pygott F: Effect of smoking on the production and maintenance of gastric and duodenal ulcers. *Lancet* 1:657, 1958.
33. Rogot E, Murray JL: Smoking and causes of death among US veterans: 16 years of observation. *Pub Health Rep* 95:213, 1980.
34. Collen MJ, Stanczak VJ, Ciarleglio CA: Refractory duodenal ulcers (non-healing duodenal ulcers with standard doses of antisecretory medication). *Dig Dis Sci* 34:233, 1989.
35. Reynolds JC: Famotidine therapy for active duodenal ulcers. A multivariate analysis of factors affecting early healing. *Ann Intern Med* 111:7, 1989.
36. Conn HO, Blitzer BL: Nonassociation of adrenocorticosteroid therapy and peptic ulcer. *N Engl J Med* 294:433, 1976.
37. Bonnevie O: Causes of death in duodenal and gastric ulcer. *Gastroenterology* 73:1000, 1977.
38. Stemmerman GN, Marcus EB, Buist AS et al: Relative impact of smoking and reduced pulmonary function on peptic ulcer risk. *Gastroenterology* 96:1419, 1989.
39. Kirk AP, Dooley J, Hunt RH: Peptic ulceration in patients with chronic liver disease. *Dig Dis Sci* 25:10, 1980.
40. Langman MJS, Cooke AR: Gastric and duodenal ulcer and their associated diseases. *Lancet* 1:680, 1976.
41. Cohen MM: Treatment and mortality of perforated peptic ulcer: A survey of 852 cases. *Can Med Assoc J* 105:263, 1971.

42. Jordan GL Jr, DeBakey ME, Duncan J Jr: Surgical management of perforated peptic ulcer. *Ann Surg* 179:628, 1974.

43. Boey J, Lee NW, Wong J et al: Perforation in acute duodenal ulcers. *Surg Gynecol Obstet* 155:193, 1982.

44. McGee GS, Sawyers JL: Perforated gastric ulcers. *Arch Surg* 122:555, 1987.

45. Steed DL, Brown B, Reilly J et al: General surgical complications in heart and lung transplantation. *Surgery* 98:739, 1987.

46. Fernandez JA, Rosenberg JC: Posttransplantation pancreatitis. *Surg Gynecol Obstet* 143:695, 1976.

47. Greenstein RJ, McElhonny AJ, Ruben D et al: Colonic vascular ectasias and aortic stenosis: Coincidence or causal relationship? *Am J Surg* 151:347, 1986.

48. Bardenheier JA, Kaminski DL, William VL: Pancreatitis after biliary tract surgery. *Am J Surg* 16:773, 1968.

49. Peterson LM, Collins JJ, Wilson RE: Acute pancreatitis occurring after operation. *Surg Gynecol Obstet* 127:23, 1968.

50. White TT, Morgan A, Hopton D: Postoperative pancreatitis: A study of seventy cases. *Am J Surg* 120:132, 1970.

51. Feiner H: Pancreatitis after cardiac surgery. *Am J Surg* 131:684, 1976.

52. Johnson WC, Nasbeth DC: Pancreatitis in renal transplantation. *Ann Surg* 171:309, 1969.

53. Crepps JT, Foster JH: Clinical significance of postoperative elevation of the serum amylase. *Conn Med* 52:7, 1988.

54. Gross J, Levitt MD: Postoperative elevation of amylase/creatinine ratio in patients without pancreatitis. *Gastroenterol* 77:497, 1979.

55. Cooperberg PL, Burhenne HJ: Real-time ultrasonography. Diagnostic technique of choice in calculous gallbladder disease. *N Engl J Med* 302:1277, 1980.

56. van der Linden W, Suneel H: Early versus delayed operation for acute cholecystitis: A controlled clinical trial. *Am J Surg* 120:7, 1970.

57. McArthur P, Cuschieri A, Sells RA et al: Controlled clinical trial comparing early with interval cholecystectomy for acute cholecystitis. *Br J Surg* 62:850, 1978.

58. Johnson LB: The importance of early diagnosis of acute acalculus cholecystitis. *Surg Gynecol Obstet* 164:197, 1987.

59. Gerding DN, Olson MM, Peterson LR et al: *Clostridium difficile*–associated diarrhea and colitis in adults. *Arch Intern Med* 146:95, 1986.

60. Lashner BA, Todorczuk JT, Sahm DF et al: *Clostridium difficile* culture–positive toxin–negative diarrhea. *Am J Gastroenterol* 81:940, 1986.

61. Young G, Barley N, Ward P et al: Antibiotic-associated colitis caused by *Clostridium difficile*: Relapse and risk factors. *Med J Aust* 144:303, 1986.

62. Teasley DG, Olson MM, Gebhard RL et al: Prospective randomized trial of metronidazole versus vancomycin for *Clostridium difficile*–associated diarrhoea and colitis. *Lancet* 2:1043, 1983.

63. Moore Jr WM, Hollier LH: Mesenteric artery occlusive disease. *Cardiol Clin* 9:535, 1991.

64. Eisenberg RL, Heineken P, Hedgcock MW et al: Evaluation of plain abdominal radiographs in the diagnosis of abdominal pain. *Ann Surg* 197:464, 1983.

68 POSTOPERATIVE GASTROINTESTINAL BLEEDING

Gary M. Levine

Gastrointestinal bleeding is a serious life-threatening event in postoperative patients. Bleeding often occurs suddenly without a prior history of gastrointestinal disease. There may be confusion at first as to whether or not bleeding is related to the operative procedure. Wound pain, postoperative ileus, and narcotic administration all compound the difficulty of evaluation and treatment. These impediments must be overcome in order to determine the cause of bleeding and reduce morbidity and mortality.

Postoperative gastrointestinal bleeding occurs most often in patients with multisystem failure, sepsis, severe burns, and central nervous system (CNS) injury or surgery. The incidence of upper gastrointestinal bleeding may exceed 25 percent in these patients.[1] Mortality in high-risk patients, directly attributed to or associated with bleeding, ranges up to 50 percent in patients with stress ulcer and may exceed 90 percent for patients with mesenteric vascular disease.[2,3] The advent of accurate endoscopic and radiographic diagnostic techniques has improved our understanding of the causes of bleeding. Advances in medical treatment and prophylaxis as well as nonsurgical invasive therapy offer new hope for salvage of these critically ill patients.

UPPER GASTROINTESTINAL BLEEDING

Upper gastrointestinal bleeding has an ominous prognosis in postoperative patients. In a nationwide study of 2225 patients with acute upper gastrointestinal bleeding, the mortality rate was 22 percent in individuals who bled after undergoing major surgery within the prior month, more than twice the rate in nonsurgical patients. When upper gastrointestinal bleeding occurred in trauma patients with shock, 33 percent died; in the presence of respiratory failure, 59 percent died.[1]

The etiology of gastrointestinal bleeding in postoperative patients differs from that in the general population. Stress-induced erosive disease is the most important cause of bleeding in patients with sepsis, burns, head injury, and multiorgan failure. In postoperative patients, there is a direct correlation between the number of

failing organ systems and the incidence of bleeding.[1,3] The pathogenesis and prophylaxis of acute stress-related bleeding is discussed in Chap. 46.

Stress-related bleeding is common, and its natural history is well known. Within 12 hours of admission to an intensive care unit, patients with trauma, sepsis, or shock develop erosions.[4] Within 24 hours of a severe burn, the gastric and duodenal mucosa begin to develop microscopic hemorrhagic lesions that progress to erosions and frank ulceration from which 25 percent of the patients subsequently bleed.[5] The degree of ulceration is directly proportional to the severity of the burn. Patients with burns involving less than 30% of the total body surface rarely develop stress ulcers, but 86 percent of patients with burns covering more than 50% of body surface develop mucosal abnormalities. Overall, 25 percent of burn patients develop a gastric ulcer at the site of the most intense superficial erosions. Bleeding is greatest in those patients who clinically deteriorated. Duodenal ulcer often accompanies gastric lesions and further complicates management.[5]

Harvey Cushing first described gastrointestinal bleeding after intracranial injury or neurosurgical intervention in 1932.[6] The incidence of gastrointestinal bleeding after CNS injury may exceed 25 percent in patients who do not receive prophylaxis.[7] Patients with CNS injury and additional extracranial trauma have the highest risk of bleeding. The erosive mucosal disease follows a course similar to that seen in burn patients. Patients who bleed from stress-related lesions in spite of adequate prophylaxis tend to be those with the highest trauma scores who require assisted ventilation, vasopressors, and dialysis.[1]

Other causes of upper gastrointestinal bleeding should also be considered. Postoperative patients have an increased risk of developing Mallory-Weiss esophageal tears from repeated wretching, emesis, and coughing.[8] These maneuvers generate intraabdominal pressures in excess of 200 torr, creating a shearing force on the mucosa that can cause laceration and bleeding.[9] The diagnosis of the Mallory-Weiss syndrome is easily made endoscopically. If bleeding is observed, the tear can be treated through the endoscope. Bleeding from most tears is self-limited and has stopped by the time endoscopy is performed. However, when bleeding is observed or rebleeding occurs, the patient should undergo endoscopic therapy with a heater probe or mono- or bipolar cautery. A small number of patients may fail endoscopic therapy and require angiographic control or surgical intervention.

Peptic ulcer is a common disease with a prevalence rate of four percent in healthy asymptomatic individuals.[10] Although unproven, it seems clear that patients with silent ulcers are liable to hemorrhage in the perioperative period. One survey of 72 patients undergoing major elective surgery showed that 14 percent had erosions or ulcers, and another 10 percent had gastroduodenitis.[11] Peptic ulcer is also commonly encountered in patients after kidney transplantation.[12] They are usually asymptomatic but frequently bleed. Peptic ulcer is not as prevalent after cardiac transplantation, but, when an ulcer develops, it presents suddenly with hemorrhage.[13,14] Prophylaxis with H_2 antagonists is recommended for all patients with a history of peptic ulcer disease and for those undergoing organ transplantation.

Bleeding from esophagitis in postoperative patients is a consequence of either reflux of gastric contents through the lower esophageal sphincter or infection. Nasogastric intubation, prolonged bed rest in the supine position, and recent abdominal surgery may all exacerbate reflux.[15] Reflux makes the mucosa erythematous, friable, and prone to focal areas of peptic ulceration. Surgical stress and the use of antibiotics or immunosuppressive agents facilitate mucosal invasion with candida, cytomegalovirus, and herpes virus. Candidiasis produces a characteristic endoscopic appearance of whitish plaques varying in size from several millimeters to large confluent areas with surrounding erythema.[16] In viral esophagitis, the appearance varies from focal punched-out ulcers to diffuse ulceration.[17,18] Unfortunately, symptoms of esophagitis may be minimal in these patients. In some reports, fewer than half the patients complain of significant substernal burning, dysphagia, or odynophagia.[16,18]

Initial therapy of esophagitis is aimed at eliminating the causes of reflux. The nasogastric tube should be removed, and the patient should be encouraged to sit upright. High doses of H_2 antagonists or omeprazole are effective for reflux,[19] and antacids are useful for symptomatic relief of pyrosis. Most patients with candidiasis who are not immunosuppressed respond to oral nystatin. In severely affected patients, especially those with hematologic disease or those receiving immunosuppressive therapy for transplantation, fluconazole or ketoconazole is recommended.[20] Serious herpes infections may respond to acyclovir.[21] Cytomegalovirus infection should be treated with gancyclovir.[22]

Postoperative patients on anticoagulants have an increased risk of bleeding into the intestinal lumen or bowel wall. When bleeding occurs in those with therapeutic levels of anticoagulation, it is usually caused by a structural lesion.[23] However, those who bleed as a result of excessive anticoagulation are less likely to have a demonstrable cause. Reversal or better regulation of anticoagulation usually controls bleeding in the latter group.

Patients who have undergone gastric resection with a gastroduodenal or gastrojejunal anastomosis occasionally bleed from the suture line in the immediate postoperative period. A bleeding site is usually identified at endoscopy and is amenable to endoscopic therapy.[1]

Bleeding from an aorto-enteric fistula is a postoperative complication that can occur months to years after abdominal aortic surgery. This condition is due to an infected prosthetic graft or pseudoaneurysm formation at the anastomosis between the aorta and the graft.[24,25] Since the duodenum crosses the aorta, it is the most likely site of bleeding. A history of aortic surgery therefore merits serious consideration of this diagnosis if no other obvious site of bleeding is found. If endoscopy is not diagnostic, either because the fistula is not seen or the diagnosis is not considered initially, angiography should be performed. If a fistula is found, immediate reparative surgery is indicated.[24]

LOWER GASTROINTESTINAL BLEEDING

Initial evaluation of postoperative lower gastrointestinal bleeding is facilitated by noting the presence or absence of abdominal pain. Although this distinction may be difficult in postoperative patients complaining of generalized discomfort, the presence of new localized pain suggests that an inflammatory or ischemic process is responsible for the bleeding. Antibiotic-associated pseudomembranous colitis is probably the most frequent cause of lower gastrointestinal bleeding in postoperative patients. Within days to weeks after receiving antibiotic treatment, patients usually develop diarrhea that may be followed by passage of bloody mucopurulent stools. However, this disorder has not been reported with the usual antibiotics used for preoperative bowel cleansing. Other features include fever, abdominal pain, rebound tenderness, bloody diarrhea, and leukocytosis. Pseudomembranous colitis is caused by the toxin elaborated by *Clostridium difficile*, which is allowed to overgrow when antibiotics induce changes in bowel flora.[26] If possible, the responsible antibiotics should be discontinued, and therapy with metronidazole or vancomycin should be initiated. Seriously ill patients with an ileus should receive intravenous metronidazole.[27] Pseudomembranous colitis is further discussed in Chap. 67.

One of the most serious causes of postoperative lower gastrointestinal bleeding is mesenteric vascular insufficiency. Severity ranges from localized ischemic colitis to extensive bowel infarction. Bleeding may not be a prominent part of the presentation but is invariably present.[3] The two major causes of mesenteric vascular disease in postoperative patients are emboli and nonocclusive infarction. Patients with recent cardiac or vascular surgery, a history of rheumatic heart disease, or atrial fibrillation have the highest risk of developing emboli. When clot embolizes to the abdominal vessels, the superior mesenteric artery is most commonly involved and it results in small-bowel infarction. Nonocclusive ischemia is seen in patients with severe congestive heart failure, sepsis, hypoxia, and shock. It is associated with underlying arteriosclerotic vascular disease, diabetes, hypertension, and digitalis administration.[28]

Since there is no characteristic presentation of mesenteric ischemia, the physician must suspect the disease in postoperative patients with unexplained abdominal pain, hypotension, hemoconcentration, acidosis, or signs of an acute abdomen. Abdominal x-rays may show an "airless" abdomen, thickened mucosal folds, or air in the bowel wall. The presence of air within the intestinal wall is a late finding characteristic of bowel infarction.[3]

Acute mucosal necrosis of the colon occurs in 1 to 2 percent of patients after aortic aneurysm surgery.[29] Resection of an aneurysm or reconstruction of the aortoiliac vessels usually includes interruption of the inferior mesenteric artery for technical reasons. Half to two-thirds of patients who develop colonic ischemia in this setting require partial colectomy with a postoperative mortality rate approaching 50 percent. Operative injury to the superior mesenteric artery can rarely occur, producing small-bowel ischemia. Patients usually require intestinal resection and, if they survive, may suffer from the short-bowel syndrome.[3]

Patients who have undergone organ or bone marrow transplantation have a high risk of developing lower gastrointestinal bleeding from colonic ischemia and infectious colitis.[22,30,31] Opportunistic infection of the bowel with cytomegalovirus or herpes virus is common after bone marrow transplantation. The transmural ulcerations caused by these pathogens may lead to severe bleeding or perforation of the distal ileum and cecum.

When postoperative patients develop painless rectal bleeding, a noninflammatory process such as a bleeding colonic diverticulum or angiodysplasia should be considered.[32,33] Although surgery does not increase the risk of bleeding from these lesions, they are a frequent cause of bleeding and commonly occur in elderly patients. Diverticular bleeding is thought to result from the stretching of an arteriole over the dome of the diverticulum causing erosion of the vessel.[34] Small acquired arteriovenous malformations are seen in angiodysplasia. Lesions may be multiple and are usually located in the right colon and terminal ileum. Patients with aortic stenosis may have a higher risk of developing these lesions.[35]

Diversion colitis is a cause of lower gastrointestinal bleeding encountered in patients with defunctionalized distal colon. The endoscopic appearance of the bowel is similar to that of ulcerative colitis and improves after treatment with enemas containing short-chain fatty acids[36] or restoration of normal bowel continuity. Rectal bleeding is a rare complication of anorectal surgery. Massive bleeding can be encountered after hemorrhoidectomy. Treatment by local tamponade or suturing of the bleeding site is usually effective.[37]

MANAGEMENT OF UPPER GASTROINTESTINAL BLEEDING

The first priority is to stabilize the patient. Multiple large-bore intravenous lines should be placed for fluid resuscitation. Although crystalloid solutions can maintain blood pressure transiently, they quickly leave the intravascular space. Therefore, hetastarch or albumin should be used initially until blood is available. The severity of bleeding should be rapidly assessed, and a large nasogastric tube such as an Ewald tube should be inserted to confirm or exclude active upper gastrointestinal bleeding. The presence of hematemesis, orthostatic hypotension, or bright red blood in the lavage that does not clear strongly suggests massive bleeding with a loss of at least 25% of the blood volume.[1] In about 10 percent of patients with duodenal ulcers, bloody duodenal contents do not reflux into the stomach. However, if nasogastric lavage is stained with bile but free of blood, upper gastroduodenal bleeding is essentially excluded. Nasogastric lavage is successful in stopping one-half to two-thirds of bleeding episodes.[1]

Saline irrigation may lead to absorption of large quantities of salt and water, and volume overload may occur. Irrigation with tap water is preferable because absorbed free water is usually more easily excreted by the kidneys. Iced or cold solutions should be avoided since they lead to considerable discomfort, shivering, and possible hypothermia. Although these solutions may cause tempo-

rary vasoconstriction, reactive hyperemia occurs on rewarming. Vigorous nasogastric suction should be avoided during lavage because injury to the gastric mucosa may enhance bleeding or produce artifacts that may prove confusing to the endoscopist.

Endoscopy should be performed for diagnosis and possible treatment of the bleeding site. There is no role for barium contrast studies in the bleeding patient. Endoscopy provides a diagnosis in over 90 percent of patients, and, when performed for evaluation of bleeding, the risk of perforation, aspiration, or arrhythmia is only about 0.5 percent.[38] Respiratory distress may result from aspiration or the effects of sedative drugs. Endoscopy is contraindicated in uncooperative patients and in those with cardiorespiratory instability. Continued massive bleeding may necessitate immediate angiography or laparotomy without endoscopy.

Most endoscopists agree that when a bleeding site is seen during endoscopy, attempts should be made to achieve hemostasis during the procedure. Several methods to treat bleeding from ulcers, Mallory-Weiss tears, and angiodysplasia have been developed, ranging from injection of dilute (1:10,000) epinephrine into and around the bleeding site to the use of thermal cautery.[40] Thermal ("heater") probes and monopolar and bipolar (bicap) coagulators have all proven effective, although injection of epinephrine may be easiest and most cost-effective to perform.[41] Endoscopic treatment of peptic ulcers should be guided by the presence or absence of active bleeding or a visible vessel.[42] H_2 antagonists and antacids have not proven effective in the treatment of active gastrointestinal bleeding or in preventing rebleeding.[43,44] Patients in whom esophageal varices are found should be treated with either esophageal banding or sclerotherapy.[45]

Angiography should be performed if the patient continues to bleed. This technique may demonstrate extravasation of contrast material into the lumen of the gastrointestinal tract.[39] Intermittent or venous bleeding such as that from varices is difficult to demonstrate by this method. If a bleeding site is demonstrated, an angiographic catheter should be selectively placed into the appropriate vessel for infusion of vasopressin in a dose of 0.2 to 0.4 units/min.

Intraarterial vasopressin is recommended for acute gastric mucosal hemorrhage unresponsive to conventional medical therapy. In a retrospective analysis of 50 patients with gastric bleeding of various etiologies, therapeutic angiography controlled hemorrhage in 84 percent of patients, and only 10 percent required surgery. In comparison, 80 percent of patients who did not receive vasopressin required surgery.[46] When vasopressin infusion is not feasible or effective, autogenous clot or Gelfoam can be embolized into the bleeding vessel.[47] The complications of therapeutic angiography include hematomas at the site of catheterization and bowel ischemia or infarction. Over the past decade, the number of patients requiring angiography has declined, probably because of the efficacy of stress ulcer prophylaxis and the advent of therapeutic endoscopy.

MANAGEMENT OF LOWER GASTROINTESTINAL BLEEDING

The evaluation of lower gastrointestinal bleeding should begin with sigmoidoscopy as soon as the patient is stable. Inflammatory or ischemic lesions may produce characteristic mucosal abnormalities visible through the sigmoidoscope and obviate the need for further diagnostic studies. For example, the picture of pseudomembranous colitis is one of innumerable small raised whitish plaques adherent to the mucosa.[48] Sigmoidoscopic findings in the patient with ischemic colitis range from friability and erythema of the mucosa to more characteristic dusky cyanosis in the rectosigmoid area.[3]

If a diagnosis is not established by sigmoidoscopy and hemorrhage continues, a bleeding scan should be performed. This technique utilizes intravenous injection of 99m-technetium-labeled red blood cells and is rapid and noninvasive. Extravasation of labeled blood into the intestinal lumen can be established by gamma camera imaging.[49] Although bleeding scans may be limited, they are at least as sensitive as angiography, if not more so, in localizing the source of bleeding. In most cases, angiography is not performed without a prior positive bleeding scan.[50]

Urgent colonoscopy has been advocated in evaluating the cause of severe lower gastrointestinal bleeding after an upper gastrointestinal source has been excluded. When performed as an initial diagnostic study, colonoscopy can establish a diagnosis in over two-thirds of patients.[51] At the time of colonoscopy, many lesions such as angiodysplasia can be treated immediately. However, the utility of urgent colonoscopy may be reduced in postoperative patients because they may not tolerate the repeated enemas or oral ingestion of electrolyte lavage solutions necessary to cleanse the bowel.

SUMMARY

1. Postoperative gastrointestinal bleeding occurs most frequently in severely ill patients with sepsis, extensive burns, central nervous system injury, and multisystem failure and carries significant mortality.

2. Stress-induced erosive disease is the most frequent cause of postoperative upper gastrointestinal bleeding. Endoscopy is the most effective diagnostic tool and should be performed as soon as the patient is stable. When bleeding cannot be controlled endoscopically, angiography with vasopressin infusion may be required.

3. Although helpful in prevention of mucosal ulceration, H_2 antagonists and antacids are not effective in controlling upper gastrointestinal bleeding or preventing recurrence.

4. Postoperative lower gastrointestinal disease is frequently the result of antibiotic-induced pseudomembranous colitis or ischemic disease, but bleeding from diverticular disease is common, especially in elderly patients. Sigmoidoscopy allows rapid diagnosis in many cases, but bleeding scans and angiography may be necessary.

REFERENCES

1. Silverstein FE, Gilbert DA, Tedesco FJ et al: The national ASGE survey on upper gastrointestinal bleeding: II. Clinical prognostic factors. *Gastrointest Endosc* 27:80–93, 1981.
2. Hastings PR, Skillman JJ, Bushnell LS et al: Antacid titration in the prevention of acute gastrointestinal bleeding: A controlled, randomized trial in 100 critically ill patients. *N Engl J Med* 298:1041–1045, 1978.
3. Ottinger LW, Austen WG: A study of 136 patients with mesenteric infarction. *Surg Gynec Obstet* 124:251–261, 1967.
4. Peura DA, Johnson LF: Cimetidine for prevention and treatment of gastroduodenal mucosal lesions in patients in an intensive care unit. *Ann Int Med* 103:173–177, 1985.
5. Czaja AJ, McAlhany JC, Pruitt BA Jr: Acute gastroduodenal disease after thermal injury. *N Engl J Med* 291:925–929, 1974.
6. Cushing H: Peptic ulcer and the interbrain. *Surg Gynec Obstet* 55:1–34, 1932.
7. Halloran LG, Fas AM, Goyle WE et al: Prevention of acute gastrointestinal complications after severe head injury: A controlled trial of cimetidine prophylaxis. *Am J Surg* 139:44–48, 1980.
8. Mallory GK, Weiss S: Hemorrhages from lacerations of cardiac orifice of the stomach due to vomiting. *Am J Med Sci* 178:506–515, 1929.
9. Knauer CM: Mallory-Weiss syndrome. Characterization of 75 Mallory-Weiss lacerations in 528 patients with upper gastrointestinal hemorrhage. *Gastroenterology* 71:5–8, 1976.
10. Akdamar K, Ertan A, Agrawal NM et al: Upper gastrointestinal endoscopy in normal asymptomatic volunteers. *Gastrointest Endosc* 32:78–80, 1986.
11. Rypins EB, Sarfeh IJ, Collins-Irby D et al: Asymptomatic peptic ulcer disease in patients undergoing major elective operations: A prospective endoscopic study. *Am J Gastroenterol* 83:927–929, 1988.
12. Feduska NJ, Amend WJC, Vincenti F et al: Peptic ulcer disease in kidney transplant recipients. *Am J Surg* 148:51–57, 1984.
13. Lebovics E, Lee SS, Dworkin BM et al: Upper gastrointestinal bleeding following open heart surgery: Predominant finding of aggressive duodenal ulcer disease. *Dig Dis Sci* 36:757–760, 1991.
14. Johnson R, Peitzman AB, Webster MW et al: Upper gastrointestinal endoscopy after cardiac transplantation. *Surgery* 103:300–304, 1988.
15. Dent J, Dodds WJ, Hogan WJ et al: Factors that influence induction of gastroesophageal reflux in normal human subjects. *Dig Dis Sci* 33:270–275, 1988.
16. Mathieson R, Dutta SK: Candida esophagitis. *Dig Dis Sci* 28:365–370, 1983.
17. McBane RD, Gross JB: Herpes esophagitis: Clinical syndrome, endoscopic appearance and diagnosis in 23 patients. *Gastrointest Endosc* 37:600–603, 1991.
18. Alexander JA, Brouillette DE, Chien MC et al: Infectious esophagitis following liver and renal transplantation. *Dig Dis Sci* 33:1121–1126, 1988.
19. Collen MJ, Strong RM: Comparison of omeprazole and ranitidine in the treatment of refractory gastroesophageal reflux disease in patients with gastric acid hypersecretion. *Dig Dis Sci* 37:897–903, 1992.
20. Saag MS, Dismukes WE: Azole antifungal agents: Emphasis on new triazoles. *Antimicrob Agents Chemother* 32:1–8, 1988.
21. Kadakia SC, Oliver GA, Peura DA: Acyclovir in endoscopically presumed viral esophagitis. *Gastrointest Endosc* 33:33–35, 1987.
22. Kaplan CS, Petersen FA, Icenogle TB et al: Gastrointestinal cytomegalovirus infection in heart and heart-lung transplant recipients. *Arch Int Med* 149:2095–2100, 1989.
23. Tabibian N: Acute gastrointestinal bleeding in anticoagulated patients: A prospective evaluation. *Am J Gastroenterol* 84:10–12, 1989.
24. Champion MC, Sullivan SN, Coles JC: Aortoenteric fistulae. Incidence, presentation, recognition and management. *Ann Surg* 195:314–317, 1982.
25. Reilly LM, Ehrenfeld WK, Goldstone J et al: Gastrointestinal tract involvement by prosthetic graft infection. *Ann Surg* 202:342–348, 1985.
26. Bartlett JG, Chang TW, Gurwith M et al: Antibiotic-associated pseudomembranous colitis due to toxin-producing clostridia. *N Engl J Med* 298:S31–S34, 1978.
27. Teasley DG, Gerding DN, Olson MM et al: Prospective randomized trial of metronidazole versus vancomycin for *Clostridium difficile*-associated diarrhea and colitis. *Lancet* 2:1043–1046, 1983.

28. Bounous G: Acute necrosis of the intestinal mucosa. *Gastroenterology* 82:1447–1467, 1982.
29. Brewster DC, Franklin DP, Cabria RP et al: Intestinal ischemia complicating abdominal aortic surgery. *Surgery* 109:447–454, 1991.
30. Misra MK, Pinkus GS, Birtch AG et al: Major colonic diseases complicating renal transplantation. *Surgery* 73:942–948, 1973.
31. Stratta RJ, Schaeffer MS, Markin RS et al: Cytomegalovirus infection and disease after liver transplantation: An overview. *Dig Dis Sci* 37:673–678, 1992.
32. Almy TP, Howell DA: Diverticular disease of the colon. *N Engl J Med* 302:324–331, 1980.
33. Richter JM, Christensen MR, Colditz GA et al: Angiodysplasia: Natural history and efficacy of therapeutic interventions. *Dig Dis Sci* 34:1542–1546, 1989.
34. Meyers MA, Volberg F, Katzen B et al: Angioarchitecture of colonic diverticula: Significance in bleeding diverticulosis, *Radiology* 108:249–261, 1973.
35. Imperiale TF, Ransohoff DF: Aortic stenosis, idiopathic gastrointestinal bleeding, and angiodysplasia: Is there an association? A methodologic critique of the literature. *Gastroenterology* 95:1670–1676, 1988.
36. Harig JM, Soergel KH, Komorowski RA et al: Treatment of diversion colitis with short-chain fatty acid irrigation. *N Engl J Med* 320:23–28, 1989.
37. Ferguson EF Jr, Houston CH: Postoperative anorectal bleeding. *Surg Gyn Obstet* 149:506–508, 1979.
38. Gilbert DA, Silverstein FE, Tedesco FJ et al: The national ASGE survey on upper gastrointestinal bleeding: III. Endoscopy in upper gastrointestinal bleeding. *Gastrointest Endosc* 27:94–102, 1981.
39. Ng BL, Thompson JN, Adam A et al: Selective visceral angiography in obscure postoperative bleeding. *Ann R Coll Surg* 69:237–240, 1987.
40. Cook DJ, Guyatt GH, Salena BJ et al: Endoscopic therapy for acute nonvariceal upper gastrointestinal hemorrhage: A meta-analysis. *Gastroenterology* 102:139–148, 1992.
41. Chung SCS, Leung JWC, Sung JY et al: Injection or heat probe for bleeding ulcer. *Gastroenterology* 100:33–37, 1991.
42. Chang-Chien G-S, Wu C-S, Chen P-C et al: Different implications of stigmata of recent hemorrhage in gastric and duodenal ulcers. *Dig Dis Sci* 33:400–404, 1988.
43. Collins R, Langman M: Treatment with histamine H_2 antagonists in acute upper gastrointestinal hemorrhage. Implications of randomized trials. *N Engl J Med* 313:660–666, 1985.
44. Daneshmend TKK, Hawkey CJ, Langman MJS et al: Omeprazole versus placebo for acute upper gastrointestinal bleeding; randomized double blinded controlled trial. *Brit Med J* 304:143–147, 1992.
45. Steigmann GV, Goff JS, Michaletz-Onody PA et al: Endoscopic sclerotherapy as compared with endoscopic ligation for bleeding esophageal varices. *N Engl J Med* 326:1527–1532, 1992.
46. Athanasoulis CA, Baum S, Waltman AC et al: Control of acute gastric mucosal hemorrhage. *N Engl J Med* 290:597–603, 1974.
47. Bookstein JJ, Chlosta EM, Foley D et al: Transcatheter hemostasis of gastrointestinal bleeding using modified autogenous clot. *Radiology* 113:277–285, 1974.
48. Tedesco FJ, Bacton RW, Aleers DH: Clindamycin-associated colitis. A prospective study. *Ann Intern Med* 81:429–433, 1974.
49. Markisz JA, Front D, Royal HD et al: An evaluation of Tc-labeled red blood cell scintigraphy for the detection and localization of gastrointestinal bleeding sites. *Gastroenterology* 83:394–398, 1982.
50. Fiorito JJ, Brandt LJ, Kozicky O et al: The diagnostic yield of superior mesenteric angiography: Correlation with the pattern of gastrointestinal bleeding. *Am J Gastroenterol* 84:878–881, 1989.
51. Jensen DM, Machicado GA: Diagnosis and treatment of severe hematochezia. *Gastroenterology* 95:1569–1574, 1988.

69 POSTOPERATIVE JAUNDICE

Raymond A. Rubin

Clifford A. Brass

The differential diagnosis of postoperative jaundice is extensive and includes etiologies of extrahepatic duct obstruction, intrahepatic cholestasis, hepatocellular dysfunction, and bilirubin overproduction. Frequently, postoperative jaundice represents dysfunction of other organs rather than intrinsic liver disease. A single cause of postoperative hyperbilirubinemia is not always determined and there are often several concurrent etiologies. While most patients can be managed conservatively, it is important to identify those in whom invasive intervention is indicated. In adults, bilirubin itself is not toxic and is cleared slowly from the circulation. Therefore, it is more important to identify an underlying etiology than to focus on small changes in serum bilirubin levels and slow resolution of established jaundice. Postoperative jaundice often resolves spontaneously without establishment of a clear cause.

BILIRUBIN METABOLISM

An outline of bilirubin metabolism is shown in Fig. 69–1. About 80 percent of bilirubin is derived from degradation of hemoglobin from senescent erythrocytes in the liver, spleen, and bone marrow. The remainder originates from ineffective erythropoiesis and the breakdown of nonhemoglobin hemoproteins such as myoglobin and various cytochromes.[1] In the circulation, unconjugated bilirubin is reversibly bound to albumin. In the liver, bilirubin is transported into hepatocytes and conjugated with glucuronic acid, forming direct bilirubin. Water-soluble direct bilirubin is secreted by a carrier-mediated mechanism across the canalicular membrane into the biliary tree. Bilirubin excretion is dependent on the presence of bile salts, and alteration of the hepatic bile salt pool may alter the process. The liver conjugates and excretes 250 to 350 mg of bilirubin daily.[2] In patients with normal hepatic function, larger bilirubin loads can be accommodated easily without an appreciable rise in the serum bilirubin concentration.

The liver normally excretes bilirubin into the bile, and in healthy individuals only trace amounts of conjugated bilirubin escape into the plasma.[3,4] Theoretically, a direct reacting bilirubin level of more than 3% to 5% of total bilirubin levels represents conjugated hyperbilirubinemia due to a hepatobiliary disorder. However, the standard diazo method of measuring low concentrations of direct and indirect bilirubin is unreliable. Clinical experience has therefore dictated that direct bilirubin levels greater than 0.3 mg/dl or exceeding 20% of the total plasma bilirubin concentration defines conjugated hyperbilirubinemia.[5] This distinction may become less important as improved diagnostic tests become more widely available.[4] Unconjugated hyperbilirubinemia usually due to hemolysis may be accompanied by slight increases in direct bilirubin levels.

A third clinically measurable type of bilirubin is the delta fraction. It represents the monoconjugated fraction of direct bilirubin covalently linked to albumin. Its serum level may rise after prolonged conjugated hyperbilirubinemia.[6] Because of its irreversible link to albumin, it has a half-life of two to three weeks, and its clearance significantly lags behind that of the diglucuronide conjugated fraction.

Accumulation of bilirubin or its conjugates is not visible in the sclera, skin, and mucosal membranes until the plasma concentration exceeds three mg/dl. The clinical appearance of jaundice may lag behind elevation in serum values by a few days as tissue levels accumulate.

INCIDENCE

The incidence of postoperative jaundice varies depending on the specific surgical population studied, the method employed to measure the serum bilirubin concentration, the definition of jaundice used, and the length of follow-up. Hyperbilirubinemia is distinctly uncommon in healthy patients undergoing elective surgery who do not receive blood transfusions.[7] However, mild jaundice with serum bilirubin levels between 1.4 and 4.0 mg/dl has been reported in 16 percent of patients undergoing major procedures.[8] Up to 24

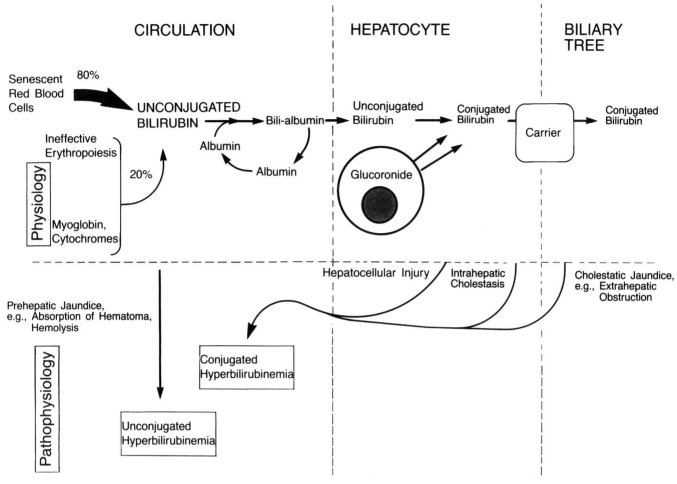

FIGURE 69–1. Bilirubin metabolism.

percent of those with normal preoperative bilirubin levels undergoing cardiac surgery develop postoperative concentrations exceeding three mg/dl.[9]

Although the use of specific anesthetic agents and the type or duration of the procedure do not independently predict the development of jaundice, preexisting liver disease, right heart failure, hypoxemia, hypotension, and the quantity of blood transfused are important risk factors.[9,10] Changes in anesthetic technique (e.g., decreased use of halothane) and perioperative care may alter the incidence of postoperative jaundice in future studies.

ASSESSMENT OF THE PATIENT

Assessment of the jaundiced postoperative patient requires review of the prior medical history, medications, intraoperative course, temporal sequence and pattern of liver function test abnormalities, and physical examination. This evaluation is often complemented by radiologic imaging of the right-upper quadrant.

A history of congestive heart failure, pulmonary hypertension, or chronic pericardial disease suggests passive congestion of the liver, while a history of glucose-6-phosphate-dehydrogenase deficiency or immune-mediated hemolytic anemia may point to a medication causing hemolysis. Those with a history of pancre-

aticobiliary disease may have choledocholithiasis or strictures causing extrahepatic obstruction. Underlying chronic liver disease is suggested by past history of alcohol abuse, blood transfusions, intravenous drug abuse, or other percutaneous exposures. The onset of jaundice after surgery may signal the compromised hepatic reserve of previously unrecognized cirrhosis. A history of preexisting liver disease is often more important in estimating surgical risk than in narrowing the differential diagnosis of postoperative jaundice. Poor hepatic synthetic function, ascites, or encephalopathy escalates the morbidity and mortality of otherwise relatively low-risk procedures.[11] In particular, active hepatitis markedly increases operative risk.

Medication-induced hepatotoxicity accounts for a significant percentage of cases of jaundice in hospitalized patients, especially among the elderly.[12] Drug-induced jaundice may be cholestatic, indicative of hepatocellular injury, or both (see Table 69–1). It is therefore imperative to review the medications received before, during, and after surgery. Hepatotoxic agents and drugs may be classified as predictable (intrinsic) or unpredictable (idiosyncratic) toxins. Intrinsic hepatotoxins may directly injure liver cells (e.g., chloroform) or indirectly damage them by selective interference with specific metabolic pathways (e.g., estrogen). An example of the latter is the production of a toxic metabolite from acetaminophen and its binding to protein thiols.

TABLE 69–1. Predominant Pattern of Liver Injury Related to Medications Commonly Prescribed in the Perioperative Setting

I. *Cholestatic*
- Cardiovascular: angiotensin-converting enzyme (ACE) inhibitors (e.g., captopril), thiazides
- Psychotropic: phenothiazines (especially chlorpromazine), imipramine, haloperidol
- Antibiotics: erythromycin, nitrofurantoin, oxacillin, dicloxacillin
- Oral hypoglycemics: chlorpropamide, tolbutamide, glyburide
- Total parenteral nutrition

II. *Hepatocellular Inflammation*
- Cardiovascular: alpha-methyldopa, amiodarone, calcium channel blockers (e.g., verapamil), hydralazine, procainamide, quinidine
- Antimicrobials: isoniazid, ketoconazole, nifedipine, sulfonamides, sulfones
- Anti-epileptic: phenytoin, valproic acid
- Anesthetics: halothane, other halogenated anesthetics (e.g., enflurane, methoxyflurane)

III. *Prehepatic, i.e., hemolysis*
- Related to G-6-PD deficiency: sulfas, aspirin, probenecid, quinidine
- Autoimmune phenomena: alpha-methyldopa
- Binding to red blood cells: penicillins
- Binding to plasma proteins: sulfonamides, phenothiazines, quinidine

IV. *Mixed cholestatic–hepatocellular*
- Amrinone, disopyramide, azathioprine, H_2 antagonists, diazepam, trazodone, chloroquine nitrofurantoin, penicillin, trimethoprim-sulfamethoxazole

---

Most drug-induced liver disease reflects unpredictable idiosyncratic hepatic injury. Idiosyncratic hepatotoxins are subdivided into two groups: (1) those that cause an immunologic hypersensitivity reaction associated with fever, rash, arthralgias, and eosinophilia; and (2) those that occur because of a metabolic aberration in a susceptible patient. Immunologic reactions caused by drugs like halothane or sulfonamides usually occur within one to five weeks. However, it may take from one week to 12 months of exposure to agents like isoniazid or valproic acid for liver injury to occur. In addition, response to rechallenge may be delayed for days to weeks in the latter group.

Even if temporal relationships are clear, proving that jaundice is due to a particular medication usually involves exclusion of other etiologies. This problem can be difficult in the perioperative period when clinical status is continuously changing and several medications are introduced simultaneously. In addition, drug-induced cholestasis may continue for many months after withdrawal of the offending agent[13] and in rare instances may lead to complete liver failure.[14]

In evaluating postoperative jaundice, it is important not only to consider the particular procedures but also to focus on intraoperative details including the choice of anesthetic agents and complications like hemodynamic instability and excessive bleeding. The specific surgical procedure can provide clues to the etiology of postoperative jaundice. Cardiac surgery requiring bypass and multiple blood transfusions is often associated with postoperative jaundice.[15] Extrahepatic duct obstruction due to choledocholithiasis may develop after cholecystectomy despite unrevealing preoperative cholangiography or common bile duct exploration. When jaundice appears shortly following cholecystectomy, particularly after laparoscopic resection, it may signify inadvertent common bile duct ligation.[16] Other procedures in the region of the common bile duct or duodenum may be complicated by postoperative stricture or functional extrahepatic obstruction from local inflammation. Abdominal operations may also be complicated by vascular thrombosis and resultant hepatocellular necrosis.

Although anesthesia and general surgery are accompanied by decreased hepatic oxygen consumption, they may be complicated by significant decreases in hepatic blood flow and result in liver ischemia. The liver normally receives 25 percent of cardiac output.[17] As portal blood flow is reduced, hepatic arterial flow increases. Anesthetic agents may compromise hepatic blood flow by decreasing cardiac output (halothane, enflurane, spinal and epidural anesthesia), increasing splanchnic resistance (cyclopropane), or both (methoxyflurane).[10] Sympathetic activation in response to surgical stimulation increases splanchnic vascular resistance and decreases splanchnic blood flow.[18]

The liver is well protected against ischemia by its dual blood supply and autoregulation of hepatic arterial blood flow that compensates for changes in portal blood supply. However, regions of relative ischemia may develop during surgery. Within hepatic lobules, hepatocytes adjacent to central veins and farthest from portal triads are most susceptible to injury. Perioperative hypotension, decreased cardiac output, and hypoxemia increase the possibility of ischemic liver injury. Hematoma formation and transfusion of blood products may cause hyperbilirubinemia as a result of increased bilirubin load or transmission of viral hepatitis.

When assessing jaundice in postoperative patients, there are three specific areas of importance on physical examination: (1) localizing signs like rebound tenderness, involuntary guarding, and Murphy's, Cullen's, or Turner's sign that may indicate the need for reoperation; (2) findings associated with extrahepatic causes of jaundice such as decreased cardiac output, congestive heart failure, pulmonary hypertension, or localized infections; and (3) stigmata of chronic liver disease such as palmar erythema, spider telangiectasias, gynecomastia, testicular atrophy, ascites, splenomegaly, or caput medusae. However, none of these latter signs need be present in patients with cirrhosis.

PATTERNS OF LIVER FUNCTION TEST ABNORMALITIES

The differential diagnosis of jaundice is facilitated by using the clinical presentation and pattern of liver function test abnormalities to classify patients into three categories: "cholestatic" jaundice, jaundice due to hepatocellular inflammation, and "prehepatic" jaundice. These categories can be roughly correlated with three pathophysiologic mechanisms: extrahepatic or intrahepatic cholestasis, hepatocellular injury, and bilirubin overproduction (see Table 69–2). While individual patients may not neatly fall into one of these categories, the framework is useful in guiding diagnostic and therapeutic strategies. Extrahepatic obstruction may require antibiotics and endoscopic or surgical intervention. However, hepatocellular injury and bilirubin overproduction are usually managed by correcting the underlying process or supporting the patient after withdrawing an offending agent.

TABLE 69–2. Etiologies of Postoperative Jaundice

Type	Mechanism	Example	Serum Alkaline Phosphatase	% Direct Bilirubin	Serum ALT/AST	Synthetic Function
A. Cholestatic						
Extrahepatic	obstruction of extrahepatic bile duct	choledocholithiasis bile duct ligation/ transection bile duct stricture	elevated, $> 2\times$	$> 15\%$	normal/slightly abnormal	normal
Intrahepatic	decreased secretion and/or processing of bilirubin	infection/sepsis acalculous cholecystis benign postoperative jaundice medications total parenteral nutrition	slightly abnormal, $< 2\times$	$> 15\%$	normal/slightly abnormal	normal
B. Hepatocellular	injury to hepatocytes with decreased ability to secrete bilirubin and/or secondary injury to intrahepatic biliary system	ischemia viral hepatitis chronic liver disease toxins/drugs	slightly abnormal, $< 2\times$	$> 15\%$	elevated up to $1000 \times$	may be decreased
C. Prehepatic	increased bilirubin load	hemolysis resorption of hematoma intravascular hemolysis drug, immune-mediated Gilbert's disease	normal	low	normal	normal

"CHOLESTATIC" JAUNDICE

Cholestatic jaundice is the result of extrahepatic bile duct obstruction or impaired hepatic bile excretion ("intrahepatic" cholestasis). It is usually characterized by direct hyperbilirubinemia, at least a doubling of the levels of alkaline phosphatase, gamma-glutamyltranspeptidase (GGT), and 5'-nucleotidase (5'NT), and only minor increases in serum transaminase concentrations. In acute obstruction, the serum transaminase levels may increase immediately, but elevation in serum alkaline phosphatase concentration lags behind by 24 to 48 hours during which synthesis of the enzyme is induced.[19,20] While GGT and 5'NT are useful tests to confirm that the alkaline phosphatase elevation is related to liver disease, they are less helpful thereafter. In fact, the great sensitivity of many currently used assays for GGT may lead to overinterpretation of the data.

Extrahepatic Duct Obstruction

Postoperative extrahepatic duct obstruction may require endoscopic or surgical intervention. Given this possibility, diagnostic efforts should be directed toward confirming or excluding underlying causes of obstruction. In the immediate postoperative period, bile duct obstruction is usually related to choledocholithiasis or inadvertent intraoperative bile duct ligation or transection. While choledocholithiasis may be relatively asymptomatic, bile duct injury may present with peritoneal signs. Bile duct stricture due to postoperative pancreatitis or inflammation following common bile duct exploration or other abdominal procedures usually becomes apparent sometime after surgery. Bile duct strictures from preexisting malignancy or sclerosing cholangitis may become evident at any point in the perioperative period.

Radiologic evaluation of postoperative jaundice is useful in demonstrating the patency and caliber of the biliary tree, determin-

ing the presence of gallstones in the gallbladder or bile ducts, assessing structures adjacent to the liver and biliary tree, and searching for evidence of localized infections. Ultrasound is usually the initial test of choice in view of its relatively low cost, availability, and safety. It provides excellent visualization of the gallbladder and gallstones. In patients with extrahepatic ductal dilatation and severe jaundice with bilirubin levels over 10 mg/dl, its sensitivity exceeds 90 percent.[21] However, in those with ductal dilatation and less severe jaundice or incomplete ductal obstruction without dilatation, its sensitivity drops considerably. The sensitivity of ultrasound is operator-dependent, and visualization may be compromised by adipose tissue, bowel gas from postoperative ileus, and surgical clips. The addition of color flow doppler imaging provides valuable information concerning the patency of the hepatic and portal veins as well as the inferior vena cava and hepatic artery.

Computerized axial tomography (CT) is a useful alternative for imaging the abdomen, especially in obese patients. Visualization may be obscured by surgical clips but not by bowel gas, fat, or ascites. It may provide better images of the distal bile duct and pancreas. Its sensitivity as a diagnostic tool in obstructive jaundice is highly variable.[22–24] However, its use may be limited by the potential nephrotoxicity of intravenous contrast agents. Like ultrasound, CT cannot absolutely exclude choledocholithiasis or subtle but clinically significant bile duct strictures.

Hepatobiliary scintigraphy (HIDA, PIPIDA, TcIDA) takes advantage of the ability of the hepatocyte to take up and to excrete a radiopharmaceutical into the biliary tree. This functional test is most useful in looking for obstruction of the cystic duct as in acute cholecystitis, or in screening for biliary complications of laparoscopic cholecystectomy including bile leaks and complete transection of the extrahepatic duct.[25,26] Scintigraphy requires intact hepatocyte function to take up tracer material, and its utility is therefore limited in patients with diffuse hepatocellular disease. In acute biliary obstruction, hepatocyte uptake of the tracer is normal, but there is no excretion into the biliary system. Although these findings may precede the development of ductal dilatation detectable on ultrasound or CT, scintigraphy does not provide information regarding the etiology of the blockage.

In patients with postoperative jaundice in whom there is a reasonable pre-test probability of extrahepatic duct obstruction, endoscopic retrograde cholangiopancreatography (ERCP) is the definitive technique to assess choledocholithiasis, stricture, or other bile duct pathology. ERCP can be used to extract impacted bile duct or ampullary stones, obtain tissue for diagnosis in cases of suspected malignancy, and place stents in partially obstructed bile ducts. Gaining access to the bile duct for such purposes may require endoscopic sphincterotomy. ERCP can also be used to evaluate the pancreas for anatomic abnormalities, to explain pancreatitis, or to diagnose malignancy. Air insufflation needed to perform ERCP may pose a problem for fresh operative wounds. ERCP may also be complicated by perforation or pancreatitis. The risk of perforation and significant bleeding is increased when the diagnostic procedure is accompanied by endoscopic sphincterotomy. However, in cases of common bile duct obstruction with cholangitis, emergency ERCP may provide definitive intervention with significantly less morbidity and mortality than surgery.[27]

Percutaneous transhepatic cholangiography (PTC) may provide better access to the proximal common hepatic duct than ERCP and can be used to extract bile duct stones, bypass strictures, and diagnose biliary malignancies. It does not provide visualization of the pancreatic duct. It requires a percutaneous puncture of the liver to gain access to the biliary tree and may be complicated by bleeding, especially in patients with coagulopathy or infection. Difficulty in performing this procedure and related morbidity are inversely related to the degree of ductal dilatation. The choice of ERCP or PTC may depend on institutional expertise. While either can be used effectively to exclude and in many cases treat extrahepatic obstruction, they carry significant risks and should be reserved for patients who fail conservative management.

Intrahepatic Cholestasis Due to Infection

The important differential diagnosis in patients with postoperative cholestatic jaundice lies between extrahepatic obstruction and intrahepatic cholestasis caused by localized and systemic infections, "benign" cholestasis, or medication-induced liver disease. Localized infections like cholangitis usually cause right upper quadrant pain, fever, and conjugated hyperbilirubinemia. In the absence of obstruction, cholestatic jaundice can also complicate severe systemic infections, particularly those caused by gram-negative bacteria.[28–30] Hypotension, decreased cardiac output, regional or systemic hypoxia, or hemolysis associated with sepsis may all contribute to postoperative liver dysfunction. However, conjugated hyperbilirubinemia may be caused in part by endotoxin-induced reduction of bile salt–independent bile flow.[31] In sepsis complicated by hypotension, decreased blood flow through the peribiliary plexus may lead to ischemic damage and impair excretory cholangiolar function.[32]

Jaundice associated with sepsis usually develops a few days after bacteremia. While the serum bilirubin level ordinarily peaks at three to five mg/dl, values of 30 to 50 mg/dl have been reported.[29] Rarely, the serum alkaline phosphatase and GGT levels can rise disproportionately to that of bilirubin.[33] Successful treatment of the underlying infection usually results in rapid resolution of the liver function test abnormalities. Although the severity of the underlying infection often contributes to significant morbidity and mortality, cholestasis itself does not appear to affect overall prognosis. The diagnosis of sepsis-associated cholestatic jaundice is supported by a compatible clinical history and exclusion of other etiologies of cholestasis. Liver biopsy in patients with infection-related jaundice demonstrates nonspecific pathologic changes.[32]

Acalculous Cholecystitis

Cholecystitis is an unusual cause of postoperative jaundice when surgery is unrelated to the biliary tree but should be suspected when jaundice is accompanied by fever, pain, and right-upper-quadrant tenderness. It is most commonly accompanied by leukocytosis, a two- to fourfold rise in serum bilirubin concentration, and mild elevations in serum alkaline phosphatase and transaminase levels. Although ultrasound may be useful, up to 50 percent of patients in this setting have no visible stones. Making an early diagnosis of acute acalculous cholecystitis is clinically important since the risk of gallbladder perforation increases significantly if the diagnosis is delayed more than 48 hours.[34] Since 30 percent of these patients may have gangrene of the gallbladder,[35] a "rim sign" on radionucleotide scan can be highly sensitive (88 percent) but nonspecific (44 percent) for gallbladder necrosis.[36,37] Although variable, ultrasonography and CT can be very sensitive (> 90 percent) in detecting findings that accompany cholecystitis including gallbladder sludge, gallbladder wall thickening, gallbladder dilatation, and pericholecystic fluid.[38] Unfortunately, ascites, hypoalbuminemia, and biliary sludge may also produce or mimic some of these findings.[34,39] Fasting itself is associated with dilatation of the gallbladder. An ultrasonographic Murphy's sign and pericholecystic fluid in the absence of ascites are more specific findings suggesting acalculous cholecystitis, but certain diagnosis of this entity is often difficult despite appropriate history, physical examination, and radiologic evaluation.

"Benign" Postoperative Jaundice

Benign postoperative jaundice or cholestasis is not a specific disease but a syndrome with multiple etiologies characterized by a self-limited rise in bilirubin after surgery requiring no specific intervention. It is therefore a diagnosis of exclusion. The term cholestasis in this syndrome may be somewhat misleading because morphologic evidence of cholestasis is variable.[40] Benign intrahepatic cholestasis was first described in patients undergoing abdominal surgery.[41,42] Subsequently, it was documented in patients with extensive burns, severe trauma, and large hematomas.[42–47] It is most common in patients undergoing major abdominal surgery under general anesthesia who receive multiple blood transfusions.

Jaundice usually develops in the first or second postoperative day, and serum bilirubin levels peak on the third to tenth. However, hyperbilirubinemia may begin as late as the tenth day. The increased bilirubin is primarily conjugated and may infrequently reach levels as high as 40 mg/dl, especially in patients undergoing major cardiac surgery requiring bypass. Although alkaline phosphatase, 5'NT, and GGT levels may be elevated two- to fourfold, serum transaminase and albumin levels and prothrombin time are only mildly abnormal. All abnormalities disappear by the third week after surgery.

Although the etiology of this syndrome is unknown, it is thought to be related to three distinct processes: (1) increased bilirubin production subsequent to blood transfusions during surgery, hemolysis, or absorption of large hematomas or intraperitoneal blood; (2) decreased clearance of bilirubin by the liver induced by intraoperative hypoxemia, shock, release of toxins, or postoperative sepsis; and (3) decreased renal clearance of bilirubin. Although benign postoperative jaundice has been associated with an increased bilirubin load, it is primarily an intrahepatic cholestatic disease marked by direct hyperbilirubinemia.

Although biopsy is not indicated in most patients, histopathology shows intrahepatic cholestasis, bile staining of hepatocytes, and elongation of bile duct canaliculi but little or no inflammation or necrosis of hepatocytes.[48] These findings, although not invariable, tend to confirm the notion of a mild decrement in bilirubin clearance due to intraoperative factors like hypoxia, shock, and toxins that have not been fully characterized.

Jaundice occurring after cardiac surgery is often marked. Higher serum bilirubin and transaminase levels representing more extensive hepatocellular injury are related to more pronounced hypoxia, hypotension, higher transfusion requirements, and hemolysis induced by extracorporeal circulation.

Invasive testing, including liver biopsy, is rarely indicated in patients who have had multiple blood transfusions, perioperative hypoxia, or hypotension. Serum chemistries including creatinine concentration should be performed. If abdominal pain or fever is present or serum transaminase levels are unusually high, an ultrasound may be required to exclude obstruction. Elevation in the serum bilirubin level is itself benign in adults. Management should focus on exclusion of serious treatable underlying disease.

Medications

Drug-induced hepatotoxicity should be considered in the differential diagnosis of cholestatic jaundice in the absence of extrahepatic obstruction (Table 69–1). Adverse reactions to medications usually occur shortly after initiating therapy but may be delayed, making identification of the offending hepatotoxin difficult. Drugs commonly used in the perioperative setting associated with cholestasis include cardiovascular drugs such as angiotensin-converting enzyme inhibitors, thiazides, and verapamil; psychotropics such as phenothiazines, tricyclic antidepressants, and haloperidol; antibiotics such as erythromycin and carbenicillin; and oral hypoglycemic agents.[12,49]

The mechanisms by which these drugs alter secretion of bile have not been fully elucidated. Some may affect bile canaliculi only (e.g., chlorpromazine) while others injure hepatocytes as well (e.g., anabolic and contraceptive steroids).[13] Proposed mechanisms include changes in the physical and chemical properties of hepatocyte membranes and immunologic attack on hepatocytes or bile ducts.[50]

The diagnosis of medication-induced cholestasis is suggested by circumstantial temporal evidence and exclusion of other etiologies of cholestasis. Liver biopsy is rarely useful in diagnosis.[51] Histology usually demonstrates bile pigment accumulation and bile duct proliferation, nonspecific features consistent with both extrahepatic duct obstruction and intrahepatic cholestasis.

The prognosis in drug-induced cholestasis is favorable, and liver function tests usually return to normal after the offending agent has been withdrawn. However, cholestatic reactions may occasionally persist for several months, and in rare instances cholestasis may continue indefinitely and can lead to liver failure.[14]

Patients with acute drug-induced hepatic injury may demonstrate features of both cholestatic and hepatocellular injury.[11] Drugs implicated in such cases include cardiovascular agents such as amrinone and disopyramide; azathioprine; H_2 antagonists; neuropsychotropics such as diazepam and trazodone; and the antibiotics chloramphenicol, nitrofurantoin, penicillins, and trimethoprimsulfamethoxazole.[11]

Total Parenteral Nutrition (TPN)

Liver function test abnormalities are a well-recognized complication in patients receiving total parenteral nutrition.[52] While serum transaminase levels may increase transiently in the first few weeks after therapy is initiated, alkaline phosphatase and conjugated bilirubin levels typically peak after two to four weeks.[53–55] A minority of adults on TPN will experience either progressive cholestatic hepatitis or a steatohepatitis indistinguishable from that seen in alcoholic liver disease.[56] Severe disease leading to cirrhosis has been most notably associated with massive small-bowel resection and prolonged TPN.

Possible etiologies for TPN-induced cholestasis include bacterial overgrowth,[57] excess caloric load,[58] abnormalities in bile salt composition,[55] and nutritional imbalances.[53,59–61] TPN-induced cholestasis can often be treated by decreasing caloric load, altering protein/carbohydrate ratios, and cycling administration.[24] In addition, metronidazole or cholecystokinin may be effective.[57,61,62]

HEPATOCELLULAR INFLAMMATION

Postoperative jaundice may mimic acute hepatitis with marked (five- to twentyfold) elevations in serum transaminase levels, conjugated hyperbilirubinemia greater than 15 to 20% of the total bilirubin level, and only modest increases in serum alkaline phosphatase concentration. Jaundice associated with hepatocellular injury is usually the result of hepatic ischemia, viral hepatitis, and medication-induced liver disease.

Hepatic Ischemia

Perioperative hypovolemia, cardiac ischemia, arrhythmias, pulmonary embolism, congestive heart failure, and sepsis can contribute to systemic hypotension and hypoxemia and subsequent liver ischemia. The incidence is especially high after trauma and open heart surgery.[9] Postoperative portal vein or hepatic arterial occlusion are uncommon causes of ischemic liver injury.

Ischemic hepatitis is usually characterized by abrupt dramatic elevations in serum transaminase levels to more than 1000 IU. The prothrombin time is less commonly elevated. Several days later, conjugated hyperbilirubinemia develops.[63] These laboratory abnormalities usually resolve rapidly when normal hemodynamic parameters and oxygenation are restored. Fulminant hepatic failure has only rarely been associated with ischemic hepatitis.[64]

Viral Hepatitis

Viral hepatitis contracted in the perioperative period does not manifest itself immediately after surgery. The two major parenterally transmitted viruses causing hepatitis, hepatitis B and C, both have an incubation period of several weeks. Moreover, the risk of transfusion-associated hepatitis has been reduced dramatically over the last several years with the sequential introduction of screening for HBsAg, ALT, anti-HBc, anti-HIV, and most recently anti-HCV. The incidence of hepatitis B in this setting is now very low, and the overall risk of acquiring transfusion-related hepatitis has decreased from 10 percent to less than one percent in the last five years.[65,66]

Although patients may have viral hepatitis from parenteral exposure several weeks before surgery, the ability to make a diagnosis is limited by the long period of time before antibody to hepatitis C can be detected. Hepatitis C antibody, as measured by standard ELISA I procedures, does not develop for several months. Newer assays like RIBA II and ELISA II methods and more widespread use and improved specificity of assays measuring hepatitis C viral RNA (e.g., polymerase chain reaction techniques) should allow detection of viremia at the time of clinically apparent infection. Using tests for hepatitis B surface antigen and antibody and IgM core antibody, one can detect hepatitis B infection within six weeks of infection.

Viral hepatitis is notable for high elevations in transaminase levels similar to those in ischemic hepatitis and toxic injury. These elevations resolve more slowly than those seen with ischemia, but it may be difficult to distinguish them from those seen in massive necrosis due to toxins. Moreover, the later rise in bilirubin level seen in viral hepatitis usually marks resolution of the disease.

Chronic Liver Disease

Cirrhosis is difficult to diagnose in clinically compensated patients and may first become apparent during or after surgery. Patients with well-compensated cirrhosis may not demonstrate any of the usual clinical signs of chronic liver disease and may have normal or near-normal synthetic function as indicated by serum albumin level and prothrombin time. However, any major stress like surgery may tax minimal hepatic reserve and lead to clinically apparent liver disease with ascites or encephalopathy or aberrant laboratory studies in the postoperative period. This situation requires a complete evaluation of all causes of chronic liver disease. A liver biopsy is often required and is most expeditiously performed during surgery if the liver appears grossly abnormal. With supportive care, patients in this setting may often return to their preoperative status.

Medications

Drug-induced hepatotoxicity may present with features resembling viral hepatitis. Clinical jaundice due to hepatocellular injury is associated with a higher morbidity and mortality than drug-induced cholestatic jaundice.[12] Medications commonly used in the perioperative period associated with predominantly hepatocellular reactions include cardioactive agents such as alpha-methyldopa, amiodarone, calcium channel blockers, hydralazine, procainamide, and quinidine; antimicrobials such as isoniazid, ketoconazole, rifampin, sulfonamides, and sulfones; and the antiepileptics phenytoin and valproic acid.[12]

The role of halothane in the development of postoperative liver disease has been controversial for decades. Hepatitis associated with halothane is rare with an incidence of approximately 1:10,000.[10] Obese middle-aged females have an increased risk, but preexisting liver disease does not predispose patients to halothane hepatotoxicity. Halothane-related hepatitis is characterized by fever, malaise, and eosinophilia occurring within one to several weeks after initial exposure, and jaundice following 3 to 10 days later.[67–70] Laboratory studies usually demonstrate conjugated hyperbilirubinemia, high serum transaminase levels, and a modestly elevated serum alkaline phosphatase concentration. An immunologic mechanism for halothane-induced liver damage is supported by the increased risk of recurrence, shortened asymptomatic period after repeat exposures, and cross-sensitization to other halogenated anesthetics.[71–74] There is no specific therapy for halothane-related hepatitis, and it is treated with supportive care.[75] When complicated by jaundice, mortality approaches 20 percent.[76] Other poor prognostic signs are a prolonged prothrombin time and the development of hepatic encephalopathy.[76]

As in other drug-related hepatotoxicity, there are no specific laboratory tests or liver biopsy findings pathognomonic of medication-induced hepatocellular injury from halothane or other medications. In suspected cases, the most likely offending agent(s) should be withdrawn while other etiologies are excluded.

"PREHEPATIC" JAUNDICE

The term "prehepatic" jaundice refers to conditions in which the capacity of the liver to conjugate bilirubin is exceeded. It is characterized by indirect hyperbilirubinemia of less than five to six mg/dl and normal or slightly elevated levels of alkaline phosphatase and ALT. Precipitating events can often be identified and corrected without endoscopic or surgical intervention. Bilirubin overproduction results from hemolysis of circulating red blood cells or phagocytic breakdown of extravasated red blood cells in an extravascular collection. The normal liver can conjugate and excrete more than the 250 mg of bilirubin produced daily, and only acute or massive red cell destruction results in clinical jaundice. Laboratory evidence of red cell breakdown is manifested by reticulocytosis, increased levels of AST and lactate dehydrogenase, and consumption of serum haptoglobin. Direct bilirubin levels may rise proportionally to those of indirect unconjugated bilirubin.[1] Hemoglobinuria may occur as a result of rapid intravascular hemolysis.

Red Cell Hemolysis

Acquired hemolytic disorders, precipitated by transfusions, medications, and trauma to red blood cells, are often suggested by their temporal relationship to the development of postoperative jaundice. Bilirubin overproduction related to hemolysis after blood transfusions is the most common cause of jaundice in the first week after surgery.[77,78] Hemolysis of senescent red cells in stored whole blood can result in significant bilirubin overload when patients receive multiple transfusions. Alternatively, massive hemolysis can occur within minutes to hours after transfusion of incompatible blood products. Finally, an amnestic antibody response, undetected by routine compatibility testing, can occur approximately one week after transfusion.

Numerous medications may be associated with acquired hemolytic anemia. Immune hemolysis can be the result of autoimmune phenomena after taking drugs like alpha-methyldopa. Antibodies can also bind to red blood cells (e.g., penicillins) or plasma proteins (e.g., sulfonamides, phenothiazines, and quinidine) and cause hemolysis. Red cells can be mechanically destroyed by shear forces induced by valvular prosthesis or cardiopulmonary bypass equipment and by microvascular thrombi in disseminated intravascular coagulation complicating sepsis. Hemolysis due to congenital red cell disorders may also cause postoperative jaundice. While a history of sickle cell disease or thalassemia is usually easily obtained in adults, dramatic intravascular hemolysis from unsuspected glucose-6-phosphate-dehydrogenase deficiency may be precipitated by infection or challenge with oxidant drugs like azulfidine, sulfonamides, sulfones, nitrofurantoin, chloramphenicol, or acetylsalicylic acid.[79]

Resorption of Hematomas

In trauma surgery or procedures complicated by significant hematoma formation, bilirubin production from resorption of extravasated erythrocytes can cause "prehepatic" jaundice. This is often suspected because of the specifics of the surgical procedure. On physical examination, blue periumbilical discoloration (Cullen's sign) or purple or grey-brown flank discoloration (Turner's sign) reflect hemoperitoneum and catabolism of hemoglobin.

Gilbert's Syndrome

Bilirubin overload or the stress of anesthesia and surgery may unmask Gilbert's syndrome, a benign congenitally acquired impairment in bile pigment clearance affecting three to seven percent of otherwise healthy adults.[80–82] This disorder most likely reflects an inherited conjugating enzyme defect.[84] Patients may provide a positive family history or describe prior episodes of transient jaundice following prolonged fasting, strenuous exercise, or significant infection. The diagnosis of Gilbert's syndrome is made by excluding other causes of prehepatic jaundice and structural liver disease rather than by actually measuring hepatic bilirubin clearance or glucuronyltransferase activity. Elevations in unconjugated bilirubin levels usually resolve as the patient resumes feeding, and further evaluation is not necessary.

SUMMARY

1. A careful history, physical examination, and liver function studies allow classification of patients with postoperative jaundice into three categories: cholestatic (extrahepatic or intrahepatic), hepatocellular, and prehepatic.

2. Diagnostic testing may include evaluation of the hepatobiliary tree by ultrasound or other means (ERCP, CT, PTC), but liver biopsy is rarely helpful in acute management. The goal of diagnosis is to identify the small subset of patients who may require invasive interventions like ERCP or surgery for extrahepatic obstruction and those who may benefit from drug withdrawal, antibiotic therapy, or improvement in cardiovascular and pulmonary function.

3. Because bilirubin is not toxic in adults and clears slowly, general supportive care and observation usually suffice after correctable etiologies are excluded. Jaundice frequently resolves with overall clinical improvement without conclusive diagnosis.

REFERENCES

1. Blankaert N, Fevery J: Physiology and pathophysiology of bilirubin metabolism, in Zakim D, Boyer TD (eds): *Hepatology*. Philadelphia, Saunders, 1990, pp 254–302.
2. Berk PD, Howe RB, Bloomer JR et al: Studies of bilirubin kinetics in normal adults. *J Clin Invest* 48:2176, 1969.
3. Brodersen R: Bilirubin diglucuronide in normal human blood serum. *Scand J Clin Lab Invest* 18:361, 1966.
4. Blankaert N, Kabra PM, Farina FA et al: Measurement of bilirubin and its monoconjugates and diconjugates in human serum by alkaline methanolysis and high-performance liquid chromatography. *J Lab Clin Med* 96:198, 1980.
5. Capron JP, Gineston JL, Herve MA et al: Metronidazole in the prevention of cholestasis associated with total parenteral nutrition. *Lancet* 1:446, 1983.
6. Weiss JS, Gautam A, Lauff JJ et al: The clinical importance of a protein-bound fraction of serum bilirubin in patients with hyperbilirubinemia. *N Engl J Med* 309:147–150, 1983.
7. Clarke RSJ, Doggart JR, Lavery T: Changes in liver function after different types of surgery. *Br J Anaesth* 48:119–127, 1976.
8. Evans C, Evans M, Pollack AV: The incidence and causes of postoperative jaundice: A prospective study. *Br J Anaesth* 46:520–529, 1974.
9. Chu C-M, Chang C-H, Liaw Y-F et al: Jaundice after open heart surgery: A prospective study. *Thorax* 39:52–56, 1984.
10. Cooperman LH, Wollman H, Marsh ML: Anesthesia and the liver. *Surg Clin N Am* 57:421–428, 1977.
11. Garrison RN, Cryer HM, Howard DA et al: Clarification of risk factors for abdominal operations in patients with hepatic cirrhosis. *Ann Surg* 199:649–655, 1984.
12. Lewis JH, Zimmerman HJ: Drug-induced liver disease. *Med Clin N Am* 73:775–792, 1989.
13. Zimmerman HJ: *Hepatotoxity: The Adverse Effects of Drugs and Other Chemicals on the Liver*. New York, Appleton-Century-Crofts, 1978.
14. Zimmerman HJ, Lewis JH: Drug-induced cholestasis. *Med Toxicol* 2:112–160, 1982.
15. Lockey E, McIntyre H, Ross DN et al: Early jaundice after open heart surgery. *Thorax* 22:165–169, 1967.
16. Davidoff AM, Pappas TN, Murray EA et al: Mechanisms of major biliary injury during laparoscopic cholecystectomy. *Ann Surg* 215:196–202, 1992.
17. Greenway CV, Lautt WW: Blood volume, the venous system, pre-load, and cardiac output. *Can J Phys Pharm* 64:383, 1986
18. Ngal SH: Effects of anesthetics on various organs. *N Engl J Med* 302:564, 1980.
19. Seetharam S, Sussman NL, Komoda T et al: The mechanism of elevated alkaline phosphatase activity after bile duct ligation in the rat. *Hepatology* 6:374–380, 1986.
20. Patwardhan RV, Smith OJ, Framelant MH: Serum transaminase levels and cholescintigraphic abnormalities in acute biliary tract obstruction. *Arch Int Med* 147:1249, 1987.
21. Lapis JL, Orlando RC, Mittelstaedt CA et al: Ultrasonography in the diagnosis of obstructive jaundice. *Ann Int Med* 89:61, 1978.
22. Jeffrey RB et al: Computed tomography of choledocholithiasis. *AJR* 140:1179, 1983.
23. Pedrosa CS et al: Computed tomography in obstructive jaundice: The level of obstruction. *Radiology* 139:635, 1981.
24. Baker AL, Rosenberg IH: Hepatic complications of total parenteral nutrition. *Am J Med* 82:489–497, 1987.

25. Estrada WN, Zanzi T, Ward R et al: Scintigraphic evaluation of post-operative complications of laparoscopic cholecystectomy. *J Nucl Med* 32:1910–1911, 1991.

26. Walker AT, Shapiro AW, Brooks DC et al: Bile duct disruption and biloma after laparoscopic cholecystectomy: Imaging evaluation. *AJR* 158:785–789, 1992.

27. Neoptolemos JP, Carr-Locke DL, London NJ et al: Controlled trial of urgent endoscopic retrograde cholangiopancreatography and endoscopic sphincterotomy versus conservative treatment of acute pancreatitis due to gallstones. *Lancet* 2:9879–9883, 1988.

28. Vermillon SE, Greff JA, Baggenstoss AH et al: Jaundice associated with bacteremia. *Arch Int Med* 124:611–616, 1969.

29. Miller DJ, Keeton GR, Webber BL et al: Jaundice in severe bacterial infection. *Gastroenterology* 71:94–97, 1976.

30. Zimmerman HJ, Fang F, Utili R et al: Jaundice due to bacterial infection. *Gastroenterol* 77:362–374, 1979.

31. Utili R, Abernathy CO, Zimmerman HJ: Cholestatic effects of *Escherichia coli* endotoxin on the isolated perfused rat liver. *Gastroenterology* 70:248–253, 1976.

32. Banks JG, Foulis AK, Ledingham AMcA et al: Liver function in septic shock. *J Clin Path* 35:1249–1252, 1982.

33. Fang MH, Ginsberg AL, Dobbins WO: Marked elevation in serum alkaline phosphatase activity as a manifestation of systemic infection. *Gastroenterology* 78:592–597, 1980.

34. Johnson LB: The importance of early diagnosis of acute acalculous cholecystitis. *Surg Gynecol Ob* 164:197–203, 1987.

35. Howard RJ, Delaney JP: Postoperative cholecystitis. *Am J Dig Dis* 17:213–218, 1972.

36. Bushnell DL et al: The rim sign: Association with acute cholecystitis. *J Nucl Med* 27:353, 1986.

37. Brachman MB et al: Acute gangrenous cholecystitis: Radionuclide diagnosis. *Radiology* 151:209, 1984.

38. Freeze RC, Nogorney DM, Mucha P: Acute acalculous cholecystitis. *Mayo Clin Proc* 64:163, 1989.

39. Mirvis SE, Vainright JR, Nelson AW et al: The diagnosis of acute acalculous cholecystitis: A comparison of sonography, scintigraphy, and CT. *AJR* 147:1171–1175, 1986.

40. Editorial: The spectrum of jaundice. *N Engl J Med* 276:635, 1967.

41. Caroli J, Paraf A, Champeau J et al: Les icterese de la gastrectomie. *Arch Mal App Dig* 39:1057–1085, 1950.

42. Sevett S: Hepatic jaundice after blood transfusion in injured and burned subjects. *Br J Surg* 46:68–74, 1958.

43. Schmid M, Hefti ML: Benign postoperative jaundice, a form of intrahepatic cholestasis. *Gastroenterology* 4:89, 1966.

44. Schniefers KH, Wenn B: Icterus following operative interventions. *Dtsch Med Wochenschr* 92:540, 1967.

45. Pichimayr I, Stich W: Der bilirubenostatische ikterus, eine neue ikterusform beim zusammentraffen von operation, narkose und bluttransfusion. *Klin Wochenschr* 13:665, 1962.

46. Hartley S, Scott AJ, Spence M: Benign postoperative jaundice complication in severe trauma. *NZ Med J* 86:174–178, 1977.

47. Stasberg SM, Silver MD: Postoperative hepatogenic jaundice. *Surg Gynecol Obstet* 1:81–86, 1971.

48. Kantrowitz PA, Jones WA, Greenberger NG et al: Severe postoperative hyperbilirubinemia simulating obstructive jaundice. *N Engl J Med* 276:591–598, 1967.

49. King PD, Blitzer BL: Drug-induced cholestasis: Pathogenesis and clinical features. *Sem Liv Dis* 10:316–321, 1990.

50. Kaplowitz N: Drug-induced hepatotoxicity. *Ann Int Med* 104:826–839, 1986.

51. Snover DC: *Biopsy Diagnosis of Liver Disease*. Baltimore, Williams & Wilkins, 1992.

52. Fisher RL: Hepatobiliary abnormalities associated with total parenteral nutrition. *Gastroenterol Clin N Am* 18:645–666, 1989.

53. Sheldon GF, Peterson SR, Sanders R: Hepatic dysfunction during hyperalimentation. *Arch Surg* 113:504–508, 1978.

54. Leaseburge LA, Winn NJ, Schloerb PR: Liver test alterations with total parenteral nutrition and nutritional status. *JPEN* 16:348–352, 1992.

55. Fouin-Fortunet H, LeQuernec L, Erlinger S et al: Hepatic alterations during total parenteral nutrition in patients with inflammatory bowel disease: A possible consequence of lithocholate toxicity. *Gastroenterology* 82:932–937, 1982.

56. Craig RM, Neuman T, Jeipebhoy RN et al: Severe hepatocellular reaction resembling alcoholic hepatitis with cirrhosis after massive small bowel resection and prolonged total parenteral nutrition. *Gastroenterology* 79:131–137, 1980.

57. Buzby GP, Mullen JL, Stein TP et al: Manipulation of TPN caloric substrate and fatty infiltration of the liver. *J Surg Res* 31:46–54, 1981.

58. Allardyce DB: Cholestasis caused by lipid emulsions. *Surg Gynecol Obstet* 54:641–647, 1982.

59. Burt ME, Hanin I, Brennan MF: Choline deficiency associated with total parenteral nutrition. *Lancet* 2:638–639, 1980.

60. Worthley LG, Fishlock RC, Snoswell AW: Carnitine deficiency with hyperbilirubinemia, a generalized skeletal muscle weakness and reactive hypoglycemia in a patient on long-term TPN treatment with intravenous L-carnitine. *JPEN* 7:176–180, 1983.

61. Doty JE, Pitt HA, Porter-Fink V: Cholecystokinin prophylaxis of parenteral nutrition–induced gallbladder disease. *Ann Surg* 210:76–80, 1985.

62. Sitzmann JV, Pitt HA, Steinborn PA et al: Cholecystokinin prevents parenteral nutrition–induced biliary sludge in humans. *Surg Gynecol Obstet* 170:25–31, 1990.

63. Cohen JA, Kaplan MM: Left-sided heart failure presenting as hepatitis. *Gastroenterology* 74:583–587, 1978.

64. Kaymakcalan H, Dourdourekas D, Szanto PB et al: Congestive heart failure as cause of fulminant hepatic failure. *Am J Med* 65:384–388, 1978.

65. Genesca J, Esteban JI, Alter HT: Blood-borne non-A, non-B hepatitis: Hepatitis C. *Sem Liver Dis* 11:147–164, 1991.

66. Alter HJ: Clinical, virological, and epidemiological basis for the treatment of chronic non A, non B hepatitis. *J Hepatol* 11(Suppl 1):S19–S25, 1990.

67. Bottiger LE, Dalen E, Hallen B: Halothane-induced liver damage: An analysis of the material reported to the Swedish Adverse Drug Reaction Committee, 1966–1973. *Acta Anaesth Scand* 20:40–46, 1976.

68. Wright R, Chisholm M, Lloyd B et al: Controlled prospective study of the effect on liver function of multiple exposures to halothane. *Lancet* 1:817–820, 1975.

69. Fee JPH, Black GW, Dundee JW: A prospective study of liver enzyme and other changes following repeat administration of halothane and enflurane. *Br J Anaesth* 51:1133–1139, 1979.

70. Sherlock S: Halothane hepatitis. *Lancet* 1:364–365, 1978.

71. Schlippert W, Anuras S: Recurrent hepatitis following halothane exposures. *Am J Med* 65:25–30, 1978.

72. Reynolds ES, Brown BR, Vandam LD: Massive hepatic necrosis after fluroxene anesthesia—a case of drug interaction? *N Engl J Med* 286:530, 1972.

73. Joshi PH, Conn HO: The syndrome of methoxyflurane-associated hepatitis. *Ann Int Med* 80:395–401, 1974.

74. Neuberger J, Williams R: Halothane anesthesia and liver damage. *Br Med J* 289:1136–1139, 1984.

75. Becker SD, Lamont JT: Postoperative jaundice. *Sem Liv Dis* 8:183–190, 1988.

76. Moult PJA, Sherlock S: Halothane-related hepatitis. *Q J Med* 173:99–114, 1975.

77. Evans C, Evans M, Pollack AV: The incidence and causes of postoperative jaundice: A prospective study. *Br J Anaesth* 46:520–529, 1974.

78. Menitove JE: Blood transfusion, in Wyngaarden JB, Smith LH, Bennett JC (eds): *Textbook of Medicine*. Philadelphia, Saunders, 1992, pp 893–898.

79. Arese P, DeFlora A: Pathophysiology of hemolysis in glucose-6-

phosphate-dehydrogenase deficiency. *Sem Hematol* 27:1, 1990.

80. Quinn NW, Gollan JL: Jaundice following oral surgery: Gilbert's syndrome. *Br J Oral Surg* 12:285, 1975.

81. Berthelot P, Dhumeaux D: New insights into the classification of hereditary, chronic, non-hemolytic hyperbilirubinemias. *Gut* 19:474–480, 1978.

82. Berk PD, Bloomer JR, Howe RB et al: Constitutional hepatic dysfunction (Gilbert's syndrome): A new definition based on kinetic studies with unconjugated radiobilirubin. *Am J Med* 49:296, 1970.

83. Feisher BF, Craig JR, Carpio N: Hepatic bilirubin glucuronidation in Gilbert's syndrome. *J Lab Clin Med* 81:829, 1973.

70 POSTOPERATIVE DELIRIUM

James L. Stinnett

Loren M. Freimuth

Steven A. Silber

Patients may exhibit changes in affect, behavior, and thinking after surgery. In many cases these are manifestations of delirium, a mental disorder due to organic impairment in brain function. Physiological and behavioral changes accompanying delirium can complicate the postoperative course and significantly increase morbidity. Delirium may be the first sign of a systemic disorder unmasked by the stress of surgery. This chapter focuses on the recognition, causes, and treatment of postoperative delirium.

INCIDENCE AND DEFINITION

The incidence of postoperative delirium varies with the type of surgery performed and various risk factors. In a group of 57,600 surgical patients, the incidence of severe postoperative mental changes was 1 in 1600.[1] Of 36 cases of severe psychiatric disturbance, 12 to 33 percent were classified as confusional states. In another study of 150 consecutive psychiatric consultations on a teaching hospital surgery service over a two-year period, 20.7 percent of the patients were diagnosed with delirium with 87.1 percent occurring in the postoperative period.[2] Significant mental status changes including delirium have been observed in patients following cardiac, ophthalmologic, orthopedic, abdominal, and gynecological procedures.

Specific operative procedures are associated with a high incidence of postoperative delirium. Although the incidence of delirium among general surgical patients is less than 0.19 percent, the rate of postcardiotomy delirium at one time was 38 to 59 percent[3] but has decreased to 24 to 32 percent as operative techniques have improved.[4,5] The rate is higher in aortic or multiple valve replacement than in mitral valve replacement.[4] However, postoperative psychosis is more common in valvular surgery of any type than in coronary artery bypass procedures.[6]

The recent Diagnostic and Statistical Manual of Mental Disorders (DSM-III-R) of the American Psychiatric Association lists five specific criteria for the diagnosis of delirium:[7]

A. Reduced ability to maintain attention to external stimuli (e.g., questions must be repeated because attention wanders) and to appropriately shift attention to new external stimuli (e.g., perseverates answer to a previous question)

B. Disorganized thinking, as indicated by rambling, irrelevant or incoherent speech

C. At least two of the following:
   1. Reduced level of consciousness, e.g., difficulty keeping awake during examination
   2. Perceptual disturbances, e.g., misinterpretations, illusions, or hallucinations
   3. Disturbance of sleep-wake cycle with insomnia or daytime sleepiness
   4. Increased or decreased psychomotor activity
   5. Disorientation to time, place, or person
   6. Memory impairment, e.g., inability to learn new material such as the names of several unrelated objects after five minutes or to remember past events such as history of current episode of iilness

D. Clinical features develop over a short period of time (usually hours to days) and tend to fluctuate over the course of a day

E. Either 1. or 2.:
   1. Evidence from the history, physical examination, or laboratory tests of a specific organic factor or factors judged to be etiologically related to the disturbance
   2. In the absence of such evidence, an etiologic organic factor can be presumed if the disturbance cannot be accounted for by a nonorganic mental disorder, e.g., manic episode accounting for agitation and sleep disturbance

The DSM-III-R criteria present a rather narrow definition of delirium in comparison with others that include psychologic as well as organic factors. Unlike functional or psychogenic psycho-

699

sis, delirium includes deficits in higher cortical functioning such as decreased memory, disorders of consciousness, and disorientation in addition to alterations in normal metabolic and physiologic processes, correction of which results in return to baseline mental status.

Delirium should also be distinguished from dementia, another organic brain disorder with multiple causes. Although the hallmark of dementia is a decrease in memory and cognitive functioning, it differs from delirium in several ways. Unless severe, dementia does not impair the level of consciousness or orientation. Dementia develops gradually and follows a chronically progressive time course while delirium develops acutely with fluctuating levels of alertness and disorientation. In any case, when mental status is altered, dementia should always be considered.

The central feature of delirium is a clouded state of consciousness or change in level of awareness.[8,9] Patients find it hard to shift, focus, and sustain attention and have difficulty in screening out irrelevant and distracting stimuli. This can be tested by asking the patient to pick a certain letter from a group, subtract serial sevens, or repeat a series of digits forward and backward.

The most common variant of psychomotor abnormality in delirium is characterized by aroused, agitated, or poorly organized behavior which is not goal-directed. Occasionally, patients demonstrate purposeless stereotyped movements such as repetitive picking at their bedclothes. In some cases, agitation progresses to destructive activities including jumping out of bed or pulling out intravenous lines. Delirium tremens due to abstinence from alcohol is the prototype of hyperactive delirium.

Hypoactive or "quiet" delirium is characterized by stupor and apathy. It is often overlooked because it is rarely accompanied by overtly abnormal behavior. On an inpatient unit, the quiet "good" patients are assumed to have normal cerebral function. However, one need only ask them a few questions to realize that they are delirious.

Altered perceptions in delirium may be expressed as illusions or hallucinations. A shadow on the wall interpreted as an attacking animal is an example of an illusion. Seeing threatening people when in fact no one is present is an example of an hallucination. The reality of the hallucination to the patient may lead to emotional and behavioral responses consistent with the altered perception.

Hallucinations are usually visual but may be auditory, tactile, gustatory, olfactory, or proprioceptive. The clinician should specifically ask patients about any unusual perceptions such as hearing voices or seeing things. Sometimes they deny these experiences because they are frightened or confused by them. However, behavior usually serves to alert the clinician to active hallucination. For example, a patient may turn his head from side to side in response to perceived voices.

Delirious patients may exhibit disorganized and tangential thinking and difficulty in relating to the environment. They may be disoriented to time, place, or person and suffer loss of short- and long-term memory. Short-term memory loss is common and can be tested by asking the patient independently verifiable questions. If the patient's concentration and attention are seriously impaired, testing of orientation or memory may be impossible. Delirious patients occasionally manifest a reversal of the sleep-wakefulness cycle with nighttime insomnia and daytime drowsiness.

Delirium develops over a short period of time and fluctuates in severity. Patients may appear lucid at one point during the day and disoriented several hours later. During a lucid interval, the clinician may conclude that initial diagnostic impressions may have been erroneous or the process causing the initial change in mental status may have been corrected. The patient should therefore be evaluated at various times during the day. The "sundowning syndrome" is an example of the fluctuating nature of delirium. In the evening, formerly lucid patients may suddenly become confused and agitated because of sensory deprivation. The same behavior can be precipitated by drugs, particularly central nervous system (CNS) depressants, which alter sensory input or interfere with cognitive integration.

Delirium causes significant morbidity, particularly in postoperative or intensive care settings. It is difficult for delirious patients to cooperate with and participate in their care. Agitation and increased motor activity may interfere with vital monitoring functions or life support systems, occasionally with catastrophic results. Those who are extremely agitated sometimes need to be restrained and sedated. These treatments carry their own morbidity in increasing the risk of atelectasis, thrombophlebitis, and pulmonary embolism.

Clinical lore suggests that there may be long-term morbidity from episodes of delirium. Some patients who have been delirious and recover have varying degrees of recollection and sometimes remember the experience as a frightening or confusing time in their life. The episode may have significant impact on their self-image and make them wonder if they will "go crazy" at some time in the future. It is therefore important to discuss the event with the patient after recovery.

Unfortunately, delirium is still variably defined and only incompletely understood. Many clinical studies are retrospective in nature, lack precision, and are limited in their application. With wider acceptance of the DSM-III-R diagnostic criteria, increased understanding of delirium should follow.

BIOLOGICAL CAUSES OF POSTOPERATIVE DELIRIUM

Postoperative delirium is the result of interaction among various biological, psychological, and socioenvironmental factors and is rarely caused by one factor alone. Although any of these factors can alter mental status, some are more common after surgery. Previously occult or compensated pathophysiologic processes may be exacerbated by the stress of the operation. The physician should therefore approach the delirious postoperative patient as any other with acute alteration in mental status, with special attention to factors specific to the preoperative setting and intraoperative events.

Preoperative Factors

Any pathophysiologic process directly or indirectly affecting brain function before surgery can predispose a patient to postoperative delirium. Age itself is a critical factor. The incidence of postoperative delirium increases markedly in patients over the age of

45.[3,5,10] In one study, the prevalence of postoperative delirium was approximately five times greater in those over 60. Medical illness and physical complications are often associated with delirium.[11]

Organic brain syndrome is the most common antecedent medical condition in patients with postoperative changes in mental status. The differential diagnosis of organic brain syndrome is extensive but can be divided into several broad categories:

1. *Vascular disease.* Patients with disorders affecting the cerebral circulation usually have focal neurological signs. However, if vascular disease affects only certain areas of the cortex, it may only cause a deficit in higher cortical functions such as orientation, memory, and ability to think in abstract terms. So-called "multi-infarct dementia" is characterized by a stuttering progression of language difficulty, confusion, and occasionally transient sensory and motor deficits.

2. *Infections and inflammatory processes.* Bacterial, fungal, and viral infections and the inflammatory processes seen in disorders like lupus cerebritis should all be considered. Of particular note is the encephalopathy seen with HIV infection.

3. *Neoplasm.* Many tumors of the central nervous system may present initially with deficits of higher cortical functioning. Some like meningiomas may be amenable to surgical correction which may reverse the organic brain disorder.

4. *Degenerative disorders.* These include senile dementia, Alzheimer's disease, and Pick's disease.

5. *Normal pressure hydrocephalus.* This disorder of cerebral spinal fluid circulation is characterized by the triad of dementia, urinary incontinence, and gait disturbance.

6. *Congenital.* A number of congenital abnormalities may be seen in adults, including Huntington's chorea.

7. *Trauma.* Closed-head trauma and the possibility of epidural or subdural hematoma should always be considered. Elderly patients, alcoholics, and those taking anticoagulants have a higher risk of trauma and intracranial bleeding.

8. *Intoxication or withdrawal.* The effects of drugs and their withdrawal may constitute the most common cause of delirium and dementia in hospitalized patients. Many medications have central nervous system effects even in small doses and include cardiac drugs like digoxin and procainamide, CNS drugs like bromocriptine and anticonvulsants, and gastrointestinal drugs like anticholinergic agents and H_2 antagonists. Withdrawal of drugs and alcohol also commonly contributes to CNS dysfunction.

9. *Vitamin deficiency.* Deficiencies of folate and B_{12} are among the most well-known causes of delirium and dementia. Thiamine deficiency can result in the acute confusional state of Wernicke's syndrome. Pyridoxine and niacin deficiency can also produce dementia.

10. *Endocrine/metabolic.* Excessive or deficient levels of thyroid, parathyroid, and adrenal hormones as well as hypoglycemia and hyperglycemia commonly cause CNS dysfunction. Common metabolic etiologies include hypoxia, hypercarbia, electrolyte abnormalities, hypo- or hyperosmolarity, acid-base abnormalities, and hepatic dysfunction. Rare forms of liver disease include Wilson's disease and acute intermittent porphyria.

Intraoperative Factors

Several intraoperative factors play a role in the development of postoperative delirium. Unexpected transient hypotension or hypoxemia can cause cerebral anoxia and lead to postoperative changes in mental status. When the etiology of postoperative mental changes is unclear, a thorough review of the surgical record in consultation with the anesthesiologist may be rewarding.

Drugs administered in the perioperative period may cause mental status changes. In patients with underlying cardiac, renal, or hepatic disease, metabolism and elimination of sedatives, narcotics, and barbiturates may be impaired, leading to high serum levels and prolonged effects. These drugs have all been associated with dose-dependent paradoxical reactions, especially in elderly patients with intrinsic brain disease.

The type of surgical procedure may be related to the development of delirium. As noted above, postcardiotomy delirium has been extensively studied. The duration of surgery and the degree of hypothermia may be predisposing factors.[6,12] The length of time on cardiopulmonary bypass may correlate with the incidence of development of postcardiotomy delirium, but this remains controversial.[5,6,10,13,14] Although older patients and men have an increased risk of developing it, children under 14 rarely do so. Occult cerebrovascular disease and intraoperative cerebral ischemia may contribute to the syndrome.[5,12,14] The severity of preoperative illness and the presence of antecedent organic brain disease or chronic psychiatric illness are probably contributing factors.[5,15]

In one study, autopsies of patients who had developed inappropriate behavior or abnormal neurologic changes after cardiac surgery demonstrated definite CNS lesions in 90 percent.[13] The most common findings were anoxic changes in the hippocampus, diffuse foci of infarction in the gray matter, and areas of perivascular tissue damage in the white matter. The authors found that the presence of neurologic dysfunction strongly correlated with age and the degree and duration of intraoperative hypotension on bypass. Inadequate cerebral perfusion during bypass may also result from microemboli that form as blood passes through the oxygenator. In animal studies, this microembolic encephalopathy has been avoided by blood filtration.[16] Emboli generated during intracardiac manipulations in valvular heart surgery may explain the increased incidence of postoperative psychosis in these procedures as compared to coronary artery bypass.

"Black-patch delirium," frequently seen in elderly patients after ophthalmologic surgery, may be due to sensory deprivation, underlying organic brain syndrome, and in some cases toxicity from anticholinergic agents.[17,18] Parathyroid surgery has been associated with psychosis even when serum calcium and magnesium levels are normal. It may be due to fluctuating levels of calcium and magnesium levels in the brain that are not reflected in the serum.[19,20] Surgery perceived as particularly mutilating such as extensive head and neck dissection or procedures viewed as altering sexual function such as hysterectomy, mastectomy, or orchiectomy are associated with an increased incidence of postoperative depression.[21,22]

Postoperative Factors

Several important factors in the development of delirium after surgery require special attention. Myocardial depression and inappropriate volume replacement during surgery may lead to congestive heart failure and inadequate cerebral perfusion. Severe hypoxemia or hypercarbia may develop because of central hypoventilation, upper-airway obstruction, atelectasis, aspiration, pulmonary embolism, or splinting. A detailed neurologic exam should be performed to exclude the possibility of a perioperative cerebrovascular accident. Patients with abnormal mental status but no focal neurologic deficits always require further investigation.

Drug withdrawal can cause dramatic mental status changes in patients who chronically ingest alcohol, barbiturates, benzodiazepines, narcotics, or hypnotics. The physician is often unaware of the extent of preoperative drug or alcohol use either because the patient withholds information or an adequate drug and alcohol history could not be obtained. When drug withdrawal is suspected, it is important to review the drug history with family or friends.

Many drugs used in the perioperative period may cause or exacerbate delirium. Lidocaine, cimetidine, xanthine derivatives, atropine, alpha-methyldopa, propranolol, L-dopa, steroids, and digoxin have all been associated with toxic delirium. Drugs with anticholinergic activity are especially important in the development of postoperative delirium.[23,24] Obtaining serum drug levels is sometimes useful, but some medications like digoxin may cause toxicity at therapeutic levels. Patients may infrequently obtain illicit drugs from outside the hospital, and in such cases serum and urine toxicology screens may be useful.

Many metabolic abnormalities arising in the postoperative period can alter CNS function. Hyponatremia often accompanies edematous states or can result from adrenal insufficiency unmasked by the stress of surgery or injudicious use of hypotonic fluids when levels of antidiuretic hormone (ADH) are high. After surgery, pain itself stimulates the secretion of ADH from the hypothalamus. Drugs implicated in the syndrome of inappropriate ADH (SIADH) include morphine, chlorpropamide, vincristine, carbamazepine, and amitriptyline. The type and severity of neurological dysfunction vary with the degree of hyponatremia and the rapidity with which it develops. Lethargy, confusion, and coma occur with gradually progressive hyponatremia while agitation, irritability, and seizures accompany more rapid changes. Symptoms should not be ascribed to hyponatremia unless the serum sodium concentration is below 125 meq/liter.

Hyperosmolarity causes alterations in brain metabolism. Hypernatremia can result from excessive free water losses and salt administration in patients who have impairment of thirst or no access to water and is commonly seen with prolonged tube feeding or intravenous hyperalimentation. Hyperosmolar nonketotic coma may occur in volume-depleted patients with maturity-onset diabetes stressed by surgery. The CNS signs of hyperosmolarity are similar to those of hyponatremia, ranging from agitation and confusion to seizure and coma.

Hypoglycemia with its attendant alterations in mental status may occur in insulin-dependent diabetics in the perioperative period when exogenous insulin requirements vary markedly. It rarely occurs in patients with advanced renal or hepatic failure and in those with large retroperitoneal tumors in whom it is unmasked by decreased oral intake after surgery.

Hypercalcemia due to hyperparathyroidism, multiple myeloma, occult neoplasm, or immobilization may be exacerbated by mild volume depletion in the perioperative period and lead to a variety of psychiatric syndromes. Severe hypophosphatemia with serum phosphate concentrations of less than one mg/dl in malnourished or debilitated patients causes weakness, lethargy, confusion, and

sometimes even coma. Encephalopathy has been associated with increased D-lactate levels after gastrointestinal procedures like jejunoileal bypass.[25] Increased serum beta-endorphin and cortisol levels may also correlate with delirium after surgery.[26] Acid-base disturbances due to a variety of causes may contribute to postoperative changes in mental status.

Delirium may be the first sign of impending sepsis. Fever and leukocytosis may be absent in elderly, debilitated, or catabolic surgical patients. Postoperative CNS infections are uncommon except after specific neurosurgical or head and neck procedures. However, altered mental status and other signs of systemic infection without an identifiable source necessitate diagnostic lumbar puncture.

Psychologic and Environmental Causes

There is controversy concerning the role of anxiety in the pathogenesis of postoperative psychologic changes. Some contend that anxiety generated by a realistic appraisal of what surgery involves is associated with good psychologic adaptation in the postoperative period. Others stress the role of denial as the dominant mechanism for coping with the stress of surgery. In such cases, anxiety levels are low, and the postoperative course is often smooth.[10,14]

The patient's perception of the real and symbolic meaning of the organ or part of the body involved in surgery is an important factor. Patients undergoing cardiac surgery may be especially anxious because they perceive the heart to be the basis for life. Patients undergoing brain surgery may fear injury to the organ that contains the biologic substrate of all that is special and unique in being human. A woman undergoing a mastectomy or hysterectomy may feel that surgery will affect her body image and identity as a woman. A man undergoing an orchiectomy or other genitourinary procedure may feel that his manhood will be irrevocably altered. A person receiving an organ transplant may feel that his body has been invaded and is no longer entirely his own. Some patients with ostomies may suffer losses in self-esteem and changes in their sense of body integrity. Each of these reactions is highly individual, and there is a wide spectrum of responses to a given procedure.

The ability of the patient to adjust to the sick role is another factor that may contribute to the development of postoperative psychiatric illness. Relinquishing autonomy and becoming dependent on others for help with basic biologic functions such as eating, bathing, and toileting can be extremely stressful for some patients. Postoperative pain contributes to the overall psychologic burden, especially when inadequate amounts of analgesics are prescribed.[27] By increasing anxiety and sapping psychologic reserve, chronic unrelieved pain may lead to delirium in the immediate postoperative period.

Sleep deprivation is an important component of postoperative delirium. After surgery, many patients experience a sense of heightened vigilance and are afraid to fall asleep for fear of catastrophe or death. The constant high noise and activity levels and lack of light-dark cycles in intensive care units prevent patients from sleeping adequately. Studies of normal volunteers have shown that definite psychologic changes begin to occur after two to three days of total sleep deprivation,[28] and similar changes may develop in postoperative patients.[5,29,30] Some studies have found sleep loss to be a consequence and not a cause of postcardiotomy delirium.[31]

Others postulate fundamental impairment in the sleep-wake cycle after surgery.[32]

Environment plays a major role in the development of postoperative delirium. Most recovery rooms and intensive care units are frightening places in which sensory experience is markedly abnormal and characterized by deprivation of stimuli, overstimulation, or sensory monotony. Monitors and ventilators emit a constant monotonous sound. Time-orienting cues are absent, and lights are on around the clock. Modulated sensory input without extremes of sensory deprivation and overload are necessary for normal psychologic function. Patients who exhibit signs of postoperative delirium often improve when they are transferred to a regular hospital floor.

MANAGEMENT

Early recognition and treatment of patients with postoperative delirium is aimed at controlling behavior that might significantly interfere with postoperative care and uncovering and correcting underlying pathophysiologic processes. Preventive steps before surgery significantly decrease the incidence of postoperative delirium. Preoperative counseling by nurses and psychiatrists significantly decreases postoperative psychiatric complications.[33] Most surgical centers involved in open-heart surgery provide preoperative counseling to orient patients to the environment of the recovery room and intensive care unit and to the monitors, life-support systems, and therapeutic procedures to be used.

Once signs of delirium appear, neuroleptic drugs like haloperidol can be used. Haloperidol, a butyrophenone, is effective and safe in postoperative patients because it has little effect on blood pressure or respiratory drive. The drug is given in doses of 1 to 5 mg intramuscularly at a frequency determined by the response. In elderly or debilitated patients, the starting dose should be 0.5 mg. It should not be prescribed on a straight-order basis, since individual responses are difficult to predict. The patient should be reevaluated every one to two hours to allow appropriate dosage adjustments until adequate behavioral control is achieved. The most important target symptoms are hallucinations and confused thinking, and the therapeutic endpoint should be adequately controlled behavior conducive to good postoperative care. The medication should be continued until hallucinations have ceased and thought processes have returned to normal. Care should be taken to avoid neuroleptic-induced stupor.

Occasionally, marked psychomotor activity can constitute an emergency if a patient attempts to extubate himself or pulls out vital monitors or arterial lines. In these situations, immediate control of behavior is necessary. Cassem and Sos administered intravenous doses of haloperidol ranging from 5 to 185 mg over a 24-hour period to postcardiotomy patients in a surgical intensive care unit.[34] The usual intravenous dose of haloperidol is 2 to 5 mg every 30 to 60 minutes titrated to an endpoint of behavioral control. The drug had no significant effect on blood pressure, heart rate, or ventilation. Neurologic side effects including extrapyramidal signs were infrequent and mild. Dudley et al. used intravenous haloperidol in doses of up to 20 mg and achieved resolution of severe psychomotor agitation without significant cardiovascular or CNS toxicity.[35] Thus, intravenous haloperidol acts within two to five minutes in acute delirium and avoids the pain and inconvenience of repeated intramuscular injections.

Extrapyramidal signs, including acute dystonic reactions, parkinsonism-bradykinesia syndrome, and akathisia are documented side effects of haloperidol. Acute dystonia, also known as oculogyric crisis, is more frequently seen in men and occurs more often than parkinsonism. It is usually limited to muscle spasm of the face, tongue, jaw, or neck but occasionally causes painful flexion of the limbs. Dystonic reactions are rapidly reversed by parenteral administration of an anticholinergic drug such as benztropine in a dose of 1 to 3 mg. The parkinsonism-bradykinesia syndrome, consisting of decreased spontaneous movement, cog-wheel rigidity, and increased salivation with drooling can also be reversed by anticholinergic agents.

Akathisia is one of the most common and troubling side effects of the neuroleptic drugs. It is difficult to document because its manifestations consist of a subjective sense of anxiety, restlessness, tension, and an irresistible urge to move. The discomfort of these sensations is heightened in patients who must remain immobile after surgery. Akathisia responds to anticholinergic drugs, although less readily than acute dystonic reactions and parkinsonism. If anticholinergic drugs are ineffective, decreasing the dose of a neuroleptic or prescribing low doses of a beta-blocker like propranolol is often helpful.

Postoperative drug withdrawal can be life-threatening. If possible, the drug should be identified and restarted, especially in the case of barbiturate withdrawal which leads to agitation, delirium, weakness, hypotension, and seizures after 48 to 96 hours. For alcohol or other drug withdrawal syndromes, benzodiazepines like diazepam, chlordiazepoxide, and oxazepam are the treatment of choice. When given intramuscularly, they are poorly absorbed and produce unpredictable plasma levels,[36] and they should therefore be given orally or intravenously. In patients with liver disease who do not metabolize drugs normally, oxazepam is best because it has a short half-life and no pharmacologically active metabolites. Unlike other benzodiazepines, it is directly conjugated with glucuronide and does not require demethylation, deamination, and hydroxylation that may be impaired in those with hepatic dysfunction.[37] Phenothiazines should be avoided because they lower the seizure threshold.

Varying and controlling sensory input is important. Attempts should be made to enable postoperative patients to get uninterrupted sleep. Nursing procedures at night should be deferred if they are not critical for patient care. If the patient is in an intensive care unit, curtains should be drawn and lights dimmed at night to decrease sensory stimulation.

Sometimes simple interventions like a radio or television can have a salutary effect. Placing a calendar within view and marking off the days help patients to orient themselves in time. Familiar objects and pictures of family and friends provide significant comfort. Nursing personnel and family should be encouraged to keep the patient oriented frequently to time and place. Seeing the same nurses regularly helps the patient to develop a sense of trust and familiarity with the staff.

Nurses and physicians should reassure the patient that his confusing experience is temporary and does not signify mental illness. Staff should not assume that the delirious patient has no insight or awareness. After recovery, some patients reveal that they were aware of their confusion and were extremely frightened. If the experience is not acknowledged and explained by the staff, apprehension may increase and delirium may worsen.

SUMMARY

1. Delirium is a syndrome of higher cortical function deficits with acute onset and a fluctuating course. The major clinical features are alterations in consciousness, perception, attention, memory, orientation, and psychomotor behavior.

2. Advanced age, underlying intrinsic neurologic deficits, acute or chronic medical illnesses, and chronic psychiatric syndromes predict the development of postoperative delirium. The stress of surgery in patients with these conditions may be enough to produce delirium.

3. Hypoxemia, hypercarbia, hypotension, metabolic abnormalities, sepsis, and acute cerebrovascular accident must be excluded in patients with postoperative delirium.

4. Drug withdrawal must always be considered as a cause of postoperative delirium.

5. Haloperidol in appropriate doses is the drug of choice for the treatment of delirium.

REFERENCES

1. Knox SJ: Severe psychiatric disturbances in the postoperative period—a five-year survey of Belfast Hospital. *J Ment Sci* 107:1078, 1961.
2. Golinger, RC: Delirium in surgical patients seen at psychiatric consultation. *Surg Gyn Obs* 163(2):104–106, 1986.
3. Blachy PH, Starr A: Post-cardiotomy delirium. *Am J Psych* 121:371, 1964.
4. Heller SS, Frank KA, Malm JR et al: Psychiatric complications of open-heart surgery. *N Engl J Med* 283:1015, 1970.
5. Dimsdale, JE: Postcardiotomy delirium: Conclusions after 25 years? *Am J Psych* 146:4, 1989.
6. Rabiner CJ, Wallner AE, Fishman J et al: Psychiatric complications following coronary bypass surgery. *J Nerv Ment Dis* 160:342, 1975.
7. *Diagnostic and Statistical Manual of Mental Disorders*, 3d revision. Washington DC, American Psychiatric Association, 1987.
8. Lipowski ZJ: Delirium, clouding of consciousness and confusion. *J Nerv Ment Dis* 145:227, 1967.
9. Engel GL, Romano J: Delirium: A syndrome of cerebral insufficiency. *J Chron Dis* 9:260, 1959.
10. Morse RM, Litin E: Post-operative delirium: A study of etiologic factors. *Am J Psych* 126:388, 1969.
11. Millar HR: Psychiatric morbidity in elderly surgical patients. *Br J Psych* 138:17–20, 1981.
12. Kornfeld DS, Zimberg S, Malm JR et al: Psychiatric complications of open-heart surgery. *N Engl J Med* 273:287, 1965.
13. Tufo HM, Ostfeld AM, Shekelle R: Central nervous system dysfunction following open-heart surgery. *JAMA* 212:1333, 1970.
14. Layne OL, Yudofsky SC: Post-operative psychosis in cardiotomy patients. *N Engl J Med* 284:518, 1971.
15. Rubenstein D, Thomas K: Psychiatric findings in cardiotomy patients. *Am J Psych* 126:360, 1969.
16. Brennan RW, Patterson RH, Kessler J: Cerebral blood flow and metabolism during cardiopulmonary bypass: Evidence of microembolic encephalopathy. *Neurology* 21:665, 1971.
17. Summers WK, Reich TC: Delirium after cataract surgery: Review and two cases. *Am J Psych* 136:386, 1979.
18. Ziskind E, Jones H, Folante W: Observations and mental symptoms in eye patched patients: Hypnogogic symptoms in sensory deprivation. *Am J Psych* 116:893, 1960.
19. Mikkelsen EJ, Reider AA: Post-parathyroidectomy psychosis: Clinical and research implications. *J Clin Psych* 40(8):352–357, 1979.
20. Lawlor BA: Hypocalcemia, hypoparathyroidism, and organic anxiety syndrome. *J Clin Psych* 49(8):317–318, 1988.
21. Anath J: Hysterectomy and depression. *Obst Gyn* 52:724, 1978.
22. Lindemann E: Observations on psychiatric sequelae to surgical operations in women. *Am J Psych* 98:132, 1941.
23. Golinger RC: Association of elevated plasma anticholinergic activity with delirium in surgical patients. *Am J Psych* 144(9):1218–1220, 1987.
24. Tune LE, Holland H, Folstein M et al: Association of postoperative delirium with raised serum levels of anticholinergic drugs. *Lancet* 2(8248):651–653, 1981.
25. Thurn JR, Pierpont GL, Ludvigsen CW et al: D-lactate encephalopathy. *Am J Med* 79(6):717–721, 1985.
26. McIntosh TK, Bush HL, Yeston NS et al: Beta-endorphin, cortisol and postoperative delirium: A preliminary report. *Psychoneuroendocrinology* 10(3):303–313, 1985.
27. Marks RM, Sacher EJ: Undertreatment of medical inpatients with narcotic analgesics. *Ann Intern Med* 78:173, 1973.
28. Johnson LC: Psychological and physiological changes following total sleep deprivation, in Kales A (ed): *Sleep Physiology and Pathology: A Symposium*. Philadelphia, Lippincott, 1969, p 206.
29. Johns W, Large AA, Masterson JP et al: Sleep and delirium after open heart surgery. *Br J Surg* 61:377, 1974.
30. Sveinsson I: Postoperative psychosis after heart surgery. *J Thorac Cardiovasc Surg* 70:717, 1975.
31. Harrell RG: Postcardiotomy confusion and sleep loss. *J Clin Psychiatry* 48(11):445–446, 1987.
32. Aurell J, Elmqvist D: Sleep in the surgical intensive care unit: Continuous polygraphic recording of sleep in nine patients receiving postoperative care. *Br Med J* 290:1029–1032, 1985.
33. Lazarus HR, Hagens JH: Prevention of psychosis following open heart surgery. *Am J Psychiatry* 124:1190, 1968.
34. Cassem NH, Sos J: Intravenous use of haloperidol for acute delirium in intensive care settings (abstract). Presented at the 131st annual meeting of the American Psychiatric Association, Atlanta, GA, May 8–12, 1978.
35. Dudley DL, Rowlett DB, Loebel PJ: Emergency use of intravenous haloperidol. *Gen Hosp Psych* 1:240, 1979.
36. Greenblatt DJ, Shader RI, Koch-Weser J et al: Slow absorption of intramuscular chlordiazepoxide. *N Engl J Med* 291:116, 1974.
37. Greenblatt DJ, Shader RI: Pharmacokinetic understanding of antianxiety drug therapy. *South Med J* 71(Suppl):2, 1978.

71 NEUROLOGIC PROBLEMS IN THE POSTOPERATIVE PERIOD

Eric C. Raps

Steven L. Galetta

Michael E. Selzer

A wide variety of neurological complications may arise during or after surgery. These may involve the peripheral or central nervous systems and may result from the procedure itself, the anesthesia, exacerbation of preexisting conditions, or postoperative infection. This chapter discusses status epilepticus, malignant hyperthermia, neuroleptic malignant syndrome, peripheral nerve injury, infections of the nervous system, perioperative stroke, and brain death. Cerebrovascular complications are discussed extensively in Chap. 35.

STATUS EPILEPTICUS

Individual seizures occur infrequently in the perioperative period. They have several etiologies including the effects of certain anesthetics and analgesics.[1–5] Isolated seizures do not require treatment beyond immediate physical protective measures.

Status epilepticus is defined as the repetitive occurrence of seizures with sufficient frequency or duration to produce a prolonged continuous state of neurological dysfunction, often arbitrarily set at more than 30 minutes. Patients with seizure disorders that are otherwise well controlled may develop status epilepticus as a result of an acute febrile illness, head trauma, or an abrupt cessation of or change in anticonvulsant regimen. Consequently, there is increased risk of developing status epilepticus in the perioperative period. In addition, status epilepticus may result from cerebral ischemia due to episodes of hypotension, even in patients with no history of epilepsy. Whatever the etiology, status epilepticus can result in permanent neurological damage or even death. The mortality rate of status epilepticus is 10 to 12 percent even with treatment.[6] From a practical standpoint, patients with persistent seizures for 10 minutes should be treated emergently for status epilepticus.

The term status epilepticus usually refers to major motor or generalized tonic-clonic seizures following which seizures recur before the patient has regained full consciousness. However, other forms of seizures may be prolonged and repetitive. Focal status epilepticus refers to continuous partial seizures like focal motor or sensory seizures. Complex partial status epilepticus refers to continual complex partial seizures for more than 30 minutes. Patients may exhibit automatisms and clouding of consciousness that may fluctuate in a cyclical pattern. Petit mal status epilepticus refers to prolonged absence seizure activity accompanied by a continual three-per-second spike-wave abnormality on the electroencephalogram (EEG). In patients with severe encephalopathies, either traumatic or toxic/metabolic, the motor component may be very subtle, consisting of small focal movements that are often unilateral and nonrhythmic.[7] However, the EEG confirms generalized seizure activity and is often helpful in diagnosing otherwise mysterious postoperative obtundation.

During major motor seizures, patients may have prolonged periods of apnea. Vigorous muscular contractions and apnea result in lactic acidosis. Although a single seizure probably produces no lasting consequences unless the patient is injured by falling, the metabolic consequences of prolonged major motor seizure activity can be severe and result in permanent neurologic damage.[6,8] The extent to which the metabolic consequences of continual epileptic electrical activity in the brain contributes to this morbidity is controversial, but systemic hypoxia and lactic acidosis pose the earliest threat. Other forms of status epilepticus are less threatening because they are not associated with systemic lactic acidosis or hypoxia. However, local brain metabolic overactivity may cause neurologic damage and should be treated promptly.

The treatment of status epilepticus has been well summarized in various therapeutic manuals and is summarized in Table 71–1.[7,9] The first step is to establish the diagnosis. Although an EEG may be required in unusual circumstances, the diagnosis is usually obvious by history and examination. Patients in status epilepticus must be supported metabolically. It is essential to establish an airway and an intravenous line to obtain blood samples and administer medication. Blood serum concentrations of calcium, magnesium, sodium, urea nitrogen (BUN), and glucose should be measured to exclude common metabolic causes of seizures. Hy-

TABLE 71–1. Treatment of Status Epilepticus

1. Establish an airway.
2. Start intravenous line with normal saline.
3. Draw blood for CBC, serum glucose, BUN, sodium, calcium, magnesium, and anticonvulsant levels.
4. Inject 100 mg thiamine and then 50 ml glucose by IV push.
5. Inject lorazepam (Ativan) 0.1 mg/kg IV at a rate no greater than 2 mg/min.
6. Concomitantly, infuse phenytoin (Dilantin) 18–25 mg/kg IV at a rate no faster than 50 mg/min. Use cardiac monitor and check blood pressure every five minutes.
7. If seizures persist, try phenobarbital 5 mg/kg IV at a rate no faster than 50 mg/min checking blood pressure every five minutes. Intubation is advisable before administration. Give another 5 mg/kg after 20 min if seizures persist.
8.* Lidocaine 3–10 mg/kg/hr IV in D_5W until seizures stop. Monitor BP and ECG. Give additional doses of 50–100 mg to keep seizure-free for 12–24 hr.
9.* Paraldehyde 4% in saline IV at 50 ml/hr. Increase rate by 50 ml/hr every five minutes until seizures stop or BP falls. Continue for 12 hr at decreasing doses, maintaining flow just fast enough to keep seizures from restarting. Monitor BP and EEG and keep patient intubated.
10. Barbiturate coma
    a. Keep patient intubated and monitor BP and EEG.
    b. Pentobarbital 5 mg/kg IV loading dose.
    c. Infuse at 1–3 mg/kg/hr until seizures cease or until burst suppression pattern appears on EEG.
    d. The infusion rate should keep patient seizure-free for 12–24 hr.

*Not used frequently but may be considered instead of phenobarbital in patients who are allergic to it or who are otherwise intolerant of barbiturates.

poxia should be excluded. A complete blood count (CBC) should be done since infection can sometimes precipitate status epilepticus in an otherwise well-controlled patient. If the patient is receiving an anticonvulsant, a serum level should be measured to determine whether more of the drug should be administered. If medication history is unknown, blood should be sent for immediate measurement of phenytoin, phenobarbital, and carbamazepine.

Opinions differ with regard to the order in which anticonvulsant medications should be administered. The need to terminate seizure activity as soon as possible has led most neurologists to favor initial use of benzodiazepines. However, since they are not usually effective in long-term treatment, it is common practice to begin an infusion of phenytoin concomitantly. This strategy allows ongoing treatment with a longer-acting less sedating anticonvulsant to be initiated by the time benzodiazepines have terminated the seizure.

The choice of benzodiazepine is also controversial. Diazepam is the most widely used, but its short duration of action requires repeated doses before phenytoin loading is complete, increasing the already substantial risk of respiratory depression. Lorazepam has a longer duration of action than diazepam but similarly carries the risk of respiratory depression.[10] Administering benzodiazepines to patients who have already been medicated with barbiturates increases the risk of respiratory arrest. If one benzodiazepine is not effective in terminating status epilepticus, other benzodiazepines should not be used subsequently.

Phenytoin precipitates in solutions of glucose and water and should therefore be dissolved in saline for administration. The loading dose is 18 mg/kg intravenously, equivalent to 1000 to 1400 mg in adults. An additional 7 mg/kg may be given if seizures do not stop. These doses may result in serum levels of 25 to 30 μg/ml, which are above the usual therapeutic range of 10 to 20 μg/ml. Although some toxic side effects like drowsiness or vertigo may develop, cessation of status epilepticus should be given priority. Phenytoin should not be given at a rate greater than 50 mg/min. The main hazards of intravenous phenytoin are hypotension and heart block, especially in frail elderly patients with preexisting heart disease. Hypotension is due mainly to the propylene glycol diluent,[11] while cardiac arrhythmias are probably the result of direct action of the drug on the conduction system.[12] Frequent blood pressure determinations and electrocardiographic monitoring should be performed during phenytoin loading. If complications arise, the drug should be stopped until blood pressure and heart rhythm return to normal. Maintenance doses of 4 to 6 mg/kg/day, equivalent to 200 to 400 mg/day in adults, may be resumed in 24 hours.

If lorazepam and phenytoin do not terminate the seizures, phenobarbital should be given in a dose of 5 mg/kg, equivalent to 200 to 400 mg in adults, intravenously over 10 to 15 minutes. This can be repeated every 30 minutes until the seizure activity stops or until a full loading dose of 15 mg/kg or about 1000 mg has been administered. Respiratory depression and somnolence are frequent side effects. Patients should be intubated before phenobarbital is administered in case assisted ventilation is required. If phenobarbital is used as a long-term anticonvulsant, maintenance doses of 1 to 3 mg/kg/day, equivalent to 90 to 240 mg/day in adults, can be resumed after 24 hours.

In refractory patients and particularly those intolerant to phenobarbital, paraldehyde may be useful. It can be given as a 4% solution in saline intravenously as indicated in Table 71–1 or as a rectal enema by mixing 0.3 ml/kg in an equal volume of mineral oil that can be repeated in 20 to 30 minutes. Although absorption is not always predictable when given rectally, toxic effects may include respiratory depression, pulmonary hemorrhage, and congestive heart failure. Paraldehyde is also associated with hepatic and renal toxicity. Because of its high volatility and unpleasant odor, it is difficult to use in a recovery room or intensive care setting. Lidocaine in a dose of 3 to 10 mg/kg/hr intravenously, mixed in a dextrose and water solution, is another alternative to phenobarbital. However, it can cause paradoxical seizures and cardiac arrest if given too rapidly. It should therefore never be administered at a rate above 50 mg/min.

When all else fails, general anesthesia can be used to treat refractory status epilepticus. Although halothane can be used, the most popular agent is intravenous pentobarbital.[13] Patients are anesthetized for 12 to 24 hours and then allowed to emerge from anesthesia to determine if seizures return while on maintenance anticonvulsant therapy. Pressor support may be necessary.

MALIGNANT HYPERTHERMIA

Malignant hyperthermia is a familial autosomal dominant disorder in which patients develop muscle rigidity and high fever following administration of certain general anesthetics like halothane and depolarizing neuromuscular blockers like succinylcholine.[14] Although the pathogenetic mechanisms are not completely understood, the sarcoplasmic reticulum of skeletal muscle leaks calcium, leading to excessive activation of the contractile mechanism and metabolic overload.[15,16] Prolonged muscle contraction can lead to myoglobinuria, hyperkalemia, and lactic acidosis. Serum levels of creatine phosphokinase (CPK) are markedly elevated. Death occurs in a high proportion of cases.

Anesthesiologists now routinely question patients about prior experiences with anesthesia and family history suggestive of malignant hyperthermia, but negative histories do not prevent all cases. The anesthetic should be discontinued as soon as the syndrome is recognized. The body should be cooled with a cooling blanket or ice packs, and cold fluids should be administered orally or through a nasogastric tube. Fluid and electrolyte loss should be appropriately replaced intravenously as detailed in Chap. 6.

In recent years, dantrolene sodium in a dose of 2.5 mg/kg by rapid intravenous push has been found life-saving.[17] The dose should be repeated until muscle rigidity resolves or until a total dose of 10 mg/kg has been reached. Thereafter, a dose of 1 to 2 mg/kg should be administered orally four times daily for the next several days until the symptoms stop. Dantrolene is a muscle relaxant that blocks release of calcium by the sarcoplasmic reticulum. Overmedication can cause respiratory failure by paralyzing respiratory muscles.[18]

NEUROLEPTIC MALIGNANT SYNDROME

A clinical picture similar to that of malignant hyperthermia has been observed in some patients receiving neuroleptic drugs like phenothiazines.[19,20] However, it is not an inherited disorder and is characterized by extrapyramidal movements such as dystonic posturing and choreoathetosis as well as fever and muscle rigidity. These features suggest that the primary disorder affects the central rather than the peripheral nervous system and may involve block-

ade of dopamine receptors. Treatment is the same as for malignant hyperthermia.[21] In addition, the dopamine agonist bromocriptine may be given orally[22,23] or through a nasogastric tube every six hours. The dose may be increased gradually to a maximum of 60 mg daily.

PERIOPERATIVE NERVE INJURIES

During surgery, peripheral nerves may be injured in several ways. They can be lacerated or compressed at the operative site. Ischemic damage may occur if the arterial supply to the nerve is interrupted. After surgery, a hematoma may develop and compress a nerve. In all cases, careful examination is required to determine the territory of the neurological deficit and the level at which the nerve has been injured. Computerized tomography or magnetic resonance imaging is helpful in identifying a large hematoma requiring evacuation. The various types of perioperative nerve injuries have been reviewed by Dawson and Krarup.[24] Subclavian central venous line placement may rarely result in injury to adjacent nerves including the brachial plexus, phrenic nerve, cervical sympathetic trunk, and recurrent laryngeal nerve.[25]

Peripheral nerves may also be injured by compression or traction at a site remote from the surgical field. The two most common examples are ulnar and brachial plexus palsies. The ulnar nerve is often compressed against the edge of the operating table or by a tourniquet, blood pressure cuff, or bandage, especially if the arm is adducted and pronated. Intraoperative ulnar nerve damage tends to occur in patients predisposed to compression neuropathy as judged clinically or by the fact that electrical conduction abnormalities are found not only in the affected nerve but also in the contralateral ulnar nerve.[26]

Brachial plexus palsy results from stretching of the plexus when the arm is abducted and extended during anesthesia.[27] The

TABLE 71–2. Perioperative Compressive and Traction Neuropathies

Surgical Position	Nerve	Sign
Dorsal decubitus	C4–8 or brachial plexus	Upper plexus: Weak biceps, deltoid, shoulder, external rotation. Lower plexus: Weak hand; Horner's syndrome
	Long thoracic	Scapular winging
	Radial	Wrist drop; inability to extend at M-P joints
	Median	Numb digits 1 and 2; inability to make tight ring between thumb and another finger
	Ulnar	Claw hand; numb digits 4 and 5
Lateral decubitus	Suprascapular	Shoulder pain; weak shoulder abduction and external rotation
	Long thoracic	Scapular winging
	Peroneal	Foot drop
Ventral decubitus	Brachial plexus	Upper plexus: Weak biceps, deltoid, shoulder, external rotation. Lower plexus: Weak hand; Horner's syndrome. Aggravation of thoracic outlet syndrome
	Ulnar	Claw hand; numb digits 4 and 5
	Radial	Wrist drop; inability to extend at M-P joints
Sitting with knees extended	Sciatic	Foot drop; large territory numbness

contiguity of the plexus to bony prominences like the head of the humerus may contribute to the traction. The upper plexus is most commonly involved, resulting in neurological deficits seen in the distribution of the C5–7 roots. Weakness is more prominent than sensory loss or pain. Thin patients are more likely to be affected. A more complete description of the effects of positioning on the distribution of deficits in intraoperative brachial plexus palsies can be found in the review by Britt et al.[28] Different surgical positions are associated with different compressive nerve injuries (see Table 71–2).[29]

The prognosis of perioperative nerve injuries depends on the type and severity of the lesion. Deficits due to lacerations of nerves far from their target muscles are unlikely to resolve. Even after surgical repair, regenerating axons do not grow into their original endoneural sheaths and are misrouted into the wrong nerve branches. However, compression or traction injuries leave the endoneural tubes intact, allowing regenerating axons to follow their original paths and reinnervate their normal target muscles and organs.[30]

The time course of recovery depends on the duration and severity of the compression. Mild compression of short duration can cause conduction block without producing degeneration of the distal axon stump, and recovery of function can occur in minutes, hours, or within three days. With severe prolonged compression, distal degeneration of the axon slows recovery. Regeneration proceeds at a rate of one to two mm/day. When this occurs in the brachial plexus, recovery can take as long as three months to a year. Intermediate degrees of compression or stretch probably cause focal demyelination without loss of axonal continuity. In this case, remyelination and functional recovery can take place in six to eight weeks. Electromyography and nerve conduction studies are helpful in locating the point of conduction failure. However, because signs of denervation do not appear for 10 to 14 days, electromyography should be repeated after two weeks to assess the degree of axonal degeneration.

POSTOPERATIVE HEADACHE

Postoperative headache is often ascribed to the effects of anesthetic agents. However, headache due to migraine, sinus disease, dental disease, and myofacial spasm may occur in the perioperative period. Fennelly et al. recently suggested that caffeine withdrawal may be a significant factor in patients with unexplained postoperative headache.[31] They found that the risk of postoperative headache strongly correlated with the level of caffeine consumption before surgery.

Patients who develop headache after epidural anesthesia should be questioned for symptoms of low cerebrospinal fluid pressure syndrome. In this case, headache is present in the upright posture and is dramatically relieved when supine. Other symptoms include lightheadedness, doubt vision, and "ear-popping." These headaches usually resolve in 24 to 72 hours, but occasionally an epidural blood patch is necessary to alleviate symptoms.

Rare causes of headache like intracranial hemorrhage or carotid occlusion should be considered in vasculopathic, hypertensive, or anticoagulated patients. These patients invariably develop focal neurological signs. Noninvasive studies including computed tomography of the head or carotid ultrasonography should readily confirm these diagnostic possibilities.

Most postoperative headaches spontaneously resolve, particularly when sleep patterns return to normal. Some patients may require symptomatic therapy with a low-potency narcotic or a nonsteroidal anti-inflammatory agent to alleviate pain.

POSTOPERATIVE INFECTIONS OF THE CENTRAL NERVOUS SYSTEM

Surgical patients may develop infections in the postoperative period which are directly related to the surgical site or more commonly to invasive tubes, catheters, and lines. Systemic bacteremia can readily lead to fulminant sepsis, particularly in patients who are immunocompromised by chronic illness, age, and immunosuppressive medications. Patients undergoing organ transplantation are treated with high doses of immunosuppressive therapy and are susceptible not only to the typical bacterial pathogens but also to many opportunistic infections listed in Table 71–3.

Bacterial and fungal sepsis are well-recognized causes of encephalopathy.[32] In a study of twelve cases of encephalopathy associated with sepsis,[33] Jackson et al. found that eight patients had disseminated microabscesses in the brain at autopsy, suggesting an anatomic explanation for diffuse cerebral dysfunction in at least some patients with fulminant sepsis. Indirect encephalopathic effects of bacterial endotoxins and secondary perturbations on plasma and brain amino acids and neurotransmitters may contribute to mental status changes in infected postoperative patients.[32-35] More recently, gamma-aminobutyric acid (GABA), GABA-like endogenous substances, and instability of the blood-brain barrier have been implicated in both hepatic and septic encephalopathy.[35-37] These investigations further support the recommendation that long-acting GABA agonists like diazepam should be avoided in encephalopathic patients with multisystem failure and associated septicemia.

Postoperative mental changes should therefore prompt a vigorous search for infection. Lumbar puncture should be obtained after exclusion of intracranial mass lesion by computerized axial tomography. Such an evaluation is especially important in immunosuppressed patients.

TABLE 71–3. Opportunistic Infections Seen in Immunosuppressed Postoperative Patients

A. *Viral*
    Cytomegalovirus
    Epstein-Barr virus
    Varicella zoster virus
    Papovavirus
    Adenovirus
    Herpes simplex virus

B. *Bacterial*
    Listeria
    Tuberculosis

C. *Fungal/Parasitic*
    Aspergillus
    Nocardia
    Toxoplasmosis
    Mucormycosis

Source: Adapted from Conti DJ, Rubin RH: Infection of the central nervous system in organ transplant recipients. *Neurol Clin* 6:241–260, 1988.

PERIOPERATIVE STROKE

Acute cerebral infarction may complicate surgery, particularly if the procedure involves cardiac or neurovascular manipulation or cardiopulmonary bypass is required. In valve replacement surgery or septal defect repair, opening the heart predisposes patients to air embolism that can cause seizures and/or cerebral infarction.

Several patterns of brain injury are associated with cardiopulmonary bypass. Global hypoperfusion sometimes occurs and may result in watershed infarction in territory near areas supplied by two major vessels. Alternatively, diffuse cortical, hippocampal, and cerebellar injury can occur since these regions are particularly sensitive to ischemia. Finally, focal ischemic injury can occur as a result of embolization. Moody et al. have described the pathology of the cerebral microvasculature in patients subjected to proximal aortography or cardiopulmonary bypass.[39]

Postoperative arrhythmias, particularly atrial fibrillation, predispose patients to distal embolization and stroke. Prompt attention should be given to chemical or electrical cardioversion with appropriate anticoagulation as needed.

BRAIN DEATH

Brain death results from irreversible neurologic damage and is characterized by the absence of brainstem and cerebral function.[40,41] The patient remains unresponsive without cognitive function or purposeful movements. Lack of brainstem function is established by the absence of pupillary, oculovestibular, gag, and corneal reflexes. Spinal reflexes and plantar-extensor responses can be preserved in brain death.

Apnea can be demonstrated by removing the patient from the respirator, delivering a continuous flow of oxygen through the endotracheal tube and observing for a spontaneous ventilatory response to hypercarbia. The PCO_2 rises approximately three mmHg for every minute of nonventilation, but the rise may be more erratic depending on the baseline PCO_2 and the duration of apnea.[42] The PCO_2 should be allowed to reach 60 mmHg before apnea is considered definite.[43]

Complicating conditions such as severe hypothermia, circulatory collapse, sedative or other drug intoxication, and significant metabolic derangements should be excluded since they may alter the clinical examination.[44,45] Laboratory confirmation of brain death includes an isoelectric electroencephalogram or the demonstration of absent cerebral blood flow.[40,46] When organ transplantation is a consideration, most authorities believe that the criteria for brain death should be met for a period of at least six hours. Since barbiturates and some other drugs can reversibly produce an isoelectric EEG, the presence of these drugs in the serum requires a longer period of observation.[40,45] Cardiovascular collapse usually follows brain death within several days.[46]

SUMMARY

1. Postoperative status epilepticus may occur in patients with or without a history of seizures and may be due to intercurrent illness or an abrupt change in anticonvulsant medications.

2. Evaluation of postoperative seizures should include careful examination, laboratory evaluation including metabolic parameters, and complete blood count and anticonvulsant drug levels. Electroencephalogram and other neurologic studies may or may not be necessary.

3. Treatment of status epilepticus after surgery consists of airway protection, a longer-acting benzodiazepine like lorazepam and a loading dose of phenytoin (18 mg/kg intravenously). If status cannot be terminated, phenobarbital in a dose of 5 mg/kg intravenously can be given. Paraldehyde and general anesthesia are alternatives when other agents are ineffective or cannot be tolerated.

4. Malignant hyperthermia is a familial disorder of muscle rigidity and high fever following general anesthesia, requiring early recognition and treatment with fluids, cooling measures, and dantrolene in a dose of 2.5 mg/kg intravenously.

5. Neuroleptic malignant syndrome is similar to malignant hyperthermia but follows administration of neuroleptic agents and is often accompanied by extrapyramidal signs. Treatment is the same as for malignant hyperthermia with the addition of bromocriptine in increasing doses to 60 mg daily in divided doses every six hours.

6. Perioperative nerve injuries are the direct result of surgery or due to positioning during surgery. The time course of recovery and prognosis depend upon the nature and duration of the injury. Careful examination and electromyography are helpful in defining neurologic dysfunction.

7. The etiologies of postoperative headache are similar to those in nonsurgical patients. Postoperative headache correlates with caffeine consumption before surgery and may be due to withdrawal. Headache related to spinal or epidural anesthesia is present in the upright and absent in the supine position. It usually resolves spontaneously in 24 to 72 hours but may require placement of an epidural patch.

8. Postoperative CNS dysfunction in sepsis can be due to direct involvement of the brain or to septic encephalopathy. Patients who are elderly, chronically ill or immunosuppressed are especially susceptible. Postoperative mental status changes in the setting of systemic infection should prompt evaluation for CNS infection with lumbar puncture after exclusion of an intracranial mass by computerized axial tomography.

9. Postoperative stroke may be the result of intraoperative hypotension, manipulation of the heart or neurovascular structures, cardiopulmonary bypass, or embolization due to postoperative arrhythmias. Treatment should be directed at the underlying etiology.

10. Brain death is the result of irreversible neurologic damage and is characterized by the absence of brainstem and cerebral function. In the absence of barbiturates, an isoelectric electroencephalogram or demonstration of absent cerebral blood flow are confirmatory. Apnea should be documented off mechanical ventilation when the PCO_2 rises to 60 mmHg or above.

REFERENCES

1. Modica PA, Tempelhoff R, White PF: Pro- and anticonvulsant effects of anesthetics (part I). *Anesth Analg* 70:303–315, 1990.

2. Modica PA, Tempelhoff R, White PF: Pro- and anticonvulsant effects of anesthetics (part II). *Anesth Analg* 70:433–444, 1990.

3. Christys AR, Moss E, Powell D: Retrospective study of early postoperative convulsions after intracranial surgery with isoflurane or enflurane anesthesia. *Br J Anaesth* 62:624–627, 1989.

4. Collier C, Kelly K: Propofol and convulsions—the evidence mounts. *Anesth Intens Care* 19:573–575, 1991.

5. Tempelhoff R, Modica PA, Bernardo KL et al: Fentanyl-induced electrocorticographic seizures in patients with complex partial epilepsy. *J Neurosurg* 77:201–208, 1992.

6. Delgado-Escueta AV, Wasterlain CG, Treiman DM et al (eds): *Status Epilepticus: Mechanisms of Brain Damage and Treatment (Advances in Neurology, vol 34)*. New York, Raven Press, 1983, pp 537–543.

7. Treiman DM: Status Epilepticus, in Johnson RT (ed): *Current Therapy in Neurologic Disease II*. Toronto, Decker, 1987, pp 38–42.

8. Meldrum BS, Vigouroux RA, Brierly JB: Systemic factors and epileptic brain damage: Prolonged seizures in paralyzed, artificially ventilated baboons. *Arch Neurol* 28:82–87, 1973.

9. Samuels MA, Fernandez RF: Epilepsy, in Samuels MA (ed): *Manual of Neurologic Therapeutics*, 3d ed. Boston, Little Brown, 1986, pp 81–118.

10. Treiman DM: Pharmacokinetics and clinical use of benzodiazepines in the management of status epilepticus. *Epilepsia* 30(Suppl 2):S4–S10, 1989.

11. Al-Khudhairi D, Whitwam JG: Autonomic reflexes and the cardiovascular effects of propylene glycol. *Br J Anaesth* 58:897–902, 1986.

12. Louis S, Kutt H, McDowell F: The cardiocirculatory effects of Dilantin and its solvent. *Am Heart J* 74:523–529, 1967.

13. Goldberg M, McIntyre H: Barbiturates in the treatment of status epilepticus, in Delgado-Escueta AV, Wasterlain CG, Treiman DM et al (eds): *Status Epilepticus: Mechanisms of Brain Damage and Treatment (Advances in Neurology, vol 34)*. New York, Raven Press, 1983, pp 499–503.

14. Gronert GA: Malignant hyperthermia. *Anesthesiology* 53:395–423, 1980.

15. Endo M, Yagi S, Ishizaka T et al: Changes in the Ca-induced Ca release mechanism in the sarcoplasmic reticulum of the muscle from a patient with malignant hyperthermia. *Biomed Res* 4:83–92, 1983.

16. Takagi A, Sunohara N, Ishihara T et al: Malignant hyperthermia and related neuromuscular diseases: Caffeine contracture of the skinned muscle fibers. *Muscle Nerve* 6:510–514, 1983.

17. Larew RE: Malignant hyperthermia. Quick recognition and treatment to avoid death. *Postgrad Med* 85:117–129, 1989.

18. Britt BA (ed): *Malignant Hyperthermia*. Boston, Martinus Nijhoff, 1987.

19. Delay J, Deniker P: Drug-induced extrapyramidal syndromes, in Vinken PJ, Bruyn GW (eds): *Handbook of Clinical Neurology: Diseases of the Basal Ganglia*. New York, Elsevier, 1968, vol 6, p 248.

20. Kurland R, Hamill R, Shoulson I: Neuroleptic malignant syndrome. *Clin Neuropharmacol* 7:109–120, 1984.

21. May DC, Morris SW, Stewert RM et al: Neuroleptic malignant syndrome: Response to dantrolene sodium. *Ann Int Med* 98:183–184, 1983.

22. Mueller PS, Vester JW, Fermaglich J: Neuroleptic malignant syndrome. Successful treatment with bromocriptine. *JAMA* 249:386–388, 1983.

23. Grantano JE, Stern BJ, Ringel A et al: Neuroleptic malignant syndrome: Successful treatment with dantrolene and bromocriptine. *Ann Neurol* 14:89–90, 1983.

24. Dawson DM, Krarup C: Perioperative nerve lesions. *Arch Neurol* 46:1355–1360, 1989.

25. Mihm FG, Rosenthal MH: Central venous catheterization, in Benumof JL (ed): *Clinical Procedures in Anesthesia and Intensive Care*. Philadelphia, Lippincott, 1992, pp 339–373.

26. Alvine FG, Schurrer ME: Postoperative ulnar nerve palsy: Are there predisposing factors? *Am J Bone Joint Surg* 69:255–259, 1987.

27. Kwaan JHM, Rappoport I: Postoperative brachial plexus palsy. *Arch Surg* 101:612–615, 1970.

28. Britt BA, Joy N, Mackay MB: Positioning trauma, in Orkin FK, Cooperman LH (eds): *Complications in Anesthesiology*. Philadelphia, Lippincott, 1983, pp 646–670.

29. Martin JT: Patient positioning, in Barash PG, Cullen BF, Stoelting RK (eds): *Clinical Anesthesia*. Philadelphia, Lippincott, 1992, pp 709–736.

30. Selzer ME: Regeneration of peripheral nerve, in Sumner AJ (ed): *The Physiology of Peripheral Nerve Disease*. Philadelphia, Saunders, 1980, pp. 358–431.

31. Fennelly M, Galletly DC, Purdie GI: Is caffeine withdrawal the mechanism of postoperative headache? *Anesth Analg* 72:449–453, 1971.

32. Hasselgren PO, Fischer JE: Septic encephalopathy: Etiology and management. *Intens Care Med* 12:13–16, 1986.

33. Jackson AC, Gilbert JJ, Young GB: The encephalopathy of sepsis. *Can J Neurol Sci* 2:303–307, 1985.

34. Freund HR, Muggia-Sullam M, LaFrance R: Regional brain amino acid and neurotransmitter derangements during abdominal sepsis and septic encephalopathy in the rat. *Arch Surg* 121:209–216, 1986.

35. Winder TR, Minuk GY, Sergeant EJ: GABA and sepsis-related encephalopathy. *Can J Neurol Sci* 15:23–25, 1988.

36. Takezawa J, Taenaka N, Nishijima MK: Amino acids and thiobarbituric reactive substances in cerebrospinal fluid and plasma of patients with septic encephalopathy. *Crit Care Med* 11:876–879, 1983.

37. Jeppsson B, Freund H, Gimmar Z: Blood-brain barrier derangement in sepsis: Cause of septic encephalopathy. *Am J Surg* 141:136–142, 1981.

38. Conti DJ, Rubin RH: Infection of the central nervous system in organ transplant recipients. *Neurol Clin* 6:241–260, 1988.

39. Moody DM, Bell MA, Challa VR et al: Brain microemboli during cardiac surgery or aortography. *Ann Neurol* 28:477–486, 1990.

40. Guidelines for determination of death: Report of the medical consultants on the diagnosis of death to the President's Commission on the Study of Ethical Problems in Medicine and Biomedical and Behavioral Research. *JAMA* 246:2184–2186, 1981.

41. Black PM: From heart to brain, the new definitions of death. *Am Heart J* 99:279–281, 1980.

42. Benzel EC, Gross CD, Hadden JA: The apnea test for the determination of brain death. *J Neurosurg* 71:191–194, 1989.

43. Schaffer JA, Caronna JJ: Duration of apnea needed to confirm brain death. *Neurology* 28:665–668, 1978.

44. Molinari GF: Review of clinical criteria of brain death, in Korein T (ed): Brain death: Interrelated medical and social issues. *Ann NY Acad Sci* 315:62–69, 1978.

45. Walker AE: An appraisal of the criteria of cerebral death. A summary statement. A collaborative study. *JAMA* 237:982–986, 1977.

46. Black PM: Brain death. *N Engl J Med* 299:338–344, 393–401, 1978.

72 MANAGEMENT OF POSTOPERATIVE PAIN

Wilhelmina C. Korevaar

ACUTE PAIN AND THE RESPONSE TO TISSUE INJURY

Tissue trauma results in a well-characterized injury response that includes increased sympathetic efferent activity, increased release of epinephrine and norepinephrine from the adrenal glands, decreased pancreatic release of insulin with resultant hyperglycemia, metabolic consumption of proteins and fats, and a centrally mediated response to primary afferent neurogenic stimuli resulting in increased serum cortisol and ADH levels. Catabolism following acute tissue injury increases oxygen consumption and respiratory demands. Compromise of respiratory function, often seen following upper-abdominal and thoracic surgery, can aggravate catabolism. The extent of tissue damage determines the severity of the injury response, and the magnitude of the response affects postoperative morbidity and mortality.[1]

Acute pain is often associated with tissue trauma and represents an adverse psychological event that cannot be measured objectively. It is not clear to what extent pain itself, independent of the neuroendocrine stress response to injury, affects postoperative morbidity or mortality.[1,2] The pain experience is subject to multifactorial inputs and modifications.[3] Some of these modifications coincidentally attenuate stress responses,[4] but none has been conclusively shown to reduce morbidity or mortality.[5]

Increased responsiveness of peripheral nociceptors follows tissue injury because of mechanoreceptor stimulation due to chemoreceptor threshold changes caused by altered physical stimuli; a change in chemical environment (pH); and the release or synthesis of endogenous algesic substances like prostaglandins, serotonin, histamine, bradykinin, and substance P. Nociceptor activity is perpetuated by local changes in the microcirculation. Nerve fibers of different sizes are activated, allowing the first perception of pain to be rapidly localized and a delayed second perception of pain to be more diffuse, throbbing, and generally disturbing.

Within the spinal cord, pain transmission depends on complex chemically mediated interactions between inhibitory and facilitating pathways. Substance P may play a role in primary afferent trans-

mission. Neurotensin, another algesic substance, excites primary afferent neurons. The gut peptides, VIP and CCK, may also be instrumental in the transmission of pain. In addition, there are several endogenous inhibitory substances. Noradrenergic and serotonergic pathways in the spinal cord inhibit pain transmission. Enkephalins operate locally within the dorsal horn and centrally in the nervous system to enhance release of monoamines and stimulate the gamma-aminobutyric (GABA) system. Stress and pain cause release of endogenous opioids, and levels of these peptides can be correlated with variations in pain response among patients.[6]

Pain and stress activate descending pathways from the periaqueductal gray matter in the brainstem, producing naloxone-reversible analgesia mediated by norepinephrine and serotonin and suppressing spinal cord activity. The thalamus biases the entry of noxious impulses to the cerebral cortex probably based on an overall pattern of anticipated input or body image.[7] There is no correlation between cortical evoked potentials and painful stimuli.

The neuroendocrine stress response can be blocked only by abolition of both the primary afferent impulse activation and the sympathetic efferent response to tissue injury. Using conventional regional anesthetic techniques, attenuation of the stress response to lower-extremity or lower-abdominal surgery has been more easily achieved than that following upper-abdominal or thoracic procedures.[8]

MODIFICATION OF THE PAIN EXPERIENCE

The pain experience can be modified in a variety of ways, ranging from inhibition of synthesis or release of algesic substances at the tissue level to alterations in cortical responses. Numerous subjective measures have been used to evaluate the extent of acute pain control. The most frequently used pain scale is the nonnumeric visual analog scale (VAS). The scale consists of a 10-cm line with the words "no pain" at one end and "worst pain" at the other. Numbers are not presented to the patient since they may bias response. Quantitative responses are derived by measuring the distance in centimeters from the words "no pain" to a mark made by the patient. Other investigators rely on questionnaires designed to test the effects of mood and affect on pain and vice versa.[9,10] Quantification of narcotic use is considered by some to be a more objective measure of the efficacy of pain control modalities. However, when using continuous intravenous narcotic infusions, the minimum effective analgesic blood concentration may vary fourfold for postoperative pain caused by the same surgical procedure.[11] No measure of pain has been found to correlate with surgical outcome or measurements of the neuroendocrine stress response.

Despite the difficulty in quantifying pain, there are several factors that appear to influence its intensity. In many cases, the pain experience is largely predetermined by ethnic and socioeconomic variables. There is a growing body of literature that supports central modulation of the pain experience, and one surgeon has even popularized his observations that pain and hemostasis respond to intraoperative suggestion.[12] The duration of pain experienced after a particular operation correlates best with the location of the incision. Procedures involving incisions to either side of the midline cause more prolonged postoperative pain than those involving vertical midline incisions. The potential for peripheral nerve damage associated with lateral incisions increases the likelihood that chronic pain will develop after thoracotomies, flank incisions, inguinal hernia repairs, appendectomies, and procedures requiring lower-abdominal transverse incisions.

The respiratory effects of surgery also depend on the site of the incision. As noted in Chap. 22, upper-abdominal and thoracic incisions result in a decrease in vital capacity (VC) and an altered relationship of closing volume (CV) to functional residual capacity (FRC). As the FRC declines in relation to the CV, there is an increase in the alveolar-to-arterial oxygen gradient. The FRC falls more than the CV in the first 48 hours after surgery due to alterations in diaphragmatic activity, and the reduction in FRC may be proportional to pain. Any form of analgesia helps to restore VC and causes measurable improvements in effort-dependent pulmonary function tests. However, there are no data to confirm that analgesia restores the normal ratio of FRC to CV.[13–16]

In summary, the pain experience and its modification are difficult to measure directly. However, modification of the pain experience by a number of modalities also attenuates various components of the stress response that are sometimes more easily quantified.[17] Therefore, these modalities are discussed in the context of their effect in modulating the injury stress response at various levels of pain perception and transmission.

Anti-Inflammatory Drugs

Pain accompanying tissue inflammation can be modified by systemic drugs that alter the responsiveness of nociceptors. Acetylsalicylic acid and nonsteroidal anti-inflammatory agents inhibit cyclooxygenase and thereby reduce the synthesis of prostaglandins. Indomethacin has been used to decrease postoperative narcotic requirements.[17] Corticosteroids inhibit the metabolism of a precursor of prostaglandins. Capsaicin depletes fine cutaneous nerve endings of substance P. Antihistamines and local anesthetics modify changes in the microcirculatory blood supply in injured tissue.

The decreased platelet adhesiveness caused by acetylsalicylic acid and nonsteroidal anti-inflammatory drugs may limit their use-

fulness in the perioperative setting. Nonsteroidal anti-inflammatory drugs may affect platelet adhesion for 48 hours after their discontinuation; the residual effect of aspirin can last more than a week.

Peripheral Nerve Blocks

Local anesthetic infiltration of the operative site has been shown to diminish postoperative pain as recorded subjectively and corroborated by decreased narcotic requirements.[18] Peripheral nerve blocks are useful in a variety of settings. Following upper-abdominal or thoracic procedures, intercostal nerve blocks improve effort-dependent pulmonary function test results.[19] Ilioinguinal and iliohypogastric nerve blocks provide analgesia and improve ambulation after inguinal procedures.[20] Penile blocks are used to minimize pain following circumcision. Brachial plexus blocks provide analgesia and increase blood flow after surgery involving the upper extremities.

Improvement in recovery time and outcome in patients receiving peripheral nerve blocks and infiltration of the incision with local anesthetic provides evidence that the experience of pain and the neuroendocrine stress response are functionally distinct. The stress response to tissue injury cannot be attenuated unless noxious input to the central nervous system is blocked by establishing a sensory level of anesthesia at least 30 minutes before injury occurs. Moreover, continued attenuation of the stress response depends on maintaining a sensory level corresponding with the highest visceral afferent stimulation anticipated for a given procedure. Local anesthetic infiltration and peripheral nerve blocks provide more effective postoperative analgesia when executed before the incision,[21] allowing for significant modification of effort-dependent outcome. Patients with less pain ambulate better, cough more effectively, and exhibit higher vital capacities, all of which translate into a lower incidence of postoperative complications.

Interpleural Bupivacaine

Instillation of relatively large volumes and nearly toxic doses of bupivacaine into the potential space between the parietal and visceral pleura has been used to provide analgesia after thoracic and upper-abdominal procedures. Success requires that no chest tube be left in place to drain away the local anesthetic before it acts completely. The incidence of complicating pneumothorax may equal that associated with intercostal nerve block.[22]

Study of this technique has provided new insight into regional anatomy.[23] Interpleural instillation of bupivacaine as a single injection or through a catheter may anesthetize multiple intercostal nerves but does not affect more proximal portions of the spinal nerve.[24]

Cryoanalgesia

Tissue freezing to $-70°C$ to remove oral cancers was noted to have a beneficial effect on postoperative pain in the 1960s. Freezing of intercostal nerves during thoracotomy to provide postoperative analgesia was proposed in the mid 1970s.[25] The epineurium is maintained after cryoneurolysis and provides an anatomically intact pathway for eventual regeneration of the nerve. Under direct visualization during surgery, the intercostal nerves are frozen at and two segments above and below the level of the incision. Although incisional pain is decreased, patients experience discomfort from pleural irritation, especially when a chest tube is left in place. Loss of intercostal muscle function is not usually a problem. Incomplete neurolysis can result in neuritis-like pain, and several freeze-thaw cycles are recommended to prevent incomplete neural destruction. Nerve regeneration occurs in 6 to 12 months. Although patients may experience some sensory loss corresponding to the area of freezing in the interim, the technique decreases the incidence of chronic postthoracotomy pain syndrome.[26]

Spinal or Epidural Block Using Local Anesthetic

In the 1930s, O'Shaughnessy et al. noted improved survival in dogs following blunt hind-limb trauma if spinal anesthesia was administered before the trauma.[27] There have been numerous subsequent attempts to document diminished stress responses to surgery when spinal or epidural anesthesia is included in the anesthetic management of patients undergoing thoracic and abdominal operations.[28] The effect of intraoperative thoracic epidural anesthesia on cardiac performance does not favor enhancement of tissue oxygen delivery.[29] The most obvious benefit of combined regional and general anesthetic technique is the postoperative use of the epidural catheter to reduce pain and the respiratory and vascular consequences of immobility.[30]

"Intraspinal" Narcotics

In the last decade, there has been significant interest in providing segmental analgesia without sympathetic, sensory, or motor block. Opioids have an affinity for certain receptors located in the dorsal horn of the spinal cord, the periaqueductal gray matter, the reticular activating system, and the hypothalamic-limbic system. Since selective spinal opioid analgesia was first demonstrated in the rat in 1976, clinicians have used it extensively, even before prospective studies of its action, efficacy, and risk could be completed.

Unlike local anesthetics, epidural or intrathecal narcotics do not produce sympathetic block or significantly diminish the endocrine response to surgery.[31] Attenuation of the catabolic response to tissue injury by epidural morphine was demonstrated in one comparative study of patients undergoing cholecystectomy.[32] Modification of postoperative hypertension by epidural morphine was postulated to be the result of attenuation of sympathetic hyperactivity in another study.[33] Otherwise, there has been little evidence to support the attenuation of stress responses or improved outcome following surgery using "intraspinal" narcotics without local anesthetics.[34,35]

Before safe and effective dose ranges were established, "intraspinal" administration of morphine sometimes resulted in delayed respiratory depression 6 to 12 hours after administration and rarely in death due to unrecognized apnea.[36] The incidence of delayed respiratory depression is associated with the dose and lipophilicity of the narcotic and patient variables including age over 65 and the use of sedatives, other narcotics, or other centrally acting medications.[37] Epidural and intrathecal narcotics are administered with increasing frequency and safety to patients upon return to the general wards after surgery.[38] Greater attention is now paid to obtaining maximum efficacy from minimal doses of narcotics and their combination with low doses of local anesthetics.[39] A greater understanding of the "pharmacokinetics" of epidural drug administration allows a greater margin of safety in their use.[40] Morphine in an epidural dose of 5 mg is safe and effective. Current intrathe-

cal doses of morphine range from 0.1 to 0.25 mg. The risk of respiratory depression is greater after intrathecal administration and extends beyond 12 hours after surgery. Intrathecal morphine provides analgesia for an average of 22 hours compared with 16 hours provided by a single epidural morphine dose.[41]

"Intraspinal" opioids, whether hydrophilic or lipophilic, can produce pruritis, urinary retention, nausea, vomiting, and somnolence. Indwelling epidural catheters in place for more than three days predispose patients to infection. The pruritis, nausea, vomiting, and urinary retention can be treated with naloxone in doses of approximately 0.1 mg intravenously or intramuscularly without affecting analgesia.[42]

Patient-Controlled Analgesia (PCA)

Patient-controlled analgesia devices are widely used for control of pain caused by surgery, trauma, and chronic cancer.[43] Intermittent bolus therapy is most effective as an adjunct to narcotic infusion, especially after a steady-state level has been attained with a loading dose. Narcotics are most often administered intravenously to control postoperative pain, but patient-controlled devices also function effectively in delivering opiates subcutaneously or into the epidural space.

Self-administered dosing can be instituted immediately upon emergence from anesthesia in the recovery room if patients have been instructed in the proper use of the PCA device by the anesthesiologist before surgery. The anesthetic can be tailored to include an intravenous loading dose of narcotic to achieve a steady state in which the rate of delivery equals the rate of elimination. Opioids are rapidly redistributed after intravenous administration, but several hours are required for equilibration between blood and tissues. Clearance of opioids is obviously dependent upon hepatic and renal function.

The use of narcotics to treat postoperative pain has been limited by fear of addiction regardless of the underlying circumstances. With the understanding that addiction is a specific biochemical disease, health care providers have become more willing to administer narcotics to patients with acute pain. The dose and frequency of narcotic administration should be carefully determined and frequently reviewed to assure individual analgesia. Ordering narcotics on an "as needed" basis using "standard" doses frequently results in inadequate analgesia.[62]

The patient-controlled analgesia device provides patients with a sense of control over the pain. Relative narcotic overdose resulting in respiratory depression can occur if the bolus dose is too high or the interval is too short. There have been occasional reports of death from equipment failure or improper concentrations of narcotic in the device. The degree of analgesia obtained with PCA is slightly less than that with epidural narcotic, but patients clearly prefer it.[45,46] There are no data to support the impression that analgesia provided by PCA-delivered narcotics is superior to that obtained with intramuscular narcotics in adequate doses offered on a schedule.

Other Narcotic Applications

There is renewed interest in less-invasive methods for delivering narcotics. Using iontophoresis, lipophilic narcotics like fentanyl can be delivered through the skin. Beneath the medication patch, a reservoir of drug is established to provide a stable blood level.

However, rapid regulation of dose is limited using existing transdermal delivery systems.

Since the veins of distal two-thirds of the rectum drain into the systemic circulation, narcotics administered rectally at first bypass the liver to achieve higher initial blood levels. Rectal administration of narcotics has not gained widespread acceptance in the perioperative setting but has been popular for cancer patients.

Long-acting oral morphine preparations are available as enterically-coated pills. Opiate is slowly released as the tablet passes through the gastrointestinal tract. Regular function of the gastrointestinal tract is required for effective and safe use of these drugs. Even patients in whom there has been no manipulation of internal organs experience problems with unpredictable gastrointestinal function in the early postoperative period. These preparations are most problematic in elderly patients who may remain constipated until the second or third postoperative day when they request a cathartic. A bolus of morphine might be absorbed quickly into the systemic circulation during a bowel movement.

T.E.N.S.

T.E.N.S. units deliver small electrical impulses to the skin and enhance peripheral input to the spinal cord. The use of these units in the early postoperative period was initially limited by an increased incidence of wound infection following the application of unsterile pads under the surgical dressing. Now sterile pads are placed along the incision in the operating room before the final dressing is applied. Following preoperative instruction and immediate use after surgery, T.E.N.S. results in effective postoperative analgesia more than 30 percent of the time.[47] The most effective applications are along lateral incisions used for thoracotomy, nephrectomy, and inguinal hernia. High-frequency low-intensity stimulation is recommended for management of acute pain.

Positive Imagery and Therapeutic Relationships

The efficacy of utilizing placebo response, therapeutic in 30 to 35 percent of patients, and hypnosis suggests that the cortex is an untapped resource in managing posttraumatic pain and stress.[48] Centrally acting alpha$_2$-adrenergic agonists are presently under investigation. In addition, increased awareness of the significance of preoperative interviews underlines the importance of patient-physician relationships in pain control. There is no doubt that hyperactivity of the sympathetic nervous system, often manifested as anxiety, has a tremendous impact on surgical morbidity. There is a close relationship between analgesia and preoperative sympathetic tone and subsequent control of pain. Simple reassurance that postoperative pain can be controlled postoperatively is often therapeutic, and acknowledgment of the importance of comfort frequently results in improved patient acceptance of invasive procedures. Thus, provision of adequate postoperative analgesia includes a comprehensive preoperative interview, judicious use of preoperative medications, careful choice of intraoperative anesthetic agents, and management of a variety of analgesic modalities in the first 48 hours after surgery.

SUMMARY

1. Tissue trauma causes a well-characterized neuroendocrine stress response that correlates poorly with subjective postoperative pain.

2. In addition to traditional parenteral opiates, modalities for control of postoperative pain include nonsteroidal anti-inflammatory agents, peripheral nerve blocks, interpleural bupivacaine when appropriate, cryoanalgesia, spinal or epidural block with local anesthetics, epidural and intrathecal narcotics, patient-controlled devices for delivery of analgesics, and T.E.N.S. units.

3. Optimal management of postoperative pain includes good communication between the patient and physician before surgery, appropriate medication to control preoperative anxiety, an intraoperative anesthetic plan that anticipates postoperative analgesic need, and frequent monitoring of the analgesic regimen in the 48 hours following the procedure.

REFERENCES

1. Cousins MJ, Phillips GD (eds): *Acute Pain Management*. New York, Churchill Livingstone, 1986.
2. Taenzer P, Melzack R, Jeans ME: Influence of psychological factors on postoperative pain, mood and analgesic requirements. *Pain* 24:331–342, 1986.
3. Melzack R, Wall PD, Ty TC: Acute pain in an emergency clinic: Latency of onset and descriptor patterns related to different injuries. *Pain* 14:33–43, 1982.
4. Kehlet H: Surgical stress: The role of pain and analgesia. *Br J Anaesth* 63:189–195, 1989.
5. Dershwitz M, Sherman EP: Acute myocardial infarction symptoms masked by epidural morphine? *J Clin Anesth* 3:146–148, 1991.
6. Tamsen A, Sakurada T, Wahlstrom A et al: Postoperative demand for analgesics in relation to individual levels of endorphins and substance P in cerebrospinal fluid. *Pain* 13:171–183, 1982.
7. Melzack R, Loeser JD: Phantom body pain in paraplegics: Evidence for central "pattern generating mechanisms" for pain. *Pain* 4:195–210, 1978.
8. Vedrinne C, Vedrinne JM, Guirand M et al: Nitrogen-sparing effect of epidural administration of local anesthetics in colon surgery. *Anesth Analg* 69:354–359, 1989.
9. Chapman CR: Measurement of pain: Problems and issues, in Bonica JJ, Albe-Fessard D (eds): *Advances in Pain Research and Therapy*. New York, Raven Press, 1976, vol I, pp 345–353.
10. Margoles MS: The pain chart: Spatial properties of pain, in Melzack R (ed): *Pain Measurement and Assessment*. New York, Raven Press, 1983, pp 215–225.
11. Austin KL, Stapleton JV, Mather LE: Relationship between blood meperidine concentrations in analgesic response. *Anesthesiology* 53:460, 1980.
12. Siegel BS: *Love, Medicine & Miracles*. New York, Harper & Row, 1986.
13. McKenzie PJ, Wishart HY, Dewar KMS et al: Comparison of the effects of spinal anaesthesia and general anaesthesia on postoperative oxygenation and perioperative mortality. *Br J Anaesth* 52:49–53, 1980.
14. Rawal N, Sjostrand U, Christoffersson E et al: Comparison of intramuscular and epidural morphine for postoperative analgesia in the grossly obese: Influence on postoperative ambulation and pulmonary function. *Anesth Analg* 63:583–592, 1984.

15. Shulman M, Sandler AN, Bradley JW et al: Post-thoracotomy pain and pulmonary function following epidural and systemic morphine. *Anesthesiology* 61:569–575, 1984.

16. Ullman DA, Fortune JB, Greenhouse BB et al: The treatment of patients with multiple rib fractures using continuous thoracic epidural narcotic infusion. *Regional Anesth* 14:43–47, 1989.

17. Rigamonti G, Zanella E, Lampugnani R et al: Dose-response study with indoprofen IV as an analgesic in postoperative pain. *Br J Anaesth* 55:513, 1983.

18. Reid MF, Harris R, Phillips PD et al: Day-case herniotomy in children. A comparison of ilio-inguinal nerve block and wound infiltration for postoperative analgesia. *Anaesthesia* 42:658–661, 1987.

19. Rawal N, Sjostrand UH, Dahlstrom B et al: Epidural morphine for postoperative pain relief: A comparative study with intramuscular narcotic and intercostal nerve block. *Anesth Analg* 61:93–98, 1982.

20. Hinkle AJ: Percutaneous inguinal block for the outpatient management of post-herniorrhaphy pain in children. *Anesthesiology* 67:411–413, 1987.

21. Ejlersen E, Andersen HB, Eliasen K et al: A comparison between preincisional and postincisional lidocaine infiltration and postoperative pain. *Anesth Analg* 74:495–498, 1992.

22. Reiestad F, Stromskag KE: Interpleural catheter in the management of postoperative pain. *Regional Anesth* II:89–91, 1989.

23. Covino BG: Interpleural regional analgesia. *Anesth Analg* 67:427–429, 1988.

24. Ferrante FM, Chan VWS, Arthur GR et al: Interpleural analgesia after thoracotomy. *Anesth Analg* 72:105–109, 1991.

25. Nelson KM, Vincent RG, Bourke RS et al: Intraoperative intercostal nerve freezing to prevent post-thoracotomy pain. *Ann Thorac Surg* 18:280–284, 1974.

26. Maiwand MO, Makey AR, Rees A et al: Cryoanalgesia after thoracotomy. Improvement of technique and review of 600 cases. *J Thorac Cardiovasc Surg* 92:291–295, 1986.

27. O'Shaughnessy L, Stome D: Etiology of traumatic shock. *Br J Surg* 22:589, 1934.

28. Yeager MP, Glass DD, Neff RK et al: Epidural anesthesia and analgesia in high-risk surgical patients. *Anesthesiology* 66:728–736, 1987.

29. Reinhart K, Floerhing U, Kersting T et al: Effects of thoracic epidural anesthesia on systemic hemodynamic function and systemic oxygen supply-demand relationship. *Anesth Analg* 69:360–369, 1989.

30. Baron J-F, Bertrand M, Barre E et al: Combined epidural and general anesthesia versus general anesthesia for abdominal aortic surgery. *Anesthesiology* 65:611–618, 1991.

31. Rutberg H, Hakanson E, Anderberg B et al: Effects of the extradural administration of morphine, or bupivacaine, on the endocrine response to upper abdominal surgery. *Br J Anaesth* 56:233–237, 1984.

32. Hakanson E, Rutberg H, Jorfeldt L et al: Effects of the extradural administration of morphine or bupivacaine on the metabolic response to upper abdominal surgery. *Br J Anaesth* 57:394–399, 1985.

33. Breslow MJ, Jordan DA, Christopherson R et al: Epidural morphine decreases postoperative hypertension by attenuating sympathetic nervous system hyperactivity. *JAMA* 261:3577–3581, 1989.

34. Hjortso NC, Christensen NJ, Andersen T et al: Effects of the extradural administration of local anesthetic agents and morphine on the urinary excretion of cortisol, catecholamines and nitrogen following abdominal surgery. *Br J Anaesth* 57:400–406, 1985.

35. Tuman KJ, McCarthy RJ, March RJ et al: Effects of epidural anesthesia and analgesia on coagulation and outcome after major vascular surgery. *Anesth Analg* 73:696–704, 1991.

36. Bromage PR, Camporesi EM, Durant PAC et al: Rostral spread of epidural morphine. *Anesthesiology* 56:431–436, 1982.

37. Rawal N, Arner S, Gustafsson LL et al: Present state of extradural and intrathecal opioid analgesia in Sweden. *Br J Anaesth* 59:791–799, 1987.

38. Ready LB, Loper KA, Nessly M et al: Postoperative epidural morphine is safe on surgical wards. *Anesthesiology* 75:452–456, 1991.

39. Cousins MJ: Comparative pharmacokinetics of spinal opioids in humans: A step toward determination of relative safety. *Anesthesiology* 67:875–876, 1987.

40. Sjostrom S, Hartvig P, Persson MP, Tamsen A: Pharmacokinetics of epidural morphine and meperidine in humans. *Anesthesiology* 67:877–888, 1987.

41. Chadwick HS, Ready LB: Intrathecal and epidural morphine sulfate for postcesarean analgesia—a clinical comparison. *Anesthesiology* 68:925–929, 1988.

42. El-Baz NMI, Faber LP, Jensik RJ: Continuous epidural infusion of morphine for treatment of pain after thoracic surgery: A new technique. *Anesth Analg* 63:757–764, 1984.

43. White PF: Patient-controlled analgesia: A new approach to the management of postoperative pain. *Sem Anesth* IV:255–266, 1985.

44. Austin KL, Stapleton JV, Mather LE: Multiple intramuscular injections: A major source of variability in analgesic response to meperidine. *Pain* 8:47, 1980.

45. Eisenach JC, Grice SC, Dewan DM: Patient-controlled analgesia following cesarean section: A comparison with epidural and intramuscular narcotics. *Anesthesiology* 68:444–448, 1988.

46. Harrison DM, Sinatra R, Morgese L et al: Epidural narcotic and patient-controlled analgesia for post-cesarean section pain relief. *Anesthesiology* 68:454–457, 1988.

47. Tyler E, Caldwell C, Ghia JN: Transcutaneous electrical nerve stimulation: An alternative approach to the management of postoperative pain. *Anesth Analg* 61:449–456, 1982.

48. Lasagna L: The placebo effect. *J Allergy Clin Immunol* 78:161–165, 1986.

INDEX

Page numbers in *italics* indicate figures; page numbers followed by t indicate tables.